Morson and Dawson's Gastrointestinal Pathology

Morson and Dawson's Gastrointestinal Pathology

David W. Day
Jeremy R. Jass
Ashley B. Price
Neil A. Shepherd
James M. Sloan
Ian C. Talbot
Bryan F. Warren
Geraint T. Williams

FOURTH EDITION

Blackwell
Science

A Blackwell Publishing Company
Blackwell Publishing, Inc., 350 Main Street, Malden, Massachusetts 02148-5018, USA
Blackwell Publishing Ltd, Osney Mead, Oxford OX2 0EL, UK
Blackwell Publishing Asia Pty Ltd, 550 Swanston Street, Carlton, Victoria 3053, Australia
Blackwell Verlag GmbH, Kurfürstendamm 57, 10707 Berlin, Germany

First published 1972
Revised reprint 1974
Second edition 1979
Reprinted 1985
Third edition 1990
Reprinted 1991
Fourth edition 2003

Library of Congress Cataloging-in-Publication Data

Morson and Dawson's gastrointestinal pathology.—4th ed./
David W. Day . . . [et al.].
p. ; cm.
Includes bibliographical references and index.
ISBN 0-632-04204-4 (alk. paper)
1. Gastrointestinal system—Diseases.
[DNLM: 1. Gastrointestinal Diseases—pathology.
WI 140 M886 2003]
I. Title: Gastrointestinal pathology. II. Day, David W.
III. Morson, Basil C. (Basil Clifford). Gastrointestinal pathology.
RC802.9.M67 2003
616.3′307—dc21

2002011931

ISBN 0-632-04204-4

A catalogue record for this title is available from the British Library

Set in 9/12 Palatino by SNP Best-set Typesetter Ltd., Hong Kong
Printed and bound in Slovenia by Mladinska knjiga tiskarna d.d.

Commissioning Editor: Alison Brown
Editorial Assistant: Elizabeth Callaghan
Production Editor: Fiona Pattison
Production Controller: Kate Wilson

For further information on Blackwell Publishing, visit our website:
www.blackwellpublishing.com

Contents

Contributors

David W. Day
MB BChir FRCPath
Consultant Histopathologist
Royal Devon and Exeter Hospital
Barrack Road
Exeter
EX2 5DW

Jeremy R. Jass
MD DSc FRCPath FRCPA
Professor of Gastrointestinal Pathology
Department of Pathology
McGill University
Montreal
Quebec, W3A 2B4
Canada

Ashley B. Price
MA BM BCh FRCPath
Professor of Gastrointestinal Pathology
Imperial College Faculty of Medicine
Consultant Histopathologist
Northwick Park and St. Mark's Hospitals
Watford Road
Harrow, HA1 3UJ
UK

Neil A. Shepherd
MB BS FRCPath
Consultant Histopathologist and Head of Department
Department of Histopathology
Gloucestershire Royal Hospital
Great Western Road
Gloucester, GL1 3NN
UK

James M. Sloan
MB BCh MD FRCPath
Consultant Histopathologist Royal Victoria Hospital
Formerly Reader in Pathology Queen's University Belfast
Institute of Pathology
Grosvenor Road
Belfast, BT12 6BL
UK

Ian C. Talbot
MD FRCPath
Professor of Histopathology
Imperial College School of Medicine
and Consultant Histopathologist
Academic Department of Pathology
St Mark's Hospital
Watford Road
Harrow, HA1 3UJ
UK

Bryan F. Warren
MB ChB FRCPath
Consultant Gastrointestinal Pathologist
Department of Cellular Pathology
John Radcliffe Hospital
Headington
Oxford, OX3 9DU
UK

Geraint T. Williams
MD FRCP FRCPath F Med Sci
Professor of Pathology
Department of Pathology
University of Wales College of Medicine
Heath Park
Cardiff, CF14 4XN
UK

Foreword

Until about the time of World War II knowledge of Gastrointestinal Pathology was largely based on autopsy studies which were often erroneous because of tissue autolysis. Although the years beteeen the two World Wars saw the beginnings of an increase in the number of surgically resected specimens, after the second World War there was a huge increase in the number of gastrectomies and intestinal resections. New techniques of gastric biopsy, small bowel biopsy and colonoscopic biopsy followed and added to the abundance of tissue available to pathologists for the diagnosis and the study of the pathogenesis of gastrointestinal disease. Today gastrointestinal pathology is accepted as one of the largest sub-specialties within general histopathology. There has been a steady movement away from old style morbid anatomy and histology during the past 50 years to a greater appreciation of cellular pathology. This has been particularly fruitful in the study of mucosal infiltrates and malignant tumours especially lymphomas and connective tissue tumours. Although new techniques, in particular immunocytochemistry and molecular analysis, have become popular, especially in research, it is remarkable how the old technique of haematoxylin and eosin staining remains the standard for diagnostic purposes.

This book was conceived during the late 1950s by myself and the late Professor I.M.P. Dawson. We were a happy and productive partnership but it took many years before the first edition was published in 1972. A second edition came out in 1979 but it was becoming clear that the scope of gastrointestinal pathology was increasing so fast that additional authors were essential for a third edition, published in 1990. That trend has continued. It is a real pleasure for me to see so many of my former trainees, research fellows and visitors to the Pathology Department of St Marks Hospital contributing to this fourth edition.

This book was conceived at its very beginning as a source of reference to both pathologists and gastroenterologists. It is patient orientated in the sense that it aims to provide information of value in the clinical management of gastrointestinal disorders.

Comparison of this edition with previous ones illustrates how the revolution in the technology of publishing, both text and illustrations, has advanced. The quality of illustrations is particularly important as they add so much to a reading of the text.

Basil C. Morson
August 2002

Preface to Fourth Edition

It is twelve years since the last edition of *Morson and Dawson* was published, and during this period there have been considerable advances in our knowledge and understanding of the pathology of gastrointestinal diseases. Some of these advances have resulted from developments in basic science that have allowed molecular diagnostics on fixed tissue to become a reality or the armamentarium of monoclonal antibodies for immunohistochemical diagnosis and classification to be continually expanded. Changes in our approaches to gastrointestinal lymphomas and stromal tumours are good examples. However, other important advances have come from more careful observation and clinico–pathological correlation, either of routine histological sections (such as the identification of new forms of colitis) or of resection specimens (such as the recognition of the clinical relevance of circumferential margin involvement in rectal cancer). Concomitant advances in therapy have produced 'new' pathological lesions induced by drugs, radiotherapy, or surgery. The scope of *Gastrointestinal Pathology* has therefore enlarged significantly since the last edition of this book.

The twelve year interval has also seen the retirement of Dr Basil Morson from clinical practice at St Mark's Hospital and the sad death of Professor Ian Dawson. This edition therefore represents the first in which the two original authors have played no direct part in the revision. Their four 'disciples' from the third edition have been joined by four additional authors, Professor Neil Shepherd, Dr Jimmy Sloan, Professor Ian Talbot and Dr Bryan Warren, all of whom have had a special interest in gastrointestinal pathology for many years, and it is a great pleasure to welcome them to the team. Dr Basil Morson and the late Professor Ian Dawson have had a profound influence on the professional lives of all eight of us, and we all feel privileged to be entrusted with this new edition. We are delighted that the names Morson and Dawson continue to be incorporated into the title of the book, and we are especially grateful to Dr Basil Morson for his unfailing interest and encouragement, and for honouring us by writing the foreword to this edition.

The overall structure of this fourth edition is similar to the last three, in that diseases are considered in relation to the anatomical regions of the gut. However, within these sections we have made changes to the way we deal with tumours. Our increasing understanding of the relationships between benign and malignant tumours makes it inappropriate to deal with them any longer in separate chapters. Tumour-like lesions, on the other hand, have been given their own chapters in the stomach, small and large intestines. We have not included a section on the pathology of the peritoneum in this edition, because many of the diseases affecting this structure fall outside the purview of gastroenterology, and a number of excellent publications covering this area have appeared during the last twelve years. The chapters covering gastritis, peptic ulcer disease and gastric neoplasia have been completely re-written, as have those on inflammatory disorders of the small intestine and non-epithelial tumours in all parts of the gut. Many others have been extensively modified, but we have endeavoured to maintain the style of the previous editions. It is probably the inclusion of a large number of colour illustrations for the first time that has made the greatest impact on the overall appearance of the book. There were eight in the last edition, we now have 402. Nevertheless, we have retained about 150 black-and-white figures, mainly because we have been unable to better them in colour, and the overall number of figures has increased by more than 120.

We would like to place on record our gratitude to all our colleagues and friends, too numerous to mention individually, who have supplied us with the material on which this book is based. We do, however, give special thanks to Dr Nick Francis for providing many of the illustrations of the more 'exotic' infectious diseases. A book of this kind is inevitably dependent on the skills of very many laboratory staff, medical photographers, secretaries and experts in information technology. To them all we offer our sincere thanks, but we would like to acknowledge particularly Mr R. Roberts-Gant, Mr R. Creighton, Mr N. Garraghan, and Mrs B. Kelly. Andrew Robinson, Alison Brown, Elizabeth Callaghan, Fiona Pattison and the staff of Blackwell Publishing have carefully and patiently steered us through the various stages of the publication process and it is a pleasure to express our gratitude for their huge efforts on our behalf.

David W. Day
Jeremy R. Jass
Ashley B. Price
Neil A. Shepherd
James S. Sloan
Ian C. Talbot
Bryan F. Warren
Geraint T. Williams
October 2002

Preface to First Edition

Gastroenterology is a rapidly developing and expanding branch of medicine in which histopathology plays an important role in diagnosis and treatment no less than in research. Surgical specimens and biopsy material from the gastrointestinal tract account for a considerable proportion of all the material seen in any department of general histopathology. This book is the outcome of our special interest in both the histopathology and histochemistry of the gastrointestinal tract over the last 20 years during which we have been fortunate enough to have access to a large amount of surgical and biopsy material related to our earlier appointments at the Bland-Sutton Institute of Pathology, the Middlesex Hospital, London, the Department of Pathology in the University of Leeds, and particularly to our current posts at St Mark's Hospital and within the Westminster Hospital Group. We have directed our attention particularly to pathologists who require a reference book for use in the laboratory but we hope this book will also be useful to those studying for the final MRCPath or its equivalent. It contains sufficient related clinical and radiological detail, with references, to interest physicians, surgeons and radiologists who either require ready access to information on pathology for diagnostic, teaching or research purposes, or are interested in pathology for its own sake.

Progress in gastroenterology has been so rapid that a textbook can become out of date in some aspects between writing and publication. We have provided lists of references for diseases or groups of diseases at the end of each chapter which are reasonably comprehensive up to the end of 1970; where possible we have selected those references which themselves contain valuable reviews or give a more detailed account of the subject. No one, however, can entirely encompass the rapidly growing literature in gastroenterology and there may inevitably be some omissions.

We would like to record our sincere thanks to all those clinical colleagues without whose help we could not have documented our experience; and we are grateful to all the pathologists, physicians and surgeons who have referred difficult or interesting material to us over the years, providing experience of a special character. We owe particular thanks to Dr Arthur Spriggs who has contributed the chapter on Cytology from his own vast experience; to Dr H.J.R. Bussey who has given such stalwart support over many years and to Mr Norman Mackie, Senior Photographer at St Mark's Hospital whose technical and artistic skill is evident in many of the photographs. Every histopathologist and histochemist is dependent on the skill of his laboratory technicians and we would like to thank all those who have helped, especially Mr Lloyd Soodeen, AIMLT, Mrs Bhanu Patel, AIMLT, and Miss Jane Hepple.

We are grateful to the following for providing illustrations: Dr R.J. Sandry, Dr Barbara Smith, Dr R. Whitehead, Dr Jane Burnett, Dr H. Lederer, Dr D. Spencer and the photographic department of Westminster Hospital Medical School. Dr J. Gleeson kindly advised us on the value of radiology in malabsorption syndromes. The photographs and charts of carcinoma of the stomach are reproduced by permission of the Editor of the *British Journal of Surgery*. If we have inadvertently omitted any acknowledgement we offer our apologies. Our special thanks must go to Miss Jill Ashby (now Mrs Griffith Jones) who typed and retyped the seemingly endless pages of semilegible manuscript efficiently and cheerfully; and to Mrs Marion Cook who compiled the index for us. We are indebted to Mr Per Saugman and Mr J.L. Robson of Blackwell Scientific Publications for their courteous and enthusiastic cooperation. Finally, as our dedication appropriately indicates, we thank our wives and children who will be no less glad than we are that 12 years of reading, writing and proof reading have come to an end.

London B.C.M.
1972 I.M.P.D.

PART

1 Examination and reporting

1 Reception and examination of biopsy and surgical specimens

Pathology reporting procedures

The primary aim of examining pathology specimens is to provide physicians and surgeons with essential diagnostic and prognostic information allowing the best clinical management of the individual patient. However, this is not the only purpose of pathological examination. Biopsy and surgical resection specimens are a very important source of material for research into disease processes and for teaching. Moreover, advances in information technology and word processing in recent years have meant that pathology records are being used more and more for epidemiological studies and for medical audit. It is important therefore that valuable pathological material is dealt with in such a way as to give as much information as possible for each of these purposes.

The best clinical pathology service can only be obtained when there is close co-operation and understanding between the pathologist and the laboratory staff on the one hand, and physicians and surgeons with their paramedical staff on the other. In order to report on gastrointestinal specimens the practising pathologist should not only have a good basic knowledge of clinical gastroenterology but also know the various clinical procedures used for obtaining specimens, so that difficulties in obtaining adequate biopsies are appreciated. Similarly, the clinical gastroenterologist, surgeon, endoscopist or radiologist should have an understanding of the fundamentals of histopathological diagnosis so that they not only know which tissue samples are most likely to yield the most useful information but also appreciate the limitations of histopathology. Recent advances have made this even more important. Endoscopy, diagnostic imaging and therapeutic instrumentation have each made a great impact on the management of gastrointestinal disease and have provided pathologists with biopsy material from sites that hitherto were inaccessible without major surgery. Similarly, in the pathology laboratory, new techniques in enzyme histochemistry, immunocytochemistry, morphometry, flow cytometry and molecular biology have provided important new methods for diagnosis, which are of great relevance to all physicians and surgeons. More than ever before, the way in which tissue is resected, handled and presented to the laboratory determines and limits the information potentially available.

We believe that there should be an agreed routine between physicians and surgeons, pathologists and technical staff as to how all the common suspected conditions should be handled, in both resected and biopsied material. Regular meetings and discussions are essential to explain what the pathologist can and cannot demonstrate given the optimal material, and to permit the pathologist to appreciate more fully what physicians and surgeons need to know. In few fields of medicine will such co-operation pay greater dividends. In particular, suspected unusual or rare conditions should always be discussed *before* any tissue is removed.

General principles

Each specimen for pathological examination must be accompanied by a request form which, apart from the obvious details of the patient's name, age, sex, hospital number, ward or outpatient clinic, date and the name of the clinician, should give a summary of the *relevant* clinical information and an indication of what specific information the physician or surgeon is seeking. For biopsies it is essential to know the site of biopsy and the endoscopic appearances, while for surgical specimens it is necessary to know the type of operation carried out and, for any non-routine procedure, a diagram illustrating the surgical anatomy of the specimen. Details of previous biopsies and previous treatment, such as radiotherapy, are invaluable. The importance of the information given on the request form in diagnostic interpretation cannot be underestimated—frequently it provides the only information available to the pathologist. All too often the filling in of forms is regarded as a chore by clinical staff, so that the information given is either sketchy, incomplete or indecipherable; or the job is delegated to a junior member of the paramedical staff who is unfamiliar with the patient and unaware of the reason why pathological examination is being requested. Unless the pathologist goes to some considerable length to get the necessary information in such cases, there is always the possibility of diagnostic misinterpretation and serious harm to the patient.

It is also important that the pathologist be allowed to examine the *whole* of any specimen submitted for pathological diagnosis, in order that tissue blocks for histology may be selected from those areas which are known by experience to yield the greatest amount of information. No prior interference should be allowed and specimens should most certainly not be divided, or samples taken for some other purpose such as research, without the pathologist's express agreement. On the other hand, the pathologist should always endeavour to co-operate with the requirements of any reasonable research project.

Generally speaking, therefore, it is best that all surgical specimens for pathological examination reach the laboratory in the fresh, unfixed and unopened state. Because of their small size, gastrointestinal biopsies dry out quickly and should be orientated and placed in an appropriate fixative as soon as possible. Knowledge and understanding of pathological techniques by those submitting the specimen to the laboratory is particularly important here, because whilst most specimens may be fixed in a standard formaldehyde-based laboratory fixative, those needing special study with enzyme histochemistry or electron microscopy may require quenching or immersion in a special fixative (see p. 8).

Laboratory investigation of gastrointestinal biopsies

Most gastrointestinal mucosal biopsies are just tiny samples of a large surface area of suspected disease or volume of abnormal tissue. It is important therefore that they are taken from the right place, and are of sufficient size, number and quality to be representative of the lesion under investigation. Care must be taken to minimize crushing of tissues by biopsy forceps or coagulation during diathermy, since these artefacts make interpretation difficult or impossible.

The vast majority of diagnostic biopsies will be conventionally orientated, fixed, processed and sectioned. In this section we comment on these. Special techniques are described in Chapter 2.

Orientation, fixation and embedding

Biopsies that include muscularis mucosae are usually orientated easily with the naked eye or using a hand lens since the muscularis contracts and the mucosal surface becomes convex. To avoid this phenomenon of curling up, the clinician or endoscopy assistant taking the biopsy should place it mucosal surface upwards onto a flat sheet to which it can adhere during fixation. Some units use either a piece of frosted glass or smooth-surfaced card. Strips of cellulose nitrate ('Millipore') filter material are particularly useful because they can be sectioned without removing the biopsy tissue and permit a series of up to eight or even 10 endoscopic biopsies to be sectioned and mounted in one procedure on a single microscope slide, thus saving time and laboratory resources and easing the task of the pathologist in reviewing the whole series [1]. The normal serum exudate will stick the biopsy to the mounting vehicle, provided that the latter is dry. The biopsy is then placed in a standard fixative, according to the preference of the individual pathologist; 10% aqueous formal saline, buffered at neutral pH, is widely used. However, some laboratories claim better preservation of morphology with unbuffered formal saline, despite the fact that different batches of fixative may vary quite considerably in their pH. Improved nuclear preservation is often obtained when 2% acetic acid is added to the formal saline, or when Bouin's fixative is used. However, the latter suffers the disadvantage of destroying Paneth cell granules, and acid fixatives cause fragmentation of DNA and RNA, seriously hampering molecular biological investigation. Examination with a dissecting microscope, which provides a three-dimensional view of the mucosal architecture of small intestinal biopsies, is rarely done nowadays.

Smaller biopsies, particularly those taken at upper gastrointestinal endoscopy, do not always contain muscularis mucosae and can be impossible to orientate in the operating theatre or clinic. They should be placed in a square of porous non-soluble paper tissue (not gauze), wrapped and placed in fixative. Specimens from different sites must always be kept separate and specifically labelled.

The pathologist or a trained technician should check the orientation of large biopsies before embedding in paraffin wax, using a dissecting microscope if necessary. Tiny biopsies can sometimes be correctly orientated in this way; they should ideally be embedded singly since this allows reorientation if necessary, which is impracticable in a whole block containing three or four specimens in different planes. When biopsies are particularly badly curled and distorted they may be flattened for orientation by embedding in heated 1% aqueous agar precooled to 5°C, keeping the biopsy flat while the agar sets [2]. Processing and double embedding in paraffin wax can then be undertaken.

Sectioning and staining

It is a wise precaution, when sectioning a paraffin block of a small mucosal biopsy, to mount and stain one section as soon as the knife begins to cut into the tissue, so that the orientation may be checked before the block is partly cut through or any step-sectioning is done. At this early stage, reorientation is still possible if sections prove to be transverse or tangential. Biopsies of any size should always be step-sectioned at three different levels and stained routinely with haematoxylin and eosin (H&E). Intervening sections should be kept for further investigation if necessary. With gastric biopsies, in addition to staining with H&E, we routinely stain for *Helicobacter*-like organisms, using either crystal-fast violet or a modified toluidine blue. We do not use any special stains routinely on other biopsies, since occasionally they result in valuable sections being 'wasted' on inappropriate stains. When serial or semiserial sections are being stained using a number of techniques, however, it is wise to stain the first and last with H&E to check that any lesion is present at the beginning and end of a run.

Laboratory examination of surgical specimens

All surgical specimens should be received in the laboratory fresh, unfixed and unopened by operating room staff, including the surgeon. If a specimen has been removed outside normal laboratory working hours it can be safely placed unfixed in a plastic bag in a refrigerator (not in a deep freeze compartment) overnight for examination next morning. It is important that specimens be examined in the fresh, untouched state so that they may be prepared, if necessary, for colour photography and samples taken for special histological techniques such as electron microscopy or histochemistry. Photography of fresh, unfixed specimens has a number of disadvantages. Their shiny, glistening surfaces give rise to 'highlights' and reflections which detract from the quality of photographs obtained, and the delay in fixation, along with the drying effect of photographic lights, has a detrimental effect on tissues which may compromise good histology. It should therefore be confined to cases whose special appearances may become lost or modified by the process of specimen preparation or fixation.

Fresh specimens should be opened and examined carefully, using a hand lens if necessary, in a good light. The specimen is then fixed in 10% formal saline in such a way as to preserve the normal and pathological anatomy for photography. No amount of macroscopic description is any substitute for good photographs, which are easily reproducible for records and teaching purposes. The advent of digital cameras has greatly simplified the photography of specimens and permits the incorporation of a printout of a photograph to be incorporated in the computer-generated report. Although colour can be restored by immersing fixed specimens in 70% ethyl alcohol, we find this unnecessary in most cases.

Most gastrointestinal specimens are best prepared by opening them longitudinally with scissors, gently washing the mucosal surface with cold water or formal saline to remove any blood or excess mucus, and pinning them out flat on a cork board, mucosal surface uppermost. In the case of rectal tumours situated below the pelvic peritoneal reflection, where it is important to preserve the anatomy of the circumferential resection plane for assessment of completeness of excision, it is recommended that the lower rectum is left to fix unopened, so that serial 5-mm slices can be cut in a horizontal plane once the specimen is well fixed. This avoids disturbance by the pathologist of the anterior resection plane, which could obscure its true position. When in such circumstances the lumen of the lower rectum is stenosed, it is helpful to place a wick of formalin-soaked paper tissue, to speed penetration of the fixative. After the specimen has been carefully labelled, the board is then floated, face downwards, for 24 h in a tank of 10% formal saline covered by a close-fitting lid. The specimen is then unpinned, and kept in fixative until blocks for histology are taken. However, if the disease has produced an annular, tight, thick-walled stricture, or if there are diverticula or there is an intussusception, it is better that the specimen be distended with formalin and tied off at both ends as close to the limits of excision as possible; after 24 h fixation it can then be cut longitudinally over a probe passed through the lumen of the stricture so that the pathology is demonstrated at the correct level. Gastrectomy specimens should usually be opened by cutting along the greater curve because this will avoid most gastric pathology which is centred on the lesser curve; small intestinal and colonic specimens opened by cutting along the antimesenteric border; and rectal specimens (other than those removed for carcinoma) opened anteriorly. Specimens from Whipple's operation for tumours of the ampulla of Vater, common bile duct and carcinomas of the head of the pancreas include the duodenal loop which can be opened along its lateral aspect, thus leaving the ampulla intact. Cannulae may be passed through the ampulla in the fresh specimen as far as possible into the common bile duct and pancreatic duct to enable the anatomy of the fixed specimen to be easily assessed.

Before blocks for histological study are taken it is important to make a macroscopic description of every resection specimen and, if necessary, a diagram on which the site of each tissue block can be marked. We use photocopies of a set of simplified diagrams for this purpose, an example of which is shown in Fig. 1.1. The advent of more sophisticated computer systems for handling histopathology data will permit incorporation of such diagrams in printouts of reports. The description should give the length of the specimen, including both greater and lesser curvatures of gastrectomy specimens, and a concise account of all pathological lesions to include their size and appearance, and their position relative to the resection lines, the gastric curvatures, the mesenteric attachments, or other anatomical landmarks such as the ileocaecal valve for right hemicolectomy specimens or the dentate (pectinate) line for abdominoperineal excisions of the rectum and anus. With rectal specimens removed by anterior resection, when

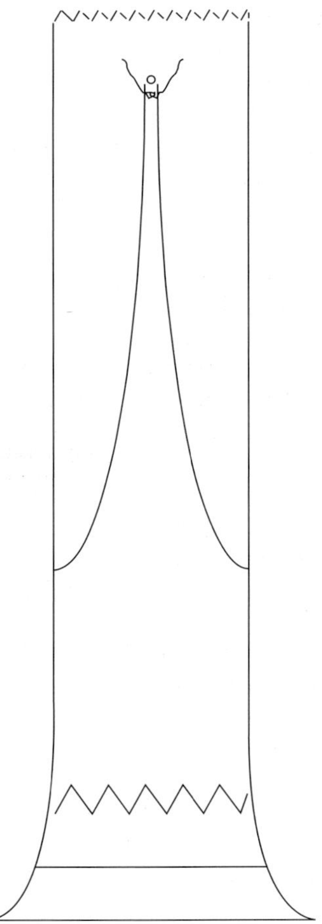

Fig. 1.1 An example of a simplified diagram of an abdominoperineal resection of rectum on which the site of the tumour and of tissue blocks taken for histology can be marked.

the anus is not included in the specimen, a useful anatomical landmark is provided by the pelvic peritoneal reflection, which lies on the anterior surface at approximately the midpoint of the rectum (the average length of the rectum being 15 cm). When the peritoneal reflection is present, it is therefore possible to judge that approximately 7.5 cm above it the colon ends and the rectum begins.

The taking of blocks for histology is obviously a very important step in the examination of any pathology specimen, and it is essential that sufficient samples are taken so that the maximum possible amount of information about the disease process under study can be obtained from the specimen. Nowadays the great majority of gastrointestinal resections are for tumours, polyps or inflammatory bowel disease and the methods used for these will be described in some detail.

Resections for neoplasia

The gross description of macroscopic appearances should include the position of the tumour relative to anatomical landmarks, its size and morphology, and its distance from the surgical limits of excision. The selection of blocks is geared towards assessing the nature of the tumour, the extent of local spread, involvement of the peritoneal surface, the presence of vascular invasion and the degree of lymphatic spread. It is usual to take between two and four blocks of the tumour, making sure that any parts with different macroscopic appearances are sampled, and also the junction between the tumour and the adjacent mucosa. Blocks should also be taken to establish the extent of spread through the bowel wall and, for advanced tumours, whether or not there is invasion of adjacent serosal surfaces, omentum, mesentery, soft tissues or other organs.

It is also important to establish that the tumour has been excised completely, since this is obviously a predictor of local recurrence. Transverse sections through both proximal and distal resected ends of oesophagectomy or gastrectomy specimens should always be examined for direct spread or lymphatic permeation; experience shows that for resections for colorectal cancer this is only necessary when the tumour is within 3 cm of one end [3]. In recent years the use of stapling devices for surgical anastomoses provides two 'doughnuts' of tissue, which represent the resection ends. Histological examination of transverse sections of these provides an excellent method of assessing the completeness of excision in the longitudinal plane. Assessment of the deep (so-called circumferential) planes of excision, around the advancing margin of the tumour, is also important when dealing with excisions of oesophageal and colorectal carcinomas because they may predict local recurrence. This is most easily done by cutting 5-mm slices transversely through the tumour to identify macroscopically the slice with the deepest penetration and least surgical clearance. This slice should then be subjected to histological examination for confirmation or otherwise of total excision [4,5]. It may be helpful to paint the deep or circumferential excision plane with Indian ink or some other marker that withstands tissue processing.

Venous invasion, especially when present in extramural vessels, has a profound effect upon the prognosis of gastrointestinal carcinoma and should always be sought macroscopically and microscopically The veins in the neighbourhood of a tumour should be carefully inspected by dissection of the adjacent mesentery or omentum, and any suspicious vessels examined histologically. More frequently venous invasion is occult and is best discovered in blocks taken from adjacent to the tumour, and tangentially to it.

For cancers of the gastrointestinal tract from the oesophagus to anus it is an important principle that all regional lymph nodes, however small, should be removed for microscopic examination. There is ample evidence that prognosis after surgical treatment of both gastric and colorectal cancer is profoundly altered not only by the presence of lymph node metastases but also by the numbers of nodes involved. There is evidence that the effect on prognosis is in direct proportion to the distance of involved nodes from the primary tumour, it therefore being important to examine all lymph nodes in the field of drainage between the primary tumour and the surgeon's vascular tie [6]. The 'highest' lymph node (the one nearest the tied vascular pedicle) in resections for colorectal cancer should be taken separately, as this allows proper Dukes' classification into C1 or C2 cases. Careful dissection of the omentum or mesentery adjacent to gastric or colorectal cancers usually allows the lymph nodes to be identified, but in difficult cases, when they are obscured by abundant adipose tissue or situated around the lower rectum, an alcohol-xylene clearance technique may be useful [7]. As an alternative, blocks of perigastric or perirectal fat from places where lymph nodes would be expected to lie can be processed and sectioned for microscopic examination. Charts showing the anatomical position of the primary growth and the position of regional lymph nodes may be helpful to the surgeon and useful for the concise presentation of data at multidisciplinary cancer management meetings.

Polypectomy specimens

Resected polyps of any substantial size are usually adenomas of the large bowel, which are preinvasive neoplasms in which it is vital to establish whether or not invasive malignancy has developed and total excision has been achieved. Although polyps from other sites and of different types exist, it is best to deal with them all in the same way. It is first necessary to identify the stalk of the polyp because this gives a guide to the correct plane for trimming and must be sectioned so that it is correctly orientated in relationship to the head of the polyp. It is also the only place where completeness of excision can be established histologically. If the stalk cannot be identified it will be necessary to trim all the more carefully so that multiple step-sections into the lesion will display it satisfactorily. Trimming of a polyp should be minimal and confined to two sides of the lesion so that it can rest on either side with the intact stalk projecting from one end. One should never cut across a polyp but, as far as is possible, embed the whole lesion in one wax block and then cut multiple step-sections (keeping spares for special stains) through the head until the level of the stalk is reached.

Resections for inflammatory bowel disease

The examination of these specimens can be a laborious and time-consuming task because of the considerable amount of tissue that may be resected and because of the complicated surgical anatomy, with strictures, fistulae and abscesses, that may result from the inflammatory process, especially in Crohn's disease. Preparation of the specimens, either by opening or by inflating with fixative, is a particularly important step in identifying the various complicated lesions that occur and good specimen photographs often make a much more informative record than lengthy macroscopic descriptions. When taking blocks, it is important to sample areas representative of the different macroscopic features. It is preferable to take them all from the same plane, usually along the longitudinal axis of the intestine, since these allow a better survey of the extent of the disease process. It is also important to label the blocks accurately and, in complicated cases, to make a diagram of the sites from which each is taken, so that macroscopic and microscopic appearances may be correlated. It is difficult to generalize as to how many blocks should be taken. For a total colectomy anything less than six blocks from different parts of the colon is probably insufficient and as many as 12 may be essential for accurate diagnosis. The regional lymph nodes should also be sampled, although it is unnecessary and probably impracticable to remove all of them.

When colonic resection is undertaken for dysplasia or carcinoma in chronic inflammatory bowel disease the examination must be particularly exhaustive. Blocks should be taken from all recognizable mucosal lesions, and numerous random samples taken from the background 'flat' mucosa. If they are taken from the entire length of the large bowel in two parallel 'tramlines', foci of dysplasia can be mapped. It is vital to establish whether invasive malignancy has developed at any of the sites of dysplasia, and if so, its extent of spread should be assessed as described above for carcinoma specimens.

References

1 Sheffield JP, Talbot IC. ACP Broadsheet 132. Gross examination of the large intestine. *J Clin Pathol*, 1992; 45: 751.

2 Blewitt ES, Pogmore T, Talbot IC. Double embedding in agar/paraffin wax as an aid to orientation of mucosal biopsies. *J Clin Pathol*, 1982; 35: 365.

3 Cross SS, Bull AD, Smith JH. Is there any justification for the routine examination of bowel resection margins in colorectal adenocarcinoma? *J Clin Pathol*, 1985; 42: 1040.

4 Chan KW, Boey J, Wong SKC. A method of reporting radial invasion and surgical clearance of rectal carcinoma. *Histopathology*, 1985; 9: 1319.

5 Quirke P, Durdey P, Dixon MF, Williams NS. Local recurrence of rectal adenocarcinoma due to inadequate surgical resection. Histopathological study of lateral tumour spread and surgical excision. *Lancet*, 1986; ii: 996.

6 Murphy J, Ueno H, O'Sullivan GC, Lee G, Shepherd NA, Talbot IC. Prognostic value of mapping nodal metastases in Dukes' C rectal cancer. *J Pathol*, 2001; 195: 5A.

7 Cawthorn SJ, Gibbs NM, Marks CC. Clearance technique for the detection of lymph nodes in colorectal cancer. *Br J Surg*, 1986; 73: 58.

2 Special investigations

The days are now past when the only way to process a biopsy or a tissue block from a resected specimen was to fix it in formalin, embed it in paraffin wax, stain the sections with haematoxylin and eosin and examine them under the light microscope. Many new and sophisticated techniques are now available which, when correctly chosen, provide valuable additional information, and most hospital laboratories are equipped to undertake at least some of them. A number require other than conventional processing and handling of tissues and it is vital to establish, *before* a biopsy or a resected specimen is immersed in fixative, what the clinician considers the likely diagnosis to be, whether a particular investigation is required and which techniques the pathologist should use to provide the most useful information. Closer co-operation has led to a surge of interest in gastrointestinal problems and a higher standard of diagnosis. This chapter affords a brief description of the more important techniques available and their value. Details of methodology are available in standard textbooks and reviews [1–8].

Gastrointestinal biopsies, except for those from the small intestine, are now normally taken under direct vision and visible lesions can be sampled directly. The various biopsy techniques and the orientation of specimens are described in Chapter 1.

Preservation of tissues

There are two principal and two subsidiary techniques for tissue preservation [1–3].

Fixation and embedding

This, followed by light microscopy, is still the most widely used and valued technique. Fixation is usually in 10% buffered formaldehyde. There are three possible embedding techniques (Figs 2.1–2.3).

1 *Embedding in paraffin wax.* This is easy, all laboratories are equipped for it, pathologists are used to it, and it allows large blocks to be taken from resected specimens and some crude electron microscopy is possible after reprocessing thick sections. It allows some special investigations but precludes others (Fig. 2.1).

2 *Embedding in acrylic resin.* This is suitable only for small pieces of tissue; it is technically more difficult to cut the thin 2-μm sections, is expensive and the material cannot be used for electron microscopy as acrylic resin disintegrates in the electron beam. It has the advantage that much cellular and intracellular detail can be made out (Fig. 2.2).

3 *Embedding in epoxy resin.* This, normally preceded by fixation in freshly prepared buffered glutaraldehyde, is the method of choice for electron microscopy. Tissue blocks are small, but semithin 1-μm sections can be taken from them, stained with toluidine blue and examined by light microscopy. This provides a fine-detail image of cellular structure that bridges the gap between light and electron microscopy (Fig. 2.3).

Quenching without prior fixation

This technique involves plunging small pieces of fresh tissue into an inert liquid such as isopentane, precooled in liquid

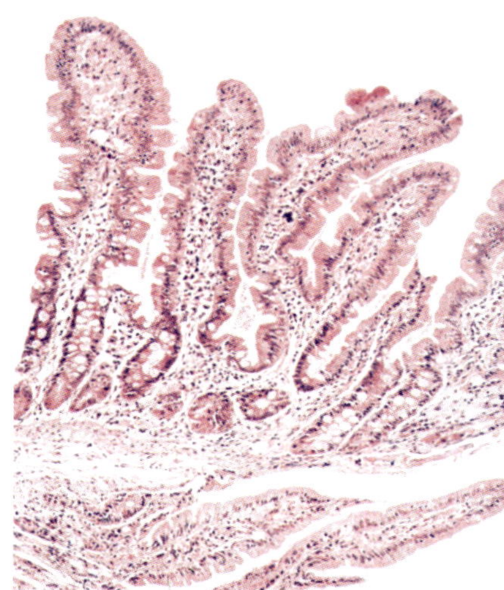

Fig. 2.1 Normal jejunum. Tissue fixed in buffered formaldehyde, followed by embedding in paraffin wax. Villous outlines are well preserved and the nuclear staining is crisp and clear; cell boundaries are distinct. The villi have, however, probably undergone some shrinkage.

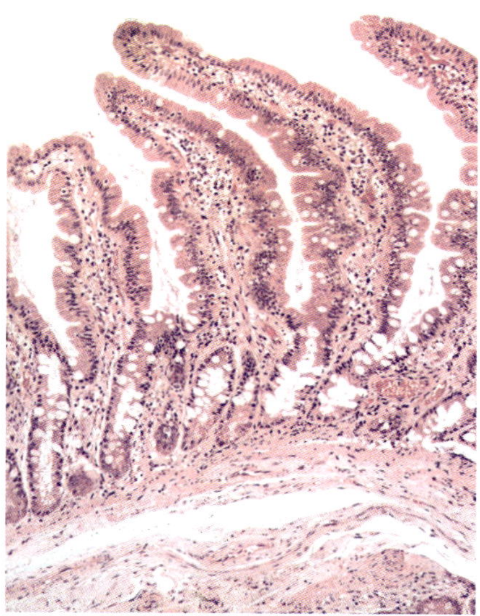

Fig. 2.2 Normal jejunum. Tissue fixed in formal calcium, followed by embedding in acrylic resin (JB4 glycol methacrylate, section 2 μm). Appearances are comparable with Fig. 2.1, but the thinner section allows more nuclear and cytoplasmic detail to be recognized.

nitrogen, followed by the cutting of sections at 5–6 μm in a cryostat at about –25°C, thus avoiding the use of a fixative. Once cut, sections can be postfixed if necessary. It allows the histochemical demonstration of those enzymes that do not tolerate fixation and the identification by immunocytochemical methods of antigenic components that are altered by routine fixatives. It may also provide a rapid answer for the surgeon in

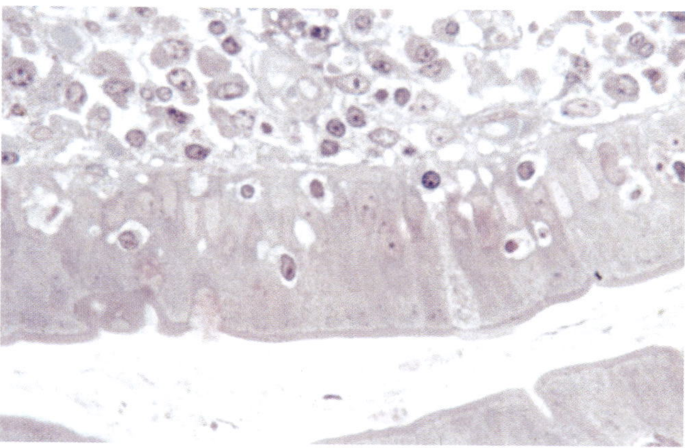

Fig. 2.3 Normal jejunal villus. Tissue fixed in buffered glutaraldehyde followed by embedding in epoxy resin (araldite, section 1 μm, toluidine blue). Cell outlines are perhaps slightly less clear than in Fig. 2.2 but there is further improvement in the intracellular nuclear and cytoplasmic detail and the brush border can be clearly seen.

problems such as Hirschsprung's disease. The technique's principal disadvantages are the need for constant supply of liquid nitrogen for quenching, difficulty with subsequent storage of the quenched tissue, and a certain loss of fine cellular detail after staining, though this can be improved by postfixing the section. It is often useful to divide a sufficiently large sample to allow both conventional fixation and quenching.

Refrigeration at 4°C

This method is useful when tissue is being retained for biochemical analysis. Unfixed surgically resected specimens can be stored in this way overnight when removed after laboratory hours.

Freeze drying

This technique, followed by vapour fixation, is a valuable research method particularly for the identification of biological amines. It has little place in routine diagnosis.

Choice of technique

This depends on three factors.

1 *The nature of the information required.* Are there specific factors to be looked for, and if not how can the tissue be best preserved so that as wide a range of investigations as possible can be done later if necessary?

2 *The size of the piece of tissue available.* Is it divisible and if so, will each piece be representative of the whole?

3 *The laboratory facilities available.* What can be offered locally or through access to more specialized facilities elsewhere, provided that the tissue is initially properly preserved?

If there is a particular problem to be solved—e.g. a survey of mucosal nerves in Hirschsprung's disease—this clearly governs the technique of preparation used. When there is no such indication, the size of the piece of tissue is likely to be the determining factor. If it is divisible into three, it is probably best to fix one piece in formaldehyde, one in fresh buffered glutaraldehyde and quench the third. If divisible only into two, omit the glutaraldehyde; if indivisible the pathologist must choose between formaldehyde fixation and quenching (with postfixing for haematoxylin staining) according to preference; the first is probably the preferred technique for biopsies as rebiopsy is often possible.

Morphometry, quantification and stereology

Morphometry is the measurement of the size and shape of objects. It allows calculation of area, perimeter and other variables.

Quantification is the measurement of the number of structures or features per area or length of tissue or the amount of a particular material present using microdensitometry techniques.

Stereology is the calculation of three-dimensional properties of an object from two-dimensional planes.

Such studies can be performed on paraffin- or resin-embedded sections and to some extent on postfixed cryostat sections.

Three types of morphometric technique are available for direct light microscopy without automation. All of them can be applied to photomicrographs, electron micrographs, projected slides or transparencies. They are:

1 the use of a camera lucida attachment or a projection microscope to project an image onto standard thickness paper or card. A tracing is then made of the cells under study and their areas are either measured using a planimeter or calculated by cutting out the shapes of individual cells and weighing them;

2 the use of either a linear intercept eyepiece graticule to express the area of a particular tissue component as a percentage of the total tissue area or a hexagonal line graticule to give a surface : volume ratio; and

3 the use of a point counting graticule.

Many laboratories now possess some form of image analysing equipment. Simpler quantification can be undertaken using tracings and photomicrographs as above. More sophisticated versions allow automated analysis of size, shape, texture or staining intensity from images captured on monitor screens. Such techniques (which may be used to measure villus height and thickness, determine the relative numbers of cell types present, or assess nuclear changes in epithelia showing disordered growth and differentiation) have an important place in research and evidence-based practice [7,8] and will be referred to in appropriate chapters. Certain basic principles must be observed to ensure that valid and reproducible results are obtained.

1 There must be sufficient tissue to provide an adequate number of microscopic fields for sampling.

2 The biopsy must be representative of any lesion present; not all disease processes are evenly distributed throughout a section.

3 Section orientation must be accurate and avoid factors such as tangential cutting which distort surface areas and volumes.

4 There must be no artefacts such as those produced in a small bowel biopsy which does not include muscularis mucosae, as a result of which 'spreading' of villi can occur.

5 Sections must be of uniform thickness.

Electron microscopy

Electron microscopic techniques fall under the following two headings.

Scanning electron microscopy

A scanning electron microscope creates three-dimensional representations of unsectioned specimens which have been fixed, dried and coated (Fig. 2.4). This is predominantly a research technique [5] and it will not be further discussed here.

Transmission electron microscopy

Light microscopes cannot resolve particles smaller than about 2 µm. Transmission electron microscopes allow resolution down to about 2 nm (about × 1000 that of their light counterparts). They are used diagnostically to evaluate changes in microvilli, to demonstrate subcellular particles such as mitochondria, lysosomes and Golgi apparatus, to show

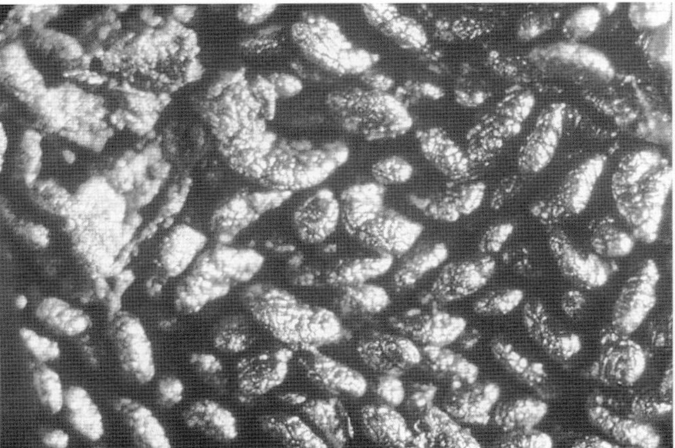

Fig. 2.4 Normal jejunum. Scanning electron micrograph, gold sputter coated. This provides a three-dimensional surface view of villi but does not yield a great deal of useful diagnostic information.

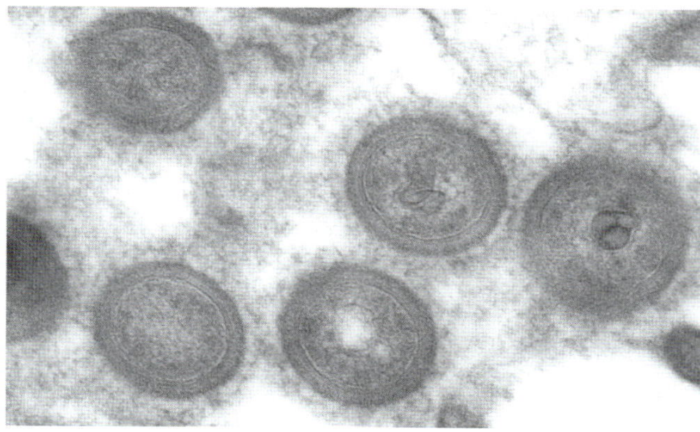

Fig. 2.5 Transmission electron micrograph in Whipple's disease showing the causative bacillary organism (*Tropheryma whipelii*) in cross-section.

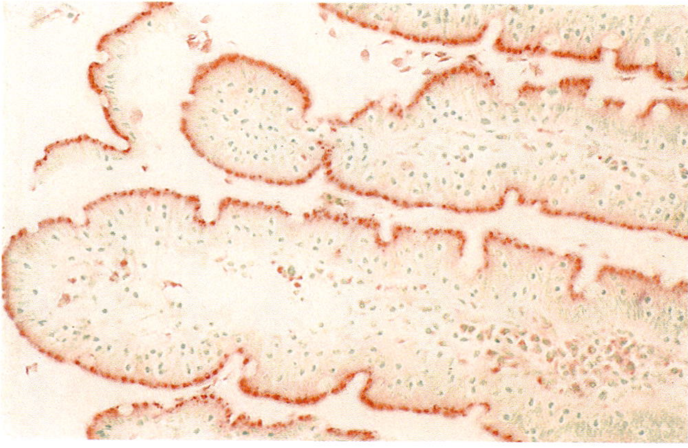

Fig. 2.6 Normal jejunum. Acid phosphatase, cryostat section (6 μm) postfixed in buffered formaldehyde, pararosanilin technique, methylene blue counterstain. The location of the enzyme within digestive sacs and lysosomes is clearly visible. Some is also present in macrophages in the lamina propria.

cytoplasmic inclusions such as bacteria, and to demonstrate intracellular granules [6] (Fig. 2.5). Some techniques for histochemistry and immunocytochemistry are possible at ultrastructural level.

Histochemistry

Histochemistry is the use of chemical techniques on tissue sections, usually to identify specific substances within cells or to define sites of enzyme activity. In gastrointestinal pathology they are of value in three main fields: (i) the identification of particular enzymes within cells or nerve fibres; (ii) the detailed investigation of mucosubstances; and (iii) as a method for identifying and partially classifying intracellular cytoplasmic granules.

Enzyme histochemistry

Histochemical techniques for enzymes do not stain them directly. When a section is incubated with a substrate specific for a particular enzyme under controlled conditions and the enzyme is present in active form in the section, a breakdown product (the primary reaction product or PRP) is formed (or, in the case of oxidoreductases, an electron transfer takes place). The PRP (or the electrons) are 'captured' by the addition of a suitable chemical to produce an insoluble coloured end-product, the location of which indicates the site of enzyme activity. Methods of tissue preservation are particularly important since some enzymes are relatively unaffected by fixatives while others are inactivated. Examples of useful techniques are those for alkaline and acid phosphatases, aminopeptidases, disaccharidases (particularly lactase and sucrase; Fig. 2.6), and cholinesterase (Fig. 2.7). However, as monoclonal or polyclonal antibodies directed at enzymic epitopes have become available, many of these often capricious histochemical techniques have been superseded by immunohistochemistry.

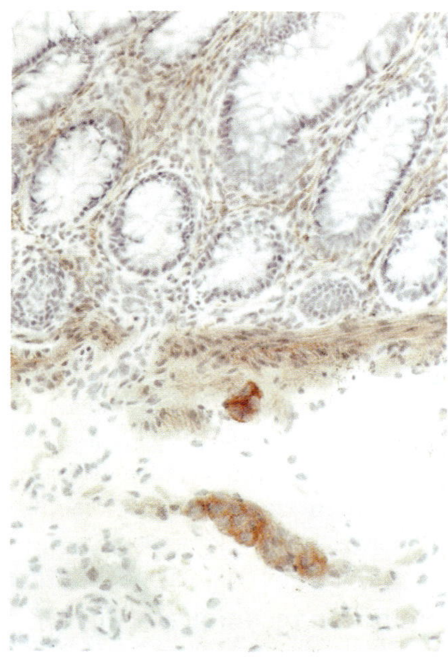

Fig. 2.7 Normal large intestine. Acetylcholinesterase (AChE), formaldehyde fixation, gum sucrose impregnation, cryostat section (6 μm). Individual cholinesterase-positive nerve fibres can be seen in the lamina propria and there is heavy 'staining' of ganglion cells. Some AChE-positive material is also present in the muscularis mucosae.

Mucin (glycoprotein) histochemistry

Reliable techniques, which can be performed in any routine laboratory on formalin-fixed material, allow the separation of

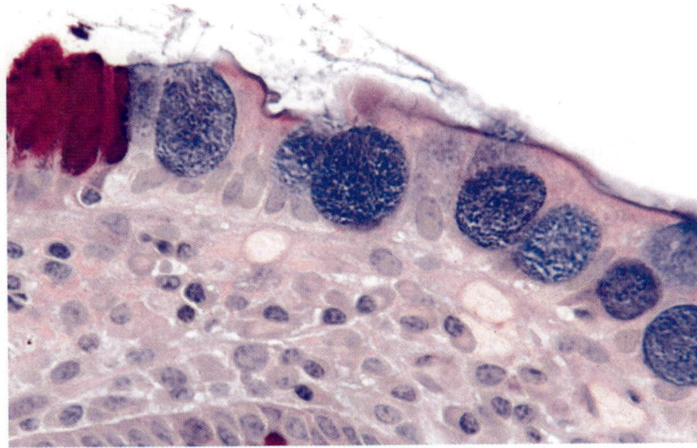

Fig. 2.8 Intestinal metaplasia of gastric mucosa. Goblet cells stain deep blue with alcian blue/dPAS, being reactive with both alcian blue (due to the presence of sialic acid) and dPAS. Residual gastric columnar cells are dPAS reactive (magenta), secreting only neutral mucins.

mucosubstances into *neutral mucins* (diastase digestion, followed by a periodic acid–Schiff (dPAS) technique); *acid non-sulphated* sialomucins (stained by alcian blue at pH 2.5); and *acid sulphated* sulphomucins (stained by alcian blue at pH 0.5 or by high iron diamine, or Gomori's aldehyde fuchsin) [9–11]. These techniques can be combined to demonstrate more than one pattern of mucin in a single section (Fig. 2.8). They can be made more discriminating by pretreatment of sections with selected enzymes such as neuraminidase, by the use of saponification methods for deacylation, by the use of alternative oxidizing agents to periodic acid, and by varying the concentrations of magnesium chloride in the incubating medium. More precise identification of glycoproteins can also be obtained by the use of specific lectins in a peroxidase technique. Their use and value have been critically discussed [12], and they are referred to where appropriate in subsequent chapters.

Silver precipitation techniques

Most silver 'stains' consist of aqueous or alcoholic solutions of silver nitrate which probably bind to anionic side-chains and disulphide groups. They must then be reduced to visible silver, either by a reducing substance already present in particular cells (argentaffin reaction) or by the addition of a reducing agent (argyrophil reaction). The only intracellular reducing agents capable of giving an argentaffin reaction in ordinary preparations of gut tissues are the compounds formed between 5-hydroxytryptamine (5-HT) and aldehyde fixatives. Other biological amines such as histamine or noradrenaline, which are capable of forming reducing complexes, diffuse away rapidly in aqueous fixatives. A positive argentaffin reaction can therefore be regarded as demonstrating 5-HT. The granules of other endocrine cells are, by contrast, argyrophil. However, different argyrophil techniques have different sensitivities for the granules of the various cell types. For example, the Grimelius technique, probably the most widely used, does not consistently identify somatostatin-containing D cells, while the Sevier–Munger technique does. One study has suggested that the Churukian–Schenk technique is the most sensitive overall [13].

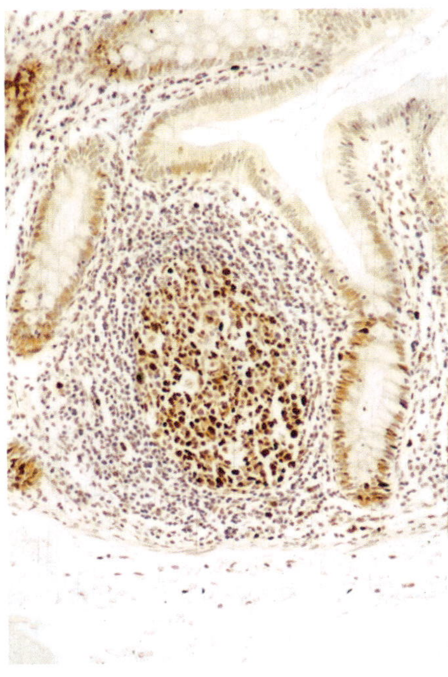

Fig. 2.9 Lymphoid aggregate within normal colorectum. Proliferative cell nuclear antigen (PCNA) immunohistochemistry reveals nuclear positivity in germinal centres and within crypt bases.

Basic and metachromatic dyes

These cationic dyes bind to anionic side-chains in polypeptides and staining is often improved by acid hydrolysis; they can be used, along with lead haematoxylin, as alternative staining methods for endocrine cell granules.

Immunocytochemical techniques

All of these depend on the ability to raise and purify a specific antibody to an antigenic component of a cell. Examples of diagnostically useful antigens that can be recognized include endocrine cell and neuronal granules, vesicles and peptides, cytokeratins and intermediate filaments, leucocyte markers, immunoglobulins, oncofetal antigens, proliferation markers [4], mucin core proteins and numerous enzymes (Fig. 2.9). Suitable methods of tissue preservation that do not alter antigen combining power, antigen retrieval protocols and adequate controls are essential. These techniques are reliable and are continually being improved and extended; they represent one of the great advances in histopathology in the last 25 years.

Investigation of the innervation of the gut

Modern concepts of the innervation of the gut have stemmed from the ability of histochemists and immunocytochemists to classify different types of nerve fibres and ganglia by demonstrating the polypeptides that they contain and the enzymes that they synthesize.

Pioneer studies in the 1970s showed that satisfactory demonstration of the distribution of nerve fibres and ganglia in myenteric and submucosal plexuses requires thick (20–100-μm) sections cut in the plane of the plexuses, parallel to the bowel wall, from large (20–100-mm) blocks of tissue, fixed for a week in 10% formaldehyde [14]. It is clear that such studies can have no place in routine work, but the results obtained from them can be applied by practising pathologists once the experimentalist has indicated which fibres or ganglia are important in which disorders. A classic example is the use of cholinesterase techniques on mucosal biopsies from suspected Hirschsprung's disease (Fig. 2.10).

Five main groups of neurotransmitters are now recognized: acetylcholine, the biological amines adrenaline and noradrenaline, gamma aminobutyric acid, neuropeptides (an ever expanding family that includes substance P, vasoactive intestinal polypeptide (VIP), somatostatin and bombesin) and nitric oxide. These may be identified using appropriate histochemical or immunocytochemical techniques [15], and are likely to prove of increasing importance as our knowledge of gastrointestinal innervation increases. The functions of these neurotransmitters and the independence of the gut-associated intrinsic nervous system are more fully discussed in the appropriate sections of this book.

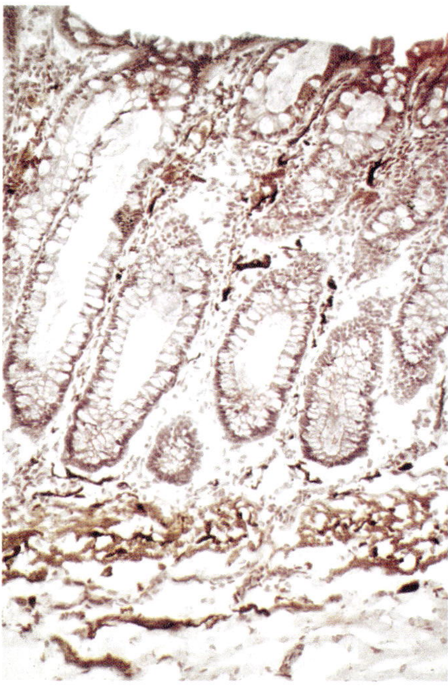

Fig. 2.10 Rectal biopsy in Hirschsprung's disease showing the more numerous, thickened fibres present in the lamina propria. Compare with Fig. 2.7, same technique.

Flow cytometry

Until recently, histopathologists have been content to rely on the microscopic examination of tissue sections for diagnosis, supplemented when necessary by those special techniques already described above. Techniques that do not rely on tissue sections are now being increasingly used for both research and diagnosis. Examples are flow cytometry which provides a rapid quantitative means of measuring a variety of cell constituents and can be adapted to analyse the cell cycle, and the measurement of nuclear DNA content which can provide important insight into the nature and behaviour of precancerous and cancerous lesions [16]. Flow cytometry can be modified to sort and count cells labelled with a fluorescent antibody.

DNA technology in gastrointestinal pathology

Recombinant DNA technology has provided an important investigative tool in the field of gastrointestinal pathology. Its value has been most obvious in explaining the pathogenesis of neoplastic disorders, but DNA technology will increasingly be employed to augment tissue diagnosis. Important examples are the hereditary disorders that happen to involve the gastrointestinal tract. For a number of these the underlying gene has been cloned, allowing affected persons to be identified through germline mutation analysis. Of particular relevance in gastrointestinal pathology are methods that can be applied directly to tissue sections such as *in situ* hybridization and methods that utilize DNA or mRNA extracted from tissue samples. Small groups of cells or even single cells can be isolated from tissues by laser capture microdissection [17]. Such methods have been of particular value in uncovering the genetic basis of neoplasia, for which bowel cancer has served as an important model for solid tumours. The principles and practical uses of recombinant DNA technology are described briefly below.

Restriction endonucleases

Around 500 different restriction endonucleases are available. These bacterially derived enzymes recognize particular base sequences and cut the DNA molecule at specific sites determined by the presence of the relevant base sequences. The ability to cut DNA at specific sites is crucial for many aspects of recombinant DNA technology. Being of different length and physical structure, restriction fragments will have a characteristic electrophoretic mobility in agarose gel and may therefore be separated. However, each individual carries maternally and paternally derived chromosomes that are not identical, so that 'equivalent' restriction fragments may not be of identical length or electrophoretic mobility. This difference or polymorphism has been used for linkage analysis and to demonstrate loss of heterozygosity (LOH) [18,19].

Southern blotting

This refers to the transfer of electrophoretically separated fragments of denatured DNA from agarose gel to a nitrocellulose membrane. Fragments of special interest are detected with radiolabelled probes of complementary DNA. This classical approach has been used for linkage analysis and to demonstrate loss of heterozygosity [18,19], but has been largely superseded by PCR-based methodologies (see below).

DNA microsatellite markers

Non-coding repetitive tracts known as microsatellites may show considerable variability and have been used to establish an individual's DNA fingerprint. DNA probes to these regions provide a powerful approach to haplotyping (i.e. characterizing and distinguishing maternally and paternally derived alleles) and demonstrating loss of heterozygosity.

Polymerase chain reaction (PCR)

Molecular biological analysis of DNA derived from tissue is limited by the amount and quality of the extractable DNA. Viral DNA may have integrated with a fraction of the cells and/or be present as a small number of copies. Mutation detection requires analysis of relatively large amounts of DNA of a particular quality. However, if the structure of the DNA sequence is known, single-stranded DNA can be replicated within the laboratory by means of a pair of primers and the enzyme DNA polymerase. The process can be repeated until the DNA has been replicated a millionfold, hence the designation polymerase chain reaction (PCR) [20]. PCR bridges the gulf between histopathology and molecular genetics by allowing DNA to be extracted from formalin-fixed paraffin-embedded tissues that may be merely selected, microdissected or extracted at the level of individual cells by laser capture microdissection [17]. For example, human papilloma virus has been demonstrated within amplified DNA samples obtained from fixed tissues [21]. The method has also been used to detect subtle mutations within oncogenes and loss of tumour suppressor genes, and for the demonstration of DNA microsatellite instability (see below). Messenger RNA expression can be studied by means of reverse transcriptase (generating cDNA) PCR (RT-PCR) using a commonly expressed housekeeping gene (e.g. glyceraldehyde 3-phosphate dehydrogenase) as an internal control. The prospect of developing *in situ* PCR marks the total integration of histopathology and molecular biology [22].

Linkage analysis

The ability to distinguish between equivalent but genetically polymorphic fragments of DNA of maternal and paternal origin allows the inheritance of a particular restriction fragment length polymorphism (RFLP) or haplotype determined by DNA microsatellite markers to be traced through a family. Linkage means that a gene causing a disease is on the same chromosome and physically close to the fragment of DNA that is being traced, i.e. that the disease and the linked DNA marker or haplotype are consistently coinherited. Demonstration of linkage of a disease to an inherited RFLP or haplotype proves that the disease is genetically determined and identifies the approximate locus of the disease causing gene. It was on the basis of linkage analysis that genetic loci for familial adenomatous polyposis [18], hereditary non-polyposis colorectal cancer [23] and Peutz–Jeghers syndrome [24] were identified.

Demonstration of loss of heterozygosity (LOH) and DNA microsatellite instability (MSI)

An individual shows heterozygosity when maternally and paternally derived allelic pairs can be resolved into bands with differing electrophoretic mobility. Tumours may show loss of heterozygosity (LOH), meaning that one or other band has been lost. The loss is generally due to a mitotic error leading to loss of the entire chromosome or a part of the chromosome containing the DNA fragment. It has been established that when LOH for a particular locus occurs on a consistent basis in a particular type of tumour, then the chromosome involved will contain a tumour suppressor gene that is implicated in the pathogenesis of that tumour [19]. Colorectal cancer shows consistent LOH for chromosomes 5, 17 and 18 corresponding to the tumour suppressor genes *APC*, *TP53* and possibly *DCC* [25]. Tumour suppressor genes act recessively at the somatic level, meaning that both genes need to be non-functioning before there is a full transforming effect. The first gene may be non-functioning because of an acquired somatic mutation or as a result of an inherited mutation.

Using DNA microsatellite markers, tumour DNA may sometimes show not band loss, but additional bands (bandshifts) indicating mutation of the microsatellite region. This serves as a marker of defective DNA mismatch repair that may be inherited or acquired [26] (Fig. 2.11).

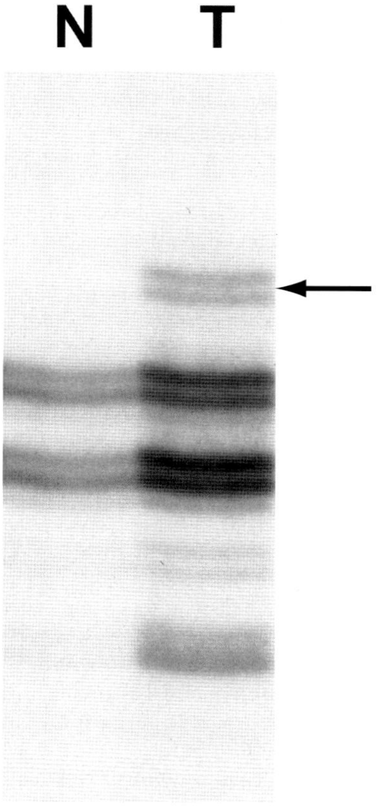

Fig. 2.11 Bandshifts (arrow) in tumour DNA indicating DNA microsatellite instability (MYCL).

Demonstration of clonality

In order to demonstrate changes at the DNA level, a certain amount of DNA is required and the change must therefore implicate a population of cells. The fact that a population of cells shows loss of heterozygosity or an identical point mutation is evidence of its clonality or origin from a single cell [27]. The demonstration of clonality is of diagnostic importance in lymphomas. Here one exploits specific, naturally occurring gene rearrangements (for example of the T-cell receptor) to show a clonal or neoplastic expansion of T cells. More recently, PCR-based strategies have been employed to demonstrate clonality using DNA extracted from formalin-fixed lymphomas [28].

Dot blot hybridization

This allows quantitative information to be obtained such as the presence of gene amplification or an indication of the number of copies of a viral gene, for example *HPV*, within a DNA sample. Measured amounts of DNA or RNA are applied to moistened nitrocellulose membrane, denatured and hybridized with a specific, labelled probe. The intensity of the labelling of each dot is proportional to the content of specific DNA sequences and calibration is achieved by comparison with dots prepared from standards [29].

In situ hybridization

The demonstration of specific DNA or mRNA sequences within tissue sections can be achieved with labelled probes consisting of DNA or mRNA. 'Antisense' RNA is ideal for localizing mRNA because a labelled 'sense' strand serves as a negative control and test of specificity. The overall principle is similar to that of immunohistochemical staining. Radiolabelled probes are highly sensitive and can detect one or two copies of a particular DNA sequence per cell. Non-radioactive labels are less sensitive but are more acceptable for routine diagnostic use. The main diagnostic value of *in situ* hybridization lies in the detection of viral DNA. Loss or gain of DNA sequences derived from neoplastic versus normal sources (labelled with different fluorochromes) may be demonstrated by comparing patterns of hybridization with normal metaphase chromosomal spreads (comparative genomic hybridization) [30].

Mass testing for gene expression

Microchip arrays of many thousands of genes (cDNA) likely to be expressed in normal tissues can be used to test for reduced or increased expression of mRNA derived from counterpart neoplastic tissues. This powerful research tool will accelerate understanding of the role of known genes in carcinogenesis [31].

DNA methylation

Evidence is increasing that gene inactivation in the course of tumorigenesis occurs not only by structural alteration of genes but by epigenetic mechanisms including methylation of the promoter region [32].

References

1 Kiernan JA. *Histological and Histochemical Methods, Theory and Practice*, 3rd edn. Oxford: Butterworth-Heinemann, 1999.
2 Filipe MI, Lake BD. *Histochemistry in Pathology*, 2nd edn. Edinburgh: Churchill Livingstone, 1990.
3 Bancroft JD, Stevens A. *Theory and Practice of Histological Techniques*, 4th edn. Edinburgh: Churchill Livingstone, 1995.
4 Dobbs DJ. *Diagnostic Immunohistochemistry*. Edinburgh: Churchill Livingstone, 2001.
5 Carr KE, Toner PG, Saleh KM. Scanning electron microscopy. *Histopathology*, 1982; 6: 3.
6 Toner PG, Carr KE, Wyburn GM. *The Digestive System. An Ultrastructural Atlas and Review*. London: Butterworths, 1971.
7 Aherne WA, Dunnill MS. *Morphometry*. London: Edward Arnold, 1987.

8 Baak JP, Oort JA. *A Manual of Morphometry in Diagnostic Pathology*. Berlin: Springer-Verlag, 1983.

9 McFadden DE, Owen DA, Reid PA, Jones EA. The histochemical assessment of sulphated and non-sulphated sialomucin in intestinal epithelium. *Histopathology*, 1985; 9: 1129.

10 Williams GT. Commentary: transitional mucosa of the large intestine. *Histopathology*, 1985; 9: 1237.

11 Shah KA, Deacon AJ, Dunscombe P, Price AB. Intestinal metaplasia subtyping: evaluation of Gomori's aldehyde fuchsin for routine use. *J Clin Pathol*, 1997; 51: 277.

12 Brooks SA, Leathem AJC, Schumacher U. *Lectin Histochemistry*. Oxford: BIOS Scientific Publishers, 1996.

13 Smith DM Jr, Haggitt RC. A comparative study of generic stains for carcinoid secretory granules. *Am J Surg Pathol*, 1983; 7: 61.

14 Smith B. *The Neuropathology of the Alimentary Tract*. London: Edward Arnold, 1972.

15 Krishnamurthy S, Schuffler MD. Pathology of neuromuscular disorders of the small intestine and colon. *Gastroenterology*, 1987; 93: 610.

16 Quirke P, Dyson DED. Flow cytometry: methodology and applications in pathology. *J Pathol*, 1986; 149: 79.

17 Sirivatanauksorn Y, Drury R, Crnogorac-Jurcevic T, Sirivatanauksorn V, Lemoine NR. Laser-assisted microdissection: applications in molecular pathology. *J Pathol*, 1999; 189: 150.

18 Bodmer WF, Bailey CJ, Bodmer J *et al*. Localization of the gene for familial adenomatous polyposis on chromosome 5. *Nature*, 1987; 328: 614.

19 Solomon E, Voss R, Hall V *et al*. Chromosome 5 allele loss in human colorectal carcinomas. *Nature*, 1987; 328: 616.

20 Erlich HA, Gelfand DH, Saiki RK. Specific DNA amplification. *Nature*, 1988; 331: 461.

21 Shibata DK, Arnheim N, Martin WJ. Detection of human papilloma virus in paraffin-embedded tissue using the polymerase chain reaction. *J Exp Med*, 1988; 167: 225.

22 O'Leary JJ, Chetty R, Graham AK, McGee J O'D. In situ PCR. Pathologist's dream or nightmare? *J Pathol*, 1996; 178: 11.

23 Peltomäki P, Aaltonen LA, Sistonen P *et al*. Genetic mapping of a locus predisposing to human colorectal cancer. *Science*, 1993; 260: 810.

24 Amos CI, Bali D, Thiel TJ *et al*. Fine mapping of genetic locus for Peutz–Jeghers syndrome on chromosome 19p. *Cancer Res*, 1997; 57: 3653.

25 Vogelstein B, Fearon ER, Hamilton SR *et al*. Genetic alterations during colorectal-tumor development. *N Engl J Med*, 1988; 319: 525.

26 Aaltonen LA, Peltomaki PS, Leach FS *et al*. Clues to the pathogenesis of familial colorectal cancer. *Science*, 1993; 260: 812.

27 Vogelstein B, Fearon ER, Hamilton SR, Feinberg AP. Use of restriction fragment length to determine the clonal origin of human tumours. *Science*, 1984; 227: 642.

28 Pan LX, Diss TC, Isaacson PG. The polymerase chain reaction in histopathology. *Histopathology*, 1995; 26: 201.

29 Spandidos DA, Kerr IB. Elevated expression of the human *ras* oncogene family in premalignant and malignant tumours of the colorectum. *Br J Cancer*, 1984; 49: 681.

30 Meijer GA, Hermsen MAJA, Baak JPA *et al*. Progression from colorectal adenoma to carcinoma is associated with non-random chromosomal gains as detected by comparative genomic hybridisation. *J Clin Pathol*, 1998; 51: 901.

31 Schena M, Shalon D, Davis RW, Brown PO. Quantitative monitoring of gene expression patterns with complementary DNA microarray. *Science*, 1995; 270: 467.

32 Toyota M, Ahuja N, Ohe-Toyota M *et al*. CpG island methylator phenotype in colorectal cancer. *Proc Natl Acad Sci USA*, 1999; 96: 8681.

3 The autopsy

The value of the autopsy examination in general has been under threat in recent years for several reasons, and its importance in medical education and in monitoring diagnostic techniques and refining clinical skills ('medical audit') has been highlighted in recent publications [1–5]. Apart from this, careful autopsy studies can provide very valuable epidemiological data relating to the prevalence and time trends of disease in different geographical areas. Examples of this in connection with the gastrointestinal tract include dysplasia [6] and carcinoma [7] in the oesophagus, studies of intestinal metaplasia and gastric cancer [8–10], peptic ulcer prevalence [11], and the epidemiology of diverticular disease [12–14] and of adenomas [15–17] in the large bowel. Guidelines for the retention of tissues and organs at postmortem examination have recently been published in the United Kingdom [18].

Postmortem examination of the gastrointestinal tract

When the primary disease killing a patient is not obviously in the gastrointestinal tract, the oesophagus and stomach are opened for inspection but the small bowel and colorectum are seldom carefully examined throughout their length. This is unfortunate as careful external and internal examination often reveal unexpected pathology, such as leukaemic ulceration, or the presence of polyps and drug-related lesions [19]. If no external examination is made, the bowel should be described either as 'externally normal' or as 'unexamined'; a description of an unexamined bowel as 'normal' only falsifies statistics based on necropsy reports. All pathologists have their own techniques for examining the tract but the following has proved satisfactory in our hands, and is described in order of performance.

Oesophagus

Separate the oesophagus with the heart and lungs from the vertebral column from above downwards so that it remains attached to the trachea anteriorly. Separate any basal adhesion between lungs and diaphragm and examine the diaphragm carefully for hiatus hernia. Examine the oesophagus for external abnormality; then divide it as high up as possible and dissect the lower segment free to be removed later with the stomach and diaphragm (*see* below). This technique preserves a lower oesophagus lined by columnar epithelium or one involved with varices. Carcinoma may make such dissection difficult. Open the upper segment from behind before opening the trachea. Varices are often difficult to demonstrate at postmortem because they collapse when the oesophagus is opened. A way to avoid this is by passing a piece of string attached to a rod from the stomach up through the oesophagus. The string is untied from the rod and fastened around the outside of the upper oesophagus. Gentle traction of the lower end of the string will then evert the oesophagus so that the mucosa may be carefully examined in continuity with the stomach.

Intestines (including rectum and anus)

Locate the fourth part of the duodenum as it receives its mesenteric attachment, tie off in two places, and cut between the ties. Examine the peritoneum and mesentery and note any enlargement of lymph nodes. Using a sharp knife or scissors separate the mesentery from the small bowel as near the bowel wall as possible (this makes subsequent opening of the bowel easier). If local mesenteric nodes are enlarged, excise the involved nodes with bowel, so that location is preserved. Note the presence or absence of the appendix and whether the mesenteric attachments of caecum and ascending, transverse, descending and sigmoid colon are normal. It is comparatively easy, with a little practice, to free the rectum from surrounding structures by blunt dissection with the fingers and then to cut around the anus and remove the rectum and anus together; but some mortuary technicians do not take kindly to the procedure! Decide whether you need to take cultures, and if so from where, and take them at this stage. Open the small intestine along the antimesenteric border using a large pair of ball-pointed scissors; do not cut but pull the bowel over the half-opened blades with the ball inside the bowel lumen. The caecum and large bowel can be opened in the same way; if obvious diverticular disease is present you will see it more clearly by tying the bowel off above and below the involved segment, washing out thoroughly and distending with fixative. Wash the opened bowel in cold water and look for polyps, ulcers, etc. Specimens to be preserved may be pinned out for fixation.

Stomach and duodenum

These are more easily dissected free, usually with the liver, pancreas and spleen, when the intestine has been removed. Decide whether you need to retain the gastric content or culture the duodenal fluid. Open the oesophagus along the left lateral aspect with scissors and continue downwards along the greater curve of the stomach up into the anterior aspect of the pylorus and along the anterior aspect of the duodenum. This allows inspection of the ampulla of Vater and the bile and pancreatic ducts. Look carefully for old duodenal ulcer scars. Specimens to be preserved should be pinned out for fixation as already described.

References

1 Cameron HM, McGoogan E. A prospective study of 1152 hospital autopsies. I. Inaccuracies in death certification. *J Pathol*, 1981; 133: 273.
2 Cameron HM, McGoogan E. A prospective study of 1152 hospital autopsies. II. Analyses of inaccuracies in clinical diagnoses and their significance. *J Pathol*, 1981; 133: 285.
3 Goldman L, Sayson R, Robbins S, Cohn LH, Bettmann M, Weisberg M. The value of the autopsy in three medical eras. *N Engl J Med*, 1983; 308: 1000.
4 Sarode VR, Datta BN, Banerjee AK *et al*. Autopsy findings and clinical diagnoses: a review of 1,000 cases. *Hum Pathol*, 1993; 24: 194.
5 Start RD, Firth JA, Macgillivray F, Cross SS. Have declining clinical necropsy rates reduced the contribution of necropsy to medical research? *J Clin Pathol*, 1995; 48: 402.
6 Auerbach O, Stout AP, Hammond EC, Garfinkel L. Histologic changes in esophagus in relation to smoking habits. *Arch Environ Health*, 1965; 11: 4.
7 Mandard AM, Chasle J, Marnay J *et al*. Autopsy findings in 111 cases of esophageal cancer. *Cancer*, 1981; 48: 329.
8 Correa P, Cuello C, Duque E. Carcinoma and intestinal metaplasia of the stomach in Colombian migrants. *J Natl Cancer Inst*, 1970; 44: 297.
9 Correa P, Sasano N, Stemmermann GN, Haenszel W. Pathology of gastric carcinoma in Japanese populations: comparisons between Miyagi prefecture, Japan and Hawaii. *J Natl Cancer Inst*, 1973; 51: 1449.
10 Imai T, Murayama H. Time trend in the prevalence of metaplasia in Japan. *Cancer*, 1983; 52: 353.
11 Watkinson G. The incidence of chronic peptic ulcer found at necropsy. *Gut*, 1960; 1: 14.
12 Hughes LE. Post-mortem survey of diverticular disease of the colon. *Gut*, 1969; 10: 336.
13 Stemmerman GN, Yatani R. Diverticulosis and polyps of the large intestine. *Cancer*, 1973; 31: 1260.
14 Lee Y-S. Diverticular disease of the large bowel in Singapore. An autopsy survey. *Dis Colon Rectum*, 1986; 29: 330.
15 Eide TJ, Stalsberg H. Polyps of the large intestine in northern Norway. *Cancer*, 1978; 42: 2839.
16 Rickert RR, Auerbach O, Garfinkel L, Hammond EC, Frasca JM. Adenomatous lesions of the large bowel. An autopsy survey. *Cancer*, 1979; 43: 1847.
17 Williams AR, Balasooriya BAW, Day DW. Polyps and cancer of the large bowel: a necropsy study in Liverpool. *Gut*, 1982; 23: 835.
18 Royal College of Pathologists. *Guidelines for the Retention of Tissues and Organs at Post-Mortem Examination*. London: Royal College of Pathologists, 2000.
19 Allison MC, Howatson AG, Torrance CJ, Lee FD, Russell RI. Gastrointestinal tract damage associated with the use of nonsteroidal antiinflammatory drugs. *N Engl J Med*, 1992; 327: 749.

PART 2 Oesophagus

4 Normal oesophagus

Anatomy

The adult oesophagus is a muscular tube some 25 cm long, which extends from the pharynx at the cricoid cartilage opposite the 6th cervical vertebra to the cardia, about 2.5 cm to the left of the midline, opposite the 10th or 11th thoracic vertebra. For endoscopists, the distance from the incisor teeth to its upper end is about 15 cm and to the cardia about 40 cm. It pierces the left crus of the diaphragm and has an intra-abdominal portion about 1.5 cm in length. Its principal relations, important to the pathologist in assessing the local spread of cancer, are with the trachea, the left main bronchus, the aortic arch and descending aorta, and the left atrium. It is supplied by the inferior thyroid, bronchial, left phrenic and left gastric arteries and by small twigs directly from the aorta. Its veins form a well developed submucous plexus draining into thyroid, azygos, hemiazygos and left gastric veins, and so provide an important link between systemic and portal venous systems. Lymphatic channels from the pharynx and upper third of the oesophagus drain to the deep cervical lymph nodes, either directly or through the paratracheal nodes, and also to infrahyoid nodes; from the lower two-thirds they drain to posterior mediastinal (para-oesophageal) nodes and thence to the thoracic duct; and from the infradiaphragmatic portion to the left gastric nodes and to a ring of nodes around the cardia. Some lymph vessels may drain directly into the thoracic duct. In its upper part the oesophagus receives a nerve supply from the glossopharyngeal nerve, and throughout its length it is supplied by fibres from the vagus and from local sympathetic ganglia.

The lower end of the oesophagus is anchored posteriorly to the preaortic fascia and is surrounded by the phreno-oesophageal ligament which blends with the muscle coats. This arrangement allows some degree of movement and rebound. Dissection studies seem to indicate that no discrete anatomical sphincter is present but there are differences of opinion as to whether, and if so, how, the muscle at the oesophagocardiac junction is modified. One careful anatomical study [1] denies that there is any thickening of the muscularis mucosae or of the circular muscle coat but describes a separation of obliquely arranged inner circular muscle fibres into fascicles which continue into the stomach to form the middle circular coat; another equally thorough investigation [2] describes a definite thickening of the inner circular muscle coat. Both authors are agreed that the arrangements which they describe could, and probably do, act as a functional sphincter.

Cineradiography shows that, following a single swallow, there is a hold-up at the oesophagogastric junction associated with a rise in intraoesophageal pressure; this relaxes to allow emptying before the peristaltic wave reaches the junction. In continuous drinking this hold-up does not occur, which also suggests a functional sphincteric mechanism, active during swallowing but inhibited during drinking, perhaps by preliminary diaphragmatic movement. There is doubt as to how much the angle at which oesophagus and stomach meet contributes to the control of reflux. Many aspects of the problem have been extensively reviewed [3–7]; the mechanisms are important in the understanding of reflux and achalasia.

Histology (Fig. 4.1)

The oesophagus is lined by squamous epithelium except for a small segment at its lower end which consists of surface mucin-secreting columnar epithelium with underlying mucous glands. The latter continues a short but variable distance into the stomach where it is usually referred to as cardiac mucosa. Since it is common to both sites the term junctional mucosa has been proposed [8]. The squamocolumnar junction occurs at about diaphragmatic level. It is recognized endoscopically as a serrated line (ora serrata, Z-line) with four to six long or short extensions, with the pink-coloured columnar epithelium standing slightly proud of the paler, smooth and shiny squamous epithelium.

The squamous-lined mucosa is some 500–800 μm thick and is composed of non-keratinizing stratified squamous epithelium with subjacent lamina propria (Fig. 4.2), which rests on the underlying muscularis mucosae. The squamous epithelium has a basal zone consisting of several layers of cuboidal or oblong basophilic cells, with dark nuclei, in which glycogen is absent. It occupies some 10–15% of the thickness of the normal epithelium, although it may be increased in the last 2 cm or so of the squamous-lined oesophagus (see Chapter 7, p. 39).

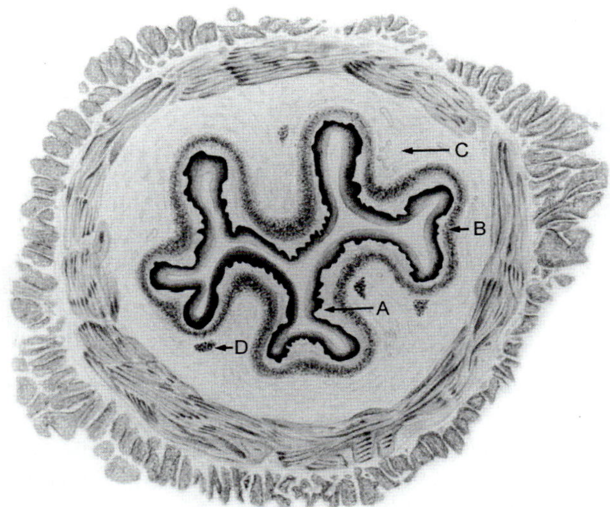

Fig. 4.1 Microanatomy of the wall of the oesophagus. In this cross-section, A is the squamous epithelial-lined mucosa; the muscularis mucosae is B which is separated from the mucous membrane by the lamina propria. The circular and longitudinal layers of the muscularis propria surround the submucosa (C). In the submucosa there are mucous glands (D).

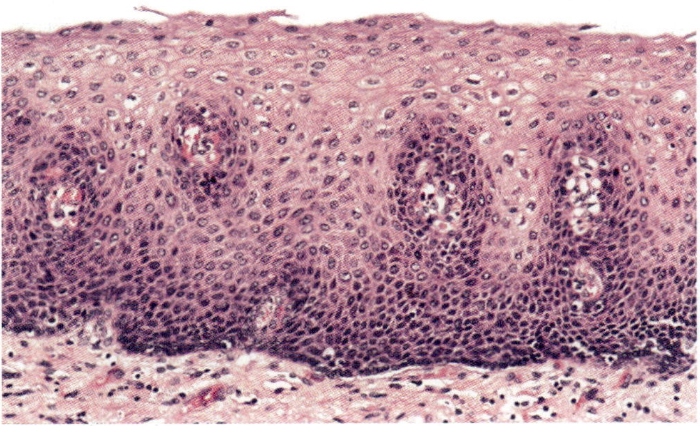

Fig. 4.2 Normal oesophageal squamous epithelium. Note the thickness of the basal cell layer and the height of the papillae. Compare with Fig. 7.1.

Occasional mitoses are seen in the basal cell layer. Above the basal zone the epithelial cells are larger and become progressively flattened, but even on the surface retain their nuclei. Keratohyalin granules are not usually present in the surface cells of normal epithelium. Glycogen is abundant. Single intraepithelial lymphocytes lying between the squamous cells are common ('squiggle' cells) particularly in the lower half of the mucosa, and in this situation their convoluted nuclei may be confused with the nuclei of neutrophils. Characterization using monoclonal antibodies has shown them to be T lymphocytes [9]. Langerhans cells are antigen-presenting cells which are demonstrable by electron microscopy and metal impregnation techniques as sparsely distributed ovoid forms with radiating dendritic processes, and occurring in all layers of the oesophageal epithelium [10]. They stain positively with antibodies to S-100 protein and react with monoclonal antibodies against HLA-DR (MHC Class II) and OKT6 (CD1) and also contain calcitonin gene-related peptide (CGRP), which may serve as an immunomodulator. The number of Langerhans cells and the intensity of their immunoreactivity for CGRP are increased in reflux oesophagitis [11].

Both melanocytes and non-melanocyte argyrophil cells can occur randomly distributed in the basal layer of the epithelium, the former usually as small groups and the latter singly [12,13]. These cell types are presumably the source of the rare primary malignant melanomas and oat cell carcinomas that occur at this site.

Transmission electron microscopic and histochemical studies have amplified the histological picture [14–19]. Basal cells are cuboidal or columnar with large, centrally placed nuclei and relatively simple cytoplasm containing few organelles. They are attached to the basement membrane by frequent hemidesmosomes. Prickle cells show numerous tonofilaments, relatively abundant glycogen, a prominent Golgi apparatus and more numerous desmosomes. The squames of the superficial or functional zone become increasingly flattened towards the lumen, contain some phospholipid material, and have a coating of acid mucosubstance which may be protective. Scanning electron microscopy shows a complex pattern of microridges on their luminal aspects. Membrane-coating granules 0.1–0.3 μm in diameter are present in intermediate and superficial zones of the oesophageal epithelium. As well as the source of mucosubstances they also contain acid hydrolases and these, when secreted into the intercellular space, may be responsible for the desmosomal reduction present in squamous cells as they approach the lumen of the oesophagus.

The lower border of the squamous epithelium is irregular because of the presence of numerous vascular papillae of connective tissue which project upwards from the lamina propria to reach as far as two-thirds of the way into the total thickness of the epithelium. Cell proliferation studies have shown a slower cell cycle time in basal cells overlying papillae compared with the interpapillary basal cells [20]. The lamina propria consists of loose connective tissue in which there are a sprinkling of lymphocytes, mostly helper T cells, plasma cells and an occasional eosinophil and mast cell. Focal collections of lymphocytes and plasma cells may be aggregated around the ducts of the submucosal glands.

At the cardiac end of the oesophagus, papillae and rete pegs become arranged longitudinally to form visible surface ridges. There is a sudden change from stratified squamous epithelium to mucin-secreting columnar epithelium which dips down at intervals to form pits or foveolae, into which compound or branched tubular glands open. At the upper end of this zone, groups of these glands which branch freely and

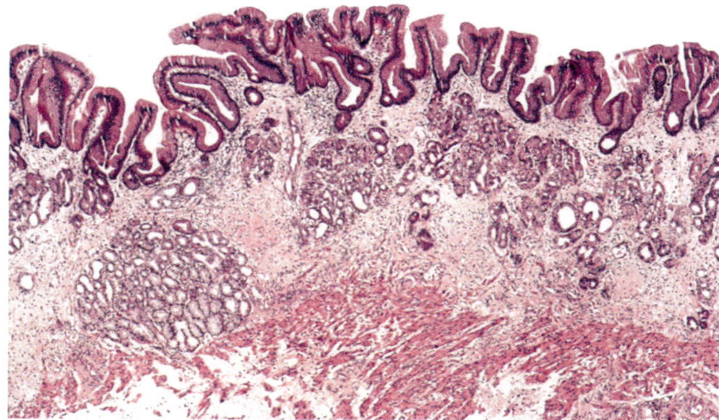

Fig. 4.3 Cardiac mucosa. Mucous gland lobules are present. A few parietal cells are seen in gland lobules at right.

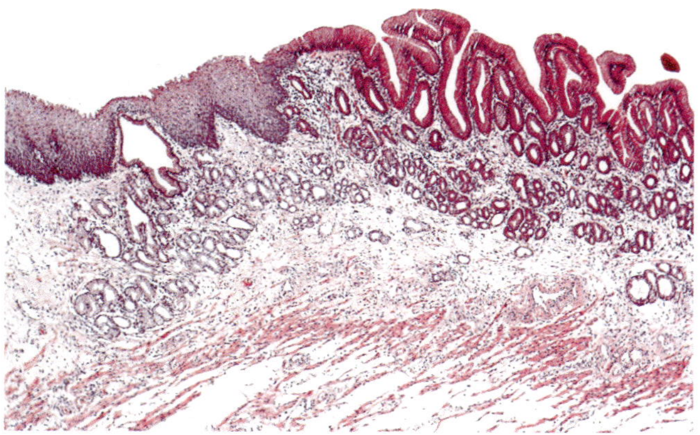

Fig. 4.4 Cardio-oesophageal junctional mucosa. At left mucous glands are seen deep to oesophageal squamous epithelium, so-called superficial oesophageal glands.

pursue a tortuous course are aggregated into lobules by thin septa of collagen and fibres derived from the muscularis mucosae (Fig. 4.3). This lobular arrangement disappears distally, with glands becoming less branched, and here the mucosa is thinner. The transition from this zone to the fundic glands is gradual. The junctional glands often extend a short distance deep to the oesophageal squamous epithelium or occur in small groups just above the squamocolumnar junction, and have been referred to as superficial glands of the oesophagus or as oesophageal cardiac glands (Fig. 4.4). The extension of the junctional mucosa distally varies considerably, usually being of the order of 0.5–1.5 cm but can be as much as 3–4 cm.

In cardiac mucosa, the majority of the gland cells are mucous and stain strongly with the periodic acid–Schiff (PAS) method. Occasional cells near the upper ends of the glands close to the squamous junction may secrete both sialo- and sulphomucins [21]. Parietal cells, morphologically identical to those in the fundic glands, are present in small numbers, and

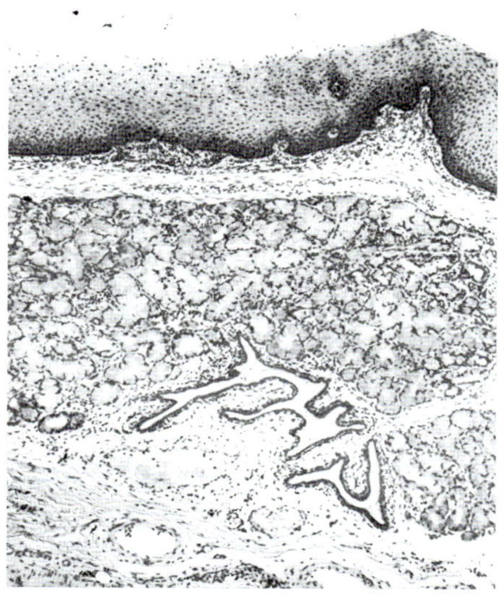

Fig. 4.5 Normal submucosal oesophageal mucous gland and duct.

occasionally chief cells as well. Numerous endocrine cells, some of which are argentaffin and others argyrophil, are found in this region [22]. Cystic change is common, particularly near the squamous junction, and can occur close to the opening of the glands into the foveolae or deeper. Lymphoid follicles are also common in the deeper part of the mucosa or extending through the muscularis mucosae into the submucosa.

A recently described change in gastro-oesophageal mucosa has been the presence of variably sized nests or lobules of acinar tissue (0.2–1.6 mm) admixed with cardiac glands and composed of cells with basally located, small, round and uniform nuclei and abundant cytoplasm. This is eosinophilic and granular in the apical and middle portions and basophilic in the basal area. Some mucous cells may be intermingled [23]. Because of their resemblance to pancreatic exocrine cells and their positivity for lipase on immunohistochemical staining the term pancreatic acinar metaplasia has been used to describe these appearances. In the original description there appeared to be an association with gastritis, but a subsequent study has shown that it is a common finding in patients attending for elective upper gastrointestinal endoscopy, and is not specifically associated with any clinical or histological abnormalities of the oesophagus or stomach [24]. It is likely that so-called pancreatic acinar metaplasia is a constituent of normal mucosa at this site. Similar foci have been described in gastric antral and body mucosa but appear to be much less common at these sites, although they have been reported in some 3% of children in antral biopsies [25]. The function of this tissue is unclear.

The muscularis mucosae has a variable pattern. In the upper part it commonly consists of isolated or irregularly arranged muscle bundles rather than forming a continuous sheet, but in the middle and lower thirds it forms a continuum of longitudinal and transverse fibres and may reach up to 300 μm in thickness at the squamocolumnar junction.

The submucosa is wide; it contains the deep oesophageal glands and a ramifying lymphatic plexus in a loose connective tissue network, which accounts for the early and extensive submucosal spread of oesophageal carcinoma. The glands tend to be arranged in rows parallel to the long axis [26] and, although scattered, are relatively concentrated at the upper and lower ends of the oesophagus. They are tubuloalveolar in type and resemble labial salivary glands, containing both mucous and serous secretory cells together with surrounding myoepithelial cells, which anchor them to underlying basement membrane. The mucous cells contain sulphomucins. From two to five lobules drain into a common duct lined by a flattened cuboidal epithelium initially, which becomes stratified squamous in type and surrounded by lymphocytes and plasma cells after passing obliquely through the muscularis mucosae (Fig. 4.5).

The main muscle layer consists of well developed circular and longitudinal coats. In its upper part these are striated, and both oxidative (fast-twitch) and glycolytic (slow-twitch) fibres are present [27]. There is a gradual change to smooth muscle in the middle third, while in the lower third both coats are entirely smooth muscle without evidence of sphincter formation. A well marked myenteric nerve plexus is present at all levels but there does not appear to be a well formed submucosal plexus. Three types of neurone are identifiable [28,29]. One is argyrophilic, multiaxonal and probably sympathetic, sends out numerous dendrites and axones to surround other neurones in the same and adjacent ganglia, but does not directly supply muscle; a second type is not argyrophilic, is cholinergic and probably parasympathetic; it supplies the muscle. It is probable that the first is co-ordinating, the second motor (see general discussion on gut innervation on p. 245). A third type of fibre, probably a part of the communicating system, is rich in vasoactive intestinal polypeptide (VIP); such fibres are commonly associated with sphincteric mechanisms [29]. There are also numerous intrinsic fibres containing neuropeptide Y [30]. Ganglion cells decrease in number with age [31] but the smooth muscle does not appear to undergo a corresponding atrophy.

There are two sets of lymphatic channels, one in the submucosa, one in the muscle coats; their importance in the spread of oesophageal cancer has already been noted.

References

1 Jackson AJ. The spiral constrictor of the gastro-esophageal junction. *Am J Anat*, 1978; 151: 265.

2 Liebermann-Meffert D, Allgower M, Schmid P, Blum AL. Muscular equivalent of the lower esophageal sphincter. *Gastroenterology*, 1979; 76: 31.

3 Castell DO. Oesophageal motility and its disorders. *Curr Opin Gastroenterol*, 1986; 2: 504.

4 Cohen S, Harris LD. The lower esophageal sphincter. *Gastroenterology*, 1972; 63: 1066.

5 Meyer GW, Castell DO. Physiology of the oesophagus. *Clin Gastroenterol*, 1982; 11: 439.

6 Paterson WG, Goyal RK. Oesophageal motility and its disorders. *Curr Opin Gastroenterol*, 1985; 1: 549.

7 Mittal RK, Balaban DH. The esophagogastric junction. *N Engl J Med*, 1997; 336: 924.

8 Hayward J. The lower end of the oesophagus. *Thorax*, 1961; 16: 36.

9 Mangano MM, Antonioli DA, Schnitt SJ, Wang HH. Nature and significance of cells with irregular nuclear contours in esophageal mucosal biopsies. *Mod Pathol*, 1992; 5: 191.

10 Geboes K, DeWolf-Peeters C, Rutgeerts C *et al*. Lymphocytes and Langerhans cells in the human oesophageal epithelium. *Virchows Arch Pathol Anat*, 1983; 401: 45.

11 Singaram C, Sengupta A, Stevens C, Spechler SJ, Goyal RK. Localization of calcitonin gene-related peptide in human esophageal Langerhans cells. *Gastroenterology*, 1991; 100: 560.

12 de la Pava S, Nigogosyan G, Pickren JW, Cabrera A. Melanosis of the esophagus. *Cancer*, 1963; 16: 41.

13 Tateishi R, Taniguchi H, Wada A, Horai T, Tanaguchi K. Argyrophil cells and melanocytes in esophageal mucosa. *Arch Pathol*, 1974; 98: 87.

14 Hopwood D, Logan KR, Coghill D, Bouchier IAD. Histochemical studies of mucosubstances and lipids in normal human oesophageal epithelium. *Histochem J*, 1977; 9: 153.

15 Logan KR, Hopwood D, Milne G. Ultrastructural demonstration of cell coat on the cell surface of normal human oesophageal epithelium. *Histochem J*, 1977; 9: 495.

16 Al Yassin TM, Toner PG. Fine structure of squamous epithelium and submucosal glands in human oesophagus. *J Anat*, 1977; 123: 705.

17 Hopwood D, Logan KR, Bouchier IAD. The electron microscopy of normal human oesophageal epithelium. *Virchows Arch B*, 1978; 26: 345.

18 Hopwood D, Logan KR, Milne G. The light and electron microscopic distribution of acid phosphatase activity in normal human oesophageal epithelium. *Histochem J*, 1978; 10: 159.

19 Logan KR, Hopwood D, Milne G. Cellular junctions in human oesophageal epithelium. *J Pathol*, 1978; 126: 157.

20 Jankowski J, Austin W, Howat K *et al*. Proliferating cell nuclear antigen in oesophageal mucosa: comparison with autoradiography. *Eur J Gastroenterol Hepatol*, 1992; 4: 579.

21 Gad A. A histochemical study of human alimentary tract mucosubstances in health and disease. I. Normal and tumours. *Br J Cancer*, 1969; 23: 52.

22 Krause WJ, Ivey KJ, Baskin WN, MacKercher PA. Morphological observations on the normal human cardiac glands. *Anat Rec*, 1978; 192: 59.

23 Doglioni C, Laurino L, Dei Tos AP *et al*. Pancreatic (acinar) metaplasia of the gastric mucosa: histology, ultrastructure, immunocytochemistry and clinicopathologic correlation of 101 cases. *Am J Surg Pathol*, 1993; 17: 1134.

24 Wang HH, Zeroogian JM, Spechler SJ, Goyal RK, Antonioli DA. Prevalence and significance of pancreatic acinar metaplasia at the gastroesophageal junction. *Am J Surg Pathol*, 1996; 20: 1507.

25 Krishnamurthy S, Integlia MJ, Grand RJ, Dayal Y. Pancreatic acinar cell clusters in pediatric gastric mucosa. *Am J Surg Pathol*, 1998; 22: 100.

26 Goetsch E. The structure of the mammalian esophagus. *Am J Anat*, 1910; 10: 1.

27 Whitmore I. Oesophageal striated muscle arrangement and histochemical fibre types in guineapig, marmoset, macaque and man. *J Anat*, 1982; 134: 685.

28 Smith B. The neurological lesion in achalasia of the cardia. *Gut*, 1970; 11: 388.

29 Alumets J, Schaffalitzky de Muckadell O, Fahrenkrug J *et al*. A rich VIP nerve supply is characteristic of sphincters. *Nature*, 1979; 280: 155.

30 Aggestrup S, Emson P, Uddman R *et al*. Distribution and content of neuropeptide Y in the human lower esophageal sphincter. *Digestion*, 1987; 36: 68.

31 Eckardt V, Le Compte PM. Esophageal ganglia and smooth muscle in the elderly. *Am J Dig Dis*, 1978; 23: 443.

5 Normal embryology and fetal development; developmental abnormalities of the oesophagus

Embryology and fetal development

There are a number of excellent accounts of the development of the trachea and oesophagus [1–6] and its relation to various malformations.

Between the 23rd and 26th day of embryonic development (3 mm, 10–11 somite stage) a bud develops on the ventral (anterior) aspect of the foregut at the caudal end of the primitive pharynx, grows to become a diverticulum and develops a lumen. This diverticulum will form the larynx, trachea, bronchi and lung buds. It grows caudally and becomes separated from the oesophagus posteriorly by the craniocaudal ingrowth of two lateral folds which fuse in the midline and separate the tracheal lumen from that of the oesophagus. As separation proceeds the oesophagus elongates, mainly due to a rapid increase in growth at its cranial end rather than a primary caudal positioning of the stomach. Separation is complete at 35–40 days, by which time the stomach has been carried down below the developing diaphragm. Interesting anatomical studies [5] suggest that the tracheo-oesophageal septum may in fact be the primitive floor of the respiratory outgrowth.

The epithelial lining is initially stratified columnar; ciliated cells develop in it by the 70-mm stage [7–9]. The ciliated epithelium in the middle third then changes to stratified squamous and this change extends both upwards and downwards [10] to form a complete squamous lining at term, though small islands of ciliated epithelium may remain in postnatal life [11]. Submucosal glands, which probably develop from the original columnar epithelium, appear late in pregnancy and much of their development is postnatal [8].

The circular muscle coat is present at 8 weeks, but the longitudinal coat does not become apparent until approximately 13 weeks of gestation. Neurones can be recognized concomitantly with the circular muscle at 8 weeks, and their density increases up to 16–20 weeks, when there is a rapid decrease, with further reduction towards adult levels during infancy. Ganglion cells and nerve fibres in the myenteric plexus are also maximal at 16–20 weeks, with subsequent decline in their density to 30 weeks, when the numbers become constant despite further oesophageal growth [12,13]. The ontogeny and distribution of neuropeptide expression in the human oesophagus from 8 weeks gestation to 28 months postnatally has shown immunoreactivity appearing progressively in myenteric plexus fibres at 11 weeks and in cell bodies at 13–15 weeks, with patterns of expression of hormones and peptides comparable to those in mature newborns and infants by 22 weeks of gestation [14].

Anomalies of development

Duplications, diverticula and cysts

A detailed discussion on the mode of genesis of duplications, diverticula and cysts throughout the alimentary tract and their relationship with vertebral defects is given on p. 256. In some descriptions of oesophageal varieties the three conditions are separated, but many embryologists and pathologists, ourselves included, now regard the majority of them as differing degrees of manifestation of a single embryological defect. A number of subgroups have been defined [15]. The most common are *duplication cysts* [16–18], which represent a doubling of the oesophagus in some degree; they can be spherical or tubular and even triplication has been described [19,20]. The lining epithelium may be ciliated or non-ciliated columnar, squamous or a mixture of these types, and there are usually two muscle coats present. *Bronchogenic cysts* are anterior in position, contain intramural cartilage and are usually lined by respiratory-type epithelium. Although generally related to the bronchial tree, rare cases have been reported in the abdomen [21] or subcutaneous tissues of the neck or chest [22]. There are other *inclusion cysts* also lined by respiratory or squamous epithelium which do not contain cartilage but are probably of similar origin. *Gastric cysts*, which have a gastric mucosal lining and can secrete hydrochloric acid, are also described. *Neurenteric cysts*, which are usually associated with detectable neurenteric and/or vertebral defects [23–26], may be incorporated into or secondarily fused with the oesophageal wall; they are posterior and lined by squamous or ciliated columnar epithelium.

Most of these developmental cysts are found in children who present with respiratory distress or feeding difficulties. In adults, foregut duplication cysts are uncommon and may be an incidental finding on routine radiological studies. Endoscopic ultrasonography has been found valuable in diagnosis and may eliminate the need for surgery in asymptomatic individuals [27].

Atresia and stenosis

A knowledge of the normal development of the trachea and oesophagus and the mode of separation of their lumina (see above) suggests a number of potential defects, some of which are found in practice [28]. There may be complete failure of division resulting in a single common trachea and oesophagus [29]. Division may be so unequal that the oesophagus is absent or is represented only by a thin fibrous cord of variable length without a lumen or fistulous communication of the trachea. Part or all of the upper trachea may similarly be absent, though this extremely rare malformation is usually associated with distal tracheo-oesophageal [30] or broncho-oesophageal [31] fistula and a single umbilical artery. Tracheal dominance with oesophageal stenosis or atresia is the more common form of unequal division and a fistula is much more commonly present than absent.

Pure oesophageal atresia without fistula is extremely rare; however, stenosis without fistula occurs in about 13–16% of all infants with some form of oesophageal maldevelopment [32,33], is usually found in the mid-oesophageal region opposite the tracheal bifurcation and can be associated with maternal hydramnios [34]. There are occasional cases reported of fusiform stenosis, usually occurring in the distal oesophagus and resulting from tracheobronchial remnants (chondro-epithelial choristoma, cartilaginous oesophageal ring) deep to normal squamous-lined mucosa [35–37]. Oesophageal atresia with tracheo-oesophageal fistula is a relatively common congenital anomaly with an incidence varying from 1 in 800 to 1 in 10 000 live births in different studies [38,39]. The atresia may extend over a variable length or, rarely, may consist of a single transverse diaphragm which may or may not be totally imperforate. It has occasionally been described in siblings [40] but hereditary factors probably do not normally play a part. Other congenital malformations are common [41]; some of these are described under the VATER syndrome which links together *v*ertebral defects, *a*nal atresia and *t*racheo-*e*sophageal and *r*enal dysplasias [42], and has been subsequently expanded (VACTERL) to include *c*ardiac anomalies and *l*imb, especially radial defects [43]. Congenital heart defects also are common [44], as is duodenal atresia with gastric distension [45,46]. When any of these are present in a neonate the others should be searched for. Infantile pyloric stenosis has been described as developing after surgical treatment [47]. There is no significant difference in sex incidence, and maternal hydramnios is more common in association with pure atresia.

A number of anatomical varieties of oesophageal atresia are described [48] (Fig. 5.1). In the most common, accounting for some 85–90% of cases, the upper end of the oesophagus ends in a blind pouch. All coats of the oesophagus are present and the muscle is usually hypertrophied. The anterior wall of the pouch often fuses with the trachea but only rarely communicates with it. The lower oesophagus is normal at the cardia but becomes progressively narrowed proximally. It usually communicates with the trachea within 2 cm of the bifurcation, but occasionally ends in one or other main bronchus, more often the right. The opening is slit-shaped or funnel-like and oesophageal and tracheal muscle are intimately blended. The gap between the blind upper pouch and the lower end varies from 1 to 5 cm, and there is sometimes a fibrous cord uniting the two. Surgical operation is usually feasible but subsequent stenosis leading to recurrent respiratory infection is common. This may be due to stricture consequent upon operation or to an alteration in normal oesophageal physiological activity.

The pathogenesis of oesophageal atresia is uncertain. The most probable explanation is that, as dorsal structures elongate rapidly in the 4th and 5th weeks, cell proliferation in the

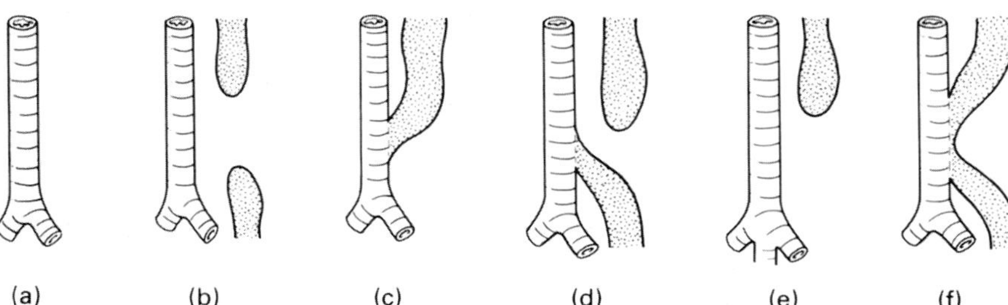

Fig. 5.1 Types of oesophageal and tracheo-oesophageal fistula. The most common is (d).

foregut does not keep pace and both dorsally and ventrally situated cells differentiate into tracheal rather than oesophageal tissue. Failure of recanalization is inherently unlikely since the oesophageal lumen is probably never occluded, and the condition has been described in a 9-mm embryo [49]. The presence of abnormal vessels running between the upper and lower parts of the oesophagus has been implicated, but these are not present in the majority of cases [50]. The lateral septa which separate trachea from oesophagus may meet on the posterior rather than the anterior wall of the foregut, or the posterior wall may be drawn forward with partial incorporation of the oesophagus into the trachea. The radiological evidence of additional thoracic or lumbar vertebrae, often with supernumerary ribs in many of these babies, supports the idea of a disturbance of growth at this period of development [51]. The possibility of genetic factors or viral infection [39] has also been mooted, but is open to criticism in favour of a non-specific action of several teratogenic processes [52].

Deficiencies in Auerbach's (myenteric) plexus with an extra plexus in the membranous part of the trachea in some patients have been reported, which the authors ascribe to incomplete separation of trachea from oesophagus [53,54]. There is also clinical evidence that disorders of motility can be a problem after surgical repair [55].

Occasional examples of fistula without atresia have been recorded and are compatible with survival to adult life. In many the fistula is between oesophagus and bronchus rather than trachea. Oesophageal webs and rings are described on p. 86.

Oesophagobronchial fistula and pulmonary sequestration

A small number of cases have been reported in which a supernumerary lung bud appears to arise from the lower part of the foregut in association with a congenital diaphragmatic hernia; its bronchus may or may not retain a patent communication with the oesophagus [56–58].

Heterotopias

The islands of ciliated epithelium, found sometimes in premature infants, more rarely in full-term babies [11] and very occasionally in adults [59] in any part of the oesophagus, are remains of the ciliated epithelium normally present at an early stage of development. They are therefore not true heterotopias.

The presence and frequency of heterotopic gastric mucosa in the upper oesophagus has long been appreciated from post-mortem studies [60–62] but only recently observed at endoscopy, where surveys have shown these lesions, when carefully looked for, in up to 10% of patients [63,64]. They are present as deep pink, translucent, velvety patches which contrast sharply with adjacent pearl-grey squamous oesophageal mucosa and occur just below the upper oesophageal sphincter ('the inlet patch'), with occasional lesions straddling it. Anything from 0.2 to 5 cm in maximum dimension, they are typically oval with the greatest diameter in the longitudinal oesophageal plane. Rarely, lateral extension may involve the whole circumference of the oesophagus. Multiple lesions are not uncommon. The histology is of body-type gastric mucosa of normal appearance or of a thinned body mucosa with equal proportions of foveolae and glands. Less commonly, a transitional type of mucosa and an antral pattern may be present. Very occasional intestinal metaplasia of complete type has been documented [65]. Inflammation is not usually a feature, although adjacent oesophageal squamous epithelium may show basal cell hyperplasia and elongation of papillae. Despite their ability to secrete acid [63] these lesions are rarely associated with clinical complications or even symptoms. There are occasional reports of high oesophageal stricture [66,67], oesophagotracheal fistula [68], upper oesophageal web [69] and adenocarcinoma of the cervical oesophagus [70–72] attributed to heterotopic gastric mucosa. The current consensus favours a congenital origin, and suggested associations with oesophageal reflux disease and Barrett's oesophagus have not been substantiated [64].

Heterotopic gastric epithelium has also been described in the lower oesophagus as islands surrounded by squamous epithelium [73], but in practice such changes are virtually always an acquired metaplasia (Barrett's oesophagus, see p. 40) as a result of reflux of gastric contents. Heterotopic pancreas has also been described in the lower oesophagus [74].

Heterotopic sebaceous glands were first described at autopsy where they were present in 2% of cases when the whole of the oesophagus was examined using a 'swiss-roll' technique [75]. There have been subsequent reports in the endoscopy literature describing yellow, papular, oval and rounded lesions, sometimes multiple and 1–5 mm in dimension, at different levels of the oesophagus [76,77]. Histologically, mature sebaceous glands are present deep to oesophageal epithelium which open via a duct to the surface (Fig. 5.2). There can be associated chronic inflammatory cells [78].

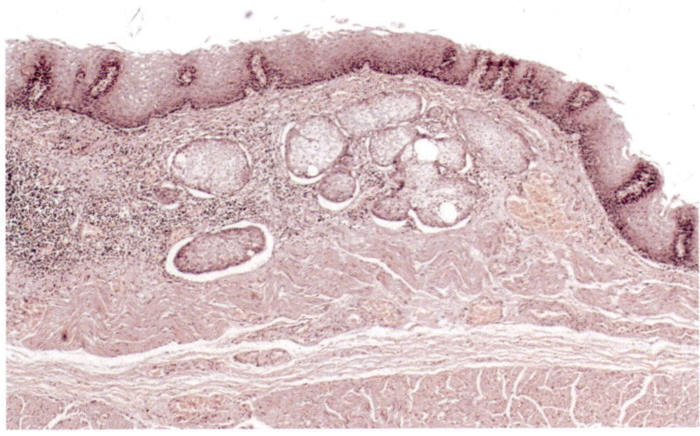

Fig. 5.2 Sebaceous glands deep to oesophageal squamous epithelium.

Congenital diaphragmatic hernia

Congenital maldevelopment of the diaphragm may give rise to herniation of abdominal contents into the thoracic cavity [79].

The ventral part of the diaphragm is derived from the septum transversum, which in the early embryo separates the heart from the abdominal contents. Normally it fuses with the rib cage and sternum, but small canals, the foramina of Morgagni, remain lateral to the sternum on either side. The dorsal part is formed from the dorsal mesentery but there are persistent posterolateral communications on either side, the canals of Bochdalek, between the pleural and peritoneal membranes; later they are further separated by an ingrowth of muscle from the body wall. The oesophagus passes through a hiatus posterior and to the left of the central part.

Four main types of hernia occur in association with imperfectly closed foramina or with the oesophageal hiatus. They are as follows.

1 *Left posterolateral* (through the left Bochdalek canal). Stomach, intestine and spleen herniate.

2 *Right posterolateral* (through the right Bochdalek canal). The liver and intestine herniate.

3 *Retrosternal* (through Morgagni's canals). These are much less common. Liver and intestine herniate.

4 *Hiatus hernia.* The oesophageal hiatus enlarges and the stomach herniates. Rarely the central tendon of the diaphragm is absent.

There is a high incidence of congenital malrotations of midgut with all types of congenital diaphragmatic hernia.

Anterior and posterior rachischisis

These conditions are associated with anomalies of cervical and thoracic vertebrae which are completely or partially divided into halves. There may be anomalies of diaphragm formation with herniation of abdominal contents into the thorax [80] and of the gastrointestinal tract taking the form of short oesophagus or of neurenteric cysts lying between the tract and vertebrae, spinal cord or even dorsal skin. The condition is more fully discussed on p. 222.

References

1 Lewis FT. Separation of the esophagus from the trachea. In: Keibel F ed. *Manual of Human Embryology*, Vol. 2. Philadelphia: Lippincott, 1912: 473.

2 Smith EI. The early development of the trachea and esophagus in relation to atresia of the esophagus and tracheo-esophageal fistula. *Embryology*, 1957; 36: 41.

3 Gray SW, Skandalakis JE. *Embryology for Surgeons*. London: W.B. Saunders, 1972: 63.

4 Moore KL. *The Developing Human. Clinically Orientated Embryology*. London: W.B. Saunders, 1974: 167 & 175.

5 Zaw-Tun HA. The tracheo-esophageal septum—fact or fantasy? Origin and development of the respiratory primordium and esophagus. *Acta Anat (Basel)*, 1982; 114: 1.

6 Montgomery RK, Mulberg AE, Grand RJ. Development of the human gastrointestinal tract: twenty years of progress. *Gastroenterology*, 1999; 116: 702.

7 Johnson FP. The development of the mucous membrane of the esophagus, stomach and small intestine in the human embryo. *Am J Anat*, 1910; 10: 521.

8 Johns BAE. Developmental changes in the oesophageal epithelium in man. *J Anat*, 1952; 86: 431.

9 Botha GSM. Organogenesis and growth of the gastroesophageal region in man. *Anat Rec*, 1959; 133: 219.

10 Menard D, Arsenault P. Maturation of human fetal esophagus maintained in organ culture. *Anat Rec*, 1987; 217: 348.

11 Rector LE, Connerley ML. Aberrant mucosa in the esophagus in infants and in children. *Arch Pathol*, 1941; 31: 285.

12 Smith RB, Taylor IM. Observations on the intrinsic innervation of the human fetal esophagus between the 10 mm and 140 mm crown–rump length stages. *Acta Anat*, 1972; 81: 127.

13 Hitchcock RJ, Pemble MJ, Bishop AE, Spitz L, Polak JM. Quantitative study of the development and maturation of human oesophageal innervation. *J Anat*, 1992; 180: 175.

14 Hitchcock RJI, Pemble MJ, Bishop AE, Spitz L, Polak JM. The ontogeny and distribution of neuropeptides in the human fetal and infant esophagus. *Gastroenterology*, 1992; 102: 840.

15 Arbona JL, Figueroa-Fazzi JG, Mayoral J. Congenital esophageal cysts: case report and review of literature. *Am J Gastroenterol*, 1984; 79: 177.

16 Langston HT, Tuttle WM, Patton TB. Esophageal duplications. *Arch Surg*, 1950; 61: 949.

17 Maier HC. Intramural duplication of the esophagus. *Ann Surg*, 1957; 145: 395.

18 Borrie J. Duplication of the oesophagus. *Br J Surg*, 1961; 48: 611.

19 Sherman NJ, Morrow D, Asch M. A triple duplication of the alimentary tract. *J Pediatr Surg*, 1978; 13: 187.

20 Milsom J, Unger S, Alford BA, Rodgers BM. Triplication of the esophagus with gastric duplication. *Surgery*, 1985; 98: 121.

21 Sumiyoshi K, Shimazu S, Enjoji M, Iwashita A, Kawakami K. Bronchogenic cyst in the abdomen. *Virchows Arch Pathol Anat*, 1985; 408: 93.

22 Bagwell CE, Schiffman RJ. Subcutaneous bronchogenic cysts. *J Pediatr Surg*, 1988; 23: 993.

23 Rhaney K, Barclay GP. Enterogenous cysts and congenital diverticula of the alimentary canal with abnormalities of the vertebral column and spinal cord. *J Pathol Bacteriol*, 1959; 77: 457.

24 Fallon M, Gordon ARG, Lendrum AC. Mediastinal cysts of foregut origin associated with vertebral abnormalities. *Br J Surg*, 1953; 41: 520.

25 Smith JR. Accessory enteric formations. Classification and nomenclature. *Arch Dis Child*, 1960; 35: 87.

26 Superina RA, Ein SH, Humphreys RP. Cystic duplications of the esophagus and neurenteric cysts. *J Pediatr Surg*, 1984; 19: 527.

27 Geller A, Wang KK, Dimagno EP. Diagnosis of foregut duplication cysts by endoscopic ultrasonography. *Gastroenterology*, 1995; 109: 838.

28 De Lorimier AA, Harrison MR. Esophageal atresia: embryogenesis and management. *World J Surg*, 1985; 9: 250.

29 Zachary RB, Emery JL. Failure of separation of larynx and trachea from the esophagus: persistent esophago-trachea. *Surgery*, 1961; 49: 525.
30 Sankaran K, Bhagirath CP, Bingham ET, Hjeertas R, Haight K. Tracheal atresia, proximal esophageal atresia and distal tracheo-esophageal fistula; a report of 2 cases and review of the literature. *Pediatrics*, 1983; 71: 821.
31 Parameswaran A, Krishnaswami, Walter A. Congenital broncho-oesophageal fistula associated with tracheal agenesis. *Thorax*, 1983; 38: 551.
32 Guthrie KJ. Congenital malformations of the oesophagus. *J Pathol Bacteriol*, 1945; 57: 363.
33 Rosenthal AH. Congenital atresia of the esophagus with tracheo-esophageal fistula. Report of 8 cases. *Arch Pathol*, 1931; 12: 756.
34 Scott JS, Wilson JK. Hydramnios as an early sign of oesophageal atresia. *Lancet*, 1957; ii: 569.
35 Fonkalsrud EW. Esophageal stenosis due to tracheo-bronchial remnants. *Am J Surg*, 1972; 124: 101.
36 Sneed WF, LaGarde DC, Kogutt MS, Arensman RM. Esophageal stenosis due to cartilaginous tracheobronchial remnants. *J Pediatr Surg*, 1979; 14: 786.
37 Shoshany G, Bar Maor JA. Congenital stenosis of the esophagus due to tracheobronchial remnants: a missed diagnosis. *J Pediatr Gastroenterol Nutr*, 1986; 5: 977.
38 Belsey RHR, Donnison CP. Congenital atresia of the oesophagus. *Br Med J*, 1950; ii: 324.
39 Ozimek CD, Grimson RC, Aylsworth RS. An epidemiologic study of tracheo-esophageal fistula and esophageal atresia in North Carolina. *Teratology*, 1982; 25: 53.
40 Hausmann PF, Close AS, Williams LP. Occurrence of tracheo-esophageal fistula in three consecutive siblings. *Surgery*, 1957; 41: 542.
41 Holder TM, Cloud DT, Lewis JR Jr, Pilling GP. Esophageal atresia and tracheo-esophageal fistula. A survey of its members by the surgical section of the American Academy of Pediatrics. *Pediatrics*, 1964; 34: 542.
42 Quan L, Smith DW. The VATER Association: *V*ertebral defects, *A*nal atresia, *T-E* fistula with oesophageal atresia, *R*adial and *R*enal dysplasia. A spectrum of associated defects. *Pediatrics*, 1973; 34: 542.
43 Baumann W, Greinacher I, Emmrich P *et al*. VATER- oder VACTERL-syndrom. *Klin Padiatr*, 1976; 188: 328.
44 Barry JE, Auldist AW. The VATER association: one end of a spectrum of anomalies. *Am J Dis Child*, 1974; 128: 769.
45 McCook TA, Felman AH. Esophageal atresia, duodenal atresia, and gastric distention. Report of two cases. *Am J Roentgenol*, 1978; 131: 167.
46 Crowe JE, Sumner TE. Combined esophageal and duodenal atresia without tracheobronchial fistula; characteristic radiographic changes. *Am J Roentgenol*, 1978; 130: 167.
47 Ovist N, Rasmussen L, Hansen LP, Pedersen SA. Development of infantile hypertrophic pyloric stenosis in patients treated for oesophageal atresia. *Acta Chir Scand*, 1986; 152: 237.
48 Willis RA. Oesophageal atresia. In: *Borderland of Embryology and Pathology*, 2nd edn. London: Butterworths, 1962: 186.
49 Fluss Z, Poppen KJ. Embryogenesis of tracheo-esophageal fistula and esophageal atresia: a hypothesis based on associated vascular anomalies. *Arch Pathol*, 1951; 52: 168.
50 Gruenwald P. A case of atresia of the esophagus combined with tracheo-esophageal fistula in a 9-mm human embryo, and its embryological explanation. *Anat Rec*, 1940; 78: 293.
51 Stevenson RE. Extra vertebrae associated with esophageal atresia and tracheo-esophageal fistula. *J Pediatr*, 1972; 81: 1123.
52 David TJ. The epidemiology of esophageal atresia. *Teratology*, 1983; 28: 479.
53 Nakazato Y, Landing BH, Wells TR. Abnormal Auerbach plexus in the esophagus and stomach of patients with esophageal atresia and tracheo-esophageal fistula. *J Pediatr Surg*, 1986; 10: 831.
54 Nakazato Y, Wells TR, Landing BH. Abnormal tracheal innervation in patients with esophageal atresia and tracheo-esophageal fistula: study of the intrinsic nerve plexuses by a microdissection technique. *J Pediatr Surg*, 1986; 10: 838.
55 Romeo G, Zuccarello B, Porietto F, Romeo C. Disorders of the esophagus motor activity in atresia of the esophagus. *J Pediatr Surg*, 1987; 22: 120.
56 Louw JH, Cywes S. Extralobar pulmonary sequestration communicating with the oesophagus and associated with a strangulated congenital diaphragmatic hernia. *Br J Surg*, 1962; 50: 102.
57 Halasz NA, Lindskog GE, Liebow AA. Esophago-bronchial fistula and broncho-pulmonary sequestration. Report of a case and a review of the literature. *Ann Surg*, 1962; 155: 215.
58 Frater RWM, Dowdle EB. Congenital esophago-bronchial fistula. Report of a case and review of the literature. *Surgery*, 1964; 89: 949.
59 Raeburn C. Columnar ciliated epithelium in the adult oesophagus. *J Pathol Bacteriol*, 1951; 26: 399.
60 Schmidt FA. *De mammalium oesophago atque ventriculo*. Inaugural dissertation, Halle, 1805.
61 Hewlett AW. The superficial glands of the oesophagus. *J Exp Med*, 1901; 5: 319.
62 Taylor AL. The epithelial heterotopias of the alimentary tract. *J Pathol Bacteriol*, 1927; 30: 415.
63 Jabbari M, Goresky CA, Lough J *et al*. The inlet patch: heterotopic gastric mucosa in the upper esophagus. *Gastroenterology*, 1985; 89: 352.
64 Borhan-Manesh F, Farnum JB. Incidence of heterotopic gastric mucosa in the upper oesophagus. *Gut*, 1991; 32: 968.
65 Bogomoletz WV, Geboes K, Feydy P *et al*. Mucin histochemistry of heterotopic gastric mucosa of the upper esophagus in adults: possible pathogenic implications. *Hum Pathol*, 1988; 19: 1301.
66 Steadman C, Kerlin P, Teague C, Stephenson P. High esophageal stricture: a complication of 'inlet patch' mucosa. *Gastroenterology*, 1988; 94: 521.
67 McBride MA, Vanagunas AA, Breshnahan JP, Barch DB. Combined endoscopic thermal electrocoagulation with high dose omeprazole therapy in complicated heterotopic gastric mucosa of the esophagus. *Am J Gastroenterol*, 1995; 90: 2029.
68 Kohler B, Kohler G, Riemann JF. Spontaneous esophagotracheal fistula resulting from ulcer in heterotopic gastric mucosa. *Gastroenterology*, 1988; 95: 828.
69 Weaver GA. Upper esophageal web due to a ring formed by a squamocolumnar junction with ectopic gastric mucosa (another explanation of the Paterson–Kelly, Plummer–Vinson syndrome). *Dig Dis*, 1979; 24: 959.
70 Christensen WN, Sternberg SS. Adenocarcinoma of the upper esophagus arising in ectopic gastric mucosa; two case reports and review of the literature. *Am J Surg Pathol*, 1987; 11: 397.
71 Ishii K, Ota H, Nakayama J *et al*. Adenocarcinoma of the

cervical oesophagus arising from ectopic gastric mucosa. The histochemical determination of its origin. *Virchows Arch Pathol Anat*, 1991; 419: 159.
72 Sperling RM, Grendell JH. Adenocarcinoma arising in an inlet patch of the esophagus. *Am J Gastroenterol*, 1995; 90: 150.
73 Haque AK, Merkel M. Total columnar lined esophagus: a case for congenital origin? *Arch Pathol Lab Med*, 1981; 105: 546.
74 Razi MD. Ectopic pancreatic tissue of esophagus with massive upper gastrointestinal bleeding. *Arch Surg*, 1966; 92: 101.
75 De la Pava S, Pickren JW. Ectopic sebaceous glands in the esophagus. *Arch Pathol*, 1962; 73: 55.
76 Salgado JA, Filho JSA, Lima GF Jr *et al*. Sebaceous glands in the esophagus. *Gastrointest Endosc*, 1980; 26: 150.
77 Bambirra EA, Andrade JS, de Souza LAH *et al*. Sebaceous glands in the esophagus. *Gastrointest Endosc*, 1983; 29: 251.
78 Bertoni G, Sassatelli R, Nigrisole E, Conigliaro R, Bedogni G. Ectopic sebaceous glands in the esophagus: report of three new cases and review of the literature. *Am J Gastroenterol* 1994; 89: 1884.
79 Kiesewetter WB, Gutierrez IZ, Sieber WK. Diaphragmatic hernia in infants under one year of age. *Arch Surg*, 1961; 83: 561.
80 Dodds GS. Anterior rachischisis. *Am J Pathol*, 1941; 17: 861.

6 Muscular disorders of the oesophagus

Classification

The control of normal oesophageal motor function entailing transport of a swallowed bolus from the oesophagus to the stomach takes place at three levels: (a) intrinsic activity of oesophageal smooth and striated muscle; (b) intrinsic nerve pathways, mainly involving neurones containing neuropeptides; and (c) extrinsic nerves arising from the central nervous system and which modulate intrinsic nerve or muscle function. It is not surprising from this that the exact aetiological mechanism for most oesophageal motor disorders remains unknown and that classification is not clear cut [1]. In one [2], the main causes of motor dysfunction fall into four groups, namely, connective tissue disorders; neural, neuromuscular and primary muscular disorders; metabolic and endocrine disorders; and miscellaneous conditions. The more important are described below and good reviews of selected aspects are available [3–6]. Gastro-oesophageal reflux disease, the most clinically significant motility disorder, is considered in Chapter 7.

Progressive systemic sclerosis (scleroderma)

Scleroderma in the oesophagus occurs either as part of a generalized systemic disease or as part of a more localized systemic sclerosis confined to the alimentary tract. Oesophageal involvement is frequent in both [7]. Symptoms include dysphagia for solid foods and heartburn. Motor abnormalities of decreased or absent peristalsis are present, predominantly affecting the lower two-thirds of the oesophagus including the lower oesophageal sphincter. The resting tone of the latter is markedly decreased, with predisposition to gastro-oesophageal reflux and its complications [8] (see Chapter 7). Strictures are not uncommon and tend to be intractable, leading to severe dysphagia or even aphagia and aspiration into the lungs. Adenocarcinoma arising in metaplastic columnar-lined (Barrett's) mucosa has been described [9,10]. Candidiasis has been reported in up to 30% of patients [11].

Histologically, there is a gradual patchy atrophy with some replacement fibrosis of smooth but not striated muscle, particularly the inner circular layer, submucosal fibrosis, and some non-specific inflammatory changes [12]. There is a prominent vascular component consisting of elastosis and intimal fibrosis in the smaller arteries. The amount and degree of fibrosis vary markedly from patient to patient and may represent chronic ischaemia consequent on the arterial lesions [12,13]. Ultrastructural studies show thickening and lamination of capillary basement membranes, replacement of muscle fibres by normal collagen and the appearance of dense plaques in some fibres [14]. Local nerves are normal and ganglion cells are preserved. However, the recent detection of circulating antibodies to myenteric neurones in a considerable proportion of patients with scleroderma [15] and the association with Raynaud's phenomenon in up to 90% raise the possibility of a neural rather than a vascular pathogenesis.

Similar motility disorders and abnormalities to those occurring in scleroderma have been described in patients with Raynaud's phenomenon alone, in patients with the latter condition and lupus erythematosus or mixed connective tissue disease [16,17], rarely in association with rheumatoid arthritis [18], and in infants breast-fed by mothers with silicone breast implants [19].

Muscular dystrophies

Occasional cases of progressive non-myotonic muscular dystrophy have shown oedema and loss of smooth muscle fibres in the lower oesophagus [20–22]. The fibres that remain are disorientated, variable in size and vacuolated. There is no inflammatory reaction. The changes are less severe than those seen in scleroderma and the myenteric plexus is not involved.

Studies of radiological and pressure changes in dystrophia myotonica show an overall muscular weakness, and a considerable proportion of patients with this condition have dysphagia. The predominant motor dysfunction is a weakness of the upper oesophageal sphincter, and oesophageal striated muscle shows marked variation in fibre size with internalization of nuclei and pyknosis, focal necrosis and regeneration, and a lack of inflammatory cells [21]. By contrast, oesophageal smooth muscle appears histologically normal.

Diffuse oesophageal spasm and other motor disorders of the oesophagus

Diffuse oesophageal spasm [23] is one of a variety of poorly understood motor disorders of the oesophagus characterized manometrically by repetitive and simultaneous oesophageal body contractions in the presence of essentially normal peristalsis and a normally relaxing lower oesophageal sphincter. It affects males predominantly, and is usually associated with dysphagia and angina-type chest pain. Radiological studies show segmental spasm giving a corkscrew or curling oesophagus with the appearance of pseudodiverticula. In cases that have come to surgery the oesophagus has been reported to be normal with muscular hypertrophy in a few, although details of the latter are scanty. This condition differs from, and has been confused in the literature with, idiopathic or diffuse muscular hypertrophy, a disorder which is related to, and may coexist with, so-called oesophageal leiomyomatosis (see Chapter 8, p. 74).

Other types of abnormal oesophageal motility such as nutcracker oesophagus and hypertensive lower oesophageal sphincter have been documented on the basis of manometric studies, but their clinical significance is debated [24,25].

Acquired diverticula

Most oesophageal diverticula are acquired; congenital examples are rare. The acquired types, which are becoming less common, are divisible into *pulsion diverticula* consequent on raised intraluminal pressure and *traction diverticula* in which the oesophagus is secondarily involved from without, usually by inflammation and fibrosis or by adherent neoplastic or tuberculous lymph nodes. Traction diverticula are more common at or below the tracheal bifurcation.

Pulsion diverticula occur at either end of the oesophagus. They are most common at the upper end (pharyngo-oesophageal or Zenker's diverticulum) where increased hypopharyngeal pressure produces herniation posteriorly between the cricopharynx and the inferior pharyngeal constrictor muscles (Killian's triangle). The primary abnormality appears to be incomplete opening of the upper oesophageal sphincter, whereas neuromuscular pharyngosphincteric co-ordination and sphincter relaxation are normal [26]. Patients are generally middle-aged or elderly, and may be asymptomatic or present with dysphagia, regurgitation of undigested food often swallowed hours earlier, aspiration and voice changes [27]. The diverticula have a narrow neck and all layers of the posterior pharyngeal wall are present although the muscularis propria is attenuated. Histology of the cricopharyngeus muscle has shown marked changes, including fibro-adipose replacement and fibre degeneration [28]. An increased frequency of squamous cell carcinoma has been reported in Zenker's diverticula [29].

Epiphrenic diverticula occur within the distal third of the oesophagus and frequently accompany conditions causing functional or structural obstruction such as hiatus hernia, diffuse oesophageal spasm and achalasia [30,31]. They are usually wide-mouthed and can reach a large size. Most arise from the right posterior wall.

Intramural oesophageal diverticulosis or pseudodiverticulosis is an uncommon condition in which there is dilatation of excretory ducts of the submucosal oesophageal glands. If multiple, this gives rise to a characteristic radiological picture of flask- or collar button-shaped outpouchings projecting perpendicularly from the lumen [32,33]. When only a portion of the oesophagus is involved it tends to be the proximal third. Most cases have occurred in the 6th and 7th decades. The aetiology and pathogenesis is not clear. Similar, but less extensive, changes have been described at autopsy as a common feature in 'normal' oesophagi where they have been associated with marked chronic inflammation of the submucosal ducts and glands [34]. A non-specific oesophagitis has been present in the majority of clinical cases, often associated with disorders of oesophageal motility and stricture formation. Dilatation of the latter, or treatment of oesophagitis, has reversed the process in some cases [35–37]. *Candida* organisms have been present in some 8% of cases [33].

Acquired hiatus hernia

Most diaphragmatic hernias are acquired, and many present in late adult life. It is a common condition, being found in 1–3% of adults on routine barium examination and the prevalence rises further when the prone position is adopted or on increasing intra-abdominal pressure [38]. There is wide geographical variation in its prevalence, with the condition being uncommon in Africa [39,40].

There are two main types, which in some instances may be combined. The so-called *sliding* hiatus hernia accounts for some 95% of the total. The stomach and the lowest 1–2 cm of the oesophagus move through the oesophageal diaphragmatic hiatus which becomes enlarged, either because the diaphragm muscle has failed or because the phreno-oesophageal ligament has stretched. Sliding hernias are thought to relate to increased intra-abdominal pressure associated with chronic cough, kyphosis and obesity, but some may be familial [41]. The main complication of this type of hernia is of reflux oesophagitis, although most patients are free of symptoms and have no evidence of reflux. Conversely, the majority of patients with moderate to severe reflux disease have a hiatal hernia [42]. It is now appreciated that both the intrinsic smooth muscle of the distal oesophagus and the skeletal muscle of the crural diaphragm constitute the sphincter mechanism at the lower end of the oesophagus and contribute to the oesophagogastric junction pressure which acts as a barrier to reflux. Upward misplacement of the gastrooesophageal junction will not necessarily therefore result in its malfunction. However the presence of a large and non-reducing hernial sac may impair oesophageal emptying and acid clearance [43,44].

Para-oesophageal (sometimes called rolling) hernia accounts for the remaining cases of hiatus hernia and has a female predominance. In its pure form the oesophagogastric junction remains fixed posteriorly to the periaortic fascia, but due to a widened hiatus and a weakened phreno-oesophageal ligament the gastric fundus protrudes alongside and anterior to the oesophagus into the posterior mediastinum. However, in practice many examples are mixed hernias with some degree of a 'sliding' element [45]. Often the herniation is progressive and in extreme cases the whole stomach may enter the thorax. Other organs such as the small bowel, colon and spleen may also enter the hernia sac. Compared to sliding types of hernia, reflux oesophagitis is uncommon in the pure type of para-oesophageal hernia, but bleeding from erosions or ulcer may occur and ulcers may perforate with mediastinal inflammation and abscess [46]. With giant hernias, obstruction, incarceration and strangulation may result [47–49]. Increase in intra-abdominal pressure, as with sliding hernias, is thought to be important in pathogenesis and some have occurred following previous surgery in the region of the diaphragmatic hiatus.

Traumatic hernias following a breach of the diaphragm have also been reported [50].

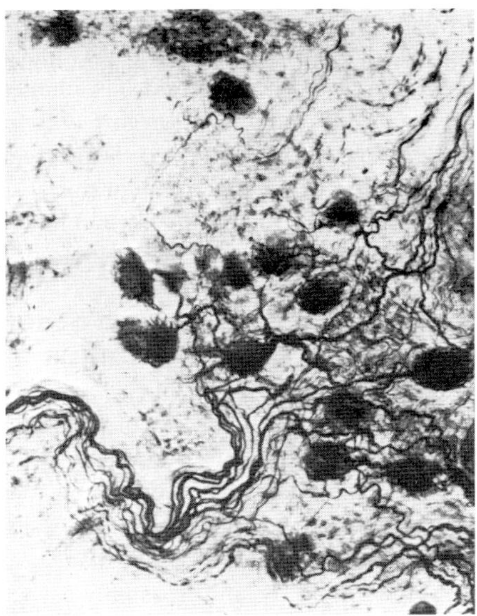

Fig. 6.1 Normal argyrophilic ganglion cells, dendrites and axons, showing arborization of fibres. Silver impregnation technique.

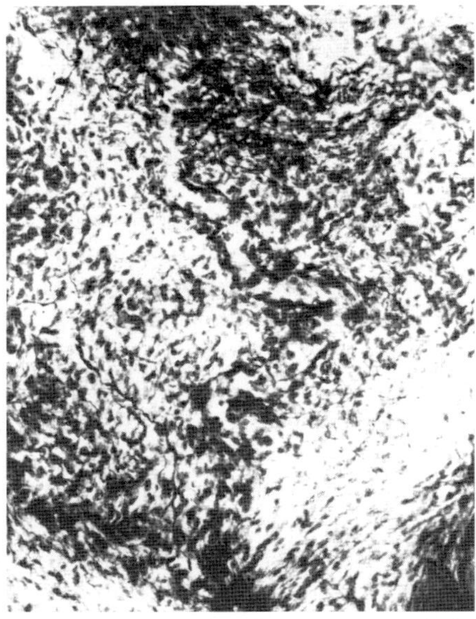

Fig. 6.2 Achalasia. There is a virtual absence of argyrophilic ganglion cells and a markedly irregular arrangement of fibres. Compare with Fig. 6.1 (silver impregnation technique).

Achalasia

In this condition there is obstruction to the onward passage of food at the level of the cardia [51,52]. The annual incidence of new cases in one survey on a stable British population was 0.5 in 10 000 and the prevalence 8 in 10 000; it is most frequent in patients over the age of 60 [53]. There is evidence of regional variations in prevalence [54]. Clinically, patients have pain, regurgitation and dyspepsia over a long period, followed by episodes of respiratory infection due to overspill, and may die from inhalation pneumonia.

Manometric studies demonstrate failure of relaxation of the lower oesophageal sphincter in response to swallowing, absence of peristalsis in the smooth muscle of the oesophageal body, low-amplitude non-peristaltic contractions, a normal or high resting lower oesophageal sphincter pressure and increased intraoesophageal pressure [1]. Radiologically, there is a narrow constricted distal segment and gross proximal dilatation, with distal beak-like narrowing.

Macroscopically, the characteristic appearance of end-stage achalasia is of an enormously dilated and lengthened oesophagus (megaoesophagus) which is filled with stagnant fluid and partially digested food and occupies the entire mediastinum, tapering down at the level of the cardio-oesophageal junction. There is considerable hypertrophy of the muscularis propria, particularly the circular layer. Histologically, there is a marked reduction or complete absence of ganglion cells in the myenteric plexus, variable infiltrates of lymphocytes and eosinophils with a patchy distribution in and around the myenteric nerves, and widespread fibrosis involving the myenteric nerves (Figs 6.1 & 6.2). Inflammatory and reactive epithelial changes are seen in the mucosa, presumably as a response to stasis, and food material, bacteria or *Candida* may be present on the luminal surface [55]. A recent study evaluating the changes in deep muscle strips obtained at oesophagomyotomy from patients with early achalasia demonstrated myenteric inflammation, predominantly in the form of T lymphocytes, even in patients with normal numbers of ganglion cells, suggesting that achalasia results from a primary inflammatory process, with destruction of myenteric ganglion cells and nerves being secondary [56]. What initiates this inflammatory process remains unknown. Achalasia has occasionally been reported in siblings [57], and there is a significant association with HLA-DR and HLA-DQ alleles [58,59]. The latter finding raises the possibility of an immunogenetic mechanism in the pathogenesis of achalasia. Viruses such as measles or varicella zoster have also been implicated as initiating agents [60,61]. Lewy bodies, identical to those seen in Parkinson's disease, have been described in the myenteric plexus neurones as well as the dorsal motor nucleus of the vagus in some patients with achalasia [62].

It appears that in achalasia nitric oxide-containing neurones are more sensitive than cholinergic nerves to the pathological insult. This is consistent with the findings of a marked reduction in nitric oxide synthase in the region of the sphincter [63], the cholinergic hyper-responsiveness of achalasic smooth muscle [64], and the recent use of botulinum toxin (a potent inhibitor of the release of acetylcholine from nerve endings) locally injected into the region of the lower oesophageal sphincter as an effective treatment for the condition in some cases [65]. The traditional treatments for this condition have been either endoscopic pneumatic dilatation or Heller's myotomy.

The most serious complication of achalasia is the development of squamous cell carcinoma. A recent prospective study of patients treated by pneumatic dilatation estimated a 33-fold increased risk compared to an age- and sex-matched population, with an average interval of 17 years from the onset of dysphagia to the diagnosis of malignancy [66]. An occasional case of adenocarcinoma arising in a columnar-lined (Barrett's) oesophagus has been reported in achalasic patients after a Heller myotomy, a procedure often associated with subsequent reflux oesophagitis [67]. Small cell carcinoma has also been reported [68].

A number of conditions may give rise to clinical, radiological and manometric features identical to those of idiopathic achalasia. The term secondary achalasia (pseudoachalasia) is applied in these cases. The most common cause is tumours at the cardio-oesophageal junction or in close proximity to it [69]. Small cell carcinoma may also produce a paraneoplastic syndrome involving neuropathy of the myenteric plexus. Other causes include truncal vagotomy [70], secondary amyloidosis [71], sarcoidosis [72], pancreatic pseudocyst [73] and involvement in multiple endocrine neoplasia type 2B [74]. Chagas' disease is described in the next chapter (see p. 49).

References

1 Cohen S. Classification of the esophageal motility disorders. *Gastroenterology*, 1983; 84: 1050.

2 Mukhopadhyay A, Graham D. Esophageal motor dysfunction in systemic diseases. *Arch Intern Med*, 1976; 136: 583.

3 Castell DO. Oesophageal motility and its disorders. *Curr Opin Gastroenterol*, 1986; 2: 504.

4 Ekberg O, Wahlgren L. Dysfunction of pharyngeal swallowing—a cineradiographic investigation in 854 dysphagic patients. *Acta Radiol*, 1985; 26: 389.

5 Gelfand MD, Botoman VA. Esophageal motility disorders; a clinical overview. *Am J Gastroenterol*, 1987; 82: 181.

6 Mittal RK, Balaban DH. The esophagogastric junction. *N Engl J Med*, 1997; 336: 924.

7 Lock G, Holstege A, Lang B, Schölmerich J. Gastrointestinal manifestations of progressive systemic sclerosis. *Am J Gastroenterol*, 1997; 92: 763.

8 Cameron AJ, Payne WS. Barrett's esophagus occuring as a complication of scleroderma. *Mayo Clin Proc* 1978; 53: 612.

9 McKinley M, Sherlock P. Barrett's esophagus with adenocarcinoma in scleroderma. *Am J Gastroenterol*, 1984; 79: 438.

10 Katzka DA, Reynolds JC, Saul SH *et al*. Barrett's metaplasia and adenocarcinoma of the esophagus in scleroderma. *Am J Med*, 1987; 82: 46.

11 Girsson AJ, Akesson A, Gustafson T *et al*. Cineradiography identifies esophageal candidiasis in progressive systemic sclerosis. *Clin Exp Rheumatol*, 1989; 7: 43.

12 Treacy WL, Bagenstoss AH, Slocum CH, Code CF. Scleroderma of the esophagus, a correlation of histologic and physiologic findings. *Ann Intern Med*, 1963; 59: 351.

13 Atkinson M, Summerling MD. Oesophageal changes in systemic sclerosis. *Gut*, 1966; 7: 402.

14 Russell ML, Friesen D, Henderson RD, Hanna WM. Ultrastructure of the esophagus in scleroderma. *Arthritis Rheum*, 1982; 25: 1117.

15 Howe S, Eaker EY, Sallustio JE *et al*. Antimyenteric neuronal antibodies in scleroderma. *J Clin Invest*, 1994; 94: 761.

16 Gutierrez F, Valenzuela JE, Ehresmann GR *et al*. Esophageal dysfunction in patients with mixed connective tissue diseases and systemic lupus erythematosus. *Dig Dis Sci*, 1982; 27: 592.

17 Lapadula G, Muolo P, Semeraro F *et al*. Esophageal motility disorders in the rheumatic diseases: a review of 150 patients. *Clin Exp Rheumatol*, 1994; 12: 515.

18 Ljubich P, Parkman HP, Fisher RS, Sorokin JJ, Conaway DC. Diffuse gastrointestinal dysmotility in a patient with rheumatoid arthritis. *Am J Gastroenterol*, 1993; 88: 1443.

19 Levine JJ, Illowite NT. Scleroderma-like esophageal disease in

infants breast fed by mothers with silicone breast implants. *JAMA*, 1994; 271: 213.
20 Bevans M. Changes in the musculature of the gastrointestinal tract and in the myocardium in progressive muscular dystrophy. *Arch Pathol*, 1945; 40: 225.
21 Eckardt VF, Nix W, Kraus W, Bohl J. Esophageal motor function in patients with muscular dystrophy. *Gastroenterology*, 1986; 90: 628.
22 Leon SH, Shuffler MD, Kettler M *et al*. Chronic intestinal pseudo-obstruction as a complication of Duchenne's muscular dystrophy. *Gastroenterology*, 1986; 90: 455.
23 Dalton CB, Castell DO, Hewson EG *et al*. Diffuse esophageal spasm. A rare motility disorder not characterized by high-amplitude contractions. *Dig Dis Sci*, 1991; 36: 1025.
24 Kahrilas PJ, Clouse RE, Hogan WJ. American Gastroenterological Association position statement and technical review on the clinical use of esophageal manometry. *Gastroenterology*, 1994; 107: 1865.
25 Leite LP, Johnston BT, Castell DO. Perspectives on esophageal manometry: 'lumpers versus splitters' (letter). *Gastroenterology*, 1995; 109: 2053.
26 Cook IJ, Gabb M, Panagopoulos V *et al*. Pharyngeal (Zenker's) diverticulum is a disorder of upper esophageal sphincter opening. *Gastroenterology*, 1992; 103: 1229.
27 Watemberg S, Landau O, Avrahami R. Zenker's diverticulum: reappraisal. *Am J Gastroenterol*, 1996; 91: 1494.
28 Cook IJ, Blumbergs P, Cash K *et al*. Structural abnormalities of the cricopharyngeus muscle in patients with pharyngeal (Zenker's) diverticulum. *J Gastroenterol Hepatol*, 1992; 7: 556.
29 Wychulis AR, Gunnlaugsson GH, Clagett OT. Carcinoma occurring in pharyngo-esophageal diverticulum: report of three cases. *Surgery*, 1969; 66: 976.
30 Evander A, Little AG, Ferguson MK, Skinner DB. Diverticula of the mid- and lower esophagus: pathogenesis and surgical management. *World J Surg*, 1986; 10: 820.
31 Rasmussen PC, Jensen BS, Winther A. Oesophageal achalasia combined with epiphrenic diverticulum: a case report. *Scand J Thorac Cardiovasc Surg*, 1988; 22: 81.
32 Mendl K, McKay JM, Tanner CH. Intramural diverticulosis of the oesophagus and Rokitansky–Aschoff sinuses in the gall-bladder. *Br J Radiol*, 1960; 33: 496.
33 Fromkes J, Thomas FB, Mekhjian H *et al*. Esophageal intramural pseudodiverticulosis. *Dig Dis*, 1977; 22: 690.
34 Medeiros LJ, Doos WG, Balogh K. Esophageal intramural pseudo-diverticulosis. a report of two cases with analysis of similar, less extensive changes in 'normal' autopsy esophagi. *Hum Pathol*, 1988; 19: 928.
35 Bender MD, Haddad JK. Disappearance of multiple esophageal diverticula following treatment of esophagitis: serial endoscopic, manometric, and radiologic observations. *Gastrointest Endosc*, 1973; 20: 19.
36 Hammon JW Jr, Rice RP, Postlethwait RW, Young WG. Esophageal intramural diverticulosis: a clinical and pathological survey. *Ann Thorac Surg*, 1974; 17: 260.
37 Dua KS, Stewart E, Arndorfer R, Shaker R. Esophageal intramural pseudodiverticulosis associated with achalasia. *Am J Gastroenterol*, 1996; 91: 1859.
38 Atkinson M. The patho-physiology of gastro-oesophageal reflux. In: Truelove SC, Ritchie JA, eds. *Topics in Gastroenterology*, Vol. 4. Oxford: Blackwell Scientific Publications, 1976: 67.
39 Burkitt DP, James PA. Low-residue diets and hiatus hernia. *Lancet*, 1973; i: 128.
40 Bassey OO, Eyo EE, Akinhanmi GA. Incidence of hiatus hernia and gastro-oesophageal reflux in 1030 prospective barium meal examinations in adult Nigerians. *Thorax*, 1977; 32: 356.
41 Carré IJ, Johnston BT, Thomas PS, Morrison PJ. Familial hiatal hernia in a large five generation family confirming true autosomal dominant inheritance. *Gut*, 1999; 45: 649.
42 Wright RA, Hurwitz AL. Relationship of hiatal hernia to endoscopically proved reflux esophagitis. *Dig Dis Sci*, 1979; 24: 311.
43 Mittal RK, Lange RC, McCallum RW. Identification and mechanism of delayed oesophageal acid clearance in subjects with hiatal hernia. *Gastroenterology*, 1987; 92: 130.
44 Sloan S, Kahrilas PJ. Impairment of esophageal emptying with hiatal hernia. *Gastroenterology*, 1991; 100: 596.
45 Wo JM, Branum GD, Hunter JG, Trus TN, Mauren SJ, Waring JP. Clinical features of type III (mixed) paraesophageal hernia. *Am J Gastroenterol*, 1996; 91: 914.
46 Meredith HC, Seymour EQ, Vujic I. Hiatal hernia complicated by gastric ulceration and perforation. *Gastrointest Radiol*, 1980; 5: 229.
47 Pearson FG, Cooper JD, Ilves R *et al*. Massive hiatal hernia with incarceration: a report of 53 cases. *Ann Thorac Surg*, 1983; 35: 45.
48 Dunn DB, Quick G. Incarcerated paraesophageal hernia. *Am J Emerg Med*, 1990; 8: 36.
49 Haas O, Rat P, Christophe M *et al*. Surgical results of intrathoracic gastric volvulus complicating hiatal hernia. *Br J Surg*, 1990; 77: 1379.
50 Sebayel MI, Qasabi QO, Katugampola W, Ahmed I. Traumatic diaphragmatic hernia: review of 15 cases. *Br J Accident Surg*, 1989; 20: 94.
51 Adams CMW, Brain RHF, Ellis FG, Kauntze R, Trounce JR. Achalasia of the cardia. *Guys Hosp Reports*, 1961; 110: 191.
52 Barrett NR. Achalasia of the cardia. Reflections on a clinical study of over 100 cases. *Br Med J*, 1964; i: 1135.
53 Mayberry JF, Atkinson M. Studies of incidence and prevalence of achalasia in the Nottingham area. *Q J Med*, 1985; 56: 451.
54 Mayberry JF, Atkinson M. Variations in the presence of achalasia in Great Britain and Ireland; an epidemiological study based on hospital admissions. *Q J Med*, 1987; 62: 67.
55 Goldblum JR, White RI, Orringer MB *et al*. Achalasia. A morphologic study of forty-two resected specimens. *Am J Surg Pathol*, 1994; 18: 327.
56 Goldblum JR, Rice TW, Richter JE. Histopathologic features in esophagomyotomy specimens from patients with achalasia. *Gastroenterology*, 1996; 111: 648.
57 Bosher P, Shaw A. Achalasia in siblings. Clinical and genetic aspects. *Am J Dis Child*, 1981; 135: 709.
58 Wong RKH, Maydonovitch CL, Metz SJ, Baker JR. Significant DQw1 association in achalasia. *Dig Dis Sci*, 1989; 34: 349.
59 Verne GN, Hahn HB, Pineau BC, Hoffman BJ, Wojciechowski BW, Wu WC. Association of HLA-DR and -DQ alleles with idiopathic achalasia. *Gastroenterology*, 1999; 117: 26.
60 Jones DB, Mayberry JF, Rhodes J, Munro J. Preliminary report of an association between measles virus and achalasia. *J Clin Pathol*, 1983; 36: 655.
61 Robertson CS, Martin BAB, Atkinson M. Varicella-zoster virus DNA in the oesophageal myenteric plexus in achalasia. *Gut*, 1993; 34: 299.

62 Qualman SJ, Haupt HM, Yang P, Hamilton SR. Esophageal Lewy bodies associated with ganglion cell loss in achalasia. Similarity to Parkinson's disease. *Gastroenterology*, 1984; 87: 848.
63 Mearin F, Mourelle M, Guarner F *et al*. Patients with achalasia lack nitric oxide synthase in the gastro-oesophageal junction. *Eur J Clin Invest*, 1993; 23: 724.
64 Holloway RH, Dodds WJ, Helm JF, Hogan WJ, Dent J, Arndorfer RC. Integrity of cholinergic innervation to the lower esophageal sphincter in achalasia. *Gastroenterology*, 1986; 90: 924.
65 Pasricha PJ, Rai R, Ravich WJ, Hendrix TR, Kalloo AN. Botulinum toxin for achalasia: long-term outcome and predictors of response. *Gastroenterology*, 1996; 110: 1410.
66 Meijssen MAC, Tilanus HW, van Blankenstein M, Hop WCJ, Ong GL. Achalasia complicated by oesophageal squamous cell carcinoma: a prospective study in 195 patients. *Gut*, 1992; 33: 155.
67 Gallez JF, Berger F, Moulinier B, Partensky C. Esophageal adenocarcinoma following Heller myotomy for achalasia. *Endoscopy*, 1987; 19: 76.
68 Proctor DD, Fraser JL, Mangano MM, Calkins DR, Rosenberg SJ. Small cell carcinoma of the esophagus in a patient with longstanding primary achalasia. *Am J Gastroenterol*, 1992; 87: 664.
69 Tucker HJ, Snape WJ Jr, Cohen S. Achalasia secondary to carcinoma: manometric and clinical features. *Ann Intern Med*, 1978; 89: 315.
70 Greatorex RA, Thorpe JAC. Achalasia-like disturbance of oesophageal motility following truncal vagotomy and antrectomy. *Postgrad Med J*, 1983; 59: 100.
71 Suris X, Moya F, Panes J, del Olmo JA, Sole M, Munoz-Gomez J. Achalasia of the esophagus in secondary amyloidosis. *Am J Gastroenterol*, 1993; 88: 1959.
72 Boruchowicz A, Canva-Delcambre Z, Guillemot F *et al*. Sarcoidosis and achalasia: a fortuitous association (letter)? *Am J Gastroenterol*, 1996; 91: 413.
73 Woods CA, Foutch PG, Waring JP, Sanowski RA. Pancreatic pseudocyst as a cause for secondary achalasia. *Gastroenterology*, 1989; 96: 235.
74 Ghosh P, Linder J, Gallagher TF, Quigley EM. Achalasia of the cardia and multiple endocrine neoplasia 2B. *Am J Gastroenterol*, 1994; 89: 1880.

7 Oesophagitis

Classification

Inflammation of the oesophagus can result from numerous causes and in an individual case may even be multifactorial. The pathological features are frequently non-specific and a careful assessment of clinical factors is often essential in determining aetiology. The somewhat arbitrary distinction of acute and chronic oesophagitis used in previous editions will not be followed here since these may coincide both temporally and pathologically.

The most common cause of oesophagitis is reflux of material from the stomach, so-called peptic oesophagitis, but inflammation may also be a consequence of various types of infection [1], follow the ingestion of injurious agents such as corrosive chemicals and certain drugs, or result from irradiation. It is often seen in the mucosa adjacent to tumours. Rarely the oesophagus may be targeted in Crohn's disease, in eosinophilic gastroenteritis, and accompanying several skin disorders. In graft-versus-host disease following allogeneic bone marrow transplantation oesophagitis may result from an immunological reaction [2] or be due to infection in this vulnerable group of patients [3]. Ischaemia has been implicated in the few reported cases of acute necrotizing oesophagitis [4,5].

Reflux oesophagitis

Pathogenesis

Some degree of gastro-oesophageal reflux is commonplace, occurring for example in healthy individuals after meals [6] and during early pregnancy [7]. The prevalence of heartburn and/or acid regurgitation experienced at least weekly was found in approximately 20% of individuals aged 25–74 years in one study [8]. The reasons why some people with gastro-oesophageal reflux disease develop oesophagitis are not fully understood and there is a poor correlation between symptoms and histological changes. It has been estimated that oesophagitis involves approximately 5% of the population aged 55 years or older [9] but it is likely that the majority have only mild to moderate inflammation [10]. Inflammatory changes of the lower oesophagus, when marked, cause erosions and ulcers, and extension of the inflammation deep into the wall with associated fibrosis can result in a stricture. In some cases of reflux oesophagitis the stratified squamous epithelium is replaced by columnar epithelium, so-called Barrett's or columnar-lined oesophagus (see below).

Gastro-oesophageal reflux disease occurs in many clinical settings and its pathogenesis is almost certainly multifactorial [11–13]. A sliding hiatus hernia is a common, although not essential, accompaniment and sometimes there is an associated duodenal ulcer [14]. It may follow nasogastric intubation, repeated vomiting, operations which interfere with the gastro-oesophageal junction, and surgical vagotomy. It can also occur in diabetic and autonomic neuropathy and in connective tissue disorders, especially scleroderma. It is common in Zollinger–Ellison syndrome [15], asthma [16] and the irritable bowel syndrome [17].

The central event for gastro-oesophageal reflux disease is contact and injury to the oesophageal epithelium by acid, and persistent or transient loss of tone of the lower oesophageal sphincter is generally accepted as the major determinant of the reflux [18], although interference with non-sphincteric anatomical mechanisms is probably also important [19]. Delay in emptying of the stomach [20,21] and duodenogastric regurgitation [22,23] have been present in some patients, with the latter mechanism being thought to be particularly important following partial gastrectomy [24]. One study found a correlation between gastric motor activity and an increase in duration and number of gastro-oesophageal reflux episodes [25]. Taken together these observations indicate the need to consider a more generalized abnormality of the upper gastrointestinal tract in the causation of this disorder.

Whether or not inflammation or reflux changes (see below) result probably depends on a number of factors, including the volume and nature of the refluxate [26,27], the efficiency of secondary peristalsis in clearing the oesophagus of refluxed material [28], the resistance of the oesophageal epithelium to injury and the neutralizing effects of bicarbonate-rich saliva [29] and secretions from the oesophageal glands, which probably also contain bicarbonate [30,31]. A retrospective cohort study has shown that severe forms of gastro-oesophageal reflux disease (GORD) associated with erosions, ulcers or stricture formation predominantly affected elderly, white male patients [32].

The macroscopic appearances of reflux oesophagitis are observed at endoscopy, and several grading systems exist or are being developed to define and classify lesions reproducibly [33]. The earliest changes appear to be diffuse or patchy hyperaemia or erythema of the distal oesophageal mucosa due to a marked widening and irregularity of small blood vessels, which are present in the normal mucosa as fine, parallel, longitudinal red lines [34]. The distinction between squamous and columnar epithelium may become indistinct or effaced. At a more advanced stage the mucosa is friable and bleeds when touched. Linear erosions, which are surrounded by a red halo and covered by a yellow exudate, initially occur on the longitudinal folds of the posterior wall some 1–2 cm proximal to the Z-line. With increasing severity, erosions are multiple and confluent and may involve the whole circumference of the lower oesophagus. Chronic disease can result in a nodular appearance of the mucosa, poor distensibility of the oesophageal wall, the presence of a stricture, and ulceration. Single or multiple inflammatory polyps can occur [35], and fibrous septum formation, resulting in a double lumen [36], and multiple oesophagogastric fistulae [37] have also been reported as complications of long-standing disease.

In the majority of cases the appearances at endoscopy, particularly when there is erosive or ulcerative disease, correlate with histological evidence of inflammation in targeted biopsies. In patients with minor or equivocal features, or those with a normal appearance but who have symptoms of reflux, or who have reflux on clinical investigation, there may be little or no evidence of inflammation on light microscopical examination (although more subtle damage with dilatation of intercellular spaces has been observed ultrastructurally [38]) but instead a number of features which have been designated as reflux changes [39].

Histology

Reflux changes

These consist of basal cell hyperplasia, with this layer making up more than 15% of the thickness of the oesophageal epithelium, and extension of the connective tissue papillae of the lamina propria more than two-thirds of the distance to the surface (Fig. 7.1). These features have been found with a random distribution over the distal 8 cm of the oesophagus [40]. Presumably the basal zone thickening reflects increased regenerative activity in response to low-grade injury. Cell kinetic studies have revealed a higher thymidine labelling index in the basal zone of patients with reflux as compared with normal controls [41]. It is generally agreed, however, that these appearances can occur normally in the lowermost 2 cm of the squamous-lined oesophageal mucosa as a result of 'physiological' reflux, and even in biopsies from higher levels. Some observers have found a poor correlation between the changes and the demonstration of reflux [42–44]. In addition, these histological features have been described in suction biopsies, which incorporate lamina propria and often muscularis mucosae as well as epithelium, and which because of their size may be easily orientated. The usual biopsies removed from intact oesophageal mucosa using fibreoptic endoscopes are small and difficult to orientate, with less than half the specimens containing lamina propria. In this type of material the presence of overlapping capillaries on tangentially cut specimens has been suggested as indicative of reflux [45], as has the finding of markedly dilated capillaries high up in the epithelium surrounded by flattened epithelial cells containing pyknotic nuclei and sometimes associated with the extravasation of red blood cells [46]. The presence of even occasional

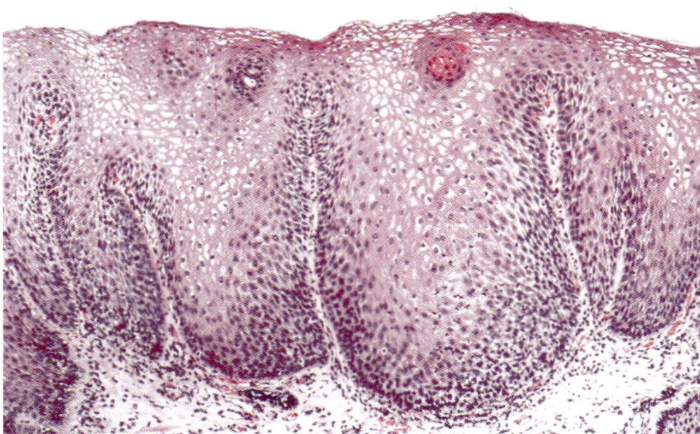

Fig. 7.1 Reflux changes. There is thickening of the basal cell layer of the oesophageal epithelium and elongation of connective tissue papillae which approach close to the surface.

eosinophils in the oesophageal epithelium of children appears to be a more specific and earlier marker of peptic injury than other features such as basal zone hyperplasia and papillary length [47]. This does not appear to be the case in adults, where occasional intraepithelial eosinophils have been identified in asymptomatic volunteers with normal oesophageal function tests [48]. The finding of larger numbers of eosinophils usually correlates with other histological and clinical changes of oesophagitis. Lymphocytes occur normally in the lamina propria and between squamous epithelial cells where they may have an elongated irregular outline and have been termed 'squiggle' cells, and their presence therefore is not informative. Morphometric studies of nuclear parameters, correlating them with acid reflux measurements or response to treatment in patients with GORD, have given conflicting results [49,50].

In summary, reflux changes reflect an increased cell turnover of the oesophageal epithelium, which in the lowermost oesophagus is probably physiological but at higher levels is abnormal. The changes are best assessed when orientated suction biopsies that include the whole thickness of the mucosa are examined. With endoscopic biopsies recognition of reflux changes is more difficult and the material should be step-sectioned and multiple biopsies taken when symptoms and/or endoscopic appearances dictate.

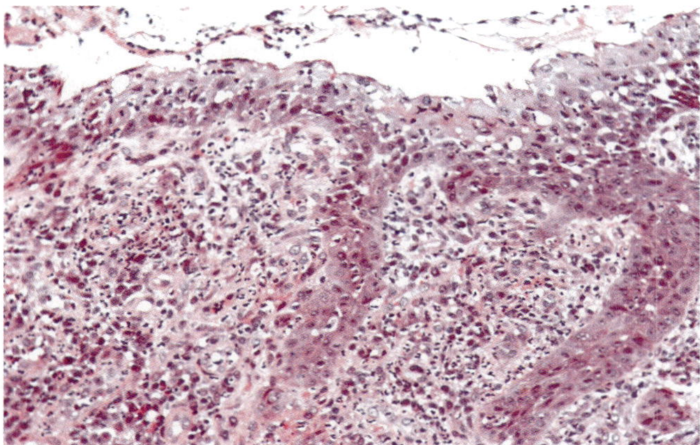

Fig. 7.2 Markedly inflamed oesophageal mucosa with regenerative epithelial changes and some epithelial detachment. Numerous acute and chronic inflammatory cells are present in the lamina propria, which shows increased vascularity.

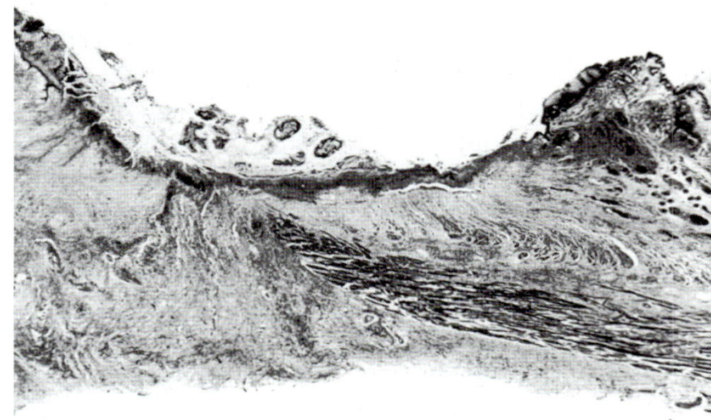

Fig. 7.3 Peptic ulceration of the lower oesophagus resulting in a stricture. Squamous epithelium is present at the margins of the ulcer and there is transmural fibrosis with interruption of the muscle layers.

Inflammatory changes

Milder forms of oesophagitis are recognized in endoscopic biopsies by the presence of small numbers of polymorphs in the lamina propria and infiltrating the squamous epithelium. There may be accompanying reflux changes. With more severe degrees of inflammation there are increased numbers of acute inflammatory cells often associated with oedema, manifest in the epithelium as widening of the intercellular spaces. Lamellar detachment may follow so that eventually only a thin layer of squamous epithelium is present, overlying an acutely inflamed lamina propria in which capillary proliferation is prominent and in which there are increased numbers of lymphocytes and plasma cells (Fig. 7.2). Groups of superficial squamous cells may show ballooning degeneration with abundant, pale, periodic acid–Schiff (PAS)-negative cytoplasm and irregular, pyknotic or karyorrhectic nuclei [51]. This change may also be seen in infectious or chemotherapy-related oesophagitis, and in inflamed or damaged squamous epithelium at other sites such as the mouth, anus and vagina. Erosions appear first over the papillae and subsequently extend to the areas between. Ulceration, by definition involving loss of tissue deep to the mucosa, is associated when severe or recurrent with extensive submucosal fibrosis. The muscle coats and perioesophageal tissues may also be involved [52]. Thickening and shortening of the involved segment may result in a stricture (Fig. 7.3). Sometimes squamous epithelial regeneration is incomplete and the lower oesophagus is lined by inflamed granulation or fibrous tissue that bleeds readily. Ulceration and inflammation are normally easy to recognize in biopsies. However, carcinomas may be surrounded by a zone of oesophagitis and it is therefore important to step-section such biopsies to exclude concomitant malignancy. At autopsy, antemortem ulceration can be distinguished from postmortem digestion by the presence of inflammatory changes.

Columnar-lined (Barrett's) oesophagus

Pathogenesis

In some individuals with reflux oesophagitis, for reasons which are not clear, the stratified squamous epithelium is replaced by columnar epithelium. The condition was first described by Barrett [53] who mistakenly considered it as a 'congenitally short oesophagus' with an attenuated intrathoracic stomach. Subsequently it was realized that the columnar epithelium present was lining the anatomical oesophagus [54,55] and, because of the common association of the condition with a history and radiological evidence of gastro-oesophageal reflux, is now considered to be an acquired disorder in which there is replacement of the squamous epithelium by columnar epithelium at the lower end of the oesophagus [56–58]. A columnar-lined oesophagus has been described in patients with scleroderma and treated achalasia [59,60], and has also developed following partial oesophagogastrectomy with anastomosis between squamous-lined oesophagus and gastric fundus [61], after total gastrectomy with oesophagojejunal anastomosis [62,63], following gastric tube reconstruction in children [64], and, as a localized change, at the site of a lye stricture [65]. In addition, it has been described as a sequel to chemotherapy [66,67]. In experimental studies, oesophageal injury has been followed by re-epithelialization with columnar epithelium under conditions of high acid exposure and when squamous barriers to proximal migration of gastric columnar epithelium had been created [68]. Oral extension of gastric epithelium to replace damaged squamous epithelium cannot explain the development of a columnar-lined oesophagus in all these situations, and alternative mechanisms proposed are metaplasia of stratified squamous epithelium or migration of columnar cells from superficial oesophageal glands. It is also possible that some cases may be congenital [69], although this is generally considered unlikely. A multilayered epithelium within Barrett's mucosa which expresses both squamous and glandular cytokeratin markers has recently been described and suggested as providing support for a multipotential cell derived from squamous epithelium which, in the abnormal milieu of ongoing reflux-induced injury, may be stimulated to give rise to columnar epithelium [70].

There are conflicting reports as to whether or not columnar mucosa may regress following a successful antireflux operation [71–76] or with medical treatment [77–80]. There is also current interest in the effects of photoablative techniques, namely laser treatment [81,82] and photodynamic therapy [83,84], combined with suppression of gastric acid secretion, to induce regression of Barrett's epithelium. This is an important question to answer because Barrett's oesophagus is a premalignant condition (see below).

Prevalence

A columnar-lined oesophagus is more frequent in males than females and has been documented in 0.5–4% of upper gastrointestinal endoscopies [85–87] and in 7.5–14% of those with macroscopic oesophagitis or reflux symptoms [88–90]. An autopsy study found an approximately 21-fold increase over that predicted from a prevalence study of clinically diagnosed cases from the same geographical area [91], highlighting the fact that most individuals with Barrett's oesophagus remain undiagnosed during life. In another study, the prevalence increased with age to reach a plateau by the seventh decade, although the mean length of involved oesophagus was similar in young, middle-aged and elderly patients and did not significantly change in those individuals followed up for several years, suggesting a fairly rapid evolution of Barrett's oesophagus to its full extent with little change subsequently [92]. There is increasing recognition of cases occurring in children with gastro-oesophageal reflux [93–95] and even in the newborn [96]. There have been occasional reports of familial cases [97,98].

Malignant potential

Since the original description by Barrett there have been numerous reports of dysplasia and carcinoma complicating this condition [71,99–104]. The estimated risk of development of adenocarcinoma has varied from 1 in 441 to 1 in 52 patient-years [103,105–109]. The extent of the change in the oesophagus is not generally thought to be a risk factor in the predisposition to malignancy [107,110] and cases of adenocarcinoma have been described arising in tongues or short segments of columnar-lined mucosa [111]. There is also evidence that a considerable proportion of tumours at the cardio-oesophageal junction arise on this basis [112–115].

Several cases have been reported of oesophageal squamous carcinoma in patients with Barrett's oesophagus [116–118]. They have occurred at the squamocolumnar junction or, more commonly, in the oesophagus, separated from columnar epithelium by normal squamous epithelium.

It is clear that epithelial dysplasia is nearly always associated with adenocarcinoma in resection specimens when these have been meticulously examined. Some reports have described multifocal or patchily distributed lesions [119,120], while in others discrete areas of variable extent have been present [121,122]. In most cases dysplasia has occurred in a flat mucosa, but a nodular or low villous pattern may be present [123]. In addition, dysplasia has been documented in long-term endoscopic surveillance studies of patients with Barrett's oesophagus, where it has increased in frequency as well as in severity during follow-up and, in some cases, progressed to adenocarcinoma [103,108,120,122,124]. Apart from difficulties in the histological assessment of epithelial dysplasia (see below), it is apparent that there is considerable variation in its progression, if at all, to adenocarcinoma in individual cases [103,122]. Other parameters which have been or are being assessed as putative markers of increased malignant potential include flow cytometry [125–128], DNA image cytometry [129], ornithine decarboxylase activity [130], p53 protein expression [131,132] and results of cellular proliferation and apoptotic studies [133–137]. The aim of surveillance programmes in patients with Barrett's oesophagus is to identify high-grade dysplasia or carcinoma at an early stage, offering these patients the possibility of curative therapy [138,139].

Surveillance can also evaluate the response to various types of treatment. It is known that in a considerable proportion of patients with adenocarcinoma complicating a columnar-lined oesophagus the diagnosis is only made at the time of symptomatic presentation [140,141]. Because the incidence of malignancy is low, considerable medical resources are required to identify a small number of cases of carcinoma, and this has led some to question of systematic endoscopic surveillance [105,107,142,143]. Current research aims to identify the subset of patients at increased risk of malignancy. It is important that, where the decision to undertake surveillance has been made, adequate histological sampling is carried out, with two or more biopsies for every 2 cm of the Barrett's segment, and additional specimens from any mucosal abnormalities seen. Cytological brushing or lavage can also be used as a complementary method of sampling [144,145]. Blind, non-endoscopically directed balloon cytology sampling, analogous to that used in China for the detection of oesophageal squamous cell carcinoma and its precursors, has been suggested as a potential cost-effective alternative for cancer surveillance in patients with Barrett's oesophagus [146].

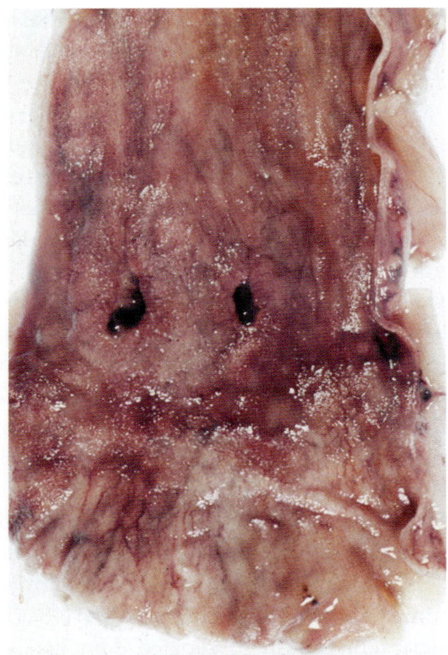

Fig. 7.4 Columnar-lined oesophagus with two well demarcated, punched-out peptic ulcers just above the gastro-oesophageal junction.

Macroscopic appearances

The appearance of Barrett's oesophagus at endoscopy [147] is of a velvety, orange-red mucosa lining the lower oesophagus and extending a variable distance proximally. The wall of the oesophagus is hypotonic and no longitudinal folds are present. The proximal margins of the gastric mucosal folds provide the only reliable endoscopic landmark in Barrett's oesophagus for identifying the junction of the muscular wall of the oesophagus and the stomach [148]. Its exact location may be somewhat subjective, especially in the presence of a hiatus hernia. In the normal situation, the squamocolumnar junction is present within 2 cm of the proximal edge of the gastric folds, so that the finding of columnar mucosa in a biopsy more than 2 cm from this margin is indicative of Barrett's oesophagus. This mucosa is often seen below a high peptic stricture accompanied by varying degrees of oesophagitis [149]. A small hiatus hernia is common. Peptic ulcers—round, oval or circumferential—may be present either at the junction of the columnar and squamous mucosa [150,151] or within the segment of columnar-lined oesophagus, so-called Barrett's ulcer [152] (Fig. 7.4). With aggressive medical therapy the complications of life-threatening haemorrhage, perforation and stenosis reported by Barrett are less frequently seen. The lower oesophagus may be completely lined by columnar mucosa or there may be residual islands of squamous mucosa. Irregular borders of columnar epithelium with tongue-like extensions (Fig. 7.5) and islands of columnar epithelium within the squamous mucosa may make precise delineation of the affected area difficult at endoscopy. Instillation of Lugol's solution, which stains the squamous mucosa black in contrast to unstained columnar mucosa, has been used in these situations [86,153]. Dysplastic areas can be visible as whitish plaques or as shallow depressions or be discovered in areas that appear inflamed or manifest increased vascularity. Occasionally, a nodular or polypoid appearance of the affected oesophagus may be present. In general, however, no specific endoscopic features are identified which enable a distinction between dysplastic and non-dysplastic epithelium to be made. The use of endoscopic laser-induced fluorescence spectroscopy to detect high-grade dysplasia is currently being evaluated [154].

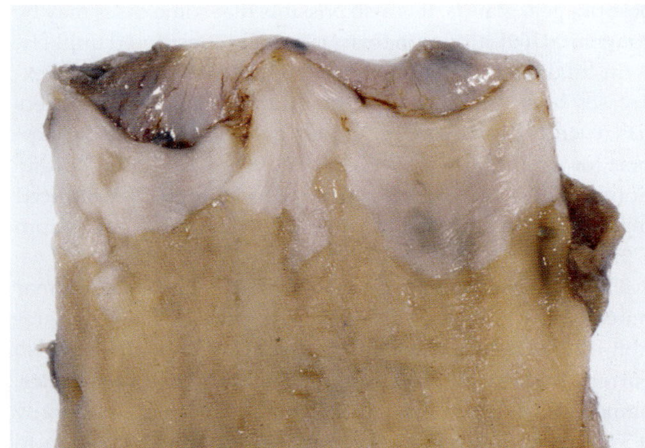

Fig. 7.5 Columnar-lined oesophagus. The junction between squamous epithelium (above) and columnar mucosa is irregular with some squamous islands at left.

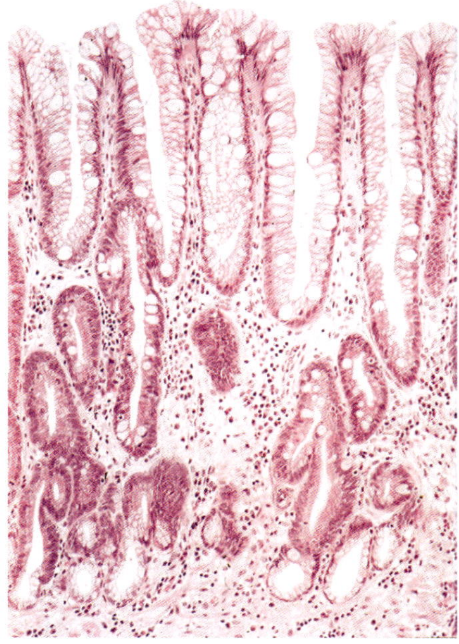

Fig. 7.6 Columnar-lined oesophagus. The mucosa has a villiform surface epithelium consisting of a mixture of goblet and columnar cells. Similar cells line the glands except at the base where mucous cells containing neutral mucin are present.

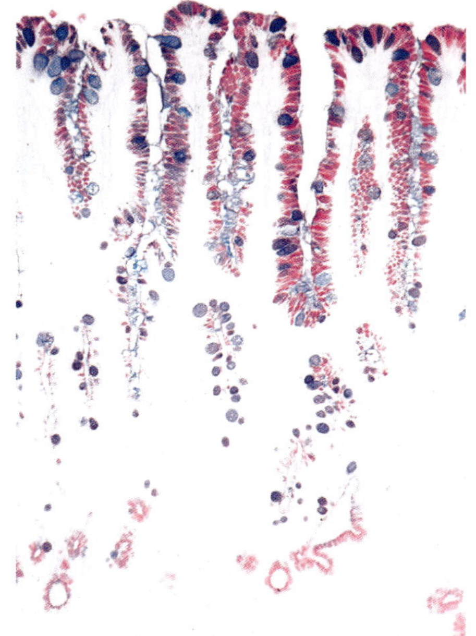

Fig. 7.7 Columnar-lined oesophagus. Neutral mucin (magenta) predominates in columnar cells with alcian blue-positive mucin in goblet cells. PAS/AB stain.

Microscopic appearances

The mucosa of the columnar-lined oesophagus shows a heterogeneous morphology regarding both gland type and surface architecture. This can often be present in the same individual [89,119,155,156]. Despite this complex histopathology, three main epithelial patterns can be identified.

The most common variety, sometimes referred to as distinctive or specialized-type mucosa, consists of epithelium with a flat or villiform surface comprising a mixture of columnar cells and intestinal-type goblet cells, with underlying crypt-like glands in which the same cell types, together with endocrine cells, are present (Fig. 7.6). The latter include cells showing immunopositivity to serotonin, somatostatin, secretin, pancreatic polypeptide and, in some studies, gastrin [157–159]. Scattered Paneth cells may be seen at the base of the glands. A few of the surface mucous columnar cells resemble those of normal gastric mucosa, although more often they have features of mucous neck cells at an ultrastructural level [160]. The majority of columnar cells, also known as intermediate [161], principal [162] or pseudoabsorptive cells, have a variably developed brush border and contain apical mucin in their cytoplasm, i.e. they have characteristics of both absorptive and secretory cells. On ultrastructural examination the mucin granule morphology resembles that of mucous neck cells and the microvilli of the brush border are of variable size and are based on poorly formed terminal webs. An increase in microvilli has been shown to correlate with decreased numbers

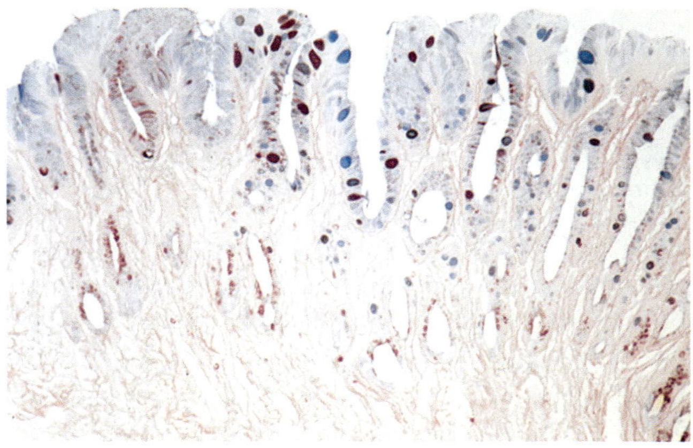

Fig. 7.8 Columnar-lined oesophagus. HID/AB stain showing sulphomucins (brown-black) in some columnar and goblet cells.

of mucous granules [160]. Mucin histochemistry demonstrates that the columnar cells, of both gastric and intestinal (intermediate) type, contain predominantly neutral mucins (PAS positive) (Fig. 7.7), but acidic mucins of both sulphated (sulphomucins) and non-sulphated (sialomucins) type may also be present in the latter. They can be demonstrated using high iron diamine–alcian blue (HID/AB) at pH2.5, which stains sulphomucins brown-black and sialomucins blue (Fig. 7.8), or by a combined Gomori's aldehyde fuchsin–alcian blue technique [163]. Goblet cells contain acidic mucins which are predominantly sialomucins, although sulphomucins are not uncommon as well [89]. An incompletely differentiated variant of intestinal metaplasia secreting sulphomucins (so-called type III intestinal metaplasia) has been associated with gastric carcinoma of intestinal type [164,165]. Although a similar association has been described with Barrett's mucosa and oesophageal adenocarcinoma [161], several studies have shown that incomplete intestinal metaplasia with sulphomucin secretion is very common in biopsies from the columnar-lined oesophagus in the absence of dysplasia or carcinoma and its finding is therefore not sufficiently discriminatory to identify a subgroup of patients at particular risk of malignant transformation [89,156,166–168]. Intestinal metaplasia appears to be age related and is less common in children with Barrett's oesophagus [169]. Although intestinal metaplasia is usually incomplete, foci of complete type (see Chapter 12) may occur, usually deep to areas showing incomplete metaplasia [89]. Recent studies have suggested that the intestinal metaplasia that occurs in Barrett's oesophagus has a distinctive immunostaining pattern with cytokeratins 7 and 20 that allows it to be distinguished from intestinal metaplasia of the stomach [170].

The second main type of mucosa present in Barrett's oesophagus is the cardiac type or junctional mucosa and is similar to that found at the normal squamocolumnar junction, although with a paucity of glands and often showing some distortion of mucosal architecture. It tends to be the usual type in children.

The third and least common type of mucosa is an atrophic gastric fundal type with parietal and chief cells and tending to occur distally in the columnar-lined oesophagus. Although zonation of the other two types has been described, with distinctive-type mucosa occurring proximal to cardiac type [155], a mosaic distribution is usual [119].

Active inflammation is common in Barrett's mucosa and can be associated with the presence of *Helicobacter pylori* when the mucosa is of cardiac type [171–173]. Occasionally, hyperplastic polyps with similar appearances to those in the stomach can arise in Barrett's oesophagus. Also described in resection specimens is a double muscularis mucosae, with the deeper part in continuity with the muscularis mucosae of the oesophagus and stomach at its proximal and distal ends, and the superficial element considered to be newly formed as part of the metaplastic process [174] (Fig. 7.9).

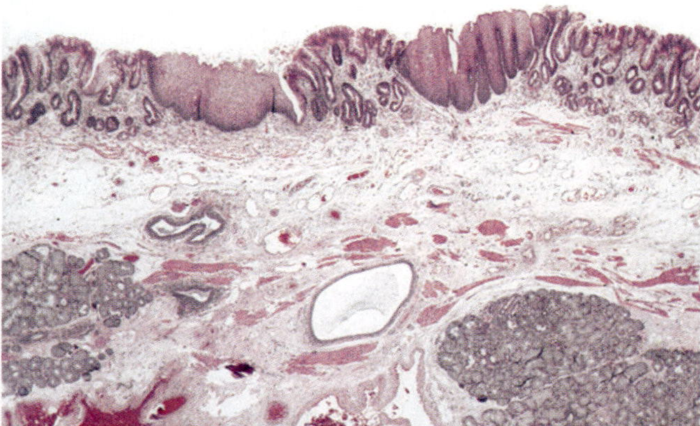

Fig. 7.9 Columnar-lined oesophagus. Note duplication of muscularis mucosae, residual islands of squamous epithelium, and submucosal oesophageal glands and ducts.

Biopsy diagnosis of columnar-lined oesophagus

The histological features described above are not in isolation sufficiently distinctive to make a diagnosis of a columnar-lined oesophagus in biopsy material. Cardiac and fundal-type mucosa are normally present at the cardio-oesophageal junction and complete or, more frequently, incomplete intestinal metaplasia in the former is common when the squamocolumnar junction is not misplaced [175]. This has recently been quantified in several studies [176,177], where the prevalence has ranged from 9 to 36%. The consensus from these studies was that there appeared to be no significant association with gastro-oesophageal reflux disease or with endoscopic and, when looked for, histological oesophagitis. Contributions from *H. pylori* infection, advancing age, race and sex were unresolved. Whilst the significance of intestinal metaplasia in the cardiac region of the gastro-oesophageal junction remains to be elucidated, particularly in relation to any association it may have to the rising incidence of carcinoma at this site (i.e. separate from the contribution of cancers arising in association with a columnar-lined oesophagus [111]), it follows that in order to diagnose a columnar-lined

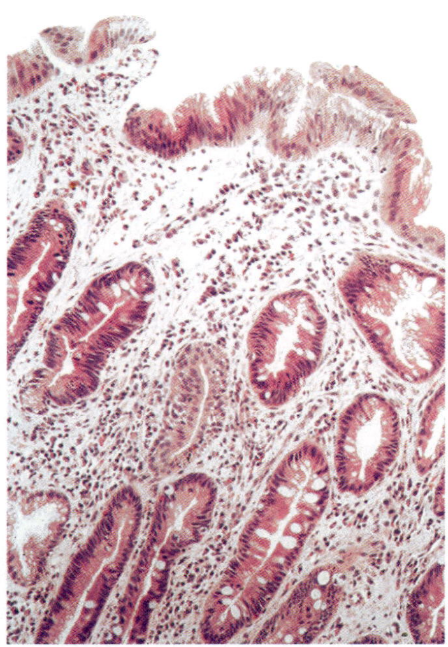

Fig. 7.10 Columnar-lined oesophagus. The duct of an oesophageal submucosal gland is seen centrally.

oesophagus it is essential to know the endoscopic appearances and the level from which biopsies have been taken. Occasionally, the duct of an oesophageal submucosal gland may be identified in a biopsy (Fig. 7.10), and this is presumptive evidence that the material has been taken from the oesophagus.

Epithelial dysplasia

Regenerative epithelial changes may be conspicuous, particularly with material removed from an ulcer edge. They have to be distinguished from dysplasia, and, as elsewhere in the gastrointestinal tract, this is not always straightforward. In both conditions there is nuclear enlargement and hyperchromasia, increased numbers of mitoses, and a decrease in intracellular mucin. Cytological features which favour repair comprise relatively uniform, evenly spaced, round to oval nuclei with smooth external contours and a lower nuclear to cytoplasmic ratio. Nuclear chromatin is granular, with single or multiple nucleoli. Apoptosis is not a feature and the usually plentiful cytoplasm characteristically stains purple as a result of increased ribosomes and decreased secretions. Active inflammation is a frequent accompaniment. Obviously dysplastic epithelium shows marked cytological and architectural abnormalities. Nuclei are enlarged and hyperchromatic, and vary in size and shape. They have a coarse chromatin pattern with prominent, often irregular, nucleoli. Apoptosis with karyorrhectic fragments may be present. Nuclei often show loss of polarity, crowding and stratification. Mitoses are often seen on the surface or in the upper parts of glands. There is a depletion of mucin. Dysplastic epithelium may be present throughout the length of the glands or be confined to their superficial portions with transitions from cardiac-type or distinctive-type epithelium in the subjacent crypts. Architectural changes are frequently present, particularly in more severe degrees of dysplasia, and consist of a prominent papillary or villous configuration of the surface and branching, complex budding, and a back-to-back arrangement of glands. Two types of dysplasia have been described by some observers [178]. In type 1, the changes have resembled those seen in adenomatous epithelium with enlarged, elongated, hyperchromatic nuclei showing crowding and stratification. In type 2 dysplasia there were rounded or pleomorphic vesicular nuclei without crowding or stratification. Type 1 dysplasia was associated with intestinalized mucosa, whereas this was not a feature with type 2 dysplasia. The two forms were frequently found together. In terms of severity, dysplasia has been categorized, in the same way as that occurring in inflammatory bowel disease [179], as high grade or low grade, and an indefinite group, where the changes are equivocal [177] (Figs 7.11–7.15). An interobserver study demonstrated a high level of agreement amongst experienced gastrointestinal pathologists in the diagnosis of high-grade dysplasia and intramucosal carcinoma when these were

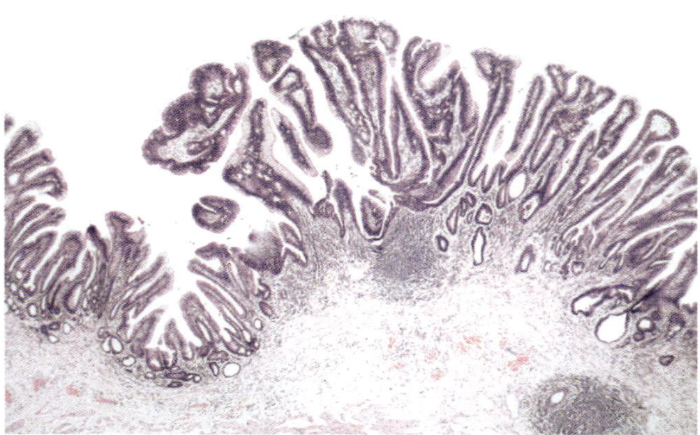

Fig. 7.11 Low-grade villous dysplasia is present on the right, contrasting with non-dysplastic, hyperplastic epithelium to the left. This dysplastic lesion was visible macroscopically.

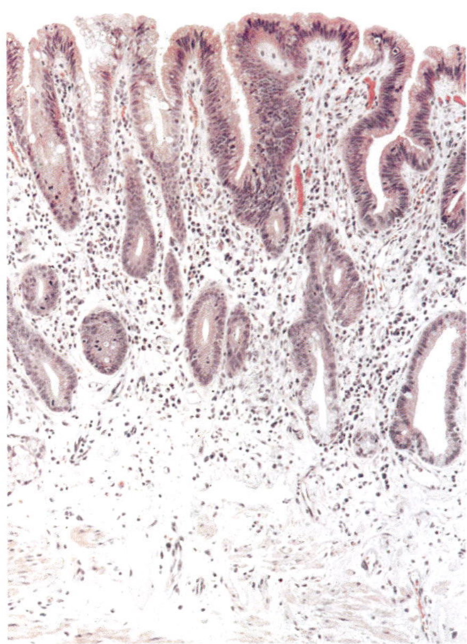

Fig. 7.12 Columnar-lined oesophagus. Low-grade dysplastic epithelium on the right is demarcated from non-dysplastic epithelium to the left.

grouped together. Disagreement was greatest in the differentiation of indefinite from low-grade dysplasia [180]. As in the stomach, distinction of high-grade dysplasia from intramucosal carcinoma may not be possible in biopsy material. However, definite evidence of malignancy may be obvious and a similar range of histological appearances is seen as with gastric cancer.

Management of dysplasia

The finding of dysplasia in endoscopic biopsies from individuals with a columnar-lined oesophagus involves difficult de-

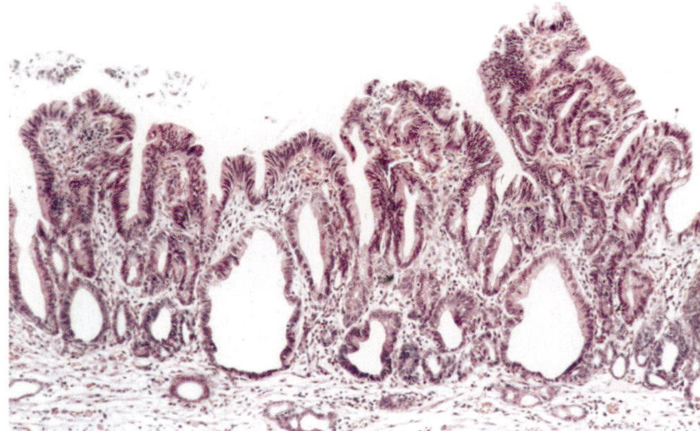

Fig. 7.13 Columnar-lined oesophagus with high-grade epithelial dysplasia. There is considerable glandular disorganization with focal dilatation.

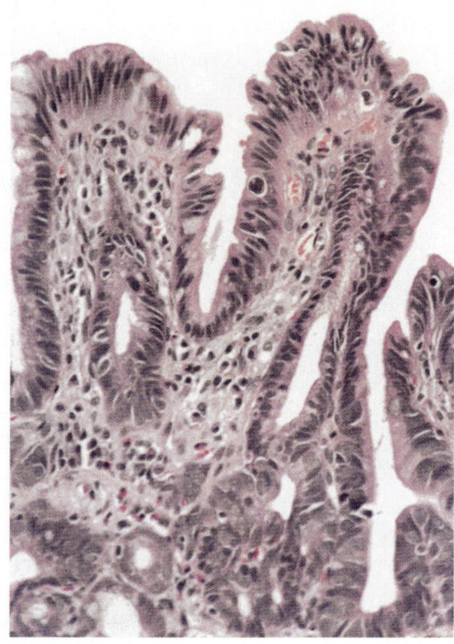

Fig. 7.14 High-grade dysplasia with nuclear stratification and loss of polarity together with abnormal mitoses. Note glandular budding at bottom right.

cisions in management, which are currently being evaluated. Follow-up examinations in individuals with low-grade dysplasia should probably be carried out at 6-monthly intervals [177]. The finding of high-grade dysplasia in biopsies has often been associated with invasive carcinoma in the subsequent resection specimen, although in some the tumour has been limited in its spread through the wall of the oesophagus. Because of the high mortality and morbidity associated with surgery in a predominantly elderly population, the decision to operate has to be considered very carefully on an individual basis [122]. In one prospective study from a referral centre for Barrett's oesophagus using a rigorous, systematic endoscopic

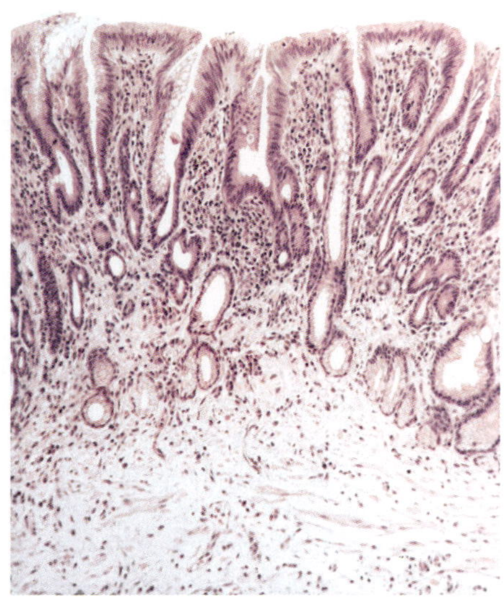

Fig. 7.15 Columnar-lined oesophagus. Indefinite for dysplasia. In this non-inflamed mucosa, areas of glandular and surface epithelium show an increased nuclear : cytoplasmic ratio. There is mild glandular distortion.

protocol, including the use of large-channel instruments and large open-span biopsy forceps, it was possible to differentiate early adenocarcinoma from high-grade dysplasia [181]. Multiple biopsy specimens were taken, particularly from endoscopically visible lesions and from sites at which high-grade dysplasia had been previously diagnosed. Samples were orientated before fixation and step-serial sections prepared. In this way individuals diagnosed as having high-grade dysplasia alone could be endoscopically followed up, without recourse to surgical resection to rule out an undiagnosed carcinoma. However, cancers arising in this situation may be very small and missed, even when a rigorous endoscopic and biopsy protocol is followed [120]. Because of this the tendency is to recommend oesophageal resection for otherwise fit patients with high-grade dysplasia [182–184].

Histopathological changes following eradication therapy

Histopathologists are likely to be seeing with increasing frequency biopsy samples from patients with Barrett's oesophagus treated with various therapies aimed at eradication of this metaplastic epithelium. They include medical treatment with proton pump inhibitors and photoablative techniques. The latter have also been used in the treatment of dysplasia and superficial carcinoma [82,84,185–188]. Squamous regeneration occurs probably from encroachment of adjacent squamous epithelium at the squamocolumnar junction and from extension of epithelium from submucosal gland ducts to form squamous islands. In addition, in cases where photodynamic therapy has been used, there is extensive squamous metaplasia present deep within Barrett's glands with no relationship

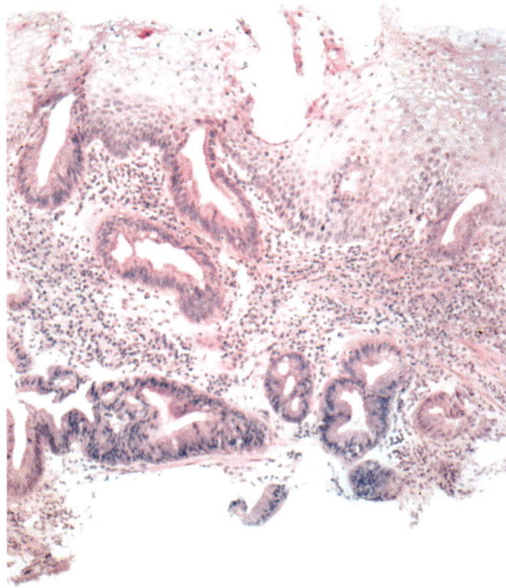

Fig. 7.16 In this biopsy from a patient treated with photodynamic therapy, there has been squamous re-epithelialization over intestinal-type columnar mucosa.

to oesophageal gland ducts and with overlying intestinalized epithelium, implying the existence of pluripotential stem cells within Barrett's mucosa [189]. A common finding is of residual glandular mucosa beneath the squamous epithelium, and the fact that this may show dysplasia highlights the need for deep biopsies to assess the changes present in this situation [82,188,190] (Fig. 7.16). Long-term follow-up studies will be needed to investigate the behaviour of this concealed glandular mucosa, but there is already one report of adenocarcinoma following complete squamous re-epithelialization after photodynamic therapy [189].

Infective oesophagitis

In the immune competent, the oesophagus is usually very resistant to infection, although an oesophagitis can occur in the course of such infectious diseases as measles, scarlet fever, diphtheria and typhoid. It follows that most individuals who have infections of the oesophagus have impaired host responses. With minor abnormalities, infection with *Candida* spp. typically results, but with more serious and prolonged derangements of immunity a variety of fungal, viral and bacterial agents may be responsible.

Candidal oesophagitis

This is far and away the commonest infective cause of oesophagitis, with *Candida albicans* the predominant agent. Other organisms such as *C. krusei*, *C. tropicalis*, *C. stellatoidea* and *C. glabrata* (formerly *Torulopsis glabrata*) [191,192] have

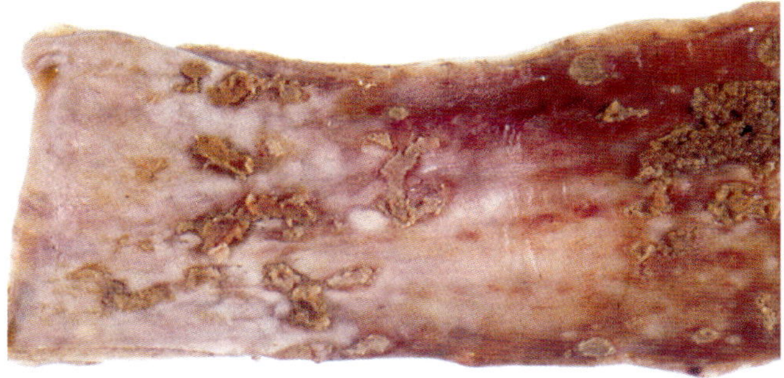

Fig. 7.17 *Candida* oesophagitis. Numerous adherent plaques are present showing focal confluence.

also been isolated. *C. albicans* is normally a saprophyte and has been found to colonize the oesophagus in up to 20% of the population [193], but may become pathogenic and invade the epithelium under a variety of circumstances. These include cases of underlying malignancy, particularly leukaemia and lymphoma [194,195], diabetes, following steroid therapy or immunosuppressive drugs and irradiation, in alcoholics, or after the use of broad-spectrum antibiotics which result in changes in the microecology of the gut flora. Human immunodeficiency virus (HIV) infection is a significant risk factor, and oesophageal candidiasis is common in the early stages of the disease or may arise in the course of treatment for other opportunistic infections. Individuals with persistently low CD4 lymphocyte counts appear most at risk [196]. Interference with oesophageal peristalsis, occurring in diseases such as achalasia and progressive systemic sclerosis, and hypochlorhydria, with acid suppressant therapy [197] or following gastric surgery and resulting in loss of the periodic acid-cleansing mechanism in the oesophagus, can both predispose to colonization and subsequent invasion by *Candida*. In chronic mucocutaneous candidiasis there are defects in cell-mediated immunity, most commonly subnormal production of lymphokines by T cells in response to candidal antigens and defective chemotaxis of leucocytes. This leads to chronic infections of the skin and mucous membranes including the oesophagus. Lastly ulcers, whether herpetic, peptic or malignant, may be colonized by *Candida*.

The characteristic macroscopic appearance of oesophageal candidiasis is of adherent white or cream patches or plaques in the middle and lower oesophagus overlying a friable, erythematous mucosa (Fig. 7.17). Confluence results in a pseudomembrane that may be accompanied by erosion or superficial ulceration. In chronic cases the mucosa may show umbilicated warty lesions, sometimes with central ulceration. On microscopic examination organisms are seen as a pseudomycelium of non-branching hyphae some 2 μm in diameter, and as oval spores up to 4 μm, often incorporated

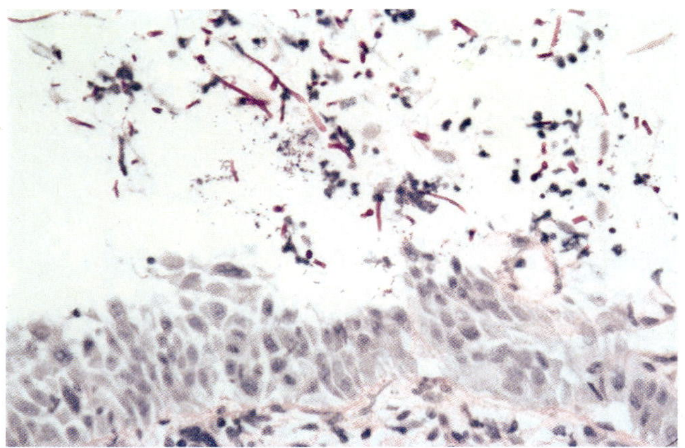

Fig. 7.18 Hyphae and spores of *Candida* are incorporated in inflammatory slough on the oesophageal epithelial surface. PAS stain.

within a pseudomembrane composed of fibrin, necrotic cells and a variable number of polymorphs (Fig. 7.18). When numerous, they are readily apparent in routinely stained sections, but when sparse are demonstrated if a PAS, Grocott or Gomori preparation is examined. In many cases invasion affects the superficial epithelium only, but deeper extension with ulceration can occur and may give rise to complications. Brushing of suspicious lesions at endoscopy followed by direct smears has resulted in a higher detection rate than examination of histological material [198].

Candida oesophagitis may be asymptomatic, particularly in immunocompetent individuals. Complications are more likely when host defences are impaired and where the infection is more extensive and deep-seated. Perforation [199] and fistula formation [200] occur occasionally and oesophageal stricture can follow chronic infection. The latter is most frequent in the upper oesophagus where it may complicate intramural oesophageal pseudodiverticulosis [201], an inflammatory disorder of unknown cause in which there is dilatation of the excretory ducts of submucosal glands (see p. 33). Disseminated candidiasis is associated with considerable morbidity and mortality and occurs in the setting of granulocytopenia, particularly involving patients with acute leukaemia during the induction of remission following chemotherapy [202–204].

Herpes simplex virus (HSV) oesophagitis

Until fairly recently herpetic oesophagitis was rarely suspected or diagnosed during life, although postmortem studies had shown up to 25% of oesophageal ulcers were due to this virus [205]. The oesophagus is in fact the most common visceral site of infection [206], which appears to result most often from reactivation of latent virus in sensory ganglion cells with axonal spread to the oesophagus [207]. Although herpes oesophagitis may occur in otherwise healthy individuals as an acute self-limiting disease [208,209], it most frequently affects immunosuppressed patients with malignant disease (particularly malignant lymphomas and leukaemias), but can also occur in a wide variety of clinical settings, e.g. following burns, in the acquired immune deficiency syndrome (AIDS) or after transplantation. Complications in unresponsive or untreated cases include extensive mucosal necrosis, coexistent opportunistic infections due to cytomegalovirus, *Candida*, *Mucor*, *Aspergillus* or *Torula* [210–212], gastrointestinal bleeding which may be severe [213,214], strictures and disseminated infection [1]. There are occasional reports of spontaneous oesophageal perforation [215].

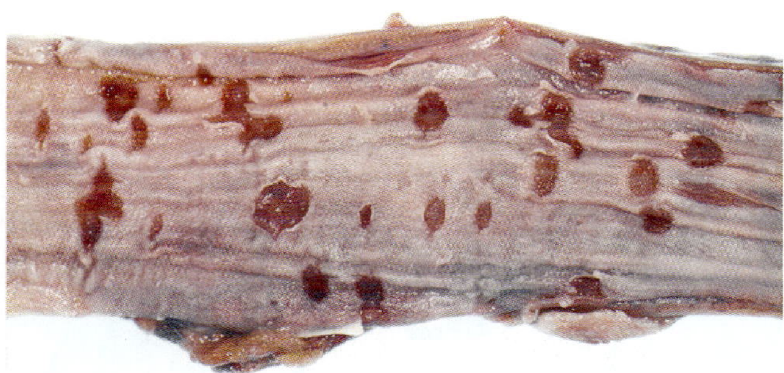

Fig. 7.19 Herpetic oesophagitis. Multiple discrete ulcers of variable size are present.

The earliest changes at endoscopy are of small discrete vesicles with an erythematous base. These subsequently break down to give rise to multiple shallow ulcers (Fig. 7.19) which can coalesce and may eventually result in a non-specific pseudomembrane [216]. The middle and distal thirds of the oesophagus are most commonly involved.

Microscopically the characteristic features of herpetic infection occur in squamous epithelium at the margin of ulcers or erosions. Infected cells contain homogeneous, ground glass, eosinophilic to amphophilic round or oval Cowdry type A intranuclear viral inclusions (Fig. 7.20). Immunohistochemical studies using specific antibodies can be used to positively identify them as HSV [207]. Multinucleated giant cells may be present. These can rarely be found in other types of oesophagitis [217], but are distinguished from them by the presence of viral inclusions. In desquamated necrotic cells the inclusions are palely basophilic with clumping of chromatin just inside the nuclear membrane. Prominent aggregates of macrophages with convoluted nuclei in adjacent tissues have been proposed as a sensitive and fairly specific marker of herpes virus infection [218]. When the diagnosis is suspected at endoscopy, biopsies from the edge of ulcers should also be sent for viral culture [215].

Cytomegalovirus (CMV) oesophagitis

This may accompany other opportunistic infections and its

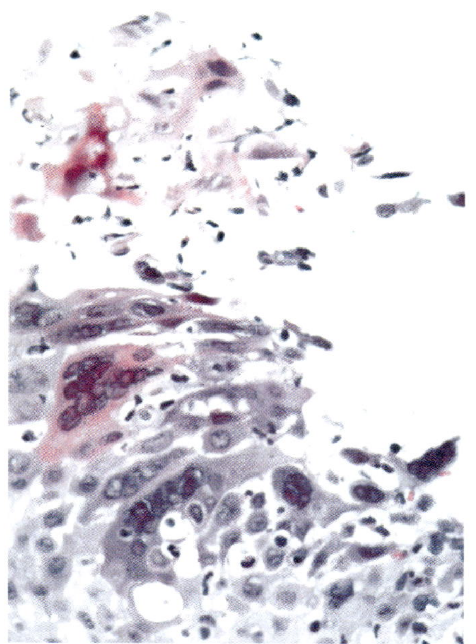

Fig. 7.20 Herpetic oesophagitis. Many of the oesophageal epithelial cells contain intranuclear inclusions and multinucleated cells are prominent.

presence usually signals immune deficiency which may be iatrogenic or, increasingly, a feature of AIDS, where it is the most common viral pathogen causing oesophageal disease [219]. CMV and *Candida* coexist in a considerable proportion of AIDS patients [220]. The endoscopic appearances vary from a diffuse oesophagitis to single or multiple ulcers, usually in the distal oesophagus, which may reach a large size [221]. The histological diagnosis is made in biopsies from the ulcer base, since CMV infects endothelial cells, pericytes, fibroblasts and smooth muscle cells and not the squamous epithelium. Increased detection of CMV infection is facilitated with immunoperoxidase techniques [222].

Other infections

Bacterial

It has recently been appreciated that a bacterial oesophagitis due to a wide range of Gram-positive and Gram-negative organisms may occur in immunocompromised patients [223,224], with bacteria demonstrable in the lamina propria and involving blood vessels in biopsy material.

Mycobacterium tuberculosis infection of the oesophagus is rare and is almost always secondary to pulmonary disease [225–227]. It results either from the swallowing of infected sputum or from direct involvement of the oesophagus by a tuberculous hilar lymph node or infected lung. More recent reports have been in patients with signs of oesophageal pathology but without significant evidence of systemic illness or radiological abnormalities. Occasional primary cases are reported in which there is ulceration with a typical caseating granulomatous reaction. The disease may mimic oesophageal carcinoma clinically [228,229]. *Mycobacterium avium* complex infection has occasionally involved the oesophagus in patients with AIDS [230,231].

There is a recent case report of bacillary angiomatosis associated with numerous polyps throughout the oesophagus in a patient with AIDS [232].

Fungal

Fungal infections, other than candidiasis, which may affect the oesophagus include aspergillosis [233,234], mucormycosis [235], blastomycosis [236], cryptococcosis [237] and histoplasmosis [238–240].

Viral

Epstein–Barr virus (EBV) has been demonstrated by DNA *in situ* hybridization techniques in biopsy material from oesophageal ulcers of homosexual men with AIDS [241]. Accompanying histological features included koilocytosis, epithelial thickening, individual cell keratinization and multinucleation. Ulceration in the absence of any identifiable pathogen has also been described in HIV infection, including small aphthoid ulcers at the time of seroconversion and large, deeper ulcers later in the course of infection [242,243]. Papova virus [244] and human herpes virus 6 [245] have also been isolated from the oesophagus in patients with AIDS.

The oesophagus may also be involved in patients with a thoracic distribution of herpes zoster [246].

Protozoal

Chagas' disease is caused by *Trypanosoma cruzi*, which is found in South and Central America, Mexico and Texas [247–251]. The main vector is the cone-nosed triatomine bug, *Panstrongylus megistus*. The trypanosomes develop in the bug's faeces. These are deposited on human skin at the time of biting, and penetrate it to enter the bloodstream and invade smooth muscle and the myocardium. They multiply as the *Leishmania*-like amastigote form which is ingested either by histiocytes adjacent to ganglion cells or by muscle and ganglion cells themselves (Fig. 7.21). The resulting pseudocysts rupture and liberate their contained parasites. Some of these release neurotoxins leading to inflammatory damage of the myenteric plexus. Others enter the bloodstream to repeat the cycle.

The disease progresses to a chronic phase, in which cardiomegaly, megaoesophagus and megacolon are the most important complications. A striking reduction in the number of ganglion cells within the myenteric plexus accompanies the gut involvement. The number of ganglion cells must be reduced by at least 50% to produce functional disturbance and by 90% to produce megaoesophagus. Patients come to surgery

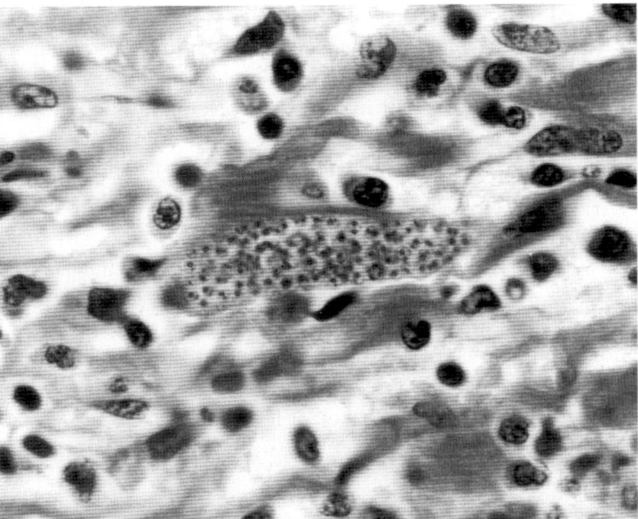

Fig. 7.21 Chagas' disease. Parasites have multiplied within a myocardial cell, forming a pseudocyst.

when the disease is chronic, inflammatory changes are minimal, and organisms are not demonstrable. A considerable proportion of individuals with chronic Chagas' disease have circulating autoantibodies to muscarinic cholinergic receptors [252].

Cryptosporidiosis has been described in biopsies from the gastro-oesophageal junction in a child with AIDS [253].

Other forms of oesophagitis

Chemical and drug-induced oesophagitis

Ingestion of corrosive chemicals may be either accidental or purposeful in a suicide attempt. The former occurs mainly in young children and usually involves small quantities, whereas the latter predominantly involves adults, when large amounts are swallowed. The degree of damage depends on the nature of the substance swallowed and its concentration, the amount and the contact time. As a general rule, effects of ingestion of strong alkalis are seen in the oesophagus, and of acids in the stomach. This is because alkalis dissolve tissue and thus penetrate more deeply, whereas acids result in coagulative necrosis, which has the effect of limiting penetration. Following ingestion, the acute phase of necrosis lasts 4 or 5 days and is associated with oedema and acute inflammation with vascular thrombosis. There may be secondary bacterial infection. A subacute phase follows sloughing of superficial necrotic tissue and ulceration, with subsequent repair by granulation and collagenous connective tissue. Perforation is most likely during the early part of this phase in the first 10–12 days after injury [254]. Re-epithelialization and fibrosis, which may or may not lead to stricture formation, occurs in the chronic phase which extends over the next 1–3 months. The strictures which commonly follow lye ingestion may be complicated many years later by squamous cell carcinoma [255,256].

A number of drugs swallowed as tablets or capsules have given rise to inflammation and ulceration of the oesophagus by a local irritative effect following hold-up [257]. This is more likely to occur when drugs are taken with little fluid prior to lying down. Those most commonly implicated have been the anticholinergic agent emepronium bromide, doxycycline, tetracycline and, more recently, the aminobiphosphonate alendronate [258], used in the treatment of osteoporosis and Paget's disease. The commonest site of damage has been in the mid-oesophagus and the ulcers are discrete, often multiple, and may be serpiginous in outline. They usually heal without stricture formation. More severe cases, associated with stricture, have occurred with slow-release potassium chloride tablets in patients with oesophageal obstruction [259], following ingestion of quinidine, and in patients on nonsteroidal anti inflammatory drugs (NSAIDs), where injury is aggravated by gastro-oesophageal reflux [260]. It has been estimated that 1 in 5 oesophageal strictures may be drug related [261].

Radiation oesophagitis

Radiation therapy to the chest may be followed by a self-limiting but rarely severe oesophagitis. In some cases, however, serious complications such as ulcer, stricture and fistula formation can occur. These changes are probably a consequence of ischaemia due to underlying arterial occlusion. Irradiation of squamous cell carcinoma of the oesophagus can result in a tracheo-oesophageal fistula and biopsies carried out to detect recurrent tumour may show radiation changes with bizarre fibroblasts, oedema and an obliterative vasculitis. Serious effects, including stricture formation, can result from even low radiation doses when adjunctive chemotherapy with Adriamycin, daunorubicin or actinomycin D has been used [262,263]. Recurrent oesophagitis can follow subsequent chemotherapy. Several cases of carcinoma of the oesophagus that may have been induced by radiation have been reported, with a latent interval ranging from 3 to 45 years [264,265].

Crohn's disease

Oesophageal involvement in patients with Crohn's disease is well recognized [266–269], and its prevalence appears to be higher in children than in adults [270]. Crohn's oesophagitis may be the presenting feature of the disease and can occur in the absence of intestinal disease. The lower third is the site of predilection. Depending on the stage of the disease there is an erosive oesophagitis with or without stricture formation. On occasion, characteristic endoscopic appearances may be visible with shallow and irregular aphthoid ulcers occurring in a normal mucosa [265], or there may be a cobblestone pattern. Filiform polyps and fistulae to adjacent viscera have also been reported [271]. Biopsies may show non-specific inflammation but, in one study, non-caseating granulomas were present in 50% of specimens [270].

Eosinophilic oesophagitis

There are a few reports of oesophageal involvement in eosinophilic gastroenteritis [272,273]. Some have been associated with motility disturbances such as diffuse spasm and achalasia. In biopsies, there is elongation of the papillae, basal cell hyperplasia and marked infiltration by eosinophils of the epithelium, lamina propria and muscularis mucosae. The infiltrate may be deep and involve the entire thickness of the oesophageal wall with maximal impact in the muscularis propria, which may be hypertrophied [274]. It has to be borne in mind that the most common cause of eosinophils in distal oesophageal biopsies is gastro-oesophageal reflux [275]. In this regard the presence or absence of tissue eosinophilia in more proximal oesophageal samples, allied with clinical data, will aid in the differential diagnosis. The presence of full-thickness infiltration of the oesophagus has been recently reported also in association with oesophageal leiomyomatosis [276].

Oesophagitis and skin diseases

The oesophagus may be involved in a number of skin diseases including pemphigus vulgaris, bullous pemphigoid, benign mucosal pemphigoid, lichen planus, epidermolysis bullosa, toxic epidermal necrolysis (Lyell's disease), Stevens–Johnson syndrome, Darier's disease, tylosis palmaris et plantaris, and acanthosis nigricans. The subject has been well reviewed [277,278]. There are rare reports of oesophageal involvement in Behçet's syndrome [279–281]. The ulcers are multiple, discrete and shallow with a punched-out appearance and the surrounding mucosa is normal. The mid-oesophagus is the commonest site. Absence of peristalsis and loss of lower oesophageal sphincter tone predispose to reflux oesophagitis in systemic sclerosis [282,283], and coexistent candidiasis is common [284]. Localized epidermolysis bullosa acquisita has been described in the oesophagus of a patient with Crohn's ileocolitis [285].

Oesophagitis in graft-versus-host disease

A desquamative oesophagitis with web formation affecting the upper and mid-oesophagus has been seen in patients with chronic graft-versus-host disease complicating allogeneic bone marrow transplantation [2]. Acute graft-versus-host disease may also involve the oesophageal mucosa in transplanted patients and in non-transplant patients after blood transfusion [286].

References

1 Baehr PH, McDonald GB. Esophageal infections: risk factors, presentation, diagnosis, and treatment. *Gastroenterology*, 1994; 106: 509.
2 McDonald GB, Shulman HM, Sullivan KM, Spencer GD. Intestinal and hepatic complications of human bone marrow transplantation. Part II. *Gastroenterology*, 1986; 90: 770.
3 McDonald GB, Sharma P, Hackman RC *et al.* Esophageal infections in immunosuppressed patients after marrow transplantation. *Gastroenterology*, 1985; 88: 1111.
4 Goldenberg SP, Wain SL, Marignani P. Acute necrotizing esophagitis. *Gastroenterology*, 1990; 98: 493.
5 Benhaim-Iseni M-C, Brenet P, Petite J-P. Acute necrotizing esophagitis: another case (letter). *Gastroenterology*, 1991; 101: 281.
6 Kaye MD. Postprandial gastroesophageal reflux in healthy people. *Gut*, 1977; 18: 709.
7 Fisher RS, Roberts GS, Grabowski CJ, Cohen S. Altered lower esophageal sphincter function during early pregnancy. *Gastroenterology*, 1978; 74: 1233.
8 Locke GR, Talley NJ, Fett SL, Zinsmeister AR, Melton LJ. Prevalence and clinical spectrum of gastroesophageal reflux: a population-based study in Olmsted County, Minnesota. *Gastroenterology*, 1997; 112: 1448.
9 Tibbling L. Epidemiology of gastro-oesophageal reflux disease. *Scand J Gastroenterol*, 1984; 19 (Suppl 106): 14.
10 Wienbeck M, Barnert J. Epidemiology of reflux disease and reflux oesophagitis. *Scand J Gastroenterol*, 1989; 24 (Suppl 156): 7.
11 Dodds WJ, Hogan WJ, Helm JF, Dent J. Pathogenesis of reflux esophagitis. *Gastroenterology*, 1981; 81: 376.
12 Timmer R, Breumelhof R, Nadorp JHSM, Smout AJPM. Recent advances in the pathophysiology of gastro-oesophageal reflux disease. *Eur J Gastroenterol Hepatol*, 1993; 5: 485.
13 Orlando RC. The pathogenesis of gastroesophageal reflux disease: the relationship between epithelial defense, dysmotility, and acid exposure. *Am J Gastroenterol*, 1997; 92: 3S.
14 Goldman MS Jr, Rasch JR, Wiltsie DS, Finkel M. The incidence of esophagitis in peptic ulcer disease. *Am J Dig Dis*, 1967; 12: 994.
15 Miller LS, Vinayek R, Frucht H *et al.* Reflux esophagitis in patients with Zollinger–Ellison syndrome. *Gastroenterology*, 1990; 98: 341.
16 Sontag SJ, Schnell TG, Miller TQ *et al.* Prevalence of oesophagitis in asthmatics. *Gut*, 1992; 33: 872.
17 Smart HL, Nicholson DA, Atkinson M. Gastro-oesophageal reflux in the irritable bowel syndrome. *Gut*, 1986; 27: 1127.
18 Dent J, Holloway RH, Toouli J, Dodds WJ. Mechanisms of lower oesophageal sphincter incompetence in patients with symptomatic gastrooesophageal reflux. *Gut*, 1988; 29: 1020.
19 Mittal RK, Rochester DF, McCallum RW. Effect of the diaphragmatic contraction on lower oesophageal sphincter pressure in man. *Gut*, 1987; 28: 1564.
20 Baldi F, Corinaldesi R, Ferrarini F *et al.* Gastric secretion and emptying of liquids in reflux esophagitis. *Dig Dis Sci*, 1981; 26: 886.
21 McCallum RW, Berkowitz DM, Lerner E. Gastric emptying in patients with gastro-esophageal reflux. *Gastroenterology*, 1981; 80: 285.

22 Gillison EW, Capper WM, Airth GR *et al*. Hiatus hernia and heartburn. *Gut*, 1969; 10: 609.

23 Kaye MD, Showalter JP. Pyloric incompetence in patients with symptomatic gastroesophageal reflux. *J Lab Clin Med*, 1974; 83: 198.

24 Vaezi MF, Richter JE. Contribution of acid and duodenogastro-oesophageal reflux to oesophageal mucosal injury and symptoms in partial gastrectomy patients. *Gut*, 1997; 41: 297.

25 Gill RC, Kellow JE, Wingate DL. Gastroesophageal reflux and the migrating motor complex. *Gut*, 1987; 28: 929.

26 Hirschowitz BI. A critical analysis, with appropriate controls, of gastric acid and pepsin secretion in clinical esophagitis. *Gastroenterology*, 1991; 101: 1149.

27 Fiorucci S, Santucci L, Chiucchiu S, Morelli A. Gastric acidity and gastroesophageal reflux patterns in patients with esophagitis. *Gastroenterology*, 1992; 103: 855.

28 Eriksen CA, Sadek SA, Cranford C *et al*. Reflux oesophagitis and oesophageal transit: evidence for a primary oesophageal motor disorder. *Gut*, 1988; 29: 448.

29 Helm JF, Dodds WJ, Pelc LR *et al*. Effect of esophageal emptying and saliva on clearance of acid from the esophagus. *N Engl J Med*, 1984; 310: 284.

30 Meyers RL, Orlando RC. *In vivo* bicarbonate secretion by human esophagus. *Gastroenterology*, 1992; 103: 1174.

31 Brown CM, Rees WDW. Human oesophageal bicarbonate secretion: a phenomenon waiting for a role (commentary). *Gut*, 1997; 40: 693.

32 El-Serag HB, Sonnenberg A. Associations between different forms of gastro-oesophageal reflux disease. *Gut*, 1997; 41: 594.

33 Lundell LR, Dent J, Bennett JR *et al*. Endoscopic assessment of oesophagitis: clinical and functional correlates and further validation of the Los Angeles classification. *Gut*, 1999; 45: 172.

34 Hattori K, Winans CS, Archer F, Kirsner JB. Endoscopic diagnosis of esophageal inflammation. *Gastrointest Endosc*, 1974; 20: 102.

35 Rabin MS, Bremner CG, Botha JR. The reflux gastroesophageal polyp. *Am J Gastroenterol*, 1980; 73: 451.

36 Mihas AA, Slaughter RL, Goldman LN, Hirschowitz BI. Double lumen esophagus due to reflux esophagitis with fibrous septum formation. *Gastroenterology*, 1976; 71: 136.

37 Raymond JI, Khan AH, Cain LR, Ramin JE. Multiple esophagogastric fistulas resulting from reflux esophagitis. *Am J Gastroenterol*, 1980; 73: 430.

38 Tobey NA, Carson JL, Alkiek RA, Orlando RC. Dilated intercellular spaces. a morphological feature of acid reflux-damaged human esophageal epithelium. *Gastroenterology*, 1996; 111: 1200.

39 Ismail-Beigi F, Horton PF, Pope CE II. Histological consequences of gastroesophageal reflux in man. *Gastroenterology*, 1970; 58: 163.

40 Ismail-Beigi F, Pope CE II. Distribution of the histological changes of gastroesophageal reflux in the distal esophagus of man. *Gastroenterology*, 1974; 66: 1109.

41 Livstone EM, Sheahan DG, Behar J. Studies of esophageal epithelial cell proliferation in patients with reflux esophagitis. *Gastroenterology*, 1977; 73: 1315.

42 Weinstein WM, Bogoch ER, Bowes KL. The normal human esophageal mucosa: a histological reappraisal. *Gastroenterology*, 1975; 68: 40.

43 Seefeld U, Krejs GJ, Siebenmann RE, Blum AL. Esophageal histology in gastroesophageal reflux. Morphometric findings in suction biopsies. *Dig Dis*, 1977; 22: 956.

44 Adami B, Eckardt VF, Paulini K. Sampling error and observer variation in the interpretation of esophageal biopsies. *Digestion*, 1979; 19: 404.

45 Kobayashi S, Kasugai T. Endoscopic and biopsy criteria for the diagnosis of esophagitis with a fibreoptic esophagoscope. *Dig Dis*, 1974; 19: 345.

46 Geboes K, Desmet V, Vantrappen G, Mebis J. Vascular changes in the esophageal mucosa. An early histologic sign of esophagitis. *Gastrointest Endosc*, 1980; 26: 29.

47 Winter HS, Madara JL, Stafford RJ *et al*. Intraepithelial eosinophils: a new diagnostic criterion for reflux esophagitis. *Gastroenterology*, 1982; 83: 818.

48 Tummala V, Barwick KW, Sontag SJ *et al*. The significance of intraepithelial eosinophils in the histologic diagnosis of gastroesophageal reflux. *Am J Clin Pathol*, 1987; 87: 43.

49 Jarvis LR, Dent J, Whitehead R. Morphometric assessment of reflux oesophagitis in fibreoptic biopsy specimens. *J Clin Pathol*, 1985; 38: 44.

50 Collins JSA, Watt PCH, Hamilton PW *et al*. Assessment of oesophagitis by histology and morphometry. *Histopathology*, 1989; 14: 381.

51 Jessurun J, Yardley JH, Giardiello FM *et al*. Intracytoplasmic plasma proteins in distended esophageal squamous cells (balloon cells). *Mod Pathol*, 1988; 1: 175.

52 Sandry RJ. The pathology of chronic oesophagitis. *Gut*, 1962; 3: 16.

53 Barrett NR. The esophagus lined with gastric mucous membrane. *Surgery*, 1957; 41: 881.

54 Allison PR, Johnstone AS. The oesophagus lined with gastric mucous membrane. *Thorax*, 1953; 8: 87.

55 Cohen BR, Wolf BS, Som M, Janowitz HD. Correlation of manometric, oesophagoscopic, and radiological findings in the columnar-lined gullet (Barrett syndrome). *Gut*, 1963; 4: 406.

56 Goldman MC, Beckman RC. Barrett syndrome. Case report with discussion about concepts of pathogenesis. *Gastroenterology*, 1960; 39: 104.

57 Mossberg SM. The columnar-lined esophagus (Barrett syndrome): an acquired condition? *Gastroenterology*, 1966; 50: 671.

58 Endo M, Kobayashi S, Kozu T *et al*. A case of Barrett epithelization followed up for five years. *Endoscopy*, 1974; 6: 48.

59 Cameron AJ, Payne WS. Barrett's esophagus occurring as a complication of scleroderma. *Mayo Clin Proc* 1978; 53: 612.

60 Jaakkola A, Reinikainen P, Ovaska J, Isolauri J. Barrett's esophagus after cardiomyotomy for esophageal achalasia. *Am J Gastroenterol*, 1994; 89: 165.

61 Hamilton SR, Yardley JH. Regeneration of cardiac type mucosa and acquisition of Barrett mucosa after esophagogastrostomy. *Gastroenterology*, 1977; 72: 669.

62 Meyer W, Vollmar F, Bär W. Barrett-esophagus following total gastrectomy. A contribution to its pathogenesis. *Endoscopy*, 1979; 11: 121.

63 Tada T, Suzuki T, Iwafuchi M *et al*. Adenocarcinoma arising in Barrett's esophagus after total gastrectomy. *Am J Gastroenterol*, 1990; 85: 1503.

64 Lindahl H, Rintala R, Sariola H, Louhimo I. Cervical Barrett's esophagus: a common complication of gastric tube reconstruction. *J Pediatr Surg*, 1990; 25: 446.

65 Spechler SJ, Schimmel EM, Dalton JW *et al*. Barrett's epithelium complicating lye ingestion with sparing of the distal esophagus. *Gastroenterology*, 1981; 81: 580.

66 Dahms BB, Greco MA, Strandjord SE, Rothstein FC. Barrett's esophagus in three children after antileukemia chemotherapy. *Cancer*, 1987; 60: 2896.

67 Sartori S, Nielsen I, Indelli M *et al*. Barrett esophagus after chemotherapy with cyclophosphamide, methotrexate and 5-fluorouracil (CMF): an iatrogenic injury? *Ann Intern Med*, 1991; 114: 210.

68 Gillen P, Keeling P, Byrne PJ, West AB, Hennessy TPJ. Experimental columnar metaplasia in the canine oesophagus. *Br J Surg*, 1988; 75: 113.

69 Stadelmann O, Elster K, Kuhn HA. Columnar-lined oesophagus (Barrett's syndrome): congenital or acquired? *Endoscopy*, 1981; 13: 140.

70 Boch JA, Shields HM, Antonioli DA, Zwas F, Sawhney RA, Trier JS. Distribution of cytokeratin markers in Barrett's specialized columnar epithelium. *Gastroenterology*, 1997; 112: 760.

71 Naef AP, Savary M, Ozzello L. Columnar-lined lower esophagus: an acquired lesion with malignant predisposition. Report on 140 cases of Barrett's esophagus with 12 adenocarcinomas. *J Thorac Cardiovasc Surg*, 1975; 70: 826.

72 Brand DL, Ylvisaker JT, Gelfand M, Pope CE II. Regression of columnar esophageal (Barrett's) epithelium after anti-reflux surgery. *N Engl J Med*, 1980; 302: 844.

73 Hamilton SR, Hutcheon DF, Ravich WJ *et al*. Adenocarcinoma in Barrett's esophagus after elimination of gastroesophageal reflux. *Gastroenterology*, 1984; 86: 356.

74 Williamson WA, Ellis FH, Gibb SP. Effect of anti-reflux operation on Barrett's mucosa. *Ann Thorac Surg*, 1990; 49: 537.

75 Hassall E, Weinstein WM. Partial regression of childhood Barrett's esophagus after fundoplication. *Am J Gastroenterol*, 1992; 87: 1506.

76 Sagar PM, Ackroyd R, Hosie KB, Patterson JE, Stoddard CJ, Kingsnorth AN. Regression and progression of Barrett's oesophagus after antireflux surgery. *Br J Surg*, 1995; 82: 806.

77 Wesdorp ICE, Bartelsman J, Schipper MEI, Tytgat GN. Effect of long-term treatment with cimetidine and antacids in Barrett's oesophagus. *Gut*, 1981; 22: 724.

78 Deviere J, Buset M, Dumonceau J-M *et al*. Regression of Barrett's esophagus with omeprazole (letter). *N Engl J Med*, 1989; 320: 1497.

79 Gore S, Healey CJ, Sutton R *et al*. Regression of columnar lined (Barrett's) oesophagus with continuous omeprazole therapy. *Aliment Pharmacol Ther*, 1993; 7: 623.

80 Sharma P, Sampliner RE, Camargo E. Normalization of esophageal pH with high-dose proton pump inhibitor therapy does not result in regression of Barrett's esophagus. *Am J Gastroenterol*, 1997; 92: 582.

81 Brandt LJ, Kauvar DR. Laser-induced transient regression of Barrett's epithelium. *Gastrointest Endosc*, 1992; 38: 619.

82 Berenson MM, Johnson TD, Markowitz NR *et al*. Restoration of squamous mucosa after ablation of Barrett's esophageal epithelium. *Gastroenterology*, 1993; 104: 1686.

83 Overholt BF, Panjehpour M. Photodynamic therapy in Barrett's esophagus: reduction of specialized mucosa, ablation of dysplasia, and treatment of superficial esophageal cancer. *Semin Surg Oncol*, 1995; 11: 372.

84 Barr H, Shepherd NA, Dix A, Roberts DJH, Tan WC, Krasner N. Eradication of high-grade dysplasia in columnar-lined (Barrett's) oesophagus by photodynamic therapy with endogenously derivated protoporphyrin IX. *Lancet*, 1996; 348: 584.

85 Savary M, Miller G. *The Esophagus. Handbook and Atlas of Endoscopy*. Solothurn: Gassmann, 1978: 160.

86 Burbige EJ, Radigan JJ. Characteristics of the columnar-cell lined (Barrett's) esophagus. *Gastrointest Endosc*, 1979; 25: 133.

87 MacDonald CE, Wicks AC, Playford RJ. Ten years' experience of screening patients with Barrett's oesophagus in a University teaching hospital. *Gut*, 1997; 41: 303.

88 Herlihy KJ, Orlando RC, Bryson JC *et al*. Barrett's esophagus: clinical, endoscopic, histologic, manometric, and electrical potential difference characteristics. *Gastroenterology*, 1984; 86: 436.

89 Rothery GA, Patterson JE, Stoddard CJ, Day DW. Histological and histochemical changes in the columnar lined (Barrett's) oesophagus. *Gut*, 1986; 27: 1062.

90 Winters C Jr, Spurling TJ, Chobanian SJ *et al*. Barrett's esophagus: a prevalent, occult complication of gastroesophageal reflux disease. *Gastroenterology*, 1987; 92: 118.

91 Cameron AJ, Zinsmeister AR, Ballard DJ, Carney JA. Prevalence of columnar-lined (Barrett's) esophagus. Comparison of population-based clinical and autopsy findings. *Gastroenterology*, 1990; 99: 918.

92 Cameron AJ, Lomboy CT. Barrett's esophagus: age, prevalence, and extent of columnar epithelium. *Gastroenterology*, 1992; 103: 1241.

93 Dahms BB, Rothstein FC. Barrett's esophagus in children: a consequence of chronic gastro-esophageal reflux. *Gastroenterology*, 1984; 86: 318.

94 Hassall E, Weinstein WM, Ament ME. Barrett's esophagus in childhood. *Gastroenterology*, 1985; 89: 1331.

95 Cooper JE, Spitz L, Wilkins BM. Barrett's esophagus in children: a histologic and histochemical study of 11 cases. *J Pediatr Surg*, 1987; 22: 191.

96 Robins DB, Zaino RJ, Ballantine TVN. Barrett's esophagus in a newborn. *Pediatr Pathol*, 1991; 11: 663.

97 Crabb DW, Berk MA, Hall TR *et al*. Familial gastroesophageal reflux and development of Barrett's esophagus. *Ann Intern Med*, 1985; 103: 52.

98 Jochem VJ, Fuerst PA, Fromkes JJ. Familial Barrett's esophagus associated with adenocarcinoma. *Gastroenterology*, 1992; 102: 1400.

99 McDonald GB, Brand DL, Thorning DR. Multiple adenomatous neoplasms arising in columnar-lined (Barrett's) esophagus. *Gastroenterology*, 1977; 72: 1317.

100 Berenson MM, Riddell RH, Skinner DB, Freston JW. Malignant transformation of esophageal columnar epithelium. *Cancer*, 1978; 41: 554.

101 Haggitt RC, Tryzelaar J, Ellis FH, Colcher H. Adenocarcinoma complicating epithelium-lined (Barrett's) esophagus. *Am J Clin Pathol*, 1978; 70: 1.

102 Witt TR, Bains MS, Zaman MB, Martini N. Adenocarcinoma in Barrett's esophagus. *J Thorac Cardiovasc Surg*, 1983; 85: 337.

103 Hameeteman W, Tytgat GNJ, Houthoff HJ, van den Tweel JG. Barrett's esophagus: development of dysplasia and adenocarcinoma. *Gastroenterology*, 1989; 96: 1249.

104 Williamson WA, Ellis FH Jr, Gibb SP *et al*. Barrett's esophagus:

prevalence and incidence of adenocarcinoma. *Arch Intern Med*, 1991; 151: 2212.

105 Spechler SJ, Robbins AH, Rubins HB *et al*. Adenocarcinoma and Barrett's esophagus: an overrated risk? *Gastroenterology*, 1984; 87: 927.

106 Cameron AJ, Ott BJ, Payne WS. The incidence of adenocarcinoma in columnar-lined (Barrett's) esophagus. *N Engl J Med*, 1985; 313: 857.

107 van der Veen AH, Dees J, Blankensteijn JD, van Blankenstein M. Adenocarcinoma in Barrett's oesophagus: an overrated risk. *Gut*, 1989; 30: 14.

108 Miros M, Kerlin P, Walker N. Only patients with dysplasia progress to adenocarcinoma in Barrett's oesophagus. *Gut*, 1991; 32: 1441.

109 Drewitz DJ, Sampliner RE, Garewal HS. The incidence of adenocarcinoma in Barrett's esophagus: a prospective study of 170 patients followed 4.8 years. *Am J Gastroenterol*, 1997; 92: 212.

110 Harle IA, Finley RJ, Belsheim M *et al*. Management of adenocarcinoma in a columnar-lined esophagus. *Ann Thorac Surg*, 1985; 40: 330.

111 Cameron AJ, Lomboy CT, Pera M, Carpenter HA. Adenocarcinoma of the esophagogastric junction and Barrett's esophagus. *Gastroenterology*, 1995; 109: 1541.

112 Wang HH, Antonioli DA, Goldman H. Comparative features of esophageal and gastric adenocarcinomas. Recent changes in type and frequency. *Hum Pathol*, 1986; 17: 482.

113 MacDonald WC, Macdonald JB. Adenocarcinoma of the esophagus and/or gastric cardia. *Cancer*, 1987; 60: 1094.

114 Hamilton SR, Smith RRL, Cameron JL. Prevalence and characteristics of Barrett esophagus in patients with adenocarcinoma of the esophagus or esophagogastric junction. *Hum Pathol*, 1988; 19: 942.

115 Pera M, Cameron AJ, Trastek VF *et al*. Increasing incidence of adenocarcinoma of the esophagus and esophagogastric junction. *Gastroenterology*, 1993; 104: 510.

116 Rosengard AM, Hamilton SR. Squamous carcinoma of the esophagus in patients with Barrett esophagus. *Mod Pathol*, 1989; 2: 2.

117 Rubio CA, Åberg B. Barrett's mucosa in conjunction with squamous carcinoma of the esophagus. *Cancer*, 1991; 68: 583.

118 Paraf F, Fléjou J-F, Potet F *et al*. Esophageal squamous carcinoma in five patients with Barrett's esophagus. *Am J Gastroenterol*, 1992; 87: 746.

119 Thompson JJ, Zinsser KR, Enterline HT. Barrett's metaplasia and adenocarcinoma of the esophagus and gastroesophageal junction. *Hum Pathol*, 1983; 14: 42.

120 Cameron AJ, Carpenter HA. Barrett's esophagus, high-grade dysplasia, and early adenocarcinoma: a pathological study. *Am J Gastroenterol*, 1997; 92: 586.

121 Hamilton SR, Smith RRL. The relationship between columnar epithelial dysplasia and invasive adenocarcinoma arising in Barrett's esophagus. *Am J Clin Pathol*, 1987; 87: 301.

122 Reid BJ, Weinstein WM, Lewin KJ *et al*. Endoscopic biopsy can detect high-grade dysplasia or early adenocarcinoma in Barrett's esophagus without grossly recognizable neoplastic lesions. *Gastroenterology*, 1988; 94: 81.

123 Lee RG. Adenomas arising in Barrett's esophagus. *Am J Clin Pathol*, 1986; 85: 629.

124 Katz D, Rothstein R, Schned A, Dunn J, Seaver K, Antonioli D. The development of dysplasia and adenocarcinoma during endoscopic surveillance of Barrett's esophagus. *Am J Gastroenterol*, 1998; 93: 536.

125 Reid BJ, Haggitt RC, Rubin CE, Rabinovitch PS. Barrett's esophagus. Correlation between flow cytometry and histology in detection of patients at risk for adenocarcinoma. *Gastroenterology*, 1987; 93: 1.

126 Fennerty MB, Sampliner RE, Way D *et al*. Discordance between flow cytometric abnormalities and dysplasia in Barrett's esophagus. *Gastroenterology*, 1989; 97: 815.

127 Garewal HS, Sampliner RE, Fennerty MB. Flow cytometry in Barrett's esophagus. What have we learned so far? *Dig Dis Sci*, 1991; 36: 548.

128 Reid BJ, Blount PL, Rubin CE *et al*. Flow-cytometric and histological progression to malignancy in Barrett's esophagus: prospective endoscopic surveillance of a cohort. *Gastroenterology*, 1992; 102: 1212.

129 James PD, Atkinson M. Value of DNA image cytometry in the prediction of malignant change in Barrett's oesophagus. *Gut*, 1989; 30: 899.

130 Garewal HS, Sampliner R, Gerner E *et al*. Ornithine decarboxylase activity in Barrett's esophagus: a potential marker for dysplasia. *Gastroenterology*, 1988; 94: 819.

131 Ramel S, Reid BJ, Sanchez CA *et al*. Evaluation of p53 protein expression in Barrett's esophagus by two-parameter flow cytometry. *Gastroenterology*, 1992; 102: 1220.

132 Fléjou J-F, Potet F, Muzeau F *et al*. Overexpression of p53 protein in Barrett's syndrome with malignant transformation. *J Clin Pathol*, 1993; 46: 330.

133 Iftikhar SY, Steele RJC, Watson S *et al*. Assessment of proliferation of squamous, Barrett's and gastric mucosa in patients with columnar lined Barrett's oesophagus. *Gut*, 1992; 33: 733.

134 Gray MR, Hall PA, Nash J *et al*. Epithelial proliferation in Barrett's esophagus by proliferating cell nuclear antigen immunolocalization. *Gastroenterology*, 1992; 103: 1769.

135 Hong MK, Laskin WB, Herman BE *et al*. Expansion of the Ki-67 proliferative compartment correlates with degree of dysplasia in Barrett's esophagus. *Cancer*, 1995; 75: 423.

136 Polkowski W, Baak JPA, Van Lanschot JJB *et al*. Clinical decision making in Barrett's oesophagus can be supported by immunoquantitation and morphometry of features associated with proliferation and differentiation. *J Pathol*, 1998; 184: 161.

137 Whittles CE, Biddlestone LR, Burton A *et al*. Apoptotic and proliferative activity in the neoplastic progression of Barrett's oesophagus: a comparative study. *J Pathol*, 1999; 187: 535.

138 Atkinson M, Iftikhar SY, James PD *et al*. The early diagnosis of oesophageal adenocarcinoma by endoscopic screening. *Eur J Cancer Prev*, 1992; 1: 327.

139 Wright TA, Gray MR, Morris AI *et al*. Cost effectiveness of detecting Barrett's cancer. *Gut*, 1996; 39: 574.

140 Streitz JM Jr, Andrews CW Jr, Ellis FH Jr. Endoscopic surveillance of Barrett's esophagus: does it help? *J Thorac Cardiovasc Surg*, 1993; 105: 383.

141 Bytzer P, Christensen PB, Damkier P, Vinding K, Seersholm N. Adenocarcinoma of the esophagus and Barrett's esophagus: a population-based study. *Am J Gastroenterol*, 1999; 94: 86.

142 Atkinson M. Barrett's oesophagus—to screen or not to screen? *Gut*, 1989; 30: 2.

143 van der Burgh A, Dees J, Hop WCJ, van Blankenstein M. Oesophageal cancer is an uncommon cause of death in patients with Barrett's oesophagus. *Gut*, 1996; 39: 5.

144 Robey SS, Hamilton SR, Gupta PK, Erozan YS. Diagnostic value of cytopathology in Barrett esophagus and associated carcinoma. *Am J Clin Pathol*, 1988; 89: 493.

145 Geisinger KR, Teot LA, Richter JE. A comparative cytopathologic and histologic study of atypia, dysplasia, and adenocarcinoma in Barrett's esophagus. *Cancer*, 1992; 69: 8.

146 Falk GW, Chittajallu R, Goldblum JR *et al*. Surveillance of patients with Barrett's esophagus for dysplasia and cancer with balloon cytology. *Gastroenterology*, 1997; 112: 1787.

147 Tytgat GNJ, Hameeteman W, Onstenk R, Schotborg R. The spectrum of columnar-lined esophagus—Barrett's esophagus. *Endoscopy*, 1989; 21: 177.

148 McClave SA, Boyce HW, Gottfried MR. Early diagnosis of columnar-lined esophagus: a new endoscopic diagnostic criterion. *Gastrointest Endosc*, 1987 ; 33: 413.

149 Atkinson M, Robertson CS. Benign oesophageal stricture in Barrett's columnar epithelialised oesophagus and its responsiveness to conservative management. *Gut*, 1988; 29: 1721.

150 Wolf BS, Marshak RH, Som ML, Winkelstein A. Peptic esophagitis, peptic ulcer of the esophagus and marginal esophagogastric ulceration. *Gastroenterology*, 1955; 29: 744.

151 Komorowski RA, Hogan WJ, Chausow DD. Barrett's ulcer: the clinical significance today. *Am J Gastroenterol*, 1996; 91: 2310.

152 Barrett NR. Chronic peptic ulcer of the oesophagus and 'oesophagitis'. *Br J Surg*, 1950; 38: 175.

153 Woolf GM, Riddell RH, Irvine EJ, Hunt RH. A study to examine agreement between endoscopy and histology for the diagnosis of columnar lined (Barrett's) esophagus. *Gastrointest Endosc*, 1989; 35: 541.

154 Panjehpour M, Overholt BF, Vo-Dinh T, Haggitt RC, Edwards DH, Buckley FP. Endoscopic fluorescence detection of high-grade dysplasia in Barrett's esophagus. *Gastroenterology*, 1996; 111: 93.

155 Paull A, Trier JS, Dalton MD *et al*. The histologic spectrum of Barrett's esophagus. *N Engl J Med*, 1976; 295: 476.

156 Zwas F, Shields HM, Doos WG *et al*. Scanning electron microscopy of Barrett's epithelium and its correlation with light microscopy and mucin stains. *Gastroenterology*, 1986; 90: 1932.

157 Banner BF, Memoli VA, Warren WH, Gould VE. Carcinoma with multidirectional differentiation arising in Barrett's esophagus. *Ultrastruct Pathol*, 1983; 4: 205.

158 Buchan AMJ, Grant S, Freeman HJ. Regulatory peptides in Barrett's oesophagus. *J Pathol*, 1985; 146: 227.

159 Griffin M, Sweeney EC. The relationship of endocrine cells, dysplasia and carcinoembryonic antigen in Barrett's mucosa to adenocarcinoma of the oesophagus. *Histopathology*, 1987; 11: 53.

160 Levine DS, Rubin CE, Reid BJ, Haggitt RC. Specialized metaplastic columnar epithelium in Barrett's esophagus. A comparative transmission electron microscopic study. *Lab Invest*, 1989; 3: 418.

161 Jass JR. Mucin histochemistry of the columnar epithelium of the oesophagus: a retrospective study. *J Clin Pathol*, 1981; 34: 866.

162 Trier JS. Morphology of the epithelium of the distal esophagus in patients with midesophageal peptic strictures. *Gastroenterology*, 1970; 58: 444.

163 Shah KA, Deacon AJ, Dunscombe P, Price AB. Intestinal metaplasia subtyping: evaluation of Gomori's aldehyde fuchsin for routine use. *J Clin Pathol*, 1997; 31: 277.

164 Jass JR. Role of intestinal metaplasia in the histogenesis of gastric carcinoma. *J Clin Pathol*, 1980; 33: 801.

165 Sipponen P. Seppälä K, Varis K *et al*. Intestinal metaplasia with colonic-type sulphomucins in the gastric mucosa; its association with gastric carcinoma. *Acta Pathol Microbiol Scand [A]*, 1980; 88: 217.

166 Lee RG. Mucins in Barrett's esophagus: a histochemical study. *Am J Clin Pathol*, 1984; 81: 500.

167 Peuchmaur M, Potet F, Goldfain D. Mucin histochemistry of the columnar epithelium of the oesophagus (Barrett's oesophagus): a prospective biopsy study. *J Clin Pathol*, 1984; 37: 607.

168 Haggitt RC, Reid BJ, Rabinovitch PS, Rubin CE. Barrett's esophagus: correlation between mucin histochemistry, flow cytometry, and histologic diagnosis for predicting increased cancer risk. *Am J Pathol*, 1988; 131: 53.

169 Qualman SJ, Murray RD, McClung J, Lucas J. Intestinal metaplasia is age related in Barrett's esophagus. *Arch Pathol Lab Med*, 1990; 114: 1236.

170 Ormsby AH, Goldblum JR, Rice TW *et al*. Cytokeratin subsets can reliably distinguish Barrett's esophagus from intestinal metaplasia of the stomach. *Hum Pathol*, 1999; 30: 288.

171 Talley NJ, Cameron AJ, Shorter RG *et al*. *Campylobacter pylori* and Barrett's esophagus. *Mayo Clin Proc* 1988; 63: 1176.

172 Paull G, Yardley JH. Gastric and esophageal *Campylobacter pylori* in patients with Barrett's esophagus. *Gastroenterology*, 1988; 95: 216.

173 Loffeld RJLF, Ten Tije BJ, Arends JW. Prevalence and significance of *Helicobacter pylori* in patients with Barrett's esophagus. *Am J Gastroenterol*, 1992; 87: 1598.

174 Takubo K, Sasajima K, Yamashita K, Tanaka Y, Fujita K. Double muscularis mucosae in Barrett's esophagus. *Hum Pathol*, 1991; 22: 1158.

175 Day DW. *Biopsy Pathology of the Oesophagus, Stomach and Duodenum*. London: Chapman & Hall, 1986: 26–7.

176 Spechler SJ, Zeroogian JM, Antonioli DA, Wang HH, Goyal RK. Prevalence of metaplasia at the gastro-oesophageal junction. *Lancet*, 1994; 344: 1533.

177 Morales TG, Sampliner RE, Bhattacharyya A. Intestinal metaplasia of the gastric cardia. *Am J Gastroenterol*, 1997; 92: 414.

178 Schmidt HG, Riddell RH, Walther B, Skinner DB, Rieman JF. Dysplasia in Barrett's esophagus. *J Cancer Res Clin Oncol*, 1985; 110: 145.

179 Riddell RH, Goldman H, Ransohoff DF *et al*. Dysplasia in inflammatory bowel disease: standardized classification with provisional clinical applications. *Hum Pathol*, 1983; 14: 931.

180 Reid BJ, Haggitt RC, Rubin CE *et al*. Observer variation in the diagnosis of dysplasia in Barrett's esophagus. *Hum Pathol*, 1988; 19: 116.

181 Levine DS, Haggitt RC, Blount PL, Rabinovitch PS, Rusch VW, Reid BJ. An endoscopic biopsy protocol can differentiate high-grade dysplasia from early adenocarcinoma in Barrett's esophagus. *Gastroenterology*, 1993; 105: 40.

182 Robertson CS, Mayberry JF, Nicholson DA *et al*. Value of endoscopic surveillance in the detection of neoplastic change in Barrett's oesophagus. *Br J Surg*, 1988; 75: 760.

183 Pera M, Trastek VT, Carpenter HA *et al*. Barrett's esophagus with high-grade dysplasia. An indication for esophagectomy? *Ann Thorac Surg*, 1992; 54: 199.
184 Clark GWB, Ireland AP, DeMeester TR. Dysplastic Barrett's: is continued surveillance appropriate? (letter). *Gastroenterology*, 1994; 106: 1128.
185 Laukka MA, Wang KK. Initial results using low-dose photodynamic therapy in the treatment of Barrett's esophagus. *Gastrointest Endosc*, 1995; 42: 59.
186 Sibille A, Lambert R, Souquet J, Sabben G, Descos F. Long-term survival after photodynamic therapy for esophageal cancer. *Gastroenterology*, 1995; 108: 337.
187 Overholt BF, Panjehpour M. Photodynamic therapy for Barrett's esophagus: clinical update. *Am J Gastroenterol*, 1996; 91: 1719.
188 Gossner L, Stolte M, Sroka R *et al*. Photodynamic ablation of high-grade dysplasia and early cancer in Barrett's esophagus by means of 5-aminolevulinic acid. *Gastroenterology*, 1998; 114: 448.
189 Biddlestone LR, Barham CP, Wilkinson SP, Barr H, Shepherd NA. The histopathology of treated Barrett's esophagus. Squamous reepithelialization after acid suppression and laser and photodynamic therapy. *Am J Surg Pathol*, 1998; 22: 239.
190 Overholt BF, Panjehpour M. Barrett's esophagus: photodynamic therapy for ablation of dysplasia, reduction of specialized mucosa, and the treatment of superficial esophageal cancer. *Gastrointest Endosc*, 1995; 42: 64.
191 Jensen KB, Stenderup A, Thomsen JB, Bichel J. Oesophageal moniliasis in malignant neoplastic disease. *Acta Med Scand*, 1964; 175: 455.
192 Tom W, Aaron JS. Esophageal ulcers caused by *Torulopsis glabrata* in a patient with acquired immune deficiency syndrome. *Am J Gastroenterol*, 1987; 82: 766.
193 Anderson LI, Frederiksen HJ, Appleyard M. Prevalence of esophageal *Candida* colonization in a Danish population, with special reference to esophageal symptoms, benign esophageal disorders, and pulmonary disease. *J Infect Dis*, 1992; 165: 389.
194 Eras P, Goldstein MJ, Sherlock P. *Candida* infection of the gastrointestinal tract. *Medicine*, 1972; 51: 367.
195 Vermeersch B, Rysselaere M, Dekeyser K *et al*. Fungal colonization of the esophagus. *Am J Gastroenterol*, 1989; 84: 1079.
196 Lopez-Dupla M, Mora-Sanz P, Pintado-Garcia V *et al*. Clinical, endoscopic, immunologic, and therapeutic aspects of oropharyngeal and esophageal candidiasis in HIV-infected patients: a survey of 144 cases. *Am J Gastroenterol*, 1992; 87: 1771.
197 Larner AJ, Lendrum R. Oesophageal candidiasis after omeprazole therapy. *Gut*, 1992; 33: 860.
198 Kodsi BE, Wickremesinghe PC, Kozinn PJ *et al*. Candida esophagitis. A prospective study of 27 cases. *Gastroenterology*, 1976; 71: 715.
199 Gonzalez-Crussi IF, Iung OS. Esophageal moniliasis as a cause of death. *Am J Surg*, 1965; 109: 634.
200 Weiss J, Epstein BS. Esophageal moniliasis. *Am J Roentgenol*, 1962; 88: 718.
201 Orringer MB, Sloan H. Monilial esophagitis: an increasingly frequent cause of esophageal stenosis? *Ann Thorac Surg*, 1978; 26: 364.
202 Myerowitz RL, Pazin GJ, Allen CM. Disseminated candidiasis. Changes in incidence, underlying diseases, and pathology. *Am J Clin Pathol*, 1977; 68: 29.
203 Maksymiuk AW, Thongprasert S, Hopfer R, Luna M, Fainstein V, Bodey GP. Systemic candidiasis in cancer patients. *Am J Med*, 1984; 77 (Suppl 4D): 20.
204 Walsh TJ, Merz WG. Pathologic features in the human alimentary tract associated with invasiveness of *Candida tropicalis*. *Am J Clin Pathol*, 1986; 85: 498.
205 Nash G, Ross JS. Herpetic esophagitis: a common cause of esophageal ulceration. *Hum Pathol*, 1974; 5: 339.
206 Buss DH, Scharyj M. Herpes virus infection of the esophagus and other visceral organs in adults: incidence and clinical significance. *Am J Med*, 1979; 66: 457.
207 Warren KG, Brown SM, Wroblewska Z, Gilden D, Koprowski H, Subak-Sharpe J. Isolation of latent herpes simplex virus from the superior cervical and vagus ganglions of human beings. *N Engl J Med*, 1978; 298: 1068.
208 McKay JS, Day DW. Herpes simplex oesophagitis. *Histopathology*, 1983; 7: 409.
209 Deshmukh M, Shah R, McCallum RW. Experience with herpes esophagitis in otherwise healthy patients. *Am J Gastroenterol*, 1984; 79: 173.
210 Moses HL, Cheatham WJ. Frequency and significance of human herpetic esophagitis: an autopsy study. *Lab Invest*, 1963; 12: 663.
211 Montgomerie JZ, Becroft DMO, Croxson MC, Doak PB, North JDK. Herpes simplex virus infection after renal transplantation. *Lancet*, 1969; i: 867.
212 Brayko CM, Kozarek RA, Sanowski RA, Lanard BJ. Type 1 herpes simplex esophagitis with concomitant esophageal moniliasis. *J Clin Gastroenterol*, 1982; 4: 351.
213 Fishbein PG, Tuthill R, Kressel H, Freidman H, Snape WJ Jr. Herpes simplex esophagitis: a cause of upper gastrointestinal bleeding. *Dig Dis Sci*, 1979; 24: 540.
214 Rattner HM, Cooper DJ, Zaman MB. Severe bleeding from herpes esophagitis. *Am J Gastroenterol*, 1985; 80: 523.
215 Cronstedt JL, Bouchama A, Hainau B, Halim M, Khouqeer F, Al Darsouny T. Spontaneous esophageal perforation in herpes simplex esophagitis. *Am J Gastroenterol*, 1992; 87: 124.
216 McBane RD, Gross JB Jr. Herpes esophagitis: clinical syndrome, endoscopic appearance, and diagnosis in 23 patients. *Gastrointest Endosc*, 1991; 37: 600.
217 Singh SP, Odze RD. Multinucleated epithelial giant cell changes in esophagitis: a clinicopathologic study of 14 cases. *Am J Surg Pathol*, 1998; 22: 93.
218 Greenson JK, Beschorner WE, Boitnott JK, Yardley JH. Prominent mononuclear cell infiltrate is characteristic of herpes esophagitis. *Hum Pathol*, 1991; 22: 541.
219 Gould B, Kory WP, Raskin JB, Ibe MJ, Redhammer DE. Esophageal biopsy findings in the acquired immunodeficiency syndrome: clinical pathological correlation in 20 patients. *South Med J*, 1988; 81: 1395.
220 Laine L, Bonacini M, Sattler F *et al*. Cytomegalovirus and Candida esophagitis in patients with AIDS. *J AIDS*, 1992; 5: 605.
221 Wilcox CM, Diehl DL, Cello JP, Margaretten W, Jacobson MA. Cytomegalovirus esophagitis in patients with AIDS. A clinical, endoscopic, and pathologic correlation. *Ann Intern Med*, 1990; 113: 589.
222 Theise ND, Rotterdam H, Dieterich D. Cytomegalovirus esophagitis in AIDS: diagnosis by endoscopic biopsy. *Am J Gastroenterol*, 1991; 86: 1123.
223 Walsh TJ, Belitsos NJ, Hamilton SR. Bacterial esophagitis in immunocompromised patients. *Arch Intern Med*, 1986; 146: 1345.

224 Ezzell JH Jr, Bremer J, Adamec TA. Bacterial esophagitis: an often forgotten cause of odynophagia. *Am J Gastroenterol*, 1990; 85: 296.
225 Dow CJ. Oesophageal tuberculosis: four cases. *Gut*, 1981; 22: 234.
226 Gordon AH, Marshall JB. Esophageal tuberculosis: definitive diagnosis by endoscopy. *Am J Gastroenterol*, 1990; 85: 174.
227 Newman RM, Fleshner PR, Lajam FE, Kim U. Esophageal tuberculosis: a rare presentation with hematemesis. *Am J Gastroenterol*, 1991; 86: 751.
228 Seivewright N, Feehalley J, Wicks ACB. Primary tuberculosis of the esophagus. *Am J Gastroenterol*, 1984; 79: 842.
229 Laajam MA. Primary tuberculosis of the esophagus: pseudotumoral presentation. *Am J Gastroenterol*, 1984; 79: 839.
230 Horsburgh CR Jr. *Mycobacterium avium* complex infection in the acquired immunodeficiency syndrome. *N Engl J Med*, 1991; 324: 1332.
231 El-Serag HB, Johnston DE. *Mycobacterium avium* complex esophagitis. *Am J Gastroenterol*, 1997; 92: 1561.
232 Chang AD, Drachenberg CI, James SP. Bacillary angiomatosis associated with extensive esophageal polyposis: a new mucocutaneous manifestation of acquired immunodeficiency disease (AIDS). *Am J Gastroenterol*, 1996; 91: 2220.
233 Young RC, Bennett JE, Vogel CL *et al*. Aspergillosis: the spectrum of the disease in 98 patients. *Medicine*, 1970; 49: 147.
234 Obrecht WF Jr, Richter JE, Olympio GA, Gelfand DW. Tracheoesophageal fistula: a serious complication of infectious esophagitis. *Gastroenterology*, 1984; 87: 1174.
235 Neame P, Ragner D. Mucormycosis. a report of twenty-two cases. *Arch Pathol*, 1960; 70: 261.
236 McKenzie R, Khakoo R. Blastomycosis of the esophagus presenting with gastrointestinal bleeding. *Gastroenterology*, 1985; 88: 1271.
237 Jacobs DH, Macher AM, Handler R *et al*. Esophageal cryptococcosis in a patient with the hyperimmunoglobulin E-recurrent infection (Job's) syndrome. *Gastroenterology*, 1984; 87: 201.
238 Lee J-H, Neumann DA, Welsh JD. Disseminated histoplasmosis presenting with esophageal symptomatology. *Dig Dis*, 1977; 22: 831.
239 Schneider RP, Edwards W. Histoplasmosis presenting as an esophageal tumour. *Gastrointest Endosc*, 1977; 23: 158.
240 Fucci JC, Nightengale ML. Primary esophageal histoplasmosis. *Am J Gastroenterol*, 1997; 92: 530.
241 Kitchen VS, Helbert M, Francis ND *et al*. Epstein–Barr virus associated oesophageal ulcers in AIDS. *Gut*, 1990; 31: 1223.
242 Rabeneck L, Popovic M, Gartner S. Acute HIV infection presenting with painful swallowing and esophageal ulcers. *JAMA*, 1990; 263: 2318.
243 Wilcox CM, Zaki SR, Coffield LM, Greer PW, Schwartz DA. Evaluation of idiopathic esophageal ulceration for human immunodeficiency virus. *Mod Pathol*, 1995; 8: 568.
244 Schechter M, Pannain VLN, Viana de Loiveria A. Papova-virus associated esophageal ulceration in a patient with AIDS. *J AIDS*, 1991; 5: 238.
245 Corbellina M, Lusso P, Gallo RC *et al*. Disseminated human herpes-virus 6 infection in AIDS (letter). *Lancet*, 1993; 342: 1242.
246 Gill RA, Gebhard RL, Dozeman RL, Sumner HW. Shingles esophagitis: endoscopic diagnosis in two patients. *Gastrointest Endosc*, 1984; 30: 26.
247 Atias A, Neghme A, Mackay LA, Jarpa S. Megaesophagus, megacolon and Chagas' disease in Chile. *Gastroenterology*, 1963; 44: 433.
248 Köberle F. Chagas' disease and Chagas' syndrome: the pathology of American typanosomiasis. *Adv Parasitol*, 1968; 6: 63.
249 Earlam RJ. Gastrointestinal aspects of Chagas' disease. *Am J Dig Dis*, 1972; 17: 559.
250 Martins-Campos JV, Tafuri WL. Progress report: Chagas' enteropathy. *Gut*, 1973; 14: 910.
251 Betarello A, Pinotti HW. Oesophageal involvement in Chagas' disease. *Clin Gastroenterol*, 1976; 5: 27.
252 Goin JC, Sterin-Borda L, Bilder CR *et al*. Functional implications of circulating muscarinic cholinergic receptor autoantibodies in chagasic patients with achalasia. *Gastroenterology*, 1999; 117: 798.
253 Kazlow PG, Shah K, Benkov KG, Dische R, LeLeiko NS. Esophageal cryptosporidiosis in a child with acquired immune deficiency syndrome. *Gastroenterology*, 1986; 91: 1301.
254 Butler C, Madden JW, Davis WM. Morphologic aspects of experimental lye strictures. I. Pathogenesis and pathophysiologic correlations. *J Surg Res*, 1974; 17: 232.
255 Kiviranta UK. Corrosion carcinoma of the oesophagus: 381 cases of corrosion and 9 cases of corrosion carcinoma. *Acta Otolaryngol*, 1952; 42: 89.
256 Appelqvist P, Salmo M. Lye corrosion carcinoma of the esophagus. A review of 63 cases. *Cancer*, 1980; 45: 2655.
257 Kikendall JW, Friedman AC, Oyewole MA *et al*. Pill-induced esophageal injury. Case reports and review of the medical literature. *Dig Dis Sci*, 1983; 28: 174.
258 Colina RE, Smith M, Kikendall JE, Wong RKH. A new probable increasing cause of esophageal ulceration: alendronate. *Am J Gastroenterol*, 1997; 92: 704.
259 Collins FJ, Mathews HR, Baker SE, Strakova JM. Drug-induced oesophageal injury. *Br Med J*, 1979; i: 1673.
260 Eng J, Sabanathan S. Drug-induced esophagitis. *Am J Gastroenterol*, 1991; 86: 1127.
261 Bonavina L, De Meester TR, McChesney L *et al*. Drug-induced esophageal strictures. *Ann Surg*, 1987; 206: 173.
262 Greco FA, Brereton HD, Kent H *et al*. Adriamycin and enhanced radiation reaction in normal esophagus and skin. *Ann Intern Med*, 1976; 85: 294.
263 Newburger PE, Cassady JR, Jaffe N. Esophagitis due to adriamycin and radiation therapy for childhood malignancy. *Cancer*, 1978; 42: 417.
264 Sherrill DJ, Grishkin BA, Galal FS *et al*. Radiation associated malignancies of the esophagus. *Cancer*, 1984; 54: 726.
265 Vanagunas A, Jacob P, Olinger E. Radiation-induced esophageal injury: a spectrum from esophagitis to cancer. *Am J Gastroenterol*, 1990; 85: 808.
266 Huchzermeyer H, Paul F, Seifert E *et al*. Endoscopic results in five patients with Crohn's disease of the esophagus. *Endoscopy*, 1976; 8: 75.
267 Degryse HRM, De Schepper AMAP. Aphthoid esophageal ulcers in Crohn's disease of ileum and colon. *Gastrointest Radiol*, 1984; 9: 197.
268 Freedman PG, Dieterich DT, Balthazar EJ. Crohn's disease of the esophagus: case report and review of the literature. *Am J Gastroenterol*, 1984; 79: 835.
269 Geboes K, Janssens J, Rutgeerts P, Vantrappen C. Crohn's disease of the esophagus. *J Clin Gastroenterol*, 1986; 8: 31.

270 Lenaerts C, Roy CC, Vaillancourt M *et al*. High incidence of upper gastrointestinal tract involvement in children with Crohn disease. *Pediatrics*, 1989; 83: 777.

271 D'Haens G, Rutgeerts P, Geboes K *et al*. The natural history of esophageal Crohn's disease: three patterns of evolution. *Gastrointest Endosc*, 1994; 296: 300.

272 Dobbins JW, Sheahan DG, Behar J. Eosinophilic gastroenteritis with esophageal involvement. *Gastroenterology*, 1977; 72: 1312.

273 Landres RT, Kuster GGR, Strum WB. Eosinophilic esophagitis in a patient with vigorous achalasia. *Gastroenterology*, 1978; 74: 1298.

274 Blei E, Gonzalez-Crussi F, Lloyd-Still JD. Eosinophilic infiltration of the esophageal muscle layer: a difficult diagnostic problem. *J Pediatr Gastroenterol Nutr*, 1992; 15: 93.

275 Lee RG. Marked eosinophilia in esophageal mucosal biopsies. *Am J Surg Pathol*, 1985; 9: 475.

276 Nicholson AG, Li D, Pastorino U, Goldstraw P, Jeffery PK. Full thickness eosinophilia in oesophageal leiomyomatosis and idiopathic eosinophilic oesophagitis. A common inflammatory allergic profile? *J Pathol*, 1997; 183: 233.

277 Geboes K, Janssens J. The esophagus in cutaneous diseases. In: Vantrappen GR, Hellemans JJ, eds. *Diseases of the Esophagus*. New York: Springer-Verlag, 1974: 823.

278 Walton S, Bennett JR. Skin and gullet. *Gut*, 1991; 32: 694.

279 Lockhart JM, McIntyre W, Caperton EM. Esophageal ulceration in Behçet's syndrome. *Ann Intern Med*, 1976; 84: 572.

280 Kaplinsky N, Neumann G, Harzahav Y, Frankl O. Esophageal ulceration in Behçet's syndrome. *Gastrointest Endosc*, 1977; 23: 160.

281 Mori S, Yoshihara A, Kawamura H, Takeuchi A, Hashimoto T, Inaba G. Esophageal involvement in Behçet's disease. *Am J Gastroenterol*, 1983; 78: 548.

282 Atkinson M, Summerling MD. Oesophageal changes in systemic sclerosis. *Gut*, 1966; 7: 402.

283 Zamost BJ, Hirschberg J, Ippoliti AF *et al*. Esophagitis in scleroderma: prevalence and risk factors. *Gastroenterology*, 1987; 92: 421.

284 Cohen S, Laufer I, Snape WJ Jr *et al*. The gastrointestinal manifestations of scleroderma: pathogenesis and management. *Gastroenterology*, 1980; 79: 155.

285 Schattenkirchner SL, Lémann M, Prost C *et al*. Localized epidermolysis bullosa acquisita of the esophagus in a patient with Crohn's disease. *Am J Gastroenterol*, 1996; 91: 1657.

286 Iwakuma A, Matsuyoshi T, Arikado T *et al*. Two cases of post-operative erythroderma: clinical and pathological investigation. *J Jpn Assoc Thorac Surg*, 1991; 39: 209.

8 Tumours and tumour-like lesions of the oesophagus

Benign epithelial tumours

Squamous cell papillomas are rare multilobulated tumours with a granular or warty surface and a firm consistency (Fig. 8.1). They are usually small (under 1.5 cm in diameter) and may be multiple [1]. The lower third of the oesophagus is the commonest site. Histologically, they have a papillary architecture with central cores of vascular connective tissue covered by thickened stratified squamous epithelium which lacks atypia and shows normal differentiation from the basal to the surface layers. Some have shown changes characteristic of human papillomavirus (HPV) infection [2,3] and variable numbers in two recent series have had the presence of HPV DNA demonstrated with the polymerase chain reaction [4,5]. Squamous cell papillomas have to be differentiated from inflammatory polyps occurring on the basis of gastro-oesophageal reflux [6,7]. These have a relatively smooth surface and show basal cell hyperplasia with varying erosion of the epithelium and usually a marked acute inflammatory cell infiltrate of the lamina propria. There is no evidence that squamous cell papillomas have any significant malignant potential.

The only examples of true adenomas have all occurred in the columnar-lined (Barrett's) oesophagus [8,9], where dysplasia in this premalignant condition may result in polypoid masses with a tubular or villous configuration. Intervening flat mucosa can also show dysplasia.

There are occasional reports of benign oesophageal epithelial neoplasms of salivary gland type with a presumptive origin from submucosal glands or ducts [10–12].

Malignant epithelial tumours

On a worldwide basis oesophageal cancer accounts for some 310 000 cases per year, with an estimate in 1980 that 50% of new cases would occur in China [13]. At least 90% of oesophageal carcinomas are squamous in type with most of the rest being adenocarcinomas, and other types such as small cell carcinoma and malignant melanoma are seen occasionally. In the USA and UK the overall incidence of all forms of oesophageal carcinoma varies from 5.2 to 10.4 per 100 000 people and accounts for 2–5% of deaths from malignant disease [14]. However, analyses of cancer incidence data have shown that in North America and Europe the incidence of oesophageal adenocarcinoma has been rising since the mid-1970s, when it accounted for some 16% of all oesophageal cancers among white men in the USA, to approach 50% of the total in the years 1988–90. The rates of adenocarcinomas of the gastric cardia have also increased, although to a lesser extent than oesophageal adenocarcinoma. Over the same period there had been a decline in the rate of oesophageal squamous cell carcinoma of 23% in one study and a smaller decline for adenocarcinomas involving more distal portions of the stomach [15–17]. A large majority of adenocarcinomas of the oesophagus and cardia have arisen from a columnar-lined (Barrett's) oesophagus.

Squamous cell carcinoma

Epidemiology

Squamous carcinoma of the oesophagus, although relatively infrequent in most of Western Europe and North America, is a major disease for a large proportion of the world's population with about 80% of cases occurring in developing countries

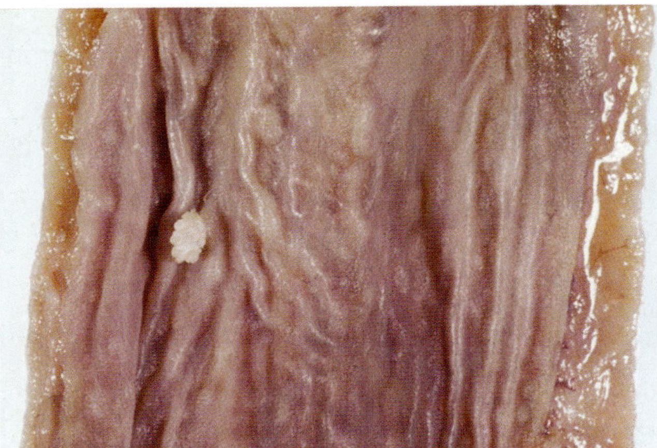

Fig. 8.1 Squamous cell papilloma. This small warty lesion was an incidental finding in the middle third of the oesophagus at postmortem.

[18]. Striking variations in its incidence occur, with approximately a 500-fold difference between the most and least affected areas. As well as this, there are sharp gradients of incidence between regions only a few hundred miles apart. Thus in northern China there is a 60-fold decrease for men and a 90-fold decrease for women between the north-east of Honan province and northern Shansi, 300 miles away [19], and in the Transkei, in South Africa and Uganda, the incidence varies so much that clearly defined adjacent localities show 10- to 20-fold differences [20]. Even in Europe, where the incidence is generally low, pockets of high incidence occur, such as in Normandy and Brittany, although there is marked variation between the different communes in these areas [21]. The increased risk here is predominantly amongst males where the incidence rises as high as 56 in 100 000, with a male to female ratio of 23 : 1. The formerly high rates of cancer in parts of Scandinavia, particularly of the postcricoid region and upper oesophagus, which predominantly affected women and were associated with anaemia, dysphagia, hypochlorhydria and other signs of iron and vitamin deficiency (Paterson–Kelly or Plummer–Vinson syndrome) [22,23], have now largely disappeared. A belt of high incidence of oesophageal cancer extends across Asia from north-east China through Soviet central Asia to the Caspian littoral, and levels of incidence in Kazakhstan and northern Iran are the highest observed for any type of cancer, in general populations, anywhere in the world [24]. The disease occurs mostly in people of Mongol or Turkic origin and, as its incidence rises, men and women are affected equally, or there may even be female preponderance.

The incidence of oesophageal cancer increases with age, and figures from China, where it is estimated that over 50% of the world total of cases occurs [18], show the peak of total oesophageal cancer deaths to be in the 60–64 age group. However, death tends to occur at an earlier age in high-risk than in low-risk areas [25].

Predisposing factors

Multiple factors seem to be involved in the aetiology of squamous oesophageal cancer and epidemiological studies have provided evidence that causative agents differ between geographical areas and may act synergistically.

Alcohol and tobacco

These have long been implicated as risk factors and it has been estimated that together they account for at least 80% of oesophageal cancer in male populations from France, the USA, Japan and some Latin American countries [26–29]. Among drinkers and smokers the risk rises considerably more with increased alcohol consumption than with rising tobacco consumption, and with the drinking of spirits rather than beer or wine [30]. In the UK, variations in the rate of oesophageal cancer have closely paralleled total alcohol consumption, with only a short lag, suggesting that the effect of alcohol is on the later stages of carcinogenesis, i.e. it is acting as a promoter [31]. It has been suggested that the distribution of high-incidence areas of oesophageal cancer in Africa correlates with the use of maize as the principal ingredient of home-made beer, which has replaced the traditional millets and sorghum [32].

There is a statistically higher incidence of oesophageal carcinomas among those who smoke or chew tobacco, and this is apparently equally true for pipe, cigar and cigarette smokers [33]. Oesophageal carcinomas are not infrequently associated with separate primary tumours in the mouth, pharynx, stomach or intestine [34,35], and it has been suggested that these are related to the ingestion of nicotine and other carcinogenic matter [36]. An autopsy study of the oesophagus of American men with a known smoking history showed some atypical nuclei in the basal layer of the epithelium in 6.6% of non-smokers and no cases of carcinoma *in situ*, whereas in smokers, basal atypia was found in 79.8% and carcinoma *in situ* in 1.9% [37]. In some high-risk populations in South Africa and India tobacco appears to play a more important role than alcohol [38–40]. Thus in South Africa the smoking of pipe tobacco had a positive association with oesophageal cancer [39], and tobacco pyrolysis products from the Transkei region have been shown to have mutagenic activity in the Ames test [41]. Unusual practices associated with pipe smoking, such as sucking out and swallowing the dottle from the stem of pipes through a straw and scraping out and then chewing the residues from the bowl of the pipe, probably increase the risk. A parallel situation is seen in north-eastern Iran where the eating of residues from opium pipes (sukhteh) is widespread in both sexes. Measurements of urinary morphine metabolites have indicated that addiction is common in the high-incidence areas, occurring in about half the men and women over 35 years old [42]. Mutagens in sukhteh and in morphine and opium pyrolysates have been identified and characterized [43–45] and are thought to be one factor involved in the aetiology of oesophageal cancer in the region.

Diet

Another factor, present in other high-incidence areas as well, is an inadequate and often unvarying diet. In northern Iran detailed dietary surveys have found clear regional variations, with the restriction of diet to home-baked bread and tea being a major factor determining the geographical distribution of oesophageal cancer. Such populations had low calorie and total protein intake and low intake of vitamin A, riboflavin and vitamin C [42].

Similar dietary deficiencies have been documented in high-risk populations in Linxian county of Henan province in China where cornbread and millet have been the staple foods until recently [46]. Contamination of these foodstuffs and pickled vegetables by fungi such as species of *Fusarium*, *Geotrichum* and *Aspergillus* occurs and induces the formation of nitrosamines [47], potent oesophageal carcinogens in the laboratory rat [48,49]. It is of interest that in these high-risk areas for human oesophageal carcinoma in China, cancers have also been found in the pharynx and upper oesophagus of domestic animals and fowls which closely resemble those in humans in clinicopathological morphology [50]. Fungal oesophagitis, mostly due to *Candida* spp., is very common in Linxian. It particularly involves the middle third of the oesophagus and has been proposed as a possible aetiological factor in oesophageal carcinogenesis [51]. Deficiency of trace elements such as zinc has been associated with oesophageal cancer [52,53]. There is a large and growing body of evidence that fruit and vegetables protect against oesophageal cancer [54].

Infectious agents

As well as the fungal agents referred to above, much recent research has focused on the role of human papillomavirus (HPV) infection in oesophageal carcinogenesis prompted by known associations of this virus with malignancies at other squamous epithelial sites, notably the anogenital tract [55–57] and skin, and by observations of histological changes in oesophageal squamous cell carcinomas identical to those of condylomatous genital lesions [58]. There have been numerous studies on the prevalence of HPV in squamous carcinoma of the oesophagus with detection rates varying from 0 to 71%. This variation is to some extent a result of the technique used (immunohistochemistry, *in situ* hybridization, polymerase chain reaction, Southern blot analysis), but more significantly appears to be related to the population studied, with a tendency towards higher rates in populations with a high incidence of cancer [59,60]. In some studies, where this has been looked for, the virus has been more easily detected in adjacent squamous mucosa than in the tumour itself [61]. The types of HPV identified have included HPV-6, -11, -16, -18, -30 and -73 [62], and more than one viral genotype has been reported in individual cases [61].

Oncogenic properties of HPVs, mainly types 16 and 18, have been confirmed in experimental studies and it is thought that protein products of early genes E6 and E7 bind to the protein products of tumour suppressor genes known to regulate the cell cycle, namely p53 and pRb (retinoblastoma), respectively [63], consequently leading to the uncontrolled proliferation of the infected cells. It appears that synergistic action with other initiating events, such as environmental factors, is required for oncogenesis [64]. The role that other viruses may play in oesophageal cancer has been recently reviewed [65].

Exogenous factors

Other suggested exogenous factors which may play a role in particular populations have included thermal irritation [66–68], the eating of bracken fern [29], and plant irritants in foods [69,70].

It has been known for many years that there is an increased risk of oesophageal carcinoma developing in the strictures which follow the ingestion of lye (crude sodium hydroxide with sodium carbonate), commonly after a time-interval which may exceed 40 years [71–73]. The evidence for their development in organic strictures from other causes is less convincing [74]. A number of cases of oesophageal cancer have been reported following therapeutic irradiation for various neck or spinal diseases [75] and after irradiation to the chest for breast carcinoma and, less frequently, for lymphoma [76].

Genetic factors

In general most of the available evidence lends no support to any hereditary basis for oesophageal carcinoma [77,78], although a study from northern Iran showed that around 47% of patients in the high-risk region of Turkoman Sahara gave a positive family history of oesophageal cancer, as compared with only 2% among the low-risk population of non-Turkoman [79]. As well as this, cases of oesophageal cancer in families associated with keratosis palmaris and plantaris (tylosis) inherited as a dominant characteristic have been described [80–82]. Recently, linkage analysis has mapped the tylosis oesophageal cancer (TOC) gene locus to chromosome 17q25 [83] and it has been shown that this locus is commonly deleted in sporadic oesophageal squamous cell carcinomas, suggesting the existence of a tumour suppressor gene for oesophageal squamous cell carcinoma at this site [84].Somatic molecular abnormalities include overexpression of epidermal growth factor receptors, amplification of cyclin D1, mutation of p53 and MTS1, allele loss in the p53, Rb and APC genes, and loss of heterogeneity (LOH) at loci on chromosomes 3p, 9q, 10p, 17q, 18q, 19q and 21q [85,86].

Associated conditions

Other conditions associated with an increased risk of oesophageal cancer include achalasia [87], diverticula [88,89], the Plummer–Vinson syndrome [90] and coeliac disease [91,92]. There is one report documenting squamous cell carcinoma arising in a duplication cyst of the oesophagus [93].

There is a well recognized association between oesophageal

cancer and cancers in adjacent organs of the aerodigestive tract [94], with tobacco, alcohol and irradiation implicated as pathogenetic factors. There is recent evidence suggesting that aspirin use may reduce the risk of developing oesophageal carcinoma [95].

Precancerous lesions

Some endoscopic studies have shown that chronic oesophagitis is very common in the population of areas where there is a high incidence of oesophageal carcinoma such as northern China and Iran. This is often symptomless and is characterized endoscopically by an irregular, friable mucosa with variable oedema and hyperaemia but without ulceration. Diffuse or scattered white patches may also be present. It usually involves the middle and lower thirds of the oesophagus whilst leaving the cardio-oesophageal junctional area free and thus differs in its distribution from the reflux-associated changes of oesophagitis found in low-risk populations which, in addition, are often complicated by erosions and ulcerations. Histologically, the commonest change, corresponding to the white patches seen at endoscopy, has been acanthosis of the epithelium due to the presence of swollen clear squamous cells which in general are periodic acid–Schiff (PAS)-negative (differing therefore from glycogenic acanthosis—see p. 74). Chronic oesophagitis often accompanies this with a lymphoplasmacytic infiltrate of the mucosa and submucosa with papillary elongation and parakeratosis of the epithelium [96]. Proliferative abnormalities have been demonstrated in the oesophageal epithelium of high-risk populations irrespective of the presence of oesophagitis on histological examination [97]. However, a more recent endoscopic survey, carried out in Linxian in a population with a previous diagnosis of dysplasia following screening by oesophageal balloon cytology, has cast doubt on the role of oesophagitis as a precursor lesion, with this diagnosis only being made in 4.6%. Epithelial atrophy was not observed at all in this study [98]. These discrepancies highlight the importance of standardized and reproducible histological criteria in epidemiological studies.

Of more import as a precancerous lesion is the presence of epithelial dysplasia. Most of the reports of oesophageal dysplasia are from countries with a high incidence of squamous carcinoma, particularly China. In one mass survey using the abrasive balloon technique to obtain cytological specimens and carried out over a 9-year period on 21 581 inhabitants aged over 30 in Linxian county, 12.7% of the subjects showed mild dysplasia, 1.2% had severe dysplasia and in 0.9% the appearances were consistent with invasive squamous carcinoma [99]. The age distribution of dysplasia and carcinoma suggested a continuous progression from mild to severe dysplasia and carcinoma *in situ*. Moreover, follow-up studies of patients with severe dysplasia showed progression to cancer in about a quarter of all cases. Another prospective follow-up study from Linxian [100] found that moderate and severe dysplasia and carcinoma *in situ* were the only histological lesions associated with a significantly increased risk of development of squamous cell carcinoma within 3.5 years of endoscopic biopsy diagnosis. Increasing grades of dysplasia were associated with increasing risk, although severe dysplasia and carcinoma *in situ* identified similar degrees of risk. This and other studies have also shown that nearly all of the biopsies with moderate dysplasia, or worse, came from endoscopically identified focal lesions [100,101]. These took the form of erosions, plaques or nodules, or areas of increased friability or redness. The data from China further suggest that dysplasia can be reversible [102]. The problems of dysplasia and carcinoma *in situ* in the oesophagus are fundamentally no different from the same changes seen, for example, in the uterine cervix. The histological criteria for dysplasia include increased cellularity of the whole thickness of the mucous membrane, hyperchromatic nuclei, pleomorphism of nuclei and increased numbers of mitotic figures. The degree of dysplasia can be graded into mild, moderate and severe. In some cases of hyperplasia and dysplasia the presence of koilocytotic change indicates an underlying human papillomavirus infection [2,3,103]. As with the cervix and other epithelial surfaces, the difficulty arises in distinguishing true dysplasia from the reactive and predominantly basal cell hyperplasia seen, for example, in gastro-oesophageal reflux [104] and glycogenic acanthosis of the oesophagus (see p. 74).

Further evidence of the role of dysplasia as a precancerous lesion comes from its frequent occurrence in areas adjacent to or distant from invasive squamous carcinoma when oesophagectomy specimens have been studied in detail [105–109]. One investigation found that the prevalence of intraepithelial carcinoma (epithelial dysplasia) at the margins of invasive carcinoma was inversely related to the depth of invasion of the main lesion [110], supporting the view that such changes are not secondary to lateral intraepithelial spread of tumour but represent a primary field transformation from which invasive carcinoma has subsequently arisen.

Studies of oesophageal carcinogenesis in animals have also established dysplasia as a precancerous lesion [111,112].

Superficial oesophageal cancer

There have been numerous reports of oesophageal cancer in which the tumour is confined to the mucosa or has spread no further than the submucosa, with or without lymph node metastasis. Most emanate from China or Japan [113–115], but series are also being reported from Europe [116–118] and the USA [119]. In China the large majority of cases have been detected in mass surveys involving balloon cytology and X-ray examinations in high-incidence areas, but other cases have been symptomatic. The Chinese have described four basic types of macroscopic appearance. Lesions may be plaque-like or consist of single or multiple map-like erosions (Fig. 8.2) which can resemble the changes in reflux oesophagitis but,

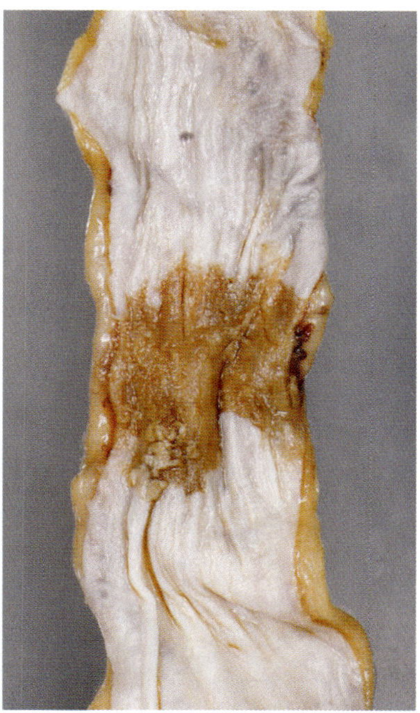

Fig. 8.2 Superficial oesophageal cancer. Extensive erosive lesion found incidentally at postmortem in middle third of oesophagus.

unlike that condition, are usually separated by normal mucosa from the gastro-oesophageal junction. Less commonly, a protuberant lesion is present. Occasionally the mucosa has looked normal apart from a colour change (occult type), and histological examination of resected specimens has shown these to be intraepithelial carcinomas. The Japanese have classified macroscopic features along the lines of their classification for early gastric cancer, namely elevated or protruded type, superficial (with three subtypes), and depressed or ulcerative. In terms of stage, however, the prognosis of early oesophageal cancer as defined above differs from that of early gastric cancer with 5-year survival rates of the order of 50–60% with infiltration of the submucosa, related to the fact that some 30–40% of patients with submucosal spread have lymph node metastasis [117,120,121]. This has led some authors to suggest that the term early oesophageal cancer is restricted to cases in which there is carcinoma *in situ* (intraepithelial carcinoma) or mucosal carcinoma only and where the prognosis approaches 100% [121,122,123]. It has been found in one study that the presence of an elevated component in superficial oesophageal cancer, the demonstration of which is facilitated at endoscopy by iodine staining of the oesophagus [124], was an important macroscopic feature suggesting submucosal invasion and a high probability of lymph node involvement. Some superficial carcinomas have occupied a large area of the oesophagus [105,125,126,127]. Endoscopic ultrasonography has been used in cases of superficial oesophageal carcinoma to assess the depth of invasion and to evaluate perioesophagogastric lymph node metastasis [128]. Observations and investigations like these are important since, increasingly, non-surgical interventions such as photodynamic therapy [129] and endoscopic mucosal resection [130] are being considered in the treatment of these lesions and their dysplastic precursors.

Whilst most reports of superficial carcinomas have been of squamous histology, adenocarcinomas arising in Barrett's oesophagus may also present in this way [131]. Like early gastric cancer, they appear to have a better prognosis compared to squamous cell carcinoma, being less likely to recur locally or to have second primary tumours [118].

Advanced squamous carcinoma

It is the custom, when assessing the site of origin of an oesophageal tumour, to divide the oesophagus arbitrarily into thirds. In males squamous growths are rare in the upper part, most common in the middle third, and less frequent in the lower third. In women, the postcricoid carcinoma used to be the most common, but with the decline of the Plummer–Vinson syndrome, the site distribution approximates to that in males. The distribution in one large series from Linxian, China, based on a combination of balloon cytology, oesophagoscopy and radiological examination, found involvement by tumour of the upper third of the oesophagus in 11.7%, the middle third in 63.3%, and the lower third in 24.9% [132].

Macroscopic appearances

Macroscopically, squamous carcinomas appear as exophytic, ulcerating or infiltrating lesions or a combination of these (Figs 8.3 & 8.4) and often result in a stricture which is usually irregular, friable and haemorrhagic. However, undermining of proximal adjacent epithelium by the tumour may give rise to a smooth, annular stenosis. True papillary or verrucous squamous cell carcinoma is uncommon and occurs usually as a large, warty, slowly growing neoplasm [133]. Most have occurred in the upper third and in some there has been a history of achalasia or the presence of a diverticulum or caustic stricture [134–136].

Rarely, a diffuse infiltrative type of growth, resembling the 'leather bottle stomach', involves a length of oesophagus. Superficial spreading carcinomas, with extensive intramucosal involvement and a propensity to permeate lymphatics and metastasize to lymph nodes, have also been described [137]. Other bizarre patterns, including spiral forms, may be seen [138].

Squamous carcinomas situated in the postcricoid region of the oesophagus do not differ appreciably from those of the middle and lower thirds. Coincident oesophageal webs, which spread across the upper oesophagus as a thin diaphragm and readily rupture on oesophagoscopy, are not uncommon. These webs consist of connective tissue covered by normal squamous epithelium, sometimes with chronic inflammatory changes in subepithelial tissues. They appear

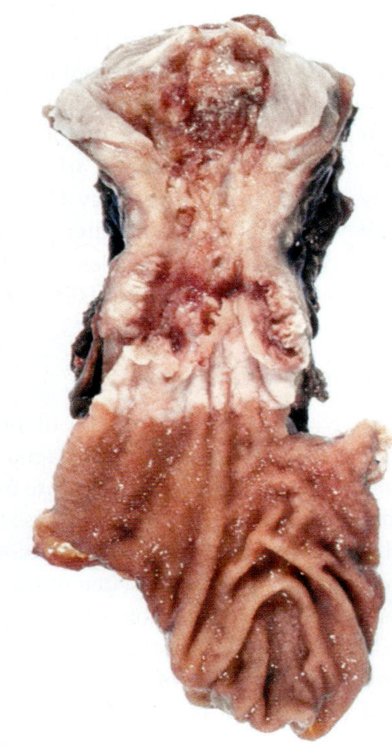

Fig. 8.3 An extensively ulcerated squamous cell carcinoma of the lower third of the oesophagus resulting in a stricture.

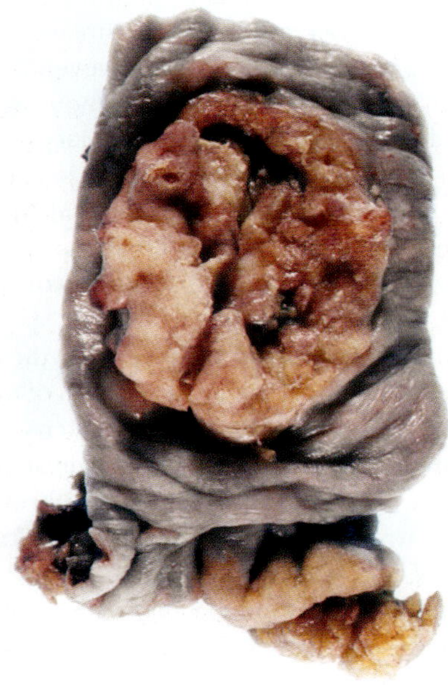

Fig. 8.4 A fungating ulcerated squamous cell carcinoma of the oesophagus.

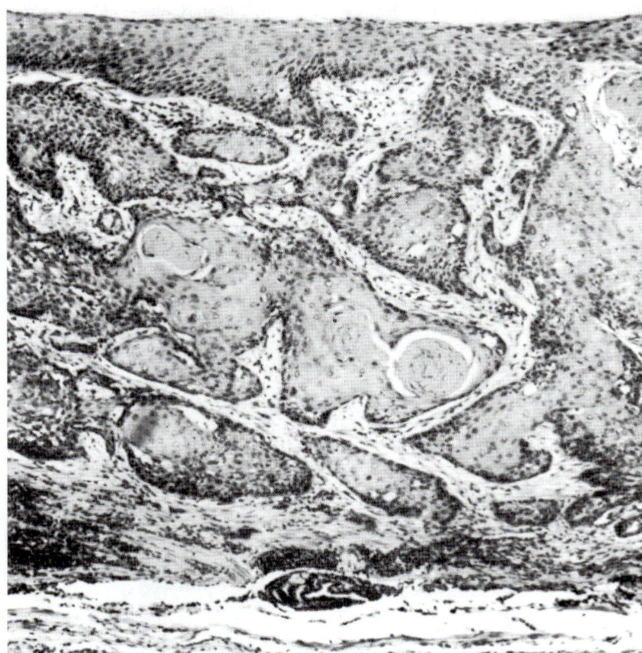

Fig. 8.5 Well differentiated, keratinizing squamous cell carcinoma.

to represent folds of oesophageal epithelium and show no evidence of premalignant change [139,140].

Not uncommonly an oesophageal carcinoma is surrounded by satellite nodules due to submucosal extension. More than one primary tumour of the oesophagus is a fairly frequent finding when detailed histopathological examination of resection specimens has been carried out and where the possibility of submucosal spread or intramural metastasis has been eliminated. It was found in 14.6% of a Japanese series of 205 patients undergoing subtotal oesophagectomy, and the prevalence rose to 25.6% when only those cases without preoperative irradiation treatment were considered [141]. A prevalence of 31% was present in another series from Yugoslavia [142]. Oesophageal carcinoma is also associated with tumours in other organs, particularly the oropharynx and larynx [143–145]. This presumably relates to shared risk factors, particularly a history of heavy smoking and high alcohol intake [146].

Microscopic appearances

These tumours show all grades of differentiation, from keratinizing squamous carcinomas with well formed cell nests (Fig. 8.5) to undifferentiated growths without recognizable keratin or prickle cells, which are difficult to identify as squamous (Fig. 8.6). Sometimes a superficial resemblance to a basal cell carcinoma may be present when cells adjoining the stroma have a palisaded arrangement. In most tumours, however, epithelial nests, pearls or intercellular bridges can be found.

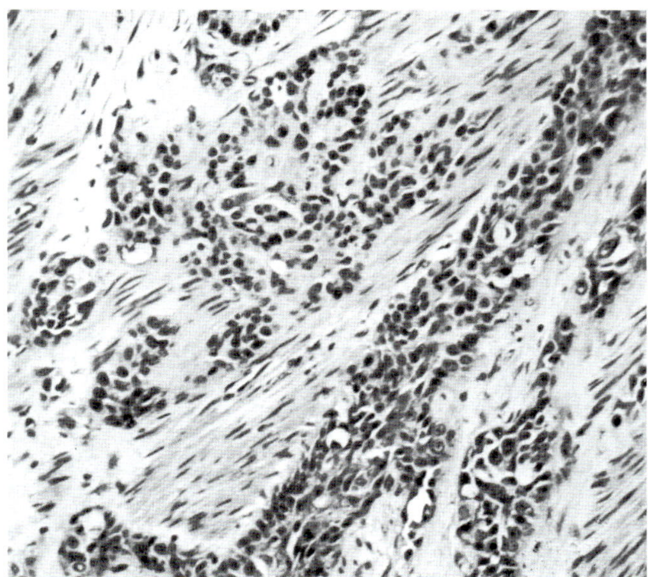

Fig. 8.6 Poorly differentiated squamous cell carcinoma.

There is a marked tendency to variations in differentiation in different parts of the growth when resected specimens are rigorously examined. As well as this, histochemical, immunohistochemical and ultrastructural studies have confirmed morphological heterogeneity, with approximately 30% of tumours showing focal adenocarcinomatous differentiation [147–149]. In most cases, the diagnosis of squamous cell carcinoma is reasonably straightforward in biopsy material, but regenerative epithelium from the edge of a benign ulcer or erosion may show considerable enlargement of the basal or parabasal cells with numerous mitoses and, particularly in poorly orientated material, give a misleading impression of malignancy. Lack of pleomorphism, uniformity of nuclear morphology, and the tendency towards normal surface maturation are all helpful pointers to a reactive, rather than a neoplastic, state. Bizarre, pleomorphic stromal cells with hyperchromatic nuclei and prominent nucleoli associated with granulation tissue are another potential source of confusion with malignancy [150], as is the cytonuclear atypia of squamous epithelial cells following irradiation [106]. Infiltration of the submucosa, not readily detectable by the naked eye, is often a conspicuous microscopic feature of squamous cell carcinoma [151]; segmental resection is therefore not often adequate [152,153] and in any surgically removed tumour a careful study should be made of the resected ends, particularly proximally, to ensure that removal has been complete [154]. Frozen section has been advocated in this situation [155]. The tumour commonly infiltrates the muscle coats and often breaches them: local extension to surrounding structures is common.

Three uncommon variants of squamous cell carcinoma—verrucous squamous cell carcinoma, so-called carcinosarcoma, and basaloid–squamous carcinoma—deserve special mention, since they may give rise to misleading appearances in biopsy material.

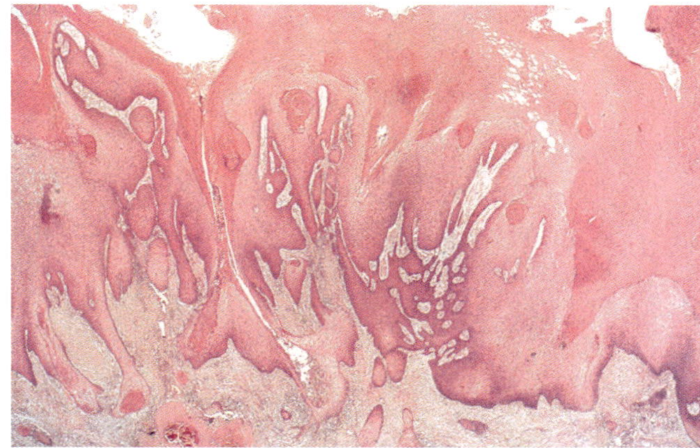

Fig. 8.7 Verrucous carcinoma. Well differentiated papillary squamous cell carcinoma with surface maturation but obvious infiltration of the deep aspect in this section from a resection specimen.

Verrucous carcinoma

Verrucous squamous cell carcinoma is usually a large, exophytic neoplasm with a shaggy papillary or warty morphology that can arise at any site in the oesophagus. Similar tumours occur at other sites, notably the oral cavity, larynx, glans penis, vulva and anal canal [156,157]. Most of the cases in the oesophagus have occurred in the upper part [134]. In some there has been a history of achalasia, diverticulum [134], postcricoid web [158] or lye stricture [135]. In a recently reported case, verrucous squamous carcinoma evolved from chronic oesophagitis, squamous papillary hyperplasia and dysplasia over a period of 16 years [159]. Histologically, verrucous carcinoma consists of papillary projections composed of well differentiated squamous cells with parakeratosis and hyperkeratosis most prominent between the papillae (Fig. 8.7). In biopsies, evidence of invasion is frequently lacking so that a pathologist unaware of the endoscopic appearances would interpret the rather bland features as a benign hyperplastic process. Despite the features of low-grade malignancy and the fact that metastasis is uncommon [133], this tumour has a poor prognosis because of its propensity to invade locally, with fistula formation being common in reported cases [160].

Carcinosarcoma (spindle cell carcinoma)

These usually occur as bulky polypoid growths in the lower oesophagus (Fig. 8.8). They consist of a 'sarcomatous' component of interlacing bundles of spindle-shaped cells in which bizarre giant cells are present, and in which osseous and cartilaginous metaplasia may occur, together with an epithelial component of squamous or undifferentiated carcinoma (Fig. 8.9). Occasionally an adenocarcinomatous [161] or adenocystic component [162] has been described and in a recent

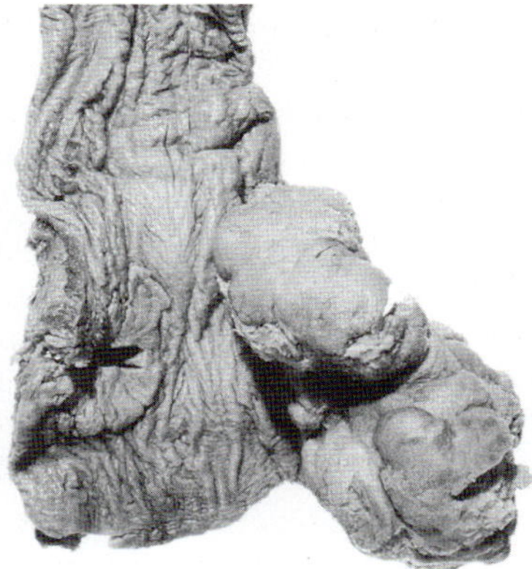

Fig. 8.8 Carcinosarcoma. A large lobulated polypoid growth is present at the lower end of the oesophagus.

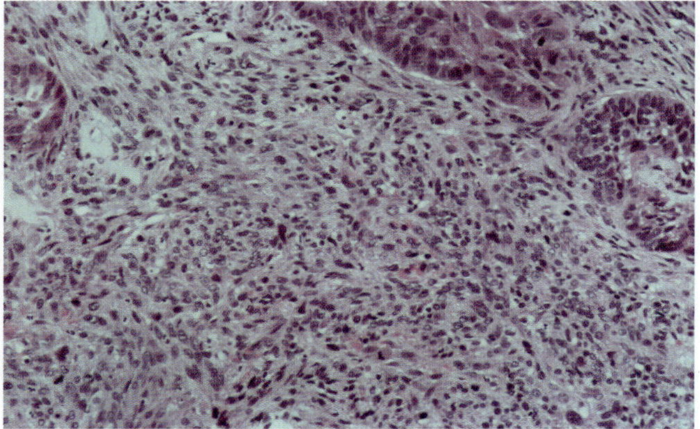

Fig. 8.9 Carcinosarcoma (spindle cell carcinoma). Interlacing spindle cells with a 'sarcomatous' morphology are seen together with two groups of poorly differentiated squamous cell carcinoma.

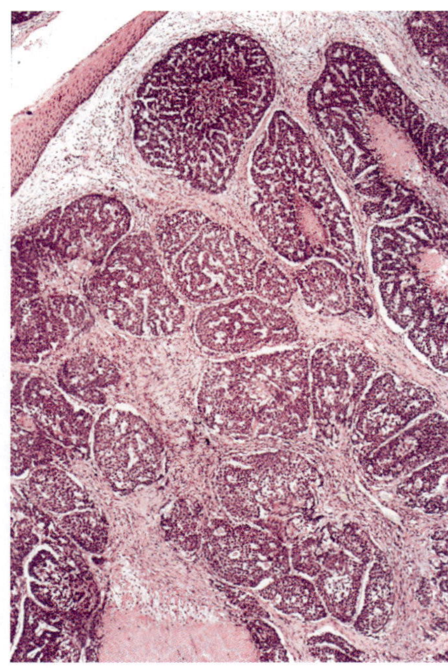

Fig. 8.10 Basaloid–squamous carcinoma. Lobules of basaloid cells with a festoon appearance peripherally are present deep to oesophageal epithelium. Central necrosis is seen in several of the tumour lobules.

case there was neuroendocrine and glandular differentiation [163]. There may be an admixture of these two elements throughout the tumour or the sarcomatous part may predominate, with often only inconspicuous intramucosal or invasive squamous cell carcinoma confined to small areas at the base of the pedicle. With this latter appearance the term pseudosarcoma has been used, in the belief that the spindle cell element represents a non-neoplastic reparative host response to the carcinoma. The finding of transition from typical squamous carcinoma to the sarcomatous component when carefully looked for in many of the resected specimens [162,164], and the demonstration ultrastructurally of tonofibrils and well developed desmosomes in some of the spindle cells [161,165], together with evidence of collagen production [166], suggests that the 'sarcomatous' cells are squamous cells which have undergone mesenchymal metaplasia. Immunohistochemical studies have demonstrated disparate findings, with some authors describing immunoreactivity to keratin in the spindle cell component [167,168] and others reporting negative reactions to keratin and variable positivity to desmin, smooth muscle actin, vimentin, alpha-1-antichymotrypsin and alpha-1-antitrypsin [163,169,170]. Recent studies on the clonality of these tumours have also led to disparate results [171,172]. Biopsy of these tumours may produce tissue suggesting a highly malignant undifferentiated sarcoma, although in the majority of reported cases squamous cell carcinoma of varying degrees of differentiation has been present. In some reports this tumour has been associated with longer survival than the usual type of squamous cell carcinoma [162], whereas in others the prognosis has appeared similar [161].

Basaloid–squamous carcinoma

These tumours usually occur in elderly males and present at an advanced stage. They show a biphasic pattern. There is an undifferentiated basaloid component in the form of solid sheets, anastomosing trabeculae, festoons or microcystic structures, and associated with a high mitotic index, frequent comedo necrosis and stromal hyalinization (Fig. 8.10). The other is a neoplastic squamous component which can be invasive or *in situ*, and which may be inconspicuous. They have comprised 1.9% and 11.3% of oesophageal squamous cell malignancies in two recent series [173,174]. Tumours with a similar histology have also occurred in the larynx, pharynx, base of tongue and hard palate [175–177]. It seems apparent that the majority of cases in the literature reported as adenoid cystic carcinomas of the oesophagus probably represent examples of basaloid–squamous carcinoma. The rare genuine examples of oesophageal adenoid cystic carcinoma have a less aggressive clinical course [178,179] (see p. 69). The prognosis of patients with basaloid–squamous carcinoma does not appear to differ from that of typical squamous cell carcinoma [174].

Adenocarcinoma arising in Barrett's oesophagus

Oesophageal adenocarcinoma, previously an uncommon (or under-recognized) disease, has assumed increasing importance in recent years. There are two main reasons for this. The first is the recognition and description of the columnar-lined oesophagus and the subsequent realization that this metaplastic epithelium was precancerous. In fact the first case of malignancy arising in this condition was reported by one of the original coauthors of this textbook [180]. It is now considered that nearly all adenocarcinomas of the oesophagus and gastro-oesophageal junction occur on this basis. The second reason for the current interest in oesophageal and junctional adenocarcinoma is due to the very large increase in reported cases in recent decades, particularly in the USA and Europe.

The pathogenesis of Barrett's oesophagus and its malignant potential have already been alluded to (see p. 40) and the following discussion will concentrate on epidemiological and pathological aspects of adenocarcinoma and its precursors. Other rare types of adenocarcinoma that occur in the oesophagus, unrelated to Barrett's metaplasia, will be considered subsequently (see p. 68).

Epidemiology

Analyses of cancer incidence data have shown that in North America and Europe the incidence of oesophageal adenocarcinomas has been rising since the mid-1970s. At that time it accounted for some 16% of all oesophageal cancers among white males in the United States, increasing to about one-third of the total by the mid-1980s [16], and constituting the majority of oesophageal malignancies during the period 1992–94, an increase of over 350% in this period. Rates also rose among black males during this period, but remained at much lower levels. The rates of adenocarcinomas of the gastric cardia also increased, although to a lesser extent, with rates in white males almost equalling those for the rest of the stomach. The upward trend for both tumours was much greater among older than younger men. Although the incidence also rose among females, rates remained much lower than in males. Analysis suggested that the increases in incidence were real and unrelated to diagnostic shifts with reference to location, specificity of cell type, or earlier endoscopy-based diagnosis [181]. Increasing rates of oesophageal adenocarcinoma have also been reported from the UK, Scandinavia, France, Switzerland, Australia and New Zealand [182–187]. A recent report from Denmark documented an eightfold increase in oesophageal adenocarcinoma over the period 1970–90, with this type now comprising 34% of all oesophageal cancers. A previous diagnosis of Barrett's oesophagus had been made in only seven of the 524 cases reported over a 6-year period when medical data were retrieved, suggesting that screening programmes were unlikely to reduce the death rate in the general population [188]. The increasing incidence of adenocarcinoma of both the oesophagus and the oesophago-gastric junction over a similar period, together with an association of the cancers in both locations with a predominance in white males and reflux symptoms, suggest that they arise on the same basis. Detailed pathological studies have lent support to this, with demonstration of a columnar-lined oesophagus in a considerable proportion of tumours centred within 2 cm of the gastro-oesophageal junction [189–191]. The likelihood of finding associated Barrett's mucosa in junctional cancers is considerably greater with smaller tumours than larger ones, implying that, in the latter situation, the specialized epithelium is overgrown and therefore not identified [191]. Small adenocarcinomas have also been described arising in tongues or short segments of columnar-lined mucosa [189,192].

Predisposing factors

Tobacco and alcohol

The role that cigarette smoking and alcohol consumption may play in the development of oesophageal adenocarcinoma has been examined in several studies and it appears that there is a two- to threefold increase in risk in smokers, although the risk does not decrease substantially after cessation of smoking [193–195]. This differs from the situation with oesophageal squamous cell carcinoma. Changing patterns of smoking may explain the changing incidence of both adenocarcinoma and squamous cell carcinoma of the oesophagus in some countries [181]. Unlike the situation with squamous cell carcinoma, alcohol appears to be a less important factor in oesophageal adenocarcinoma.

Dietary factors

Obesity has also been proposed as a risk factor for these tumours, with increased abdominal pressure predisposing to gastro-oesophageal reflux disease and involvement of dietary factors as possible mechanisms [196,197].

Genetic factors

The role that inherited factors may play in gastro-oesophageal reflux disease, Barrett's oesophagus and oesophageal adenocarcinoma based on reports of familial clustering has been recently reviewed [198], as has the spectrum of molecular abnormalities, both somatic and germline [16,199,200].

Associated conditions

Conditions which predispose to reflux oesophagitis are associated with an increased incidence of adenocarcinoma. They include treated achalasia [201,202], scleroderma [203,204] and

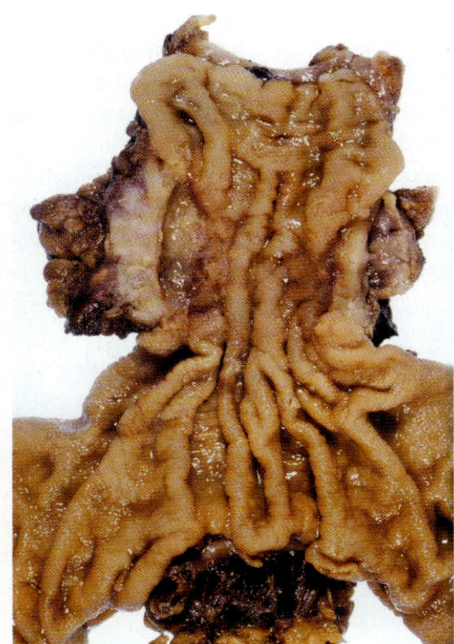

Fig. 8.11 Ulcerated adenocarcinoma arising in columnar-lined oesophagus.

the Zollinger–Ellison syndrome [205]. Unlike the situation with oesophageal squamous cell carcinoma, there does not appear to be an increased risk of extraoesophageal malignancy in patients with adenocarcinoma [206], apart from a possible modest increased risk of colorectal cancer [207].

Macroscopic appearances

The majority of adenocarcinomas are flat, ulcerating, infiltrative lesions, frequently associated with stenosis of the oesophageal lumen (Fig. 8.11). A minority are polypoid and fungating [208,209]. Rarely, a diffusely infiltrative growth resembling that of linitis plastica in the stomach [210] or a papillary lesion is apparent. Leaving aside lesions identified during surveillance programmes, most tumours are advanced at the time of diagnosis, with extensive intramural and adventitial involvement. Multiple tumours have been described [209,211]. Background metaplastic columnar mucosa is often apparent adjacent to the tumour, although in some cases an origin from Barrett's mucosa is dependent upon careful histological examination. Dysplasia, whilst frequently seen histologically adjacent to adenocarcinoma [212], is only rarely identified grossly (Fig. 8.12).

Microscopic appearances

Histologically these tumours show a similar spectrum of changes to adenocarcinomas arising in the stomach. The majority have a tubular or papillary pattern of intestinal type [213]. In some, there is prominent extracellular mucus production, but the diffuse type of signet-ring cell carcinoma is very

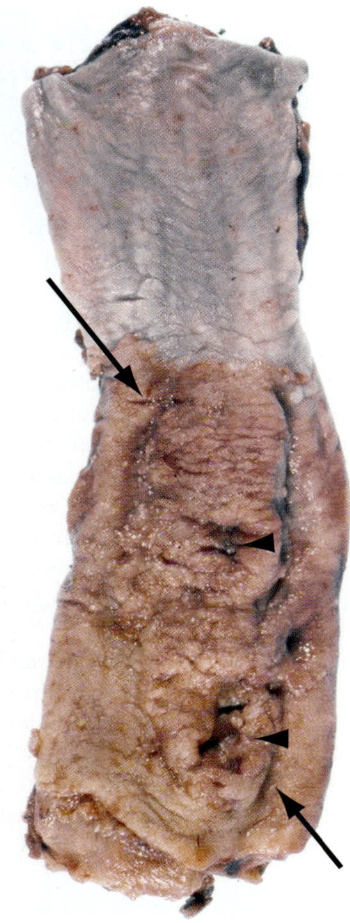

Fig. 8.12 This oesophagectomy specimen shows the upper part lined by squamous epithelium and the lower part lined by columnar epithelium, in which there is extensive raised villous dysplasia (arrows) with ulcers (arrowheads) corresponding histologically to foci of malignant change.

unusual. High-grade dysplasia is common in adjacent epithelium [208,212] (Fig. 8.13). Tumours may contain scattered argyrophil endocrine cells [214], and occasional Paneth cells. Transmission electron microscopy and immunohistochemistry have highlighted the frequent multidirectional differentiation that may be present in Barrett's adenocarcinomas [215]. Some tumours have shown squamous differentiation [209,216], and adenocarcinoid, carcinoid and mucoepidermoid carcinomas have all been described [209,217,218]. In addition, squamous cell carcinomas may arise in columnar-lined epithelium [209,219,220]. More than 80% of symptomatic tumours have shown infiltration through the oesophageal muscular coat, often with conspicuous perineural invasion. Lymph node metastases have been frequent [221].

Other adenocarcinomas

Adenocarcinomas, other than those arising on the basis of a

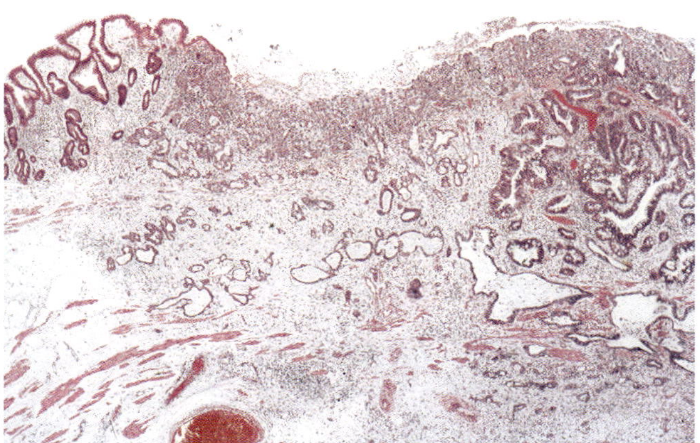

Fig. 8.13 Adenocarcinoma infiltrating oesophageal wall. Note high-grade epithelial dysplasia at upper left. There is reduplication of the muscularis mucosae.

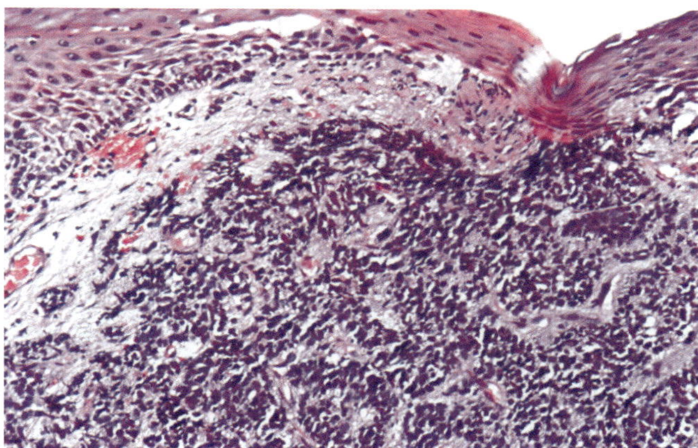

Fig. 8.14 Small cell carcinoma showing focal crush artefact is present deep to oesophageal epithelium.

columnar-lined (Barrett's) oesophagus, are uncommon. Some of those occurring in the lower oesophagus could well represent this sequence, where the tumour has overgrown any residual metaplastic epithelium [191]. Occasional reports of adenocarcinoma have described tumours arising in heterotopic gastric mucosa in the cervical oesophagus [222,223]. Apart from this, there are a few reports of tumours with a morphological resemblance to salivary gland tumours. Most have occurred in the middle third. Characteristically, they have been small, intramural lesions covered by an intact, non-neoplastic squamous epithelium, and have been associated with a relatively good prognosis. The histology has been that of either a mucoepidermoid carcinoma [224] or an adenoid cystic carcinoma [178,179]. A critical review of the literature, however, suggests that many of the published cases of oesophageal mucoepidermoid and adenoid cystic carcinoma have been of large aggressive tumours, often involving the surface epithelium and intermingled with other elements, usually classical squamous cell carcinoma (SCC) or undifferentiated carcinoma [179,224–228]. The so-called mucoepidermoid elements have often shown keratinization, and frequent necrosis has occurred in adenoid cystic areas, features not associated with classical salivary gland-type tumours. There is no doubt as well that many reported cases of adenoid cystic carcinoma represent the recently described basaloid–squamous carcinoma (see p. 66). It is not uncommon to find glandular, mucus-secreting and cribriform elements in a significant proportion of oesophageal SCCs, particularly in their more superficial parts [147,229]. From the above it would appear that adenocarcinomas of salivary gland type are extremely uncommon when strict criteria are applied, and that most of the reported cases probably represent variants of SCC showing bidirectional differentiation.

Adenosquamous carcinoma

These are uncommon aggressive tumours in which adenocarcinomatous and squamous carcinomatous components are intermingled or have a fairly clear boundary. Most cases have occurred in a columnar-lined (Barrett's) oesophagus [209,216]. They may be confused histologically with mucoepidermoid carcinoma but features such as the frequent presence of keratinization in the squamous component and the marked nuclear pleomorphism in adenosquamous carcinoma enable a differentiation to be made [230].

Small cell (oat cell) carcinoma

Since the first description of primary small cell carcinoma of the oesophagus [231], approximately 230 cases have been reported [232]. Reviews of large series of primary oesophageal carcinomas have identified 1–2.4% of the total with this morphology [233,234]. This tumour has also been described as oat cell carcinoma, argyrophil cell carcinoma, neuroendocrine carcinoma, small cell undifferentiated carcinoma and anaplastic carcinoma. In the majority of cases these tumours have been large, often protuberant and arising in the middle and lower thirds of the oesophagus. On histological examination, small, fusiform or polygonal cells with little cytoplasm, hyperchromatic nuclei and inconspicuous nucleoli are present, arranged in sheets or anastomosing cords and ribbons. Crush artefact of the tumour cells is common, particularly in biopsy material (Fig. 8.14). Rosette formation may be present. Squamous differentiation has been described, as well as foci of glandular differentiation, particularly in resection specimens when minutely examined [235]. As well as this, carcinoid-like areas have been reported occasionally [233]. If spread from the lung can be ruled out [236], confirmation that the tumour is a primary small cell carcinoma and not an undifferentiated squamous cell carcinoma depends on the demonstration of argyrophilia of the tumour cells, immunopositivity for neuroendocrine markers such as neurone specific enolase, synaptophysin and chromogranin, or the finding of neurosecretory granules on ultrastructural examination. Immunostaining of tumour cells or assay of tumour tissue has demonstrated adrenocorticotrophic hormone (ACTH) and calcitonin in some cases [235,237]. Vasoactive intestinal peptide has also been shown in one tumour which was associated with the watery diarrhoea–hypokalaemia–achlorhydria syndrome [238]. A few non-oat cell anaplastic or undifferentiated carcinomas remain uncharacterized after these techniques and have been referred to as reserve cell carcinomas [239].

Because of the heterogeneity of small cell carcinoma of the oesophagus referred to above it appears likely that these tumours arise from a totipotential stem cell rather than the differentiated argyrophilic endocrine cells which are present in the basal layer of the oesophageal epithelium [240]. The prognosis of these tumours is poor with a median survival of 8 months for patients with disease confined to the oesophagus and of 3 months with disease that has spread beyond locoregional boundaries [232]. Occasional long-term survivors have been reported [241–243]. Because of the small numbers of patients and lack of controlled data the effects of different types of treatment are difficult to assess, but as with small cell carcinomas of the lung, multidrug chemotherapy and radiation probably offer the best chance for improvement in survival, with resection reserved for the minority of tumours without evidence of distant metastasis [241,244].

Very rare cases of carcinoid tumours of the oesophagus have been reported [245,246].

Choriocarcinoma

A few cases of choriocarcinoma of the oesophagus have been reported [247–251]. They have been large, exophytic, fungating tumours with extensive haemorrhage and necrosis which have mostly involved the lower part. Some have been admixed with adenocarcinoma, and two of the tumours occurred in a columnar-lined (Barrett's) oesophagus. An admixture of syncytio- and cytotrophoblast is present on histological examination, and one tumour showed yolk-sac differentiation [251]. There have been increased serum and urinary gonadotrophin levels [247,250,251], and gynaecomastia has been present in males. All patients have been under 50 years of age. The importance of immunostaining for tumour markers in young patients with oesophageal adenocarcinoma, in order that appropriate therapy may be selected, has been highlighted in one report [251].

Malignant melanoma

Though it is now well recognized that melanocytes can be found in normal oesophageal mucosa in about 4–8% of normal people [252,253], a melanoma presenting in the oesophagus is still more likely to be secondary than primary. The criteria for a primary oesophageal melanoma are that it should be seen either to arise from, or be surrounded by, squamous epithelium showing junctional change [254]. Most of the 100 or so well documented cases in the literature have also contained demonstrable melanin. Acceptable primary melanomas have predominantly affected elderly people and involved the middle or lower thirds of the oesophagus. Characteristically, the tumours are large, polypoid and friable, and may or may not be pigmented (Fig. 8.15). In some cases the adjacent mucosa has shown patchy or diffuse melanosis, with or without melanocytic atypia [255–257], and satellite lesions may be present [258]. Histologically, spindle and/or epithelioid cells are present which contain melanin pigment demonstrable by conventional stains or immunohistochemically by antibody to S-100 protein and HMB45, the latter a monoclonal antibody with high specificity for the majority of melanomas [259].

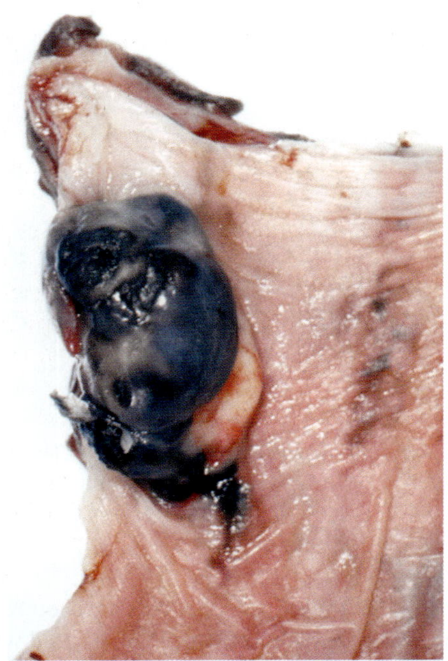

Fig. 8.15 Malignant melanoma. A protuberant, superficially ulcerated, pigmented tumour of the middle third of the oesophagus.

Involvement of the oesophagus by metastasis from a malignant melanoma usually results in compression of the lumen. At endoscopy, a smooth, projecting lesion covered by intact mucosa is seen and biopsies may not sample the tumour. Occasionally a large pigmented polypoid mass results [260], resembling a primary malignant melanoma, but distinguishable from it by the absence of junctional change in adjacent epithelium. Both primary and secondary tumours have a poor prognosis.

The spread of oesophageal carcinomas

Direct spread

The most common and extensive form of direct spread is in the wall of the viscus, particularly in the submucosa and in submucosal lymphatics [151,152]. Spread along the ducts of oesophageal glands is not uncommon and may represent an important pathway for deeper invasion in the early stages of oesophageal carcinoma [261]. Occasional cases of pagetoid spread of tumour cells within the oesophageal epithelium have been reported in association with squamous cell carcinoma [127,262,263]. In all resected specimens it is necessary to take transverse blocks from the proximal and distal ends to ensure that the line of resection is clear of any submucosal extension of the growth, even though it may well appear clear to the naked eye [154,264,265]. Downward extension of oesophageal carcinoma into the stomach is not common in our experience, despite the continuity of the submucosa. Any extension may subsequently ulcerate through the mucosa thus producing satellite growths. Once the growth has breached the muscle coats it commonly involves the trachea or main bronchi, the lung parenchyma and the superior or posterior mediastinum. Less commonly, there is direct invasion of the aorta with perforation; more rarely, the pericardium, heart and laryngeal nerves are involved.

Metastasis

By the time that the diagnosis of symptomatic oesophageal carcinoma is confirmed, metastases have occurred in 50–80% of cases [151,266–268]. Adenocarcinomas seem to metastasize earlier, and more frequently, than the squamous type.

The most common sites of metastasis are the regional lymph nodes, probably because there are two sets of lymphatics, one draining mucosa and submucosa, the other the muscle coats and adventitia. Nodes likely to be affected include paratracheal, parabronchial, paraoesophageal, posterior mediastinal, coeliac and upper deep cervical groups. Nodes below the diaphragm are frequently involved, including those in the splenic hilum. Because there is a wide intercommunication between these groups, clinical involvement of the nodes palpable in the neck does not necessarily mean that the growth is in the upper or middle oesophagus. In a detailed study [269], involving predominantly squamous cell carcinomas of the oesophagus in which radical oesophagectomy with extensive lymphadenectomy had been carried out, there was a significant difference in the number of positive lymph nodes per patient when intramural cancers (submucosal T1 and T2 tumours—TNM classification [270]) were compared with transmural tumours (T3–T4). With both adenocarcinoma and squamous cell carcinoma, metastases can occur in nodes well away from the primary tumour in the absence of regional lymph node involvement, so-called 'jumping' metastases [118,269].

Another phenomenon, which is well documented at this site and considered to be a potentially important pathway of tumour spread [271], is intramural metastasis. It has been defined as a metastatic lesion that is clearly separated from the primary tumour and invades the oesophageal or gastric wall but is not surrounded by endothelium. There is a high frequency of concurrent lymph node metastases in patients with intramural metastasis, lending support to the theory that the latter arises by intramural lymphatic spread and the establishment of secondary intramural tumour deposits. Most of the reported cases have emanated from the Far East [265,272,273].

Visceral metastases by the bloodstream occur most commonly to liver, lungs and adrenal glands. They are found in approximately 70% of all cases and would probably be more frequent were the expectation of life after diagnosis not so short [144,274–276]. Using chest or abdominal computed tomography in newly diagnosed cases of oesophageal carcinoma, distant metastases were most commonly diagnosed in abdominal lymph nodes (45%), followed by liver (35%), lung (20%), cervical/supraclavicular lymph nodes (18%), bone (9%), adrenals (5%), peritoneum (2%), brain (2%), and stomach, pancreas, pleura, skin/body wall, pericardium and spleen (each 1%) [277]. Patients with squamous cell carcinomas showed a higher rate of tumour spread to cervical/supraclavicular lymph nodes and there was a greater tendency for adenocarcinoma to spread to the liver. This probably reflected tumour location rather than histological cell type, since lower oesophageal adenocarcinomas metastasize more frequently to the liver than mid-oesophageal adenocarcinomas. Micrometastases have been detected in rib marrow by immunohistochemistry in a large proportion of patients undergoing potentially curative surgical resection of oesophageal or oesophagogastric junctional malignancy. The rate of detection was independent of histological type (squamous vs. adenocarcinoma) or of the presence or absence of nodal metastasis. Metastatic cells were viable and tumorigenic, and appeared to be resistant to neoadjuvant therapy [278]. Immunohistochemical examination of lymph nodes for cytokeratins has been used to refine the staging of oesophageal cancer and help identify patients who will not be cured by surgery alone [279], but there is as yet insufficient evidence of benefit to recommend its use routinely.

Prognosis

The prognosis of advanced carcinoma of the oesophagus of all types is poor. A review in 1980 of published results showed that of 100 patients presenting with malignant dysphagia, 39 will have a resectable tumour, 26 leave hospital, and only 4 patients will be alive at 5 years [280]. This is related to the fact that symptomatic patients present late in the course of the disease, when tumour has spread through the muscular oesophagus to involve adventitial tissue and regional lymph nodes. Because of this, local tumour recurrence is common following surgical resection [281]. Other complicating factors in patients with squamous carcinoma result from the frequent comorbidity consequent on tobacco and alcohol abuse. Surgical outcomes have improved more recently with an increased rate of curative resection, decrease in postoperative deaths, and a better 5-year survival [282].

The effects of chemotherapy and/or radiation, with or without surgery, have been the subject of numerous investigations. A clear survival advantage has been shown in randomized studies for patients treated with chemoradiotherapy when compared with those treated with radiation therapy alone [283]. In one study in patients with squamous cell carcinoma, there was no overall survival advantage of preoperative chemoradiotherapy followed by surgery compared with surgery alone, but a prolonged disease-free survival and survival free of local disease was demonstrated [284]. In another large multicentre randomized study, no survival advantage was present when surgery alone was compared with pre- and postoperative chemotherapy and surgery in patients with either squamous cell or adenocarcinoma [285]. Chemotherapy, with or without radiotherapy, can result in complete tumour regression and quantitative techniques may be useful in assessing their effects [286,287].

Meticulous examination by the pathologist of resection specimens is essential in providing diagnostic and prognostic information for the individual patient and also to enable the proper assessment of different forms of management in clinical trials so that their efficacy can be evaluated. The most important prognostic indicator, and often the only independent one on multivariate analysis, is the depth of invasion of the tumour through the wall of the oesophagus [288–291], and this is assessed using the TNM staging system [270] (Table 8.1). In terms of tumour spread, however, this does not differentiate between tumours confined to the mucosa and those involving the submucosa which, particularly with squamous cell carcinomas, has been shown to be of considerable prognostic significance (see section on 'Superficial oesophageal cancer' above). Another significant and independent indicator of prognosis, and in several studies the most significant, relates to the presence or absence of lymph node metastasis [289–292]. In addition, the number of nodes involved has frequently been found to be significant. More than four or five positive nodes, or a ratio of involved to resected nodes of more than 50%, have each been associated with a very poor prognosis [293–295]. Several studies have also shown that vascular (venous/lymphatic) invasion and the status of resection margins are important prognostic factors on univariate analysis [289,291,292,296]. With the latter, this has been most evident with proximal margin involvement increasing the likelihood of tumour recurrence [264,291,292], because of the risk of discontinuous foci of carcinoma in the proximal oesophagus [154]. As well as the proximal and distal margins the importance of circumferential margin involvement in oesophageal cancer has recently been appreciated [297,298]. The presence of tumour cells within 1 mm of the circumferential margin was found to be a significant and independent predictor of survival following potentially curative oesophageal resection in one study. Median survival in the group with circumferential margin involvement was 21 months, compared with 39 months in those where there was no such involvement. The survival advantage of those with clear circumferential margins was related to the extent of lymph node involvement, being confined to those patients with less than 25% nodes containing metastatic tumour [298].

Other potential markers of prognosis such as histological grade, lymphocytic reaction, pattern at the margin of the tumour (pushing or infiltrating), ploidy, angiogenesis, amount of tumour receptor for epidermal growth factor, and intramural metastasis have been investigated but do not appear to have independent prognostic significance. There is now general agreement for the use of standardized pathology proformas as a means of ensuring consistent incorporation of essential pathological data in the reporting of cancer resection specimens [299–301].

Table 8.1 TNM staging of oesophageal carcinoma [268].

T—Primary tumour	
pT1	Tumour invades lamina propria or submucosa
pT2	Tumour invades muscularis propria
pT3	Tumour invades adventitia
pT4	Tumour invades adjacent structures
N—Regional lymph nodes	
pN0	No regional lymph node metastasis
pN1	Regional lymph node metastasis present
*M—Distant metastasis**	
M0	No distant metastasis
M1	Distant metastasis present

*Pathological staging cannot usually comment on the presence or absence of distant metastasis, unless biopsies of distant organs have been submitted for histological examination.

Secondary tumours

Epithelial neoplasms

Secondary tumours in the oesophagus are rare; they may be the result of direct spread from adjacent organs, or of spread by the lymphatics or by the bloodstream. Direct spread occurs most commonly from carcinoma of the stomach into the lower end of the oesophagus, less commonly from the bronchus or thyroid [302–304]. Lymphatic spread has been described from carcinoma of the breast [302,303,305,306], and bloodstream metastasis from primary tumours in the testis [303], prostate [307,308], kidney [309], endometrium [310] and pancreas [302]. Examples of metastasis to the oesophagus from primary meso- and hypopharyngeal tumours are more probably examples of multiple primary tumours. Secondary deposits can cause obstruction and may mimic a primary tumour.

Leukaemias and lymphomas

Leukaemias of all types, particularly acute myelogenous and lymphoblastic forms, commonly involve the gastrointestinal tract, with gut involvement in almost half of all patients with leukaemia at postmortem [311]. This is either directly by tumour cells, or by the various complications of the disease, namely immunodeficiency, coagulation disorders and drug toxicity. In their mildest form in the oesophagus they present as subepithelial haemorrhages, which may induce secondary epithelial erosion. Infiltration of leukaemic cells occurs in the submucosa either as microscopic deposits or as macroscopic nodules which undergo necrosis and ulceration [312]. These lesions are often complicated by secondary fungal infections, especially *Candida*, particularly when irradiation or antimitotic drugs have been used. Secondary bacterial infection with formation of a pseudomembrane of debris, fibrin and bacteria also occurs. Chronic graft-versus-host disease not infrequently results in a desquamative oesophagitis in patients following allogeneic bone marrow transplantation [313].

Lymphomatous involvement of the oesophagus is mostly a secondary manifestation in the course of generalized disease. It occurs rarely in Hodgkin's disease, either by compression or due to infiltration from affected mediastinal lymph nodes [314], and dysphagia can be the presenting symptom [315,316]. It can also occur with non-Hodgkin's lymphomas. A few cases of primary Hodgkin's [316,317] and non-Hodgkin's malignant lymphoma of the oesophagus of both B-cell and T-cell phenotype have also been reported [318–321]. Some have occurred in patients with the acquired immunodeficiency syndrome [322–324]. Apparent primary extramedullary plasmacytomas of the oesophagus have also been described [325,326]. Rare cases of focal lymphoid hyperplasia [327,328] and of lymphomatoid granulomatosis in patients with HIV infection involving the oesophagus have also been reported [329].

Non-epithelial tumours

Smooth muscle tumours

Leiomyoma is the most common benign tumour of the oesophagus [330]. Unlike other segments of the gastrointestinal tract, a large majority of mesenchymal tumours at this site show smooth muscle differentiation. Leiomyomas are more common in males (1.9 : 1) and are seen in the lower more often than the upper part. Tumours are single or multiple. Careful autopsy studies have identified tiny, subclincal lesions, mostly close to the oesophagogastric junction, in almost 8% of individuals [331]. In surgical series, approximately half the cases have been asymptomatic, with symptoms of dysphagia or pain being present in the remainder. They originate either from the muscularis mucosae or muscularis propria, usually the latter, and present either as a polypoid mass projecting into the lumen or as a lobulated, intramural tumour, occasionally with crater-like ulceration of the mucosal surface [332]; flat, intramural growths are uncommon and usually undifferentiated. Occasionally, the mass is mainly extra-oesophageal in position. The cut surface is greyish-white and flecks of calcium or more general calcification may be seen.

Although most smooth muscle tumours of the oesophagus are benign and many are discovered incidentally, the distinction between leiomyoma and leiomyosarcoma histologically can be difficult, if not impossible, in some cases. The best guides to malignancy are the degree of cellularity and an excessive number of mitotic figures. It has to be said, however, that it is likely that most of the relatively small number of sarcomas of the oesophagus reported in the literature probably represent polypoid spindle cell carcinoma (carcinosarcoma—*see* above). The advent of new immunohistochemical markers such as CD34 and c-kit (CD117) is of help in the differential diagnosis of these tumours [333,334]. Benign smooth muscle tumours must be distinguished from the rare condition of diffuse leiomyomatosis (see p. 74).

Gastrointestinal stromal tumours (GISTs)

These tumours are uncommon in the oesophagus, unlike elsewhere in the gastrointestinal tract, although a series of 17 cases has recently been published [335]. All were situated in the lower third of the oesophagus and most presented with dysphagia. Their histological features mirrored those of GISTs arising in the stomach and intestines, with both spindle and epithelioid patterns. While consistently CD34 and c-kit (CD117) positive, a minority also stained for desmin or alpha smooth muscle actin. Nine tumours were fatal, including all that measured more than 10 cm and one smaller tumour with five mitoses per 50 high-power fields.

Other mesenchymal tumours

A whole range of benign and malignant connective tissue tumours of the oesophagus have been reported. Benign lesions include lipomas [336], rhabdomyomas [337], haemangiomas [338], lymphangiomas [339,340], glomus tumours [341], chondromas and osteochondromas [342]. Some of these are hamartomas, rather than true neoplasms [343].

Primary sarcomas of the oesophagus that have been reported include synovial sarcoma [344,345], malignant fibrous histiocytoma [346], rhabdomyosarcomas in childhood [347] and in adults [348], Kaposi's sarcoma in patients with immunodeficiency [349,350], liposarcoma [351], malignant mesenchymoma [352] and osteosarcoma [353]. Before such a diagnosis is made, it is important to sample a tumour extensively to exclude the possibility of sarcomatous differentiation in a spindle cell carcinoma (see p. 65).

Other oesophageal mesenchymal tumours recently reported include a benign schwannoma [354] and several autonomic nerve tumours [355–357], the latter being fairly large tumours in the upper oesophagus associated histologically with a cuff of lymphoid tissue and scattered inflammatory cells intermingled with the tumour. They have to be differentiated from inflammatory pseudotumours, a few examples of which have been reported in the oesophagus [358,359].

Granular cell tumours

Over 100 examples of this tumour have been reported in the oesophagus [360], the commonest site in the gastrointestinal tract for this uncommon lesion [361]. Most have been submucosal or subepithelial with the epithelium often showing some degree of pseudoepitheliomatous hyperplasia [362]. Most are found incidentally during upper gastrointestinal endoscopy, where they appear as sessile, yellow or yellow-white, firm nodules. Dysphagia, bleeding or abdominal discomfort have been present in symptomatic cases. There is controversy relating to the histogenesis of this lesion. An immunohistological and ultrastructural study has supported an origin from a perineural cell [363].

Tumour-like lesions

A number of different types of lesion may give rise to appearances which mimic an oesophageal tumour. Some have been considered elsewhere—namely cysts (see p. 26), heterotopias (p. 28) and inflammatory polyps as a result of reflux oesophagitis (p. 59). Here, consideration will be given to fibrovascular polyps, glycogenic acanthosis and diffuse leiomyomatosis. Other rare lesions, which have been the subject of case reports, include amyloid [364] and focal myositis [365].

Fibrous (fibrovascular) polyps

These rare and interesting lesions of unknown aetiology can reach an enormous size [366,367]. The majority are attached by a pedicle to the cricopharyngeal area and cases are reported of regurgitation of these polypoid masses into the mouth. They consist of fibrous tissue, which may be myxomatous, in which there are thin-walled blood vessels. A varying amount of adipose tissue is present and this can be the predominant component. Inflammation is usually insignificant except where ulceration of the overlying epithelium has occurred. Even when large they may be missed on endoscopic examination because their surface is similar to normal oesophageal mucosa [368]. They have to be differentiated from inflammatory fibroid polyps (inflammatory pseudotumours) [359,360].

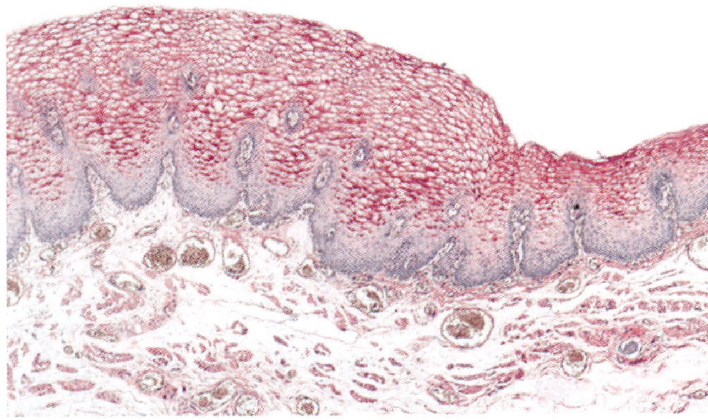

Fig. 8.16 Glycogenic acanthosis. There is focal hyperplasia of squamous epithelium with hypertrophic squamous cells containing abundant glycogen. Adjacent uninvolved oesophageal epithelium to right. PAS stain.

Glycogenic acanthosis

This term has been used to describe plaque-like rather than polypoidal areas which occur particularly in the lower oesophagus and usually on the longitudinal folds. They are discrete, white, round or oval, smooth-surfaced lesions, mostly under 5 mm maximum dimension, which have been observed in up to 15% of upper endoscopies [369,370]. At postmortem, they are almost invariable in the adult oesophagus [371]. Histologically, there is hyperplasia of the squamous epithelium with elongation of the papillae and hypertrophy of cells particularly in the superficial layers. These contain abundant glycogen, best demonstrated in alcohol-fixed biopsies (Fig. 8.16). There is no cellular atypia, keratosis or excess parakeratosis and usually no associated inflammation. Although these lesions have no relationship to malignancy, their pathogenesis and natural history is not known. One case with diffuse involvement of the oesophagus has been described in a patient with Cowden's disease [372].

Diffuse leiomyomatosis

This occurs mainly in adolescents and young adults as a marked, diffuse thickening of the oesophageal wall, with or without nodularity, and extending distally in some cases to involve the proximal stomach [373,374]. Histologically, there is diffuse hypertrophy of smooth muscle, often with a whorled pattern and a considerable amount of intermingled fibrous tissue. Neural and vascular elements may also be prominent and an infiltrate of lymphocytes and plasma cells is common. In a significant proportion of the reported cases oesophageal leiomyomatosis has been familial and associated with an Alport-type nephropathy [375–378]. Other associations have included uterine and vulvar leiomyomas, tracheobronchial leiomyomatosis, pyloric stenosis, small bowel involvement and visceral malignancies occurring at a relatively young age. Oesophageal leiomyomatosis has been separated by some authors from diffuse or giant muscular hypertrophy of the oesophagus, where nodularity is not a feature, but the finding of both patterns in the same patient, or in different members in familial examples, suggests that they represent differing manifestations of the same condition [379].

References

1 Parnell SAC, Peppercorn MA, Antonioli DA, Cohen MA, Joffe N. Squamous cell papilloma of the esophagus. Report of a case after peptic esophagitis and repeated bougienage with review of the literature. *Gastroenterology*, 1978; 74: 910.

2 Lesec G, Gogusev J, Fermaud H, Gorce D, Lemaitre J-P, Verdier A. Presence d'un antigène viral de groupe 'Papilloma' dans un condylome oesophagien chez l'homme. *Gastroenterol Clin Biol*, 1985; 9: 166.

3 Winkler B, Capo V, Reumann W *et al*. Human papillomavirus infection of the esophagus. A clinico-pathologic study with demonstration of papillomavirus antigen by the immunoperoxidase technique. *Cancer*, 1985; 55: 149.

4 Odze R, Antonioli D, Shocket D, Noble-Topham S, Goldman H, Upton M. Esophageal squamous papillomas. A clinicopathologic study of 38 lesions and analysis for human papillomavirus by the polymerase chain reaction. *Am J Surg Pathol*, 1993; 17: 803.

5 Carr NJ, Bratthauer GL, Lichy JH, Taubenberger JK, Monihan JM, Sobin LH. Squamous cell papillomas of the esophagus: a study of 23 lesions for human papillomavirus by in situ hybridization and the polymerase chain reaction. *Hum Pathol*, 1994; 25: 536.

6 Staples DC, Knodell RG, Johnson LF. Inflammatory pseudotumor of the esophagus. A complication of gastroesophageal reflux. *Gastrointest Endosc*, 1978; 24: 175.

7 Rabin MS, Bremner CG, Botha JR. The reflux gastroesophageal polyp. *Am J Gastroenterol*, 1980; 73: 451.

8 McDonald GB, Brand DL, Thorning DR. Multiple adenomatous neoplasms arising in columnar-lined (Barrett's) esophagus. *Gastroenterology*, 1977; 72: 1317.

9 Lee RG. Adenomas arising in Barrett's esophagus. *Am J Clin Pathol*, 1986; 85: 629.

10 Banducci D, Rees R, Bluett MK *et al*. Pleomorphic adenoma of the cervical esophagus: a rare tumor. *Ann Thorac Surg*, 1987; 44: 653.

11 Rouse RV, Soetikno RM, Baker RJ *et al*. Esophageal submucosal gland duct adenoma. *Am J Surg Pathol*, 1995; 19: 1191.

12 Su J-M, Hsu H-K, Hsu P-I, Wang C-Y, Chang H-C. Sialadenoma papilliferum of the esophagus. *Am J Gastroenterol*, 1998; 93: 461.

13 Parkin DM, Laara E, Muir CS. Estimates of the world-wide frequency of sixteen major cancers in 1980. *Int J Cancer*, 1988; 41: 184.

14 Day NE. The geographic pathology of cancer of the oesophagus. *Br Med Bull*, 1984; 40: 329.

15 Young JR Jr, Percy CL, Asire AJ. Surveillance, epidemiology, and end results: incidence and mortality data 1973–77. *Monogr Natl Cancer Inst*, 1981; 57: 140.

16 Blot WJ, Devesa SS, Kneller RW, Fraumeni JF Jr. Rising incidence of adenocarcinoma of the esophagus and gastric cardia. *JAMA*, 1991; 265: 1287.

17 Blot WJ, Devesa SS, Fraumeni JF Jr. Continuing climb in rates of esophageal adenocarcinoma: an update (letter). *JAMA*, 1993; 270: 1320.

18 Parkin DM, Pisani P, Ferlay J. Estimates of the world-wide incidence of eighteen major cancers in 1985. *Int J Cancer*, 1993; 54: 594.

19 Coordinating group for research on the aetiology of oesophageal cancer of north China. The epidemiology of oesophageal cancer in north China and preliminary results in the investigation of its aetiological factors. *Sci Sin*, 1975; 18: 131.

20 Rose E, McGlashan ND. The spatial distribution of oesophageal carcinoma in the Transkei, South Africa. *Br J Cancer*, 1975; 31: 197.

21 Tuyns AJ, Masse LMF. Mortality from cancer of the oesophagus in Brittany. *Int J Epidemiol*, 1973; 2: 242.

22 Jacobs A, Cavill IAJ. Pyridoxine and riboflavin status in the Paterson–Kelly syndrome. *Br J Haematol*, 1968; 14: 153.

23 Wynder EL. Etiological aspects of squamous cancer of the head and neck. *JAMA*, 1971; 215: 452.

24 Cook-Mozaffari P. The epidemiology and pathology of cancer of the oesophagus. In: Wright R, ed. *Recent Advances in Gastro-Intestinal Pathology*. London: W.B. Saunders, 1980: 267.

25 Lui BQ, Li B. Epidemiology of carcinoma of the esophagus in China. In: Huang GJ, K'ai WY, eds. *Carcinoma of the Esophagus and Gastric Cardia*. New York: Springer-Verlag, 1984: 77.

26 Wynder EL, Bross IJ. A study of etiological factors in cancers of the esophagus. *Cancer*, 1961; 14: 389.

27 Tuyns AJ, Pequignot G, Abbatucci JS. Le cancer de l'oesophage en Ile-et-Vilaine en fonction des niveaux de consommation d'alcool et de tabac. Des risques qui se multiplient. *Bull Cancer*, 1977; 64: 45.

28 Martinez I. Factors associated with cancer of the esophagus, mouth and pharynx in Puerto Rico. *J Natl Cancer Inst*, 1969; 42: 1069.

29 Hirayama T. Diet and cancer. *Nutr Cancer*, 1979; 1: 67.

30 Pottern LM, Morris LE, Blot WJ, Ziegler RG, Fraumeni JF. Esophageal cancer among black men in Washington DC. I. Alcohol, tobacco and other risk factors. *J Natl Cancer Inst*, 1981; 67: 777.

31 Chilvers C, Fraser P, Beral V. Alcohol and esophageal cancer: an assessment of the evidence from routinely collected data. *J Epidemiol Community Health*, 1979; 33: 127.

32 Cook P. Cancer of the oesophagus in Africa. *Br J Cancer*, 1971; 25: 853.

33 Paymaster JC, Sanghui LD, Gangadharan P. Cancer of the gastrointestinal tract in Western India: epidemiological study. *Cancer*, 1968; 21: 279.

34 Epstein SS, Payne PM, Shaw HJ. Multiple primary malignant

neoplasms in the air and upper food passages. *Cancer*, 1960; 13: 137.
35 Smithers DW. In: Tanner NC, Smithers DW, eds. *Tumours of the Oesophagus*. Edinburgh: Churchill Livingstone, 1961.
36 Shanta V, Krishnamurthi S. Further study in aetiology of carcinomas of the upper alimentary tract. *Br J Cancer*, 1963; 17: 8.
37 Auerbach O, Stout AP, Hammond EC, Garfinkel L. Histologic changes in esophagus in relation to smoking habits. *Arch Environ Health*, 1965; 11: 4.
38 Jussawalla DJ, Deshpande VA. Evaluation of cancer risk in tobacco chewers and smokers: an epidemiologic assessment. *Cancer*, 1971; 28: 244.
39 Bradshaw E, Schonland M. Smoking, drinking and oesophageal cancer in African males of Johannesburg, South Africa. *Br J Cancer*, 1974; 30: 157.
40 Rose EF. Patterns of occurrence of esophageal cancer with particular reference to the Transkei. In: Silver W, ed. *Carcinoma of the Esophagus*. Cape Town: Balkema, 1977.
41 Hewer T, Rose E, Ghadirian P *et al*. Ingested mutagens from opium and tobacco pyrolysis products and cancer of the oesophagus. *Lancet*, 1978; ii: 494.
42 Iran–IRAC Joint Study Group. Esophageal cancer studies in the Caspian littoral of Iran: results of population studies—a prodrome. *J Natl Cancer Inst*, 1977; 59: 1127.
43 Malaveille C, Friesen M, Camus A-M *et al*. Mutagens produced by the pyrolysis of opium and its alkaloids as possible risk factors in cancer of the bladder and oesophagus. *Carcinogenesis*, 1982; 3: 557.
44 Ghadirian P, Stein GF, Gorodetzky C *et al*. Oesophageal cancer studies in the Caspian littoral of Iran: some residual results, including opium use as a risk factor. *Int J Cancer*, 1985; 35: 593.
45 Friesen M, O'Neill IK, Malaveille C *et al*. Characterization and identification of 6 mutagens in opium pyrolysates implicated in oesophageal cancer in Iran. *Mutat Res*, 1985; 150: 177.
46 Yang CS, Sun Y, Yang Q *et al*. Vitamin A and other deficiencies in Linxian, a high esophageal cancer incidence area in northern China. *J Natl Cancer Inst*, 1984; 73: 1449.
47 Li M, Li P, Li B. Recent progress in research on esophageal cancer in China. *Adv Cancer Res*, 1980; 33: 173.
48 Levison DA, Hopwood D, Morgan RDH, Coghill G, Milne GA, Wormsley KG. Oesophageal neoplasia in male Wistar rats due to parenteral di-(2-hydroxypropyl)-nitrosamine: a combined histopathological, histochemical and electron microscopic study. *J Pathol*, 1979; 129: 31.
49 Stinson SF. Animal model of human disease: esophageal carcinoma. *Am J Pathol*, 1979; 96: 871.
50 Liu BQ, Li B. Epidemiology of carcinoma of the esophagus in China. In: Huang GJ, K'ai WY, eds. *Carcinoma of the Esophagus and Gastric Cardia*. New York: Springer-Verlag, 1984: 77.
51 Xia QJ. Carcinogenesis in the esophagus. In: Huang GJ, K'ai WY, eds. *Carcinoma of the Esophagus and Gastric Cardia*. New York: Springer-Verlag, 1984: 53.
52 Burrel RJW, Roach WA, Schadwell A. Esophageal cancer in the Bantu of the Transkei associated with mineral deficiency in garden plants. *J Natl Cancer Inst*, 1966; 36: 204.
53 Lin HJ, Chan WC, Fong YY *et al*. Zinc levels in serum, hair and tumors from patients with esophageal cancer. *Nutr Rep Internat*, 1977; 15: 635.
54 Cheng KK, Day NE. Nutrition and esophageal cancer. *Cancer Causes Control*, 1996; 7: 33.
55 Vousden KH. Human papillomaviruses and cervical carcinoma. *Cancer Cells*, 1989; 1: 43.
56 Zur Hausen H. Papillomaviruses in anogenital cancer as a model to understand the role of viruses in human cancer. *Cancer Res*, 1989; 49: 4677.
57 Bosch FX, Manos MM, Munoz N. Prevalence of human papillomavirus in cervical cancer: a worldwide perspective. *J Natl Cancer Inst*, 1995; 87: 796.
58 Syrjänen KJ. Histological changes identical to those of condylomatous lesions found in esophageal squamous cell carcinomas. *Arch Geschwulstforsch*, 1982; 52: 283.
59 Chen B, Yin H, Dhurandar N. Detection of human papillomavirus DNA in esophageal squamous cell carcinomas by the polymerase chain reaction using general consensus primers. *Hum Pathol*, 1994; 25: 920.
60 Suzuk L, Noffsinger AE, Hui YZ, Fenoglio-Preiser CM. Detection of human papillomavirus in esophageal squamous cell carcinoma. *Cancer*, 1996; 78: 704.
61 Fidalgo PO, Cravo ML, Chaves PP, Leit'o CN, Mira FC. High prevalence of human papillomavirus in squamous cell carcinoma and matched normal esophageal mucosa. Assessment by polymerase chain reaction. *Cancer*, 1995; 76: 1522.
62 West AB, Soloway GN, Lizarraga G, Tyrrell L, Longley JB. Type 73 human papillomavirus in esophageal squamous cell carcinoma. A novel association. *Cancer*, 1996; 77: 2440.
63 O'Connor DP, Bennett MA, Murphy GM, Leader MB, Kay EW. Do human papillomaviruses cause cancer? *Curr Diag Pathol*, 1996; 3: 123.
64 Howley PM. Role of the human papillomaviruses in human cancer. *Cancer Res*, 1991; 51: 5019.
65 Chang F, Syrjänen S, Wang L, Syrjänen K. Infectious agents in the etiology of esophageal cancer. *Gastroenterology*, 1992; 103: 1336.
66 de Jong UW, Breslow N, Goh Ewe Hong J, Sridharan M, Sharmuguratnam K. Aetiological factors on esophageal cancer in Singapore Chinese. *Int J Cancer*, 1974; 13: 291.
67 Segi M. Tea-gruel as a possible factor for cancer of the esophagus. *Gann*, 1975; 66: 199.
68 Ghadirian P. Thermal irritation and esophageal cancer in northern Iran. *Cancer*, 1987; 60: 1909.
69 Rose EF. The effects of soil and diet on disease. *Cancer Res*, 1968; 28: 2390.
70 O'Neill CH, Clarke G, Hodges GM *et al*. Silica fragments from millet bran in mucosa surrounding oesophageal tumours in patients in northern China. *Lancet*, 1982; i: 1202.
71 Kiviranta UK. Corrosion carcinoma of the oesophagus: 381 cases of corrosion and 9 cases of corrosion carcinoma. *Acta Otolaryngol*, 1953; 42: 89.
72 Appelqvist P, Salmo M. Lye corrosion carcinoma of the esophagus. A review of 63 cases. *Cancer*, 1980; 45: 2655.
73 Csikos M, Horvath O, Petri A, Petri I, Imre J. Late malignant transformation of chronic corrosive esophageal strictures. *Langenbecks Arch Chir*, 1985; 365: 231.
74 Benedict EB. Carcinoma of the esophagus developing in benign stricture. *N Engl J Med*, 1941; 224: 408.
75 Chudecki B. Radiation cancer of the thoracic oesophagus. *Br J Radiol*, 1972; 45: 303.

76 Fekete F, Mosnier H, Belghiti J *et al*. Esophageal cancer after mediastinal irradiation. *Dysphagia*, 1994; 9: 289.

77 Mosbech J, Videbaek A. On the etiology of esophageal carcinoma. *J Natl Cancer Inst*, 1955; 15: 1665.

78 Nasipov SN. Esophageal cancer morbidity as evidenced by the genealogy of patients registered in the Gur'ev province. *Vopr Onkol*, 1977; 23: 81.

79 Ghadirian P. Familial history of esophageal cancer. *Cancer*, 1985; 56: 2112.

80 Howel-Evans W, McConnell RB, Clarke CA, Sheppard PM. Carcinoma of the oesophagus with keratosis palmaris et plantaris (tylosis). A study of two families. *Q J Med*, 1958; 27: 413.

81 Ashworth MT, Nash JGR, Ellis A, Day DW. Abnormalities of differentiation and maturation in the oesophageal squamous epithelium of patients with tylosis: morphological features. *Histopathology*, 1991; 19: 303.

82 Marger RS, Marger D. Carcinoma of the esophagus and tylosis. A lethal genetic combination. *Cancer*, 1993; 72: 17.

83 Kelsell DP, Risk JM, Leigh IM *et al*. Close mapping of the focal non-epidermolytic palmoplantar keratoderma (PPK) locus associated with oesophageal cancer (TOC). *Hum Mol Genet*, 1996; 5: 857.

84 Iwaya T, Maesawa C, Ogasawara S, Tamura G. Tylosis esophageal cancer locus on chromosome 17q25.1 is commonly deleted in sporadic human esophageal cancer. *Gastroenterology*, 1998; 114: 1206.

85 Stemmermann G, Heffelfinger SC, Noffsinger A *et al*. The molecular biology of esophageal and gastric cancer and their precursors: oncogenes, tumor suppressor genes, growth factors. *Hum Pathol*, 1995; 25: 968.

86 Tahara E, ed. *Molecular Pathology of Gastroenterological Cancer*. Tokyo: Springer, 1997.

87 Pierce WS, MacVaugh H III, Johnson J. Carcinoma of the esophagus arising in patients with achalasia of the cardia. *J Thorac Cardiovasc Surg*, 1970; 59: 335.

88 Shin MS. Primary carcinoma arising in the epiphrenic esophageal diverticulum. *South Med J*, 1971; 64: 1022.

89 Saldana JG, Cone RO, Hopens TA. Carcinoma arising in an epiphrenic esophageal diverticulum. *Gastrointest Radiol*, 1982; 7: 15.

90 Wynder EL, Hultberg S, Jacobsson F, Bross IJ. Environmental factors in cancer of upper alimentary tract: Swedish study with special reference to Plummer–Vinson (Paterson–Kelly) syndrome. *Cancer*, 1957; 10: 470.

91 Holmes GKT, Stokes PL, Sorahan TM, Prior P, Waterhouse JAH, Cooke WT. Coeliac disease, gluten-free diet, and malignancy. *Gut*, 1976; 17: 612.

92 Cooper BT, Holmes GKT, Ferguson R, Cooke WT. Celiac disease and malignancy. *Medicine*, 1980; 59: 249.

93 Tapia RH, White VA. Squamous cell carcinoma arising in a duplication cyst of the esophagus. *Am J Gastroenterol*, 1985; 80: 325.

94 Shibuya H, Wakita T, Nakagawa T, Fukuda H, Yasumoto M. The relation between an esophageal cancer and associated cancers in adjacent organs. *Cancer*, 1995; 76: 101.

95 Funkhouser EM, Sharp GB. Aspirin and reduced risk of esophageal carcinoma. *Cancer*, 1995; 76: 1116.

96 Munoz N, Crespi M, Grassi A, Qing WG, Qiong S, Cai LZ. Precursor lesions of oesophageal cancer in high-risk populations in Iran and China. *Lancet*, 1982; i: 876.

97 Munoz N, Lipkin M, Crespi M, Wahrendorf J, Grassi A, Shih-Hsien L. Proliferative abnormalities of the esophageal epithelium of Chinese populations at high and low risk for esophageal cancer. *Int J Cancer*, 1985; 36: 187.

98 Dawsey SM, Lewin KJ, Liu F-S, Wang G-Q, Shen Q. Esophageal morphology from Linxian, China. Squamous histologic findings in 754 patients. *Cancer*, 1994; 73: 2027.

99 Coordinating Group for Research on Etiology of Esophageal Cancer in North China. The epidemiology and etiology of esophageal cancer in north China. *Chinese Med J*, 1975; 1: 167.

100 Dawsey SM, Lewin KJ, Wang G-Q *et al*. Squamous esophageal histology and subsequent risk of squamous cell carcinoma of the esophagus. A prospective follow-up study from Linxian, China. *Cancer*, 1994; 74: 1686.

101 Dawsey SM, Wang G-Q, Weinstein WM *et al*. Squamous dysplasia and early esophageal cancer in the Linxian region of China: distinctive endoscopic lesions. *Gastroenterology*, 1993; 105: 1333.

102 Coordinating Groups for the Research of Esophageal Carcinoma. Honan Province and Chinese Academy of Medical Sciences. Studies on relationship between epithelial dysplasia and carcinoma of the esophagus. *Chinese Med J*, 1975; 1: 110.

103 Hille JJ, Markowitz S, Margolius KA, Isaacson C. Human papillomavirus and carcinoma of the esophagus. *N Engl J Med*, 1985; 312: 1707.

104 Ismail-Beigi F, Horton PF, Pope CE. Histological consequences of gastroesophageal reflux in man. *Gastroenterology*, 1979; 58: 163.

105 Ushigome S, Spjut HJ, Noon GP. Extensive dysplasia and carcinoma *in situ* of esophageal epithelium. *Cancer*, 1967; 20: 1023.

106 Mandard AM, Marnay J, Gignoux M *et al*. Cancer of the esophagus and associated lesions: detailed pathologic study of 100 esophagectomy specimens. *Hum Pathol*, 1984; 15: 660.

107 Kuwano H, Morita M, Matsuda H *et al*. Histopathologic findings of minute foci of squamous cell carcinoma in the human esophagus. *Cancer*, 1991; 68: 2617.

108 Nagamatsu M, Mori M, Kuwano H *et al*. Serial histologic investigation of squamous epithelial dysplasia associated with carcinoma of the esophagus. *Cancer*, 1992; 69: 1094.

109 Morita M, Kuwano H, Yasuda M *et al*. The multicentric occurrence of squamous epithelial dysplasia and squamous cell carcinoma in the esophagus. *Cancer*, 1994; 74: 2889.

110 Kuwano H, Matsuda H, Matsuoka H, Kai H, Okudaira Y, Sugimachi K. Intra-epithelial carcinoma concomitant with esophageal squamous cell carcinoma. *Cancer*, 1987; 59: 783.

111 Adamson RH, Krolikowski FJ, Correa P. Carcinogenicity of 1-methyl-1-nitrosourea in nonhuman primates. *J Natl Cancer Inst*, 1977; 59: 415.

112 Rubio CA. Epithelial lesions antedating oesophageal carcinoma. I. Histologic study in mice. *Pathol Res Pract*, 1983; 176: 269.

113 Chinese authors. Pathology of early esophageal squamous cell carcinoma. *Chinese Med J*, 1977; 3: 180.

114 Kato H, Tachimori Y, Watanabe H *et al*. Superficial esophageal carcinoma. Surgical treatment and the results. *Cancer*, 1990; 66: 2319.

115 Yoshinaka H, Shimazu H, Fukumoto T, Baba M. Superficial esophageal carcinoma: a clinicopathological review of 59 cases. *Am J Gastroenterol*, 1991; 86: 1413.

116 Barge J, Molas G, Maillard JN *et al*. Superficial oesophageal carcinoma: an oesophageal counterpart of early gastric cancer. *Histopathology*, 1981; 5: 499.

117 Bogomoletz WV, Molas G, Gayet B, Potet F. Superficial squamous cell carcinoma of the esophagus. A report of 76 cases and review of the literature. *Am J Surg Pathol*, 1989; 13: 535.

118 Hölscher AH, Bollschweiler E, Schneider PM, Siewert JR. Prognosis of early esophageal cancer. Comparison between adeno- and squamous cell carcinoma. *Cancer*, 1995; 76: 178.

119 Schmidt LW, Dean PJ, Wilson RT. Superficially invasive squamous cell carcinoma of the esophagus. A study of seven cases in Memphis, Tennessee. *Gastroenterology*, 1986; 91: 1456.

120 Watanabe H, Tada T, Iwafuchi M *et al*. New definition and macroscopic characteristics of early carcinoma of the esophagus. *Stomach Intestine*, 1990; 25: 1075.

121 Goseki N, Koike M, Yoshida M. Histopathologic characteristics of early stage esophageal cancer. A comparative study with gastric carcinoma. *Cancer*, 1992; 69: 1088.

122 Kitamura K, Ikebe M, Morita M, Matsuda H, Kuwano H, Sugimachi K. The evaluation of submucosal carcinoma of the esophagus as a more advanced carcinoma. *Hepatogastroenterology*, 1993; 40: 236.

123 Kumagai Y, Makuuchi H, Mitomi T, Ohmori T. A new classification system for early carcinomas of the esophagus. *Dig Endosc*, 1993; 5: 139.

124 Sugimachi K, Ohno S, Matsuda H, Mori M, Kuwano H. Lugol-combined endoscopic detection of minute malignant lesions of the thoracic esophagus. *Ann Surg*, 1988; 208: 179.

125 Tsutsui S, Kuwano H, Yasuda M. *et al*. Extensive spreading carcinoma of the esophagus with invasion restricted to the submucosa. *Am J Gastroenterol*, 1995; 90: 1858.

126 Aouad K, Aubertin J-M, Bouillot J-L, Paraf F, Alexandre JH. Extensive spread of squamous cell carcinoma in situ of the esophagus: an unusual case. *Am J Gastroenterol*, 1996; 91: 2421.

127 Chu P, Stagias J, West AB, Traube M. Diffuse pagetoid squamous cell carcinoma in situ of the esophagus. A case report. *Cancer*, 1997; 79: 1865.

128 Yoshikane H, Tsukamoto Y, Niwa Y *et al*. Superficial esophageal carcinoma: evaluation by endoscopic ultrasonography. *Am J Gastroenterol*, 1994; 89: 702.

129 Sibille A, Lambert R, Souquet J-C, Sabben G, Descos F. Long-term survival after photodynamic therapy for esophageal cancer. *Gastroenterology*, 1995; 108: 337.

130 Kitamura K, Kuwano H, Yasuda M *et al*. What is the earliest malignant lesion in the esophagus? *Cancer*, 1996; 77: 1614.

131 De Baecque C, Potet F, Molas G, Flejou JF, Barbier P, Martignon C. Superficial adenocarcinoma of the oesophagus in Barrett's mucosa with dysplasia: a clinico-pathological study of 12 patients. *Histopathology*, 1990; 16: 213.

132 Liu FS. Pathology of the esophageal cancer. *Cancer Res Prev Treat*, 1976; 3: 74.

133 Meyerowitz BR, Shea LT. The natural history of squamous verrucose carcinoma of the esophagus. *J Thorac Cardiovasc Surg*, 1971; 61: 646.

134 Minielly JA, Harrison EG Jr, Fontana RS, Payne WS. Verrucous squamous cell carcinoma of the esophagus. *Cancer*, 1967; 20: 2078.

135 Parkinson AT, Haidak GL, McInerney RP. Verrucous squamous cell carcinoma of the esophagus following lye stricture. *Chest*, 1970; 57: 489.

136 Agha FP, Weatherbee L, Sams JS. Verrucous carcinoma of the esophagus. *Am J Gastroenterol*, 1984; 79: 844.

137 Soga J, Tanaka O, Sasaki K, Kawaguchi M, Muto T. Superficial spreading carcinoma of the esophagus. *Cancer*, 1982; 50: 1641.

138 Gauthier-Villars P, Dontzoff A. Anatomie macroscopique de cancer de l'oesophage (étude de pièces chirurgicales). *Presse Med*, 1947; 55: 609.

139 Shamma'a MH, Benedict EB. Esophageal webs. A report of 58 cases and an attempt at classification. *N Engl J Med*, 1958; 259: 378.

140 Entwhistle CC, Jacobs A. Histological findings in the Paterson–Kelly syndrome. *J Clin Pathol*, 1965; 18: 408.

141 Kuwano H, Ohno S, Matsuda H, Mori M, Sugimachi K. Serial histologic evaluation of multiple primary squamous cell carcinomas of the esophagus. *Cancer*, 1988; 61: 1635.

142 Pesko P, Rakic S, Milicevic M, Bulajic P, Gerzic Z. Prevalence and clinicopathologic features of multiple squamous cell carcinoma of the esophagus. *Cancer*, 1994; 73: 2687.

143 Goodner JT, Watson WL. Cancer of the esophagus: its association with other primary cancers. *Cancer*, 1956; 9: 1248.

144 Mandard AM, Chasle J, Marnay J *et al*. Autopsy findings in 111 cases of esophageal cancer. *Cancer*, 1981; 48: 329.

145 Shiozaki H, Tahara H, Kobayashi K *et al*. Endoscopic screening of early esophageal cancer with the Lugol dye method in patients with head and neck cancers. *Cancer*, 1990; 66: 2068.

146 Morita M, Kuwano H, Ohno S *et al*. Multiple recurrence of carcinoma in the upper aerodigestive tract associated with esophageal cancer. Reference to smoking, drinking and family history. *Int J Cancer*, 1994; 58: 207.

147 Kuwano H, Ueo H, Sugimachi K *et al*. Glandular or mucus-secreting components in squamous cell carcinoma of the esophagus. *Cancer*, 1985; 56: 514.

148 Takubo K, Sasajima K, Yamashita K *et al*. Morphological heterogeneity of esophageal carcinoma. *Acta Pathol Jpn*, 1989; 39: 180.

149 Newman J, Antonakopoulos GN, Darnton SJ, Matthews HR. The ultrastructure of oesophageal carcinomas: multidirectional differentiation. A transmission electron microscopic study of 43 cases. *J Pathol*, 1992; 167: 193.

150 Isaacson P. Biopsy appearances easily mistaken for malignancy in gastrointestinal endoscopy. *Histopathology*, 1982; 6: 377.

151 Burgess HM, Baggenstoss AH, Moersch HJ, Clagett OT. Cancer of the esophagus: a clinicopathologic study. *Surg Clin N Am*, 1951; 31: 965.

152 Scanlon EF, Morton DR, Walker JM, Watson WL. The case against segmental resection for esophageal carcinoma. *Surg Gynecol Obstet*, 1955; 101: 290.

153 Appelqvist P. Carcinoma of the oesophagus and gastric cardia. A retrospective study based on statistical and clinical material from Finland. *Acta Chir Scand Suppl*, 1972; 430: 1.

154 Tsutsui S, Kuwano H, Watanabe M *et al*. Resection margin for squamous-cell carcinoma of the esophagus. *Ann Surg*, 1995; 222: 193.

155 Keighley MRB, Moore J, Lee JR, Malins D, Thompson H. Preoperative frozen section and cytology to assess proximal invasion in gastro-oesophageal carcinoma. *Br J Surg*, 1981; 68: 73.

156 Kraus TK, Perez-Mesa C. Verrucous carcinoma: clinical and pathologic study of 105 cases involving oral cavity, larynx and genitalia. *Cancer*, 1966; 19: 26.
157 Prioleau PG, Santa Cruz DJ, Meyer JS, Bauer WC. Verrucous carcinoma. A light and electron microscopic, autoradiographic, and immunfluorescence study. *Cancer*, 1980; 45: 2849.
158 Jasim KA, Bateson MC. Verrucous carcinoma of the oesophagus—a diagnostic problem. *Histopathology*, 1990; 17: 473.
159 Kavin H, Yaremko L, Valaitis J, Chowdhury L. Chronic esophagitis evolving to verrucous squamous cell carcinoma: possible role of exogenous chemical carcinogens. *Gastroenterology*, 1996; 110: 904.
160 Biemond P, ten Kate FJ, van Blankenstein M. Esophageal verrucous carcinoma: histologically a low-grade malignancy but a fatal disease. *J Clin Gastroenterol*, 1991; 13: 102.
161 du Boulay CEH, Isaacson P. Carcinoma of the oesophagus with spindle cell features. *Histopathology*, 1981; 5: 403.
162 Talbert JL, Cantrell JR. Clinical and pathologic characteristics of carcinosarcoma of the esophagus. *J Thorac Cardiovasc Surg*, 1963; 45: 1.
163 Robertson NJ, Rahamim J, Smith MEF. Carcinosarcoma of the oesophagus showing neuroendocrine, squamous and glandular differentiation. *Histopathology*, 1997; 31: 263.
164 Guarino M, Reale D, Micoli G, Forloni B. Carcinosarcoma of the oesophagus with rhabdomyoblastic differentiation. *Histopathology*, 1993; 22: 493.
165 Osamura RY, Watanabe K, Shimamura K *et al.* Polypoid carcinoma of the esophagus. A unifying term for 'carcinosarcoma' and 'pseudosarcoma'. *Am J Surg Pathol*, 1978; 2: 201.
166 Battifora H. Spindle cell carcinoma. Ultrastructural evidence of squamous origin and collagen production by the tumor cells. *Cancer*, 1976; 37: 2275.
167 Kuhajda FP, Sun T-T, Mendelsohn G. Polypoid squamous carcinoma of the esophagus: a case report with immunostaining for keratin. *Am J Surg Pathol*, 1983; 7: 495.
168 Gal AA, Martin SE, Kernen JA, Patterson MJ. Esophageal carcinoma with prominent spindle cells. *Cancer*, 1987; 60: 2244.
169 Linder J, Stein RB, Roggli VL *et al.* Polypoid tumor of the esophagus. *Hum Pathol*, 1987; 18: 692.
170 Kimura N, Tezuka F, Ono I *et al.* Myogenic expression in esophageal polypoid tumors. *Arch Pathol Lab Med*, 1989; 113: 1159.
171 Thompson L, Chang B, Barsky SH. Monoclonal origins of malignant mixed tumors (carcinosarcomas). Evidence for a divergent histogenesis. *Am J Surg Pathol*, 1996; 20: 277.
172 Iwaya T, Maesawa C, Tamura G *et al.* Esophageal carcinosarcoma: a genetic analysis. *Gastroenterology*, 1997; 113: 973.
173 Abe K, Sasano H, Itakura Y, Nishihira T, Mori S, Nagura H. Basaloid-squamous carcinoma of the esophagus. A clinicopathologic, DNA ploidy, and immunohistochemical study of seven cases. *Am J Surg Pathol*, 1996; 20: 453.
174 Sarbia M, Verreet P, Bittinger F. *et al.* Basaloid squamous cell carcinoma of the esophagus. Diagnosis and prognosis. *Cancer*, 1997; 79: 1871.
175 Wain SL, Kier R, Vollmer RT, Bossen EH. Basaloid-squamous carcinoma of the tongue, hypopharynx and larynx. *Hum Pathol*, 1986; 17: 1158.
176 Tsang WYW, Chan JKC, Lee KC, Leung AKF, Fu YT. Basaloid-squamous carcinoma of the upper aerodigestive tract and so-called adenoid cystic carcinoma of the esophagus: the same tumour type? *Histopathology*, 1991; 19: 35.
177 Hellquist HB, Dahl F, Karlsson MG, Nilsson C. Basaloid squamous cell carcinoma of the palate. *Histopathology*, 1994; 25: 178.
178 Kabuto T, Taniguchi K, Iwanaga T *et al.* Primary adenoid cystic carcinoma of the esophagus: report of a case. *Cancer*, 1979; 43: 2452.
179 Bell-Thomson J, Haggitt RC, Ellis FH. Mucoepidermoid and adenoid cystic carcinoma of the esophagus. *J Thorac Cardiovasc Surg*, 1980; 79: 438.
180 Morson BC, Belcher JR. Adenocarcinoma of the oesophagus and ectopic gastric mucosa. *Br J Cancer*, 1952; 6: 127.
181 Devesa SS, Blot WJ, Fraumeni JF Jr. Changing patterns in the incidence of esophageal and gastric carcinoma in the United States. *Cancer*, 1998; 83: 2049.
182 Powell J, McConkey CC. The rising trend in oesophageal adenocarcinoma and gastric cardia. *Eur J Cancer Prev*, 1992; 1: 265.
183 Tuyns AJ. Oesophageal cancer in France and Switzerland: recent time trends. *Eur J Cancer Prev*, 1992; 1: 275.
184 McKinney PA, Sharp L, MacFarlane GJ, Muir CS. Oesophageal and gastric cancer in Scotland 1960–90. *Br J Cancer*, 1995; 71: 411.
185 Armstrong RW, Borman B. Trends in incidence rates of adenocarcinoma of the oesophagus and gastric cardia in New Zealand 1978–92. *Int J Epidemiol*, 1996; 25: 941.
186 Thomas RJ, Lade S, Giles GG, Thursfield V. Incidence trends in oesophageal and proximal gastric carcinoma in Victoria. *Aust N Z J Surg*, 1996; 66: 271.
187 Hansen S, Wiig JN, Giercksky KE, Tretli S. Esophageal and gastric carcinoma in Norway 1958–92: incidence time trend variability according to morphological subtypes and organ subsites. *Int J Cancer*, 1997; 71: 340.
188 Bytzer P, Christensen PB, Damkier P, Vinding K, Seersholm N. Adenocarcinoma of the esophagus and Barrett's esophagus: a population-based study. *Am J Gastroenterol*, 1999; 94: 86.
189 Hamilton SR, Smith RRL, Cameron JL. Prevalence and characteristics of Barrett esophagus in patients with adenocarcinoma of the esophagus or esophagogastric junction. *Hum Pathol*, 1988; 19: 942.
190 Clark GWB, Smyrk TC, Burdiles P *et al.* Is Barrett's metaplasia the source of adenocarcinoma of the cardia? *Arch Surg*, 1994; 129: 609.
191 Cameron AJ, Lomboy CT, Pera M, Carpenter HA. Adenocarcinoma of the esophagogastric junction and Barrett's esophagus. *Gastroenterology*, 1995; 109: 1541.
192 Schnell TG, Sontag SJ, Chejfec G. Adenocarcinomas arising in tongues or short segments of Barrett's esophagus. *Dig Dis Sci*, 1992; 37: 137.
193 Kabat GC, Ng SKC, Wynder EL. Tobacco, alcohol intake, and diet in relation to adenocarcinoma of the esophagus and gastric cardia. *Cancer Causes Control*, 1993; 4: 123.
194 Brown LM, Silverman DT, Pottern LM *et al.* Adenocarcinoma of the esophagus and esophagogastric junction in white men in the United States: alcohol, tobacco, and socioeconomic factors. *Cancer Causes Control*, 1994; 5: 333.
195 Gammon MD, Schoenberg JB, Ahsan H *et al.* Tobacco, alcohol, and socioeconomic status and adenocarcinomas of the esophagus and gastric cardia. *J Natl Cancer Inst*, 1997; 89: 1277.

196 Brown LM, Swanson CA, Gridley G. Adenocarcinoma of the esophagus: role of obesity and diet. *J Natl Cancer Inst*, 1995; 87: 104.
197 Chow WH, Blot WJ, Vaughan TL *et al*. Body mass index and risk of adenocarcinomas of the esophagus and gastric cardia. *J Natl Cancer Inst*, 1998; 90: 150.
198 Romero Y, Locke GR. Is there a GERD gene? (editorial). *Am J Gastroenterol*, 1999; 94: 1127.
199 Stemmerman G, Heffelfinger SC, Noffsinger A, Hui YZ, Miller MA, Fenoglio-Preiser CM. The molecular biology of esophageal and gastric cancer and their precursors: oncogenes, tumor suppressor genes, and growth factors. *Hum Pathol*, 1994; 25: 968.
200 Montesano R, Hollstein M, Hainaut P. Genetic alterations in esophageal cancer and their relevance to etiology and pathogenesis: a review. *Int J Cancer (Pred Oncol)*, 1996; 69: 225.
201 Gallez JF, Berger F, Moulinier B, Partensky C. Esophageal adenocarcinoma following Heller myotomy for achalasia. *Endoscopy*, 1987; 19: 76.
202 Goodman P, Scott LD, Verani RR *et al*. Esophageal adenocarcinoma in a patient with surgically treated achalasia. *Dig Dis Sci*, 1990; 35: 1549.
203 McKinley M, Sherlock P. Barrett's esophagus with adenocarcinoma in scleroderma. *Am J Gastroenterol*, 1984; 79: 438.
204 Katzka DA, Reynolds JC, Saul SH *et al*. Barrett's metaplasia and adenocarcinoma of the esophagus in scleroderma. *Am J Med*, 1987; 82: 46.
205 Symonds DA, Ramsey HE. Adenocarcinoma arising in Barrett's esophagus with Zollinger–Ellison syndrome. *Am J Clin Pathol*, 1980; 73: 823.
206 Achkar J-P, Post AB, Achkar E, Carey WD. Risk of extraesophageal malignancy in patients with adenocarcinoma arising in Barrett's esophagus. *Am J Gastroenterol*, 1995; 90: 39.
207 Logan RFA, Skelly MM. Barrett's oesophagus and colorectal neoplasia: scope for screening? (commentary). *Gut*, 1999; 44: 775.
208 Thompson JJ, Zinsser KR, Enterline HT. Barrett's metaplasia in adenocarcinoma of the esophagus and gastroesophageal junction. *Hum Pathol*, 1983; 14: 42.
209 Smith RRL, Hamilton SR, Boitnott JK, Rogers EL. The spectrum of carcinoma arising in Barrett's epithelium: a clinicopathologic study of 26 patients. *Am J Surg Pathol*, 1984; 8: 563.
210 Chejfec G, Jablokow VR, Gould VE. Linitis plastica carcinoma of the esophagus. *Cancer*, 1981; 51: 2139.
211 Witt TR, Bains MS, Zaman MB, Martini N. Adenocarcinoma in Barrett's esophagus. *J Thorac Cardiovasc Surg*, 1983; 85: 337.
212 Hamilton SR, Smith RRL. The relationship between columnar epithelial dysplasia and invasive adenocarcinoma arising in Barrett's esophagus. *Am J Clin Pathol*, 1987; 87: 301.
213 Lauren P. The two histological main types of gastric carcinoma: diffuse and so-called intestinal-type carcinoma. An attempt at a histoclinical classification. *Acta Pathol Microbiol Scand*, 1965; 64: 31.
214 Griffin M, Sweeney EC. The relationship of endocrine cells, dysplasia and carcinoembryonic antigen in Barrett's mucosa to adenocarcinoma of the oesophagus. *Histopathology*, 1987; 11: 53.
215 Banner BF, Memoli VA, Warren WH, Gould VE. Carcinoma with multi-directional differentiation arising in Barrett's esophagus. *Ultrastruct Pathol*, 1983; 4: 205.
216 Bosch A, Frias Z, Caldwell WL. Adenocarcinoma of the esophagus. *Cancer*, 1979; 43: 1557.
217 Pascal RR, Clearfield HR. Mucoepidermoid (adenosquamous) carcinoma arising in Barrett's esophagus. *Dig Dis Sci*, 1987; 32: 428.
218 Cary NR, Barron DJ, McGoldrick JP *et al*. Combined oesophageal adenocarcinoma and carcinoid in Barrett's oesophagitis: potential role of enterochromaffin-like cells in oesophageal malignancy. *Thorax*, 1993; 48: 404.
219 Resano CH, Cabrera N, Gonzalez-Cueto D *et al*. Double early epidermoid carcinoma of the esophagus in columnar epithelium. *Endoscopy*, 1985; 17: 73.
220 Paraf F, Fléjou J-F, Potet F *et al*. Esophageal squamous carcinoma in five patients with Barrett's esophagus. *Am J Gastroenterol*, 1992; 87: 746.
221 Potet F, Fléjou J-F, Gervaz H *et al*. Adenocarcinoma of the lower esophagus and esophagogastric junction. *Semin Diagn Pathol*, 1991; 8: 126.
222 Christensen WN, Sternberg SS. Adenocarcinoma of the upper esophagus arising in ectopic gastric mucosa; two case reports and review of the literature. *Am J Surg Pathol*, 1987; 11: 397.
223 Ishii K, Ota H, Nakayama J *et al*. Adenocarcinoma of the cervical oesophagus arising from ectopic gastric mucosa. The histochemical determination of its origin. *Virchows Arch A Pathol Anat*, 1991; 419: 159.
224 Azzopardi JG, Menzies T. Primary oesophageal adenocarcinoma. Confirmation of its existence by the finding of mucous gland tumours. *Br J Surg*, 1962; 49: 497.
225 Benisch B, Toker C. Esophageal carcinomas with adenoid cystic differentiation. *Arch Otolaryngol*, 1972; 96: 260.
226 Woodard BH, Shelburne JD, Vollmer RT *et al*. Mucoepidermoid carcinoma of the esophagus: a case report. *Hum Pathol*, 1978; 9: 352.
227 Sweeney EC, Cooney T. Adenoid cystic carcinoma of the esophagus. A light and electron microscopic study. *Cancer*, 1980; 45: 1516.
228 Epstein JI, Sears DL, Tucker RS *et al*. Carcinoma of the esophagus with adenoid cystic differentiation. *Cancer*, 1984; 53: 1131.
229 Kuwano H, Sadanaga N, Watanabe M, Yasuda M, Nozoe T, Sugimachi K. Oesophageal cancer composed of mixed histological types. *Eur J Surg Oncol*, 1996; 22: 225.
230 Bombi JA, Riverola A, Bordas JM *et al*. Adenosquamous carcinoma of the esophagus. A case report. *Pathol Res Pract*, 1991; 187: 514.
231 McKeown F. Oat-cell carcinoma of the esophagus. *J Pathol Bacteriol*, 1952; 64: 889.
232 Casas F, Ferrer F, Farrús B, Casals J, Biete A. Primary small cell carcinoma of the esophagus. A review of the literature with emphasis on therapy and prognosis. *Cancer*, 1997; 80: 1366.
233 Briggs JC, Ibrahim NBN. Oat cell carcinoma of the oesophagus: a clinico-pathological study of 23 cases. *Histopathology*, 1983; 7: 261.
234 Law SY-K, Fok M, Lam K-Y, Loke S-L, Ma L-T, Wong J. Small cell carcinoma of the esophagus. *Cancer*, 1994; 73: 2894.
235 Mori M, Matsukuma A, Adachi Y *et al*. Small cell carcinoma of the esophagus. *Cancer*, 1989; 63: 564.
236 Delpre G, Kadish U, Glanz I, Avidor I. Endoscopic biopsy diagnosis of oat cell carcinoma of the lung penetrating the esophagus. *Gastrointest Endosc*, 1980; 26: 104.
237 Tateishi R, Taniguchi K, Horai T *et al*. Argyrophil cell carcinoma

(apudoma) of the esophagus. A histopathologic entity. *Virchows Arch Pathol Anat*, 1976; 371: 283.

238 Watson KJR, Shulkes A, Smallwood RA *et al*. Watery diarrhoea–hypokalemia–achlorydria syndrome and carcinoma of the esophagus. *Gastroenterology*, 1985; 88: 798.

239 Ho K-J, Herrera GA, Jones JM, Alexander CB. Small cell carcinoma of the esophagus: evidence for a unified histogenesis. *Hum Pathol*, 1984; 15: 460.

240 Tateishi R, Taniguchi H, Wada A *et al*. Argyrophil cells and melanocytes in esophageal mucosa. *Arch Pathol*, 1974; 98: 87.

241 Nichols GL, Kelsen DP. Small cell carcinoma of the esophagus: the Memorial Hospital experience 1970–87. *Cancer*, 1989; 54: 1531.

242 Hussein AM, Feun LG, Sridhar KS, Benedetto P, Waldman S, Otrakji CL. Combination chemotherapy and radiotherapy for small-cell carcinoma of the esophagus. A case report of long-term survival and review of the literature. *Am J Clin Oncol*, 1990; 13: 369.

243 McCullen M, Vyas SK, Winwood PJ, Loehry CA, Parham DM, Hamblin T. Long-term survival associated with metastatic small cell carcinoma of the esophagus treated by chemotherapy, autologous bone marrow transplantation, and adjuvant radiation therapy. *Cancer*, 1994; 73: 1.

244 Rosenthal SN, Lemkin JA. Multiple small cell carcinomas of the esophagus. *Cancer*, 1983; 51: 1944.

245 Partensky C, Chayvialle JA, Berger F, Souquet J-C, Moulinier B. Five-year survival after transhiatal resection of esophageal carcinoid tumor with a lymph node metastasis. *Cancer*, 1993; 72: 2320.

246 Lindberg GM, Molberg KH, Vuitch MF, Albores-Saavedra J. Atypical carcinoid of the esophagus. A case report and review of the literature. *Cancer*, 1997; 79: 1476.

247 Sasano N, Abe S, Satake O. Choriocarcinoma mimickry of an esophageal carcinoma with urinary gonadotropic activities. *Tohoku J Exp Med*, 1970; 100: 153.

248 McKechnie JC, Fechner RE. Choriocarcinoma and adenocarcinoma of the esophagus with gonadotropin secretion. *Cancer*, 1971; 27: 694.

249 Trillo A, Accettullo LM, Yeiter TL. Choriocarcinoma of the esophagus. Histologic and cytologic findings. A case report. *Acta Cytol*, 1979; 23: 69.

250 Kikuchi Y, Tsuneta Y, Kawai T *et al*. Choriocarcinoma of the esophagus producing chorionic gonadotropin. *Acta Pathol Jpn*, 1988; 38: 489.

251 Wasan HS, Schofield JB, Krausz T, Sikora K, Waxman J. Combined choriocarcinoma and yolk sac tumor arising in Barrett's esophagus. *Cancer*, 1994; 73: 514.

252 De La Pava S, Nigogosyan G, Pickren JW, Cabreras A. Melanosis of the esophagus. *Cancer*, 1963; 16: 48.

253 Ohashi K, Kato Y, Kanno J, Kasuga T. Melanocytes and melanosis of the oesophagus in Japanese subjects: analysis of factors effecting their increase. *Virchows Arch Pathol Anat*, 1990; 417: 137.

254 Raven RW, Dawson I. Malignant melanoma of the oesophagus. *Br J Surg*, 1964; 51: 551.

255 Sakornpant P, Barlow D, Bevan CM. Two cases of primary malignant melanoma of the oesophagus. *Br J Surg*, 1964; 51: 386.

256 Piccone VA, Klopstock R, Leveen HH, Sika J. Primary malignant melanoma of the esophagus associated with melanosis of the entire esophagus. First case report. *J Thorac Cardiovasc Surg*, 1970; 59: 864.

257 Muto M, Saito Y, Koike T. *et al*. Primary malignant melanoma of the esophagus with diffuse pigmentation resembling superficial spreading melanoma. *Am J Gastroenterol*, 1997; 92: 1936.

258 Musher DR, Lindner AE. Primary melanoma of the esophagus. *Dig Dis Sci*, 1974; 19: 855.

259 Gown AM, Vogel AM, Hoak D *et al*. Monoclonal antibodies specific for melanocytic tumors distinguish subpopulations of melanocytes. *Am J Pathol*, 1986; 123: 195.

260 Butler ML, Vantheertum RL, Teplick SK. Metastatic malignant melanoma of the esophagus; a case report. *Gastroenterology*, 1975; 69: 1334.

261 Takubo K, Takai A, Takayama S, Sasajima K, Yamashita K, Fujita K. Intraductal spread of esophageal squamous cell carcinoma. *Cancer*, 1987; 59: 1751.

262 Yates DR, Koss LG. Paget's disease of the esophageal epithelium. *Arch Pathol*, 1968; 86: 447.

263 Norihisa Y, Kakudo K, Tsutsumi Y, Makuuchi H, Sugihara T, Mitomi T. Paget's extension of esophageal carcinoma: immunohistochemical and mucin histochemical evidence of Paget's cells in the esophageal mucosa. *Acta Pathol Jpn*, 1988; 38: 651.

264 Gall CA, Rieger NA, Wattchow DA. Positive proximal resection margins after resection for carcinoma of the esophagus and stomach—effect on survival and symptom recurrence. *Aust N Z J Surg*, 1996; 66: 734.

265 Lam KY, Ma LT, Wong J. Measurement of extent of spread of oesophageal squamous carcinoma by serial sectioning. *J Clin Pathol*, 1996; 49: 124.

266 Steiner PE. The etiology and histogenesis of carcinoma of the esophagus. *Cancer*, 1956; 9: 436.

267 Akiyama H, Tsurumaru M, Kawamura T, Ono Y. Principles of surgical treatment of carcinoma of the esophagus. Analysis of lymph node involvement. *Ann Surg*, 1981; 194: 438.

268 Sannohe Y, Hiratsuka R, Doki K. Lymph node metastases in cancer of the thoracic esophagus. *Am J Surg*, 1981; 141: 216.

269 Nishimaki T, Tanaka O, Suzuki T, Aizawa K, Hatakeyama K, Muto T. Patterns of lymphatic spread in thoracic esophageal cancer. *Cancer*, 1994; 74: 4.

270 Sobin L, Wittekind Ch, eds. *TNM Classification of Malignant Tumors*, 5th edn. New York: Wiley-Liss, 1997.

271 Watson WL. Carcinoma of the esophagus. *Surg Gynecol Obstet*, 1933; 56: 884.

272 Takubo K, Sasajima K, Yamashita K, Tanaka Y, Fujita K. Prognostic significance of intramural metastasis in patients with esophageal carcinoma. *Cancer*, 1990; 65: 1816.

273 Kato H, Tachimori Y, Watanabe H *et al*. Intramural metastasis of thoracic esophageal carcinoma. *Int J Cancer*, 1992; 50: 49.

274 Bosch A, Frias Z, Caldwell WL, Jaeschke WH. Autopsy findings in carcinoma of the esophagus. *Acta Radiol Oncol*, 1979; 18: 103.

275 Anderson LL, Lad TE. Autopsy findings in squamous-cell carcinoma. *Cancer*, 1982; 50: 1587.

276 Chan KW, Chan EYT, Chan CW. Carcinoma of the esophagus: an autopsy study of 231 cases. *Pathology*, 1986; 18: 400.

277 Quint LE, Hepburn LM, Francis IR, Whyte RI, Orringer MB. Incidence and distribution of distant metastases from newly diagnosed esophageal carcinoma. *Cancer*, 1995; 76: 1120.

278 O'Sullivan GC, Sheehan D, Clarke A *et al*. Micrometastases in

esophagogastric cancer: high detection rate in resected rib segments. *Gastroenterology*, 1999; 116: 543.
279 Izbicki JR, Hosch SB, Pichlmeier U *et al*. Prognostic value of immunohistochemically identifiable tumor cells in lymph nodes of patients with completely resected esophageal cancer. *N Engl J Med*, 1997; 337: 1188.
280 Earlam R, Cunha-Melo JR. Oesophageal squamous cell carcinoma: I. A critical review of surgery. *Br J Surg*, 1980; 67: 381.
281 Law SY, Fok M, Wong J. Pattern of recurrence after oesophageal resection for cancer: clinical implications. *Br J Surg*, 1996; 83: 107.
282 Muller JM, Erasmi H, Stelzner M, Zieren U, Pichlmaier H. Surgical therapy of oesophageal carcinoma. *Br J Surg*, 1990; 77: 845.
283 Herskovic A, Martz K, Al-Sarraf M *et al*. Combined chemotherapy and radiotherapy compared with radiotherapy alone in patients with cancer of the esophagus. *N Engl J Med*, 1992; 326: 1593.
284 Bosset J-F, Gignoux M, Triboulet J-P. Chemoradiotherapy followed by surgery compared with surgery alone in squamous-cell cancer of the esophagus. *N Engl J Med*, 1997; 337: 161.
285 Kelsen DP, Ginsberg R, Pajak TF. Chemotherapy followed by surgery compared with surgery alone for localized esophageal cancer. *N Engl J Med*, 1998; 339: 1979.
286 Darnton SJ, Allen SM, Edwards CW, Matthews HR. Histopathological findings in oesophageal carcinoma with and without preoperative chemotherapy. *J Clin Pathol*, 1993; 46: 51.
287 Mandard A-M, Dalibard F, Mandard J-C *et al*. Pathologic assessment of tumor regression after preoperative chemoradiotherapy of esophageal carcinoma. Clinicopathologic correlations. *Cancer*, 1994; 73: 2680.
288 Patil P, Redkar A, Patel SG *et al*. Prognosis of operable squamous-cell carcinoma of the esophagus. Relationship with clinicopathological features and DNA-ploidy. *Cancer*, 1993; 72: 20.
289 Ide H, Nakamura T, Hayashi K *et al*. Esophageal squamous cell carcinoma: pathology and prognosis. *World J Surg*, 1994; 18: 321.
290 Lieberman MD, Shriver CD, Bleckner S *et al*. Carcinoma of the esophagus. Prognostic significance of the histologic type. *J Thorac Cardiovasc Surg*, 1995; 109: 130.
291 Paraf F, Flejou JF, Pignon JP *et al*. Surgical pathology of adenocarcinoma arising in Barrett's esophagus. Analysis of 67 cases. *Am J Surg Pathol*, 1995; 19: 183.
292 Robey-Cafferty SS, El-Naggar AK, Sahin AA, Bruner JM, Ro JY, Cleary KR. Prognostic factors in esophageal squamous carcinoma. A study of histologic features, blood group expression, and DNA ploidy. *Am J Clin Pathol*, 1991; 95: 844.
293 Kelin S, Rugang Z, Dawei Z, Goujon H, Liangjun W. Prognostic significance of lymph node metastasis in surgical resection of oesophageal cancer. *Chinese Med J*, 1996; 109: 82.
294 Kawahara K, Maekawa K, Okabayashi K *et al*. The number of lymph node metastases influences survival in esophageal cancer. *J Surg Oncol*, 1998; 67: 160.
295 Korst RJ, Rusch VW, Venkatraman E *et al*. Proposed revision of the staging classification for esophageal cancer. *J Thorac Cardiovasc Surg*, 1998; 115: 660.
296 Theunissen P, Borchard F, Poortvliet DCJ. Histopathological evaluation of oesophageal carcinoma. The significance of venous invasion. *Br J Surg*, 1991; 78: 930.
297 Sagar PM, Johnston D, McMahon MJ, Dixon MF, Quirke P. Significance of circumferential resection margin involvement after oesophagectomy for cancer. *Br J Surg*, 1993; 80: 1386.
298 Dexter SPL, Sue-Ling H, McMahon MJ, Quirke P, Mapstone N, Martin IG. Circumferential resection margin involvement: an independent predictor of survival following surgery for oesophageal cancer. *Gut*, 2001; 48: 667.
299 Mapstone N. *Minimum Dataset for Oesophageal Carcinoma Histopathology Reports*. London: The Royal College of Pathologists, 1998.
300 Burroughs SH, Biffin AHB, Pye JK, Williams GT. Oesophageal and gastric cancer pathology reporting: a regional audit. *J Clin Pathol*, 1999; 52: 435.
301 Ibrahim NBN. Guidelines for handling oesophageal biopsies and resection specimens and their reporting. *J Clin Pathol*, 2000; 53: 89.
302 Toreson WE. Secondary carcinoma of the esophagus as a cause of dysphagia. *Arch Pathol*, 1944; 38: 82.
303 Gowing NFC. In: Tanner NC, Smithers DW, eds. *Tumours of the Oesophagus*. Edinburgh: Churchill Livingstone, 1961.
304 Hale RJ, Merchant W, Hasleton PS. Polypoidal intra-oesophageal thyroid carcinoma: a rare cause of dysphagia. *Histopathology*, 1990; 17: 475.
305 Polk HC Jr, Camp FA, Walker AW. Dysphagia and oesophageal stenosis: manifestations of metastatic mammary cancer. *Cancer*, 1967; 20: 2002.
306 Varanasi RV, Saltzman JR, Krims P, Crimaldi A, Colby J. Breast carcinoma metastatic to the esophagus: clinicopathological and management features of four cases, and literature review. *Am J Gastroenterol*, 1995; 90: 1495.
307 Gross P, Freedman LJ. Obstructing secondary carcinoma of the esophagus. *Arch Pathol*, 1942; 33: 361.
308 Gore RM, Sparberg M. Metastatic carcinoma of the prostate to the esophagus. *Am J Gastroenterol*, 1982; 77: 358.
309 Nussbaum M, Grossman M. Metastases to the esophagus causing gastrointestinal bleeding. *Am J Gastroenterol*, 1976; 66: 467.
310 Zarian LP, Berliner L, Redmond P. Metastatic endometrial carcinoma to the esophagus. *Am J Gastroenterol*, 1983; 78: 9.
311 Winton RR, Gwynn AM, Robert JC *et al*. Leukemia and the bowel. *Med J Aust*, 1975; 4: 89.
312 Kothur R, Marsh F, Posner G, Dosik H. Endoscopic leukemic polyposis. *Am J Gastroenterol*, 1990; 85: 884.
313 McDonald GB, Shulman HM, Sullivan KM, Spencer GD. Intestinal and hepatic complications of human bone marrow transplantation. Part II. *Gastroenterology*, 1986; 90: 770.
314 Bichel J. Hodgkin's disease of the oesophagus. *Acta Radiol*, 1951; 35: 371.
315 Strauch M, Martin TH, Remmele W. Hodgkin's disease of the oesophagus. *Endoscopy*, 1971; 4: 207.
316 Stein HA, Murray D, Warner HA. Primary Hodgkin's disease of the esophagus. *Dig Dis Sci*, 1981; 26: 457.
317 Loeb DS, Ribeiro A, Menke DM. Hodgkin's disease of the esophagus: report of a case. *Am J Gastroenterol*, 1999; 94: 520.
318 Nagrani M, Lavigne BC, Siskind BN *et al*. Primary non-Hodgkin's lymphoma of the esophagus. *Arch Intern Med*, 1989; 149: 193.
319 Bolondi L, de Giorgio R, Santi V *et al*. Primary non-Hodgkin's T-cell lymphoma of the esophagus: a case with peculiar endoscopic ultrasonographic pattern. *Dig Dis Sci*, 1990; 35: 1426.

320 Mengoli M, Marchi M, Rota E, Bertolotti M, Gollini C, Signorelli S. Primary non-Hodgkin's lymphoma of the esophagus. *Am J Gastroenterol*, 1990; 85: 737.

321 Pearson JM, Borg-Grech A. Primary ki-1 (CD30)-positive, large cell, anaplastic lymphoma of the esophagus. *Cancer*, 1991; 68: 418.

322 Bernal A, del Junco GW. Endoscopic and pathologic features of esophageal lymphoma: a report of four cases in patients with acquired immune deficiency syndrome. *Gastrointest Endosc*, 1986; 32: 96.

323 Chow DC, Sheikh SH, Eickhoff L, Soloway GN, Saul Z. Primary esophageal lymphoma in AIDS presenting as a nonhealing esophageal ulcer. *Am J Gastroenterol*, 1996; 91: 602.

324 Marnejon T, Scoccia V. The coexistence of primary esophageal lymphoma and *Candida glabrata* esophagitis presenting as dysphagia and odynophagia in a patient with acquired immunodeficiency syndrome. *Am J Gastroenterol*, 1997; 92: 354.

325 Morris WT, Pead JL. Myeloma of the oesophagus. *J Clin Pathol*, 1972; 25: 537.

326 Ahmed M, Ramos S, Sika S, Leveen HH, Piccone VA. Primary extramedullary esophageal plasmacytoma. First case report. *Cancer*, 1976; 38: 943.

327 Sheahan DG, West AB. Focal lymphoid hyperplasia (pseudolymphoma) of the esophagus. *Am J Surg Pathol*, 1985; 9: 141.

328 Gervaz E, Potet F, Mahé R, Lemasson G. Focal lymphoid hyperplasia of the oesophagus: report of a case. *Histopathology*, 1992; 21: 187.

329 Lin-Greenberg A, Villacin A, Moussa G. Lymphomatoid granulomatosis presenting as ulcerodestructive gastrointestinal tract lesions in patients with human immunodeficiency virus infection. *Arch Intern Med*, 1990; 150: 2581.

330 Seremetis MC, Lyons WS, De Cuzman VC, Peabody JW Jr. Leiomyomata of the esophagus. Analysis of 838 cases. *Cancer*, 1976; 38: 2166.

331 Takubo K, Nakagawa H, Tsuchiya S, Mitomo Y, Sasajima K, Shirota A. Seedling leiomyoma of the esophagus and esophagogastric junction zone. *Hum Pathol*, 1981; 12: 1006.

332 Barrett NR. Benign smooth muscle tumours of the oesophagus. *Thorax*, 1964; 19: 185.

333 Miettinen M, Virolainen M, Rikala MS. Gastrointestinal stromal tumors. Value of CD34 antigen in their identification from true leiomyomas and schwannomas. *Am J Surg Pathol*, 1995; 19: 207.

334 Sarlomo-Rikala M, Kovatich A, Barusevicius A, Miettinen M. CD117: a sensitive marker for gastrointestinal stromal tumors that is more specific than CD34. *Mod Pathol*, 1998; 11: 728.

335 Miettinen M, Sarlomo-Rikala M, Sobin LH, Lasota J. Esophageal stromal tumors: a clinicopathologic, immunohistochemical, and molecular genetic study of 17 cases with comparison with esophageal leiomyomas and leiomyosarcomas. *Am J Surg Pathol*, 2000; 24: 211.

336 Zschiedrich M, Neuhaus P. Pedunculated giant lipoma of the esophagus. *Am J Gastroenterol*, 1990; 85: 1614.

337 Pai GK, Pai PK, Kamath SM. Adult rhabdomyoma of the esophagus. *J Pediatr Surg*, 1987; 22: 991.

338 Gilbert HW, Weston MJ, Thompson MH. Cavernous haemangioma of the oesophagus. *Br J Surg*, 1990; 77: 106.

339 Castellanos D, Sebastian JJ, Larrad A *et al*. Esophageal lymphangioma: case report and review of the literature. *Surgery*, 1990; 108: 593.

340 Yoshida Y, Okamura T, Ezaki T *et al*. Lymphangioma of the oesophagus: a case report and review of the literature. *Thorax*, 1994; 49: 1267.

341 Lewin KJ, Appelman HD. Tumors of the esophagus and stomach. In: *Atlas of Tumor Pathology*. Washington: Armed Forces Institute of Pathology, Third Series, Fascicle 18, 1996.

342 Mahour GH, Harrison EG Jr. Osteochondroma (tracheobronchial choristoma) of the esophagus. Report of a case. *Cancer*, 1967; 20: 1489.

343 Saitoh Y, Inomata Y, Tadaki N *et al*. Pedunculated intraluminal osteochondromatous hamartoma of the esophagus. *J Otolaryngol*, 1990; 19: 339.

344 Bloch MJ, Iozzo RV, Edmunds LH Jr, Brooks JJ. Polypoid synovial sarcoma of the esophagus. *Gastroenterology*, 1987; 92: 229.

345 Anton-Pacheco J, Cano I, Cuadros J *et al*. Synovial sarcoma of the esophagus. *J Pediatr Surg*, 1996; 31: 1703.

346 Aagaard MT, Kristensen IB, Lund O *et al*. Primary malignant non-epithelial tumours of the thoracic oesophagus and cardia in a 25-year surgical material. *Scand J Gastroenterol*, 1990; 25: 876.

347 Willen R, Lillo-Gil R, Willen H *et al*. Embryonal rhabdomyosarcoma of the oesophagus: case report. *Acta Chir Scand*, 1989; 155: 59.

348 Vartio T, Nickels J, Hockerstedt K, Scheinin TM. Rhabdomyosarcoma of the oesophagus. *Virchows Arch Pathol Anat*, 1980; 386: 357.

349 Friedman SL, Wright TL, Altman DF. Gastrointestinal Kaposi's sarcoma in patients with acquired immunodeficiency syndrome. Endoscopic and autopsy findings. *Gastroenterology*, 1985; 89: 102.

350 Laine L, Amerian J, Rarick M *et al*. The response of symptomatic gastrointestinal Kaposi's sarcoma to chemotherapy: a prospective evaluation using an endoscopic method of disease quantification. *Am J Gastroenterol*, 1990; 85: 959.

351 Mansour KA, Fritz RC, Jacobs DM, Vellios F. Pedunculated liposarcoma of the esophagus: a first case report. *J Thorac Cardiovasc Surg*, 1983; 86: 447.

352 Haratake J, Jimi A, Horie A *et al*. Malignant mesenchymoma of the esophagus. *Acta Pathol Jpn*, 1984; 34: 925.

353 McIntyre M, Webb JN, Browning GCP. Osteosarcoma of the esophagus. *Hum Pathol*, 1982; 13: 680.

354 Prévot S, Bienvenu L, Vaillant JC, de Saint-Maur PP. Benign schwannoma of the digestive tract. A clinicopathologic and immunohistochemical study of five cases, including a case of esophageal tumor. *Am J Surg Pathol*, 1999; 23: 431.

355 Lam K-Y, Law SY-K, Chu K-M, Ma LT. Gastrointestinal autonomic nerve tumor of the esophagus. A clinicopathologic, immunohistochemical, ultrastructural study of a case and review of the literature. *Cancer*, 1996; 78: 1651.

356 Shek TW, Luk IS, Loong F, Ip P, Ma L. Inflammatory cell-rich gastrointestinal autonomic nerve tumor. An expansion of its histologic spectrum. *Am J Surg Pathol*, 1996; 20: 325.

357 Lam KY. Oesophageal mesenchymal tumours: clinicopathological features and absence of Epstein–Barr virus. *J Clin Pathol*, 1999; 52: 758.

358 LiVolsi VA, Perzin KH. Inflammatory pseudotumors (inflammatory fibrous tumors) of the esophagus: a clinicopathology study. *Am J Dig Dis*, 1975; 20: 475.

359 Wolf BC, Khettry U, Leonardi HK, Neptune WB, Bhattacharrya AK, Legg MA. Benign lesions mimicking malignant tumors of the esophagus. *Hum Pathol*, 1988; 19: 148.

360 Coutinho DSS, Soga J, Yoshikawa T *et al*. Granular cell tumors of the esophagus: a report of two cases and review of the literature. *Am J Gastroenterol*, 1985; 80: 758.

361 Johnston J, Helwig EB. Granular cell tumors of the gastrointestinal tract and perianal region. A study of 74 cases. *Dig Dis Sci*, 1981; 26: 807.

362 Gloor F, Clemencon G. Granular cell tumours ('myoblastomas') of the esophagus. *Endoscopy*, 1975; 7: 239.

363 Buley ID, Gatter KC, Kelly PMA, Heryet A, Millard PR. Granular cell tumours revisited. An immunohistological and ultrastructural study. *Histopathology*, 1988; 12: 263.

364 Solanke TF, Olurin EO, Nwakonobi F *et al*. Primary amyloid tumour of the oesophagus treated by colon transplant. *Br J Surg*, 1967; 55: 943.

365 Chiang I-P, Wang J, Tsang Y-M, Hsiao C-H. Focal myositis of esophagus: a distinct inflammatory pseudotumor mimicking esophageal malignancy. *Am J Gastroenterol*, 1997; 92: 174.

366 Patel J, Kieffer RW, Martin M, Avant GR. Giant fibrovascular polyp of the esophagus. *Gastroenterology*, 1984; 87: 953.

367 Penagini R, Ranzi T, Vellio P *et al*. Giant fibrovascular polyp of the oesophagus: report of a case and effects on oesophageal function. *Gut*, 1989; 30: 1624.

368 Burrell M, Toffler R. Fibrovascular polyp of the esophagus. *Dig Dis*, 1973; 18: 714.

369 Bender MD, Allison J, Cuartas F, Montgomery C. Glycogenic acanthosis of the esophagus: a form of benign epithelial hyperplasia. *Gastroenterology*, 1973; 65: 373.

370 Stern Z, Sharon P, Ligumsky M *et al*. Glycogenic acanthosis of the esophagus. A benign but confusing endoscopic lesion. *Am J Gastroenterol*, 1980; 74: 261.

371 Rywlin AM, Ortega R. Glycogenic acanthosis of the esophagus. *Arch Pathol*, 1970; 90: 439.

372 Kay PS, Soetikno RM, Mindelzun R, Young HS. Diffuse esophageal glycogenic acanthosis: an endoscopic marker of Cowden's disease. *Am J Gastroenterol*, 1997; 92: 1038.

373 Fernandez JP, Mascarenhas MJ, Da Costa JC, Correia JP. Diffuse leiomyomatosis of the esophagus. A case report and review of the literature. *Am J Dig Dis*, 1976; 20: 684.

374 Heald J, Moussalli H, Hasleton PS. *Histopathology*, 1986; 10: 755.

375 Guthrie KJ. Idiopathic muscular hypertrophy of esophagus, pylorus, duodenum and jejunum in a young girl. *Arch Dis Child*, 1945; 20: 176.

376 Cochat P, Guiband P, Torres R, Roussel B, Guarner V, Larbre F. Diffuse leiomyomatosis in Alport syndrome. *J Pediatr*, 1988; 113: 339.

377 Legius E, Proesmans W, van Damme B, Geboes K, Lerut T, Eggermont E. Muscular hypertrophy of the oesophagus and 'Alport-like' glomerular lesions in a boy. *Eur J Pediatr*, 1990; 149: 623.

378 Bloch P, Quijada J. Diffuse leiomyomatosis of the oesophagus. Analysis of a case and review of the literature. *Gastroenterol Clin Biol*, 1992; 16: 890.

379 Lonsdale RN, Roberts PF, Vaughan R, Thiru S. Familial oesophageal leiomyomatosis and nephropathy. *Histopathology*, 1992; 20: 127.

9 Miscellaneous conditions of the oesophagus

Trauma

Rupture and perforation

The oesophagus is relatively well protected by surrounding structures in the neck, and traumatic lesions virtually always arise from intraluminal causes. An exception is penetrating injuries from gunshot and knife wounds [1]. Most perforations are iatrogenic following intubation, dilatation or attempted extraction of foreign bodies [2–4]. Others are due to swallowed sharp foreign bodies especially bones, the impaction of foreign bodies with subsequent fistula formation, and the ulceration and inflammation that follow the swallowing of corrosive fluids [5,6]. Perforation of the oesophagus has a higher mortality than that of other sites in the gastrointestinal tract [7].

Rupture of the oesophagus can follow indirect trauma or be spontaneous (Boerhaave syndrome), often with associated haematoma [8]. It is rare and occurs as an abrupt longitudinal rent, nearly always in the left lateral wall at the lower end of a previously normal oesophagus [9]. It is much more common in males and probably results from a sudden rise in intraoesophageal pressure due to sudden compression or contraction of the stomach following a blow to the abdomen or overdistension with vomiting. A common complication is emphysema at the base of the neck.

Mallory–Weiss syndrome

Less traumatic procedures including vomiting, severe retching and even, apparently, snoring [10] can produce linear partial oesophageal tears, usually just above the cardia on the right lateral wall. The tear may extend to involve the lesser curve of the stomach in the presence of a hiatal hernia [8,11]. These usually involve mainly the mucosa and submucosa and can be associated with severe haemorrhage; they may progress to ulceration with the risk of subsequent perforation. They have been described following upper endoscopy, particularly in association with hiatus hernia [12], and account for 5–10% of all acute upper gastrointestinal bleeds [13]. They are rare, but described, in children [14]. Although most cases pursue a benign course, the bleeding may be significant and recurrent and require therapeutic endoscopy [15,16] and surgery.

Oesophageal casts

Very rarely the complete squamous lining of the oesophagus can be vomited as a cast. This can follow the ingestion of extremely hot liquids or be spontaneous [17], and can be associated with intramural rupture [18] and Mallory–Weiss syndrome [19]. Despite its apparent severity, healing with mucosal regeneration is the rule.

Varices

The normal venous drainage of the oesophagus has four components [20]. Small intraepithelial venules drain into a rich superficial submucosal venous plexus running longitudinally; this connects with a deeper plexus of fewer, larger veins, still in the submucosa. From it, perforating veins pass through the muscle coats to reach the serosal plexus. These plexuses link with those of the upper part of the stomach and drain partly into the portal, partly into the systemic venous system, forming, with the haemorrhoidal and periumbilical veins, an important linkage between the systemic and portal systems. In portal hypertension these venous plexuses dilate to form oesophageal varices, consisting of enormously distended venous channels which lie immediately beneath the mucosa and are prone to rupture [20] (Fig. 9.1). There is some evidence that venous stasis and consequent anoxia produce necrosis and ulceration of the overlying epithelium which increases this risk [21]. At autopsy the varices are collapsed and can be

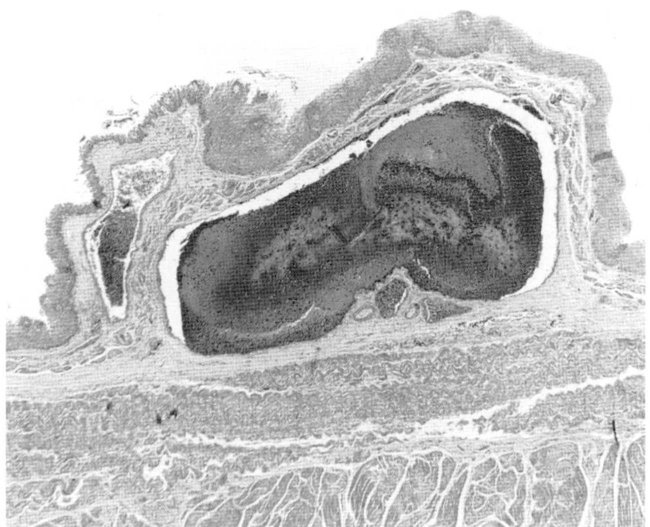

Fig. 9.1 Oesophageal varices in a patient with cirrhosis. The superficial position and liability to rupture are obvious.

difficult to detect, but they can be shown if the oesophagus and stomach are removed together by injection techniques or by everting the oesophagus (see Chapter 3).

The treatment of varices was formerly by portacaval shunt but many patients are now given endoscopic sclerotherapy or, more recently, rubber band ligation [22]. In the former situation, when such patients come to necropsy at varying times after injection, a sequence of events can be determined. Initially there is venous thrombosis, most extensive in the submucosa, less marked in muscle coats and serosa; this is accompanied by extensive superficial and less extensive deep tissue necrosis. Ulceration follows, suggesting that some of the sclerosing fluid has leaked into surrounding tissue. In those patients who survive, a degree of fibrosis and eventual re-epithelialization follows [23,24]. This can lead to stenosis with dysphagia, and there is some evidence that the greater the number of treatments and the amount of sclerosant used the greater the risk of stricture formation [25,26]. An interesting study using rabbits suggests that paravenous injection leads to perivenal fibrosis with severe venous compression and may be more effective than intravenous injection as a form of treatment [27].

An alternative treatment is to excise a full-thickness ring of oesophagus and then to staple the two ends together; this technique provides an excised ring of tissue and allows previously untreated varices to be examined histologically [28]. Such specimens show dilated vascular channels within and immediately beneath the squamous epithelium, some of which rupture into the lumen. These channels do not have a surrounding basement membrane or an endothelial cell lining, but they are probably not artefactual. They may represent a stage in the development of oesophagitis [29,30], but more probably they result from venous congestion [31].

Webs and rings

Oesophageal webs consist of single, or less commonly multiple, thin mucosal membranes that project into the oesophageal lumen. They may arise at all levels but are most frequent in the postcricoid region, where they are usually attached anteriorly and laterally and have an eccentric lumen posteriorly. A significant proportion of upper oesophageal webs have occurred in women with glossitis and iron deficiency anaemia, the Plummer–Vinson syndrome [32]. They are also seen in patients with epidermolysis bullosa, benign mucous membrane pemphigoid and pemphigus vulgaris in which they may be the end-result of scarring [33–35]. Other associations have been with heterotopic gastric mucosa [36] and with chronic graft-versus-host disease following allogeneic bone marrow transplantation [37], and after radiotherapy [38].

Histological appearances show normal squamous epithelium or there may be acanthosis and para- or hyperkeratosis. Marked basal cell hyperplasia and elongation of submucosal papillae in biopsies from all levels of the oesophagus have been described in two patients with multiple oesophageal webs [39]. There is significant association between the presence of oesophageal webs and the development of carcinoma of the buccal mucosa or oesophagus, and in the series reported by Shamma'a and Benedict [32] this occurred in nine of 58 patients.

Two types of 'ring' are found in the oesophagus. Mucosal rings are found at the lower end of the oesophagus and consist of a symmetrical concentric transverse fold of mucosa projecting into, and completely encircling, the lumen [40]. Such rings are not uncommon at autopsy [41] or endoscopy [42]. The majority of patients are asymptomatic but dysphagia may develop with decreasing diameter of the lumen. Histological studies have in general shown that the upper surface of the ring consists of normal squamous epithelium and the lower surface of junctional epithelium. The core of the ring consists of connective tissue, fibres of the muscularis mucosae and blood vessels. A sliding hiatus hernia is a frequent accompaniment.

Muscular rings are found somewhat proximal to mucosal rings and consist of a concentric thickening of the main muscle coat corresponding to the lower oesophageal sphincter and covered on both upper and lower surfaces by squamous epithelium.

Barium sulphate in the oesophagus

Barium sulphate is frequently, and on occasions repeatedly, used in the study of oesophageal stenosis and stricture, and barium is sometimes seen in histological sections [43], either as fine greenish non-refringent granules, often within vessels, or as larger birefringent rhomboid crystals in granulation tissue [44].

References

1 Horwitz B, Krevsky B, Buckman RF Jr, Fisher RS, Dabezies MA. Endoscopic evaluation of penetrating esophageal injuries. *Am J Gastroenterol*, 1993; 88: 1249.

2 Ajalat GM, Mulder DG. Esophageal perforations: the need for an individualised approach. *Arch Surg*, 1984; 119: 1318.

3 Wesdorp ECE, Bartelsman JFWM, Huitbregbe K, Jager FCAH, Tytgat GN. Treatment of instrumental oesophageal perforation. *Gut*, 1984; 25: 398.

4 Panzini L, Burrell MI, Traube M. Instrumental esophageal perforation: chest film findings. *Am J Gastroenterol*, 1994; 89: 367.

5 Rossoff L Sr, White EJ. Perforation of the esophagus. *Am J Surg*, 1974; 128: 207.

6 Michel L, Grills HC, Malt RA. Esophageal perforation. *Ann Thorac Surg*, 1982; 33: 203.

7 Berry BE, Ochsner JL. Perforation of the esophagus: a 30 year review. *J Thorac Cardiovasc Surg*, 1973; 65: 1.

8 Yeoh NTL, McNicholas T, Rothwell-Jackson RL, Goldstraw P. Intramural rupture and intramural haematoma of the oesophagus. *Br J Surg*, 1985; 72: 958.

9 Mackler SA. Spontaneous rupture of the esophagus: an experimental and clinical study. *Surg Gynecol Obstet*, 1952; 95: 345.

10 Merill JR. Snore-induced Mallory–Weiss syndrome. *J Clin Gastroenterol*, 1987; 9: 88.

11 Atkinson M, Bottrill MB, Edwards AT, Mitchell WM, Peet BG, Williams RE. Mucosal tears at the oesophago-gastric junction (the Mallory–Weiss syndrome). *Gut*, 1961; 2: 1.

12 Baker RW, Spiro AH, Trnka YM. Mallory–Weiss tear complicating upper endoscopy: case reports and review of the literature. *Gastroenterology*, 1982; 82: 140.

13 Bharucha AE, Gostout CJ, Balm RK. Clinical and endoscopic risk factors in the Mallory–Weiss syndrome. *Am J Gastroenterol*, 1997; 92: 805.

14 Powell TW, Herbst CA, Usher M. Mallory–Weiss syndrome in a 10-month old infant requiring surgery. *J Pediatr Surg*, 1984; 19: 596.

15 Harris JM, DiPalma JA. Clinical significance of Mallory–Weiss tears. *Am J Gastroenterol*, 1993; 88: 2056.

16 Bataller R, Llach J, Salmeron JL *et al*. Endoscopic sclerotherapy in upper gastrointestinal bleeding due to the Mallory–Weiss syndrome. *Am J Gastroenterol*, 1994; 89: 2147.

17 Stevens AE, Dove GAW. Oesophageal cast: oesophagitis dessicans superficialis. *Lancet*, 1960; ii: 1279.

18 Marks IN, Keet AD. Intramural rupture of the oesophagus. *Br Med J*, 1968; ii: 536.

19 Khan AA, Burkhart CR. Esophageal cast. *J Clin Gastroenterol*, 1985; 7: 409.

20 Kitano S, Terblanche J, Kahn D, Bornman PC. Venous anatomy of the lower oesophagus in portal hypertension: practical implications. *Br J Surg*, 1986; 73: 525.

21 Allison PR. Bleeding from gastro-oesophageal varices. *Ann R Coll Surg*, 1959; 25: 298.

22 Laine L, Cook D. Endoscopic ligation compared with sclerotherapy for treatment of esophageal variceal bleeding: a meta-analysis. *Ann Intern Med*, 1995; 123: 280.

23 Fabiani B, Degott C, Ramond MJ, Valla D, Benhamou JP, Potet F. Endoscopic obliteration of esophagogastric varices with bucrylate II—histopathological study in 12 post-mortem cases. *Gastroenterol Clin Biol*, 1986; 10: 580.

24 Matsumoto S. Clinicopathological study of sclerotherapy of esophageal varices. I. A review of 26 autopsy cases. *Gastroenterol Jpn*, 1986; 21: 99.

25 Evans DMD, Jones DB, Cleary BK, Smith PM. Oesophageal varices treated by sclerotherapy: a histopathological study. *Gut*, 1982; 23: 615.

26 Schellong H, v. Maercke PH, Bueb G, Pichlmaeir H. Oesophageal stenosis—a complication of sclerotherapy of oesophageal varices. *Endoscopy*, 1986; 18: 223.

27 Jensen LS, Dybdahl H, Juhl C, Nielsen TH. Endoscopic sclerotherapy of esophageal varices in an experimental animal model; a histomorphologic study. *Scand J Gastroenterol*, 1986; 21: 725.

28 Sorensen T, Burcharth F, Pedersen ML, Findahl F. Oesophageal stricture and dysphagia after endoscopic sclerotherapy for bleeding varices. *Gut*, 1984; 25: 473.

29 Spence RAJ, Sloan JM, Johnston GW, Greenfield A. Oesophageal mucosal changes in patients with varices. *Gut*, 1983; 24: 1024.

30 Geboes K, Desmet V, Vantrappen G. Esophageal histology in the early stage of gastroesophageal reflux. *Arch Pathol Lab Med*, 1979; 103: 205.

31 Geboes K, Desmet V, Vantrappen G, Mebis J. Vascular changes in the esophageal mucosa. *Gastrointest Endosc*, 1980; 26: 29.

32 Shamma'a MH, Benedict EB. Esophageal webs. A report of 58 cases and an attempt at classification. *N Engl J Med*, 1958; 259: 378.

33 Benedict EB, Lever WF. Stenosis of esophagus in benign mucous membrane pemphigus. *Ann Otol Rhinol Laryngol*, 1952; 61: 1121.

34 Marsden RA, Sambrook-Gower FJ, MacDonald AF, Main RA. Epidermolysis bullosa of the oesophagus with oesophageal web formation. *Thorax*, 1974; 29: 287.

35 Johnston DE, Koehler RE, Balfe DM. Clinical manifestations of epidermolysis bullosa dystrophica. *Dig Dis Sci*, 1981; 26: 1144.

36 Jerome-Zapadka KM, Clarke MR, Sekas G. Recurrent upper esophageal webs in association with heterotopic gastric mucosa: case report and literature review. *Am J Gastroenterol*, 1994; 89: 421.

37 McDonald GB, Shulman HM, Sullivan KM, Spencer GD. Intestinal and hepatic complications of human bone marrow transplantation. Part I. *Gastroenterology*, 1986; 90: 460.

38 Papazian A, Capron J-P, Ducroix J-P, Dupas J-L, Quenem C, Besson P. Mucosal bridges of the upper esophagus after radiotherapy for Hodgkin's disease. *Gastroenterology*, 1983; 84: 1028.

39 Janisch HD, Eckardt VF. Histological abnormalities in patients with multiple esophageal webs. *Dig Dis Sci*, 1982; 27: 503.

40 MacMahon HE, Schatski R, Gary JE. Pathology of a lower esophageal ring. *N Engl J Med*, 1958; 259: 1.

41 Goyal RK, Bauer JL, Spiro HM. The nature and location of lower esophageal ring. *N Engl J Med*, 1971; 284: 1175.

42 Arvanitakis C. Lower esophageal ring: endoscopic and therapeutic aspects. *Gastrointest Endosc*, 1977; 24: 17.

43 Womack C. Unusual histological appearances of barium sulphate—a case report with scanning electron microscopy and energy dispersive X-ray analysis. *J Clin Pathol*, 1984; 37: 488.

44 Levison DA, Crocker PR, Smith A, Blackshaw AJ, Bartram CI. Varied light and scanning electron microscopic appearances of barium sulphate in smears and histological sections. *J Clin Pathol*, 1984; 37: 481.

PART 3 Stomach

10 Normal stomach

Anatomy and physiology

The stomach develops as an unequal dilatation of the foregut. It extends as a J-shaped loop from the lower end of the oesophagus at the level of the 11th thoracic vertebra and 2 cm to the left of the midline to end in the duodenum just to the right of the first lumbar vertebra. Many workers would now include with it the first part of the duodenum, a concept with which we sympathize, but to avoid much duplication of description, we have continued to consider the duodenum under the small intestine.

The stomach is divisible into four parts. The *cardia* is a small macroscopically indistinct zone immediately distal to the gastro-oesophageal junction; it merges distally into the fundus and is distinguishable only by its histological pattern. The *fundus*, strictly speaking, is that part which lies above a line drawn horizontally through the gastro-oesophageal junction, while the *body* comprises approximately the proximal two-thirds of the remainder; in many descriptions body and fundus appear to be synonymous. The *pyloric antrum* forms the distal third, leading into the *pyloric sphincter*. The body mucosa is rugose and freely mobile on the muscle beneath, while the antral mucosa is flattened, less rugose and more firmly anchored. The boundary between them is not clearly visible to the naked eye though there is some evidence that a transverse contraction band may be present in the full stomach [1]. The incisural notch, so often used as a landmark in anatomical textbooks, is not an accurate guide. The only reliable distinguishing feature is the difference in histological appearance, for antral mucosa frequently extends far up the lesser curve and may reach almost to the cardia, particularly in women [2,3]. This is presumably a consequence of chronic gastritis with pyloric metaplasia of body mucosa [4]. The thickness of normal gastric mucosa is variable and depends to a great extent on the degree of distension of the stomach. When empty, the rugae of the body lie in predominantly longitudinal folds which in some persons are thick enough to give a curious fine cobblestone appearance, the *état mamelonné*, a variation of normal which must not be confused with the pathological hypertrophy of Ménétrier's disease (see p. 221). Along the lesser curve there are three or four relatively fixed narrow ridges which form the magenstrasse.

The stomach has a generous blood supply derived from branches of the coeliac, hepatic and splenic arteries, with an abundant anastomosis and an absence of end arteries. Some authors have described arteriovenous shunts in the submucosa or muscle coats that may be either straight connections or of glomus type. They may be important in the genesis of peptic ulcer [5–7] but do not appear to exist at the mucosal level [8]. Lymphatic channels are numerous and form a plexus in the submucosa from which many small vessels penetrate the muscularis mucosae and ramify in the deeper part of the mucosa. Their absence from the superficial mucosa correlates with the low prevalence of lymph nodal metastases in intramucosal gastric cancer [9,10]. They drain to the left gastric, right gastric and subpyloric lymph nodes and also to paracardial, pancreaticosplenic and right gastroepiploic nodes.

The nerve supply to the gastrointestinal tract is based on a regular pattern. In the stomach the parasympathetic cholinergic supply comes from the terminal branches of both vagi, the right tending to supply the posterior surface, and the left the anterior. The anterior vagus then divides into hepatic and anterior gastric branches, the posterior into coeliac and posterior gastric. This is important for the surgeon, since selective vagotomy allows preservation of hepatic and coeliac branches, which may reduce the incidence of postvagotomy diarrhoea. Sympathetic innervation comes from the lateral horns of segments D6–D10, reaching the coeliac ganglion via the greater splanchnic nerves and spreading thence to the stomach [11] where submucosal and myenteric plexuses are present. Within the myenteric plexus there is a small-meshed net of varicose axons, sometimes gathered together in bundles or fascicles, which are acetylcholinesterase (AChE) positive, as are scattered ganglia [12]. In the submucosa there are plentiful AChE-positive axons forming perivascular nerve trunks and plexuses, and a similar network is present in relation to gastric glands in the mucosa. Adrenergic nerves are scantier and tend to end adjacent to endocrine cells. There is evidence that nerves containing vasoactive intestinal polypeptide (VIP) act as interneurones between AChE-containing and adrenergic nerves [13]. Other neurones containing substance P may have a sensory function [14]. In some animals there appear to be detailed nervous connections between oesophagus and stomach [15], but we know of no descriptions of these in humans.

The stomach acts as a dilatable sac, storing food for controlled onward transmission, breaking it up to a semifluid consistency, adding secretions to it and allowing digestion to start. Little information is available about its normal size and capacity and variations of these in disease. It can probably hold about 1500 mL under conditions of normal distension. Surface areas are about 850 cm^2 in men and 750 cm^2 in women [16,17]. The greater curve is the more expansile and relatively large amounts of food can be contained in it with little rise in internal pressure. Small amounts of food, liquids and secretions probably pass down the lesser curve. There is a suggestion, based on postmortem examination of stomachs of American and Japanese men and women (in which the measurements do not seem to us entirely conclusive), that greater and lesser curve lengths may vary with race [18].

Detailed physiology is outside the scope of this book but there are good recent reviews of important practical topics, including gastric emptying [19], secretory function [20] and mucosal defence mechanisms [21].

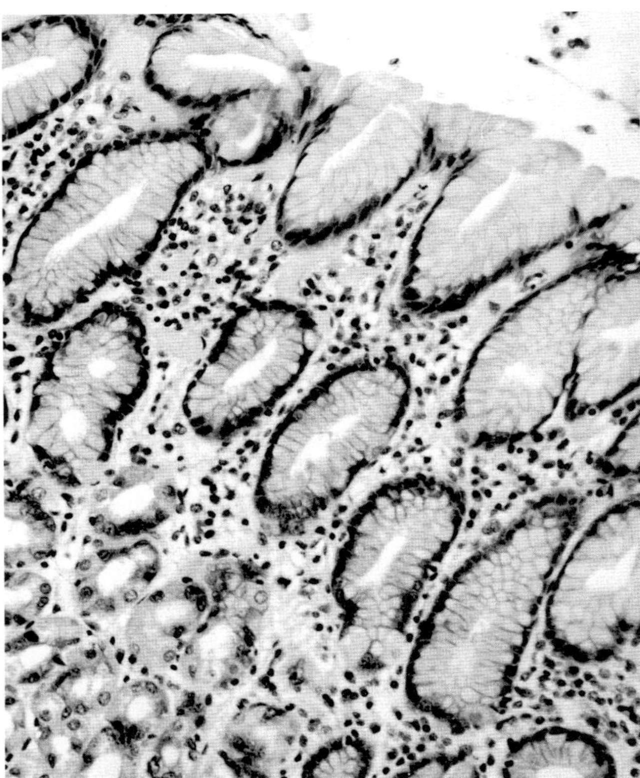

Fig. 10.1 Superficial surface layer and pits of normal body of stomach. The cells secrete neutral but not acidic mucins. The upper regions of glands are visible at lower left.

Microscopic appearances

Under the dissecting microscope the body mucosa has a 'morocco leather' appearance due to the presence of uniformly regular papillae, closely packed together and with a circular gastric gland opening at the apex of each. The antral mucosa has a coarser leaf-like pattern with several papillae aggregated to form each leaf [22]. Scanning electron micrographs of body mucosa show a 'cobblestone' pattern in which gastric pits are clearly visible [23]. Little use has so far been made of either technique in diagnostic pathology.

The surface (foveolar) epithelium

The surface (foveolar) epithelium is the same in all regions of the stomach [24]. It consists of a single layer of tall columnar mucus-secreting cells with basal nuclei that cover the surface papillae and line the gastric pits (Fig. 10.1). Individual cells are linked by junctional complexes and lateral cell membranes interdigitate. On the luminal aspect of each cell are small pleomorphic microvilli, 0.2–0.6 μm high and 0.05–0.15 μm in diameter. A glycocalyceal coat is present [25]. Within the cytoplasm are supranuclear membrane-bound granules of neutral mucin 0.1–1.0 μm in diameter. Most are uniformly electron dense but some are mottled with a denser zone beneath the limiting membrane [26]. There is a well developed Golgi complex from which the mucin granules appear to originate. The mucin gel on the surface forms a stable unstirred layer in which trapped bicarbonate ions produced by epithelial cells neutralize luminal hydrochloric acid and maintain the pH at approximately 7 at the mucosal cell surface.

The cardiac zone

The cardia lies between the end of the oesophagus and the body of the stomach; it usually extends downwards for 5–30 mm from the cardio-oesophageal junction, though there is marked individual variation [24]. Because it straddles the anatomical boundary of the oesophagus and stomach, cardiac mucosa has also been referred to as junctional mucosa. Cardiac glands are compound or branching tubular and tend to be grouped in lobules separated by connective tissue and by prolongations of the muscularis mucosae [26] (Fig. 10.2). They secrete two types of mucin, distinguishable by the use of lectin

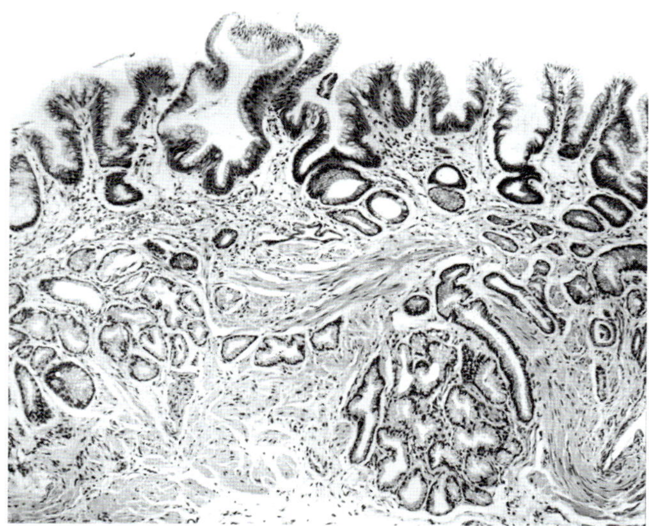

Fig. 10.2 Normal cardiac mucosa showing lobulated mucous glands with interdigitating smooth muscle fibres.

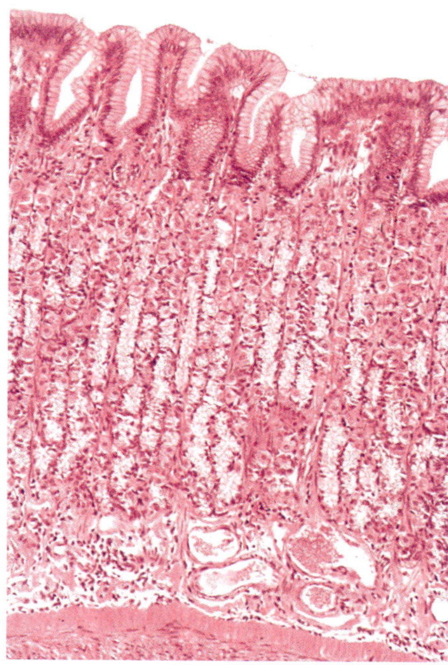

Fig. 10.3 Normal body mucosa. The crypts are lined by cells secreting neutral mucin. The deep aspect consists of glands which run perpendicular to the surface.

techniques [27], but the difference does not appear to be of diagnostic importance. Other cells present in smaller numbers include acid-secreting and endocrine cells. Pepsinogen-secreting chief cells are rare. The glands which open into pits on the surface make up about half of the total mucosal thickness. Cystic dilatation of gland elements is common enough to be regarded as a normal finding, and lymphoid follicles are also common in the deeper part of the mucosa, or extending through the muscularis mucosae into the submucosa.

The body and fundus

Body and fundal mucosa are identical and in many descriptions the two regions are not separated. The mucosal thickness varies from 400 to 1500 μm. Gastric crypts (pits, foveolae) lined by surface epithelium without specialized cells form a superficial zone comprising about 25% of the total thickness. The deep zone which forms the remaining 75% consists of straight tubules arranged perpendicularly to the surface (Fig. 10.3). They extend from the base of the crypts to the muscularis mucosae where they undergo some coiling and may appear as acini in cross-section. One to four glands open through a slight constriction or neck into the bottom of each crypt. The four types of cell present in body glands are the mucous neck cells, parietal or oxyntic cells, chief or zymogenic cells, and endocrine cells [24,28] (Fig. 10.4).

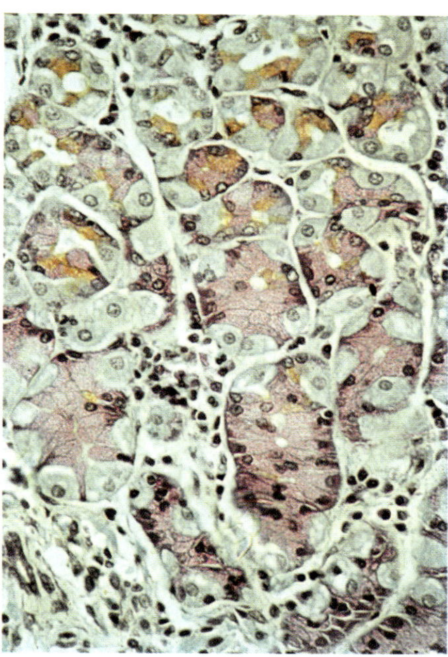

Fig. 10.4 Normal body mucosa. This preparation shows parietal cells staining green, chief cells light purple and mucous neck cells yellow. Maxwell stain.

Mucous neck cells

These cells, which occur in the regenerative zone, lie mainly in the upper part of the tubules (Fig. 10.4) where they mingle with acid-secreting cells. They differ from surface epithelial cells in being low rather than high columnar and more triangular in shape, and in not interdigitating freely with the membranes of adjacent cells. Their contained mucin granules show variable electron density. A few are present in the lower part of the tubule where they cannot readily be distinguished from pepsinogen-secreting cells on conventional staining, though they are readily recognized in thin sections after methacrylate embedding. Autoradiography using tritiated actinomycin shows a decrease in labelling from the deeper to the more superficial surface cells, indicating a switch from proliferation to maturation during the process of surface epithelial renewal [29].

Neither the mucous neck cells nor mature surface cells contain microvillous alkaline phosphatase or aminopeptidase. Their mucin content is almost entirely neutral [30] though occasional cells stain faintly for acid mucins [31]. Goblet cells are not present. These features are helpful in distinguishing normal mucosa from intestinal metaplasia.

The function of the mucous neck cell is controversial. Some, on the basis of experimental models, have regarded it as a transitional cell in the differentiation of gastric stem cells to zymogenic or chief cells [32,33]. Others, on the basis of their secretion of a number of luminally active peptides, including trefoil peptides, pancreatic secretory trypsin inhibitor and epidermal growth factor, have concluded that mucous neck cells comprise a distinctive, functional cell lineage whose role is to protect the gastric mucosa, and, in particular, adjacent parietal cells, from the effects of secreted gastric acid [34].

Acid-secreting (parietal, oxyntic) cells

These constitute the majority of cells lining the upper part of the glands of body mucosa and are the source of hydrochloric acid, blood group substances [24,35] and intrinsic factor [36]. *In vitro* receptor autoradiography has suggested that the parietal cell is the site of cholecystokinin B-gastrin receptors [37]. They are large, round or pyramidal in shape, 20–35 μm in diameter, and have a central nucleus and an eosinophilic, vacuolated cytoplasm which corresponds to the extensive secretory canaliculus seen on ultrastructural examination. Their longest side is apposed to the basement membrane and their apical end is wedged between adjoining cells. The free apical surfaces are invaginated and have numerous microvilli without any glycocalyceal coat. Within the cytoplasm are numerous mitochondria containing electron-dense granules. The cells have a high content of succinate and lactate dehydrogenases and of nicotinamide-adenine dinucleotide (NAD) tetrazolium reductase [38]. There are few intercellular junctions with either mucus-secreting or pepsinogen-secreting cells.

Pepsinogen-secreting (chief) cells

These cells are less numerous than acid-secreting cells and lie mainly in the deeper parts of the tubules. They tend to be more numerous towards the cardiac end of body mucosa, in contrast to parietal cells which are more numerous distally [39]. Chief cells probably differentiate directly from stem cells in the isthmus of glands although a derivation from mucous neck cells has also been proposed (see above). They secrete pepsinogens I and II [40] and other proteolytic proenzymes, including lipase [41,42]. They are cuboidal or low columnar and their cytoplasm is neutrophilic. Their apical surfaces bear short irregular microvilli and have a surface glycocalyx. Membrane-bound homogeneous spherical granules 0.5–3.0 μm in diameter are present in the apical supranuclear region and there is an extensive rough endoplasmic reticulum arranged as parallel cisternae. Antisera raised against pepsinogens allow their separation into groups [43] but the technique is more useful for ready identification of cells when counts are made in research projects rather than for diagnostic work.

Endocrine cells

Endocrine cells are widely and patchily distributed in the mucosa of all parts of the stomach [44,45] and their products play important regulatory roles in gastrointestinal physiology. They are recognized in haematoxylin and eosin-stained preparations as rounded clear or halo cells in the glandular layer, often wedged between the basement membrane of the glands and the epithelial cells. In some cases red or pink granules are present below the nucleus. A minority of these cells, which contain serotonin (5-hydroxytryptamine), so-called enterochromaffin (EC) or argentaffin cells, may be demonstrated by their property of reducing silver salts without exposure to a reducing substance and by a positive diazo reaction. The majority of endocrine cells are argyrophilic with the Grimelius technique on formalin-fixed tissue. Some endocrine cells fail to stain with either argentaffin or argyrophil methods but may be demonstrated immunocytochemically. Antibodies to neurone-specific enolase, synaptophysin and chromogranin have been used. Chromogranins A and B, proteins occurring in storage granules, have been found to be the most consistent markers of endocrine cells in the human gut [46]. Immunohistochemical staining techniques using antibodies specifically directed against biogenic amines or polypeptide hormones have identified in the body and antrum of the stomach D cells which produce somatostatin, EC cells which contain serotonin, D_1 cells which are VIP (vasoactive intestinal polypeptide) positive, P cells containing bombesin, and PP cells with pancreatic polypeptide. Enterochromaffin-like (ECL) cells are confined to the body of the stomach and are the most common endocrine cell at this site. They are mostly evident in the basal third of the mucosa and are particularly associated with chief cell-rich areas. They have distinctive ultrastructural granules and can be identified using antibodies against histamine and histidine decarboxylase. They play a pivotal role in the mediation of gastrin-induced parietal cell secretion [47]. No cell product has been identified in the so-called X cells which are Grimelius positive and occur principally in the oxyntic mucosa. S cells containing secretin have been identified in the lower third of the antropy-

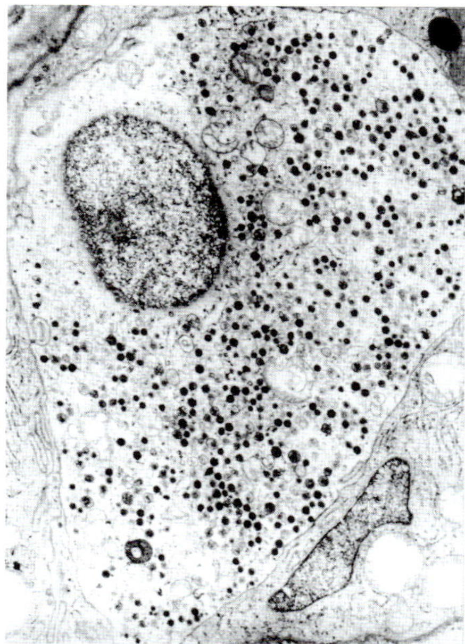

Fig. 10.5 Electron micrograph of gastrin-secreting (G) cell.

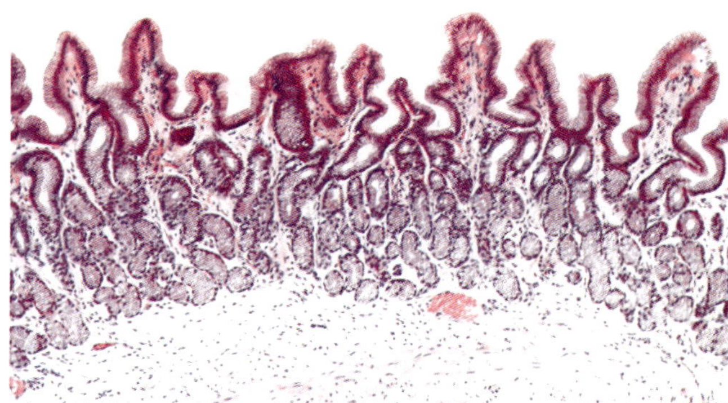

Fig. 10.6 Normal antral mucosa. The crypts form about 40% of the mucosal thickness.

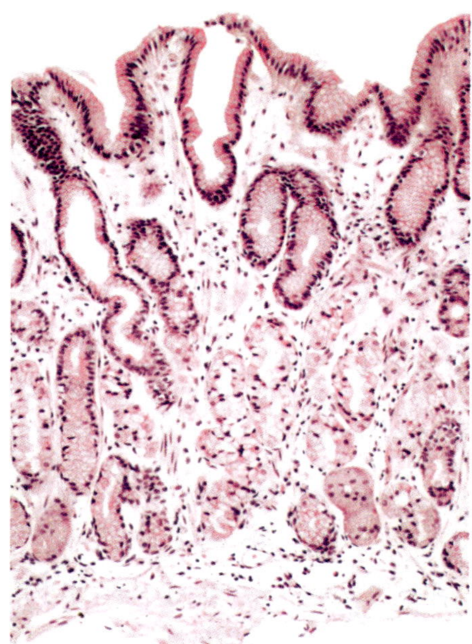

Fig. 10.7 Transitional mucosa. The pits occupy approximately half the mucosal thickness. Underlying glands are of body and antral type.

loric mucosa. G cells predominate in the lower and middle thirds of antropyloric mucosa with relatively small numbers in the crypts and Brunner's glands of the proximal duodenum. They decrease in density from the pylorus to the gastric body [48]. They are the source of gastrin, the most investigated hormone of the gastrointestinal tract, whose best-known function is its ability to stimulate gastric acid secretion. The cells are argyrophilic with the Grimelius technique. Intracytoplasmic secretory granules are spherical and membrane-bound, and have a variably electron-dense core and an average diameter of 150–250 nm (Fig. 10.5).

The antral and pyloric region

This occupies a roughly triangular area in the lower third of the stomach, with the boundary with body mucosa extending as an oblique line from a point about two-fifths of the way along the lesser curve to a point on the greater curve much nearer the pylorus. Antral mucosa varies in thickness from 200 to 1100 μm, of which the surface pits form about 40%. They branch and do not always lie perpendicular to the surface. The deep zone consists of coiled tubules; some of these are branched and separated by upgrowths of muscularis mucosae (Fig. 10.6). They are lined principally by faintly granular mucin-secreting cells with a basal nucleus, and are indistinguishable from mucous neck cells in sections stained with haematoxylin and eosin. Occasional parietal cells are present in all parts of the pyloric mucosa and may be more numerous close to the gastroduodenal junction [49]. The most useful criteria for distinguishing body from pyloric mucosa in the normal stomach are the disappearance of chief cells from the latter [50] and the change from single tubular glands in the body to branched glands in the antrum.

The intermediate (transitional) zone

The junction between the different types of gastric mucosa may be clear cut, or be occupied by a transitional type of mucosa in which the pits occupy half the mucosal thickness and the glandular zone consists of both body and pyloric or cardiac glands (Fig. 10.7).

The lamina propria

The lamina propria, as elsewhere in the gut, consists of a network of connective tissue fibres in which lie blood vessels, lymphatics, nerve fibrils and a number of cells of the immune and macrophage systems. Within the body mucosa, capillaries extend at right angles to the surface and form a network beneath the surface epithelial layer which is drained by infrequent collecting venules; there are no arteriovenous anastomoses and blood must reach the mucosal surface before it can enter the venous return [8]. Plasma cells containing immunoglobulin A (IgA) are found scattered in the lamina propria of body mucosa but are more numerous in the antral region [51]. The number of plasma cells present varies but the relation IgA : IgG : IgM is remarkably constant from patient to patient and, in sequential biopsies, from specimen to specimen [52]. IgG can be found extracellularly in 'pools' between pits in the body mucosa and between antral glands, while IgA is most obvious in the antral isthmus where it is intracellular and bound to secretory component [53]. There are also small numbers of T lymphocytes in the lamina propria, and intraepithelial lymphocytes, over 95% of which are of T-cell type [54], may be identified, although far less frequently than in the small bowel. It is debatable whether lymphoid aggregates or follicles are ever seen in the absence of gastritis; they have been described in neonates [55] but we have not seen them in an extensive experience.

Muscularis mucosae

The muscularis mucosae throughout the stomach varies in thickness from 30 to 210 μm and does not normally show fragmentation or infiltration by inflammatory cells. In the distal pylorus it grows up into and separates pyloric glands; the continuation of this process is responsible for the submucosal position of Brunner's glands in the duodenum.

Submucosa

This consists of loose connective tissue with some adipose cells in which lie blood vessels, lymphatics and ganglion cells of the submucosal plexus. There is continuity with the oesophageal submucosa, but at the gastroduodenal junction the submucosa becomes obliterated by Brunner's glands and by the encroachment of the pyloric sphincter.

Muscle coats

The stomach has three muscle coats. The *inner circular* coat is continuous with that of the oesophagus and surrounds the whole stomach. The *outer longitudinal* coat runs from the oesophagus to the duodenum and is continuous with the longitudinal fibres of each. Internal to the circular coat additional *oblique fibres* run down from the cardia more or less parallel to the lesser curve and blend with the circular coat. Ganglion cells and nerve fibres are found between the circular and longitudinal coats. At the pylorus there is a more specialized arrangement. The circular muscle thickens and forms distinct proximal and distal loops which unite in a complex or torus along the lesser curve [56,57]. There is no obvious continuity with the circular muscle of the duodenum, but we have not seen the interposed fibrous septum which is sometimes described. The longitudinal muscle splits, some fibres continuing on into the duodenum while others turn inward to blend with the sphincter. This arrangement may be significant in localized types of adult pyloric stenosis.

Serosa

This is continuous with the peritoneum and consists of loose areolar tissue containing blood vessels, lymphatics and nerve fibres, covered by a sheet of flattened mesothelial cells continuous with the serosal lining of the peritoneal cavity.

References

1 Moore JG, Dubois A, Christian PE, Elgin D, Alazraki N. Evidence for a midgastric transverse band in humans. *Gastroenterology*, 1986; 92: 92.

2 Landboe-Christensen E. Extent of the pylorus zone in the human stomach. *Acta Pathol Microbiol Scand Suppl*, 1944; 54: 671.

3 Oi M, Oshida K, Sugimura S. The location of gastric ulcer. *Gastroenterology*, 1959; 36: 45.

4 Kimura K. Chronological transition of the fundic–pyloric border determined by stepwise biopsy of the lesser and greater curvatures of the stomach. *Gastroenterology*, 1972; 63: 584.

5 Barlow TE. Arterio-venous anastomoses in the human stomach. *J Anat*, 1951; 85: 1.

6 Piasecki C. Blood supply to the human gastroduodenal mucosa with special reference to ulcer bearing areas. *J Anat*, 1974; 118: 295.

7 Anthony A. Vascular anatomy in gastrointestinal inflammation. *J Clin Pathol*, 1999; 52: 381.

8 Cannon B, Browning J, O'Brien P, Rogers P. Mucosal microvascular architecture of the fundus and body of human stomach. *Gastroenterology*, 1984; 86: 866.

9 Lehnert T, Erlandson RA, DeCosse JJ. Lymph and blood capillaries of the human gastric mucosa. A morphologic basis for metastasis in early gastric carcinoma. *Gastroenterology*, 1985; 89: 939.

10 Listrom MB, Fenoglio-Preiser CM. Lymphatic distribution of the stomach in normal, inflammatory, hyperplastic, and neoplastic tissue. *Gastroenterology*, 1987; 93: 506.

11 Smith B. *The Neuropathology of the Alimentary Tract*. London: Edward Arnold, 1972.

12 Kyosala K, Rechardt L, Veijola L, Waris T, Penttila O. Innervation of the human gastric wall. *J Anat*, 1980; 131: 453.
13 Jessen KR, Polak JM, Van Noorden S, Bloom SR, Burnstock G. Evidence that peptide-containing neurons connect the two ganglionated plexuses of the enteric nervous system. *Nature*, 1980; 283: 391.
14 Sharkey KA, Williams RG, Dockray GJ. Sensory substance P innervation of the stomach and pancreas. Demonstration of Capsaian-sensitive sensory neurones in the rat by combined immunohistochemistry and retrograde tracing. *Gastroenterology*, 1984; 87: 914.
15 Christensen J, Rick JA. Shunt fascicles in the gastric myenteric plexus in five species. *Gastroenterology*, 1985; 88: 1020.
16 Cox AJ. Variation in size of the human stomach. *Calif West Med*, 1945; 63: 1.
17 Cox AJ. Stomach size and its relation to chronic peptic ulcer. *Arch Pathol*, 1952; 54: 407.
18 Goldsmith HS, Akiyama H. A comparative study of Japanese and American gastric dimensions. *Ann Surg*, 1979; 190: 690.
19 Andrews PLR. Gastric emptying: characterization, complications and control. *Curr Opin Gastroenterol*, 1985; 1: 811.
20 Modlin IM, Sachs G. *Acid Related Diseases: Biology and Treatment*. Konstanz: Schnetztor-Verlag GmbH, 1998.
21 Scratcherd T. Gastric mucosal defence mechanisms. *Curr Opin Gastroenterol*, 1987; 3: 916.
22 Salem SN, Truelove SC. Dissecting microscope appearances of the gastric mucosa. *Br Med J*, 1964; ii: 1503.
23 Mackercher PA, Ivey KJ, Baskin WM, Krause WJ. A scanning electron microsopic study of normal human oxyntic mucosa using blunt dissection and freeze fracture. *Am J Dig Dis*, 1977; 23: 449.
24 Day DW, Morson BC. Structure and infrastructure. *Gastrointest Res*, 1980; 6: 1.
25 Stockton M, McColl I. Comparative electron microscopic features of normal, intermediate and metaplastic pyloric epithelium. *Histopathology*, 1983; 7: 859.
26 Krause WJ, Ivey KJ, Baskin WM, Mackercher PA. Morphological observations on the normal human cardiac glands. *Anat Rec*, 1978; 192: 59.
27 Suganuma T, Katsuyama T, Tsukahara M, Tatematsu M, Sakakura Y, Murata F. Comparative histochemical study of alimentary tracts with special reference to the mucus neck cells of the stomach. *Am J Anat*, 1981; 161: 219.
28 Rubin W, Ross LL, Sleisenger MH, Jeffries GH. The normal human gastric epithelia. A fine structural study. *Lab Invest*, 1968; 19: 598.
29 Staffels GL, Preumont AM, de Reuck M. Cell differentiation in human gastric gland as revealed by nuclear binding of tritiated actinomycin. *Gut*, 1979; 20: 693.
30 Dawson IMP. The value of histochemistry in the diagnosis and prognosis of gastrointestinal disease. In: Stoward PJ, Polak J, eds. *Histochemistry: the Widening Horizons*. Chichester: John Wiley, 1981: 127.
31 Gad A. A histochemical study of human alimentary tract mucosubstances in health and disease. *Br J Cancer*, 1969; 23: 52.
32 Karam SM, Leblond CP. Dynamics of epithelial cells in the corpus of the mouse stomach. III. Inward migration of neck cells followed by progressive transformation into zymogenic cells. *Anat Rec*, 1993; 236: 297.
33 Bockman DE, Sharp R, Merlino G. Regulation of terminal differentiation of zymogenic cells by transforming growth factor α in transgenic mice. *Gastroenterology*, 1995; 108: 447.
34 Hanby AM, Poulsom R, Playford RJ, Wright NA. The mucous neck cell in the human gastric corpus: a distinctive, functional cell lineage. *J Pathol*, 1999; 187: 331.
35 Kapadia A, Feizi T, Jewell D, Keeling J, Slavin G. Immunocytochemical studies of blood group A, H, I and i antigens in gastric mucosae of infants with normal gastric histology and of patients with gastric carcinoma and chronic benign peptic ulceration. *J Clin Pathol*, 1981; 34: 320.
36 Levine JS, Nakane PK, Allen RH. Immunocytochemical localization of human intrinsic factor; the non-stimulated stomach. *Gastroenterology*, 1980; 79: 493.
37 Reubi JC, Wasser B, Läderach U *et al*. Localization of cholecystokinin A and cholecystokinin B-gastrin receptors in the human stomach. *Gastroenterology*, 1997; 112: 1197.
38 Niemi M, Siurala M, Sundberg M. The distribution of cytochemically demonstrable diphosphopyridine nucleotide diaphorase and succinic and lactic dehydrogenases in the normal human gastric mucosa. *Acta Pathol Microbiol Scand*, 1960; 48: 323.
39 Hogben CAM, Kent TH, Woodward PA, Sill AJ. Quantitative histology of the gastric mucosa: man, dog, cat, guinea pig, and frog. *Gastroenterology*, 1974; 67: 1143.
40 Cornaggia M, Riva C, Capella C *et al*. Subcellular localization of pepsinogen II in stomach and duodenum by the immunogold technique. *Gastroenterology*, 1987; 92: 585.
41 Moreau H, Laugier R, Gargouri Y *et al*. Human preduodenal lipase is entirely of gastric fundic origin. *Gastroenterology*, 1988; 95: 122.
42 Ménard D, Monfils S, Tremblay E. Ontogeny of human gastric lipase and pepsin activities. *Gastroenterology*, 1995; 108: 1650.
43 Samloff IM. Cellular localization of group 1 pepsinogens in human gastric mucosa by immunofluorescence. *Gastroenterology*, 1971; 61: 185.
44 Lechago J. The endocrine cells of the digestive tract. General concepts and historic perspective. *Am J Surg Pathol*, 1987; 11 (Suppl I): 63.
45 Falkmer S, Wilander E. The endocrine cell population. In: Whitehead R, ed. *Gastrointestinal and Oesophageal Pathology*. Edinburgh: Churchill Livingstone, 1995: 63.
46 Facer P, Bishop AE, Lloyd RV *et al*. Chromogranin: a newly recognized marker for endocrine cells of the human gastrointestinal tract. *Gastroenterology*, 1985; 89: 1366.
47 Modlin IM, Tang LH. The gastric enterochromaffin-like cell: an enigmatic cellular link. *Gastroenterology*, 1996; 111: 783.
48 Voillemot N, Potet F, Mary JY, Lewin MJM. Gastrin cell distribution in normal human stomachs and in patients with Zollinger–Ellison syndrome. *Gastroenterology*, 1978; 75: 61.
49 Tominaga K. Distribution of parietal cells in the antral mucosa of human stomach. *Gastroenterology*, 1975; 69: 1201.
50 Grossman MI. The pyloric gland area of the stomach. *Gastroenterology*, 1960; 38: 1.
51 Isaacson P. Immunoperoxidase study of the secretory immunoglobulin system and lysozyme in normal and diseased gastric mucosa. *Gut*, 1982; 23: 578.

52 Kreuning P, Bosman FT, Kuiper G, van der Wal AM, Lindeman J. Gastric and duodenal mucosa in 'healthy' individuals. An endoscopic and histopathological study of 50 volunteers. *J Clin Pathol*, 1978; 31: 69.
53 Valnes K, Brandtzaeg P, Elgjo K, Stave R. Specific and nonspecific humoral defence factors in the epithelium of normal and inflamed gastric mucosa. Immunohistochemical localization of immunoglobulins, secretory component, lysozyme and lactoferrin. *Gastroenterology*, 1984; 86: 402.
54 Selby WS, Janossy G, Jewell DP. Immunohistological characterisation of intraepithelial lymphocytes of the human gastrointestinal tract. *Gut*, 1981; 22: 169.
55 Watt J. The pathology of multiple gastric ulceration in the newborn infant. *J Pathol Bacteriol*, 1966; 91: 105.
56 Torgensen J. The muscular build and movements of the stomach and duodenal bulb, especially with regard to the problem of segmental divisions of the stomach in the light of comparative anatomy and embryology. *Acta Radiol Suppl*, 1942; 45: 80.
57 McNaught GHD. Simple pyloric hypertrophy in the adult. *J R Coll Surg Edinb*, 1957; 3: 35.

11 Normal embryology and fetal development; developmental abnormalities of the stomach

Normal development

The oesophagus, stomach and first and second parts of the duodenum are all foregut derivatives.

The stomach first appears as a dilatation of the foregut at the 4-mm stage [1] and lies opposite cervical somites 3–5 in the septum transversum, which will itself develop to form the diaphragm [2]. The rapid growth of the cranial region cephalad to the stomach results in its apparent descent. By the 10-mm stage it lies at the level of T5–T10 and by the 18-mm stage at the level of T11–L4. The curvatures form at the 10-mm stage [3] and by 16 mm the rugae are developing (for the corresponding stages in weeks, see Table 19.1, p. 253).

The lining epithelium of the developing stomach is at first one or two cells thick; it proliferates and later thins again to a layer of one or two cells in depth with the cell nuclei placed apically. Crypts develop at about 9 weeks and solid masses of epithelial cells grow down from them. Recognizable gland elements develop in the 12th–13th week [4,5]; acid-secreting cells appear early, but those secreting pepsinogen are not usually seen until the 16th week [6,7]. Both types are already present in premature infants of 1000–2000 g [4]. In some embryos goblet cells are found in the surface epithelium; we have seen these in our own material but we consider that they represent a phase in normal development rather than any form of intestinal metaplasia. Endocrine cells develop early in both body and antrum [8]. Separate cells containing gastrin and somatostatin, the former in the antral region only, the latter in both antrum and fundus, are present at 8 weeks. Cells containing glucagon and indistinguishable from pancreatic A cells are present in the fundus between the 12th and 13th week [8–10] and still other cells containing 5-hydroxytryptamine (5-HT) can be detected in fundus and antrum from the 11th week onwards.

In both fundal and pyloric regions the circular muscle coat develops at the 7th–8th week followed by the longitudinal coat at the 11th–12th week. The muscularis mucosae develops much later, at about the 20th week. No lymphoid follicles are normally seen prior to term. Reviews of human gastrointestinal tract development, including molecular aspects, are available [1,11,12].

Developmental abnormalities

Complete absence of the stomach has not been described in a viable fetus.

Microgastria

This is a rare anomaly which occurs on its own or in association with asplenia and other malformations [13,14]. The stomach is small, tubular and often non-rotated, and the different regions (antrum, body, cardia) cannot be distinguished. Concomitant oesophageal dilatation and midgut malrotation are common. The primary defect is probably a failure of development of the dorsal mesogastrium.

Atresia and stenosis

A general discussion of atresias and stenoses in the gastrointestinal tract is given on p. 255. All forms, excluding pyloric stenosis, are extremely rare in the stomach, with an incidence of 0.0001–0.0003% of live births [15]. Associations with trisomy 21 and epidermolysis bullosa [16] have been reported. Atresia, in which the mucosa and muscularis mucosae were replaced by vascular connective tissue over a 10-mm length, has been described at the pylorus [17], and there are occasional descriptions of pyloric and prepyloric diaphragms which may or need not be imperforate [18–21]; these usually have a cubical or columnar-celled mucosal epithelium on each surface, though a squamous covering has also been described [19]. When perforate they may not present clinically until adult life, but are usually visible radiologically and may appear to be in the first part of the duodenum [22].

Congenital pyloric stenosis

Congenital pyloric stenosis has an incidence of between 2.8 and 4 per 1000 live births [23,24] and is between four and five times more common in males; it also affects firstborn children more commonly than those born subsequently. It is less common in Latin races than in Anglo-Saxons and is rare in African and black Americans [25]. There is some evidence that it is at least partly dependent on an autosomal recessive gene; it is disproportionately common in children of the same family [26,27], in children of parents who have suffered from it [28] and in uniovular as opposed to binovular twins [29], though it also occurs in the latter [30,31]. Other congenital anomalies may coexist and environmental as well as genetic factors are probably important in its genesis [27, 32–34].

Clinically, congenital pyloric stenosis usually presents between the 2nd and 4th weeks of life, but it has been described in stillbirths. Macroscopically there is a concentric bulbous thickening of cartilaginous consistency at the pylorus, which terminates abruptly at the first part of the duodenum and markedly narrows the pyloric canal. Microscopically the circular muscle coat hypertrophies up to four times its normal thickness [35]. Some workers have described degeneration and consequent diminution in numbers of ganglion cells in the myenteric plexus [35] while others have found these cells normal in number but immature [36]. These changes are now considered to be a consequence of compression and inflammation, rather than causal [37]. Experiments on the litters of pregnant bitches and observations on humans suggested that maternal excess of gastrin or pentagastrin could produce a similar condition [38,39], but more recent studies have indicated a role for other intestinal polypeptides with deficiency of vasoactive intestinal peptide, enkephalin, substance P and neuropeptide Y in the circular muscle, but not in the myenteric plexus of affected individuals [40–42]. A lack of nitric oxide synthetase, resulting in incoordination of pyloric sphincter activity, has also been described in infantile hypertrophic pyloric stenosis [43].

Since blood is sometimes found in the vomit of these children single mucosal biopsies taken from greater curve mucosa have also been studied [44], primarily to exclude concomitant gastritis. They have not revealed any noteworthy changes in the epithelium or lamina propria apart from small haemorrhages that may well be artefactual. Occasional examples of hypertrophy of oesophageal, pyloric, duodenal and jejunal muscle may represent a related condition [45,46].

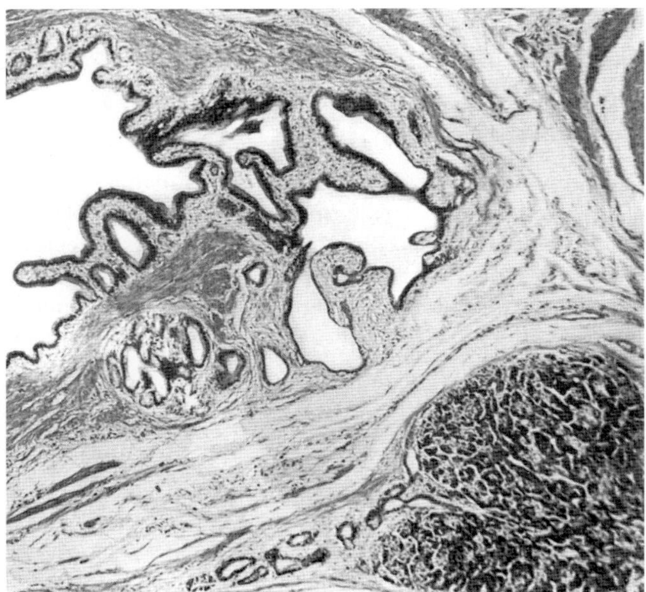

Fig. 11.1 An island of heterotopic pancreatic tissue in the submucosa of the antral region. Acinar tissue is clearly visible at the bottom right with ducts that have become cystic, interspersed with smooth muscle. Compare with Fig. 11.2.

Megaduodenum

There is a report of idiopathic megaduodenum occurring in a family [47]; we have never seen an example.

Duplications, diverticula and cysts

Duplications and diverticula of the stomach are rare [48–53].

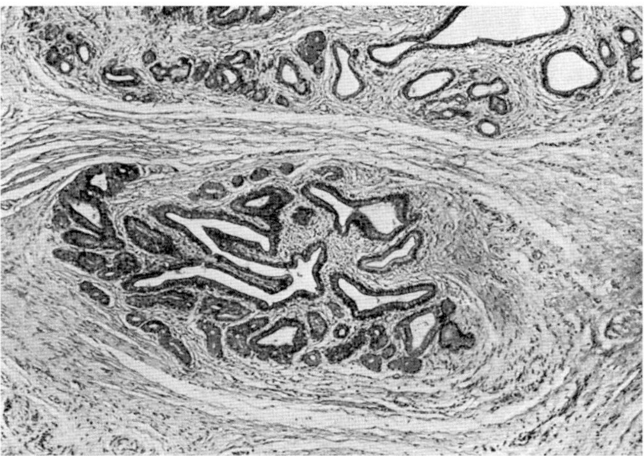

Fig. 11.2 A myoepithelial hamartoma of antral region. No pancreatic tissue is present. Compare with Fig. 11.1.

Many so-called duplications described in adults are probably an end-result of previous peptic ulceration with gastroduodenal fistula and formation of a double channel [54,55]. Congenital examples may be confined to the stomach or be associated with other anomalies which include double oesophagus [56], duodenal duplication [52], pancreatico-pleural fistula and cephalic vertebral anomalies [57], and pulmonary sequestration [58]. Cysts of congenital origin are also extremely rare [59]; in diverticula and congenital cysts there is usually a well formed mucosa of gastric type with muscularis mucosae and often submucosa, but muscle coats are less constantly present and it is rare to find well formed circular and longitudinal coats [60].

Detached cysts with a gastric epithelial lining and clearly of foregut origin are found in thoracic and abdominal cavities. Their mode of genesis is more fully discussed on p. 256.

Anomalies of position

Dextrogastria occurs in three forms—most commonly in association with total situs inversus (complete transposition), but also with dextrocardia but no other transposition and, least commonly, as the only anomaly present [61,62]. The stomach can lie completely behind the liver or above it, in which case there is eventration of the right hemidiaphragm. No structural or functional abnormalities are present in the stomach itself.

Heterotopias

Islands of heterotopic or aberrant pancreatic tissue, usually single and with (Fig. 11.1) or without a considerable smooth muscle component are not uncommon in the antrum and pyloric canal [63–65]. This is considered more fully on p. 218, Chapter 16. Clusters of pancreatic acinar cells have recently been documented in the antrum of children [66], as well as in adults [67], suggesting the possibility of a developmental rather than an acquired phenomenon (see also p. 23, Chapter 4). Very occasional cases of gastric gland heterotopia, usually in the form of intramural cysts [68], have been reported.

Heterotopic gastric mucosa has been described in some 1–3% of endoscopies, presenting as multiple small nodules, usually on the anterior wall, and almost always confined to the first part of the duodenum [69–71]. Histologically these nodules consist of normally formed body-type glands containing acid-secreting and pepsinogen cells in a normal arrangement, covered by a surface epithelium of gastric type and replacing the full thickness of the duodenal mucosa. They are to be distinguished from acquired metaplastic changes affecting the surface epithelium and the presence of occasional parietal cells and, less commonly, chief cells which have been reported particularly in association with hypersecretion of acid and duodenal ulcer [72,73].

Hamartomas

Hamartomas are not uncommon in the gastrointestinal tract where they can be composed predominantly of epithelial or connective tissue [74,75]. Those that are predominantly epithelial are described in Chapter 16.

Myoepithelial hamartomas

These are described on p. 218 in Chapter 16. Although some could be genuine hamartomas, most are considered to represent heterotopic pancreas in which glands and ducts predominate (Fig. 11.2).

Haemangiomas

Haemangiomas are extremely rare in the stomach and have the general features of similar lesions in the remainder of the bowel [76–78]. It is possible that the submucosal arterial aneurysmal malformations associated with severe bleeding which have been described are also angiomatous in nature, though some may be examples of haemorrhage from a large and superficially situated submucosal artery, usually lying on the lesser curve and adjacent to the oesophagogastric junction—the so-called Dieulafoy malformation [79]. Others may represent arteries that have failed to branch normally and in consequence retain larger lumina than normal [80].

References

1 Grand RJ, Watkins JB, Torti FM. Development of the human gastrointestinal tract. A review. *Gastroenterology*, 1976; 70: 790.

2 Gray SW, Skandalakis JE. *Embryology for Surgeons*. London: W.B. Saunders, 1972: 167 & 175.

3 Botha GSM. Organogenesis and growth of the gastro-esophageal region in man. *Anat Rec*, 1959; 133: 219.

4 Salenius P. On the ontogenesis of the human gastric epithelial cells. A histologic and histochemical study. *Acta Anat*, 1962; 50: 1 (Suppl 46).

5 Tuovinen PI. Development of the fundic and pyloric glands of the stomach. *Acta Pathol Microbiol Scand*, 1946; 23: 345.

6 Keene MFL, Hewer EE. Glandular activity in the human foetus. *Lancet*, 1924; ii: 111.

7 Werner B. Peptic and tryptic capacity of digestive glands in newborns: comparison between premature and full term infants. *Acta Paediatr (Stockh)*, 1948; 35:1 (Suppl 6).

8 Stein BA, Buchan AMJ, Morris J, Polak JM. The ontogeny of regulatory peptide-containing cells in the human fetal stomach: an immunocytochemical study. *J Histochem Cytochem*, 1983; 31: 1117.

9 Ravazzola M, Unger RH, Orci L. Demonstration of glucagon in the stomach of human fetuses. *Diabetes*, 1981; 30: 879.

10 Buchan AM, Bryant MG, Stein BA *et al*. Pancreatic glucagon in human fetal stomach. *Histochemistry*, 1982; 74: 515.

11 Andorsky M, Finley A, Davidson M. Paediatric gastroenterology

1.1.69–12.31.75. A review. Hollow viscera and pancreas. *Am J Dig Dis*, 1977; 22: 56.
12 Montgomery RK, Mulberg AE, Grand RJ. Development of the human gastrointestinal tract: twenty years of progress. *Gastroenterology*, 1999; 116: 702.
13 Shackleford GD, McAlister WH, Brodeur AE, Ragslade EF. Congenital microgastria. *Am J Roentgenol*, 1973; 118: 72.
14 Rose V, Izukawa T, Moes CAF. Syndromes of asplenia and polysplenia. A review of cardiac and non-cardiac malformations in 60 cases with special reference to diagnosis and prognosis. *Br Heart J*, 1975; 37: 840.
15 Cooke RCM, Rickham PP. *Gastric Outlet Obstruction in Neonatal Surgery*, 2nd edn. London: Butterworths, 1978.
16 Achiron R, Hamiel-Pinchas O, Engelberg O *et al*. Aplasia cutis congenita associated with epidermolysis bullosa and pyloric atresia: the diagnostic role of prenatal ultrasonography. *Prenat Diagn*, 1992; 12: 765.
17 Burnett HA, Halpert B. Perforation of the stomach of a newborn infant with pyloric atresia. *Arch Pathol*, 1947; 44: 318.
18 Bennett RJ Jr. Atresia of the pylorus. *Am J Dig Dis*, 1937; 4: 44.
19 Leichti RE, Mikkelsen WP, Snyder WH Jr. Prepyloric stenosis caused by congenital squamous epithelial diaphragm—resultant infantilism. *Surgery*, 1963; 53: 670.
20 Banks PA, Waye JD, Waitman AM, Cornell A. Mucosal diaphragm of the gastric antrum. *Gastroenterology*, 1967; 52: 1003.
21 Strange SL. Prepyloric and pyloric mucosal stenosis (four cases). *Proc R Soc Med*, 1967; 60: 1.
22 Lubbers EJC, Rijnders WPHA. Congenital stenosis of the first part of the duodenum in an adolescent. *Gastroenterology*, 1969; 57: 574.
23 Davison G. The incidence of congenital pyloric stenosis. *Arch Dis Child*, 1946; 21: 113.
24 MacMahon B, Record RG, McKeown T. Congenital pyloric stenosis. An investigation of 578 cases. *Br J Social Med*, 1951; 5: 185.
25 Swann TT. Congenital pyloric stenosis in the African infant. *Br Med J*, 1961; i: 545.
26 Gailey AAH. Congenital hypertrophic pyloric stenosis. Report of four cases in brothers. *Br Med J*, 1948; i: 100.
27 McKeown T, MacMahon B, Record RG. The familial incidence of congenital pyloric stenosis. *Ann Eugen*, 1951; 16: 260.
28 Carter CO, Powell BW. Two-generation pyloric stenosis. *Lancet*, 1954; i: 746.
29 Laubscher JH, Smith AM. Pyloric stenosis in twins. *Am J Dis Child*, 1947; 73: 334.
30 O'Connell FT, Klein JM. Pyloric stenosis in non-identical twins. *Am J Dis Child*, 1941; 62: 1025.
31 MacMahon B, McKeown T. Infantile hypertrophic pyloric stenosis: data on 81 pairs of twins. *Acta Genet Med Gemellol*, 1955; 4: 320.
32 McKeown T, MacMahon B. Infantile hypertrophic pyloric stenosis in parent and child. *Arch Dis Child*, 1955; 30: 497.
33 Scharli A, Sieber WK, Keisewetter WB. Hypertrophic pyloric stenosis at the Children's Hospital of Pittsburgh from 1912 to 1967: a critical review of current problems and complications. *J Pediatr Surg*, 1969; 4: 108.
34 Spicer RD. Infantile hypertrophic pyloric stenosis: a review. *Br J Surg*, 1982; 69: 128.
35 Belding HH III, Kernohan JW. Morphologic study of myenteric plexus and musculature of pylorus with special reference to changes in hypertrophic pyloric stenosis. *Surg Gynecol Obstet*, 1953; 97: 322.
36 Friesen SR, Boley JO, Miller DR. The myenteric plexus of the pylorus: its early normal development and its changes in hypertrophic pyloric stenosis. *Surgery*, 1956; 39: 21.
37 Challa VR, Jona JZ, Marksbery WR. Ultrastructural observations of the myenteric plexus of the pylorus in infantile hypertrophic pyloric stenosis. *Am J Pathol*, 1977; 88: 309.
38 Bleicher MA, Shandling B, Zinyg W, Karl HWA, Track NS. Increased serum immunoreactive gastrin levels in idiopathic hypertrophic pyloric stenosis. *Gut*, 1978; 19: 794.
39 Dodge JA, Karim AA. Induction of pyloric hypertrophy by pentagastrin. An animal model for infantile hypertrophic pyloric stenosis. *Gut*, 1976; 17: 280.
40 Tam PKH. An immunochemical study with neuron-specific-enolase and substance P of human enteric innervation—the normal developmental pattern and abnormal deviations in Hirschsprung's disease and pyloric stenosis. *J Pediatr Surg*, 1986; 21: 227.
41 Malmfors G, Sundler F. Peptidergic innervation in infantile hypertrophic pyloric stenosis. *J Pediatr Surg*, 1986; 21: 303.
42 Wattchow DA, Cass DT, Furness JB *et al*. Abnormalities of peptide-containing nerve fibers in infantile hypertrophic pyloric stenosis. *Gastroenterology*, 1987; 92: 443.
43 Vanderwinder JM. Nitric oxide synthase activity in infantile hypertrophic pyloric stenosis. *N Engl J Med*, 1992; 327: 511.
44 Batcup G, Spitz L. A histopathologic study of gastric mucosal biopsies in infantile hypertrophic pyloric stenosis. *J Clin Pathol*, 1979; 32: 625.
45 Guthrie KJ. Idiopathic muscular hypertrophy of oesophagus, pylorus, duodenum and jejunum in a young girl. *Arch Dis Child*, 1945; 20: 176.
46 Spencer R, Hudson TL. Idiopathic muscular hypertrophy of the gastrointestinal tract in a child. *Surgery*, 1961; 50: 678.
47 Eaves ER, Schmidt GT. Chronic idiopathic megaduodenum in a family. *Aust N Z J Med*, 1985; 15: 1.
48 Bremer JL. Diverticula and duplications of the intestinal tract. *Arch Pathol*, 1944; 38: 132.
49 Kammerer GT. Duplication of the stomach resembling hypertrophic pyloric stenosis. *JAMA*, 1969; 207: 2101.
50 McLetchie NGB, Purves JK, Saunders RL de CH. The genesis of gastric and certain intestinal diverticula and enterogenous cysts. *Surg Gynecol Obstet*, 1954; 99: 135.
51 Young HB. Juxta-oesophageal diverticula of the stomach. *Br J Surg*, 1962; 50: 150.
52 Avni F, Kalifa G, Sauvegrain J. Les duplications gastriques et duodenales chez l'enfant. *Ann Radiol*, 1980; 23: 195.
53 Weiczorec RL, Seidman I, Ranson JHC, Ruoff M. Congenital duplications of the stomach: case report and review of the English literature. *Am J Gastroenterol*, 1984; 79: 597.
54 Farack UM, Goresky CA, Jabbari M, Kinnear DG. Double pylorus: a hypothesis concerning its pathogenesis. *Gastroenterology*, 1974; 66: 596.
55 Sufian S, Ominsky S, Matsumoto T. Congenital double pylorus. A case report and review of the literature. *Gastroenterology*, 1977; 73: 154.

56 Knight J, Garvin PJ, Lewis E Jr. Gastric duplication presenting as a double esophagus. *J Pediatr Surg*, 1983; 18: 300.

57 Fitzgibbons RJ Jr, Nugent FW, Ellis FH Jr, Braasch JW, Scholz FJ. Unusual thoracico-abdominal duplication associated with pancreatico-pleural fistula. *Gastroenterology*, 1980; 79: 344.

58 Thornhill BA, Cho KC, Morehouse HT. Gastric duplication associated with pulmonary sequestration. CT manifestations. *Am J Roentgenol*, 1982; 138: 1168.

59 Potter EL. *Pathology of the Fetus and Infant*, 2nd edn. Chicago: Year Book Medical Publishers, 1961: 349.

60 Tabrisky J, Szalay G, Meade WS. Duplication of the stomach: a cause of anaemia. *Am J Gastroenterol*, 1973; 59: 327.

61 Teplick J, Wallner LH, Levine AH, Haskins ME, Teplick SK. Isolated dextrogastria. Report of two cases. *Am J Roentgenol*, 1979; 132: 124.

62 Hewlett PM. Isolated dextrogastria. *Br J Radiol*, 1982; 55: 678.

63 Barbosa JJC, Dockerty MB, Waugh JM. Pancreatic heterotopia. *Surg Gynecol Obstet*, 1946; 82: 527.

64 Palmer ED. Benign intramural tumours of the stomach. A review with special reference to gross pathology. *Medicine (Baltimore)*, 1951; 30: 81.

65 Martinez NS, Morlock CG, Dockerty MB, Waugh JM, Weber HM. Heterotopic pancreatic tissue involving the stomach. *Ann Surg*, 1958; 147: 1.

66 Krishnamurthy S, Integlia MJ, Grand RJ, Dayal Y. Pancreatic acinar clusters in pediatric gastric mucosa. *Am J Surg Pathol*, 1998; 22: 100.

67 Doglioni C, Laurino L, Dei Tos AP *et al*. Pancreatic (acinar) metaplasia of the gastric mucosa: histology, ultrastructure, immunocytochemistry and clinicopathologic correlation of 101 cases. *Am J Surg Pathol*, 1993; 17: 1134.

68 Gensler S, Seidenberg B, Rifkin H *et al*. Ciliated lined intramural cyst of the stomach: case report and suggested embryogenesis. *Ann Surg*, 1956; 163: 954.

69 Kreuning J, Bosman FT, Kuiper G, van de Wal AM, Lindeman J. Gastric and duodenal mucosa in 'healthy' individuals. An endoscopic and histopathological study of 50 volunteers. *J Clin Pathol*, 1978; 31: 69.

70 Lessells AM, Martin DF. Heterotopic gastric mucosa in the duodenum. *J Clin Pathol*, 1982; 35: 591.

71 Spiller RC, Shousha S, Barrison IG. Heterotopic gastric tissue in the duodenum. A report of eight cases. *Dig Dis Sci*, 1982; 27: 880.

72 Franzin G, Musola R, Mencarelli R. Morphological changes of the gastroduodenal mucosa in regular dialysis uraemic patients. *Histopathology*, 1982; 6: 429.

73 Carrick J, Lee A, Hazell S *et al*. *Campylobacter pylori*, duodenal ulcer, and gastric metaplasia: possible role of functional heterotopic tissue in ulcerogenesis. *Gut*, 1989; 30: 790.

74 Dawson IMP. Hamartomas in the alimentary tract. *Gut*, 1969; 10: 691.

75 Bussey HJR. Gastrointestinal polyposis syndromes. In: Anthony PP, MacSween RNM, eds. *Recent Advances in Histopathology*, Vol. 12. Edinburgh: Churchill Livingstone, 1984: 169.

76 Morton CB, Burger RE. Haemangioma of the stomach. Review of the literature and report of two cases. *Surgery*, 1941; 10: 891.

77 Taylor TV, Torrance HB. Haemangiomas of the gastrointestinal tract. *Br J Surg*, 1974; 61: 236.

78 Tedesco FJ, Hosty TA, Sumner HW. Hereditary haemorrhagic telangiectasia presenting as an unusual gastric lesion. *Gastroenterology*, 1975; 68: 384.

79 Veldhuysen van Zanten SJO, Bartelsman JFWM, Schipper MEI, Tytgat GNJ. Recurrent massive haematemesis from Dieulafoy vascular malformations—a review of 101 cases. *Gut*, 1986; 27: 213.

80 Molnar P, Miko T. Multiple arterial caliber persistence resulting in hematomas and fatal rupture of the gastric wall. *Am J Surg Pathol*, 1982; 6: 83.

12 Gastritis and related conditions

Introduction

The term 'gastritis' is often used loosely to cover any clinical condition in which upper central abdominal discomfort or pain, heartburn and nausea or vomiting are conspicuous symptoms while clinical signs and radiological examinations are negative. There is frequently poor correlation between symptoms, endoscopic appearance and histology. Thus for accurate diagnosis of gastric inflammation and of the state of the gastric mucosa, biopsy and subsequent histological examination is essential. It is preferable to reserve the term 'gastritis' for appropriate histopathological changes. With regard to terminology some authors now consider that 'gastritis' should be limited to mucosal changes associated with inflammation while non-inflammatory conditions should be designated as 'gastropathy'.

Mucosal defence mechanisms

It is usually possible to subdivide gastritis into acute and chronic forms, although the aetiology and pathogenesis of the two may overlap. Inflammation and ulceration of the gastric mucosa occurs when the balance between 'aggressive' and 'defence' factors break down. The fact that the stomach secretes hydrochloric acid and pepsinogen, which are implicated as important final mediators of gastric damage, would render this balance precarious if there were not a formidable set of defences against the continuous threat of autodigestion. Thus before detailed consideration of the various forms of gastritis and their sequelae is undertaken it seems reasonable to briefly consider gastric mucosal defence mechanisms. These can be divided into several components.

The surface mucus layer and gastric mucosal barrier

The surface mucus layer constitutes the first line of defence for surface epithelial cells and is composed of a thin layer of mucus adherent to the mucosal surface. Estimates vary but the layer is thought to be around 180 μm thick [1]. Experimental removal of this layer leads to mucosal erosion [2]. The structure of the mucus layer is not affected in the short term by exposure to bile, ethanol and very low pH. It thus limits potential damage due to such agents and facilitates epithelial repair if damage occurs [3].

The efficacy of the protective surface mucus layer is enhanced by secretion of bicarbonate by surface cells of the gastric mucosa which results in alkalinization of the overlying mucus layer with subsequent protection against luminal acid [4]. Bicarbonate secretion is stimulated by a variety of agents including acid in the gastric and duodenal lumen, cephalic stimulation and E-type prostaglandins [5]. The efficiency of the protection given by the mucus–bicarbonate layer is illustrated by a significant pH gradient across the layer resulting in almost neutral pH on the mucosal side in contrast to the very acidic levels on the luminal side [6].

The surface mucus layer is hydrophobic and this water repellent property is thought to contribute to protection of the mucosa against autodigestion. The hydrophobic property is conferred by surface-active phospholipid substances within the mucus gel. The protection afforded by the mucus gel is severely compromised by substances such as luminal aspirin with resultant damage to underlying surface mucosal cells. Prostaglandins provide some protection against such damage and maintain a hydrophobic layer of mucus gel over the damaged area and promote healing [7]. The surface-active phospholipid is produced from the lamellar bodies in parietal cells and mucous neck cells [8] and the surfactant-like phospholipid forms a multilayered surface coating which is invisible under electron microscopy using conventional aldehyde fixation [9].

Davenport proposed the existence of a gastric mucosal barrier with surface cell membranes and tight junctions between surface epithelial cells as its anatomical basis [10]. This barrier restricts the back-diffusion of hydrogen ions from acid luminal contents into gastric mucosa and also provides a transmucosal potential difference of around 50 mV [11]. It thus provides mucosal protection against low luminal pH levels. The surface-active phospholipid layer has similar properties to the barrier proposed by Davenport and is susceptible to similar barrier breakers. This layer may thus be a component of the gastric mucosal barrier [9]. In addition to providing protection, phospholipid acts as a lubricant and enhances mixing of gastric contents while minimizing mechanical damage to the mucosa [8].

Epithelial renewal

The gastric mucosa has the ability to proliferate and replace damaged surface epithelial cells very rapidly. The proliferative zone from which cells are replaced lies at the junction of the base of the surface pits and the tip of the glands [12]. Experimental studies in the rat indicate that following ethanol-induced damage to the gastric mucosa, complete restitution of mucosal integrity can occur within 15 min [4]. In other species such as the frog, restoration of normal functional activity takes approximately 6 hours [13]. Locally produced growth factors such as epidermal growth factor (EGF) synthesized in salivary glands, Brunner's glands and in small amounts in gastric mucosa, transforming growth factor alpha (TGF-α) synthesized in gastrointestinal mucosa, and gastrin are thought to facilitate mucosal repair [4,14] Mucosal injury is rapidly followed by a highly complex local sequence designed to repair injury and restore the epithelial surface. This involves up-regulation of numerous genes and expression of peptides and growth factors [15].

Mucosal blood flow

Fundamental to the protective components mentioned above is an adequate gastric mucosal blood flow. Adequate blood flow enables the mucosa to dispose of hydrogen ions diffusing in from the gastric lumen [16]. Experimental studies indicate that increased hydrogen ion concentration in the lumen causes increased gastric mucosal blood flow, which, within limits, maintains physiological levels of intramucosal pH [17]. Interruption of blood flow causes a rapid fall in intramucosal pH and subsequent ulceration. Hypovolaemic shock results in focal ulceration similar to that seen in acute erosive gastritis [18]. Duodenal mucosa appears more sensitive to minor degrees of ischaemia while gastric lesions appear only after a significant drop in mucosal blood flow [19].

Cytoprotection

Endogenous prostaglandins synthesized in the gastric mucosa from the precursor arachidonic acid provide mucosal protection against noxious agents [20]. Prostaglandins have many protective actions including stimulation of mucus secretion [21] and increase in gastric mucosal blood flow [22]. Bicarbonate production by gastric and duodenal mucosa is also stimulated [23–25] and the protective layer of hydrophobic surface-active phospholipid is maintained [24]. Adaptive cytoprotection whereby repeated exposure of the mucosa to mild irritants confers protection is also thought to be associated with prostaglandins [25].

Prostaglandins also modulate the gastric mucosal inflammatory response by inhibiting release of tumour necrosis factor (TNF) from macrophages [26] and TNF and other potentially ulcerogenic inflammatory mediators from mast cells [27,28]. There is evidence that non-steroidal anti-inflammatory drug (NSAID)-induced gastric mucosal damage is related to a reduction in endogenous prostaglandin secretion [29,30]. Exogenous prostaglandin also attenuates experimentally induced aspirin damage and maintains a hydrophobic mucus gel layer over damaged epithelium, thus aiding the healing process [7].

Nitric oxide appears to have a similar role to that of prostaglandins in cytoprotection. Suppression of endogenous nitric oxide increases susceptibility of the gastric mucosa to experimental injury [31]. The exceedingly complex effects of various cytokines in cytoprotection and wound healing are slowly becoming clarified. Both epidermal growth factor EGF and TGF-α inhibit acid secretion and protect the gastric mucosa against experimentally induced damage [14]. Removal of submandibular salivary glands, an important source of EGF which reaches the stomach via saliva, results in an increased incidence and extent of experimentally induced ulceration in rats [32]. TGF-α binds to the same receptor as EGF and is synthesized in gastric mucosa. Production is markedly increased following mucosal injury, indicating a possible role for the polypeptide in subsequent repair [33]. Lowering the concentration of TGF-α_1, which is principally derived from macrophages and activated platelets, accelerates healing of experimentally induced ulcers in rats but in contrast high concentrations of the cytokine are associated with excessive formation of extracellular matrix and scarring, a feature which may predispose to ulcer relapse [34].

Following ulceration in the stomach and elsewhere in the gut, development of a novel cell line is frequently induced from stem cells. This appears adjacent to the ulcer and grows in proliferating buds into the lamina propria and eventually reaches the mucosal surface. This ulcer-associated cell lineage (UACL) is capable of secreting EGF which may promote healing of the ulcerated mucosa [35]. The UACL also secretes trefoil peptides. These peptides, so named because of their cloverleaf-like molecular structure occur in three forms throughout the stomach and intestine: TFF1/pS2, TFF2/pSP and TFF3/ITF [15]. TFF1 is expressed by surface cells of UACL in the stomach while TFF2 is found in deeper glandular structures [36]. Some appear to promote epithelial repair following ulceration [37] while targeted gene experiments indicate that TFF1/pS2, which occurs in gastric mucosa, may promote differentiation of mucosal cells [38]. The UACL also induces TFF1/pS2 expression in adjacent goblet and neuroendocrine cells [39].

Acute gastritis

Acute gastritis is an ill-defined term which has been used to cover a wide variety of conditions ranging from life-threatening acute haemorrhagic gastritis (acute stress ulceration, acute erosive gastritis) to transient mild inflammation of the gastric mucosa. Biopsy studies are few, either because the primary disease kills the patient rapidly or because the gastritis resolves quickly. Acute haemorrhagic gastritis is associated with multiple mucosal petechiae, acute erosions and ulcers and thus is discussed in Chapter 13 under the heading of 'Gastric erosions and acute peptic ulcers'. Acute gastritis may result from ingestion of corrosives or drugs such as ferrous sulphate; milder forms are seen in patients with uraemia and in the early stages of *Helicobacter pylori* infection. The gastritis associated with chronic alcohol abuse is often termed haemorrhagic gastritis on account of the congested inflammation of the mucosa at endoscopy and is thus discussed in this section. Acute phlegmonous gastritis is a rare disease in which there is suppurative inflammation of the full thickness of the gastric wall and this is also included in this section.

Effects of corrosive poisons

A wide variety of poisons including the mineral acids, carbolic acid, lysol, sodium and potassium hydroxide, sodium hypochlorite (bleach) and sodium acid sulphate severely affect the stomach. These may be ingested accidentally or with suicidal intent. Such substances are widely used as cleaning agents, descalers and metal polish and are freely available. Ingestion causes rapid and widespread necrosis of the gastric mucosa which becomes haemorrhagic and oedematous. The antral mucosa may not be affected, depending on the amount ingested. The mucosal surface is often black due to altered blood, and necrosis frequently extends into the muscle coat resulting in friability of the wall and the likelihood of perforation. Corrosive burns also affect the mouth and surrounding skin and the oesophagus.

Acute gastritis in *Helicobacter pylori* infection

H. pylori frequently colonizes the gastric mucosa usually resulting in very long term infection and chronic gastritis. This is discussed in detail on pages 108–111. Information on the preliminary stages of the infection is sparse and is largely limited to studies on volunteers who have ingested cultures of the organism [40,41] or closely observed cases of accidental or iatrogenic infection [42,43]. These studies have yielded consistent results with regard to histological characterization of the early stages of the infection. Clinically the symptoms include epigastric pain which is sometimes severe, a bloated feeling, nausea and occasional vomiting with mild constitutional symptoms. These symptoms resolved spontaneously within a week. Achlorhydria or hypochlorhydria also occurred which persisted over several weeks [41,43].

Biopsies taken during the first 2 weeks following infection showed acute inflammation of the superficial gastric mucosa with neutrophils infiltrating between surface epithelial cells and foveolar lining cells and accumulating within gastric pits.

Neutrophils were also prominent within the lamina propria which was oedematous. The surface epithelial cells show degenerative changes with loss of mucin and increased exfoliation. The latter is supported by markedly increased DNA loss during the first week of infection [43]. This acute gastritis appeared to affect the antrum first but also involved the fundus after a few days [41,43]. Identification of *H. pylori* organisms on the mucosal surface was variable in the early stages of infection. The proportion of lymphocytes and plasma cells increased in biopsies taken after 11–14 days and typical chronic active gastritis was established after several weeks. In one case, however, following voluntary ingestion of organisms, the acute gastritis resolved spontaneously and chronic gastritis did not develop [40].

Alcohol-induced gastritis

Haemorrhagic gastritis is the descriptive term frequently used to describe the end-result of acute and chronic alcohol ingestion on the gastric mucosa. The term is not strictly accurate as there is little inflammation and the principal histological feature is intramucosal subepithelial haemorrhages [44] which impart a congested mucosal appearance on endoscopy. These small haemorrhages are often accompanied by tiny erosions and the term 'acute erosive gastropathy' has been suggested [45]. Petechial haemorrhages within the gastric mucosa have been recognized as a feature of alcoholism for many years [46]. Following short-term ingestion of large quantities of alcohol, mucosal erosions are commonly found and histology shows patchy 'necrobiosis' of the foveolar region of the mucosa with focal neutrophil infiltration. Elsewhere there is oedema of the superficial mucosa. These lesions resolved rapidly [46].

The principal histological feature of alcohol-induced gastric mucosal damage, however, is focal haemorrhage just beneath the mucosal surface. Such lesions can be induced in alcoholic patients even after a single dose [47]. Laine and Weinstein [44] carried out a detailed histological study on the gastric mucosa in alcoholics and found extensive lesions in under 20% of patients studied. On endoscopy the mucosal erythema and erosions associated with chronic alcoholism are found mainly in the proximal stomach. Histology shows focal haemorrhages within the mucosa immediately beneath the surface epithelium. Biopsies taken from adjacent non-haemorrhagic mucosa show oedema which may involve the full thickness of the mucosa and extend into the submucosa. Vascular congestion is seen in a minority of cases. Mucosal inflammation is not intense; mild epithelial cell degeneration in the form of mucus depletion and loss of nuclear polarity is seen particularly in epithelial cells overlying the haemorrhages. The risk of major upper gastrointestinal bleeding increases in proportion to the amount of alcohol consumed [48]. This may be a reflection of the intramucosal haemorrhage and vascular congestion seen histologically.

Acute phlegmonous gastritis

Acute phlegmonous gastritis is a rare condition in which there is acute suppurative transmural inflammation involving mainly the submucosa and muscularis propria of the stomach wall. The condition was more common in the preantibiotic era [49] but sporadic cases continue to occur and appear to be increasing. The condition is difficult to diagnose clinically and many cases are only identified at postmortem. Recently, cases occurring in association with human immunodeficiency virus (HIV) infection and HIV seroconversion have been reported [50,51]. A case occurring during treatment with adrenocorticotrophic hormone (ACTH) which may also cause immunosuppression has been reported [52]. Other predisposing factors include disability, gastritis and chronic alcoholism. Most cases occur in patients aged 30–70 years and present with nausea, vomiting and upper abdominal pain and tenderness. Polymorphonuclear leucocytosis is usually present and pyrexia is common but not invariable. There may be a positive blood culture [53]. On gross examination the stomach wall and especially the submucosa is thickened. Inflammation may involve the whole stomach or be localized, usually to the pyloric canal [54]. The mucosa may be intact or ulcerated, although the folds may be lost and the serosa is covered by a fibrinous exudate. Usually the inflammation and thickening of the wall do not extend beyond the cardia or pylorus (Fig. 12.1). On microscopic examination there is intense acute inflammation with abscess formation usually centred on the submucosa, which is swollen and oedematous, but extending into the muscularis propria and serosa. The mucosa is often relatively spared [54]. The most common infective organism is streptococcus [49], but

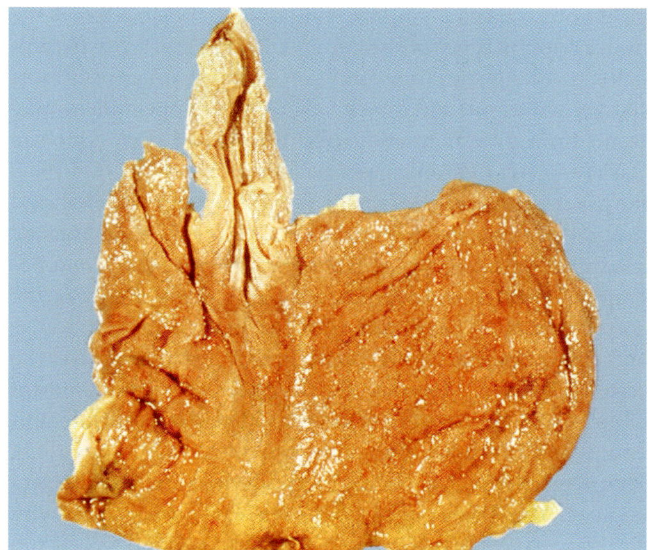

Fig. 12.1 Proximal stomach in acute phlegmonous gastritis. There is loss of mucosal folds due to submucosal oedema. Note the sharp demarcation with the distal oesophagus, which is unaffected.

staphylococcus, *Haemophilus influenzae*, *Escherichia coli* and *Proteus* have also been implicated. Emphysematous gastritis is the variant caused by gas-forming organisms.

The route of entry of the infection is often uncertain. Sometimes there is septicaemia, endocarditis [55] or pharyngitis [54]. Very rarely phlegmonous gastritis may follow endoscopic biopsy [56]. The condition is frequently fatal but patients treated surgically have a much better chance of survival [57].

Chronic gastritis

Chronic gastritis is essentially a histological diagnosis. Correlation between clinical symptoms, endoscopic appearance and histology is notoriously poor [58]. Gastric biopsy should be considered an essential part of endoscopic examination even if no specific lesion such as an ulcer is seen [45]. It is incumbent on the pathologist to provide information relevant to the correct diagnosis and subsequent treatment if at all possible. Estimates of the prevalence of chronic gastritis in biopsies taken from mucosa that is endoscopically normal vary from 30% to over 60% [59,60]. The prevalence of chronic gastritis increases with age up to around 50 years but there is evidence that in developed countries prevalence may be falling [61].

Classification

Chronic gastritis represents the non-specific histopathological sequelae to diffuse long-standing and multifactorial injury to the gastric mucosa. While most authorities sensibly separate off 'special' and relatively rare types of chronic gastritis such as granulomatous and lymphocytic gastritis, classification of the more common types of chronic gastritis has given rise to difficulty. In a long-standing condition, histological appearances change with time and similar histological appearances may result from differing aetiologies. Whitehead *et al.* advocate classification of chronic gastritis according to mucosal type, the grade of gastritis, whether it is superficial or atrophic, and the type of associated metaplasia [62]. Strickland and Mackay identified type A and type B chronic gastritis based on topography. Type A refers to chronic atrophic gastritis involving the corpus and often associated with parietal cell autoantibodies and minimal antral involvement. Type B gastritis involves the distal stomach predominantly with only patchy involvement of the corpus. This is not associated with parietal cell autoantibodies and is considerably more prevalent than type A [63]. This classification has been widely adopted and continues to be used. The discovery of *H. pylori* and its association with chronic gastritis has cast new light on the condition. Wyatt and Dixon proposed a classification based on histological features and pathogenesis. This consisted of type A (autoimmune), type B (bacterial), and reflux or chemical gastritis [64].

The most recent and now perhaps most widely used classification of chronic gastritis is the Sydney system which was devised by an international Working Party of experts and attempts to draw many previous classifications together [65]. This system combines aetiology, topography and morphology. The system relies on at least two mucosal biopsies from both the antrum and the corpus, in addition, of course, to biopsy of any specific lesions. Multiple mucosal biopsies allow assessment of extent and severity of gastritis. The overall Sydney system attempts to combine histological and endoscopic assessment [66]. Correlation between endoscopic assessment and histology, however, is poor as endoscopy is neither a sensitive nor a specific method of diagnosing gastritis [60]. Discussion here is limited to histology.

Five histological variables, chronic inflammation, activity (neutrophil infiltration), atrophy, intestinal metaplasia and *H. pylori* density are graded as mild, moderate or severe. The classification was introduced in an attempt to produce standardized interpretation of gastric biopsies and to allow semiquantitative assessment of progression or regression of histological abnormalities. The system is not difficult nor especially time-consuming to apply but interobserver variation especially with regard to grading remains an issue [67,68]. The Sydney system is now widely used but has not met with universal approval. Correa has suggested an alternative classification based on morphological and likely aetiological considerations [69].

Having been in use for a few years the Sydney system has been reappraised by a panel of experts [70]. In this reappraisal the necessity for multiple biopsies (at least five) from antrum, corpus and incisura angularis was emphasized in order to permit assessment of the distribution of gastritis, atrophy and intestinal metaplasia. In addition, the value of grading these variables as a means of monitoring progression of disease or response to treatment was emphasized, as was the use of visual analogue scales as a template for grading inflammation and atrophy. The use of standardized photomicrographs or diagrams in grading gastritis has previously been shown to be convenient and reasonably accurate [71].

Chronic gastritis associated with *Helicobacter pylori* infection

Since the association between *H. pylori* infection and chronic gastritis was first noted by Warren and Marshall [72] a huge volume of work has been published indicating that the organism is the principal cause of what was previously classified as chronic non-specific gastritis. *H. pylori* has undergone various name changes since its identification. It was first known as *Campylobacter pyloridis*, then *Campylobacter pylori* at the time of the previous edition of this book. It is not, however, a member of the *Campylobacter* genus [73]. The organism is now universally known as *H. pylori*, as suggested by Goodwin *et al.* [74].

H. pylori is a curved or spiral-shaped bacterium 2–4 μm in length with sheathed flagella at one end and occasionally at both ends [72]. The organism possesses marked urease activity, which is the basis for a number of biochemical tests for infection. There is considerable genomic diversity but pathogenicity depends to some extent on the presence of a vacuolating toxin (VacA) and cytotoxin-associated protein (CagA). Strains possessing these cytotoxins are associated with increased inflammation and mucosal damage [75].

The vast majority of cases of *H. pylori* gastritis present to clinicians and pathologists alike as chronic gastritis. There is, however, evidence that in the initial stages of infection there is acute gastritis, which has been discussed earlier in this chapter. As this is a transient condition followed by onset of chronic gastritis or by resolution, documentation is scanty. Volunteer studies indicate neutrophil polymorph infiltration of superficial gastric mucosa with mild degenerative changes in the superficial epithelium. These changes resolve or progress to chronic gastritis within 11–14 days after infection [40].

The organisms are found consistently in the antrum but many infected patients have pangastritis with organisms and inflammation in both corpus and antrum [76]. In such cases the organisms are usually present in larger numbers in the antrum and the degree of inflammation in the majority of cases is more severe in the antrum.

Since the organism was first proposed as an aetiological agent [72] in what had previously been considered as chronic non-specific gastritis, its causative role has only been slowly accepted, but numerous publications from various parts of the world support the association between *H. pylori* infection and chronic active superficial gastritis in adults and in children [77–86]. Further support for a pathogenic role for *H. pylori* in chronic gastritis is provided by studies showing a positive correlation between *H. pylori* colonization and the grade of underlying gastritis. In other words, in areas of the mucosa where large numbers of organisms are present the underlying gastritis is more intense and active. This correlation is most marked in the antrum [81]. Similarly areas of dense *H. pylori* colonization show increased damage to epithelial cells on the mucosal surface. Infection with strains of *H. pylori* which express cytotoxin-associated protein (CagA) induce an increasingly active inflammatory response with greater numbers of neutrophils [87]. This may be due to increased induction of the chemotactic agent interleukin-8 (IL-8) from gastric epithelial cells [88].

The causative role of the organism in chronic active gastritis has been further supported by eradication studies (Fig. 12.2a,b). Following eradication of the organism there is rapid improvement in gastritis. Neutrophils disappear and epithelial cell damage heals within a matter of weeks [77,89,90]. The chronic inflammatory cell infiltrate, however, regresses much more slowly, especially in the antrum. Following eradication of *H. pylori* the antral mucosa was normal in just over half of a series of patients studied 1 year later although the corpus mucosa was normal in all cases [91]. Other workers have noted a slower disappearance of the mononuclear cell infiltrate stretching over a period of 4 years [90].

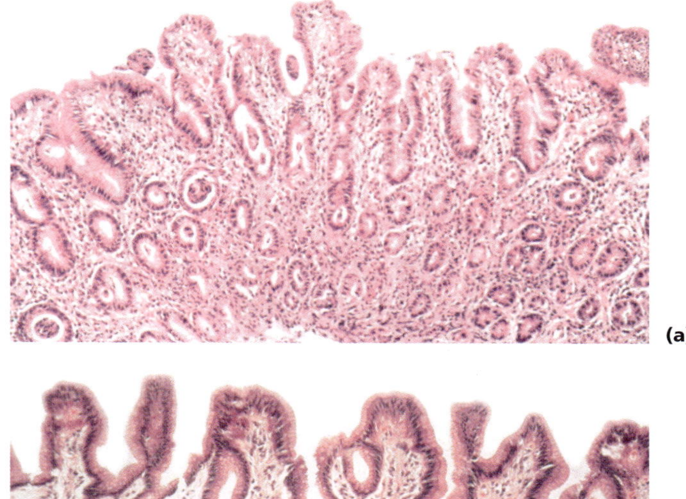

Fig. 12.2 (a) Active chronic superficial gastritis affecting the antrum in *H. pylori* infection. (b) Antral biopsy from the same patient 11 months after eradication of the organisms. There is reduced intensity of inflammation. Neutrophils have disappeared but some chronic inflammatory cells remain.

Despite the marked improvement in histological gastritis following *H. pylori* eradication, this is not necessarily paralleled by symptomatic improvement. A comprehensive review of publications relating to the effect of *H. pylori* eradication on dyspeptic symptoms indicated that while eradication leads to greater symptomatic improvement, over 25% of patients in whom the organism had been eradicated noted no improvement in dyspeptic symptoms [92]. Further studies on non-ulcer dyspepsia patients with *H. pylori* infection indicate that eradication of the organism leads to symptomatic improvement in only approximately 20% of cases [93] and that the placebo effect in untreated patients leads to symptomatic relief as often as eradication of the infection [94].

Histology

The principal and most obvious histological feature of *H. pylori* gastritis is infiltration of the lamina propria of the superficial mucosa by plasma cells, lymphocytes and small numbers of eosinophils (Fig. 12.3). The intensity of this infiltration varies considerably from patient to patient but is significantly higher in infected compared with non-infected patients [95].

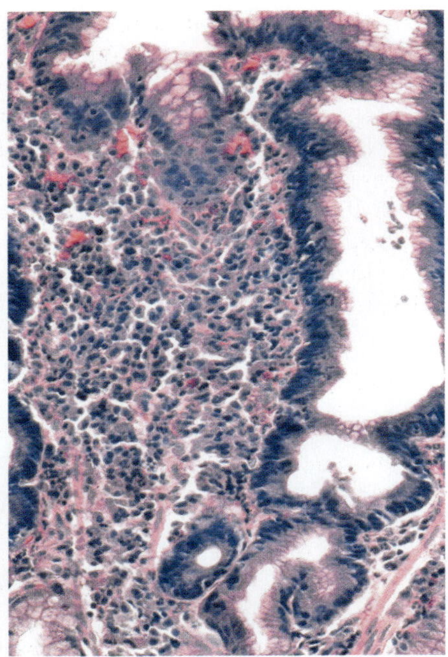

Fig. 12.3 Active antral chronic superficial gastritis in *H. pylori* infection showing intense infiltration of the lamina propria by neutrophils, lymphocytes and plasma cells. Inflammatory cells also infiltrate among surface and glandular epithelial cells.

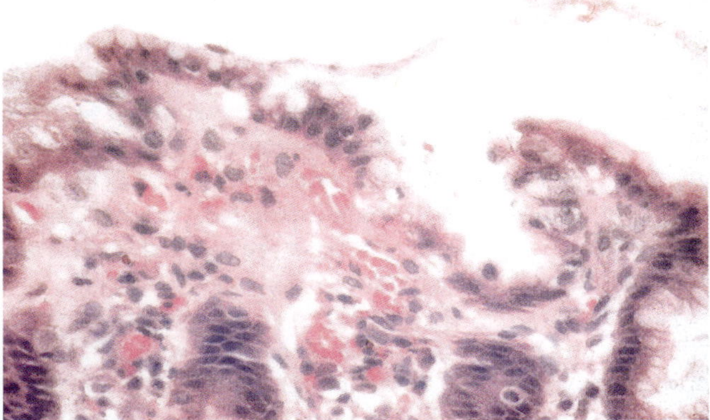

Fig. 12.4 Degenerative changes in gastric surface epithelial cells in *H. pylori* gastritis. Some cells are swollen with loss of apical mucin and there is tufting of the surface epithelial cells. A microerosion is also present.

In addition to the chronic inflammatory cell infiltration, variable numbers of neutrophils are present. These are characteristically found in and around the epithelium lining the base of gastric pits and when small numbers are present may be easily overlooked, especially if masked by a dense chronic inflammatory cell infiltrate. In cases of severe inflammation neutrophils are also present between and adjacent to the surface epithelial cells. In the terminology of the disease the term 'active' chronic superficial gastritis indicates the presence of neutrophils in addition to chronic inflammatory cells. Active inflammation in association with generalized diffuse gastritis is almost invariably associated with the presence of *H. pylori* on the surface of the mucosa and should stimulate a search for the organisms. Although in many cases of *H. pylori* gastritis the surface epithelium may show little abnormality, detailed examination indicates that degenerative changes are common. These changes include loss of apical mucus formation within epithelial cells and, less often, microerosions and ulcerations [96] (Fig. 12.4). Examination of semithin resin-embedded sections confirms this, showing cellular oedema, micropapillae, mucin loss and epithelial denudation. This is especially prominent in cells lining the upper foveolae and surface. The increased permeability of damaged surface epithelium may permit permeation of bacterial antigens and toxins and increase underlying mucosal inflammatory response and damage [97].

Lymphoid aggregates and, less often lymphoid follicles, are common features of *H. pylori* gastritis. These are located deep in the mucosa close to the muscularis mucosa and are a manifestation of local immune response [98]. They are more common in the antral mucosa than in the corpus and are also more common in cases of severe very active gastritis in comparison with mild or relatively inactive cases [99,100]. Estimates of the prevalence of lymphoid aggregates vary but one study based on multiple biopsies indicated that all patients with *H. pylori* have lymphoid follicles and that eradication of the organism leads to a slow decrease in their number [101]. The presence of lymphoid follicles or aggregates in a gastric biopsy should stimulate a search for *H. pylori*. Marked histological lymphoid hyperplasia sometimes resulting in antral nodularity on endoscopy is also a feature of *H. pylori* gastritis in children [86].

H. pylori are curved or S-shaped bacilli and in this form are often easily recognized on routine haematoxylin and eosin (H&E) staining. They are found within the surface mucus layer and are easiest to identify within gastric pits, but in cases of heavy infection are also numerous overlying the surface epithelium. Special stains are necessary when screening biopsies for *H. pylori* as they facilitate recognition, especially when small numbers are present, and help distinguish the bacteria from fibrin or debris on the mucosal surface. A variety of stains has been used. A modified Giemsa stain is simple and cheap [102] (Fig. 12.5). This is very satisfactory for routine use. The Warthin–Starry silver stain also gives satisfactory results, especially for photography, but is more difficult to carry out and more expensive. Other stains which have been used include cresyl violet, Giminez, fluorescent staining with acridine orange and the Brown–Hopps stain [103–106]. A combination of Steiner's silver stain, H&E and alcian blue has been suggested to allow good detection of the organism and simultaneously permit assessment of relevant gastric histology [107].

While recognition of *H. pylori* in the curved or S-shaped form is relatively easy, the coccoid form of the organism is

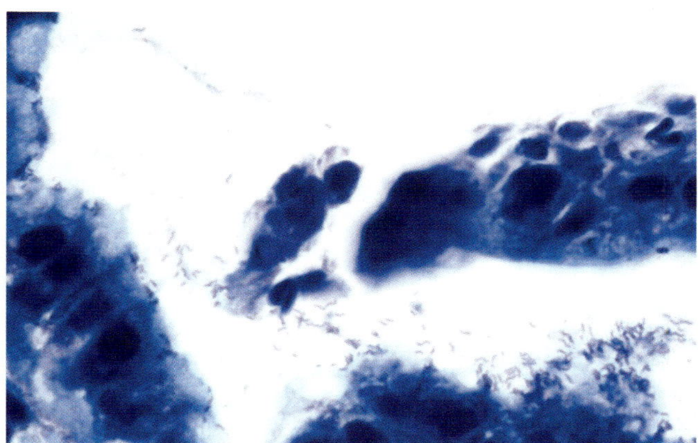

Fig. 12.5 *H. pylori* organisms on the surface of gastric mucosa showing the characteristic curved and S-shaped configuration. Giemsa, oil immersion.

much more difficult to recognize. On H&E staining it is basophilic and has a greater diameter than the bacillary form. Recognition can be enhanced by the use of special stains as the coccoid form has the same staining properties as the bacillary form [108]. Imunocytochemistry using commercially available antibody against *H. pylori* antigens is useful in problematical cases. It is highly sensitive but holds little advantage over cheaper stains in routine cases [109]. It is valuable, however, in identifying the coccoid form, especially if heat-induced antigen retrieval is used [110]. The polymerase chain reaction (PCR) has been applied to the detection of *H. pylori* in gastric biopsies. In some studies it was the most sensitive method of detection [111]. Surprisingly, in another study PCR proved less sensitive than Giemsa staining or immunocytochemistry [110].

H. pylori infection can be diagnosed clinically using a number of methods including several which are non-invasive [112]. With care a positive histological diagnosis is relatively easy and the sensitivity of histological diagnosis compares well with other methods. Histology has the added advantage of allowing assessment of the state of the gastric mucosa. *H. pylori* organisms are most numerous in the antrum in the majority of patients. The intensity of the associated gastritis is also most severe in this region. Organisms are usually more sparse in corpus biopsies and consequently more difficult to identify. In a minority of cases of long-term infection the converse is true in that the corpus is the site of maximum colonization and inflammation and the antrum is relatively spared. The organisms do not colonize normal duodenal mucosa; they are seldom found on islands of intestinal metaplasia in the stomach, except in occasional cases where the adjacent gastric epithelium is very heavily colonized. As a result where atrophic gastritis and extensive intestinal metaplasia develop after long-term infection the organisms may disappear.

The sensitivity of histological diagnosis may be affected by prior treatment with proton pump inhibitors (PPIs). These drugs appear to cause a shift of organisms proximally from antrum to corpus [113]. Thus examination of a single antral biopsy may give false-negative results. This can be avoided by examination of several biopsies from both antrum and corpus. As many patients may have received PPI therapy before coming to endoscopy, the recommendation that at least two biopsies are taken from both antrum and corpus is reinforced [65]. Long-term PPI therapy in patients with *H. pylori* infection also increases the inflammation in the gastric corpus and may accelerate development of atrophic gastritis [114].

Consequences of long-term *Helicobacter* infection

Eradication therapy is a relatively recent development and many patients are asymptomatic and do not present for treatment. Thus infection lasts for many years in large numbers of people. The evolution of the associated chronic active gastritis follows a number of different pathways. As a result the long-term effects on the gastric mucosa vary widely between different topographical regions of the stomach and between patients. It is only since the recognition of *H. pylori* as the common aetiological agent in different types of gastritis that the matter has been clarified to some extent. The variable outcomes of long-term *H. pylori* infection and the associated gastritis are considered below.

Spontaneous disappearance of the organism and subsequent regression of the chronic gastritis has been reported in approximately 10% of cases followed over several years [115–117]. It is uncertain if this is genuinely due to successful host defence mechanisms or to antibiotic therapy given for unrelated conditions.

In the great majority of patients the infection and the gastritis persist and result in a pangastritis involving both antrum and at least part of the corpus. The intensity of the inflammation and number of bacteria are usually higher in the antrum. Long-term studies indicate that the chronic gastritis changes little over the years or may decrease in intensity [116]. Other consequences of the chronic infection include atrophic gastritis, intestinal metaplasia, peptic ulceration and possibly gastric carcinoma or lymphoma. Peptic ulceration, gastric carcinoma and lymphoma are discussed in Chapters 13, 14 and 15, respectively, while atrophic gastritis and intestinal metaplasia are dealt with in the following sections.

On rare occasions *H. pylori* infection may be associated with enlargement of mucosal folds in the body of the stomach giving rise to endoscopic and radiological features suggestive of hypertrophic gastritis [118]. This so-called 'giant fold gastritis' differs histologically from true Menetrier's disease in that the mucosa is considerably thinner and foveolar hyperplasia is less marked [119]. Giant fold gastritis is also reported to be associated with histological and ultrastructural changes in parietal cells. These include dilated canaliculi, intracytoplasmic vacuole formation and loss and shortening of microvilli. Such changes revert to normal after eradication of the infection [119].

Atrophic gastritis

Chronic gastritis is a long-standing, changing condition showing progression, and, in some cases, regression with time. One of the commonest sequelae is the development of atrophic gastritis. This implies loss of mucosal glands and is frequently but not always associated with intestinal metaplasia. The aetiology of the condition is multifactorial.

Atrophic gastritis in its most extensive and severe form is seen in autoimmune atrophic gastritis which predominantly affects the corpus of the stomach leaving the antral mucosa relatively unscathed. This is discussed on p. 117. The prevalence and extent of atrophic gastritis also increases with age and with duration of chronic gastritis. The replacement of normal gastric mucosa by atrophic gastritis, intestinal metaplasia or dysplasia proceeds at a rate of about 3.3% per year in a population at high risk for gastric carcinoma [120]. Similarly in autoimmune atrophic gastritis associated with pernicious anaemia there is rapid progression from the age of 50 onwards. A similar, but much less marked trend is seen in control subjects [121].

H. pylori infection has recently emerged as a key aetiological factor in atrophic gastritis. *H. pylori* infection shows a strong association with increased risk of both atrophic gastritis and intestinal metaplasia of the gastric mucosa [82,122]. Long-term studies indicate that *H. pylori* gastritis may progress to atrophic gastritis and intestinal metaplasia and these conditions are significantly more common in patients with *H. pylori* infection in comparison with uninfected subjects [123]. Gastric acid secretion also diminishes in association with atrophic gastritis in chronic *H. pylori* infection [124]. Rugge *et al.* concluded that the increasing prevalence of intestinal metaplasia with age is due to *H. pylori* infection. They also noted that bacterial colonization of the gastric corpus mucosa is associated with extensive atrophic gastritis and intestinal metaplasia of the antrum [125]. CagA-positive strains of *H. pylori* are associated not only with increasing intensity of inflammation, but with an increased likelihood of development of atrophic gastritis and intestinal metaplasia over the long term [126].

On gross or endoscopic examination the gastric mucosa may show little change in early or mild atrophic gastritis because atrophic changes are patchy and multifocal. The lesser curvature, in the region of the incisura angularis, tends to be affected first with subsequent spread and coalescence of lesions especially in the junction between antrum and corpus [127]. The association between *H. pylori* infection, especially that involving CagA-positive strains, and antral predominant atrophic gastritis is well established. Severe atrophy affecting gastric corpus mucosa is more likely to be associated with autoimmune gastritis, manifested by parietal cell antibodies and low serum pepsinogen I levels rather than *H. pylori* infection. [128]. However in *H. pylori*-infected patients there is a subgroup in whom bacterial colonization and gastritis are more widespread and involve the corpus. This is accompanied by hypochlorhydria and increased prevalence and extent of atrophic gastritis and intestinal metaplasia in the corpus [129].

Histology

The essential histological feature of atrophic gastritis is loss of specialized glands and cells within the mucosa. The inflammatory cell content is very variable. This may range from large numbers of chronic inflammatory cells within the lamina propria together with some polymorphs in active atrophic gastritis, to a sparse infiltrate of plasma cells and lymphocytes in quiescent severe atrophic gastritis. The degree of glandular loss can be graded as mild, moderate or severe as suggested in the Sydney system [65]. Recognition and assessment of atrophy is subjective. In the gastric corpus patchy loss of parietal and chief cells is accompanied by increased space between glands occupied by inflammatory cells or later by loose connective tissue (Fig. 12.6). This is relatively easy to recognize, especially in moderate to severe cases. Antral atrophy can be more difficult to assess. As the normal mucosa in this region is composed of deep foveolae and mucus glands with a stroma of loose connective tissue, minor degrees of glandular loss are hard to appreciate. A reduction in the number of coils of mucosal glands between the base of the foveolae and the muscularis mucosa is a useful histological feature. The difficulty is compounded in the presence of an intense inflammatory cell infiltrate within the lamina propria which is often present in *H. pylori* infection. In such circumstances it is difficult to decide if there is actual glandular loss or simply separation of glands by inflammatory cells. A reticulin stain may be useful in assessing the degree of glandular atrophy [62] and

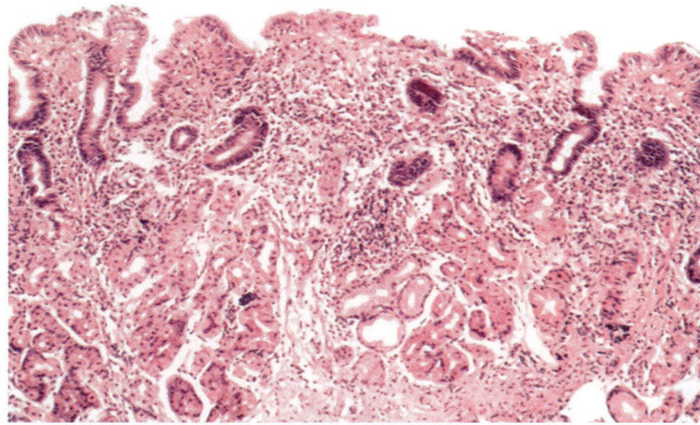

Fig. 12.6 Moderate atrophic gastritis of gastric corpus mucosa in chronic *H. pylori* infection showing loss of groups of parietal cells in association with active inflammation. Connective tissue has replaced the lost cells.

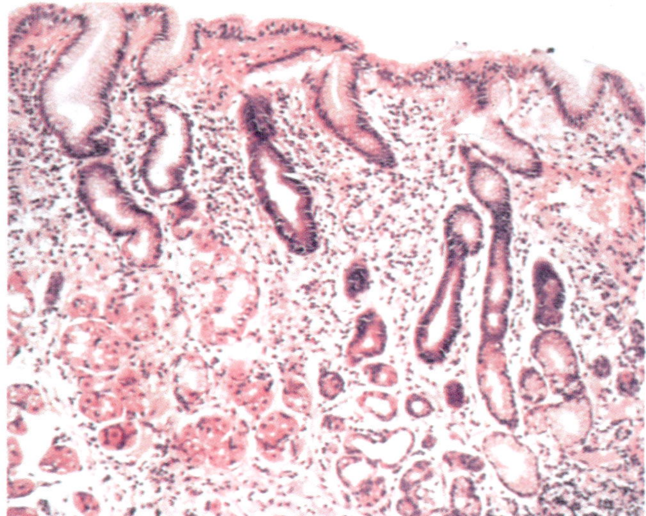

Fig. 12.7 Pyloric metaplasia in gastric corpus mucosa showing replacement of parietal cells by antral-type mucosa.

the use of a visual analogue scale using diagrams as a template for assessing the degree of atrophy may also prove helpful [130]. Nonetheless, even among experts the grading of the degrees of gastric atrophy shows considerable interobserver variation especially in mild and moderate atrophy affecting the antrum [131].

Chronic gastritis is a dynamic rather than a stable process and thus atrophic gastritis is likely to progress. Long-term studies indicate that in general, although atrophic changes in the antrum may regress, within the corpus of the stomach, atrophy tends to increase in severity. This progression slows down markedly in patients over 60 years of age [132]. Atrophic gastritis in the corpus of the stomach is accompanied by focal pyloric (sometimes called 'pseudopyloric') metaplasia. In this condition parietal and chief cells are replaced by seromucinous glands of pyloric type (Fig. 12.7). As a result biopsies taken from the body mucosa may be interpreted as coming from the antral region. It is uncertain whether this represents true metaplasia as it has been suggested that these foci of pyloric-type glands are derived from the ulcer-associated cell lineage (UACL) (see p. 106).

Foci of intestinal metaplasia commonly accompany *H. pylori*-associated atrophic gastritis. These islands of metaplastic epithelium occur in both antrum and corpus and tend to increase in extent with increasing age. *H. pylori* do not usually colonize mucosa which has undergone intestinal metaplasia. Thus as the extent of the metaplasia increases the bacteria become less obvious and may eventually disappear. It has been widely considered that bacteria are invariably absent from the surface of intestinal metaplasia and that intestinalization of the mucosa may be a defence mechanism whereby the body can eventually rid itself of this prolonged infection. This is not always the case, however, and *H. pylori* have occasionally been identified on the surface of metaplastic mucosa [133]. Recently this has been confirmed, and in a small proportion of cases *H. pylori* have been identified on the surface of incomplete intestinal metaplasia but not on complete intestinal metaplasia [134].

Pathogenesis

The reasons why there is such diversity in the evolution of chronic *H. pylori* gastritis are not fully understood. There is considerable geographical variation in the development of atrophic gastritis. Within China the prevalence of atrophy varies considerably from one region to another and correlates with a high prevalence of gastric cancer. In contrast, atrophic changes are less common in an area with a high prevalence of duodenal ulceration [135]. Acid secretion may be an important determinant factor of the course of chronic gastritis [136]. Atrophic gastritis is the most significant factor related to decreased acid secretion. As there is a strong association between *H. pylori* infection and atrophic gastritis, *H. pylori* rather than ageing *per se* is an important cause of diminished acid secretion [124]. Local acid production whether diminished or increased may determine the location of the organism within the stomach and subsequently the severity of inflammation. It is postulated that patients with predominantly antral gastritis have hypersecretion of gastric acid and are thus at a greater risk of duodenal ulcer. In contrast, patients with pangastritis predominantly affecting the corpus may develop atrophic gastritis of the corpus with hyposecretion of gastric acid and subsequently relatively mild inflammation of the antral mucosa. These patients are at greater risk of gastric ulcer and possibly gastric cancer [136,137]. There is a suggestion that prolonged therapy with proton pump inhibitors with subsequent profound suppression of acid secretion leads to increasingly active inflammation in *H. pylori* gastritis and increased development of atrophic gastritis [114]. This, however, remains unresolved.

Host factors almost certainly play an important role. Recent evidence suggests that interleukin gene cluster polymorphisms which are associated with increased production of the proinflammatory cytokine interleukin-1-beta (IL-1β) may predispose to hypochlorhydria, atrophy of corpus mucosa and increased risk of gastric cancer [138]. IL-1β is a potent inhibitor of gastric acid secretion and may facilitate spread of *H. pylori* organisms to the corpus of the stomach.

Other factors related to both host and environment which may influence progression to atrophic gastritis include salt intake and antioxidants [127]. There is little evidence that antiparietal cell antibodies play a significant part in the development of atrophic gastritis of the corpus in *H. pylori* gastritis [139]. *H. pylori* infection is rare in patients with pernicious anaemia [140,141]. However, many patients with *H. pylori*-associated atrophic gastritis are reported to have autoantibodies against surface epithelial cells and parietal cell canaliculi.

Close antigenic similarity between gastric antigens and some strains of *H. pylori* may produce cross-reacting autoantibodies which promote progression to atrophic gastritis [142].

In some patients with atrophic gastritis the lymphoid follicles described previously in association with chronic *H. pylori* gastritis are very conspicuous. This has been referred to as follicular gastritis but it is a variant of chronic gastritis and is not a separate entity. Chronic cystic gastritis is another rare variant of atrophic gastritis, though the occasional mucosal cyst is not an infrequent finding in gastrectomy specimens for cancer or benign peptic disease. Cysts may be lined by foveolar, pyloric gland, fundic gland, intestinal metaplastic or ciliated epithelium [143]. Fundic gland cysts have become much more common recently due to the association with proton pump inhibitors.

Hyperplastic (regenerative) polyps are a relatively rare complication of chronic gastritis. They may be multiple or single. When large numbers are present a state of 'gastritis polyposi' is said to have developed. There is still no adequate explanation for the development of epithelial hyperplasia, either diffuse or polypoid, in a condition that normally proceeds to a state of mucosal atrophy.

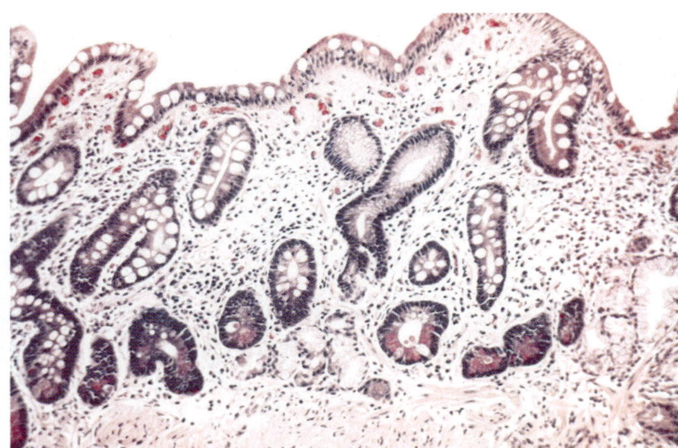

Fig. 12.8 Gastric atrophy with extensive intestinal metaplasia.

Gastric atrophy

Atrophy of the gastric mucosa can be the end-result of chronic gastritis or autoimmune gastritis or idiopathic, perhaps as an age change in the elderly. The difficulty in assessing and grading atrophic gastritis has already been mentioned. This is compounded by lack of definition and precise understanding of terms such as atrophic gastritis and gastric atrophy. Here, gastric atrophy is intended to represent the end-result of severe long-standing chronic atrophic gastritis. Most cases are associated with autoimmune gastritis. *H. pylori*-associated gastritis on account of its patchy nature only rarely gives rise to such widespread changes. Gastric atrophy is extensive rather than focal. The mucosa is greatly reduced in depth especially in the corpus and the normal mucosal folds are diminished or absent resulting in a flat mucosal surface. Parietal and chief cells are markedly reduced or absent in the corpus and in the antrum only a few pyloric glands remain. Intestinal metaplasia is extensive (Fig. 12.8). There may be cystic change within glands with extension of cystic epithelium through the muscularis mucosa. In such end-stage cases there is little or no inflammatory infiltrate in the lamina propria although there may be lymphoid aggregates. Tubules are lined by gastric crypt or intestinal epithelium.

Intestinal metaplasia (IM)

Metaplasia is the replacement of one tissue by another during postnatal life. Intestinal metaplasia within the stomach represents the replacement of gastric-type mucosa by mucosa that closely resembles that of the intestine, usually the small intestine.

In the early part of the 20th century it was argued whether intestinalized epithelium within gastric mucosa represented a congenital heterotopia or an acquired metaplasia. The latter view was supported by the failure to demonstrate foci of intestinalized mucosa within entirely normal gastric mucosa or within fetal stomachs [144] and now has universal acceptance. Numerous studies have demonstrated the association between chronic gastritis and intestinal metaplasia and have shown also that the extent of intestinalization increases with age [145–148]. IM occurs during the phase of active tissue growth, for example during regeneration following gastric injury. In long-standing conditions such as *H. pylori* infection, the chronic influence of epithelial damage and persistent neutrophil infiltration with subsequent tissue damage, coupled with reduced local concentration of antioxidants such as ascorbic acid, leads to increased regenerative activity. This persistent stimulation of regeneration associated with other mutagenic influences such as nitroso compounds and with increasing age may lead in some cases to faulty regeneration resulting in intestinal metaplasia [149,150]. Intestinalized epithelium may include all the cell types found in normal small intestine. Furthermore the change must be heritable on cell division. It is therefore clear that IM is due to an alteration at the level of the stem cell. It is not yet established whether the change in developmental commitment of the stem cell population is due to a somatic mutation or an epigenetic modulation. A non-mutational theory involving biochemical switches has been proposed [151]. Such a theory would be consistent with the possibility that IM is an adaptive phenomenon, influenced by and therefore mirroring changes in the gastric microenvironment [152].

IM arises in association with a number of different conditions that affect the gastric mucosa. It is frequently found in association with atrophic gastritis and the severity and extent of atrophic gastritis is paralleled by the severity of IM [153]. Thus it is not surprising that IM is often extensive in autoimmune gastritis where the corpus of the stomach shows extensive atrophic gastritis. IM is also associated with bile reflux and a correlation between bile reflux and prevalence and severity of IM has been demonstrated [154]. However, autoimmune gastritis and bile reflux-associated gastritis are less prevalent than *H. pylori*-related chronic gastritis and there is little doubt that the latter is an important aetiological condition associated with intestinal metaplasia. The prevalence and extent of intestinal metaplasia increases with advancing age [155]. In a high-risk population such as Japan the condition is rare before the age of 30 years but very prevalent at 60 and above [156]. However, even after adjusting for age, *H. pylori* infection is a highly significant predictor of more extensive intestinal metaplasia [125]. IM is reported to occur at a significantly younger age in *H. pylori*-infected patients than in those who are *H. pylori* negative [157] and a strong association between *H. pylori* infection and increased prevalence and extent of intestinal metaplasia has been demonstrated in several studies [122,123,125]. Even in the presence of *H. pylori* there is considerable difference in the prevalence of antral IM in different disease groups. IM is much more prevalent in patients with gastric or pyloric ulcers than in those with uncomplicated gastritis or duodenal ulceration [149]. Paradoxically *H. pylori* organisms seldom colonize foci of IM so in cases of extensive IM *H. pylori* organisms may not be present although they may have been the precipitating factor. The organisms are occasionally seen on the surface of areas of incomplete IM [134].

IM is common and is reported to occur in over 20% of gastric biopsies [158] although it should again be emphasized that it is rare in patients under 30 years of age. It is also common in Barrett's oesophagus and in biopsies taken in the region of the gastro-oesophageal junction [159]. Like atrophic gastritis, IM is patchy and arises initially on the lesser curvature in the region of the incisura angularis and may then expand both proximally and distally thus involving both antrum and corpus [70,160]. It is more common and more extensive in antral than in corpus mucosa [161,162]. On account of this patchy distribution, several biopsies from both antrum and corpus are needed to properly assess the extent of the metaplasia and it is recommended that, like other variables in the Sydney system, it should be graded as mild, moderate or severe. The use of visual analogue scales makes this easier and more reproducible [70].

Although IM is easily recognized on H&E stain by the presence of goblet cells, the use of the alcian blue/PAS stain greatly facilitates identification of small inconspicuous foci in routine biopsies. Mucin histochemistry is essential for the subtyping of intestinal metaplasia and is based on recognition of neutral or acid mucins. The latter are subdivided into sialomucins or sulphomucins. While alcian blue pH 2.5/PAS will distinguish acid from neutral mucins, it will not distinguish sialo- from sulphomucins. A combination of high iron diamine and alcian blue (HID/AB) stains can be used for this purpose. Within this combination sialomucins stain blue and sulphomucins brown. A detailed description of the mucin histochemistry of the gastrointestinal tract is given by Filipe and Ramachandra [163]. HID/AB is an overnight stain and entails the use of potentially toxic reagents. The combination of Gomori's aldehyde fuchsin and alcian blue (GAF/AB) has recently been suggested as an alternative. This stains sialomucins blue and sulphomucins purple. It is highly specific and reasonably sensitive for detection of sulphomucins in comparison with HID/AB. The colour distinction of blue and purple is subtler than the blue and brown of HID-AB and requires good colour perception. This potential disadvantage may be outweighed by the convenience of the stain in that it can be performed much more quickly and more cheaply than HID/AB [164].

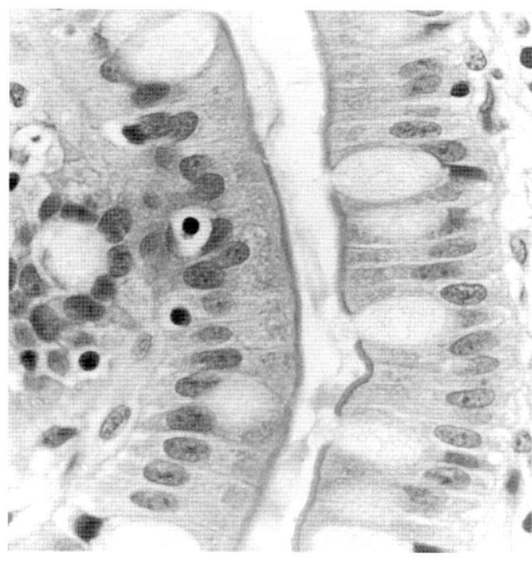

Fig. 12.9 Complete intestinal metaplasia.

Considerable heterogeneity consists within the entity of intestinal metaplasia. The variants have been classified into complete and incomplete [165,166]. The present classification consists of type I (complete) and types II and III (incomplete). Type I (complete) closely resembles normal small intestinal mucosa with goblet cells and absorptive cells with a brush border (Fig. 12.9). Paneth cells are also frequently present. In this type of metaplasia goblet cells secrete acid mucins which can be demonstrated using alcian blue/PAS stain. (Acid mucins stain blue while the normal gastric neutral mucin stains red.)

In incomplete intestinal metaplasia the typical intestinal enterocytes are replaced by a population of partially differentiated columnar mucus cells (intermediate cells) lacking a well developed brush border (Fig. 12.10) and some of the associated brush border enzymes, notably alkaline phosphatase and trehalase [167]. In addition, Paneth cells are seldom present. On the basis of the mucin histochemistry of the columnar cell

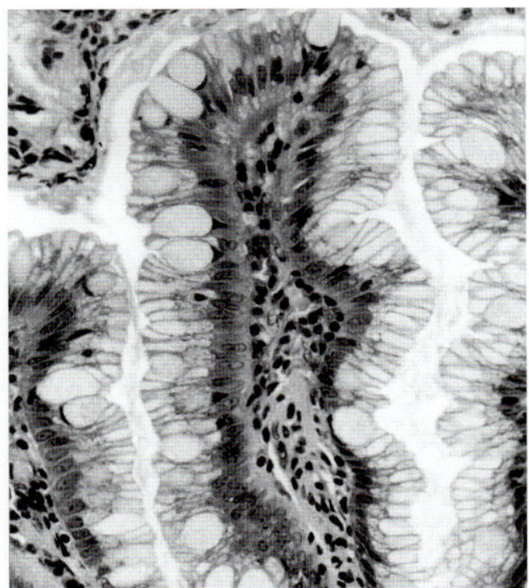

Fig. 12.10 Incomplete intestinal metaplasia.

population, incomplete metaplasia is divided into types II and III [166].

Type II shows some glandular distortion and consists of goblet cells and columnar mucus cells secreting sialomucins. The goblet cells may also occasionally secrete sulphomucins. There are few absorptive cells. Type III is the least common and is distinguished by the presence of glandular distortion and columnar mucus cells containing sulphomucins. The goblet cells secrete either sialo- or sulphomucins. This may be significant as cases containing sulphomucins in both goblet cells and columnar cells may have a higher risk of developing gastric cancer [168]. As stated above either the HID/AB or GAF/AB stain is needed to distinguish between type II and type III intestinal metaplasia (Figs 12.11a,b).

There is evidence of a hyperproliferative state in gastric mucosa showing chronic atrophic gastritis and in intestinal metaplasia [169–171]. Of the variants of intestinal metaplasia, only type III shows a selective association with gastric carcinoma and more especially with the intestinal type of carcinoma [158,165,168]. An association between type III intestinal metaplasia, dysplasia and early gastric cancer of intestinal type with evidence of p53 gene mutation in dysplasia and cancer has been demonstrated. This may indicate serious disturbance in cellular control mechanisms in this variant of intestinal metaplasia [162]. However the predictive value of type III intestinal metaplasia for gastric carcinoma is limited [172]. A very well differentiated intestinal-type carcinoma arising in a background of complete (type I) intestinal metaplasia has also been described [173]. The relationship between chronic gastritis, intestinal metaplasia and gastric carcinoma is discussed further in Chapter 14.

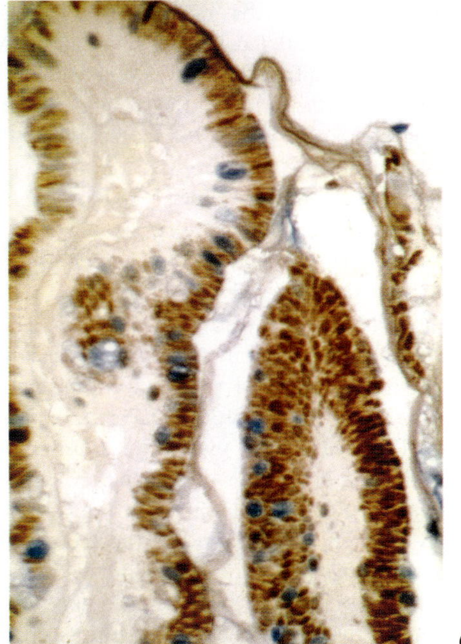

(a)

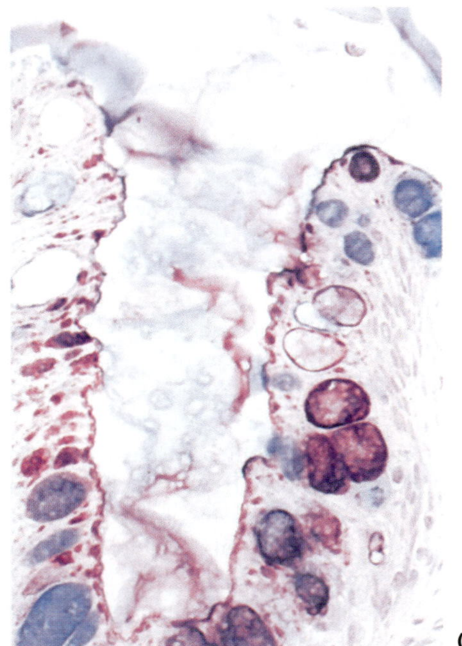

(b)

Fig. 12.11 (a) Type III intestinal metaplasia showing sulphomucin (brown) mainly in columnar cells and some goblet cells. Most goblet cells contain sialomucin (blue). (b) Type III intestinal metaplasia stained by Gomori's aldehyde fuchsin showing sulphomucins (purple) in columnar cells and in some goblet cells. Other goblet cells contain sialomucin (blue).

Pancreatic metaplasia

In addition to pyloric and intestinal metaplasia, foci of pancreatic acinar metaplasia within the stomach have been described in association with chronic gastritis [174]. These cells, showing characteristic features of acinar cells on light and electron microscopy and immunoreactivity for pancreatic lipase trypsinogen occur most frequently within pyloric mucosa affected by active chronic gastritis and atrophic gastritis. Such foci have also been noted in the cardia and fundus. The most frequent association is with *H. pylori* infection but pancreatic metaplasia was also reported in the fundus in autoimmune gastritis.

Topography of chronic gastritis and intestinal metaplasia and its relation to aetiology

The distribution of chronic gastritis varies from patient to patient but there is a pattern to this variability which is influenced by the underlying aetiology of the condition. In atrophic gastritis the mucosa may be flattened with some loss of the rugose pattern but flattening becomes more obvious in advanced gastric atrophy. In pernicious anaemia or autoimmune type A gastritis, changes are limited to the body of the stomach and are accompanied by thinning of the muscle coats. In *H. pylori*-associated chronic gastritis, especially in patients with duodenal ulcer, the changes are most commonly found in the antrum, and although a pangastritis may eventually develop the corpus is involved to a relatively minor degree with little accompanying atrophic gastritis. The reported prevalence of atrophic gastritis in *H. pylori*-infected patients is around 40% [128]. In a minority of patients, however, *H. pylori* infection can lead to extensive atrophic gastritis in the corpus of the stomach eventually leading to diminished acid output [93,175]. It is suggested that antral predominant gastritis is associated with gastric acid hypersecretion and a consequent risk of duodenal ulcer. In contrast, when *H. pylori* infection is more extensive in the corpus of the stomach, the development of atrophic gastritis in that area may lead to hypochlorhydria and increasingly more extensive IM with a subsequent increased risk of gastric carcinoma [137].

This issue is further complicated by evidence that active chronic gastritis involving the corpus of the stomach exerts a protective effect against reflux oesophagitis [176]. The likely mechanism of this is reduced acid secretion. As there is a correlation between reflux oesophagitis symptoms and subsequent development of oesophageal adenocarcinoma [177] the possibility arises that chronic gastritis affecting the gastric corpus may have a protective effect against this rapidly increasing disease.

The IM which frequently accompanies chronic atrophic gastritis is found mainly at the antrocorporal junction, at first occurring in small islands especially on the lesser curvature. Later the islands coalesce and the area of metaplasia increases and extends both proximally and distally [160,178]. Intestinal metaplasia is more generalized in stomachs harbouring a gastric cancer, often surrounding the tumour and extending into the body mucosa [146,179]. Mucosa showing intestinal metaplasia may become irregular, pebbled or even polypoid and the metaplastic areas may appear redder than the surrounding mucosa. The extent of intestinal metaplasia can be appreciated more readily by the macroscopic demonstration of small intestinal brush border enzymes *in vitro* [167,180,181].

Autoimmune gastritis and pernicious anaemia

Autoimmune or type A gastritis [63] is characterized by achlorhydria and by predominant involvement of the body mucosa with antral sparing. A high proportion of patients have circulating autoantibodies against the microsomes of (acid-secreting) parietal cells [182,183]. The parietal cells secrete, in addition to hydrochloric acid, a glycoprotein called intrinsic factor which plays a key role in the absorption of vitamin B_{12}. Intrinsic factor autoantibodies are detected in 55–60% of patients with autoimmune gastritis [184,185] and are of two types. The more common inhibits the attachment of B_{12} to intrinsic factor and the other binds the intrinsic factor/B_{12} complex, thereby interfering with its absorption within the small intestine. Thus a proportion of patients with type A chronic gastritis will develop pernicious anaemia due to vitamin B_{12} deficiency. It has been suggested that in cases where serum antibodies are not detectable, they may be present as cell-bound antibodies in the small intestinal mucosa [186]. Serum levels of pepsinogen I, which is secreted exclusively by the chief cells of the body glands, are reduced whereas serum levels of pepsinogen II, which is produced by both body and pyloric glands, remain relatively normal. An additional serum marker is a raised fasting serum gastrin level which is accompanied by G-cell hyperplasia in the gastric antrum [187]. Not uncommonly there is clinical or serological evidence of other organ-specific autoimmune diseases including Hashimoto's thyroiditis and adrenal Addison's disease [188]. In the first-degree relatives of patients with pernicious anaemia, chronic atrophic gastritis of body mucosa, achlorhydria, parietal cell antibodies and a raised serum gastrin are encountered more frequently than in control subjects [189]. This would support the view that genetic factors play an important role in the aetiology of autoimmune gastritis.

In advanced cases the body of the stomach shows severe atrophy of all coats including the muscle. The corpus mucosa is markedly flattened (Fig. 12.12). The pylorus remains relatively normal and there is a sharp line of transition between the two [190,191]. These appearances are sufficiently striking to be diagnostic to the naked eye. The thickness of the mucosa of the corpus becomes reduced by approximately 20% in advanced cases. Although the mucosa is thinned, a pebbled appearance may be apparent at endoscopy, the elevations being islands of intestinal metaplasia. The gastritis is a dynamic process in which involvement of the corpus mucosa increases in severity with age, yet the antral mucosal changes do not progress to any great extent and may even regress [121]. The corpus changes are those of superficial gastritis, atrophic gastritis or gastric atrophy in various stages as the condition

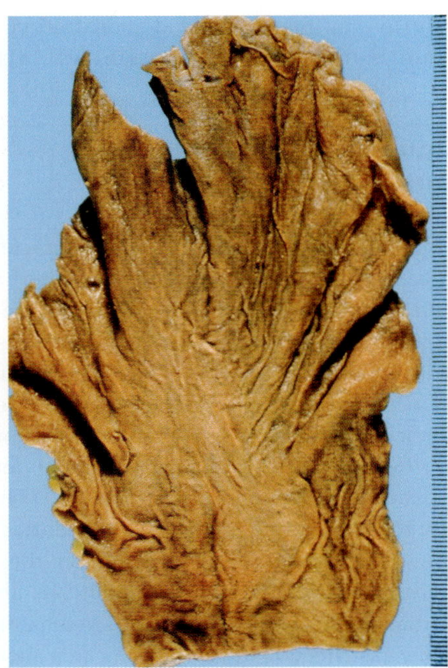

Fig. 12.12 Corpus of stomach in autoimmune atrophic gastritis. The mucosal surface is flat and featureless and the gastric wall is thinned.

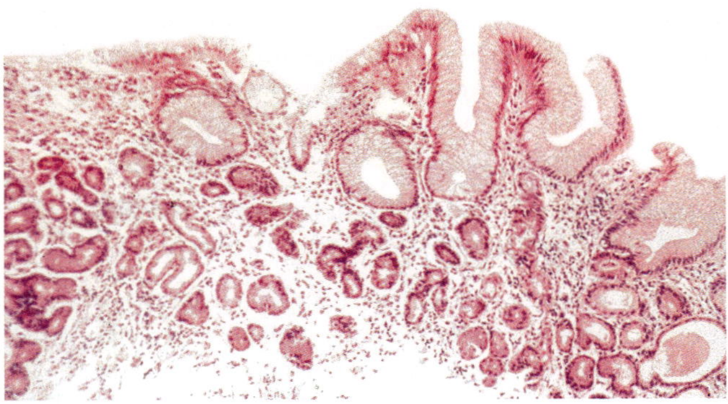

Fig. 12.13 Gastric corpus mucosa in autoimmune gastritis. There is severe atrophic gastritis with almost total loss of parietal cells and replacement by pyloric-type mucosa. Some glands show cystic dilatation and there is a lymphocytic infiltrate. Intestinal metaplasia is also focally present.

progresses. The inflammatory infiltrate, which is prominent in the earlier stages of chronic superficial gastritis and atrophic gastritis, consists mainly of lymphocytes, eosinophils and plasma cells. Neutrophils are not prominent. The inflammation involves the superficial mucosa in early stages but later the full thickness of the mucosa. Immunohistochemical studies have demonstrated an absolute increase in T and more notably B lymphocytes [192] and an increased ratio of IgG-: IgA-secreting plasma cells [193]. Superficial gastritis in corpus mucosa tends to increase with age up to around 50 years of age but then diminishes. In contrast atrophic gastritis affecting the mucosa increases in severity and extent after the age of 50 [121].

Atrophic changes are characterized by glandular loss; however, small numbers of parietal and chief cells may be present even in patients with established pernicious anaemia. Both pyloric and intestinal metaplasia are present, the former change being more frequent and extensive [194] (Fig. 12.13). Nonetheless intestinal metaplasia is seen in the corpus mucosa in around 75% of cases [195]. Retention-type cysts lined by mucus cells are common in the mucosa and may be present in the submucosa as well. In the antrum inflammatory changes in the mucosa are quite common but tend to be mild [140,195]. There is an absolute increase in the number of antral gastrin cells (G cells) in response to the hypochlorhydria and this is accompanied by raised serum levels of gastrin [187]. However, in patients with coincident antral atrophic gastritis G-cell numbers may be reduced as are the serum gastrin levels [196].

The hypergastrinaemia has a trophic effect on the enterochromaffin-like (ECL) cells which are present in the glands of body mucosa [197], leading to ECL cell hyperplasia within body mucosa. This starts within the gastric glands but later extends to include small nodules of endocrine cells in the lamina propria. Some of these nodules may bud off from adjacent glands (enteroendocrine cells) whereas others show more neural characteristics suggesting an origin from the neuroendocrine plexus of the lamina propria [198]. In addition to histamine, the latter may occasionally contain other peptides (such as gastrin, vasoactive intestinal polypeptide (VIP) and substance P) and as many as nine morphologically distinct types of granules have been identified at the ultrastructural level [198]. Single or more usually multiple neuroendocrine tumours may occasionally develop within this background of linear and nodular endocrine cell hyperplasia [199,200]. These present as small polyps which are non-functioning and grow extremely slowly. Metastases occur late in the course of the disease if at all, and are usually associated with tumours greater than 2 cm in diameter and invading the wall of the stomach. Other conditions causing hypergastrinaemia, such as the Zollinger–Ellison syndrome, may similarly predispose to ECL cell hyperplasia of the corpus and multiple carcinoids. This is discussed in more detail in Chapter 14.

Endoscopic examination of patients with pernicious anaemia leads, not infrequently, to the discovery of other types of polyp that are usually multiple, small and confined to the atrophic body mucosa in 20–37% of patients [189,201,202]. Many are hyperplastic polyps or merely represent persisting islands of body-type mucosa within a background of atrophy. The latter condition has been described as gastric pseudopolyposis and has been observed to regress with further progression of the atrophic gastritis [203]. Nevertheless, true neoplastic epithelial polyps are commoner in pernicious anaemia and one report described moderate to severe dysplasia within endoscopically visible lesions from either antrum or body of 11% of patients with pernicious anaemia [202]. The risk of gastric carcinoma developing in patients with pernicious anaemia and autoimmune gastritis is about three times that of the general population [204].

Whilst immunological factors must play an important role in the aetiology of autoimmune chronic gastritis (type A gastritis), the precise mechanisms are not understood. It has been suggested that *H. pylori* gastritis may be involved in the early stages of pernicious anaemia-associated gastritis and that autoimmune mechanisms then contribute in the progression to severe atrophic gastritis of the corpus [205]. This is difficult to prove or disprove but the prevalence of *H. pylori* infection is undoubtedly much lower in autoimmune atrophic gastritis than in the general population [140,195]. While this may be due to the extensive intestinal metaplasia or achlorhydria seen in advanced stages of the condition, it does not suggest that *H. pylori* plays a major role [206].

Juvenile forms of pernicious anaemia

These rare conditions may occur in three different forms [207]. One, occurring in later childhood and adolescence, is associated with gastric atrophy and appears to represent the adult type with an unusually early age of onset. In the second, sometimes called 'true' juvenile pernicious anaemia, intrinsic factor is not secreted by parietal cells but the mucosa is histologically normal. Acid secretion is normal when vitamin B_{12} is given, though it may be reduced without it. Vitamin B_{12} is absorbed from the small intestine if intrinsic factor is added to the diet [208–210]. The failure to secrete intrinsic factor is not explained by the presence of an autoantibody. The third type results from the failure to absorb vitamin B_{12}–intrinsic factor complex [211].

The stomach in other types of megaloblastic anaemia

Infestation with *Diphyllobothrium latum* occurs in Scandinavian countries, producing a megaloblastic anaemia. The gastric mucosa shows varying degrees of atrophic gastritis with superficial inflammation and zones of intestinal metaplasia [212]. The condition closely resembles pernicious anaemia.

Reactive gastritis

Attention was drawn to this type of gastritis by Dixon and colleagues who described a series of histological changes in the gastric mucosa of patients who had undergone previous gastric surgery for peptic ulcer [213]. The changes described were associated with reflux of bile into the stomach. Similar changes were later recognized in association with long-term ingestion of non-steroidal anti-inflammatory drugs (NSAIDs) [214,215]. Dixon and his colleagues put forward the term chemical (or type C) gastritis as the changes were associated with exposure to bile, alcohol or drugs, and they proposed a very convenient ABC classification of the commonest forms of chronic gastritis—A (autoimmune), B (bacterial) and C (chemical) [215,216]. Unfortunately the term 'chemical gastritis' has not gained universal acceptance and the alphabetical designation of different types of gastritis has been abandoned in the Sydney system of classification. The term 'reactive gastritis' is more commonly used, although synonyms which persist include reflux, NSAID or chemical gastritis. Some authorities consider that the term 'gastritis' should be reserved only for conditions characterized by inflammation. In the absence of inflammation (which is the case in reactive gastritis), the term 'gastropathy' has been suggested as being more suitable [45]. Thus the terms 'chemical gastropathy' or 'reactive gastropathy' may be added to the list of synonyms. Nonetheless 'reactive gastritis' remains widely used.

The condition is seen in its most severe form in biopsies taken from gastric mucosa proximal to a previously performed gastroenteric anastomosis. In most instances, however, changes are much more subtle. A history of NSAID ingestion may be present and if not, should be suggested in the pathologist's report. However reactive gastritis may occur in association with a variety of other conditions. It is found in some cases of heavy alcohol ingestion [215] and in almost 10% of healthy volunteers with no history of drug ingestion [217].

The histological features have been described in some detail [76,213]. They comprise foveolar hyperplasia, vascular congestion, oedema of the lamina propria, prominence of smooth muscle within the lamina propria and a reduction in numbers of inflammatory cells. There is elongation and increased tortuosity of the foveolae, otherwise known as the gastric pits, especially in the antrum. In addition there may be hyperchromatism and enlargement of the nuclei of the mucous lining cells, features that may sometimes be sufficiently marked to be confused with dysplasia (Fig. 12.14). It is possible that the oedema may serve to make normal smooth muscle cells more prominent but it has been postulated that real smooth muscle proliferation could be due to platelet-derived growth factor released by repeated leakage from vessels due to bile damage or repeated surface erosions caused by NSAIDs [76]. Oedema is especially marked in gastric mucosa adjacent to a gastroenterostomy stoma. Reduction in the number of inflammatory cells within the lamina propria in reactive gastritis may also be more apparent than real, again resulting from the accompanying oedema, but this is a consistent and often striking feature provided concomitant *H. pylori* infection is not present. Moreover, it has been noted that biopsies taken adjacent to mucosal ulcers caused by chronic salicylate use also show surprisingly

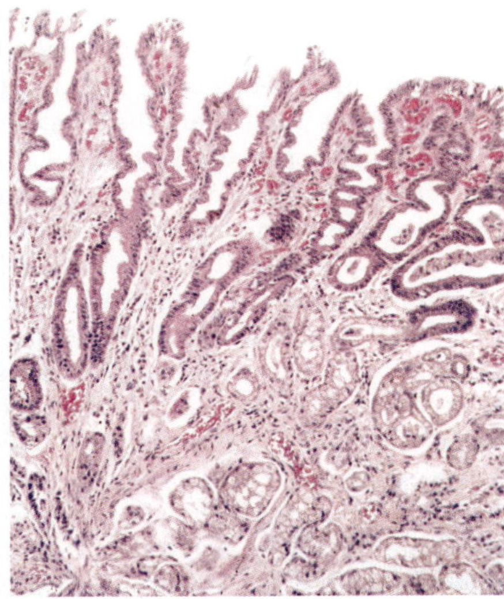

Fig. 12.14 Reactive gastritis. There is foveolar hyperplasia and tortuosity with hyperchromatism of surface epithelial cells. The lamina propria is oedematous and contains occasional elongated spindle-shaped smooth muscle cells.

little inflammation of the mucosa [218]. While many of the histological features of reactive gastritis are subjective, there is good correlation with biochemical evidence of bile reflux when formal scoring systems are used [215]. Nevertheless, it is sometimes difficult to distinguish mild changes from normality and the pathologist should be cautious of overdiagnosing this condition.

There is no doubt that *H. pylori* infection may coexist with reactive gastritis and in such cases the oedema and smooth muscle may be obscured and the paucity of inflammatory cells completely reversed. *H. pylori* infection is frequently found in patients taking NSAIDs and increases the likelihood of NSAID-induced mucosal damage [219]. In contrast, reactive gastritis in the postoperative stomach due to significant bile reflux is seldom colonized by *H. pylori* [79]. Although the association between reactive gastritis and NSAID ingestion is established, sensitivity is low. Using a semiquantitative technique based on severity of each of the histological features [213], a diagnosis of reactive gastritis was possible in only around one-third of NSAID users [217]. The most consistent abnormalities seen in mucosal biopsies in such cases were foveolar hyperplasia and prominent smooth muscle fibres in the lamina propria.

Chronic gastritis in the operated stomach

Reactive gastritis is seen in its most florid form in the operated stomach. In this situation the histological features are frequently exaggerated and foveolar hyperplasia is especially prominent. It has been suggested that duodenogastric reflux is the cause but similar histological changes are seen in the solitary ulcer syndrome of the rectum and some of the changes may be secondary to mucosal prolapse through the stoma. Cystic change of the gastric mucosa proximal to the stoma is also well recognized and may be florid such that cystically dilated glands become displaced into the submucosa or even external muscle coat. This may result in the formation of a polyp or tumour which should be distinguished carefully from adenocarcinoma. The condition has been described as gastritis cystica polyposa or profunda [220]. Typical hyperplastic polyps, either single or multiple, have been reported in about 10% of patients at long-term follow-up [221,222].

There is an increased relative risk of carcinoma developing in the gastric stump although this only becomes apparent when about 20 years has elapsed following partial gastrectomy. Epithelial dysplasia is a precancerous lesion which may help to identify patients at increased risk and while it may take the form of a sessile adenoma [223] it is more often described within flat mucosa [224]. The distinction between genuine dysplasia and the much commoner reactive atypia in foveolar hyperplasia with regenerative change can be very difficult and is almost certainly responsible for some reports claiming a high prevalence of postgastrectomy low-grade dysplasia. Such overdiagnosis of dysplasia is supported by the observation the lesion was not observed to progress to malignancy; rather it has tended to regress [225,226]. By contrast, in one large prospective series, unequivocal severe dysplasia was a rare diagnosis that progressed to, or was concomitant with, intramucosal carcinoma [227].

In addition to reactive gastritis, chronic atrophic gastritis is also common following gastroenterostomy. This is mainly limited to the mucosa around the stoma. In one study 54% of patients had developed atrophic gastritis within 2 years of surgery [228]. Atrophy may take the form of a selective loss of parietal cells leaving glands composed of mucus and chief cells [229]. Glands frequently become irregular and cystic. Pyloric and intestinal metaplasia are common.

Lymphocytic gastritis

This uncommon condition is characterized by large numbers of mature lymphocytes infiltrating among the epithelial cells lining the mucosal surface and the foveolar walls. The underlying lamina propria also contains increased numbers of lymphocytes but this is variable and is not as striking as the intraepithelial infiltration. A diagnosis of lymphocytic gastritis can only be made on histology but many cases have the endoscopic features of varioliform gastritis where there are mucosal nodules and persistent chronic erosions, often in clusters on the surface of prominent thickened mucosal folds (Fig. 12.15) that may involve the entire stomach or the corpus [230,231]. However, while patients with endoscopic features of varioliform gastritis usually have histological evidence of lymphocytic gastritis, the converse is not true and some cases

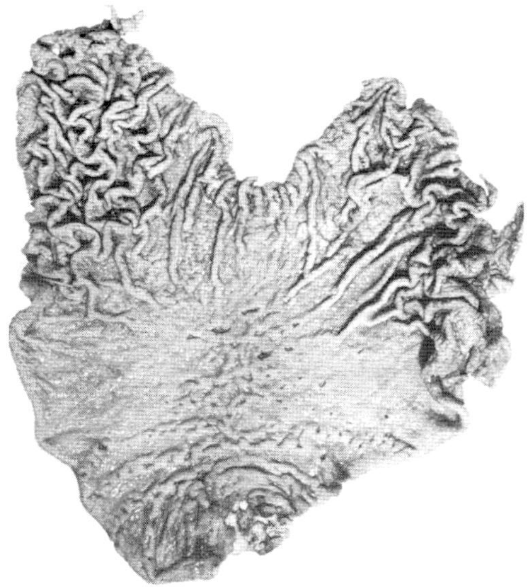

Fig. 12.15 Varioliform gastritis. Small nodules with central ulceration cluster around the junction of the antrum and body.

of lymphocytic gastritis show no distinctive endoscopic features [232]. The aetiology of lymphocytic gastritis is uncertain, though it appears to be associated with a variety of causes. Just under half of the cases identified in one series had *H. pylori* infection on biopsy, although more had serological evidence of infection, leading the authors to speculate that the condition may represent an abnormal response to an antigen such as *H. pylori* [233]. There is also an association with gluten-sensitive enteropathy (coeliac disease): in a series of patients with clinical features and small intestinal histological changes consistent with coeliac disease, 45% showed evidence of lymphocytic gastritis in gastric mucosal biopsies [234]. Further evidence supports the association between diffuse or antral predominant lymphocytic gastritis and an increase in duodenal intraepithelial lymphocytes and villous atrophy although by contrast, lymphocytic gastritis confined to the corpus is rarely associated with small bowel pathology [235]. This association with coeliac disease has been confirmed and in addition it has been noted that many patients with lymphocytic gastritis have abnormal small intestinal permeability indicating impaired function. It is possible that lymphocytic gastritis is part of a spectrum of diffuse lymphocytic gastroenteropathy representing an abnormal immunological reaction to a single or to different antigens [236].

The histological features of lymphocytic gastritis have also been noted to occur occasionally in stomachs with the gross appearances of Menetrier's disease, otherwise known as hypertrophic gastropathy (see Chapter 16). This is a rare condition in which the gastric mucosa is hypertrophied and the mucosal folds are convoluted, thickened and more prominent than normal, and which may be associated with protein loss into the gastrointestinal tract [237]. In one series of cases showing giant gastric mucosal folds and foveolar hyperplasia, over 50% showed additional features of lymphocytic gastritis [238]. The authors designated this condition hypertrophic lymphocytic gastritis, and separated it from the remaining cases that showed a much greater degree of foveolar hyperplasia but no increase in intraepithelial lymphocytes: these were designated hypertrophic gastropathy (Menetrier's disease).

Histology

The striking histological feature of lymphocytic gastritis is a marked increase in the number of intraepithelial lymphocytes (IELs) infiltrating the epithelial cells lining the mucosal surface and the foveolae, more than 25–30 IELs per 100 epithelial cells [230,236] (Fig. 12.16a). These IELs are predominantly T lymphocytes of the cytotoxic/suppressor type [236]. Intraepithelial lymphocytosis is accompanied by increased numbers of chronic inflammatory cells in the lamina propria (Fig. 12.16b) and/or oedema, and there may also be neutrophils in close proximity to erosions. The large number of IELs are best appreciated in intact mucosa, mainly in the basal part of the epithelium, and epithelial nuclear stratification may also be present [234]. Although the entire stomach may be involved the number of IELs varies from place to place [230]. Thus the condition may not be obvious in all biopsies taken from the same patient and may be missed if only a single biopsy is taken. In cases of lymphocytic gastritis associated with *H. pylori* infection and varioliform gastritis, intraepithelial lymphocytosis tends to be greater in the gastric body whereas in coeliac disease-associated cases IELs are more numerous in the antrum [235,239]. The situation is quite different from 'simple' *H. pylori*-associated chronic gastritis where an increase in IELs, if present at all, is modest and usually accompanied by much more prominent neutrophils.

Lymphocytic gastritis is a chronic condition that appears to persist over a number of years. While the number of IELs may diminish with time and fall below the diagnostic threshold, it remains higher than normal [236].

Other forms of gastritis

Varioliform gastritis (chronic erosive gastritis, verrucous gastritis)

This condition is recognized on endoscopy and double-contrast radiology [240–242]. Patients present with anorexia, weight loss, epigastric pain and sometimes a protein-losing enteropathy. At endoscopy multiple red nodules each with a shallow central ulcer are seen along prominent rugal folds of the corpus of the stomach and occasionally extending into the antrum (Fig. 12.15). The histological features of varioliform gastritis are in most cases those of lymphocytic gastritis, characterized by a marked increase in the number of

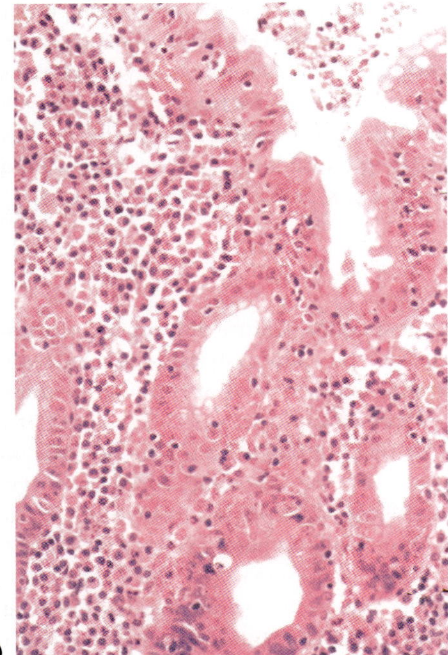

(a)

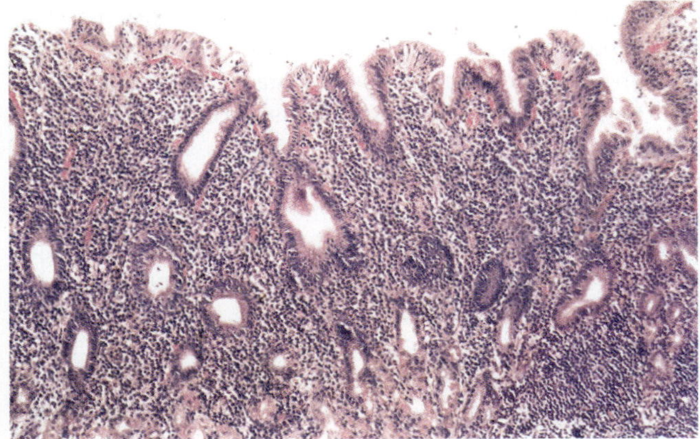

(b)

Fig. 12.16 (a) Lymphocytic gastritis showing increased numbers of intraepithelial lymphocytes among surface and foveolar epithelial cells. (b) Lymphocytic gastritis. Low-power view to show dense chronic inflammatory cell infiltrate in the lamina propria.

intraepithelial lymphocytes infiltrating the epithelial lining the surface of the mucosa and the foveolae [230]. This is discussed in more detail above. Such changes are apparent, however, only in intact mucosa and biopsy of an erosion may show a mixture of neutrophils and lymphocytes with marked regenerative atypia in adjacent surviving epithelium. In a crushed biopsy the latter appearances may simulate malignancy [243].

Eosinophilic gastritis (allergic gastroenteritis)

Allergic disease of the gastrointestinal tract may be divided into two broad groups, those affecting mainly the colon and rectum, and those with dominant or exclusive involvement of the upper gastrointestinal tract [244]. The former is a relatively harmless condition which presents in infants and results from sensitivity to milk or soya protein. The condition is cured by appropriate modification of the diet. Eosinophilic gastroenteritis may affect all age groups but mainly patients in the 30–40-year age group, many of whom have a history of asthma or allergy. There is usually peripheral blood eosinophilia and IgE levels may be raised [245–247]. The condition is defined by three criteria: (i) gastrointestinal symptoms such as abdominal pain, nausea, vomiting, diarrhoea and less often bloating and weight loss; (ii) histological evidence of marked eosinophilic infiltration of one or more parts of the gastrointestinal tract or suggestive radiological findings with peripheral eosinophilia; and (iii) no evidence of parasitic or extragastrointestinal disease [248]. Despite the latter criterion, a history of systemic allergy or asthma is present in about 25% of cases [249]. Protein-losing enteropathy, ascites and malabsorption are seen in severe cases [250].

The duodenum and proximal jejunum together with the stomach are the areas most frequently involved but any part of the gut may be affected and multiple areas of involvement are common. Within the stomach the antrum is the site most frequently affected. Endoscopic examination reveals thickening and deformity of the antrum with narrowing of the pylorus and diminished peristalsis. The mucosa may be swollen and reddened with surface erosions. Histological examination shows eosinophilic infiltration of the stomach wall accompanied by oedema [249,251]. The submucosa is affected principally (Fig. 12.17) but no layer is exempt. Gastric biopsies show infiltration of the lamina propria by eosinophils which invade the epithelium of the crypts and mucosal surface. It should be remembered that eosinophils are a common component of many inflammatory processes in the gastrointestinal tract and eosinophilic gastritis should not be overdiagnosed. While there is no agreed number of eosinophils that is considered pathognomonic of the condition, Talley *et al.* consider at least 20 eosinophils per high-power field, distributed either diffusely or multifocally, are required to be abnormal [248]. In some cases this figure is exceeded by a wide margin [252]. Within the mucosa there is focal necrosis and the epithelium shows regenerative changes. Diffuse involvement of the gastric antrum is the rule, unlike the patchy involvement of the small intestinal mucosa, and sampling error is thus less likely to occur [253]. However the eosinophilic infiltrate may predominantly affect different layers of the stomach wall [254] and a full-thickness surgical biopsy may be required to confirm the diagnosis.

Tissue eosinophilia is not specific for eosinophilic gastritis and among the differential diagnosis which should be considered are inflammatory fibroid, polyp, malignant lymphoma, parasitic infection, Langerhans cell histiocytosis, Crohn's disease, tropical sprue [255] and chronic granulomatous disease of childhood [256]. The aetiology of eosinophilic gastritis remains obscure.

Collagenous gastritis

This is a rare entity in which there is a thickened subepithelial band of collagen within gastric mucosa similar to that seen in the much more commonly recognized collagenous colitis. The condition was first described in 1989 [257]. The largest series and literature review has been reported recently [258] and indicates two subsets of affected patients. In one, comprising children and young adults, patients present with anaemia due to gastric bleeding and in some cases focal nodularity of gastric mucosa on endoscopy. In such cases the condition appears confined to the stomach. The second subset comprises adults in which there is frequently associated colitis and resultant diarrhoea. In some cases the condition occurs as an incidental finding.

The pathology is similar to that of collagenous colitis with a band of subepithelial collagen averaging 30–40 μm in thickness immediately beneath the surface of the gastric mucosa. This band varies in thickness and is not continuous. In addition there is increased inflammatory cell infiltration in the lamina propria. Lymphocytes, plasma cells and dilated capillaries are present within the collagen band. The overlying surface epithelial cells often show degenerative change with flattening and focal detachment of the epithelium.

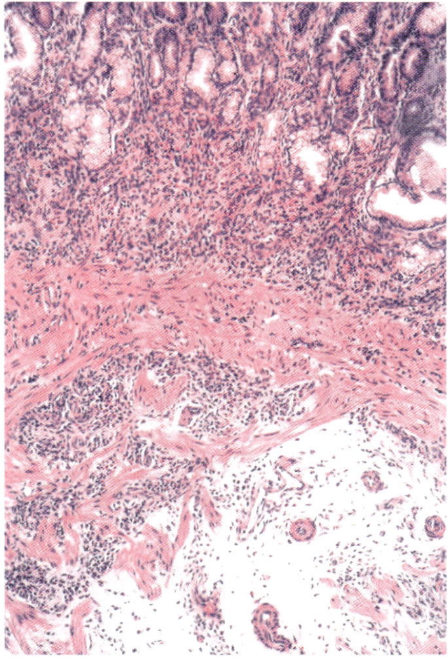

Fig. 12.17 Eosinophilic gastritis. Low-power view showing the deep mucosa and superficial submucosa. The latter is oedematous and there is diffuse infiltration of chronic inflammatory cells containing numerous eosinophils.

Other bacterial infections

Helicobacter heilmannii (*Gastrospirillum hominis*)

H. pylori is not the only bacterium to cause chronic gastritis in the human: *H. heilmannii* is another spiral organism occasionally found on the surface of the mucosa. This, too, is associated with chronic gastritis. The organism and its association with chronic active gastritis was described by Dent *et al.* [259]. The organism was originally named *Gastrospirillum hominis* by the team who first identified it [260]. This is a useful descriptive name as the organism has five to eight tight spirals which are more obvious than those of *H. pylori*. Subsequently the organism was shown to be a member of the *Helicobacter* group [261] and the name *H. heilmannii* has been suggested. Infection with *H. heilmannii* is much less common than *H. pylori* and is found in approximately 0.25% of gastric biopsies [262]. The organisms are less numerous but longer than *H. pylori* and occur in small groups or as isolated single organisms within the mucus layer on the mucosal surface or, more often, within foveolae. Thus they are easily missed on examination of a small gastric biopsy. Touch cytology with smearing of biopsies on to a slide and subsequent rapid fixation and staining resulted in a considerably higher rate of diagnosis than histological examination of the biopsy alone [263]. *H. heilmannii* is larger than *H. pylori*, measuring up to 7.5 μm in length and with five to eight prominent tight spirals (Fig. 12.18). On this basis it is usually

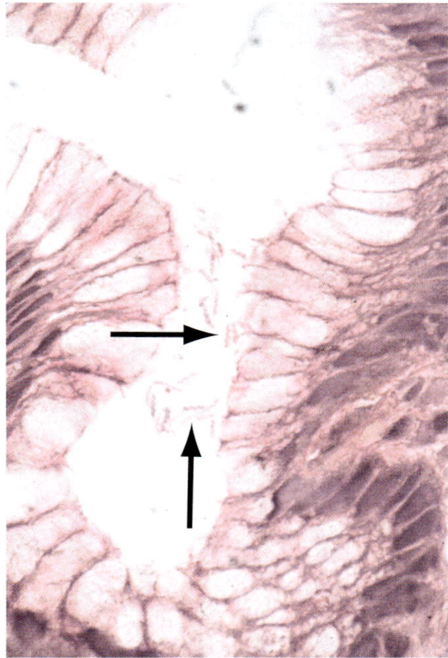

Fig. 12.18 *H. heilmannii* on the gastric mucosal surface. The organisms are larger than *H. pylori* and have several prominent spirals (arrows).

distinguishable from *H. pylori* on light microscopy. The spirals are especially well displayed on scanning electron microscopy [262]. Transmission electron microscopy shows that, like *H. pylori*, the organism possesses sheathed flagella [260,262]. Unlike *H. pylori*, *H. heilmannii* can be identified within cells of the gastric mucosa as well as on the surface [262]. Infection with *H. heilmannii* is associated with chronic active gastritis [259,262] which is usually confined to the antrum. Histologically this is similar to that seen in association with *H. pylori* but is less severe. However, in addition, the changes of reactive gastritis with foveolar hyperplasia, vasodilatation and oedema of the lamina propria have been reported in the majority of cases examined [263]. Lymphoid aggregates are rare and concomitant infection with *H. pylori* is seldom seen [262,264]. The infection may persist for years and associated symptoms include epigastric pain, vomiting and heartburn. Some cases with associated gastritis are asymptomatic [265]. The possibility that the infection is acquired from animals has been suggested [260]. Very similar organisms are found in the stomachs of various animal species [266,267] and the majority of patients infected by the organism have contact with dogs, cats and other domestic animals; it is therefore possible that transmission from pets may take place [261,264].

Other bacteria

Bacteria of a variety of species colonize the stomach in patients with hypochlorhydria due to chronic atrophic gastritis. These may be implicated in the aetiology of gastric cancer through their ability to convert nitrate to nitrite to N-nitroso compounds. Acute infection of the stomach wall by pyogenic and gas-forming organisms leading to phlegmonous or emphysematous gastritis has been described earlier in this chapter. There are rare reports of gastric anthrax [268]. Infection with tuberculosis and syphilis is described below under granulomatous gastritis.

Opportunistic infections of the stomach

The prevalence of opportunistic gastrointestinal infections in HIV-infected patients receiving effective antiretroviral therapy is declining [269]. However in those for whom such therapy is not available and those who are immunocompromised for other reasons the risk remains. The stomach is relatively rarely affected by such infections in comparison with the rest of the gut.

Fungal infections

Fungal infection of the stomach may be localized or part of a systemic infection.

Candidiasis

This has been diagnosed in 1% of patients undergoing endoscopic examination [270]. Gastric infection is not as common as oesophageal, but evidence of candidiasis has been noted in 16–18% of benign gastric ulcers [271,272]. In the majority of these cases infection is in the form of saprophytic colonization of necrotic debris in the ulcer base. The significance of such infection is uncertain but it may aggravate and perpetuate pre-existing ulcers, and in one series candidal infection was associated with a surprisingly high postoperative mortality following ulcer resection [272]. Identification of the fungal hyphae is difficult in H&E sections and PAS or Grocott stain is usually needed.

Gastric candidiasis may also occur as an opportunistic infection in immunosuppressed patients or in those with cancer or following cytotoxic or antibiotic therapy. Opportunistic infections have two endoscopic appearances. The first is that of a white or yellow plaque which can be removed to reveal a reddened underlying mucosa. Such plaques are not specific for fungal infection. More rarely chronic infection leads to the formation of warty, umbilicated nodules (Fig. 12.19).

Phycomycosis (mucormycosis)

Gastrointestinal phycomycosis is rare and usually involves terminal ileum, caecum and colon [273]. However, reports of gastric infection are fairly common [274]. Infection in infants and children has also been reported [275]. The fungal hyphae are branching and non-septate (Fig. 12.20). The organism is usually saprophytic and invariably patients with systemic involvement have underlying serious debilitating disease such as poorly controlled diabetes with acidosis, leukaemia, lym-

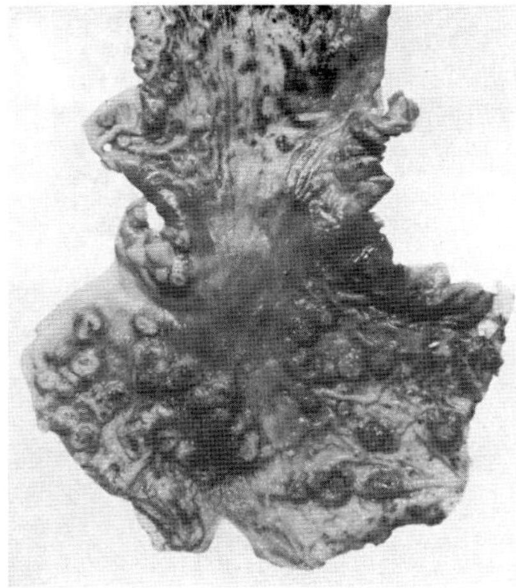

Fig. 12.19 Discrete umbilicated nodules due to candidosis. Note the ulceration and zones of surrounding haemorrhage. From a young man with Hodgkin's disease treated with cytotoxic drugs.

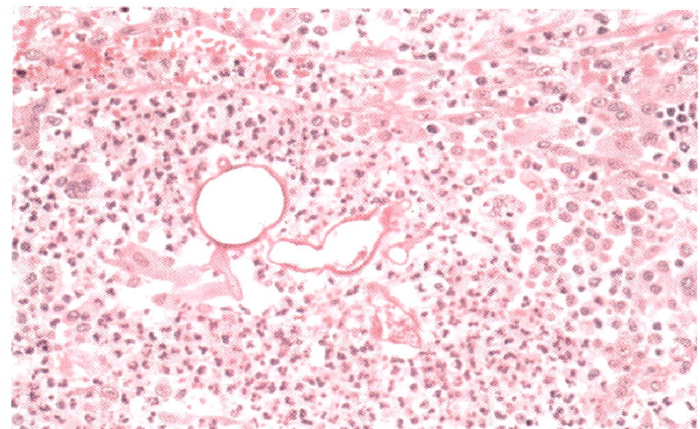

Fig. 12.20 Phycomycosis in a gastric ulcer. The fungi are branching and non-septate. Vascular invasion by fungi with subsequent thrombosis occurs frequently. PAS stain.

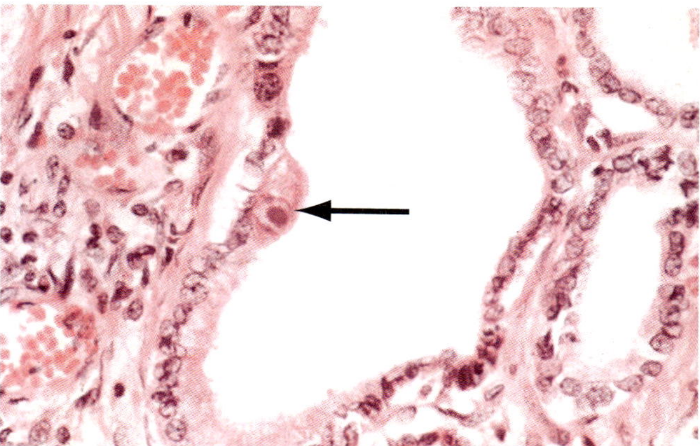

Fig. 12.21 Cytomegalovirus (CMV) infection. Characteristic inclusion body (arrow) within an infected epithelial cell in intact gastric mucosa adjacent to an ulcer in a patient who was immunosuppressed following cardiac transplantation.

phoma or other malignancy, malnutrition or immune suppression. Gastric infection results in ulceration, and invasion of adjacent blood vessel walls by the fungus with subsequent thrombosis is characteristic [274].

Other fungal infections

Gastric involvement by *Cryptococcus neoformans* is rare and is reported in conjunction with disseminated disease in immunosuppressed patients [276,277]. Infiltration of the mucosa and submucosa by *Histoplasma*-laden macrophages may produce greatly thickened gastric folds [278]. There are occasional reports of gastric involvement by *Pneumocystis carinii* in HIV-positive patients with widespread extrapulmonary pneumocystosis [279,280]. Gastroduodenal pneumocystosis is manifest by small mucosal nodules and erosions. Histology shows foamy granular exudate within the lamina propria. Organisms are difficult to identify on H&E staining, but Gomori's methenamine silver stain greatly aids diagnosis.

Viral infections

Cytomegalovirus

Cytomegalovirus (CMV) infection of the gastrointestinal tract occurs in neonates, immunologically deficient adults and occasionally apparently healthy individuals [281,282]. Oesophageal ulceration is the commonest manifestation of CMV infection of the upper gastrointestinal tract but the stomach may also be involved. Evidence of CMV infection has been identified in 13% of HIV-infected patients [283] and in a study of renal transplant patients CMV inclusions could be detected in endoscopic biopsy material from the upper gastrointestinal tract in approximately half [284]. The use of azathioprine was regarded as the major risk factor.

Gastric CMV infection takes two forms. In the first, typical intranuclear inclusions are seen in enlarged cells of the glandular epithelium without any associated tissue reaction (Fig. 12.21) and in this form of the disease the patient is frequently asymptomatic and the endoscopic appearances are often normal. In the second type of infection there is gastric ulceration and erosion causing epigastric pain and, on occasion, haemorrhage [285,286]. The ulcers are typically shallow but may be up to 5 cm in diameter, although perforation and fistula formation may also occur occasionally [287]. CMV intranuclear inclusions may be found in swollen endothelial and stromal cells in the vicinity of the ulcers, in highly vascularized granulation tissue, and in intact mucosa but their identification in biopsies may require prolonged search. Intraepithelial inclusions are much less conspicuous in this form of the disease. Infected cells are enlarged and contain large eosinophilic intranuclear inclusions, often but not always surrounded by a clear halo, and more basophilic intracytoplasmic inclusions are usually present but the former are much more conspicuous. In AIDS patients who are severely immunocompromised, histological evidence of infection may be difficult to find in small biopsies and in the absence of a normal antibody response [288]. Immunocytochemistry using anti-CMV antibody is very useful for identifying infected cells. Brush cytology to allow wider sampling of cells may also be useful. While the overall prevalence of gastroduodenal ulceration in HIV-positive patients is low, when it occurs it is associated with CMV infection of the gastric mucosa in 50% of cases [289].

Herpes virus

Occasional cases of herpes simplex and herpes zoster gastritis have been described in patients who are terminally ill [290,291]. Endoscopy shows small plaque-like or linear ulcers in the gastric mucosa or vesicles covered by a yellow exudate. The characteristic eosinophilic intranuclear inclusion bodies may be identified within epithelial cells on histological examination but these are difficult to find. Immunohistochemistry using specific antiviral antibodies is useful in identifying infected cells. Gastric infection by herpes (varicella) zoster has been reported in a bone marrow transplant patient with disseminated shingles. Multiple erosions of gastric mucosa were present and histology showed active gastritis suggestive of *H. pylori* infection. No *H. pylori* were present and no viral inclusions were seen. However varicella zoster virus was identified using PCR and electron microscopy [292].

Protozoal infections

Giardiasis

This is a common infection in which *Giardia lamblia* colonizes the small bowel, especially the duodenum. It occurs worldwide and is not confined to immunosuppressed patients. Gastric antral involvement is reported to occur in around 9% of cases [293]. There are no specific features in the accompanying gastritis and in many cases the underlying gastric mucosal histology is normal. Diagnosis is dependent on identification of the trophozoite on the mucosal surface.

Toxoplasmosis

Toxoplasmosis is a common opportunistic infection in advanced HIV infection, where central nervous system involvement is the most frequent manifestation. Gastric infection by *Toxoplasma gondii*, while very rare, has been reported in association with widely disseminated disease [294,295]. Thickening of the gastric wall and mucosal folds which may result in gastric outlet obstruction and mucosal ulceration has been described, but in some cases gastric endoscopy is normal [296]. Histological examination of biopsy material shows a corresponding spectrum of abnormalities from full-thickness mucosal necrosis to just oedema and non-specific inflammation of the mucosa. *T. gondii* cysts and tachyzoites can be found within the mucosa, and trophozoites can be identified in gastric epithelial cells, endothelial cells and smooth muscle cells and macrophages [295,296].

Cryptosporidiosis

This protozoon frequently infects the small intestine and colon in immunocompromised patients but it may be found in other sites such as the biliary tract and the stomach [297]. Indeed, detailed investigation of AIDS patients indicates that gastric infection is commoner than previously suspected [298]. Endoscopic examination frequently shows no abnormality although mucosal oedema and erosions may occur. Histology indicates that involvement of the antrum is more common than the corpus. Organisms are most frequently found on the luminal border of epithelial cells of gastric pits and infection is accompanied by non-specific active chronic inflammation. Colonization of the mucosa is patchy and examination of multiple biopsies is advisable [299]. Thus the pathologist should have a high index of suspicion of gastric cryptosporidiosis in severely immunocompromised patients.

Granulomatous gastritis

Gastric granulomas are encountered only rarely. A granuloma is a compact, organized collection of mature mononuclear phagocytes which may be accompanied by other features such as necrosis [300]. Morphologically it is composed of epithelioid macrophages and lymphoid cells with the occasional addition of neutrophils, eosinophils and giant cells and with or without necrosis. There may be a surrounding rim of lymphocytes. There are considered to be two types of granulomas: (i) those incited by inert foreign bodies; and (ii) immune granulomas in which the presence of organisms incite a T-cell immune response and the products of activated T lymphocytes transform macrophages into epithelioid cells and multinucleated giant cells [301]. Thus it is not surprising that granulomatous gastritis may be associated with a variety of conditions such as Crohn's disease, tuberculosis, reaction to foreign material, sarcoidosis, syphilis, histoplasmosis, reaction to nearby malignancy and vasculitis. The aetiology is likely to vary considerably in different parts of the world. A comprehensive survey carried out in Belgium and the UK indicated that Crohn's disease is by far the commonest cause of granulomatous gastritis in these countries, followed by idiopathic cases [302]. Less common causes were foreign body granulomas, tumour-associated granulomas and occasional cases of sarcoidosis, Whipple's disease and granulomatous vasculitis. A high prevalence of *H. pylori* infection was also found in association with granulomatous gastritis but it is unclear whether there was a causal relationship. Other causes of granulomatous gastritis include Langerhans cell histiocytosis, amyloidosis and rheumatoid nodules, and a recent review gives a comprehensive list of associated conditions [303].

In common with all granulomatous conditions, biopsy diagnosis of granulomatous gastritis is limited by sampling error and granulomas may be scarce or numerous. They are found much more frequently in the antrum than in the corpus.

Crohn's disease

Patients are usually less than 45 years old. The common presenting clinical symptoms are upper gastrointestinal pain and, less often, vomiting. A substantial minority of patients with histological evidence of gastric involvement by Crohn's disease have no gastric symptoms [304]. There may be clinical and pathological evidence of coexisting disease in the duodenum or small or large intestine [305,306]. Macroscopically

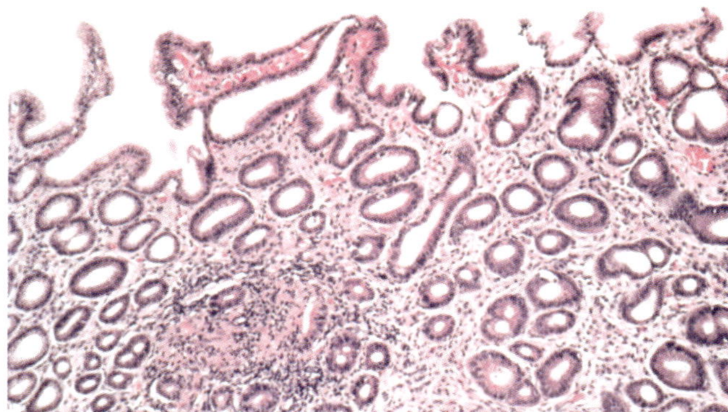

Fig. 12.22 Crohn's disease. Gastric antral biopsy from a child with small intestinal Crohn's disease. There is focal but intense gastritis with partial destruction of a gland by poorly formed granulomas.

there can be 'cobblestoning' of the mucosa with thickening of the pyloric region but most commonly endoscopy shows erosions and redness of the mucosa. The proximal stomach is involved only rarely [307]. Abnormal gastric biopsies, if taken, are found in up to 75% of cases of intestinal Crohn's disease. The characteristic feature is focal inflammation composed of lymphocytes and histiocytes usually with associated neutrophils in a background of minimally inflamed mucosa (Fig. 12.22). Although these focal lesions frequently occur deep in the mucosa they can be associated with erosion or degenerative changes in the overlying surface epithelium [304,308]. Concomitant *H. pylori* infection occurs in 10–33% of cases of Crohn's disease and the associated generalized active gastritis tends to obscure the focal inflammation of Crohn's making diagnosis very difficult. Granulomas are seen in less than 15% of gastric biopsies in Crohn's disease, and while obviously important, they are neither a sensitive diagnostic feature nor pathognomonic [302]. In children, histological evidence suggestive of mucosal involvement of the stomach and duodenum is found in one-third of cases with Crohn's ileocolitis [309].

Sarcoidosis

Sarcoidosis of the stomach can only be diagnosed when tuberculoid granulomas are found in the absence of tubercle bacilli, when there is no evidence of Crohn's disease or tuberculosis elsewhere in the gastrointestinal tract, and where there is clinical, radiological and laboratory evidence of sarcoid lesions outside the alimentary tract. In patients with sarcoidosis but no gastrointestinal symptoms, granulomas were found in 10% of gastric biopsies [310]. Symptoms of gastrointestinal involvement include haematemesis, epigastric pain, nausea, colicky abdominal pain and diarrhoea. Endoscopic examination shows changes ranging from a distal gastritis with or without nodularity, mainly affecting the greater curvature, to ulceration and pyloric stenosis [311]. In sarcoidosis the granulomas are usually well circumscribed and compact and the surrounding non-specific mucosal inflammation is absent or less marked than in Crohn's disease or tuberculosis. As stated above, supportive clinical and radiological evidence is necessary before the diagnosis can be confirmed.

Tuberculosis

The upsurge in cases of tuberculosis over the past 10–15 years in Western countries is now well recognized. Those most susceptible are the urban poor, many of whom are immigrants and/or elderly, and patients with HIV infection. Extrapulmonary tuberculosis is much more common in HIV-infected patients [312,313] and the possibility of gastrointestinal infection should always be considered in such patients. Within the gut the ileocaecal region and jejunum and ileum are the most common sites of involvement by tuberculosis. Gastric tuberculosis is rare. It is virtually never primary and it is probably unwise to make the diagnosis in the absence of demonstrable tuberculous disease elsewhere. The antrum is the most common site of involvement. Symptoms include epigastric pain, vomiting and haematemesis [314–316], and frequently there is evidence of pyloric obstruction [315–317]. On endoscopy, ulceration of the pyloric region, frequently the lesser curvature, is common and there may be a nodular hypertrophic mass which may simulate carcinoma. Diagnosis may be made on histological examination of endoscopic biopsies but more often it is made following gastric surgery. Histology shows granulomatous inflammation involving mucosa, submucosa or serosa. The granulomas may be confluent and while they are typically caseating, this is by no means always the rule [316]. Regional lymph nodes are frequently enlarged and should be carefully examined histologically as they frequently contain granulomas which may not be readily apparent in the gastric wall. Demonstration of acid-fast tubercle bacilli is pathognomonic and should always be attempted, though frequently unsuccessful. Use of PCR to identify mycobacterial DNA sequences may be helpful.

Syphilis

Syphilitic gastritis is rare and may present with diffuse enlargement of gastric folds and multiple shallow ulcers or erosions [318,319]. Less often a single large ulcer may occur, usually in the antrum. Perforation has been occasionally reported [320]. Histologically granulomas may be present but the usual finding is a dense but non-specific mucosal infiltrate of plasma cells, neutrophils and lymphocytes, often with lymphoid follicle formation. There may be destruction of mucosal glands and lymphoepithelial-like lesions strongly suggestive of malignant lymphoma [321]. The endarteritis often seen in syphilitic lesions elsewhere in the body may not be present in gastric lesions and the gummas that occur in the tertiary stage or in congenital syphilis [322] are seldom seen in the adult stomach. Diagnosis is difficult to prove as demonstration of *Treponema pallidum* within the mucosa is capricious. It can be achieved using silver stains such as Warthin–Starry, Dieterle or the modified Steiner silver stain [319,323], but identification is difficult, especially with a background of elastic or reticulin fibres. Contaminant harmless oral spirochaetes cannot be distinguished from *T. pallidum* with these stains. The presence of concomitant *H. pylori* infection and associated gastritis compounds difficulties in diagnosing syphilis [319] as both organisms stain with silver techniques. However, spirochaetes are much larger and are morphologically distinct. The use of specific immunocytochemistry, immunofluorescence or PCR to detect DNA is advisable in cases where syphilis is suspected [321].

Food granulomas

These foreign body-type, non-epithelioid, granulomas are usually distinguishable from other forms of granulomatous gastritis. Some are obviously related to visible food particles, such as vegetable matter or the insoluble coatings of cereals, in the mucosa or more deeply if there is an associated active or healed peptic ulcer. Others may be the result of small breaches in the gastric mucosa which allow gastric juice to digest the muscularis and muscle coats, producing partial necrosis and inciting a granulomatous response [324]. In both types curious amorphous eosinophilic granulomatous masses are produced which become surrounded by pallisades of histiocytes and foreign body-type giant cells (Fig. 12.23). These later undergo fibrosis, and sometimes calcification, that can be sufficiently marked to produce pyloric stenosis. When they follow perforation of an ulcer there may rarely be an associated chronic granulomatous peritonitis which can mimic malignancy. Crystalline iron material may be found in gastric mucosa in patients taking therapeutic oral iron medication [325]. This material is found in the lamina propria close to the mucosal surface (Fig. 12.24) and there is frequently erosion of the overlying surface epithelium. Other causes of foreign body granuloma in the gastric wall include kaolin, talc and suture material.

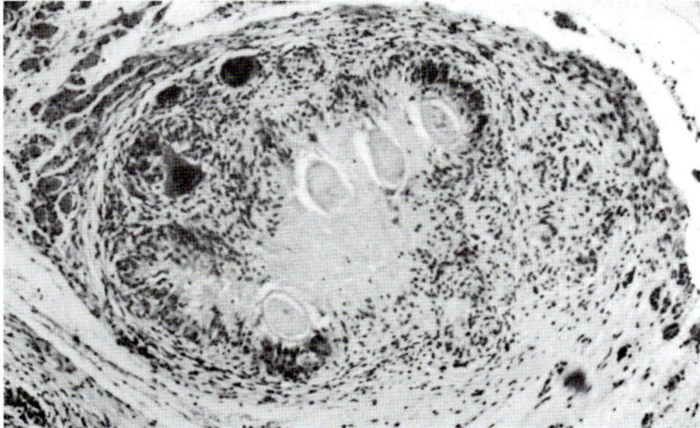

Fig. 12.23 Food granuloma.

Idiopathic granulomatous gastritis

This is an expression which can be usefully applied to the discovery of isolated sarcoid-like granulomas in the gastric mucosa when there is no evidence to incriminate tuberculosis, Crohn's disease, sarcoidosis or some other specific cause for their presence. Such granulomas are usually detected in biopsy material but may also be observed in gastrectomy specimens. The granulomas are mostly found in the mucosa and it is exceptional to see them in the deeper layers of the bowel wall and regional lymph nodes. Some degree of accompanying superficial or atrophic gastritis may be present but there is no ulceration and inflammatory cell infiltration is minimal. The granulomas are composed of histiocytes and multinucleated giant cells which can contain hyaline inclusions. The condition is clinically benign.

Anisakiasis

Gastric anisakiasis occurs mainly in Japan but some cases are reported from elsewhere such as the western United States [326]. The condition is caused by penetration of the gastric mucosa by *Anisakis* larvae. These are ingested by eating uncooked fish infested by the larvae. *Phocanema decipiens* larvae may also be involved. Ingestion may result in the larvae being coughed

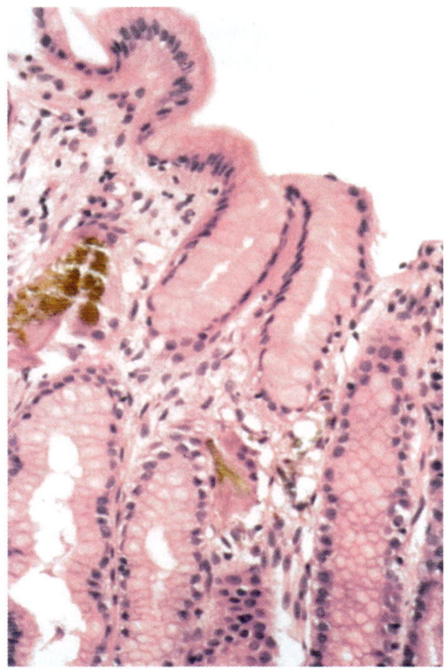

Fig. 12.24 Crystalline iron in the gastric lamina propria of a patient taking oral iron medication. Foreign body giant cells lie adjacent to iron deposits.

up or vomited but larval attachment to the gastric wall results in acute or chronic anisakiasis. The former is characterized by epigastric pain, nausea and vomiting with oedema of the gastric mucosa around the larvae. The larvae may be removed by forceps at endoscopy [327]. Chronic disease may ensue during which the larvae die and the oedematous mucosa becomes infiltrated by eosinophils and epithelioid granulomas. The larvae may disappear leaving only unidentifiable fragments [328].

Other causes of granulomatous gastritis

Rare causes of granulomatous gastritis include Whipple's disease, Langerhans cell histiocytosis and vasculitis. Involvement of the stomach in Whipple's disease is exceedingly rare although the disease may involve numerous extraintestinal sites such as lymph nodes, brain, lungs and spleen. Granulomatous gastritis with non-caseating granulomas containing macrophages with occasional PAS-positive particles has been reported in a patient with duodenal involvement by Whipple's disease [329].

Langerhans cell histiocytosis (formerly known as histiocytosis X) occasionally involves the gastrointestinal tract. Gastric involvement may manifest as multiple mucosal polyps [330]. In some cases the mucosal infiltrate of histiocytes, eosinophils and lymphocytes may take the form of distinct non-caseating giant cell granulomas leading to a diagnosis of granulomatous gastritis [331]. Gastric involvement in patients with common variable immunodeficiency and X-linked agammaglobulinaemia has also been documented [332]. A variety of abnormalities was noted in biopsies. These include single cell necrosis within glands and increased numbers of mononuclear cells within the lamina propria together with occasional ill-defined granulomas and lymphocytic infiltration of the foveolae areas of mucosal glands. The features are similar to those described in graft-versus-host disease in the stomach [333].

Vasculitis

Within the gastrointestinal tract, the small intestine and gall bladder are the sites most frequently involved by vasculitis; the stomach is seldom affected [334]. Occasional cases presenting with gastrointestinal haemorrhage [335] or refractory gastric ulcer [334] have been reported. The blood vessels show characteristic changes often with an eosinophilic fibrinoid infiltrate and occasional giant cells. Henoch–Schönlein purpura may affect small vessels of the gastric mucosa. There is focal intramucosal haemorrhage accompanied by an intense acute inflammation. Leukocytoclasis is often present. These changes often obscure the underlying eosinophilic fibrinoid degeneration in affected capillaries making biopsy diagnosis difficult without relevant clinical information (Fig. 12.25).

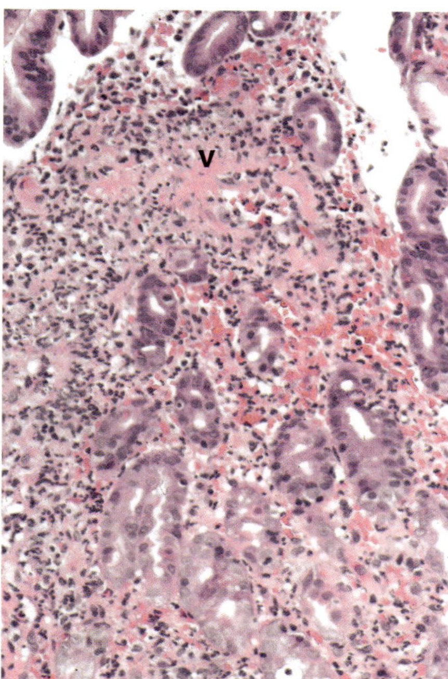

Fig. 12.25 Gastric mucosa in Henoch–Schönlein purpura. There is intense acute inflammation, and leukocytoclasis with haemorrhage around affected capillary vessels (v) which show eosinophilic fibrinoid degeneration.

Extensive necrotizing granulomatous infiltration of the submucosa, muscularis propria and serosa of the stomach with a heavy eosinophilic infiltrate has been reported in association with allergic granulomatosis (Churg–Strauss syndrome) [336].

Hypertrophic gastritis and hypertrophic gastropathy (including Menetrier's disease)

These conditions are discussed in more detail elsewhere in this book (Chapter 16). The terms hypertrophic gastritis or gastropathy imply focal or diffuse enlargement of gastric mucosa characterized histologically by tortuosity of the foveolae (gastric pits), mucosal oedema and dilatation of glands in the deeper part of the mucosa. In many cases there is associated inflammation (i.e. hypertrophic gastritis) but this is frequently not the case and in such instances hypertrophic gastropathy is the term used. There is confusion in the literature whether Menetrier's disease should be used as an overall term to describe hypertrophy of the gastric mucosa, as it frequently is, or whether it should be confined to cases without significant inflammation. Some authorities consider that Menetrier's disease should be restricted to cases of idiopathic gastric mucosal hypertrophy with massive foveolar hyperplasia without gastritis [238,337]. Others define Menetrier's disease as hypertrophic gastropathy with hypoproteinaemia, regardless of histology. Without getting deeply involved with semantics, hypertrophy of the gastric mucosa may be due to a variety of causes and different aetiologies should be considered in such cases. These include lymphocytic gastritis [237], gastric syphilis [318], CMV infection, histoplasmosis and Cronkhite–Canada syndrome [337], the Zollinger–Ellison syndrome, carcinoma and lymphoma. An association between hypertrophic gastritis and *H. pylori* infection has been identified and may represent an unusual form of *H. pylori* gastritis [338]. In some instances this *H. pylori*-associated hypertrophic gastritis is accompanied by protein-losing enteropathy [339]. The histology in *H. pylori*-associated hypertrophic gastritis differs from classical Menetrier's disease in that both mucosal thickening and foveolar hyperplasia are less marked and inflammation is more intense [119]. Such cases have been called 'enlarged fold gastritis'. The mucosa in *H. pylori*-associated hypertrophic gastritis reverts to normal following eradication of the infection. In Zollinger–Ellison syndrome thickening of the gastric corpus mucosa is due to hyperplasia and hypertrophy of acid-producing parietal cells. There is no foveolar hyperplasia [340]. By contrast, the mucosa in Menetrier's disease is thicker due to marked foveolar hyperplasia, cystic dilatation and oedema while the specialized glandular elements of the deeper mucosa are, if anything, atrophied [238].

Thus from the pathologist's viewpoint it is important to be aware of the variety of different conditions which may give rise to clinical or radiological enlargement of gastric mucosal folds. If histology supports a diagnosis of hypertrophic change, and for obvious reasons a large biopsy is necessary, pathologists should assess the degree of concomitant inflammation and the presence of lymphocytic or *H. pylori* gastritis before arriving at a diagnosis of Menetrier's disease. There is frequently a poor correlation between endoscopic or radiological findings and histology. In one series the majority of patients with large gastric folds identified radiologically or endoscopically did not have clinical or laboratory features of hypertrophic gastropathy. Most of these patients had active chronic gastritis with increased mucosal thickness due to oedema but no foveolar hyperplasia [340].

Uraemic gastropathy

In uraemia multiple small petechial haemorrhages occur in the gastric mucosa. In severe untreated cases this may give the appearance of acute haemorrhagic gastritis [341]. In patients with chronic renal failure undergoing dialysis treatment, superficial gastritis is common and gastric and duodenal erosions may be seen in some cases [342]. The reported incidence of peptic ulceration is also increased in some studies [343] but this is not always the case [344]. Such erosions and ulcers are important causes of upper gastrointestinal bleeding in patients with chronic renal failure. Concomitant use of ulcerogenic drugs such as NSAIDs may be associated with bleeding. Another significant factor is hypersecretion of acid which frequently occurs during dialysis treatment [345,346]. Apart from erosions and ulceration the gastric mucosa frequently shows superficial gastritis in the antrum and corpus [342,347]. Some patients also show severe atrophic gastritis and chronic duodenitis with gastric metaplasia [347,348]. Despite the high incidence of superficial gastritis *H. pylori* infection does not appear to be common in patients undergoing treatment for chronic renal failure. The prevalence of the infection is less than in the general population [349].

Successful kidney transplantation may frequently be associated with hypertrophic folds in mucosa of the corpus. Histology shows foveolar hyperplasia, multinucleated parietal cells and extension of parietal cells into the antrum and even the duodenum. This may be related to long-term steroid therapy and the trophic effects of hypergastrinaemia. In addition heterotopic calcification within the gastric mucosa may occur and the increased incidence of CMV infection should be considered in patients receiving immunosuppression therapy [350].

Gastric lesions associated with irradiation

Irradiation injury may take one of three forms [351–354].

1 *Irradiation gastritis.* From a few days to a few months after exposure to irradiation there is extensive mucosal necrosis and surface ulceration. Vessel walls become swollen and their lumina are reduced in size. The mucosa usually regenerates, but varying degrees of atrophy with submucosal fibrosis, mucosal and submucosal oedema and endarteritis of small arteries often persist. Fibroblasts with bizarre, hyperchromatic nuclei are characteristic.

2 *Acute ulceration.* This occurs 1–2 months after exposure. The ulcer is deep and penetrating and is often accompanied by pain and bleeding. Perforation, however, is rare, as the ulcer usually becomes walled off by surrounding structures. Histological changes characteristic of radiation damage are usually present.

3 *Chronic ulceration.* From 1 month to several years after exposure to irradiation a chronic ulcer may appear. Such ulcers are usually solitary and occur principally in the antrum. The histology of the ulcer is similar to that of the 'usual' gastric ulcer except that there are atypical fibroblasts in the ulcer base; the endothelial cells lining capillaries in granulation tissue in the ulcer base may also appear bizarre and unusually prominent [355]. In addition there may be an excessive amount of antral fibrosis which frequently has a hyalinized appearance and is accompanied by hyalinization of blood vessel walls. These features may be helpful in the diagnosis of a radiation-induced chronic ulcer.

Portal hypertensive gastropathy or congestive gastropathy

Although this entity is included in the chapter on gastritis the term 'gastritis' is not strictly accurate as mucosal inflammation is not a major component. The descriptive term gastritis has frequently been applied to gastric mucosal abnormalities associated with portal hypertension because of the endoscopic appearance of the gastric mucosa, which varies from mild hyperaemia to severe mucosal haemorrhages with 'cherry-red' spots similar to those seen in the oesophagus in varices. Histological studies show that mucosal capillary dilatation and congestion are the principal features and that inflammation is frequently absent. Thus the terms 'congestive gastropathy' [356] or more recently 'portal hypertensive gastropathy' (PHG) [357] have been suggested. The condition is very prevalent in patients with cirrhosis and affects over 60%, although less than 25% have severe lesions [358,359]. While minor lesions appear to be of little clinical significance, severe cases of PHG are of clinical importance due to the association with bleeding. This may be insidious, resulting in iron deficiency anaemia, or severe enough to warrant emergency endoscopy and blood transfusion. Bleeding from congestive gastropathy may be more common following sclerotherapy of oesophageal varices [356]. The condition may not always be apparent on gastric mucosal biopsy using routine H&E staining and immunocytochemistry may be required to highlight mucosal capillaries [360].

Histology shows focal ectasia of mucosal capillaries immediately beneath the mucosal surface, with an increase in the number and diameter of both mucosal and submucosal blood vessels. The vascular congestion and dilatation is out of proportion to any concomitant inflammatory cell infiltrate [356,360,361]. The vascular ectasia is present in both the proximal stomach and the antrum. In cases where the whole stomach has been available for examination there is marked dilatation and tortuosity of submucosal veins, especially in the corpus and cardia, possibly corresponding to gastric varices [356].

Gastric antral vascular ectasia (GAVE) (watermelon stomach)

This is characterized by similar histological and endoscopic changes to those of congestive gastropathy. Although the condition is sometimes associated with portal hypertension, in many cases this is absent. The entity is rare and was described by Jabbari *et al.* who reported three cases of severe iron deficiency anaemia due to bleeding from the lesion and applied the term 'watermelon stomach' on account of the characteristic findings at endoscopy [362]. The condition affects the middle-aged and elderly and shows marked female predominance. Iron deficiency anaemia appears to be the most common presenting symptom. Endoscopy shows characteristic longitudinal, almost parallel mucosal folds within the antrum with prominent congested vessels in the apices of the folds giving a striped appearance [362–364]. Histology of the antral mucosa shows prominent dilated, congested mucosal capillaries beneath the epithelial surface. In addition microthrombi are present within some vessels and there is fibromuscular hyperplasia in the lamina propria with prominent smooth muscle cells extending upwards perpendicular to the muscularis mucosa [363,364] (Fig. 12.26). Active inflammation is not a feature. The antral mucosa may be hypertrophic but atrophic gastritis of the corpus and hypergastrinaemia were reported to be very common in one series [365]. Many of the histological features are similar to those associated with mucosal prolapse elsewhere in the gut and antral mucosal prolapse through the pylorus has been reported at endoscopy in some cases. In antral biopsies the combination of capillary ectasia, fibrin thrombi and fibromuscular spindle cell proliferation in the lamina propria should alert the pathologist to the diagnosis [366]. The condition is important as it is increasingly recognized as a cause of gastrointestinal bleeding, especially in elderly women. Extension of lesions beyond the antrum to the proximal stomach may occur, especially in association with diaphragmatic hernia [367].

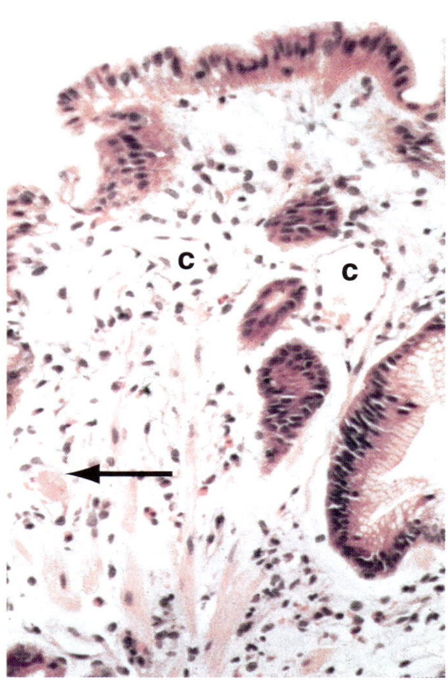

Fig. 12.26 Gastric antral vascular ectasia (GAVE). Histology shows dilated capillaries (c) in the superficial gastric mucosa with occasional thrombi (arrow). Fibromuscular spindle cells are prominent.

References

1 Allen A, Cunliffe WJ, Pearson JP, Venables CW. The adherent gastric mucus gel barrier in man and changes in peptic ulceration. *J Int Med*, 1990; 228 (Suppl 732): 83.

2 Turnberg LA. Gastric mucosal defence mechanisms. *Scand J Gastroenterol Suppl*, 1985; 110: 37.

3 Bell AE, Sellers LA, Allen A, Cunliffe WJ, Morris ER, Ross-Murphy SB. Properties of gastric and duodenal mucus: effective proteolysis, disulfide reduction, bile, acid, ethanol and hypertonicity on mucus gel structure. *Gastroenterology*, 1985; 88: 269.

4 Allen A, Flemstrom G, Garner A, Kivilaakso E. Gastroduodenal mucosal protection. *Physiol Rev*, 1993; 73: 823.

5 Hogan DL, Ainsworth MA, Isenberg JI. Review Article: Gastroduodenal bicarbonate secretion. *Aliment Pharmacol Ther*, 1994; 8: 475.

6 Williams SE, Turnberg LA. Demonstration of a pH gradient across mucus adherent to rabbit gastric mucosa: evidence for a mucus–bicarbonate barrier. *Gut*, 1981; 22: 94.

7 Goddard PJ, Kao Y-CJ, Lichtenberger LM. Luminal surface hydrophobicity of canine gastric mucosa is dependent on a surface mucus gel. *Gastroenterology*, 1990; 98: 361.

8 Hills BA. A physical identity for the gastric mucosal barrier. *Med J Aust*, 1990; 153: 76.

9 Hills BA. Gastric surfactant and the hydrophobic mucosal barrier. *Gut*, 1996; 39: 621.

10 Davenport HW. Salicylate damage to the gastric mucosal barrier. *N Engl J Med*, 1967; 276: 1307.

11 Kauffman GL. The gastric mucosal barrier: component control. *Dig Dis Sci*, 1985; 30 (Suppl): 69S.

12 Eastwood GL. Gastrointestinal epithelial renewal. *Gastroenterology*, 1977; 72: 962.

13 Svanes K, Ito S, Takeuchi K, Silen W. Restitution of the in vitro frog gastric mucosa after damage with hyperosmolar sodium chloride: morphologic and physiologic characteristics. *Gastroenterology*, 1982; 82: 1409.

14 Konturek SJ, Brzozowski T, Majka A, Dembinski A, Slomiany A, Slomiany BL. Transforming growth factor alpha and epidermal growth factor in protection and healing of gastric mucosal injury. *Scand J Gastroenterol*, 1992; 27: 649.

15 Wong W-M, Playford RJ, Wright NA. Peptide gene expression in gastrointestinal mucosal ulceration: ordered sequence or redundancy. *Gut*, 2000; 46: 286.

16 Kaufmann GL. Mucosal damage to the stomach. How, when and why? *Scand J Gastroenterol*, 1984; 19 (Suppl 105): 19.

17 Starlinger M, Schiessel R, Hung CR, Silen W. H^+ back diffusion stimulating gastric mucosal blood flow in the rabbit fundus. *Surgery*, 1981; 89: 232.

18 Kivilaakso E, Fronn D, Silen W. Relationship between ulceration and intramural pH of gastric mucosa during haemorrhagic shock. *Surgery*, 1978; 84: 70.

19 Leung FW, Itoh M, Hirabayashi K, Guth PH. Role of blood flow in gastric and duodenal mucosal injury in the rat. *Gastroenterology*, 1985; 88: 281.

20 Robert A, Nezamis JE, Lancaster C, Hanchar AJ. Cytoprotection by prostaglandins in rats. *Gastroenterology*, 1979; 77: 433.

21 Bickel M, Kauffman GL. Gastric gel mucus thickness: effect of distension 16, 16-dimethyl prostaglandin E2 and carbenoxolone. *Gastroenterology*, 1981; 80: 770.

22 Konturek SJ, Robert A. Cytoprotection of canine gastric mucosa by prostacyclin: possible mediation by increased mucosal blood flow. *Digestion*, 1982; 25: 155.

23 Konturek SJ, Tasler J, Bilski J, Kaminski A, Laskiewicz J. Role of prostaglandins in alkaline secretion from gastroduodenal mucosa exposed to acid and taurocholate. *Scand J Gastroenterol*, 1984; 19 (Suppl 92): 69.

24 Lichtenberger LM, Richards JE, Hills BA. Effects of 16, 16 dimethyl prostaglandin PGE2 on the surface hydrophobicity of aspirin-treated canine gastric mucosa. *Gastroenterology*, 1985; 88: 308.

25 Konturek SJ. Gastric cytoprotection. *Scand J Gastroenterol*, 1985; 20: 543.

26 Kunkel SL, Wiggins RC, Chensue SW, Larrick J. Regulation of macrophage tumour necrosis factor production by prostaglandin E2. *Biochem Biophys Res Commun*, 1986; 137: 404.

27 Raud J. Vasodilatation and inhibition of mediator release represent two distinct mechanisms for prostaglandin modulation of acute mast cell dependent inflammation. *Br J Pharmacol*, 1990; 99: 449.

28 Hogaboam CM, Bissonnette KY, Chin BC, Befus AD, Wallace JL. Prostaglandins inhibit inflammatory mediator release from rat mast cells. *Gastroenterology*, 1993; 104: 122.

29 Konturek SJ, Obtulowicz W, Sito E, Oleksy J, Wilkur S, Dembinski-Kiec A. Distribution of prostaglandins in gastric and duodenal mucosa of healthy subjects and duodenal ulcer patients. Effects of aspirin and paracetamol. *Gut*, 1981; 22: 283.

30 Simon LS, Mills JA. New non-steroidal anti-inflammatory drugs. *N Engl J Med*, 1980; 302: 1179 & 1237.

31 Masuda E, Kawano S, Nagano K *et al*. Endogenous nitric oxide modulates ethanol-induced gastric mucosal injury in rats. *Gastroenterology*, 1995; 108: 58.

32 Olsen PS, Poulsen SS, Kirkegaard P, Nexo EE. Role of submandibular saliva and epidermal growth factor in gastric cytoprotection. *Gastroenterology*, 1984; 87: 103.

33 Polk WH, Dempsey PJ, Russell WE *et al*. Increased production of transforming growth factor-α following acute gastric injury. *Gastroenterology*, 1992; 102: 1467.

34 Ernst H, Konturek P, Hahn EG, Brzozowski T, Konturek SJ. Acceleration of wound healing in gastric ulcers by local injection of neutralising antibody to transfoming growth factor B1. *Gut*, 1996; 39: 172.

35 Wright NA, Pike C, Elia G. Induction of a novel epidermal growth factor-secreting cell lineage by mucosal ulceration in human gastrointestinal stem cells. *Nature*, 1990; 343: 82.

36 Lalani EL, Nasir Williams P, Jayaram Y *et al*. Trefoil factor-2, human spasmolytic polypeptide promotes branching morphogenesis in MCF-7 cells. *Lab Invest*, 1999; 79: 537.

37 Plaut AG. Trefoil peptides in the defense of the gastrointestinal tract. *N Engl J Med*, 1997; 336: 506.

38 Lefebvre O, Chenard M-P, Masson R *et al*. Gastric mucosa abnormalities and tumour agenesis in mice lacking the pS2 trefoil protein. *Science*, 1996; 274: 259.

39 Wright NA, Poulsom R, Stamp G *et al*. Trefoil gene expression in gastrointestinal epithelial cells in inflammatory bowel disease. *Gastroenterology*, 1993; 104: 12.

40 Marshall BJ, Armstrong JA, McGechie DB, Glancy RJ. Attempt to

fulfil Koch's postulates for pyloric campylobacter. *Med J Aust*, 1985; 42: 436.

41 Morris A, Nicholson G. Ingestion of *Campylobacter pyloridis* causes gastritis and raised fasting gastric pH. *Am J Gastroenterol*, 1987; 82: 192.

42 Sobala GM, Crabtree JE, Dixon MF, Schorah CJ. Acute *Helicobacter pylori* infection: clinical features, local and systemic immune response, gastric mucosal histology, gastric juice, ascorbic acid concentrations. *Gut*, 1991; 32: 1415.

43 Graham DY, Alport LC, Smith JL, Yoshimura HH. Iatrogenic *Campylobacter pylori* infection is a cause of epidemic achlorhydria. *Am J Gastroenterol*, 1988; 83: 974.

44 Laine L, Weinstein WM. Histology of alcoholic haemorrhagic gastritis: a prospective evaluation. *Gastroenterology*, 1988; 94: 1254.

45 Carpenter HA, Talley NJ. Gastroscopy is incomplete without biopsy: clinical relevance of distinguishing gastropathy from gastritis. *Gastroenterology*, 1995; 108: 917.

46 Palmer ED. Gastritis: a re-evaluation. *Medicine*, 1954; 33: 199.

47 Gottfried EB, Korsten MA, Lieber CS. Alcohol-induced gastric and duodenal lesions in man. *Am J Gastroenterol*, 1978; 70: 587.

48 Kelly JP, Kaufman DW, Koff RS, Laszlo A, Wiholm B-E, Shapiro S. Alcohol consumption and the risk of major upper gastrointestinal bleeding. *Am J Gastroenterol*, 1995; 90: 1058.

49 Eliason EL, Wright VWM. Phlegmonous gastritis. *Surg Clin N Amer*, 1938; 18: 1553.

50 Mittleman RE, Suarez RV. Phlegmonous gastritis associated with the acquired immunodeficiency syndrome pre-acquired immunodeficiency syndrome. *Arch Pathol Lab Med*, 1985; 109: 765.

51 Zazzo J-F, Troche G, Millat B, Aubert A, Bedossa P, Keros L. Phlegmonous gastritis associated with HIV-I seroconversion. *Dig Dis Sci*, 1992; 37: 1454.

52 Ross DA, Vincenti AC. Acute phlegmonous gastritis: a rare condition with a potentially common cause. *Br J Hosp Med*, 1994; 52: 115.

53 O'Toole PA, Morris JA. Acute phlegmonous gastritis. *Postgrad Med J*, 1988; 64: 315.

54 Nevin NC, Eakins D, Clarke SD, Carson DJL. Acute phlegmonous gastritis. *Br J Surg*, 1969; 56: 268.

55 LaForce FM. Diffuse phlegmonous gastritis. *Arch Int Med*, 1967; 120: 230.

56 Lifton LJ, Schlossberg D. Phlegmonous gastritis after endoscopic polypectomy. *Ann Intern Med*, 1982; 197: 373.

57 Miller AI, Smith B, Rogers AI. Phlegmonous gastritis. *Gastroenterology*, 1975; 68: 231.

58 Gear MWL, Truelove SC, Whitehead R. Gastric ulcer and gastritis. *Gut*, 1971; 12: 639.

59 Taor RE, Fox B, Ware J, Johnson AG. Gastritis—gastroscopic and microscopic. *Endoscopy*, 1975; 7: 209.

60 Khakoo SI, Lobo AJ, Shepherd NA, Wilkinson SP. Histological assessment of the Sydney classification of endoscopic gastritis. *Gut*, 1994; 35: 1172.

61 Sipponen P, Helske T, Jarvinen P, Hyuarinen H, Seppala K, Siurala M. Fall in the prevalence of chronic gastritis over 15 years: analysis of outpatient series in Finland from 1977, 1985 and 1992. *Gut*, 1994; 35: 1167.

62 Whitehead R, Truelove SC, Gear MWL. The histological diagnosis of chronic gastritis in fibreoptic gastroscopic biopsy specimens. *J Clin Pathol*, 1972; 25: 1.

63 Strickland RG, Mackay IR. A reappraisal of the nature and significance of chronic atrophic gastritis. *Am J Dig Dis*, 1973; 18: 426.

64 Wyatt JI, Dixon MF. Chronic gastritis—a pathogenetic approach. *J Pathol*, 1988; 154: 113.

65 Price AB. The Sydney system: histological division. *J Gastroenterol Hepatol*, 1991; 6: 209.

66 Misiewicz JJ. The Sydney system. A new classification of gastritis. Introduction. *J Gastroenterol Hepatol*, 1991; 6: 207.

67 Andrew A, Wyatt JI, Dixon MF. Observer variation in the assessment of chronic gastritis according to the Sydney system. *Histopathology*, 1994; 25: 317.

68 Genta RM, Dixon MF. The Sydney system revisited: the Houston International Gastritis Workshop. *Am J Gastroenterol*, 1995; 90: 1039.

69 Correa P. Chronic gastritis. In: Whitehead R, ed. *Gastrointestinal and Oesophageal Pathology*, 2nd edn. Edinburgh: Churchill Livingstone. 1995: 485.

70 Dixon MF, Genta RM, Yardley JH, Correa P. Classification and grading of gastritis. The updated Sydney system. *Am J Surg Pathol*, 1996; 20: 1161.

71 Collins JSA, Watt PCH, Hamilton PW, Sloan JM, Love AHG. Grading of superficial antral gastritis: comparison of cell counting and photographic-based methods. *J Pathol*, 1991; 163: 251.

72 Warren JR, Marshall B. Unidentified curved bacilli on gastric epithelium in active chronic gastritis. *Lancet*, 1983; 1: 1273.

73 Editorial. *Campylobacter pylori* becomes *Helicobacter pylori*. *Lancet*, 1989; 2: 1019.

74 Goodwin CS, Armstrong JA, Chilvers T *et al*. Transfer of *Campylobacter pylori* and *Campylobacter mustelae* to *Helicobacter* gen. nov. as *Helicobacter pylori*, comb. nov. and *Helicobacter mustelae* comb nov. respectively. *Int J Syst Bacteriol*, 1989; 39: 397.

75 Crabtree JE. Gastric mucosal inflammatory responses to *Helicobacter pylori*. *Aliment Pharmacol Ther*, 1996; 10 (Suppl 1): 29.

76 Dixon MF. Recent advances in gastritis. *Curr Diag Pathol*, 1994; 1: 80.

77 Rauws EAJ, Langenberg W, Houthoff HJ, Zanen HC, Tytgat GNJ. *Campylobacter pyloridis*-associated chronic active antral gastritis. *Gastroenterology*, 1988; 94: 33.

78 Lambert JR, Dunn KL, Eaves ER, Korman MG, Hansky J. *Campylobacter pyloridis* in diseases of the upper gastrointestinal tract. *Gastroenterology*, 1986; 90: 1509.

79 O'Connor HJ, Wyatt JI, Dixon MF, Axon ATR. *Campylobacter*-like organisms and reflux gastritis. *J Clin Pathol*, 1986; 39: 531.

80 Rawles JW, Paull G, Yardley JH *et al*. Gastric *Campylobacter*-like organisms in a US hospital population. *Gastroenterology*, 1986; 90: 1599.

81 Bayerdörffer EB, Lehn N, Hatz R *et al*. Difference in expression of *Helicobacter pylori* gastritis in antrum and body. *Gastroenterology*, 1992; 102: 1575.

82 Gilvarry J, Leen E, Sant S, Sweeney E, O'Morain C. The long-term effect of *Helicobacter pylori* on gastric mucosa. *Irish J Med Sci*, 1992; 30 (Suppl 10): 30.

83 Rouvroy D, Bogaerts J, Nsengiumwa O, Omar M, Versailles L, Haot J. *Campylobacter pylori*, gastritis and peptic ulcer disease in Central Africa. *Br Med J*, 1987; 295: 1174.

84 Drumm B, O'Brien A, Cutz E, Sherman P. *Campylobacter pylori* are

associated with primary antral gastritis in the paediatric population. *Gastroenterology*, 1986; 90: 1379.

85 Hill R, Pearman J, Worthy P, Carusa V, Goodwin S, Blingow E. *Campylobacter pyloridis* and gastritis in children. *Lancet*, 1986; 1: 387.

86 Hassall E, Dimmick JE. Unique features of *Helicobacter pylori* disease in children. *Dig Dis Sci*, 1991; 36: 417.

87 Crabtree JE, Taylor JD, Wyatt JI. Mucosal IgA recognition of *Helicobacter pylori* 120K Da protein, peptic ulceration and gastric pathology. *Lancet*, 1991; 338: 332.

88 Crabtree JE, Farmery SM, Lindley IJD, Figura N, Peichl P, Tompkins DS. Cag A / cytotoxin strains of *Helicobacter pylori* and interleukin-8 in gastric epithelial cell lines. *J Clin Pathol*, 1994; 47: 945.

89 Witteman EM, Mravunac M, Becx MJCM *et al*. Improvement of gastric inflammation and resolution of epithelial damage one year after eradication of *Helicobacter pylori*. *J Clin Pathol*, 1995; 48: 250.

90 Tepes B, Kavcic B, Zaletel L *et al*. Two- to four-year histological follow-up of gastric mucosa after *Helicobacter pylori* eradication. *J Pathol*, 1999; 188: 24.

91 Valle J. Seppälä K, Sipponen P, Kosunen T. Disappearance of gastritis after eradication of *Helicobacter pylori*. *Scand J Gastroenterol*, 1991; 26: 1057.

92 Laheij RJF, Jansen JMBJ, Van De Lisdonk EH, Severens JL, Verbeek ALM. Review article: symptom improvement through eradication of *Helicobacter pylori* in patients with non-ulcer dyspepsia. *Aliment Pharmacol Ther*, 1996; 10: 843.

93 McColl K, Murray L, el-Omar E *et al*. Symptomatic benefit from eradicating *Helicobacter pylori* infection in patients with nonulcer dyspepsia. *N Engl J Med*, 1998; 339: 1869.

94 Talley NJ, Janssens J, Lauritsen K *et al*. Eradication of *Helicobacter pylori* in functional dyspepsia: randomised double blind placebo controlled trial with 12 months' follow up. *Br Med J*, 1999; 318: 833.

95 Collins JSA, Hamilton PW, Watt PCH, Sloan JM, Love AHG. Superficial gastritis and *Campylobacter pylori* in dyspeptic patients—a quantitative study using computer linked image analysis. *J Pathol*, 1989; 158: 303.

96 Hui PK, Chan WY, Cheung PS *et al*. Pathological changes of gastric mucosa colonised by *Helicobacter pylori*. *Hum Pathol*, 1992; 23: 548.

97 Fiocca R, Lumetti O, Villani L *et al*. Epithelial cytotoxicity, immune responses and inflammatory components of *Helicobacter pylori* gastritis. *Scand J Gastroenterol*, 1994; 29 (Suppl 205): 11.

98 Wyatt JI, Rathbone BJ. Immune response of the gastric mucosa to *Campylobacter pylori*. *Scand J Gastroenterol*, 1988; 23 (Suppl 142): 44.

99 Eidt S, Stolte M. Prevalence of lymphoid follicles and aggregates in *Helicobacter* gastritis in antral and body mucosa. *J Clin Pathol*, 1993; 46: 832.

100 Zaitoun AM. Prevalence of lymphoid follicles in *Helicobacter pylori* associated gastritis in patients with ulcer and non-ulcer dyspepsia. *J Clin Pathol*, 1995; 48: 325.

101 Genta RN, Hamner HW, Graham DY. Gastric lymphoid follicles in *Helicobacter pylori* infection. *Hum Pathol*, 1993; 24: 577.

102 Gray SF, Wyatt JI, Rathbone BJ. Simplified technique of examining *Campylobacter pyloridis*. *J Clin Pathol*, 1986; 39: 1279.

103 Burnett RA, Brown IL, Findlay J. Cresyl fast violet staining method for *Campylobacter*-like organisms. *J Clin Pathol*, 1987; 40: 353.

104 McMullen L, Walker MM, Bain LA, Karim QM, Barren JH. Histological identification of *Campylobacter* using Gimenez technique in gastric antral mucosa. *J Clin Pathol*, 1987; 40: 464.

105 Walters LL, Budin RE, Paull G. Acridine-orange to identify *Campylobacter pyloridis* in formalin fixed paraffin embedded gastric biopsies. *Lancet*, 1986; 1: 42.

106 Westblom TU, Madan E, Kemp J, Subik MA, Tseng J. Improved visualisation of mucus penetration by *Campylobacter pylori* using a Brown–Hopps stain. *J Clin Pathol*, 1988; 41: 232.

107 Genta RN, Robason GO, Graham DY. Simultaneous visualisation of *Helicobacter pylori* and gastric morphology: a new stain. *Hum Pathol*, 1994; 25: 221.

108 Chan W-Y, Hui P-K, Leung K-N *et al*. Coccoid forms of *Helicobacter pylori* in the human stomach. *Am J Clin Pathol*, 1994; 102: 503.

109 Loffeld RJLF, Stobberingh E, Flendrig JA, Arends JW. *Helicobacter pylori* in gastric body specimens. Comparison of culture, modified Giemsa stain and immunohistochemistry. A retrospective study. *J Pathol*, 1991; 165: 69.

110 Ashton-Key M, Diss TC, Isaccson PG. Detection of *Helicobacter pylori* in gastric biopsy and resection specimens. *J Clin Pathol*, 1996; 49: 107.

111 Fabre R, Sobhani I, Laurent-Puig P *et al*. Polymerase chain reaction assay for the detection of *Helicobacter* in gastric biopsy specimens: comparison with culture, rapid urease test and histopathological tests. *Gut*, 1994; 35: 305.

112 van Zwet AA, Thijs JC, Roosendaal R *et al*. Practical diagnosis of *Helicobacter pylori* infection. *Eur J Gastroenterol Hepatol*, 1996; 8: 501.

113 Dickey W, Kenny BD, McConnell JB. Effect of proton pump inhibitors on the detection of *Helicobacter pylori* in gastric biopsies. *Aliment Pharmacol Ther*, 1996; 10: 289.

114 Kuipers EJ, Lundell L, Kukenberg-Knol EC, Havu N. Atrophic gastritis and *Helicobacter pylori* infection in patients with reflux oesophagitis treated with omeprazole or fundoplication. *N Engl J Med*, 1996; 334: 1018.

115 Tham TCK, Collins JSA, Sloan JM. Long-term effects of *Helicobacter pylori* on gastric mucosa: an 8 year follow-up. *Am J Gastroenterol*, 1994; 89: 1355.

116 Niemala S, Karttunen T, Kerola T. *Helicobacter pylori*-associated gastritis. Evolution of histologic changes over 10 years. *Scand J Gastroenterol*, 1995; 30: 542.

117 Villako K, Kekki M, Maaroos H-I *et al*. A 12 year follow-up study of chronic gastritis and *Helicobacter pylori* in a population-based random sample. *Scand J Gastroenterol*, 1995; 30: 964.

118 Stolte M, Datz CH, Eidt S. Giant fold gastritis: a special form of *Helicobacter pylori* associated gastritis. *Z Gastroenterol*, 1993; 31: 289.

119 Murayama Y, Mayagawa J, Shinomura Y *et al*. Morphological and functional restoration of parietal cells in *Helicobacter*-associated enlarged fold gastritis after eradication. *Gut*, 1999; 45: 653.

120 Correa P, Haenszal W, Cuello C *et al*. Gastric pre-cancerous process in high risk population: cohort follow-up. *Cancer Res*, 1990; 50: 4737.

121 Kekki M, Varis K, Pohjanpalo H, Isokoski M, Ihamaki T, Siurala M. Course of antrum and body gastritis in pernicious anaemia families. *Dig Dis Sci*, 1983; 28: 698.

122 Fontham ETH, Ruiz B, Perez A, Hunter F, Correa P. Determinants of *Helicobacter pylori* infection on chronic gastritis. *Am J Gastroenterol*, 1995; 90: 1094.

123 Kuipers EJ, Uyterlinde AN, Pena AS *et al*. Long term sequelae of *Helicobacter pylori* gastritis. *Lancet*, 1995; 345: 1525.

124 Katelaris PH, Seow F, Lin BPC, Napoli J, Ngu MC, Jones DB. Effect of age, *Helicobacter pylori* infection and gastritis with atrophy on serum gastrin and gastric acid secretion in healthy men. *Gut*, 1993; 34: 1032.

125 Rugge M, DiMario F, Cassaro M *et al*. Pathology of the gastric antrum and body associated with *Helicobacter pylori* infection in non ulcerous patients: is the bacterium a promoter of intestinal metaplasia? *Histopathology*, 1993; 22: 9.

126 Kuipers EJ, Perez-Perez GI, Meuwissen SGM, Blaser MJ. *Helicobacter pylori* and atrophic gastritis: importance of the Cag A status. *J Natl Cancer Inst*, 1995; 87: 1777.

127 Correa P. Chronic gastritis. In: Whitehead R, ed. *Oesophageal and Gastrointestinal Pathology*, 2nd edn. Edinburgh: Churchill Livingstone, 1995: 485.

128 Oksanen A, Sipponen P, Karttunen R *et al*. Atrophic gastritis and *Helicobacter pylori* infection in outpatients referred for gastroscopy. *Gut*, 2000; 46: 460.

129 El Omar EM, Oien K, El-Nujumi A *et al*. *Helicobacter pylori* infection and chronic gastric acid secretion. *Gastroenterology*, 1997; 113: 15.

130 Genta RM. Recognising atrophy: another step toward a classification of gastritis. *Am J Surg Pathol*, 1996; 20 (Suppl 1): S23.

131 Offerhaus GJA, Price AB, Haot J *et al*. Observer agreement on the grading of gastric atrophy. *Histopathology*, 1999; 34: 320.

132 Ihamaki T, Kekki M, Sipponen P, Siurala M. The sequelae and course of chronic gastritis during a 30–34 year bioptic follow-up study. *Scand J Gastroenterol*, 1985; 20: 485.

133 Steadman C, Teague C, Kerlin P, Nimmo G. *Campylobacter pylori* in gastric antral intestinal metaplasia. *Gastroenterology*, 1988; 95: 258.

134 Genta RM, Gurer IE, Graham DY *et al*. Adherence of *Helicobacter pylori* to areas of incomplete intestinal metaplasia in the gastric mucosa. *Gastroenterology*, 1996; 111: 1206.

135 Hu PJ, Li YY, Lin HL *et al*. Gastric atrophy and regional variation in upper gastrointestinal disease. *Am J Gastroenterol*, 1995; 90: 1102.

136 Sipponen P, Kekki M, Seppala K, Siurala M. The relationship between chronic gastritis and gastric acid secretion. *Aliment Pharmacol Ther*, 1996; 10 (Suppl 1): 103.

137 Lee A, Dixon MF, Danon SJ *et al*. Local acid production and *Helicobacter pylori*: a unifying hypothesis of gastroduodenal disease. *Eur J Gastroenterol Hepatol*, 1995; 7: 461.

138 El Omar EM, Carrington M, Chow W-H *et al*. Interleukin-1 polymorphisms associated with increased risk of gastric cancer. *Nature*, 2000; 404: 398.

139 Villaka K, Kekki M, Maarooas H-I *et al*. Chronic gastritis: progression of inflammation and atrophy in a six year endoscopic follow-up of a random sample of 142 Estonian urban subjects. *Scand J Gastroenterol*, 1991; 26 (Suppl 186): 135.

140 Flejou J-F, Bahame P, Smith AC, Stockbrugger RW, Rode I, Price AB. Pernicious anaemia and *Campylobacter*-like organisms: is the gastric antrum resistant to colonisation? *Gut*, 1989; 30: 60.

141 Haruma K, Komoto K, Kawaguchi H *et al*. Pernicious anaemia and *Helicobacter pylori* infection in Japan. Evaluation in a country with a high prevalence of infection. *Am J Gastroenterol*, 1995; 90: 1107.

142 Negrini R, Savio A, Poiesi C *et al*. Antigenic mimicry between *Helicobacter pylori* and gastric mucosa in the pathogenesis of body atrophic gastritis. *Gastroenterology*, 1996; 111: 655.

143 Kato Y, Sugano H, Rubio CA. Classification of intramucosal cysts of the stomach. *Histopathology*, 1983; 7: 931.

144 Magnus HA. Observations on the presence of intestinal epithelium in the gastric mucosa. *J Pathol Bacteriol*, 1937; 44: 389.

145 Stout AP. *Atlas of Tumour Pathology*, Vol. VI. Washington: Armed Forces Institute of Pathology, 1953.

146 Morson BC. Intestinal metaplasia of the gastric mucosa. *Br J Cancer*, 1955; 9: 377.

147 Cornet A, Pagniez G, Guerre J, Delavierre P. La muqueuse gastrique des sujets agés. *Arch Fr Mal Appareil Dig*, 1964; 53: 365.

148 Suirala M, Isokoski M, Varis K, Kekki M. Prevalence of gastritis in a rural population. Bioptic study of subjects selected at random. *Scand J Gastroenterol*, 1968; 3: 211.

149 Eidt S, Stolte M. Antral intestinal metaplasia in *Helicobacter pylori* gastritis. *Digestion*, 1994; 55: 13.

150 Stemmermann GN. Intestinal metaplasia of the stomach. A status report. *Cancer*, 1994; 74: 556.

151 Slack JMW. Homoeotic transformations in man: implications for the mechanism of embryonic development and for the organization of epithelia. *J Theor Biol*, 1985; 114: 463.

152 Jass JR, Filipe MI. Disorders of differentiation and their pathobiological significance. New insights from functional probes. In: Filipe MI, Jass JR, eds. *Gastric Carcinoma*. Edinburgh: Churchill Livingstone, 1986: 273.

153 Correa P, Haenszel W, Cuello C *et al*. Gastric precancerous process in a high risk population: cross-sectional studies. *Cancer Res*, 1990; 50: 4731.

154 Sobala GM, O'Connor HJ, Dewar EP, King RJG, Axon ATR, Dixon MF. Bile reflux and intestinal metaplasia in gastric mucosa. *J Clin Pathol*, 1993; 46: 235.

155 Sipponen P, Kekki M, Siurala M. Age related trends of gastritis and intestinal metaplasia in gastric carcinoma patients and in controls representing the population at large. *Br J Cancer*, 1984; 49: 521.

156 Imai T, Murayama H. Time trend in the prevalence of intestinal metaplasia in Japan. *Cancer*, 1983; 52: 353.

157 Craanen ME, Dekker W, Blok P, Ferwerda J, Tytgat GNJ. Intestinal metaplasia and *Helicobacter pylori*: an endoscopic bioptic study of the gastric antrum. *Gut*, 1992; 33: 16.

158 Silva S, Filipe MI. Intestinal metaplasia and its variants in the gastric mucosa of Portugese subjects. *Hum Pathol*, 1986; 17: 988.

159 Spechler SJ, Zeroogian JN, Antonioli DA, Wang HH, Goyal RK. Prevalence of metaplasia at the gastro-oesophageal junction. *Lancet*, 1994; 344: 1533.

160 Correa P, Cuello C, Duque E. Carcinoma and intestinal metaplasia in Colombian migrants. *J Natl Canc Inst*, 1970; 44: 297.

161 Rothery GA, Day DW. Intestinal metaplasia in endoscopic specimens of gastric mucosa. *J Clin Pathol*, 1985; 38: 618.

162 Solcia E, Fiocca R, Luinetti O *et al*. Intestinal and diffuse gastric

cancers arise in a different background of *Helicobacter pylori* gastritis through different gene involvement. *Am J Surg Pathol*, 1996; 20 (Suppl 1): S8.
163 Filipe MI, Ramachandra S. The histochemistry of intestinal mucins; changes in disease. In: Whitehead R, ed. *Gastrointestinal and Oesophageal Pathology*, 2nd edn. Edinburgh: Churchill Livingstone, 1995: 73.
164 Shah KA, Deacon AJ, Dunscombe P, Price AB. Intestinal metaplasia subtyping: evaluation of Gomori's aldehyde fuchsin for routine diagnostic use. *Histopathology*, 1997; 31: 277.
165 Jass JR. Role of intestinal metaplasia in the histogenesis of gastric carcinoma. *J Clin Pathol*, 1980; 33: 801.
166 Filipe MI, Jass JR. Intestinal metaplasia subtypes and cancer risk. In: Filipe MI, Jass JR, eds. *Gastric Carcinoma*. Edinburgh: Churchill Livingstone, 1986: 87.
167 Matsukura N, Suzuki K, Kawachi T *et al*. Distribution of marker enzymes and mucin in intestinal metaplasia in human stomachs and relation of complete and incomplete types of intestinal metaplasia to minute gastric carcinomas. *J Natl Cancer Inst*, 1980; 65: 231.
168 Filipe MI, Munoz N, Matko I *et al*. Intestinal metaplasia types and the risk of gastric cancer: a cohort study in Slovenia. *Int J Cancer*, 1994; 54: 324.
169 Lipkin M, Correa P, Mikol YB *et al*. Proliferative and antigenic modifications in human epithelial cells in chronic atrophic gastritis. *J Natl Cancer Inst*, 1985; 75: 613.
170 Fraser AG, Sim R, Sankey EA, Dhillon AP, Pounder RE. Effect of eradication of *Helicobacter pylori* on gastric epithelial cell proliferation. *Aliment Pharmacol Ther*, 1994; 8: 167.
171 Wong W-M, Wright NA. Cell proliferation in gastrointestinal mucosa. *J Clin Pathol*, 1999; 52: 321.
172 Ectors N, Dixon MF. The prognostic value of sulphomucin positive intestinal metaplasia in the development of gastric cancer. *Histopathology*, 1986; 10: 1271.
173 Endoh Y, Tamura G, Motoyama T *et al*. Well differentiated adenocarcinoma mimicking complete-type intestinal metaplasia in the stomach. *Hum Pathol*, 1999; 30: 826.
174 Doglioni C, Laurino L, Deitos AP *et al*. Pancreatic (acinar) metaplasia of the gastric mucosa. *Am J Surg Pathol*, 1993; 17: 1134.
175 Maaroos H-I, Salupere V, Uibo R, Kekki M, Sipponen P. 17 year follow-up study of chronic gastritis in gastric ulcer patients. *Scand J Gastroenterol*, 1985; 20: 198.
176 El-Serag HB, Sonnenberg A, Jamal MM *et al*. Corpus gastritis is protective against reflux oesophagitis. *Gut*, 1999; 45: 181.
177 Lagergren J, Bergström R, Lindgren A, Nyren O. Symptomatic gastro-oesophageal reflux as a risk factor for esophageal adenocarcinoma. *N Engl J Med*, 1999; 340: 825.
178 Fenoglio-Preiser CM, Noffsinger AE, Belli J, Stemmermann GN. *Semin Oncol*, 1996; 23: 292.
179 Jass JR, Filipe MI. A variant of intestinal metaplasia associated with gastric carcinoma: a histochemical study. *Histopathology*, 1979; 3: 191.
180 Goldman H, Ming S-C. Fine structure of intestinal metaplasia and adenocarcinoma of the human stomach. *Lab Invest*, 1968; 18: 203.
181 Stemmermann GN, Hayashi T. Intestinal metaplasia of the gastric mucosa: a gross and microsocopic study of its distribution in various disease states. *J Natl Canc Inst*, 1968; 61: 693.
182 Taylor KB, Roitt IM, Doniach D, Couchman KG, Shapland C. Autoimmune phenomena in pernicious anaemia: gastric antibodies. *Br Med J*, 1962; ii: 1347.
183 Taylor KB. Immune phenomena in pernicious anaemia. *Gastroenterology*, 1963; 45: 670.
184 Ardeman S, Chanarin I. A method for the assay of human gastric intrinsic factor and for the detection and titration of antibodies against intrinsic factor. *Lancet*, 1963; ii: 1350.
185 Ardeman S, Chanarin I. Intrinsic factor antibodies and intrinsic factor mediated vitamin B_{12} absorption in pernicious anaemia. *Gut*, 1966; 6: 436.
186 Chanarin I, Ardeman S. The significance of gastric antibodies. *Proc R Soc Med*, 1966; 59: 690.
187 Polak JM, Hoffbrand AV, Reed PI, Bloom S, Pearse AGE. Qualitative and quantitative studies of antral and fundic G cells in pernicious anaemia. *Scand J Gastroenterol*, 1973; 8: 361.
188 Doniach D, Roitt IM, Taylor KB. Autoimmune phenomena in pernicious anaemia: serological overlap with thyroiditis, thyrotoxicosis and systemic lupus erythematosus. *Br Med J*, 1963; 1: 1374.
189 Varis K, Ihamaki T, Harkonen M, Samloff IM, Siurala M. Gastric morphology, function and immunology in first degree relatives of probands with pernicious anaemia and controls. *Scand J Gastroenterol*, 1979; 14: 129.
190 Cox AJ. The stomach in pernicious anaemia. *Am J Pathol*, 1943; 19: 491.
191 Magnus HA. A reassessment of the gastric lesion in pernicious anaemia. *J Clin Pathol*, 1958; 11: 289.
192 Kaye MD, Whorwell PJ, Wright R. Gastric mucosal lymphocyte populations in pernicious anaemia (PA). *Gastroenterology*, 1982; 82: 1097.
193 Odgers RJ, Wangel AG. Abnormalities in IgA containing mononuclear cells in the gastric lesion of pernicious anaemia. *Lancet*, 1968; ii: 846.
194 Lewin KJ, Dowling F, Wright JP, Taylor KB. Gastric morphology and serum gastrin levels in pernicious anaemia. *Gut*, 1976; 17: 551.
195 Fong T-L, Dooley CP, Dehesa M *et al*. *Helicobacter* infection in pernicious anaemia: a prospective control study. *Gastroenterology*, 1991; 100: 328.
196 Stockbrugger RW, Larsson L-T, Lundqvist G, Angervall L. Antral gastrin cells and serum gastrin in achlorhydria. *Scand J Gastroenterol*, 1977; 12: 209.
197 Solcia E, Fiocca R, Villani L, Luinetti O, Capella C. Hyperplastic, dysplastic, and neoplastic enterochromaffin-like cell proliferations of the gastric-mucosa—classification and histogenesis. *Am J Surg Pathol*, 1995; 19: S1.
198 Rode J, Dhillon AP, Papadiki L, Stockbrugger R, Thompson RJ, Moss E, Cotton PB. Pernicious anaemia and mucosal endocrine cell proliferation of the non-antral stomach. *Gut*, 1986; 27: 789.
199 Hodges JR, Isaacson P, Wright R. Diffuse enterochromaffin-like (ECL) cell hyperplasia in multiple gastric carcinoids: a complication of pernicious anaemia. *Gut*, 1981; 22: 237.
200 Moses RE, Frank BB, Leavitt M, Miller R. The syndrome of type A chronic atrophic gastritis, pernicious anaemia and multiple gastric carcinoids. *J Clin Gastroenterol*, 1986; 8: 61.
201 Elsborg L, Andersen D, Myhre-Jensen O, Bastrup-Madsen P. Gastric mucosal polyps in pernicious anaemia. *Scand J Gastroenterol*, 1977; 12: 49.

202 Stockbrugger RW, Menon GG, Beilby JOW *et al*. Gastroscopic screening in 80 patients with pernicious anaemia. *Gut*, 1983; 24: 1141.

203 Ikeda T, Senoue I, Hara M, Tsutsumi Y, Harasawa S, Miwa T. Gastric pseudopolyposis: a new clinical manifestation of type A gastritis. *Am J Gastroenterol*, 1985; 80: 82.

204 Hsing HW, Hansson L-E, McLaughlin JK *et al*. Pernicious anaemia and subsequent cancer. A population-based cohort study. *Cancer*, 1993; 71: 745.

205 Varis O, Valle J, Siurala M. Is *Helicobacter pylori* involved in the pathogenesis of gastritis characteristic of pernicious anaemia? *Scand J Gastroenterol*, 1993; 28: 705.

206 Haruma K, Komoto K, Kawaguchi H *et al*. Pernicious anaemia and *Helicobacter pylori* infection in Japan: evaluation in a country with a high prevalence of infection. *Am J Gastroenterol*, 1995; 90: 1107.

207 Lillibridge CA, Brandborg LL, Rubin CE. Childhood pernicious anaemia. Gastrointestinal, secretory, histological and electron microscopic aspects. *Gastroenterology*, 1967; 52: 792.

208 Benjamin B. Infantile form of pernicious (Addisonian) anaemia. Report of a long term study of a case. *Am J Dis Child*, 1948; 75: 143.

209 Mollin DJ, Baker SJ, Doniach I. Addisonian pernicious anaemia without gastric atrophy in a young man. *Br J Haematol*, 1955; 1: 278.

210 Rubin CE. Observations on the pathogenesis of juvenile pernicious anaemia. *J Clin Invest*, 1957; 36: 925.

211 Imerslund O, Bjorrstad P. Familial vitamin B12 malabsorption. *Acta Haematol*, 1963; 30: 1.

212 Siurala M. Gastric lesions in some megaloblastic anaemias with special reference to the mucosal lesions in pernicious tapeworm anaemia. *Acta Med Scand*, 1954; 151 (Suppl 299): 1.

213 Dixon MF, O'Connor HJ, Axon ATR, King RFJG, Johnston D. Reflux gastritis: a distinct histopathological entity? *J Clin Pathol*, 1986; 39: 524.

214 Quinn CM, Bjarnason I, Price AB. Gastritis in patients on non-steroidal anti-inflammatory drugs. *Histopathology*, 1993; 23: 341.

215 Sobala GM, King RFG, Axon ATR, Dixon MF. Reflux gastritis in the intact stomach. *J Clin Pathol*, 1990; 43: 303.

216 Dixon MF. Progress in the pathology of gastritis and duodenitis. In: Williams GT, ed. *Current Topics in Pathology*, No. 81. Berlin: Springer-Verlag, 1990: 1.

217 El-Zimiaty HMT, Genta RM, Graham DY. Histological features do not define NSAID-induced gastritis. *Hum Pathol*, 1996; 27: 1348.

218 Hamilton SR, Yardley JH. Endoscopic biopsy of aspirin-associated chronic gastric ulcers. *Gastroenterology*, 1980; 78: 1178.

219 Huang J-Q, Sridhar S, Hunt RH. Role of *Helicobacter pylori* infection and non-steroidal anti-inflammatory drugs in peptic ulcer disease: a meta-analysis. *Lancet*, 2002; 359: 14.

220 Franzin G, Novelli P. Gastritis cystica profunda. *Histopathology*, 1981; 5: 535.

221 Janunger K-G. Domellof L. Gastric polyps and precancerous mucosal changes after partial gastrectomy. *Acta Chir Scand*, 1978; 144: 293.

222 Savage A, Jones S. Histological appearances of the gastric mucosa 15–27 years after partial gastrectomy. *J Clin Pathol*, 1979; 32: 179.

223 Domellof L, Erisson J, Janunger K-G. The risk for gastric carcinoma after partial gastrectomy. *Am J Surg*, 1977; 73: 462.

224 Schrumpf E, Serck-Hanssen A, Stadaas J, Aunesmynen J, Osnes M. Mucosal changes in the gastric stump 20–25 years after partial gastrectomy. *Lancet*, 1977; 2: 467.

225 Farrands PA, Blake JRS, Ansell ID *et al*. Endoscopic review of patients who have had gastric surgery. *Br Med J*, 1983; 286: 755.

226 Watt PCH, Sloan JM, Spencer A, Kennedy TL. Changes in the gastric mucosa after vagotomy and gastrojejunostomy for duodenal ulcer. *Br Med J*, 1983; 287: 1407.

227 Offerhaus GJA, Stadt J, van der Huibregste K, Tytgat GNJ. Endoscopic screening for malignancy in the gastric remnant. The clinical significance of dysplasia in gastric mucosa. *J Clin Pathol*, 1984; 37: 748.

228 Pulimood BM, Knudson A, Coghill NF. Gastric mucosa after partial gastrectomy. *Gut*, 1976; 17: 463.

229 Sipponen P, Hakkiluoto A, Kalimi TV, Siurala M. Selective loss of parietal cells in the gastric remnant following antral resection. *Scand J Gastroenterol*, 1976; 11: 813.

230 Haot J, Hamichi L, Wallez I, Mainguet P. Lymphocytic gastritis: a newly described entity: a retrospective endoscopic and histological study. *Gut*, 1988; 29: 1258.

231 Haot J, Berger F, Andre C, Moulinier B, Mainguet P, Lamber R. Lymphocytic gastritis versus varioliform gastritis. A histological series revisited. *J Pathol*, 1989; 158: 19.

232 Haot J, Jouret A, Willette M, Gossuin J, Mainguet P. Lymphocytic gastritis, a prospective study of its relationship with varioliform gastritis. *Gut*, 1990; 31: 282.

233 Dixon MF, Wyatt JI, Burke DA, Rathbone BJ. Lymphocytic gastritis—relationship to *Campylobacter pylori* infection. *J Pathol*, 1988; 154: 125.

234 Wolber R, Owen D, Del Buono L, Appelman H, Freeman H. Lymphocytic gastritis in patients with coeliac sprue or sprue-like intestinal disease. *Gastroenterology*, 1990; 98: 310.

235 Hayat M, Arora DS, Wyatt JI *et al*. The pattern of involvement of the gastric mucosa in lymphocytic gastritis is predictive of the presence of duodenal pathology. *J Clin Pathol*, 1999; 52: 815.

236 Lynch DAF, Sobala GM, Dixon MF *et al*. Lymphocytic gastritis and associated small bowel disease: a diffuse lymphocytic gastroenteropathy. *J Clin Pathol*, 1995; 48: 939.

237 Haot J, Bogomoletz WV, Jouret A, Mainguet P. Menetrier's disease with lymphocytic gastritis. An unusual association with possible pathogenic implications. *Hum Pathol*, 1991; 22: 379.

238 Wolfsen HL, Carpenter HA, Talley NJ. Menetrier's disease. A form of hypertrophic gastropathy or gastritis. *Gastroenterology*, 1993; 104: 1310.

239 Wu T-T, Hamilton SR. Lymphocytic gastritis: association with aetiology and topology. *Am J Surg Pathol*, 1999; 23: 153.

240 Morgan AG, McAdam WAF, Pyrah RD, Tinsley EGF. Multiple recurring gastric erosions (aphthous ulcers). *Gut*, 1972; 19: 67.

241 Lambert R, Andre C, Moulinier B *et al*. Diffuse varioliform gastritis. *Digestion*, 1978; 17: 159.

242 Clarke AC, Lee SP, Nicholson GI. Gastritis varioliformis: chronic erosive gastritis with a protein-losing enteropathy. *Am J Gastroenterol*, 1977; 68: 599.

243 Isaacson P. Biopsy appearances easily mistaken for malignancy in gastrointestinal endoscopy. *Histopathology*, 1982; 6: 377.

244 Goldman H, Proujansky R. Allergic proctitis and gastroenteritis

in children. Clinical and mucosal biopsy features in 53 cases. *Am J Surg Pathol*, 1986; 10: 75.

245 Katz AJ, Goldman H, Grand RJ. Gastric mucosal biopsy in eosinophilic (allergic) gastroenteritis. *Gastroenterology*, 1977; 73: 705.

246 Caldwell JH, Sharma HM, Hurtubise PE, Colwell DL. Eosinophilic gastroenteritis in extreme allergy. Immunopathological comparison with non-allergic gastrointestinal disease. *Gastroenterology*, 1979; 77: 560.

247 Lucak BK, Sansaricq C, Snyderman SE, Alba Greco M, Fazzini EP, Bazaz GR. Disseminated ulcerations in allergic eosinophilic gastroenterocolitis. *Am J Gastroenterol*, 1982; 77: 248.

248 Talley NJ, Shorter MG, Phillips SF, Zinsmeister AR. Eosinophilic gastroenteritis: a clinicopathological study of patients with disease of the mucosa, muscle layer and subserosal tissues. *Gut*, 1990; 31: 54.

249 Johnstone JM, Morson BC. Eosinophilic gastroenteritis. *Histopathology*, 1978; 2: 335.

250 Harmon WA, Helman CA. Eosinophilic gastroenteritis and ascites. *J Clin Gastroenterol*, 1981; 3: 371.

251 Blackshaw AJ, Levison DA. Eosinophilic infiltrates of gastrointestinal tract. *J Clin Pathol*, 1986; 39: 1.

252 Walker NI, Croese J, Clouston AD, Loukas A, Prociv P. Eosinophilic enteritis in Northern Eastern Australia. *Am J Surg Pathol*, 1995; 19: 328.

253 Leinbach GE, Rubin CE. Eosinophilic gastroenteritis: a simple reaction to food allergens? *Gastroenterology*, 1970; 59: 874.

254 Klein NC, Hargrove RL, Sleisenger MH, Jeffries GH. Eosinophilic gastroenteritis. *Medicine*, 1970; 49: 299.

255 Floch MH, Thomassen RW, Cox RS Jr, Sheahy TW. The gastric mucosa in tropical sprue. *Gastroenterology*, 1963; 44: 567.

256 Griscom NT, Kirkpatrick JA Jr, Girdany BR *et al*. Gastric antral narrowing in chronic granulomatous disease of childhood. *Paediatrics*, 1974; 54: 456.

257 Colletti RB, Trainer TD. Collagenous gastritis. *Gastroenterology*, 1989; 97: 1552.

258 Lagorce-Pages C, Fabiani B, Bouvier R *et al*. Collagenous gastritis. A report of 6 cases. *Am J Surg Pathol*, 2001; 25: 1174.

259 Dent JC, McNulty CAM, Uff JC, Wilkinson SP, Gear MWL. Spiral organisms in the gastric mucosa. *Lancet*, 1987; 2: 96.

260 McNulty CAM, Dent JC, Curry A *et al*. New spiral bacterium in gastric mucosa. *J Clin Pathol*, 1989; 42: 585.

261 O'Rourke J, Solnick J, Lee A, Tomkins L. *Helicobacter heilmannii* (previously *Gastrospirillum*): a new species of *Helicobacter* in animals. *Irish J Med Sci*, 1992; 161 (Suppl 10): 31.

262 Heilmann KL, Brochard F. Gastritis due to spiral-shaped bacteria other than *Helicobacter pylori*: clinical, histological and ultrastructural findings. *Gut*, 1991; 32: 137.

263 Debongnie JC, Donnay M, Manesse J. *Gastrospirillum hominis* (*Helicobacter heilmannii*). A cause of gastritis, sometimes transient, better diagnosed by touch cytology? *Am J Gastroenterol*, 1995; 90: 411.

264 Stolte M, Wellens E, Bethke B, Ratter M, Eidt H. *Helicobacter heilmannii* (formerly *Gastrospirillum hominis*) gastritis. An infection transmitted by animals. *Scand J Gastroenterol*, 1994; 29: 1061.

265 Mazzucchelli L, Wilder-Smith CH, Ruchti C, Meyer-Wyss B, Merki HS. *Gastrospirillum hominis* in asymptomatic healthy individuals. *Dig Dis Sci*, 1993; 38: 2087.

266 Weber AF, Hase O, Sautter JH. Some observations concerning the presence of spirilla in the fundic glands of dogs and cats. *Am J Vet Res*, 1958; 18: 677.

267 Lee A, Dent J, Hazell S, McNulty C. Origin of spiral organisms in human gastric antrum. *Lancet*, 1988; 1: 300.

268 Dutz W, Saidl F, Kohout E. Gastric anthrax with massive ascites. *Gut*, 1970; 11: 352.

269 Monkemuller KE, Call SA, Lazenby A, Wilcox CM. Declining prevalence of opportunistic gastrointestinal disease in the era of combination antiretroviral therapy. *Am J Gastroenterol*, 2000; 95: 457.

270 Minoli G, Terruzzi V, Butti G *et al*. Gastric candidiasis: an endoscopic and histological study in 26 patients. *Gastrointest Endosc*, 1982; 28: 59.

271 Scott BB, Jenkins D. Gastro-oesophageal candidiasis. *Gut*, 1982; 23: 137.

272 Katzenstein A-LA, Maksem J. Candidial infection of gastric ulcers. *Am J Clin Pathol*, 1979; 71: 137.

273 Calle S, Klatsky S. Intestinal phycomycosis (mucormycosis). *Am J Clin Pathol*, 1966; 45: 264.

274 Deal WB, Johnson JE. Gastric phycomycosis. Report of a case and review of the literature. *Gastroenterology*, 1969; 57: 579.

275 Gatling RR. Gastric mucormycosis in a newborn infant. *Arch Pathol*, 1959; 67: 249.

276 Washington K, Gottfried MR, Wilson MI. Gastrointestinal cryptococcosis. *Mod Pathol*, 1992; 4: 707.

277 Bonacini M, Nussbaum J, Ahluwalia C. Gastrointestinal, hepatic and pancreatic involvement with *Cryptococcus neoformans* in AIDS. *J Clin Gastroenterol*, 1990; 12: 295.

278 Fisher JR, Sanowski RA. Disseminated histoplasmosis producing hypertrophic gastric folds. *Dig Dis*, 1978; 23: 282.

279 Matsuda S, Urata Y, Shiota T *et al*. Disseminated infection of *Pneumocystis carinii* in a patient with the acquired immunodeficiency syndrome. *Virchows Arch A Pathol Anat*, 1989; 414: 523.

280 Dieterich DT, Lew EA, Bacon DJ *et al*. Gastrointestinal pneumocystosis in HIV-related patients on aerosolized pentamidine: report of five cases and literature review. *Am J Gastroenterol*, 1992; 87: 1763.

281 Arnar Do, Gudmundsson G, Theodors A *et al*. Primary cytomegalovirus infection and gastric ulcers in normal host. *Dig Dis Sci*, 1991; 36: 108.

282 Yoshinaga M, Nakate S, Motmura S, Sugimara T, Sasaki I, Tsuneyoshi M. Cytomegalovirus-associated gastric ulcerations in normal host. *Am J Gastroenterol*, 1994; 89: 448.

283 Francis ND, Boylston AW, Parkin JN, Pinching AJ. Cytomegalovirus inclusion bodies in gastrointestinal tract of patients infected with HIV-I or AIDS. *J Clin Pathol*, 1989; 42: 1055.

284 Franzin G, Muolo A, Griminelli T. Cytomegalovirus inclusions in the gastroduodenal mucosa of patients after renal transplantation. *Gut*, 1981; 22: 698.

285 Henson D. Cytomegalovirus inclusion bodies in the gastrointestinal tract. *Arch Pathol*, 1972; 93: 477.

286 Strayer DS, Phillips DB, Barker KH *et al*. Gastric cytomegalovirus infection in bone marrow transplant patients. *Cancer*, 1981; 48: 1478.

287 Aqel NM, Tanner P, Drury A, Francis MD, Henry K. Cytomegalovirus gastritis with perforation and gastrocolic fistulae formation. *Histopathology*, 1991; 18: 165.

288 Gazzard BG. HIV in disease and the gastroenterologist. *Gut*, 1988; 29: 1497.

289 Varsky CG, Correa MC, Sarmiento M *et al*. Prevalence and etiology of gastroduodenal ulcer in HIV positive patients: a comparative study of 497 symptomatic subjects evaluated by endoscopy. *Am J Gastroenterol*, 1998; 93: 935.

290 Sperling HV, Reed WG. Herpetic gastritis. *Dig Dis*, 1977; 22: 1033.

291 Khilnani MT, Keller RJ. Roentgen and pathological changes in the gastrointestinal tract in herpes zoster generalizata: a unique case and brief review. *Mt Sinai J Med*, 1971; 38: 303.

292 McCluggage WG, Fox JD, Baillie KEM *et al*. Varicella zoster gastritis in a bone marrow transplant recipient. *J Clin Pathol*, 1994; 47: 1054.

293 Oberhuber G, Kastner N, Stolte M. Giardiasis: a histologic analysis of 567 cases. *Scand J Gastroenterol*, 1997; 32: 48.

294 Smart PE, Weinfield A, Thompson ME, Defortuna SM. Toxoplasmosis of the stomach: a cause of antral narrowing. *Radiology*, 1990; 174: 369.

295 Alpert L, Miller M, Alpert E, Satin R, Lamoureux E, Trudel L. Gastric toxoplasmosis in acquired immunodeficiency syndrome. Antemortem diagnosis with histopathologic characterisation. *Gastroenterology*, 1996; 110: 258.

296 Peraire J, Vidal F, Mayayo E, Razquin S, Richart C. Gastric toxoplasmosis in the acquired immunodeficiency syndrome. *Am J Gastroenterol*, 1993; 88: 1464.

297 Guarda LA, Stein SA, Cleary KA, Ordonez NG. Human cryptosporidiosis in the Acquired Immune Deficiency Syndrome. *Arch Pathol Lab Med*, 1983; 107: 562.

298 Rossi P, Rivasi F, Codeluppi M *et al*. Gastric involvement in AIDS-associated cryptosporidiosis. *Gut*, 1999; 43: 476.

299 Ravasi F, Rossi P, Righi E, Pozio E. Gastric sporidiosis: correlation between intensity of infection and histological alterations. *Histopathology*, 1999; 34: 405.

300 Adams DO. The granulomatous inflammatory response. *Am J Pathol*, 1976; 84: 164.

301 Cotran RS, Kumar V, Robbins SL. Granulomatous inflammation. In: *Robbins Pathologic Basis of Disease*, 5th edn (Schoen FJ, ed). Philadelphia: W B Saunders Co, 1994: 80.

302 Ectors NL, Dixon MF, Geboes KJ, Rutgeerts PJ, Desmet VJ, Vantrappen CR. Granulomatous gastritis: a morphological and diagnostic approach. *Histopathology*, 1993; 23: 55.

303 Fenoglio-Preiser C. Creating a framework for diagnosing the benign gastric biopsy. *Curr Diag Pathol*, 1998; 5: 2.

304 Oberhuber G, Puspok A, Oesterreicher C *et al*. Focally enhanced gastritis: a frequent type of gastritis in patients with Crohn's disease. *Gastroenterology*, 1997; 112: 698.

305 Pryse-Davies J. Gastroduodenal Crohn's disease. *J Clin Pathol*, 1964; 17: 90.

306 Johnson OA, Hoskins DW, Todd J, Thorbjarnason B. Crohn's disease of the stomach. *Gastroenterology*, 1966; 50: 571.

307 Finder CA, Doman DB, Steinberg WM, Lewcki AM. Crohn's disease of the proximal stomach. *Am J Gastroenterol*, 1984; 79: 494.

308 Wright CL, Riddell RH. Histology of the stomach and duodenum in Crohn's disease. *Am J Surg Pathol*, 1998; 22: 383.

309 Ruuska T, Vaajalahti P, Arajarvi P, Maki M. Prospective evaluation of upper gastrointestinal mucosal lesions in children with ulcerative colitis and Crohn's disease. *J Pediatr Gastroenterol Nutr*, 1994; 19: 181.

310 Palmer ED. Note on silent sarcoidosis of the gastric mucosa. *J Lab Clin Med*, 1958; 52: 231.

311 Gould SR, Handley AJ, Barnardo BE. Rectal and gastric involvement in a case of sarcoidosis. *Gut*, 1973; 14: 971.

312 Braun MM, Byers RH, Heyward WL *et al*. Acquired immunodeficiency syndrome and extrapulmonary tuberculosis in the United States. *Arch Intern Med*, 1990; 150: 1913.

313 Marshall JB. Tuberculosis of the gastrointestinal tract and peritoneum. *Am J Gastroenterol*, 1993; 88: 989.

314 Chazan BL, Aithison JD. Gastric tuberculosis. *Br Med J*, 1960; II: 1288.

315 Tromba JL, Inglese R, Rieders B, Todaro R. Primary gastric tuberculosis presenting as pyloric outlet obstruction. *Am J Gastroenterol*, 1991; 86: 1820.

316 Gupta B, Mathew S, Bhalla S. Pyloric obstruction due to gastric tuberculosis—an endoscopic diagnosis. *Postgrad Med J*, 1990; 66: 63.

317 Subei I, Attar B, Schmitt G, Levendoglu H. Primary gastric tuberculosis: a case report and literature review. *Am J Gastroenterol*, 1987; 82: 769.

318 Morin ME, Tan A. Diffuse enlargement of gastric folds as a manifestation of secondary syphilis. *Am J Gastroenterol*, 1980; 74: 170.

319 Rank EL, Goldenberg SA, Hasson J, Cartun RW, Grey N. *Treponema pallidum* and *Helicobacter pylori* recovered in a case of chronic gastritis. *Am J Clin Pathol*, 1992; 97: 116.

320 Winters HA, Notar-Francesco V, Bromberg K, *et al*. Gastric syphilis: five recent cases and a review of the literature. *Ann Intern Med*, 1992; 116: 314.

321 Inagaki H, Kawai T, Miyata M, Nagaya S, Tateyama H, Eimoto T. Gastric syphilis: polymerase chain reaction detection of treponemal DNA in pseudolymphomatous lesions. *Hum Pathol*, 1996; 27: 761.

322 Willeford G, Childers JH, Hepner WR Jr. Gumma of the stomach in congenital syphilis. *Paediatrics*, 1952; 10: 162.

323 Fyfe B, Poppiti RJ, Lubin J, Robinson MJ. Gastric syphilis. Primary diagnosis by gastric biopsy. *Arch Pathol Lab Med*, 1993; 117: 820.

324 Sherman FE, Moran TJ. Granulomas of the stomach. 1. Response to injury of muscle and fibrous tissue of human stomach. *Am J Clin Pathol*, 1954; 24: 415.

325 Abraham SC, Yardley JH, Wu T-T. Erosive injury to the upper gastrointestinal tract in patients receiving iron medication. *Am J Surg Pathol*, 1999; 23: 1241.

326 Kliks MM. Anisakiasis: four new cases from California. *Am J Trop Med Hyg*, 1983; 32: 526.

327 Sugimachi K, Inokuchi K, Ooiwa T, Fujino T, Ishii Y. Acute gastric anisakiasis. *JAMA*, 1985; 253: 1012.

328 Fontaine RE. Anisakiasis from the American perspective. *JAMA*, 1985; 253: 1024.

329 Ectors N, Geboes K, Wynants P, Desmet V. Granulomatous gastritis and Whipple's disease. *Am J Gastroenterol*, 1992; 87: 509.

330 Wada R, Yagihashi S, Konta R, Ueda T, Izumiyama T. Gastric polyposis caused by multifocal histiocytosis X. *Gut*, 1992; 33: 994.

331 Groisman GM, Rosh JR, Harpaz N. Langerhans' cell histiocytosis of the stomach. A cause of granulomatous gastritis in gastric polyposis. *Arch Path Lab Med*, 1994; 118: 1232.

332 Washington K, Stenzel T, Buckley RH, Gottfried MR. Gastrointestinal pathology in patients with common variable immunode-

ficiency and X-linked agammaglobulinaemia. *Am J Surg Pathol*, 1996; 20: 1240.

333 Snover DC, Weisdorf SA, Vercellotti GM, Rank B, Hutton S, McGlave P. A histopathologic study of gastric and small intestinal graft-versus-host disease following allogeneic bone marrow transplantation. *Hum Pathol*, 1985; 16: 387.

334 Burke A, Sobin LH, Virmani R. Localised vasculitis of the gastrointestinal tract. *Am J Surg Pathol*, 1995; 19: 338.

335 Lee HC, Kay S. Primary polyarteritis nodosa of the stomach and small intestine as a cause of gastrointestinal haemorrhage. *Am Surg*, 1958; 147: 714.

336 Abell MR, Limond RV, Blamey WE, Martel W. Allergic granulomatosis with massive gastric involvement. *N Engl J Med*, 1970; 282: 665.

337 Hendrix TR, Yardley JH. Menetrier's disease (letter). *Gut*, 1995; 36: 945.

338 Lepore MJ, Smith FB, Bonanno CA. *Campylobacter*-like organisms in a patient with Menetrier's disease. *Lancet*, 1988; 1: 466.

339 Bayerdörffer E, Ritter MM, Hatz R, Brooks W, Ruckdeschel G, Stolte N. Healing of protein-losing gatropathy by eradication of *Helicobacter pylori*. Is *Helicobacter pylori* a pathogenic factor in Menetrier's disease. *Gut*, 1994; 35: 701.

340 Komorowski RA, Gaya JG. Hyperplastic gastropathy. Clinicopathologic correlation. *Am J Surg Pathol*, 1991; 15: 577.

341 Mason EE. Gastrointestinal lesions occurring in uraemia. *Ann Intern Med*, 1952; 37: 96.

342 Franzin GN, Musola R, Mencarelli R. Morphological changes of the gastroduodenal mucosa in regular dialysis uraemic patients. *Histopathology*, 1982; 6: 429.

343 Boyle JM, Johnston B. Acute upper gastrointestinal haemorrhage in patients with chronic renal failure. *Am J Med*, 1983; 75: 409.

344 Kang JY, Wu AYT, Sutherland IH, Vathsala A. Prevalence of peptic ulcer in patients undergoing maintenance haemodialysis. *Dig Dis Sci*, 1988; 33: 774.

345 McConnell JB, Thjodleifsson B, Stewart WK, Wormsley KG. Gastric function in chronic renal failure. *Lancet*, 1975; 2: 1121.

346 Doherty CC. Gastric secretion in chronic uraemia and after renal transplantation. *Irish J Med Sci*, 1980; 149: 5.

347 Cheli R, Dodero M. Etude biopique et secretoire de la muqueuse gastrique au cours de l'urémie chironique. *Acta Gastroenterol Belg*, 1958; 21: 193.

348 Shousha S, Keen C, Parkins RA. Gastric metaplasia and *C. pylori* infection of duodenum in patients with chronic renal failure. *J Clin Pathol*, 1989; 42: 348.

349 Jaspersen D, Fassbinder W, Heinkele P *et al*. Significantly lower prevalence of *Helicobacter pylori* in uraemic patients than in patients with normal renal function. *J Gastroenterol*, 1995; 30: 585.

350 Franzin G, Musola R, Mencarelli R. Changes in the mucosa of the stomach and duodenum during immunosuppressive therapy after renal transplantation. *Histopathology*, 1982; 6: 439.

351 Doig RK, Funder JF, Weiden S. Serial gastric biopsy studies in a case of duodenal ulcer treated by deep X-ray therapy. *Med J Aust*, 1951; 1: 828.

352 Goldgraber MB, Rubin CE, Palmer WL, Dobson RL, Massey BW. The early gastric response to irradiation. A serial biopsy study. *Gastroenterology*, 1954; 27: 1.

353 Wood IJ, Ralston M, Kurrie GR. Irradiation injury to gastrointestinal tract: clinical features, management and pathogenesis. *Aust Ann Med*, 1963; 12: 143.

354 Sell A, Jensen TS. Acute gastric ulcers induced by irradiation. *Acta Radiol*, 1966; 4: 289.

355 Berthrong M, Fajardo LF. Radiation injury in surgical pathology. Part II. Alimentary Tract. *Am J Surg Pathol*, 1981; 5: 153.

356 McCormack TT, Sims J, Eyre-Brook I *et al*. Gastric lesions in portal hypertension: inflammatory gastritis or congestive gastropathy? *Gut*, 1985; 26: 1226.

357 Pérez-Ayuso RM, Piqué JM, Bosch J *et al*. Propranolol in prevention of recurrent bleeding from severe portal hypertensive gastropathy in cirrhosis. *Lancet*, 1991; 337: 1431.

358 Piqué JM. Portal hypertensive gastropathy. *Baillière's Clin Gastroenterol*, 1997; 11: 257.

359 Zaman A, Hapke R, Flora K *et al*. Prevalence of upper and lower gastrointestinal tract findings in liver transplant candidates undergoing screening endoscopic evaluation. *Am J Gastroenterol*, 1999; 94: 895.

360 Foster PM, Wyatt JI, Bullimore DW, Losowsky MS. Gastric mucosa in patients with portal hypertension: prevalence of capillary dilatation and *Campylobacter pylori*. *J Clin Pathol*, 1989; 42: 919.

361 Quintero E, Pique JM, Bombi JA *et al*. Gastric mucosal vascular ectasias causing bleeding in cirrhosis. *Gastroenterology*, 1987; 93: 1054.

362 Jabbari M, Cherry R, Lough JO, Daly DS, Kinnear DG, Goresky CA. Gastric antral vascular ectasia: the watermelon stomach. *Gastroenterology*, 1984; 87: 1165.

363 Gardiner GW, Murray D, Prokipchuk EJ. Watermelon stomach or antral gastritis. *J Clin Pathol*, 1985; 38: 1317.

364 Suit PF, Petras RE, Bauer TW, Petrini JL. Gastric antral vascular ectasia. *Am J Surg Pathol*, 1987; 11: 750.

365 Gostout CJ, Viggiano TR, Ahlquist DA *et al*. Clinical and endoscopic spectrum of the watermelon stomach. *J Clin Gastroenterol*, 1992; 15: 256.

366 Gilliam JH, Geisinger KR, Wallace CW, Weidner N, Richter JE. Endoscopic biopsy is diagnostic in gastric antral vascular ectasia. *Dig Dis Sci*, 1989; 34: 885.

367 Gretz JE, Achem SR. The watermelon stomach: clinical presentation, diagnosis and treatment. *Am J Gastroenterol*, 1998; 93: 890.

13 Peptic ulcer disease

Introduction

Peptic ulcers, or the scars of healed ulcers, can be found in the lowest part of the oesophagus or along the lesser curvature (magenstrasse) of the stomach, but they are most common in the antral and prepyloric regions, at the pylorus itself, and on the anterior and posterior walls of the first part of the duodenum. They may also be seen following gastroenterostomy, either at the line of anastomosis or in the small bowel immediately distal; in the second, third or fourth parts of the duodenum or upper jejunum in the Zollinger–Ellison syndrome; and they can occur within or immediately distal to a Meckel's diverticulum if the lining heterotopic mucosa is acid secreting.

Peptic ulcers are usually classified as acute or chronic on the basis of depth of penetration or degree of healing rather than their duration, and it is generally assumed that all chronic ulcers originate in an acute ulcer that failed to heal. There is loss of the full thickness of the mucosa with a variable degree of penetration into the underlying coats. Erosions, by contrast, are defined as shallower defects that involve less than the full thickness of the mucosa so that some basal gland elements remain. Acute ulcers and erosions tend to heal rapidly and seldom recur if the underlying cause is treated. Chronic peptic ulcers are long standing and are characterized histologically by the presence of fibrous tissue in the ulcer base.

Gastric erosions and acute peptic ulcers (acute stress ulceration of the stomach, acute haemorrhagic gastritis, acute erosive gastritis)

Erosions are acute shallow lesions, oval or circular in shape, with fresh or altered blood in the base and sharply defined edges. They are almost invariably multiple in the gastric mucosa and most measure 1–3 mm in diameter although some extend up to 3 cm. The lesions are found mainly in the fundus and corpus of the stomach although they may extend into the antrum and duodenum (Fig. 13.1). The intervening mucosa appears congested and contains petechial haemorrhages. The distribution of erosions differs with the clinical circumstances. Following trauma or sepsis they are first observed in the fundus near the greater curve and with time develop distally, only involving the antrum when the lesions in the body are widespread and severe. This contrasts with erosions caused by non-steroidal anti-inflammatory drugs (NSAIDs) and alcohol which, although most frequent in the antrum, can affect all segments of the stomach and the duodenum, and do not have a proximal to distal progression. The latter lesions also tend to be smaller and to heal quicker [1,2].

Microscopically erosions show necrosis of a small area of mucosa of variable depth but not extending down to the muscularis mucosae. The crater of the erosion contains necrotic slough, polymorphs and red blood cells. There is a variable, usually minor, degree of acute inflammation in the adjacent lamina propria with dilatation and congestion of nearby capillaries. On healing most erosions show complete mucosal regeneration and there is no visible residual scarring.

An acute ulcer is simply extension of an erosion through the full thickness of the mucosa into the submucosa or deeper into underlying tissues. Acute ulcers tend to be larger than erosions and they frequently occur in areas of intense erosion and mucosal congestion, especially on the greater curvature of the stomach. Like erosions they are often multiple. The ulcer bed is similar to that of an erosion and fibrous scar tissue is not prominent in the base. Acute ulcers are considerably less common in the duodenum but in that site they tend to be single. Haemorrhage is a frequent complication of acute ulcer due to ulceration of submucosal vessel walls.

Care must be taken not to mistake granulation tissue in the base of an erosion or acute ulcer for infiltrating carcinoma. This may cause considerable diagnostic difficulty in biopsy material, especially on frozen section, as granulation tissue may contain prominent and sometimes bizarre endothelial cells and

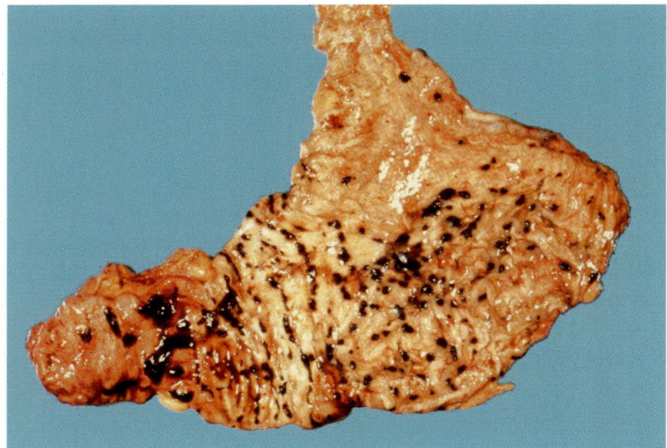

Fig. 13.1 Acute erosive gastritis. Multiple erosions with bleeding on the mucosal surface, especially in the fundus of the stomach.

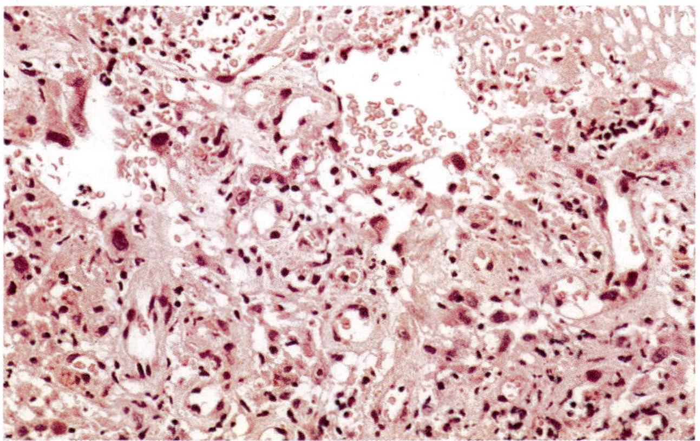

Fig. 13.2 Histology of gastric erosion. Necrotic slough is present (top) with underlying granulation tissue containing some bizarre endothelial cells and fibroblasts which may simulate carcinoma.

fibroblasts that may simulate poorly differentiated infiltrating carcinoma [3] (Fig. 13.2). Marked regenerative atypia of the epithelium adjacent to the ulcer margin can similarly cause confusion with adenocarcinoma. Good communication with the endoscopist, knowledge of the endoscopic appearances, and awareness of this difficult diagnostic problem are important to avoid overdiagnosis of carcinoma.

Incidence and pathogenesis

Acute erosive gastritis or ulceration occurs in three situations.

1 Severe stress following trauma, major surgery, sepsis, respiratory insufficiency, head injury (Cushing's ulcer) or extensive burns (Curling's ulcer).

2 Following ingestion of aspirin or other NSAIDs or alcohol.

3 In association with a variety of other conditions.

Stress-related erosions and acute ulcers

Following severe trauma or sepsis, endoscopic studies indicate that mucosal petechiae and erosions appear in the corpus of the stomach within 24 hours. They then spread distally and may involve the antral mucosa [4]. The incidence of such lesions is very high and approaches 100% in seriously ill patients [4,5]. Clinical manifestations are much less common and usually occur 3–10 days after the stressful event. Significant bleeding occurs in 5–20% of cases although this can be significantly reduced by prophylactic antacids or acid suppression therapy [6]. Recent analysis indicates that with modern intensive care treatment the risk of significant bleeding, although associated with high mortality, has decreased and is lower than previously thought, except in patients with coagulopathy or respiratory failure [7].

Curling's ulcer

Curling's ulcer is the term applied to acute gastroduodenal ulceration following burns. After extensive burns, gastric mucosal erosions are very common. They develop within 24–72 hours, predominantly within the proximal stomach as in other cases of stress gastritis, but the antrum and duodenum are also frequently involved [8]. In areas of intense mucosal erosion there may be progression to gastric ulcer, especially in burns cases complicated by sepsis or haemoconcentration, even despite prophylactic antacid therapy [9]. Duodenal ulceration occurs with approximately the same frequency as gastric ulcer [8,10] and is particularly common in children [11].

Cushing's ulcer

Cushing described a series of cases of mucosal erosions and perforation of oesophagus, stomach and duodenum following surgery for intracranial tumours [12], and the term Cushing's ulcer is used to described acute gastroduodenal ulceration associated with disease of or injury to the central nervous system. Again, endoscopic studies indicate a high incidence of visible lesions soon after severe head injury [13] although clinically significant complications are considerably less common. In contrast to other forms of stress-associated gastroduodenal disease, Cushing's ulcer is relatively commoner in the duodenum and tends to be solitary and deep. Accordingly, perforation is more common [14].

The pathogenesis of stress-related erosive gastritis is not fully understood and is likely to be due to a variety of factors related to the mucosal defence mechanisms outlined in Chapter 12. The importance of gastric acid is indicated by a significant reduction in clinical manifestations of erosive gastritis following prophylactic antacid or acid suppression therapy [6]. However, luminal acid appears to be only one pathogenic factor. Hypovolaemia in rabbits causes focal ischaemia in gastric mucosa that subsequently ulcerates when blood volume is restored, giving lesions resembling erosive gastritis [15]. Similar lesions can be produced in dogs [16]. The mucosa of the gastric corpus has a high energy requirement and it is suggested that hypovolaemic shock causes an energy deficit leading to depletion of adenosine triphosphate (ATP) levels which particularly affects the proximal stomach [17]. A further consequence of haemorrhagic shock is to alter intramucosal acid–base balance and to impair the capacity to buffer luminal acid [18]. Another possible aetiological factor concerns the role of oxygen-derived free radicals. Experimental evidence indicates that mucosal damage occurs during reperfusion following ischaemia and that this damage is reduced by agents that inhibit and scavenge free radicals [19].

NSAID- and alcohol-related erosions and acute ulcers

NSAID ingestion is regarded as the commonest cause of acute erosive gastritis [20]. Mucosal haemorrhages and erosions are extremely common in individuals taking these drugs, but in most cases there are no significant clinical manifestations. However, acute gastric ulcers have been reported in almost 7% of healthy volunteers taking therapeutic doses of aspirin for 1 week [21]. In this study, non-aspirin NSAIDs caused lesser degrees of mucosal damage. A similar endoscopic study showed that variable degrees of gastric and duodenal mucosal haemorrhage are common following aspirin therapy, but that enteric-coated tablets reduced the damage [22]. These studies investigated the acute effects of NSAIDs. It is likely that with long-term therapy mucosal adaptation occurs and the mucosal damage may diminish. The distribution of erosions caused by NSAIDs differs from that of stress-induced lesions in that they do not show a predilection for the proximal stomach, they tend to be less florid and they are relatively more common in the antrum [23].

Heavy alcohol ingestion is also associated with haemorrhagic gastritis. On gastroscopy, mucosal haemorrhages are seen in the proximal part of the stomach [24]. The haemorrhages are found in a distribution similar to that of stress-related lesions. Histology shows focal haemorrhage in the subepithelial region of the mucosa with oedema of adjacent mucosa. There is little inflammation and thus the term 'haemorrhagic gastritis' is not strictly accurate from the histological point of view. Indeed this is the case in most examples of acute erosive gastritis regardless of the underlying cause. The lesions occur in approximately 15% of heavy drinkers and it has been shown that they can be induced in healthy volunteers after acute alcohol ingestion [25]. There is evidence from experimental animal studies that exposure to high concentrations of alcohol leads to exfoliation and necrosis of the superficial gastric mucosa and that mucosal damage may be mediated via neutrophils [26]. Exposure to high concentrations of ethanol also leads to rapid reduction in gastric mucosal blood flow [27]. Nitric oxide released from vascular endothelial cells following alcohol ingestion may exert a protective vasodilator effect by preserving mucosal blood flow [28].

Other erosions and acute ulcers

Gastric erosions may also occur in association with underlying disorders such as Crohn's disease, amyloidosis, hypertrophic gastropathy and infiltrating carcinoma or lymphoma. Acute peptic ulceration occasionally occurs in the distal parts of the duodenum and jejunum in patients with Zollinger–Ellison syndrome, in the intestinal mucosa adjacent to a gastroenterostomy, and within the lining mucosa of, or in the intestinal mucosa immediately distal to, a Meckel's diverticulum if the latter contains functional gastric body-type mucosa. Haemorrhage and perforation are again recognized complications.

Chronic peptic ulcers

An ulcer may be regarded as chronic clinically when it has failed to heal over a reasonable period of time, and pathologically when attempts at repair have led to the formation of collagenous fibrohyaline tissue in the base of the ulcer to such a degree that a restoration to normal of the submucosa and muscularis propria is no longer possible; there is often concomitant failure of the mucosa to regenerate satisfactorily. Chronic peptic ulcers occur at the lower end of the oesophagus commonly in association with hiatus hernia or reflux oesophagitis, along the magenstrasse bounded by the lesser curve of the stomach, in the antral and prepyloric regions, and on the anterior and posterior walls of the first part of the duodenum. It can be difficult on occasion to decide whether a chronic ulcer with much scarring is prepyloric or duodenal.

Chronic gastric ulcers

In contradistinction to erosions and acute ulcers, chronic gastric ulcers are comparatively rare in the body mucosa [29,30]. Histological examination shows that many arise at the junction of antral and corpus mucosa surrounded mainly by pyloric-type mucosa or metaplastic mucosa of intestinal type, while others arise entirely in antral mucosa [29,31]. Chronic gastric ulcers are usually single, although large studies indicate that multiple ulcers occur in 6–13% of cases [29,32]. They are usually less than 2 cm in diameter, often smaller than 1 cm, and are round or oval. Smaller ulcers tend to occur near the pylorus [33]. They occur predominantly on the lesser curvature and less often on the posterior wall. The anterior wall and greater curvature are seldom involved [34]. They may lie across the lesser curve in a saddle-shaped form (Fig. 13.3) and are commonly found higher up on the lesser curve in women than in men, which may reflect the greater extent of antral-type mucosa in females or the increase of antral over body mucosa which occurs with advancing age [35]. The edges are clear cut but not raised or rolled and overhang, producing a flask-like appearance. The base is grey, and either blood clot or an

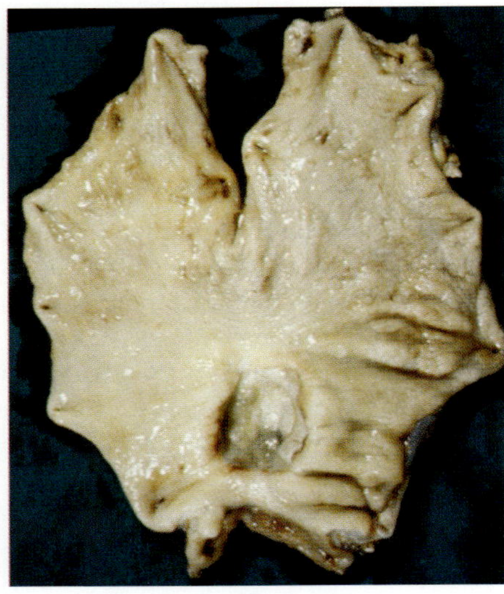

Fig. 13.3 Characteristic peptic ulcer on the lower part of the lesser curvature. The edges are clean cut but not raised or rolled. Note the flat, featureless, atrophic-appearing background mucosa.

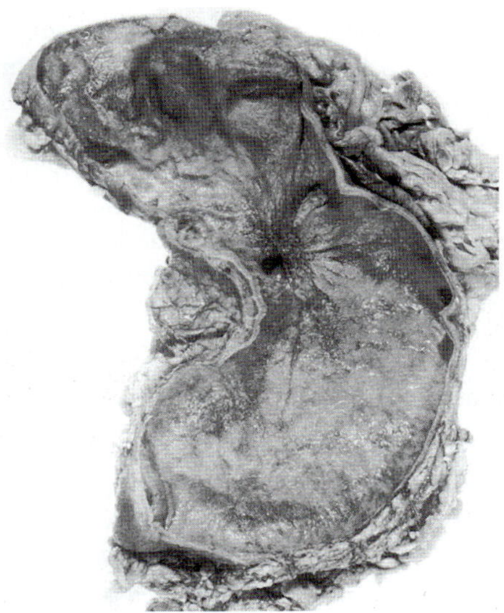

Fig. 13.4 Two chronic gastric ulcers high on the lesser curvature which caused an 'hour-glass' deformity.

eroded vessel can occasionally be seen within the crater. Chronic ulcers have by definition penetrated the mucosa and involved submucosa and muscle coats to a variable degree with resulting fibrosis, which in turn sometimes produces distortion in the form of pyloric stenosis or an 'hour-glass' constriction (Fig. 13.4). The overlying serosa is often thickened and opaque and the ulcer base adheres to underlying or overlying strictures, particularly pancreas. Adjacent lymph nodes commonly show non-specific inflammatory enlargement. The surrounding mucosa often appears flat and atrophic to the naked eye and at gastroscopy [36], and the presence of

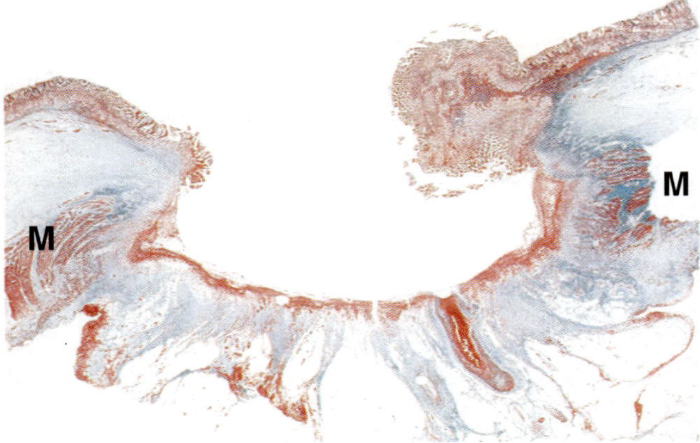

Fig. 13.5 Gastric ulcer. Histology shows interruption of the muscle coat (M) by fibrous tissue and extensive fibrosis of the ulcer base. An eroded blood vessel is present in the ulcer base. Masson trichrome.

gastritis, either local or more generalized, can be confirmed on microscopy.

Occasionally simple gastric ulcers reach extreme sizes. Lesser curve ulcers tend to enlarge in a saddle-shaped manner and may reach 10 cm or more in diameter [37]. They can also extend longitudinally as 'trench ulcers' along the lesser curve from cardia to incisura [38]; this type shows less fibrosis and the ulceration appears more acute. All large ulcers have to be distinguished from carcinomas and examined closely for carcinomatous change developing in them; distinction can usually be made by the clear-cut overhanging edges and absence of thickening in adjacent mucosa, but multiple biopsies should be taken from the base and circumference to exclude malignancy.

Microscopically all chronic peptic ulcers have a characteristic structure. In the stage of active necrosis the base has four recognizable layers. On the luminal aspect there is a narrow zone of fibrinopurulent exudate; underlying this a layer of acidophilic necrotic tissue; then a zone of granulation tissue of variable vascularity containing young fibroblasts and mononuclear inflammatory cells; which blends with the deepest layer of more dense scar tissue which interrupts and replaces the muscularis propria (Fig. 13.5). While the morphological structure of an ulcer has been recognized for many years, the importance of vascularized granulation tissue in the ulcer base in relation to subsequent healing has largely gone unrecognized. However experimental studies indicate that stimulation of angiogenesis in this area results in acceleration of ulcer healing [39]. The circular, longitudinal and oblique muscle coats are interrupted and replaced in varying degree and tend to curl upwards at the edges of the ulcer to fuse with the muscularis mucosae [40]. Many small veins show organizing or organized thrombus, and arteries in the base of the ulcer can show organizing thrombus or endarteritis obliterans or may be eroded (Fig. 13.5). Mucosal replacement begins from the edges initially as a single layer of cells; in ulcers of 2 cm diameter or less this ingrowth can extend to cover the whole ulcerated surface with a single layer of epithelium, but in larger ulcers complete surface coverage may be impossible. At the ulcer margin proliferating mucosa may grow downwards as well as extending over the ulcer, giving rise to islands of mucosa trapped in granulation or fibrous tissue; these must not be mistaken for carcinomatous change [40]. The problem of mistaking granulation tissue in the base of an active gastric ulcer or erosion for carcinoma has already been discussed earlier in this chapter.

The mucosa surrounding gastric ulcers shows varying changes. In the rare ulcer lying wholly in body mucosa, there is some degree of preceding gastritis [41] but without total destruction of acid- or pepsinogen-secreting cells. In the much more common antral and lesser curve ulceration there is usually local gastritis surrounding the ulcer or, more commonly, regional gastritis involving the whole antral-type mucosa. This is active chronic superficial gastritis with or without atrophic gastritis. *Helicobacter pylori* infection is present in 60–70% of gastric ulcers so the organisms are frequently present on the surface of intact mucosa adjacent to the ulcer. Chronic gastric ulcers associated with NSAID ingestion and without concomitant *H. pylori* infection often have little or no inflammation in the adjacent mucosa [42,43]. Intestinal metaplasia of mucosa surrounding ulcers is common especially in the antrum [31] and ulcers often arise in metaplastic epithelium at the junction of corpus and antrum [44]. Hyperaemic congestion of mucosal capillaries, especially those close to the surface is very common adjacent to ulcer margins. Occasionally inflammatory pseudopolypoid proliferation takes place at an ulcer edge during healing [45].

Chronic duodenal ulcers

Most chronic duodenal ulcers occur in the first part of the duodenum, usually immediately distal to the pylorus [46] (Fig. 13.6). The anterior wall is a more common site than the posterior wall. Approximately 2% of ulcers occur distal to the first part (postbulbar). Endoscopic studies have shown that in some 10–15% of cases the ulcers are multiple [47,48] (Fig. 13.7), not uncommonly paired on the anterior and posterior walls. They are punched out in appearance, and scarring often produces considerable distortion.

Chronic duodenal ulcers show a similar histological pattern to their gastric counterparts but we have not observed so marked a tendency for the muscularis propria to fuse with the muscularis mucosae at the ulcer edge; there is often some degree of surrounding duodenitis with shortening and thickening of villi and an increased cellular infiltration in the lamina propria. Chronic antral gastritis in the stomach is almost invariable [49]. This antral gastritis is usually associated with *H. pylori* infection and the high prevalence of infection is similar in duodenal ulcer sufferers of different races [50]. The mucosa

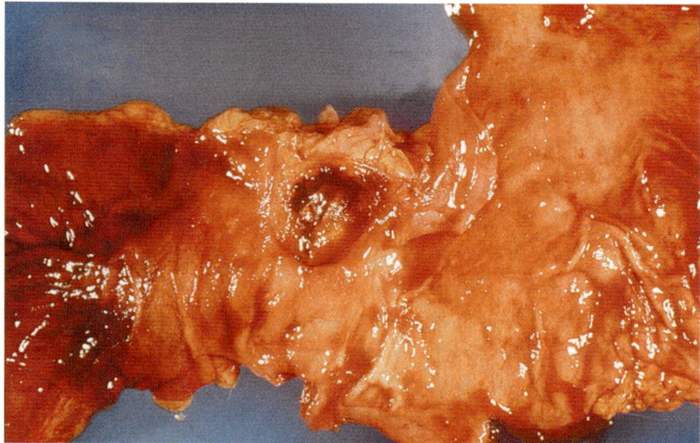

Fig. 13.6 Chronic duodenal ulcer. A large ulcer is seen immediately distal to the pylorus.

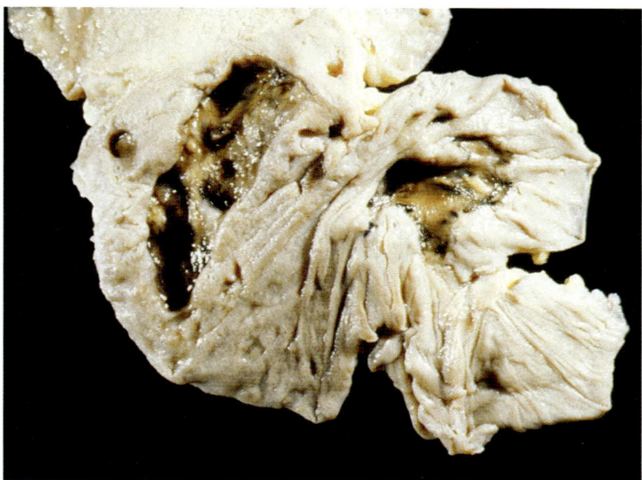

Fig. 13.7 Two large, well demarcated peptic ulcers situated on the anterior and posterior walls of the duodenum.

adjacent to the ulcer crater shows increased inflammation by polymorphs and mononuclear inflammatory cells and active mucosal inflammation is also present some distance from the ulcer, even though the mucosa in this area may appear endoscopically normal [51]. Gastric metaplasia is common in the mucosa adjacent to a duodenal ulcer. The true prevalence of metaplasia is difficult to assess on account of its patchy nature and the subsequent need to take adequate numbers of biopsies, but reports indicate that it is found in 69–90% of cases of duodenal ulcer [52–54]. The metaplasia is most often seen at the tips of duodenal villi and is often associated with some blunting of the villi [55].

Cell biological aspects of ulcer healing

Ulceration in the stomach and elsewhere in the gut is followed by development of a cell line derived from stem cells which promotes repair. This unique ulcer-associated cell lineage (UACL), which corresponds morphologically to what has previously been termed pseudopyloric metaplasia, appears adjacent to the ulcerated area and grows in proliferating buds into the lamina propria eventually reaching the mucosal surface [56]. UACL secretes or induces expression of a variety of peptides which promote cell proliferation, repair, healing and differentiation. In the stomach these peptides include epidermal growth factor (EGF) [56] and trefoil peptides TFF1/pS2 and TFF2/pSP [57,58]. In a detailed review of gene expression and gene products involved in the response to gastrointestinal ulceration Wong *et al*. [59] indicate that there is up-regulation of numerous genes following ulceration with production of a cascade of gene products that act in an integrated fashion to promote restitution and healing of the mucosa. In the stomach trefoil peptides such as TFF2/pSP are involved in the early response to injury. TFF2/pSP expression may be mediated by luminal EGF and stimulates migration of epithelial cells from the ulcer edge to cover the ulcerated area. This is followed by increased expression of EGF and transforming growth factor alpha (TGF-α) which stimulate healing and repair. Later a variety of other growth factors produced by mesodermal cells stimulate proliferation and differentiation of epithelial cells. This is accompanied by increased expression of angiogenic gene products such as platelet-derived growth factor (PDGF) and vascular endothelial growth factor (VEGF) and their receptors.

There is also evidence of alteration in cadherin expression in epithelial cells in association with ulcer healing. Cadherin molecules are important in maintaining cell–cell adhesion and polarity. They occur on the cell surface and are linked via catenins to the actin microfilaments in the cell cytoskeleton. The flattened regenerating epithelial cells on the surface of the ulcer base show decreased E-cadherin expression in comparison with that seen in normal gastric mucosa [60]. It is proposed that this promotes loss of cell adhesiveness and facilitates cell migration thus enhancing restoration of epithelial coverage of the ulcerated area.

Complications of peptic ulcer

Perforation

Acute and chronic gastric and duodenal ulcers, particularly those on the anterior wall, which are not readily walled off by surrounding structures, are liable to perforate. In reported series duodenal and pyloroduodenal ulcer perforation is much commoner than perforation of gastric ulcers [61,62]. Despite the fall in prevalence of peptic ulcer, the reduction in the number of hospital admissions for the condition and the use of effective medical treatment, several studies have shown a considerable rise in recent years in hospital admissions for perforated ulcer, especially duodenal ulcer among the elderly, particularly elderly women [63–65]. This may well be related to widespread use of NSAIDs in this group of patients. Concomitant use of NSAIDs is associated with a marked increase of bleeding or perforation in patients with a history of peptic ulcer [66]. Cigarette smoking also appears to be a significant risk factor in peptic ulcer perforation, the risk of perforation increasing with the number of cigarettes smoked [67].

The appearance of a perforated peptic ulcer is characteristic. There is a neat, round hole in the floor of the ulcer and the serosa around this perforation is hyperaemic and lustreless and partly covered by white flakes of fibrinous exudate. There are fine fibrinous adhesions between the region of the lesion and neighbouring organs, and commonly the hole is plugged by the greater omentum.

Any delay in surgical treatment of a perforated peptic ulcer will lead to diffuse peritonitis, at first the result of chemical irritation but from an early stage associated with secondary infection from bacterial contamination. Later complications include the formation of local abscesses at the site of perforation and pelvic and subdiaphragmatic abscesses. 'Food granulomas' are occasionally found in the tissues around the lower end of the stomach and first part of the duodenum in association with an active or healed peptic ulcer.

Haemorrhage

This is the commonest complication of chronic peptic ulcers (Fig. 13.8). A 15-year study carried out in general practice before the advent of efficient acid suppression therapy indicated that haemorrhage occurred in 16% of peptic ulcer patients [68]. Postbulbar duodenal ulcers and stomal ulcers are particularly prone to bleed. In a prospective study comparing two groups of patients with peptic ulcers presenting primarily with pain or bleeding, patients in the latter group were older, more likely to have taken NSAIDs within the preceding 4 weeks, and more

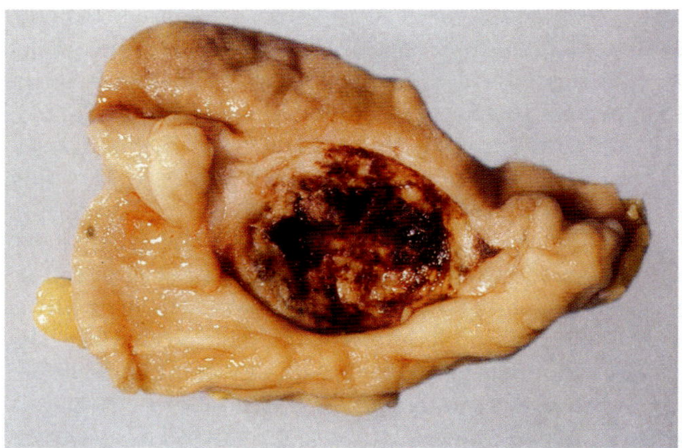

Fig. 13.8 Bleeding in a gastric ulcer. Gastric ulcer resected following severe haemorrhage. An eroded artery with fresh blood clot is visible in the ulcer base.

likely to have had a previous ulcer complication and to have an ulcer diameter greater than 2 cm [69]. The association between bleeding peptic ulcers and NSAID ingestion is emphasized by a further study indicating that the risk of bleeding is increased two to three times in patients taking these drugs compared with controls. The risk is greater in elderly patients and applies to both gastric and duodenal ulcers. Whether the bleeding is from existing chronic ulcers or acute mucosal damage is uncertain [70]. It is likely that the antihaemostatic effect of aspirin, in addition to its ulcerogenic effect, contributes to the increased risk of bleeding [71]. Non-aspirin NSAIDs are also associated with increased risk of peptic ulcer bleeding. In a British study the authors calculated that around 60% of episodes of ulcer bleeding in the elderly are associated with recent use of aspirin or other NSAIDs [72].

Erosions and acute ulcers are also liable to be associated with extensive acute haemorrhage, since the lamina propria is extremely vascular and gastric and duodenal submucosal vessels are thin walled, numerous and of wide calibre. Peptic ulceration is found in only about 50% of cases admitted for acute upper gastrointestinal bleeding [73]. A further large study reported similar findings and indicates that bleeding is more commonly associated with chronic duodenal ulcer than gastric. The incidence of upper gastrointestinal bleeding increases markedly with age and is more common in men. Overall mortality in this study was 14% [74]. Other conditions associated with increased risk of bleeding from peptic ulcers include oral anticoagulant therapy, previous history of peptic ulcer, heart failure, diabetes and oral corticosteroid therapy [75].

Pathological examination of resection specimens from individuals with bleeding gastric ulcers requiring urgent gastrectomy has shown that in the majority of cases bleeding resulted from erosion of a single artery in the floor of an ulcer (Fig. 13.5). More than half of the bleeding ulcers were acute in nature with penetration only as far as the submucosa. Aneurysmal dilatation of the artery at the bleeding point was very common and an intense arteritis was present in the wall of the vessel adjacent to the floor of the ulcer in most. Recanalized thrombus or loose intimal proliferation was seen in the bleeding artery in a minority, but endarteritis obliterans was observed only once in 27 cases [73]. As endarteritis is common in chronic ulcers resected at elective surgery, its rarity in cases of acute bleeding may indicate that it is effective in prevention of haemorrhage.

Fibrosis and stenosis

Peptic ulceration in the region of the pyloric sphincter or cardia will lead to local fibrosis and stenosis, with signs of obstruction. If there is considerable submucosal fibrosis around an ulcer in the middle part of the stomach, the deformity known as hour-glass stomach may develop (Fig. 13.4). When gastrectomy is performed for this condition it is often found that the ulcer has healed, leaving an area of intramural fibrosis radiating from its site on the lesser curvature and partially constricting the lumen. The complex role of cytokines in peptic ulcer healing and subsequent fibrosis is becoming recognized. Transforming growth factor beta 1 (TGF-β_1) derived from macrophages and platelets plays an important part in tissue repair and stimulates the production of extracellular matrix. Animal experiments indicate that increased local levels of TGF-β_1 leads to increased scarring and fibrosis in the ulcer base and greater architectural disturbance after healing [76].

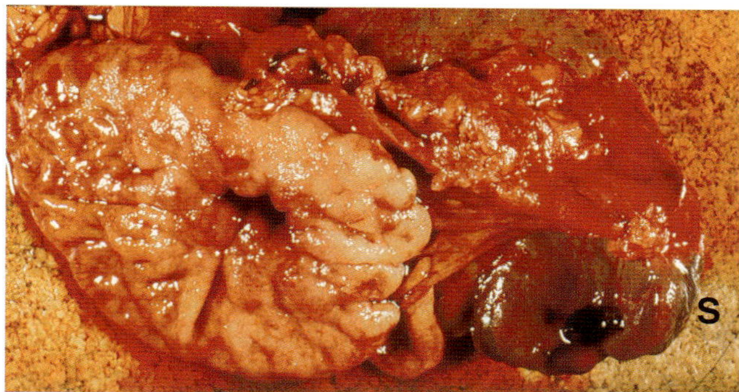

Fig. 13.9 Active chronic gastric ulcer which eroded into and was firmly adherent to the spleen (S).

Involvement of adjacent organs

A peptic ulcer in the stomach or duodenum is liable to become adherent to the pancreas or spleen (Fig. 13.9) and may erode its substance. Localized pancreatitis develops at the site of the penetration but important complications are unusual: these include haemorrhage from erosion of the splenic artery and, very rarely, acute haemorrhagic pancreatic necrosis. If a peptic ulcer leads to adhesion between the stomach or duodenum and the transverse colon the ulcer may eventually perforate into the latter, giving rise to a gastrocolic or duodenocolic fistula. Occasionally, a peptic ulcer results in adherence of the stomach or duodenum to the liver: no special complications result. However, endoscopic biopsies from the base of a deeply excavated peptic ulcer in which cords of liver cells are present may be misinterpreted as carcinoma unless this possibility is borne in mind. Rarely, benign peptic ulcers penetrate to the heart and pericardium [77,78].

Acquired diverticula

Occasionally, in association with pyloric stenosis or with a peptic ulcer that has penetrated muscle coats but excited little fibrosis, a diverticulum develops. These are usually single and arise from the posterior wall just below the cardia presenting as an outpouching in which all coats of the stomach are intact [79]. Pseudodiverticula also occur following surgical operation.

Development of carcinoma

The incidence of so-called 'ulcer cancer', i.e. carcinoma developing in a pre-existing chronic peptic ulcer, has been debated hotly for many years. There are two essential criteria for the diagnosis.

1 There must be definite evidence of a pre-existing ulcer (complete destruction of a zone of muscle, fibrous and granulation tissue in the floor of the lesion, endarteritis and thrombophlebitis in surrounding vessels, fusion of muscle coats and muscularis mucosae at the edge of the lesion).

2 There must be definite evidence of malignant change at the edge of the ulcer quite distinct from any attempt at epithelial regeneration.

Ulcer cancers undoubtedly do occur, particularly when the ulcer is a large one, but the incidence of cancer developing in a proven peptic ulcer and the presence of unequivocal evidence of previous peptic ulcer at the site of a proven carcinoma are both probably less than 1%. Accurate assessment of the true incidence of ulcer cancer is very difficult and earlier reports almost certainly included cases of pre-existing cancer presenting as an ulcer (cancer ulcer). It is generally accepted that the risk of malignant transformation applies only to chronic gastric ulcers and in these the risk is very low [80,81]. Nevertheless, careful histological examination is necessary to exclude unsuspected malignancy in all gastric ulcers that appear benign on radiological or endoscopic examination and a substantial number of biopsies from and around the ulcer must be taken to ensure diagnostic accuracy [80,82]. A diagnostic error to be avoided at all costs is to mistake as malignant small elements of regenerating epithelium at the edge of an ulcer that have either become embedded within a fibrinous inflammatory exudate or have grown down into the submucosa and become secondarily entangled in, and often distorted by, reparative fibrous tissue. Although distorted, these elements usually do not have the pleomorphism, hyperchromatism and multiple layers of cells of an adenocarcinoma and can usually be readily distinguished once the possibility of their presence is appreciated. A useful rule is never to diagnose carcinoma on the basis of dissociated islands of atypical epithelium that are only surrounded by inflammatory exudate.

A further aspect to be considered is the risk of cancer developing elsewhere in the stomach in patients with chronic peptic ulcer. Here, most studies indicate that the risk of gastric malignancy developing in association with chronic duodenal ulcer is not increased or is less than in the general population [83–85]. Results with regard to chronic gastric ulcer are less clear. Some studies indicate no increased risk [83,84]. However, a study based on prolonged follow-up of a very large number of cases indicates that in patients with chronic gastric ulcer, although not prepyloric ulcer, there is almost double the risk of gastric cancer in comparison with the general population [85]. The authors considered that while ulcers rarely cause cancer, gastric ulcer and gastric cancer might share common aetiological factors. *H. pylori* infection, which is present in up to 70% of gastric ulcer patients, is also considered to play a role in gastric carcinogenesis. It predisposes to multifocal atrophic gastritis and intestinal metaplasia (see Chapter 12) which in turn may predispose to both gastric ulcer and gastric cancer. This hypothesis is in accord with that put forward by other authorities [86,87]. Chronic *H. pylori* infection may evolve in different ways. In patients with acid hypersecretion, gastritis is predominant in the antrum and atrophic changes are limited to that area. Such patients are at risk of developing duodenal ulcer. In contrast, patients with acid hyposecretion develop more generalized pangastritis with subsequent more widespread multifocal atrophic changes throughout the gastric antrum and corpus. These patients are at greater risk of gastric ulcer and gastric cancer but are unlikely to develop duodenal ulcer. This attractive hypothesis emphasizes the significance of acid secretion in the course of chronic gastritis while acknowledging that other factors are almost certainly involved.

Incidence, aetiology and pathogenesis

Over the past 15 years a radical change has taken place regarding consideration of the aetiological agents in peptic ulceration. Chronic peptic ulcer is undoubtedly a multifactorial disease and factors such as genetic influence, smoking, diet and stress are still considered to play some contributory role. However, as in chronic gastritis, *H. pylori* is now thought to be the principal aetiological factor in the majority of cases [88,89]. The other common aetiological agents are NSAIDs, while the Zollinger–Ellison syndrome (ZES) accounts for only a tiny proportion of cases. These factors are now considered in more detail following a brief discussion of prevalence and incidence.

Prevalence and incidence

There are no wholly satisfactory estimates for the prevalence of peptic ulcer, and the reasons for this have been well reviewed [90,91]. There has been marked variation in peptic ulcer disease with time. In the latter part of the 19th century and early part of the 20th century, gastric ulcer appears to have been more common than duodenal. The disease at that time predominantly affected young women in whom perforation was a common occurrence. In the early part of the 20th century, death rates from perforation among young women fell dramatically while those in older women and men rose [92]. Some idea of the prevalence of the disease in the 1950s has come from necropsy studies which suggest that between 1 in 4 and 1 in 6 males in England over the age of 35 are likely to have had an active or healed peptic ulcer that was duodenal, both gastric and duodenal, or purely gastric in a ratio of 7:2.5:1. Duodenal ulcer frequency was estimated in middle-aged and elderly women at about 1 in 13 and gastric ulcer frequency at 1 in 21 [93]. An estimate of prevalence in the 1970s has come from an endoscopic study in Finland, which demonstrated active duodenal and gastric ulcers in 1.4% and 0.28%, respectively, of control adult subjects participating in a study of gastric carcinoma. In a further 4.2% there was evidence of gastric or duodenal scarring or a history of ulcer surgery indicating an estimated lifetime prevalence of at least 5.9% [94]. Over the last 30 years hospital admissions for peptic ulcer disease have fallen considerably [65,95,96] and this may well reflect a true decline in incidence [97]. While the introduction of H_2 receptor antagonists in the mid-1970s, followed later by proton pump inhibitors, has dramatically changed the course of peptic ulcer disease and has resulted in a significant reduction in the number of patients undergoing surgical treatment [64,65,98], the fall in hospital admissions in an area of high prevalence such as Scotland commenced before the advent of H_2 receptor antagonists [97].

In most European countries and the USA, duodenal ulcer is at least twice as common as gastric ulcer and in some areas this ratio reaches 5:1. In contrast, gastric ulcer in Japan occurs five to 10 times more often than duodenal ulcer [99]. In some countries a significant seasonal fluctuation in the frequency of peptic ulcer complications has been reported, with the number of cases falling during hot summer months [100]. Interestingly, a similar seasonal trend has been noted in the incidence of *H. pylori* infection [101].

Helicobacter pylori infection and chronic peptic ulcer

Since Marshall and Warren first noted the association between *H. pylori* infection of the stomach and peptic ulceration [102] many other reports have confirmed this important observation [103–105]. *H. pylori* infection has been found in over 90% of patients with duodenal ulcer and almost 70% of patients with gastric ulcer [106–109]. A similar association has been noted between *H. pylori* infection and duodenal ulcer in children [110], although the association is not as strong as in adults [111] and in a recent series only around 30% of children with peptic ulcer were found to have *H. pylori* infection [112].

The presence of the organism in a high proportion of cases of peptic ulcer disease does not prove a causative effect and the causal role has been questioned [113,114]. However, further incriminating evidence has been provided by numerous studies indicating that although peptic ulcers can be healed by acid suppression therapy, there is a high risk of ulcer recurrence unless *H. pylori* is eradicated. In contrast, if the organism is eradicated, no recurrence takes place in the great majority of cases. This observation was first reported with regard to duodenal ulcers in 1987 [115] and has been supported by numerous studies since [116,117]. In duodenal ulcer patients in whom *H. pylori* has been successfully eradicated, recurrence is very uncommon and is usually related to NSAID ingestion or rare causes such as Crohn's disease or gastrinoma [118], although it may occur if there is reinfection [119]. Most modern therapies for duodenal ulceration combine short-term administration of antibiotics to eliminate *H. pylori* with long-term acid suppression. Provided eradication is successful, long-term acid suppression does not appear necessary for continued healing [120]. This is a further indication that eradication is more important than acid suppression.

Although the association between *H. pylori* infection and chronic gastric ulcer is not as strong as that with duodenal ulcer, estimates indicate that the organism is present in 60–80% of cases of chronic benign gastric ulcer [50,106,121]. When the organism is present, eradication appears to promote and maintain healing of gastric as well as duodenal ulcers [122–124].

It is likely that a variety of factors take part in the pathogenesis of *H. pylori*-associated gastric ulceration. The layer of surface mucus is the first line of defence of the gastric mucosa against potentially harmful luminal agents. While there is little evidence that *H. pylori* infection alters mucus synthesis, lipopolysaccharides in the cell wall of the organism may alter the structure of the mucus [125]. There is experimental evidence that stimulated exocytosis of mucus is impaired in *H. pylori* infection [126]. Serum pepsinogen I levels are raised in the presence of *H. pylori* infection and correlate well with increased inflammation of the gastric mucosa [127] and this may indicate further means whereby the gastric mucous barrier is compromised as pepsin is capable of breaking down the mucus gel. Growth factors such as epidermal growth factor (EGF) and transforming growth factor alpha (TGF-α) have already been mentioned as playing important roles in maintaining gastric mucosal integrity (Chapter 12). *H. pylori* infection has been shown to be associated with a significantly lower concentration of EGF in the gastric juice. It is uncertain whether this reflects diminished production or increased degradation but it may lead to mucosal injury due to loss of protective effect [128]. The degenerative effects of *H. pylori* infection on surface epithelial cells resulting in mucus depletion and microerosions have been discussed in Chapter 12. This damage to the surface epithelium of the mucosa may permit permeation of acid, pepsin, bacterial antigens and toxins into the underlying mucosa, which may eventually lead to ulceration [129,130]. Indirect effects of *H. pylori* infection may also play a part in the pathogenesis of chronic gastric ulcer. The infection is associated with increased prevalence and extent of intestinal metaplasia within the stomach. Intestinal metaplasia appears to be more prevalent in patients with gastric ulcer than in other common gastric disorders [131] and antral intestinal metaplasia is much more prevalent in gastric ulceration than in duodenal ulceration [132].

A causative role for *H. pylori* infection in chronic gastric ulcer may be explained by mucosal inflammation and subsequent damage caused by bacteria colonizing the surface of the gastric mucosa. The pathogenesis of duodenal ulcer, however, is more difficult to explain. Although there is a very strong association between duodenal ulcer and *H. pylori* infection of the stomach, the organism is not found on normal duodenal mucosa and thus ulceration is not due to a direct effect of bacterial colonization of duodenal mucosa. Several mechanisms may explain the pathogenesis of *H. pylori*-associated duodenal ulcer.

1 *H. pylori*-associated antral gastritis is associated with hypergastrinaemia leading to increased gastric acid output thus increasing the risk of duodenal ulceration.

2 Islands of gastric metaplasia form in the duodenum, possibly due to increased acid flow from the stomach, may become colonized by *H. pylori* and the consequent inflammation may predispose to ulceration.

3 Strains of *H. pylori* that carry the CagA gene are more likely to be associated with peptic ulcer than CagA-negative strains.

These pathogenetic mechanisms are now considered in more detail.

Hypergastrinaemia. Basal and stimulated serum gastrin levels are increased in patients with *H. pylori* infection [133,134]. Similarly, 24-hour gastrin secretion is increased in infected patients and this may contribute to the increased parietal cell mass found in duodenal ulcer patients [135]. McColl's group found that gastrin-releasing peptide (GRP)-stimulated acid output is increased threefold in *H. pylori*-infected patients without duodenal ulcer and sixfold in infected patients with duodenal ulcer. This increased acid response to GRP reverted to normal following eradication of *H. pylori* [136]. It is suggested that *H. pylori* infection interferes with the normal control of gastrin and acid release at low gastric pH [137,138] through an effect on somatostatin-producing D cells. These cells, which are found principally in the antrum, exert a paracrine inhibitory effect on neighbouring gastrin cells. Both the number of antral somatostatin-immunoreactive D cells and mucosal levels of somatostatin are reduced in the presence of *H. pylori* infection [139,140] and D-cell numbers increase following eradication of the infection. The decrease in antral mucosal somatostatin occurs in both *Helicobacter*-associated antral gastritis and in pangastritis [141]. Further evidence that *H. pylori* infection blocks inhibition of gastric acid release is provided by a study on the effect of antral distension, which normally inhibits gastric acid release: the effect is absent in *H. pylori*-infected subjects [142].

Gastric metaplasia. A further likely pathogenetic link between *H. pylori* infection and duodenal ulcer concerns foci of gastric metaplasia within duodenal mucosa and subsequent colonization of such foci by bacteria. While gastric metaplasia in the duodenum occurs in normal subjects, it is more extensive in patients with *H. pylori* infection and duodenitis [55] and is also more prevalent in patients with duodenal ulcer [53,143,144]. Duodenal gastric metaplasia is thought to develop as a result of high levels of acidity within the duodenum. It is more extensive in patients with low pH values in gastric juice [145] and both the prevalence and the extent of metaplasia correlate with gastric acid output [53]. It also occurs in the distal duodenum in the Zollinger–Ellison syndrome [143,146]. *Helicobacter pylori* infection of the stomach *per se* does not appear to correlate with duodenal gastric metaplasia [53,54] but infection may indirectly increase the extent and prevalence of metaplasia via the increased acid secretion that it stimulates and which has been discussed above. It seems unlikely that hyperacidity is the sole aetiological factor. The circadian gastric acidity of duodenal ulcer patients is higher than that of healthy controls but shows no difference between patients with or without gastric metaplasia. Metaplasia is likely to be a non-specific response to a variety of mucosal insults, and chronic inflammation is probably another of these factors [52]. Studies indicate that foci of gastric metaplasia in the duodenum are the result of expansion of the surface component of Brunner's glands [147,148] and they appear to be related to the ulcer-associated cell lineage.

Gastric metaplasia occurs almost exclusively in the first part of the duodenum and distribution is patchy [55]. It is frequently found at the edge of a duodenal ulcer and the patches of metaplasia are frequently colonized by *H. pylori* [149]. In the absence of duodenal Crohn's disease or other relatively rare conditions, inflammation of the duodenal mucosa is seldom seen unless gastric metaplasia is present and the extent of gastric metaplasia correlates with the degree of duodenal inflammation [55]. This lends support to the proposal that colonization of islands of gastric metaplasia by *H. pylori* (Fig. 13.10) may lead to inflammation of these islands and

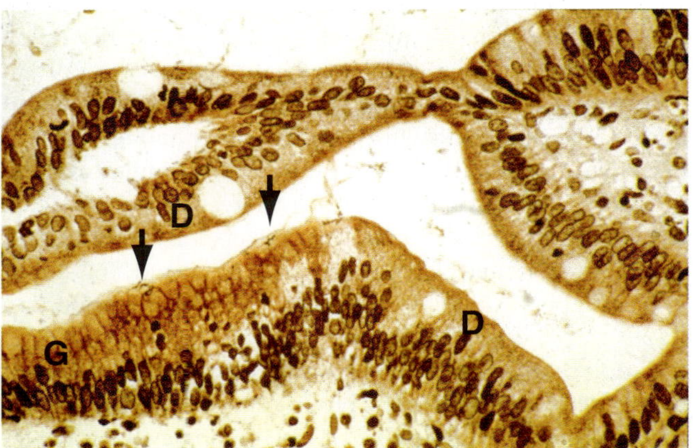

Fig. 13.10 Colonization of gastric metaplasia by *H. pylori*. Small groups of *H. pylori* organisms (arrows) are present on the surface of an area of gastric metaplasia (G), but not on the surface epithelium of duodenal epithelium (D). Warthin–Starry stain

the surrounding duodenal mucosa, which in turn renders the mucosa more susceptible to acid attack and ulceration. The likely sequence of *H. pylori* infection of the stomach, hyperacidity, gastric metaplasia in the duodenum, colonization of foci of metaplasia by *H. pylori*, duodenitis and ultimately duodenal ulceration has been termed the 'leaking roof' concept [150].

CagA positivity. There is evidence that some strains of *H. pylori* are more virulent than others and more likely to be associated with peptic ulceration. Strains of *H. pylori* can be divided into those that express the cytotoxin-associated protein (CagA) and/or the vacuolating toxin (VacA) and those that do not [151]. It was first noticed that patients with *H. pylori* infection showing a gastric mucosal IgA response to the 120 kDa CagA protein had more active gastritis, mucosal surface degeneration and peptic ulceration [152] and subsequently it was found that CagA-positive strains of *H. pylori* were more strongly associated with intense mucosal inflammation, duodenal ulceration and atrophic gastritis [152–155]. CagA-positive strains of *H. pylori* induce increased expression of interleukin-8 (IL-8) protein and mRNA in gastric mucosal epithelial cells in culture in comparison with CagA-negative strains [156], and this may lead to increased chemotaxis and accumulation of polymorphs and mononuclear inflammatory cells within the mucosa *in vivo*, which in turn leads to increased and prolonged inflammation [151,155]. There is more heterogeneity among *H. pylori* strains with regard to the vacuolating cytotoxin VacA, but some of these strains are associated with increased mucosal inflammation and are more ulcerogenic than others. However most are also CagA positive and for practical purposes identification of Cag A positivity indicates strains likely to be associated with peptic ulceration [157].

The pathogenic role of *H. pylori* infection in peptic ulceration has been supported by many studies, only a few of which have been cited here. However, many unanswered questions and some doubts remain. It has been pointed out that while Koch's postulates for determining a causal relationship between a disease and a microorganism have been fulfilled for gastritis, this is not the case for *H. pylori* infection and peptic ulcer [114].

Chronic peptic ulcer and drugs

Non-steroidal anti-inflammatory drugs (NSAIDs)

The role of aspirin and other NSAIDs in the aetiology of acute gastric lesions has been discussed earlier in this chapter. There is, however, little doubt that their ingestion also plays an important role in chronic peptic ulceration. This important side-effect of these very widely used drugs has been recognized for many years but the scale of the problem has been highlighted more recently by reports indicating increased and dose-related risk of peptic ulcer in patients taking aspirin and other NSAIDs [158,159]. Although aspirin has been supplemented or replaced by a large number of newer NSAIDs all of these, while less damaging to the gastric mucosa than aspirin, are nonetheless gastric irritants [160,161]. Adverse reactions to NSAIDs are one of the most commonly reported drug side-effects and of these, problems related to the gastrointestinal tract are the most common [162]. NSAIDs accounted for over 20 million prescriptions per year in the UK in 1986 [163]. The use of aspirin (albeit in low doses) for prophylaxis of cardiovascular disease is now widespread, and in addition, very large amounts of NSAIDs are bought without prescription for self-medication. Thus, to keep the problem in perspective, in view of the vast quantities of aspirin and other NSAIDs consumed, the increased risk of serious upper gastrointestinal complications is relatively modest at three- to four-fold [164]. A large multinational survey indicated that the incidence of peptic ulcers and/or gastrointestinal bleeding associated with non-aspirin NSAIDs is around 1% [165]. A meta-analysis of 16 studies showed that the overall risk of serious gastrointestinal events in NSAID users is approximately three times greater than in non-users but that the risk is increased in elderly patients and with concomitant use of corticosteroids. It is highest during the first 3 months of drug therapy [166]. Despite this, it is remarkable that in the USA the majority of the population who regularly take NSAIDs, especially those using non-prescription over-the-counter drugs, are not aware of or are not concerned about the risk of complications [167]. An indication of the magnitude of the problem is given by recent statistics from the USA that the number of deaths among patients with rheumatoid or osteoarthritis due to NSAID-related gastrointestinal damage is similar to the number of deaths from HIV infection.

Aspirin and non-aspirin NSAID ingestion appears to be more strongly associated with chronic gastric ulcers rather than duodenal ulcers [168–170] and there is also increased risk of upper gastrointestinal bleeding. Whether this is due to drug-induced mucosal damage or bleeding from a pre-existing ulcer is unclear. There is a three- to fourfold increase in the risk of gastric ulceration and upper gastrointestinal bleeding associated with aspirin consumption [164].

Repeated studies show that patients at greatest risk from upper gastrointestinal complications of NSAIDs are the elderly, especially women [171] and those who have had previous upper abdominal pain, peptic ulcer disease, or side-effects with NSAID use [172]. Studies on the comparative safety of individual drugs have produced rather confusing conclusions, but a recent meta-analysis indicates that ibuprofen carries a relatively low risk, although this may be because it is normally used in comparatively low doses [173]. Azapropazone carries a comparatively high risk of serious upper gastrointestinal tract side-effects [174]. The risk of NSAID complications in the elderly is compounded by the fact that NSAID-induced gastroduodenal damage in this age group is often 'silent' in that patients frequently do not complain of dyspepsia and thus the diagnosis of peptic ulceration may be delayed [170]. Indeed, among patients suffering NSAID-associated gastrointestinal complications, only a small minority report preceding gastrointestinal symptoms [175]. These clinical studies are supported by a postmortem study mainly involving elderly subjects which found a significantly increased risk of gastric ulcers in those taking NSAIDs in the 6 months prior to death [176]. Although the actual prevalence of duodenal ulcer was not increased NSAID users had a higher incidence of fatal complications of duodenal ulcer. This study also found an increased prevalence of small intestinal ulceration in association with NSAID use. In addition to advanced age and previous peptic ulcer, other risk factors for NSAID-induced peptic ulceration include concomitant use of steroids or anticoagulants, high dosage of NSAIDs or serious systemic disease [177].

In view of the widespread prevalence of *H. pylori* infection, especially in the middle-aged and elderly population, it seems reasonable to consider any synergistic association between *H. pylori* and NSAID ingestion. NSAID use does not appear to increase susceptibility to *H. pylori* infection [178] and some studies indicate that the presence of *H. pylori* infection does not increase the risk of ulceration in NSAID users or of visible gastric mucosal lesions on endoscopy [179,180]. Indeed, NSAID ingestion is reportedly associated with less inflammation around the rim of gastric ulcers in the presence of *H. pylori* infection [181]. However, other work suggests that *H. pylori* infection does increase NSAID-associated gastrotoxicity [182] and also the ulcer risk associated with at least some NSAIDs [183]. NSAID users who have *H. pylori* infection and mucosal erosions, especially duodenal erosions, are at increased risk of ulceration [184]. A recent meta-analysis involving 25 studies indicated a significantly increased risk of peptic ulcer disease and ulcer bleeding in patients taking NSAIDs who have *H. pylori* infection compared with those without the infection [185]. A study carried out in Hong Kong indicated that eradication of *H. pylori* infection in patients taking NSAIDs reduced the risk of peptic ulceration [186].

Thus it is likely that *H. pylori* infection acts synergistically on NSAID gastrotoxicity. However, anti-inflammatory drugs are independent risk factors for peptic mucosal damage and ulceration and are not dependent on *H. pylori* infection for ulcerogenesis [181]. Importantly, the presence of chemical (reactive) gastritis which is frequently associated with NSAID ingestion carries an increased risk of peptic ulceration in NSAID users [187].

Detailed discussion of the mechanisms of NSAID-induced gastroduodenal mucosal damage is beyond the scope of this book and only an overview is presented. At low pH aspirin is in a lipid soluble non-ionized form which can be transported across cell membranes. Following absorption it can lead to increased cell membrane permeability with resulting influx of sodium, calcium and water resulting in cell swelling and death [188]. Death of surface epithelial cells allows back-diffusion of acid, pepsin and aspirin into the mucosa, as first suggested by Davenport [189]. The resulting injury to mast cells, endothelial cells and neutrophils may result in release of inflammatory mediators leading to capillary leakage, neutrophil adherence to endothelial cells, vasoconstriction and subsequent local mucosal ischaemia and cellular necrosis [190]. The importance of neutrophils as mediators of NSAID-induced mucosal damage has recently been emphasized by experimental studies which indicate that inhibition of adherence of neutrophils to capillary endothelial cells protects rabbit gastric mucosa against indomethacin-induced damage [191]. This is supported by histological studies indicating that in indomethacin-induced gastric antral ulceration in rats, neutrophil infiltration precedes widespread mucosal ulceration [192]. In rats, NSAIDs induce an early and rapid increase in expression of the endothelial intracellular adhesion molecule ICAM-1 in the gastric mucosa. This may be an important precursor to neutrophil adherence [193]. Wallace has proposed that NSAID-induced adherence of neutrophils to vascular endothelium reduces mucosal perfusion which enhances injury induced by back-diffusion of luminal acid. In addition, activated neutrophils may increase local mucosal damage by release of oxygen-derived free radicals [194].

The protective effect of prostaglandins on gastric mucosa is relevant with regard to NSAID-induced gastrotoxicity. Prostaglandins are synthesized by the gastric mucosa from precursor arachidonic acid. They have a variety of protective actions including stimulation of mucus secretion [195], increasing gastric mucosal blood flow [196], and stimulation of both gastric and duodenal bicarbonate secretion [197,198]. In addition, the NSAID-induced increased expression of the endothelial adhesion molecule ICAM-1 discussed above is inhibited by prostaglandin analogues [193]. Prostaglandins also protect gastric mucosa from aspirin-induced damage in the experimental situation [199]. Endogenous prostaglandin synthesis by gastric mucosa is inhibited by NSAIDs [160] and subsequent reduction in the protection afforded is likely to leave the mucosa more susceptible to damage. This is supported by the finding that cotreatment with a synthetic prostaglandin analogue misoprostol markedly reduces the development of gastric ulcers in patients receiving long-term NSAID therapy [200].

The gastrointestinal toxicity of the present generation of NSAIDs may be mitigated by the advent of a new family of such drugs known as COX-2 inhibitors. Cyclooxygenase (COX) is an important enzyme in the production of prostaglandins and is inhibited by aspirin and other commonly used NSAIDs. There are at least two forms of this enzyme, COX-1 and COX-2. The theory that COX-1 is expressed predominantly in the stomach and plays an important part in the production of protective prostaglandins while

COX-2 is induced at sites of inflammation has led to the possibility that specific COX-2 inhibitors may exhibit an anti-inflammatory effect without concomitant gastrotoxicity [201]. This attractive theory is an oversimplification and there are numerous question marks over the efficacy and safety of such drugs [202]. Nonetheless, the potential for more 'gut-friendly' anti-inflammatory drugs is considerable and is being actively pursued. The effect of COX-2 inhibition on decreasing colonic adenoma formation and subsequent risk of colonic carcinoma is also clearly important [203,204].

Corticosteroids

There is conflicting evidence over the possible relationship between corticosteroid treatment and development of peptic ulcer disease. Although these drugs have been often incriminated, a meta-analysis of a large number of studies found no association [205]. Recent data have indicated that elderly patients receiving both steroid therapy and concomitant NSAID therapy are at risk of peptic ulcer [206], and an association between oral corticosteroids and bleeding from peptic ulcer has recently been demonstrated [75].

Other factors in the pathogenesis of peptic ulceration

Peptic ulcer is a multifactorial disease. The discovery of *H. pylori* infection and recognition of its importance in pathogenesis of peptic ulcer has dominated this topic since the mid-1980s, especially as it has led to successful medical treatment in many cases. This has tended to overshadow other factors which remain significant, although they are less important than the factors outlined above.

Stress

Although psychological stress has been proposed as an important factor to explain the occurrence or recurrence of duodenal ulcer, direct evidence for a causal role is lacking. A major problem has been the difficulty in scientifically defining and measuring an individual's stress. Patients with dyspepsia have been reported to have had increased stress levels [207] but this has not been confirmed [208,209]. The association of severe psychological stress with markedly increased gastric acid secretion and development of gastric ulceration has been documented [210]. However, a prospective study on air traffic controllers [211]—a stressful occupation—did not, after close evaluation, indicate any increase in incidence of peptic ulcer, although the incidence of hypertension was significantly increased. Despite this, the association between psychological stress, dyspepsia and chronic peptic ulcer is widely considered to be valid. With recognition of the importance of other factors such as *H. pylori* infection and NSAID ingestion, this view may change but it is premature to suggest that it should be dismissed.

Smoking

A causal relationship between peptic ulceration and smoking has long been suspected but remains unproven [212]. Before the recognition of the importance of *H. pylori*, studies indicated that smoking has an adverse effect on ulcer healing [213,214]. If *H. pylori* is eradicated, however, cigarette smoking appears to have little effect on ulcer healing although it is associated with a slightly lower bacterial eradication rate [122]. The complex effects of smoking on gastric mucosal function have been reviewed in detail [215]. There is evidence that gastric mucosal defence mechanisms such as prostaglandin and EGF secretion and mucosal blood flow are impaired in smokers. The evidence with regard to aggressive factors is often conflicting but some reports indicate that smoking is associated with increased acid and pepsin secretion and free radical production and that the incidence of *H. pylori* infection is higher in smokers. Experimental studies indicate that cigarette smoke inhibits ulcer healing and attenuates hyperaemia in the mucosa at the ulcer edge [216].

Genetic factors

The association of blood group O and duodenal ulceration was first reported in 1954 and has been confirmed on numerous occasions since then [217]. Those within that group who are in addition incapable of secreting their AB(O)H blood group substances in water-soluble form have a two to three times greater risk of developing a duodenal ulcer [218]. No association between secretor status and *H. pylori* infection has been demonstrated and non-secretor status remains an independent risk factor for gastritis, duodenitis or peptic ulcer disease [219]. Relatives of duodenal ulcer patients have two to three times the expected prevalence of ulcer in that site [220].

A number of genetic syndromes are associated with peptic ulceration [221]. These rare syndromes include multiple endocrine neoplasia (MEN) type I, an autosomal dominant disorder characterized by tumours, usually adenomas of pituitary, parathyroid and endocrine pancreas. The latter may secrete gastrin, resulting in a severe form of ulcer diathesis, the Zollinger–Ellison syndrome (ZES). Type I MEN cases constitute about one-third of Zollinger–Ellison syndrome cases and unlike sporadic cases, the gastrin-secreting tumours are usually situated in the duodenum, multiple, and frequently behave in a benign fashion [222]. Systemic mastocytosis is another inherited multisystem syndrome which may be complicated by duodenal ulceration due to high levels of histamine released from mast cells which may stimulate gastric acid secretion [223].

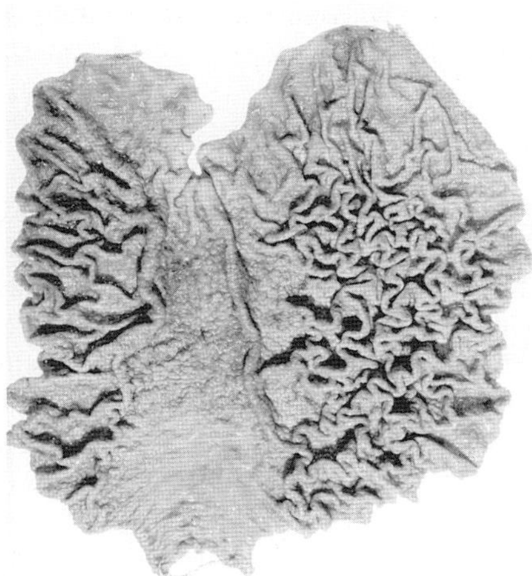

Fig. 13.11 Rugose hypertrophy of body mucosa in a patient with Zollinger–Ellison syndrome.

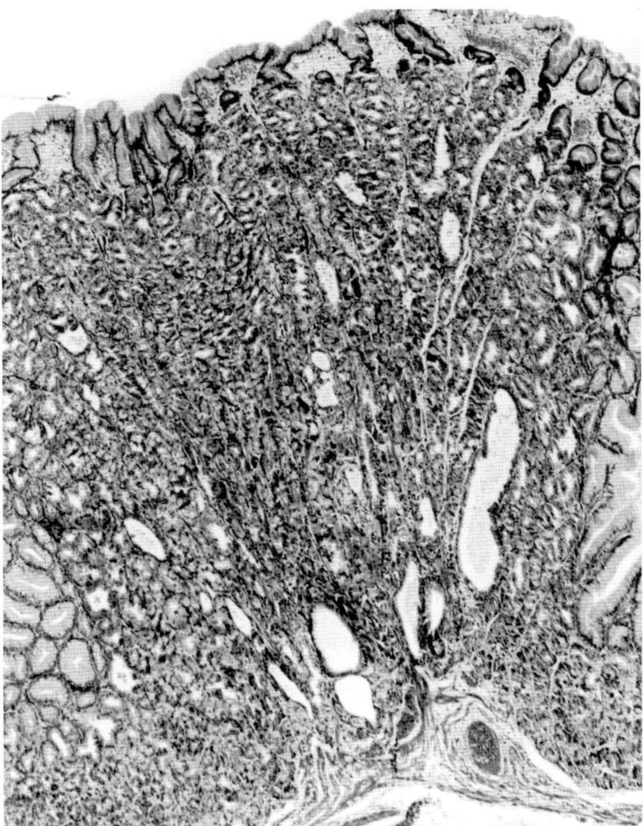

Fig. 13.12 Increase in parietal cell mass in Zollinger–Ellison syndrome with shortening of gastric pits.

Chronic renal disease

There are reports of increased frequency of chronic peptic ulcer (mainly duodenal) in patients undergoing chronic dialysis [224]. More recent reports, however, indicate little or no increase [225,226]. Increased risk of peptic ulceration may be due to the high levels of gastric acid secretion and hypergastrinaemia seen in some patients with chronic renal failure following the onset of dialysis treatment [224,227]. The levels often fall following successful renal transplantation [226,227].

Gastroduodenal reflux

It has been suggested that reflux of duodenal contents into the stomach plays an important part in the pathogenesis of gastric ulcer [228,229] and experimental studies indicate that bile salts may damage the gastric mucosa [230,231]. The importance of reflux in the human is uncertain, however, and most studies have failed to take account of *H. pylori* infection. A recent exception that did consider concomitant *H. pylori* infection found that although bile reflux was increased in peptic ulcer patients, this was not statistically significant [232]. The authors showed that bile reflux was associated with reduction in the numbers of *H. pylori* organisms, together with increased reactive and atrophic gastritis and intestinal metaplasia. They concluded that repeated bile reflux may damage gastric mucosa leading to erosions, regeneration and intestinal metaplasia.

The stomach in the Zollinger–Ellison syndrome

The majority of patients who develop the Zollinger–Ellison syndrome [233] have a primary gastrin-secreting tumour (gastrinoma) in the pancreas that stimulates the acid-secreting cells of the corpus of the stomach to maximal activity with consequent liability to duodenal or even jejunal ulceration. The most useful diagnostic feature is marked elevation of fasting serum gastrin levels [222]. The syndrome is characterized by severe and refractory peptic ulceration which may be multiple and may occur in atypical sites such as the distal duodenum and jejunum. The oesophagus may also be involved. The incidence of the syndrome is very low [234]. In approximately 10% of cases the tumours arise in the duodenum, most commonly in the second part [235,236]. While most cases are sporadic, in about 20–30% of cases the syndrome is associated with the autosomal dominant syndrome of multiple endocrine neoplasia (MEN) type I, in which case there are often multiple small gastrinomas in the duodenum, and primary tumours in other endocrine organs, notably the parathyroids and the pituitary [222,237]. In such cases the trophic effects of prolonged hypergastrinaemia on fundal enterochromaffin-like (ECL) cells induces multiple small gastric carcinoid tumours (gastric carcinoidosis) [238]. In a few patients no tumour is detectable and there is localized hyperplasia of antral G cells which results in a similar clinical picture [239,240]. Such primary G-cell hyperplasia must be distinguished from secondary forms,

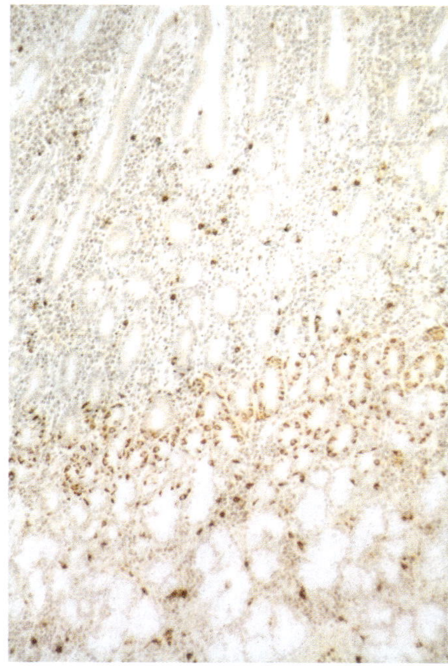

Fig. 13.13 Antral G-cell hyperplasia in a patient with Zollinger–Ellison syndrome. PAP method using antigastrin antibody.

which represent a physiological response to hypochlorhydria due to autoimmune atrophic gastritis, truncal vagotomy or occasionally prolonged treatment with H_2 receptor antagonists or proton pump inhibitors [241], and which are not associated with hyperacidity, peptic ulceration or the Zollinger–Ellison syndrome.

Grossly, the stomach in the Zollinger–Ellison syndrome shows very prominent folds in the body (Fig. 13.11), not unlike the appearance in Menetrier's disease. Histologically, a number of abnormalities can be present. Full-thickness biopsy of body mucosa shows the thickening to be due to marked expansion of the specialized glands as a result of proliferation of parietal cells (Fig. 13.12). This specialized glandular mucosa may extend into the antrum so that virtually the entire gastric mucosa is of fundal or corpus type [242]. Foveolae are normal and there is no associated inflammation. There may also be linear or nodular proliferation of ECL cells in the gastric body as described above [240], sometimes with multiple small carcinoids [243]. The duodenal mucosa shows features of nonspecific duodenitis in which gastric metaplasia of the surface epithelium is a prominent feature [143]. When the Zollinger–Ellison syndrome is due to primary antral G-cell hyperplasia the antral endocrine cells are significantly increased in number, sometimes forming small clusters or microadenomas (Fig. 13.13) [244,245]. Conversely when the cause is a discrete gastrinoma of the pancreas or duodenum the antral G cells become suppressed and their numbers may be normal or decreased [246].

Zollinger–Ellison syndrome is a rare but potent cause of severe recurrent and often multiple peptic ulcers. It appears that the marked increase in gastric acid output secondary to hypergastrinaemia alone is sufficient to cause the extensive ulceration, and *H. pylori* infection appears to play little part. Indeed the prevalence of infection is diminished in Zollinger–Ellison syndrome patients in comparison with the general population [247], probably because the sustained hyperacidity restricts bacterial colonization and growth.

References

1 Sugawa C, Lucas CE, Rosenberg B, Riddle JM, Walt AJ. Differential topography of acute erosive gastritis due to trauma or sepsis, ethanol and aspirin. *Gastrointest Endosc*, 1973; 19: 127.

2 Hoftiezer JW, O'Laughlin JC, Ivey KJ. Effects of 24 hours of aspirin, buffering, paracetamol and placebo on normal gastroduodenal mucosa. *Gut*, 1982; 23: 692.

3 Isaacson P. Biopsy appearances easily mistaken for malignancy in gastrointestinal biopsy. *Histopathology*, 1982; 6: 377.

4 Lucas CE, Sugawa C, Riddle J, Rector F, Rosenberg B, Walt AJ. Natural history and surgical dilemma of 'stress' gastric bleeding. *Arch Surg*, 1971; 102: 266.

5 Bank S, Misra P, Mausner D *et al*. The incidence, distribution and evolution of stress ulcers in surgical intensive care units. *Am J Gastroenterol*, 1980; 74: 76.

6 Shuman RB, Schuster DP, Zuckerman GR. Prophylactic therapy for stress ulcer bleeding? A reappraisal. *Ann Intern Med*, 1987; 106: 562.

7 Cook DJ, Fuller HD, Guyatt GH *et al*. Risk factors for gastrointestinal bleeding in critically ill patients. *N Engl J Med*, 1994; 330: 377.

8 Czaja AJ, McAlhany CJ, Pruitt BA. Acute gastroduodenal disease after thermal injury. *N Engl J Med*, 1974; 291: 925.

9 Nordström H, Nettelbad H. Curling's ulcer—a serious complication of the burned patient. *Scand J Gastroenterol*, 1984; 19 (Suppl 105): 14.

10 Pruitt BA, Goodwin CW. Stress ulcer in the burned patient. *World J Surg*, 1981; 5: 209.

11 Sevitt S. Duodenal and gastric ulceration after burning. *Br J Surg*, 1967; 54: 32.

12 Cushing H. Peptic ulcers and the interbrain. *Surg Gynecol Obstet*, 1932; 55: 1.

13 Browne TH, Davidson BF, Terrell S *et al*. Gastritis occurring within 24 hours of severe head injury. *Gastrointest Endosc*, 1987; 33: 150.

14 Cheung LY. Pathogenesis, prophylaxis and treatment of stress gastritis. *Am J Surg*, 1988; 156: 437.

15 Harjola P-T, Sivula A. Gastric ulceration following experimentally induced hypoxia and haemorrhagic shock: in vivo study of pathogenesis in rabbits. *Ann Surg*, 1966; 163: 21.

16 Shirazi SS, Mueller TM, Hardy BM. Canine gastric acid secretion and blood flow measurement in haemorrhagic shock. *Gastroenterology*, 1977; 73: 75.

17 Menguy R, Masters YF. Mechanism of stress ulcer. *Gastroenterology*, 1974; 66: 509.

18 Kivilaakso E, Fronn D, Silen W. Relationship between ulceration and intramural pH of gastric mucosa during haemorrhagic shock. *Surgery*, 1978; 84: 70.

19 Perry MA, Wadhwa S, Parks DA, Pickard W, Granger DN. Role of oxygen radicals in ischaemia-induced lesions in the cat stomach. *Gastroenterology*, 1986; 90: 362.

20 Chamberlain CE. Acute haemorrhagic gastritis. *Gastroenterol Clin N Am*, 1993; 22: 843.

21 Lanza FL. A review of gastric ulcer and gastroduodenal injury in normal volunteers receiving aspirin and other non-steroidal anti-inflammatory drugs. *Scand J Gastroenterol*, 1989; 24 (Suppl 163): 24.

22 Petroski D. A comparison of enteric-coated aspirin: a report of two studies. *Am J Gastroenterol*, 1986; 81: 26.

23 Silvoso GR, Ivey KJ, Butt JH *et al*. Incidence of gastric lesions in patients with rheumatic disease on chronic aspirin therapy. *Ann Intern Med*, 1979; 91: 517.

24 Laine L, Weinstein WM. Histology of alcoholic haemorrhagic 'gastritis': a prospective evaluation. *Gastroenterology*, 1988; 94: 1254.

25 Gottfried ED, Korsten MA, Lieber CS. Alcohol-induced gastric and duodenal lesions in man. *Am J Gastroenterol*, 1978; 70: 587.

26 Kvietys PR, Twohig B, Danzell J, Specian RD. Ethanol-induced injury to the rat gastric mucosa. *Gastroenterology*, 1990; 98: 909.

27 Bou-Abboud CF, Wayland H, Paulsen G, Guth PH. Microcirculatory stasis precedes tissue necrosis in ethanol-induced gastric mucosal injury in the rat. *Dig Dis Sci*, 1988; 33: 872.

28 Masuda E, Kawano S, Nagano K *et al*. Endogenous nitric oxide modulates ethanol-induced gastric mucosal injury in rats. *Gastroenterology*, 1995; 108: 58.

29 Oi M, Oshida K, Sugimora S. The location of gastric ulcer. *Gastroenterology*, 1959; 36: 45.

30 Findley JW Jr. Ulcers of the greater curve of the stomach. *Gastroenterology*, 1961; 40: 183.

31 Stadelmann O, Elster K, Stolte M *et al*. The peptic gastric ulcer—histotopographic and functional investigations. *Scand J Gastroenterol*, 1971; 6: 613.

32 Magnus HA. The pathology of peptic ulceration. *Postgrad Med J*, 1954; 30: 131.

33 Sun DCH, Stempien SJ. Site and size of the ulcer as determinants of outcome. *Gastroenterology*, 1971; 61: 576.

34 Thomas J, Greig M, McIntosh J, Hunt J, McNeil D, Piper DW. The location of chronic gastric ulcer. *Digestion*, 1980; 20: 79.

35 Kimura K. Chronological transition of the fundic–pyloric borders determined by stepwise biopsy of the lesser and greater curvatures of the stomach. *Gastroenterology*, 1972; 63: 584.

36 Tanner NC. Surgery of peptic ulceration and its complications. *Postgrad Med J*, 1954; 30: 448, 523, 577.

37 Jennings DA, Richardson JE. Giant lesser curve gastric ulcers. *Lancet*, 1954; ii: 343.

38 Kamada T, Fusamoto H, Masuzawa M, Hiramatsu K, Fukui O. 'Trench ulcer' of the stomach. *Am J Gastroenterol*, 1975; 63: 486.

39 Szabo S, Folkman J, Vattay P, Morales RE, Pinkus GE, Kato K. Accelerated healing of duodenal ulcers by oral administration of a mutein of basic fibroblastic growth factor in rats. *Gastroenterology*, 1994; 106: 1106.

40 Newcomb WD. The relationship between peptic ulceration and gastric carcinoma. *Br J Surg*, 1932–33; 20: 279.

41 Tatsuta M, Okuda S. Location, healing and recurrence of gastric ulcers in relation to fundal gastritis. *Gastroenterology*, 1975; 69: 897.

42 McDonald WC. Correlation of mucosal histology and aspirin intake in chronic gastric ulcer. *Gastroenterology*, 1973; 65: 381.

43 Hamilton SR, Yardley JH. Endoscopic biopsy diagnosis of aspirin-associated chronic gastric ulcers. *Gastroenterology*, 1980; 78: 1178.

44 Stemmermann GN. Intestinal metaplasia of the stomach. A status report. *Cancer*, 1994; 74: 556.

45 Mori K, Shiriya H, Wolff WI. Polypoid reparative mucosal proliferation at the site of a healed gastric ulcer; sequential gastroscopic, radiological and histological observation. *Gastroenterology*, 1971; 61: 523.

46 Kirk RN. Site and localisation of duodenal ulcers: a study at operation. *Gut*, 1968; 9: 414.

47 Kang JY, Nasiry R, Guan R *et al*. Influence of the site of a duodenal ulcer on its mode of presentation. *Gastroenterology*, 1986; 90: 1874.

48 Classen M. Endoscopy in benign peptic ulcer. *Clin Gastroenterol*, 1973; 2: 315.

49 Earlam RJ, Amerigo J, Kakavoulis T, Pollock DJ. Histological appearances of oesophagus, antrum and duodenum and their correlation with symptoms in patients with a duodenal ulcer. *Gut*, 1985; 26: 95.

50 Kang JY, Wee A, Math MV *et al*. *Helicobacter pylori* and gastritis in patients with peptic ulcer and non-ulcer dyspepsia: ethnic differences in Singapore. *Gut*, 1990; 31: 850.

51 Collins JSA, Hamilton PW, Watt PCH, Sloan JM, Love AHG. Quantitative histological study of mucosal inflammatory cell densities in endoscopic duodenal biopsy specimens from dyspeptic patients using computer-linked analysis. *Gut*, 1990; 31: 858.

52 Savarino V, Mela GS, Zentilin P *et al*. Circadian gastric acidity in *Helicobacter pylori*-positive ulcer patients with and without gastric metaplasia in the duodenum. *Gut*, 1996; 39: 508.

53 Harris AW, Gummett PA, Walker MM, Misiewicz JJ, Baron JH. Relations between gastric acid output, *Helicobacter pylori* and gastric metaplasia in the duodenal bulb. *Gut*, 1996; 39: 513.

54 Noach LA, Rolf TM, Bosma NB *et al*. Gastric metaplasia and *Helicobacter pylori* infection. *Gut*, 1993; 34: 1510.

55 Wyatt JI, Rathbone BJ, Sobala GM *et al*. Gastric epithelium in the duodenum: its association with *Helicobacter pylori* and inflammation. *J Clin Pathol*, 1990; 43: 981.

56 Wright NA, Pike C, Elia G. Induction of a novel epidermal growth factor-secreting cell lineage by mucosal ulceration in human gastrointestinal stem cells. *Nature*, 1990; 343: 82.

57 Wright NA, Poulsom R, Stamp G *et al*. Trefoil gene expression in gastrointestinal epithelial cells in inflammatory bowel disease. *Gastroenterology*, 1993; 104: 12.

58 Plaut AG. Trefoil peptides in the defense of the gastrointestinal tract. *N Engl J Med*, 1997; 336: 506.

59 Wong W-M, Playford RJ, Wright NA. Peptide gene expression in gastrointestinal mucosal ulceration: ordered sequence or redundancy? *Gut*, 2000; 46: 286.

60 Hanby AM, Chinery R, Poulsom R *et al*. Downregulation of E-cadherin in the regenerative epithelium of the human gastrointestinal tract. *Am J Pathol*, 1996; 148: 723.

61 Dean ACB, Clark CG, Sinclair-Gieben AH. The late prognosis of perforated duodenal ulcer. *Gut*, 1962; 3: 60.
62 Cohen MM. Treatment and mortality of perforated peptic ulcer: a survey of 852 cases. *Can Med Assoc J*, 1971; 105: 263.
63 Walt R, Katschinski B, Logan R, Ashley J, Langman M. Rising frequency of ulcer perforation in elderly people in the United Kingdom. *Lancet*, 1986; 1: 489.
64 Bardhan KD, Cust G, Hinchliffe RFC, Williamson FM, Lyon C, Bose K. Changing pattern of admissions and operation for duodenal ulcer. *Br J Surg*, 1989; 76: 230.
65 Jibril JA, Redpath A, MacIntyre IMC. Changing pattern of admission and operation for duodenal ulcer in Scotland. *Br J Surg*, 1994; 81: 87.
66 Rodriguez LAG, Jick H. Risk of gastrointestinal bleeding and perforation associated with individual non-steroidal antiinflammatory drugs. *Lancet*, 1994; 343: 769.
67 Svanes C, Sereide JA, Skarstein A *et al*. Smoking and ulcer perforation. *Gut*, 1997; 41: 177.
68 Fry J. Peptic ulcer: a profile. *Br Med J*, 1964; 2: 809.
69 Matthewson K, Pugh S, Northfield TC. Which peptic ulcer patients bleed? *Gut*, 1988; 29: 70.
70 Faulkner G, Prichard P, Somerville K, Langman MJS. Aspirin and bleeding peptic ulcers in the elderly. *Br Med J*, 1988; 297: 1311.
71 Hawkey CJ. Review article: aspirin and gastrointestinal bleeding. *Aliment Pharmacol Ther*, 1994; 8: 141.
72 Langman MJS, Weil J, Wainwright P *et al*. Risks of bleeding peptic ulcer associated with individual non-steroidal anti-inflammatory drugs. *Lancet*, 1994; 343: 1075.
73 Swain CP, Storey DW, Bown SG *et al*. Nature of the bleeding vessel in recurrently bleeding gastric ulcers. *Gastroenterology*, 1986; 90: 595.
74 Rockall TA, Logan RFA, Devlin HB, Northfield TC. Incidence of and mortality from acute upper gastrointestinal haemorrhage in the United Kingdom. *Br Med J*, 1995; 311: 222.
75 Weil J, Langman MJS, Wainwright P *et al*. Peptic ulcer bleeding: accessory risk factors and interactions with non-steroidal anti-inflammatory drugs. *Gut*, 2000; 46: 27–31.
76 Ernst H, Konturek P, Hahn EG, Brzozowski T, Konturek SJ. Acceleration of wound healing in gastric ulcers by local injection of neutralising antibody to transforming growth factor B_1. *Gut*, 1996; 39: 172.
77 Porteous C, Williams D, Foulis A, Sugden BA. Penetration of the left ventricular myocardium by benign peptic ulceration: two cases and a review of the published work. *J Clin Path*, 1984; 37: 1239.
78 West AB, Nolan N, O'Briain DS. Benign peptic ulcers penetrating pericardium and heart: clinicopathological features and factors favoring survival. *Gastroenterology*, 1988; 94: 1478.
79 Palmer ED. Gastric diverticula. *Int Abstr Surg*, 1951; 92: 417.
80 Rollag A, Jacobsen CD. Gastric ulcer and risk of cancer. *Acta Med Scand*, 1984; 216: 105.
81 Montgomery RD, Richardson BP. Gastric ulcer and cancer. *Q J Med*, 1975; 44: 591.
82 Graham DY, Schwartz JT, Cian GD, Gyoekwy F. Prospective evaluation of biopsy number in the diagnosis of oesophageal and gastric carcinoma. *Gastroenterology*, 1982; 82: 228.
83 Hole DJ, Quigley EMM, Gillis CR, Watkinson G. Peptic ulcer and cancer: an examination of the relationship between chronic peptic ulcer and gastric carcinoma. *Scand J Gastroenterol*, 1987; 22: 17.
84 Lee S, Iida M, Yao T *et al*. Risk of gastric carcinoma in patients with non-surgically treated peptic ulcer. *Scand J Gastroenterol*, 1990; 25: 1223.
85 Hansson L-E, Nyrén O, Hsing AW *et al*. The risk of stomach cancer in patients with gastric or duodenal ulcer disease. *N Engl J Med*, 1996; 335: 242.
86 Lee A, Dixon MF, Danon SJ *et al*. Local acid production and *Helicobacter pylori*: a unifying hypothesis of gastroduodenal disease. *Eur J Gastroenterol Hepatol*, 1995; 7: 461.
87 Sipponen P, Kekki M. Seppälä K, Siurala M. The relationships between chronic gastritis and gastric acid secretion. *Aliment Pharmacol Ther*, 1996; 10 (Suppl 1): 103.
88 Axon AR. Duodenal ulcer: the villain unmasked? Eradicating *Helicobacter pylori* will cure most patients. *Br Med J*, 1991; 302: 919.
89 NIH Consensus Conference. *Helicobacter pylori* in peptic ulcer disease. *JAMA*, 1994; 272: 65.
90 Langman MJS. Epidemiology. In: Carter DC, ed. *Peptic Ulcer*. Edinburgh: Churchill Livingstone, 1983.
91 Kurata JH, Haile BM. Epidemiology of peptic ulcer disease. *Clin Gastroenterol*, 1984; 13: 289.
92 Jennings D. Perforated peptic ulcer. Changes in the age-incidence and sex distribution in the last 150 years. *Lancet*, 1940; 1: 395 & 444.
93 Watkinson G. The incidence of chronic peptic ulcer found at necropsy. *Gut*, 1960; 1: 14.
94 Ihamaki T, Varis K, Siurala M. Morphological, functional and immunological state of the gastric mucosa in gastric carcinoma families. Comparison with a computer-matched family sample. *Scand J Gastroenterol*, 1979; 14: 801.
95 Coggon D, Lambert P, Langman MJS. Twenty years of hospital admission for peptic ulcer in England and Wales. *Lancet*, 1981; i: 1302.
96 McIntosh JH, Byth K, Tsang N, Berman K, Holliday FM, Piper DW. Trends in peptic ulcer mortality in Sydney from 1971 to 1987. *J Clin Gastroenterol*, 1993; 16: 346.
97 Brown RC, Langman MJS, Lambert PM. Hospital admissions for peptic ulcer during 1958 to 1972. *Br Med J*, 1976; 1: 35.
98 Wylie JH, Alexander-Williams J, Kennedy TL *et al*. Effect of cimetidine on surgery for duodenal ulcer. *Lancet*, 1981; 1: 1307.
99 Sonnenberg A. Geographic and temporal variations in the occurrence of peptic ulcer. *Scand J Gastroenterol*, 1985; 20 (Suppl 110): 11.
100 Bendahan J, Gilboa S, Paran H *et al*. Seasonal pattern in the incidence of bleeding caused by peptic ulcer in Israel. *Am J Gastroenterol*, 1992; 87: 733.
101 Moshkowitz M, Konikoff FM, Arber N *et al*. Seasonal variation in the frequency of *Helicobacter pylori* infection: a possible cause of the seasonal occurrence of peptic ulcer disease. *Am J Gastroenterol*, 1994; 89: 731.
102 Marshall BJ, Warren JR. Unidentified curved bacilli in the stomach of patients with gastritis and peptic ulceration. *Lancet*, 1984; 1: 1311.
103 Rathbone BJ, Wyatt JI, Heatley RV. *Campylobacter pyloridis*, a new factor in peptic ulcer disease. *Gut*, 1986; 27: 635.
104 Blaser MJ. Gastric *Campylobacter*-like organisms, gastritis and peptic ulcer disease. *Gastroenterology*, 1987; 93: 371.

105 Price AB, Levi J, Dolby JM *et al*. *Campylobacter pyloridis* in peptic ulcer disease: microbiology, pathology and scanning electron microscopy. *Gut*, 1985; 26: 1183.

106 Lambert JR, Dunn KL, Eaves ER, Korman MG, Hansky J. *Campylobacter pyloridis* in diseases of the human upper gastrointestinal tract. *Gastroenterology*, 1986; 90: 1509.

107 Rauws EAJ, Langenberg W, Houthouff HJ, Zanen HC, Tytgat GNJ. *Campylobacter pyloridis*-associated chronic active antral gastritis. *Gastroenterology*, 1988; 94: 33.

108 O'Connor HJ, Dixon MF, Wyatt JI, Axon ATR, Dewar EP, Johnston D. *Campylobacter pylori* and peptic ulcer disease. *Lancet*, 1987; 2: 633.

109 Rouvroy D, Bogaerts J, Nsengiumwa O, Omar M, Versailles L, Haot J. *Campylobacter pylori*, gastritis and peptic ulcer disease in Central Africa. *Br Med J*, 1987; 295: 1174.

110 Drumm B, Sherman P, Cutz E, Karmali M. Association of *Campylobacter pylori* on the gastric mucosa with antral gastritis in children. *N Engl J Med*, 1987; 316: 1557.

111 Oderda G, Vaira D, Holton J *et al*. *Helicobacter pylori* in children in peptic ulcer and their families. *Dig Dis Sci*, 1991; 36: 572.

112 Chang SKF, Lou Q, Asnicar MA *et al*. *Helicobacter pylori* infection in recurrent abdominal pain in childhood: comparison of diagnostic tests and therapy. *Paediatrics*, 1995; 96: 211.

113 Kalogeropoulos NK, Whitehead R. *Campylobacter*-like organisms and candida in peptic ulcer and similar lesions of the upper gastrointestinal tract: a study of 242 cases. *J Clin Pathol*, 1988; 41: 1093.

114 Graham JR. *Helicobacter pylori*: human pathogen or simply an opportunist. *Lancet*, 1995; 345: 1095.

115 Coghlan JG, Gilligan D, Humphries H *et al*. *Campylobacter pylori* and recurrence of duodenal ulcers—a 12-month follow-up study. *Lancet*, 1987; 2: 1109.

116 Marshall BJ, Goodwin CS, Warren JR *et al*. Prospective double-blind trial of duodenal ulcer relapse after eradication of *Campylobacter pylori*. *Lancet*, 1988; 2: 1437.

117 Hentschel E. Brandstätter G, Dragosics B *et al*. Effect of ranitidine and amoxycillin plus metronidazole on the eradication of *Helicobacter pylori* and the recurrence of duodenal ulcer. *N Engl J Med*, 1993; 328: 308.

118 Buckley M, O'Morain C. *Helicobacter pylori* eradication—a surrogate marker for duodenal ulcer healing. *Eur J Gastroenterol Hepatol*, 1996; 8: 415.

119 Patchett S, Beattie S, Leen E, Keane C, O'Morain C. *Helicobacter pylori* and duodenal ulcer recurrence. *Am J Gastroenterol*, 1992; 87: 24.

120 Goh K-L, Navaratnam P, Peh S-C *et al*. *Helicobacter pylori* eradication with short term therapy leads to duodenal ulcer healing without the need for continued acid suppression therapy. *Eur J Gastroenterol Hepatol*, 1996; 8: 421.

121 Humphreys H, Bourke S, Dooley C, McKenna D. Effect of treatment on *Campylobacter pylori* in peptic disease: a randomised prospective trial. *Gut*, 1988; 29: 279.

122 O'Connor HJ, Kanduru C, Bhutta AS, Meehan JM, Feeley KM, Cunnane K. Effect of *H. pylori* eradication on peptic ulcer healing. *Postgrad Med J*, 1995; 71: 90.

123 Labenz J, Börsch G. Evidence for the essential role of *Helicobacter pylori* in gastric ulcer disease. *Gut*, 1994; 35: 19.

124 Seppälä K, Pikkarainen P, Sipponen P *et al*. Cure of peptic gastric ulcer associated with eradication of *Helicobacter pylori*. *Gut*, 1995; 36: 834.

125 Moran AP. The role of lipopolysaccharides in *Helicobacter pylori* pathogenesis. *Aliment Pharmacol Ther*, 1996; 10 (Suppl 1): 39.

126 Micots I, Augeron C, Laboisse CL, Muzeau FM, Mégraud F. Mucin exocytosis: a major target for *Helicobacter pylori*. *J Clin Pathol*, 1993; 46: 241.

127 Oderda G, Vaira D, Dell'olio D, Holton J. Serum pepsinogen I and gastrin concentrations in children positive for *Helicobacter pylori*. *J Clin Pathol*, 1990; 43: 762.

128 Marcinkiewicz M, Van Der Linden B, Peura DA, Goldin G, Parolisi S, Sarosiek J. Impact of *Helicobacter pylori* colonisation on immunoreactive epidermal growth factor and transforming growth factor alpha in gastric juice. *Dig Dis Sci*, 1996; 41: 2150.

129 Hui PK, Chan WY, Cheung PS *et al*. Pathological changes of gastric mucosa colonised by *Helicobacter pylori*. *Hum Pathol*, 1992; 23: 548.

130 Fiocca R, Luinetti O, Villani L *et al*. Epithelial cytotoxicity, immune responses and inflammatory components of *Helicobacter pylori* gastritis. *Scand J Gastroenterol*, 1994; 29 (Suppl 205): 11.

131 Stemmerman GN, Haenszel W, Locke F. Epidemiologic pathology of gastric ulcer and gastric carcinoma among Japanese in Hawaii. *J Natl Cancer Inst*, 1977; 58: 13.

132 Eidt S, Stolte M. Antral intestinal metaplasia in *Helicobacter pylori* gastritis. *Digestion*, 1994; 55: 13.

133 Levi A, Beardshall K, Haddad G, Playford R, Ghosh P, Calam J. *Campylobacter pylori* and duodenal ulcer: the gastrin link. *Lancet*, 1989; 1: 1167.

134 Katelaris PH, Seow F, Lin PBC, Napoli J, Ngu MC, Jones DB. Effect of age, *Helicobacter* infection and gastritis with atrophy on serum gastrin and gastrin acid secretion in healthy men. *Gut*, 1993; 34: 1032.

135 Smith JTL, Pounder RE, Nwokolo CU *et al*. Inappropriate hypergastrinaemia in asymptomatic healthy subjects infected with *Helicobacter pylori*. *Gut*, 1990; 31: 522.

136 El-Omar EM, Penman ID, Ardill JES, Chittgalli RS, Howie C, McColl KEL. *Helicobacter pylori* infection and abnormalities of acid secretion in patients with duodenal ulcer disease. *Gastroenterology*, 1995; 109: 681.

137 Tarnasky PR, Kovacks TOG, Sytnik B, Walsh JH. Asymptomatic *H. pylori* infection impairs pH inhibition of gastrin and acid secretion during the second hour of peptone meal stimulation. *Dig Dis Sci*, 1993; 38: 1681.

138 Peterson WL. Gastrin and acid in relation to *Helicobacter pylori*. *Aliment Pharmacol Ther*, 1996; 10 (Suppl 1): 97.

139 Moss SF, Lagon S, Bishop AE, Polak JM, Calam J. Effect of *Helicobacter pylori* on gastric somatostatin in duodenal ulcer disease. *Lancet*, 1992; 340: 930.

140 Ødum L, Petersen HD, Andersen IB, Hansen BF, Rehfeld JF. Gastrin and somatostatin in *Helicobacter pylori* infected antral mucosa. *Gut*, 1994; 35: 615.

141 Gotz JM, Veenendaal RA, Biemond I, Muller ESM, Veselic M, Lamers CBHW. Serum gastrin and mucosal somatostatin in *Helicobacter pylori*-associated gastritis. *Scand J Gastroenterol*, 1995; 30: 1064.

142 Olbe L, Hamlet A, Palenbäck J, Fändriks L. A mechanism by which *Helicobacter pylori* infection of the antrum contributes to

the development of duodenal ulcer. *Gastroenterology*, 1996; 110: 1386.

143 James AH. Gastric epithelium in the duodenum. *Gut*, 1964; 5: 285.

144 Steer HW. Surface morphology of the gastroduodenal mucosa in duodenal ulceration. *Gut*, 1984; 25: 1203.

145 Wyatt JI, Rathbone BJ, Dixon MF, Heatley RV, Axon ATR. *Campylobacter pylori* and development of duodenal ulcer. *Lancet*, 1988; 1: 118.

146 Parrish JA, Rawlins DC. Intestinal metaplasia in Zollinger–Ellison syndrome. *Gut*, 1965; 6: 286.

147 Hanby AM, Poulsom R, Elia G *et al*. The expression of the trefoil peptide pS2 and human spasmolytic polypeptide (hSP) in gastric metaplasia of the proximal duodenum: implications for the nature of 'gastric metaplasia'. *J Pathol*, 1993; 169: 355.

148 Kushima R, Manabe R, Hattori T, Borchard F. Histiogenesis of gastric foveolar metaplasia following duodenal ulcer: a definite reparative lineage of Brunner's gland. *Histopathology*, 1999; 35: 38.

149 Marshall BJ, Goodwin CS, Warren JR *et al*. Prospective double blind trial of duodenal ulcer relapse after eradication of *Campylobacter pylori*. *Lancet*, 1988; 2: 1437.

150 Goodwin CS. Duodenal ulcer, *Campylobacter pylori* and the leaking roof concept. *Lancet*, 1988; 2: 1467.

151 Crabtree JE. Gastric mucosal inflammatory responses to *Helicobacter pylori*. *Aliment Pharmacol Ther*, 1996; 10 (Suppl 1): 29.

152 Crabtree JE, Taylor JD, Wyatt JI *et al*. Mucosal IgA recognition of *Helicobacter pylori* 120 kDa protein, peptic ulceration and gastric pathology. *Lancet*, 1991; 338: 332.

153 Blaser MJ. The role of Vac A and the Cag A locus of *Helicobacter pylori* in human disease. *Aliment Pharmacol Ther*, 1996; 10 (Suppl 1): 73.

154 Atherton JC, Peek RM, Tham KT, Perez-Perez GI, Blaser MJ. Quantitative culture of *H. pylori* in the gastric mucosa: association of bacterial density with duodenal ulcer status and infection with Cag A-positive bacterial strains and negative association with IgG levels. *Am J Gastroenterol*, 1994; 89: 1322.

155 Yamaoka Y, Kita M, Kodama T, Sawai N, Imanishi J. *Helicobacter pylori Cag A* gene and expression of cytokine messenger RNA in gastric mucosa. *Gastroenterology*, 1996; 110: 1744.

156 Crabtree JE, Farmery SM, Lindley IJD, Figura N, Peichl P, Tompkins DS. Cag A/cytotoxic strains of *Helicobacter pylori* and interleukin-8 in gastric epithelial cell lines. *J Clin Pathol*, 1994; 47: 945.

157 Atherton C, Peek RM, Tham KT, Cover TL, Blaser MJ. Clinical and pathological importance of heterogeneity in Vac A, the vacuolating cytotoxin gene of *Helicobacter pylori*. *Gastroenterology*, 1997; 112: 92.

158 Sun DC, Roth SH, Mitchell CS *et al*. Upper gastrointestinal disease in rheumatoid arthritis. *Am J Dig Dis*, 1974; 19: 405.

159 Griffin MR, Piper JM, Daugherty JR, Snowden M, Ray WA. Non-steroidal anti-inflammatory drug use and increased risk of peptic ulcer disease in elderly persons. *Ann Intern Med*, 1991; 114: 257.

160 Simon LS, Mills JA. New non-steroidal anti-inflammatory drugs. *N Engl J Med*, 1980; 302: 1179 & 1237.

161 Roth SH. Non-steroidal anti-inflammatory drug gastropathy. *Arch Intern Med*, 1986; 146: 1075.

162 Brooks PM. Clinical management of rheumatoid arthritis. *Lancet*, 1993; 341: 286.

163 CSM Update. Non-steroidal anti-inflammatory drugs and serious gastrointestinal adverse reactions. *Br Med J* 1986; 292: 614.

164 Hawkey CJ. Review article: aspirin and gastroduodenal bleeding. *Aliment Pharmacol Ther*, 1994; 8: 141.

165 Meisel AD. Clinical benefits and comparative safety of Piroxicam. *Am J Med*, 1986; 81 (Suppl 5B): 15.

166 Gabriel SE, Jaakkimainen L, Bombardier C. Risk for serious gastrointestinal complications related to use of non-steroidal anti-inflammatory drugs. *Ann Intern Med*, 1991; 115: 787.

167 Singh G, Triadafilopoulus G. Epidemiology of NSAID-induced gastrointestinal complications. *J Rheumatol*, 1999; 26 (Suppl 56): 18.

168 Hawkey CJ. Non-steroidal anti-inflammatory drugs and peptic ulcers. *Br Med J*, 1990; 300: 278.

169 Taha AS, Dahill S, Sturrock RD, Lee FD, Russell RI. Predicting NSAID-related ulcers—assessment of clinical and pathological risk factors and importance of differences in NSAID. *Gut*, 1994; 35: 891.

170 Skander MP, Ryan FP. Non-steroidal anti-inflammatory drugs and pain free peptic ulceration in the elderly. *Br Med J*, 1988; 297: 833.

171 Clinch JR, Banerjee AK, Ostick G, Levy DW. Non steroidal anti-inflammatory drugs and gastrointestinal adverse effects. *J R Coll Phys Lond*, 1983; 17: 228.

172 Fries JF, Miller SR, Spitz PW, Williams CA, Hubert HB, Bloch DA. Identification of patients at risk for gastropathy associated with NSAID use. *J Rheumatol*, 1990; 17 (Suppl 20): 12.

173 Henry D, Lim L-Y, Garcia LA *et al*. Variability of gastrointestinal complications with individual non-steroidal anti-inflammatory drugs: results of collaborative study. *Br Med J*, 1996; 312: 1563.

174 Anon *Current problems in pharmacovigilance*. 1994; 20: 9.

175 Singh G, Ramey DR, Morfield D *et al*. Gastrointestinal tract complications of non-steroidal anti-inflammatory drug treatment in rheumatoid arthritis. *Arch Intern Med*, 1996; 156: 1530.

176 Allison MC, Howatson AG, Torrance CJ, Lee FD, Russell RI. Gastrointestinal damage associated with the use of non-steroidal anti-inflammatory drugs. *N Engl J Med*, 1992; 327: 749.

177 Wolfe MM, Lichenstein DR, Singh GL. Gastrointestinal toxicity of non-steroidal anti-inflammatory drugs. *N Engl J Med*, 1999; 340: 1888.

178 Graham DY, Lidsky MD, Cox AM *et al*. Longterm non-steroidal anti-inflammatory drug use and *Helicobacter pylori* infection. *Gastroenterology*, 1991; 100: 1653.

179 Kim JG, Graham DY and the Misoprostol Study Group. *Helicobacter pylori* infection and development of gastric or duodenal ulcer in arthritic patients receiving chronic NSAID therapy. *Am J Gastroenterol*, 1994; 89: 203.

180 Loeb DS, Talley NJ, Ahlquist DA, Carpenter HA, Zinsmeister AR. Longterm non-steroidal anti-inflammatory drug use and gastroduodenal injury: the role of *Helicobacter pylori*. *Gastroenterology*, 1992; 102: 1899.

181 Laine L, Marin-Sorensen N, Weinstein WM. Non steroidal anti-inflammatory drug-associated gastric ulcers do not require *H. pylori* for their development. *Am J Gastroenterol*, 1992; 87: 1398.

182 Heresbach D, Raoul JL, Bretagne JF *et al*. *Helicobacter pylori*: a risk and severity factor of non-steroidal anti-inflammatory drug induced gastropathy. *Gut*, 1992; 33: 1608.

183 Taha AS, Dahill S, Sturrock RD, Lee FD, Russell RI. Predicting NSAID related ulcers—assessment of clinical and pathological risk factors and importance of differences in NSAID. *Gut*, 1994; 35: 891.

184 Taha AS, Sturrock RD, Russell RI. Mucosal erosions in longterm non-steroidal anti-inflammatory drug users: predisposition to ulceration and relation to *Helicobacter pylori*. *Gut*, 1995; 36: 334.

185 Huang J-Q, Sridhar S, Hunt RH. Role of *Helicobacter pylori* infection and non-steroidal anti-inflammatory drugs in peptic-ulcer disease: a meta-analysis. *Lancet*, 2002; 359: 14.

186 Chan FKL, To KF, Wu JCY *et al*. Eradication of *Helicobacter pylori* and risk of peptic ulcers in patients starting long-term treatment with non-steroidal anti-inflammatory drugs: a randomised trial. *Lancet*, 2002; 359: 9.

187 Taha AS, Nakshabendi I, Lee FD, Sturrock RD, Russell RI. Chemical gastritis and *Helicobacter pylori*-related gastritis in patients receiving non-steroidal anti-inflammatory drugs: comparison and correlation with peptic ulceration. *J Clin Pathol*, 1992; 45: 135.

188 Szabo S, Goldberg I. Experimental pathogenesis: drugs and chemical lesions in the gastric mucosa. *Scand J Gastroenterol*, 1990; 25 (Suppl 174): 1.

189 Davenport HW. Salicylate damage to the gastric mucosal barrier. *N Engl J Med*, 1967; 276: 1307.

190 Jacobson ED. Circulatory mechanism of gastric mucosal damage and protection. *Gastroenterology*, 1992; 102: 1788.

191 Wallace JL, Arfols K-E, McKnight GW. A monoclonal antibody against the CD18 leukocyte adhesion molecule prevents indomethacin-induced gastric damage in the rabbit. *Gastroenterology*, 1991; 100: 878.

192 Trevethick MA, Clayton NM, Strong P, Harman IW. Do infiltrating neutrophils contribute to the pathogenesis of indomethacin-induced ulceration of the rat gastric antrum? *Gut*, 1993; 34: 156.

193 Andrews FJ, Malcontenti-Wilson C, O'Brien PE. Effect of non-steroidal anti-inflammatory drugs on LFA-1 and ICAM-1 expression in gastric mucosa. *Am J Physiol*, 1994; 266: G657.

194 Wallace JL. Non steroidal anti-inflammatory drug gastropathy and cytoprotection: pathogenesis and mechanisms re-examined. *Scand J Gastroenterol*, 1992; 27 (Suppl 192): 3.

195 Bickel M, Kauffman GL. Gastric gel mucus thickness: effect of distension, 16,16-dimethyl prostaglandin E2 and carbenoxolone. *Gastroenterology*, 1981; 80: 770.

196 Konturek SJ, Robert A. Cytoprotection of canine gastric mucosa by prostacyclin: possible mediation by increased mucosal blood flow. *Digestion*, 1982; 25: 155.

197 Forssell H, Olbe L. Continuous computerised determination of gastric bicarbonate secretion in man. *Scand J Gastroenterol*, 1985; 20: 767.

198 Hogan DL, Ainsworth MA, Isenberg JI. Review article: gastroduodenal bicarbonate secretion. *Aliment Pharmacol Ther*, 1994; 8: 475.

199 Konturek SJ, Piastuki I, Brzozowski T *et al*. Role of prostaglandins in the formation of aspirin-induced gastric ulcers. *Gastroenterology*, 1981; 80: 4.

200 Graham DY, Agraal NM, Roth SH. Prevention of NSAID-induced gastric ulcers with misoprostol: multicentric double blind placebo-controlled trial. *Lancet*, 1988; 2: 1277.

201 Khan Z, Playford RJ. The new NSAIDs—gains, pains and financial strains. *Gastroenterol Today*, 1999; 9: 48.

202 Hawkey CJ. COX-2 inhibitors. *Lancet*, 1999; 353: 307.

203 Keller JJ, Offerhaus GJA, Polak M *et al*. Rectal epithelial apoptosis in familial adenomatous polyposis patients treated with sulindac. *Gut*, 1999; 45: 822.

204 Wu GD. A nuclear receptor to prevent colon cancer. *N Engl J Med*, 2000; 342: 651.

205 Conn HO, Blitzer BL. Non association of adrenocorticosteroid therapy and peptic ulcer. *N Engl J Med*, 1976; 294: 473.

206 Piper JM, Ray WA, Daugherty JR, Griffen MA. Corticosteroid use and peptic ulcer disease: role of non-steroidal anti-inflammatory drugs. *Ann Intern Med*, 1991; 114: 735.

207 Jorgensen LS, Bonlokke L, Christensen NJ. Life strain, life events and autonomic response to psychological stressors in patients with chronic upper abdominal pain. *Scand J Gastroenterol*, 1986; 21: 605.

208 Talley NJ, Piper DW. Major life events, stress and dyspepsia of unknown cause: a case control study. *Gut*, 1986; 27: 127.

209 Hafeiz HBA, Al-Quorian A, Mangoor SA, Karin AA. Life events, stress in functional dyspepsia: a case control study. *Eur J Gastroenterol Hepatol*, 1997; 9: 21.

210 Peters MN, Richardson CT. Stressful life events, acid hypersecretion and ulcer disease. *Gastroenterology*, 1983; 84: 114.

211 Feldman EJ, Elashoff JD, Samloff IM, Grossman MI. Psychological stress and duodenal ulcer (letter). *N Engl J Med*, 1980; 302: 1206.

212 Wormsley KG. Smoking and duodenal ulcer. *Gastroenterology*, 1978; 75: 139.

213 Piper DW, Greig M, Coupland GAE, Hobbin E, Shinners J. Factors relevant to the prognosis of chronic peptic ulcer. *Gut*, 1975; 16: 714.

214 Korman MG, Hansky J, Eaves ER, Schmidt GT. Influence of cigarette smoking on healing and relapse in duodenal ulcer disease. *Gastroenterology*, 1983; 85: 871.

215 Endoh K, Leung FW. Effects of smoking and nicotine on the gastric mucosa: a review of clinical and experimental evidence. *Gastroenterology*, 1994; 107: 864.

216 Iwata F, Leung FW. Tobacco cigarette smoke aggravates gastric ulcer in rats by attenuation of ulcer margin hyperaemia. *Am J Physiol*, 1995; 268: G153.

217 Aird I, Bentall HH, Mehigan JA, Roberts JAF. Blood groups in relation to peptic ulceration and carcinoma of the colon, rectum, breast and bronchus. *Br Med J*, 1954; 2: 315.

218 Clarke CA, Edwards JW, Haddock DRW, Howell-Evans AW, McConnell RB, Sheppard P. ABO blood groups and secretor character in duodenal ulcer. *Br Med J*, 1956; 2: 275.

219 Dickey W, Collins JSA, Watson RGP, Sloan JM, Porter KG. Secretor status and *Helicobacter pylori* infection are independent risk factors for gastroduodenal disease. *Gut*, 1993; 34: 351.

220 Doll R, Kellock TD. The separate inheritance of gastric and duodenal ulcers. *Ann Eugen*, 1951; 16: 231.

221 Ellis A. The genetics of peptic ulcer. *Scand J Gastroenterol*, 1985; 20 (Suppl 110): 25.

222 Buchanan KD, Sloan JM, O'Hare MMT, Kennedy TL. Zollinger–Ellison syndrome. In: Bouchier IAD, ed. *Textbook of Gastroenterology*. London: Bailliere Tindall, 1984: 1339.

223 Ammann RW, Vetter D, Deyhle P, Tschen H, Sulser H, Schmid M. Gastrointestinal involvement in systemic mastocytosis. *Gut*, 1976; 17: 107.

224 Shepherd AMM, Stewart WK, Wormsley KG. Peptic ulceration in chronic renal failure. *Lancet*, 1973; 1: 1357.

225 Franzin G, Musola R, Mencarelli R. Morphological changes of the gastroduodenal mucosa in regular dialysis uraemic patients. *Histopathology*, 1982; 6: 429.

226 Kang JY, Wu AYT, Sutherland IH, Vathsala A. Prevalence of peptic ulcer in patients underlying maintenance dialysis. *Dig Dis Sci*, 1988; 33: 774.

227 Doherty CC. Gastric secretion in chronic uraemia and after renal transplantation. *Irish J Med Sci*, 1980; 149: 5.

228 Ritchie WP Jr, Delaney JP. Gastric ulcer: an experimental model. *Surg Forum*, 1968; 19: 312.

229 du Plessis DJ. Pathogenesis of gastric ulceration. *Lancet*, 1965; 1: 974.

230 Duane WC, Wiegand DM. Mechanism by which bile salts disrupt the gastric mucosal barrier in the dog. *J Clin Invest*, 1980; 66: 1044.

231 Robbins PL, Broadie TA, Sosin H, Delaney JP. Reflux gastritis: the consequences of intestinal juice in the stomach. *Am J Surg*, 1976; 131: 23.

232 Sobala GM, O'Connor HJ, Dewar EP, King RFG, Axon ATR, Dixon MF. Bile reflux and intestinal metaplasia in gastric mucosa. *J Clin Pathol*, 1993; 46: 235.

233 Zollinger RM, Ellison EH. Primary peptic ulceration of the jejunum associated with islet cell tumors of the pancreas. *Ann Surg*, 1955; 142: 709.

234 Watson RGP, Johnston CF, O'Hare MMT *et al*. The frequency of gastrointestinal endocrine tumours in a well defined population—Northern Ireland 1970–1985. *Q J Med New Series*, 1989; 72: 647.

235 Oberhelman HA Jr. Excisional therapy for ulcerogenic tumors of the duodenum. Long-term results. *Arch Surg*, 1972; 104: 447.

236 Stamm B, Hedinger CE, Saremaslani P. Duodenal and ampullary carcinoid tumours. A report of 12 cases with pathological characteristics, polypeptide content and relationship to the MEN1 syndrome and von Recklinghausen's disease (neurofibromatosis). *Virchows Arch A*, 1986; 408: 475.

237 Newsome HH. Multiple endocrine adenomatosis. *Surg Clin N Am*, 1974; 54: 387.

238 Solcia E, Capella C, Fiocca R, Rindi G, Rosai J. Gastric argyrophil carcinoidosis in patients with Zollinger–Ellison syndrome due to Type I multiple endocrine neoplasia. *Am J Surg Pathol*, 1990; 14: 503.

239 Friesen SR, Tomita T. Pseudo-Zollinger–Ellison syndrome. Hypergastrinemia, hyperchlorhydria without tumor. *Ann Surg*, 1981; 194: 481.

240 Bordi C, Cocconi G, Togni R, Vezzadini P, Missale G. Gastric endocrine cell proliferation. Association with Zollinger–Ellison syndrome. *Arch Pathol*, 1974; 98: 274.

241 Lechago J. Gastrointestinal neuroendocrine cell proliferations. *Hum Pathol*, 1994; 25: 1114.

242 Neuburger PH, Lewin M, de Recherche C, Bonfils S. Parietal and chief cell populations in four cases of the Zollinger–Ellison syndrome. *Gastroenterology*, 1972; 63: 937.

243 Creutzfeldt W. The achlorhydria carcinoid sequence: role of gastrin. *Digestion*, 1988; 39: 61.

244 Lewin KJ, Elashoff JD, Yang K, Walsh J, Ulich T. Primary gastrin cell hyperplasia. *Am J Surg Pathol*, 1984; 8: 821.

245 Polak JM, Stagg B, Pearse AGE. Two types of Zollinger–Ellison syndrome; immunofluorescent, cytochemical and ultrastructural studies of the antral and pancreatic gastrin cells in different clinical states. *Gut*, 1972; 13: 501.

246 Arnold R, Hulst MV, Neuhof C, Schwarting H, Becker HD, Creutzfeldt W. Antral gastrin-producing G-cells and somatostatin-producing D-cells in different states of gastric acid secretion. *Gut*, 1982; 23: 285.

247 Weber HC, Venzon DJ, Jensen RJ, Metz DC. Studies on the inter-relation between Zollinger–Ellison syndrome, *Helicobacter pylori* and proton pump inhibitor therapy. *Gastroenterology*, 1997; 112: 84.

14 Epithelial tumours of the stomach

This chapter deals with benign and malignant gastric epithelial tumours. Non-neoplastic polyps and polyp-like lesions are discussed in Chapter 16.

Benign epithelial tumours

These are known as adenomas. Gastric adenomas are uncommon and are much less frequent than hyperplastic (regenerative) polyps (see p. 214) which they resemble on gross appearance. The important distinction between adenomas and other polyps in the stomach is that the former are composed of tubular or villous structures lined by *dysplastic* epithelium [1]. Adenomas occur predominantly in patients over 50 years of age and most are soft velvety exophytic masses that are sessile or broad-based (Fig. 14.1). In early publications they are often described as large with an average diameter of 4 cm [2], but more recent studies based on endoscopy show a wide variation in size ranging from 8 mm upwards [3,4]. Gastric adenomas are usually solitary lesions that occur mostly in the antrum or at the boundary between the antrum and gastric body. In general they are asymptomatic, and their importance lies in the fact that they have a significant potential for malignant change [4,5]. Flat and depressed adenomas also exist, although they are less common than the protuberant type. They are often considered to be early gastric cancers on endoscopy and present as small shallow circumscribed lesions measuring up to 2 cm in diameter with irregular margins [6]. Recently some authors have advocated that the term 'adenoma' be confined to raised dysplastic lesions and that non-raised dysplasia be classified as GED (gastric epithelial dysplasia) [7].

Histologically gastric adenomas may have a tubular, villous or tubulovillous architecture. Small tumours are usually tubular adenomas while the larger are more likely to be villous. The epithelium consists of crowded columnar cells with large hyperchromatic, elongated nuclei and amphophilic to slightly basophilic cytoplasm in which mucus is scanty. Pseudostratification of nuclei is extensive and mitoses may be frequent. In sessile tubular adenomas and in depressed adenomas a distinct two-layer structure may be apparent in which hyperplastic pyloric-type glands, often showing cystic dilatation, lie deep to dysplastic epithelium on the surface [8] (Fig. 14.2). There is usually a sharp demarcation between the dysplastic adenomatous epithelium and the adjacent mucosa, which often shows atrophic gastritis with intestinal metaplasia. This, and the frequent 'intestinal' features of the lesions themselves, suggest that some, at least, may originate from metaplastic glands [9]. The dysplastic epithelium contains a variety of cell types. Most commonly it resembles dysplastic colonic epithelium, sometimes with differentiation towards goblet cells, Paneth cells and enterochromaffin cells [3,10]. Less often it is composed of gastric foveolar-type epithelium with apical mucin vacuoles. Some lesions appear to exhibit a mixture of the two [10]. In adenomas with a predominantly villous architecture the villi show considerable branching resulting in a papillary surface. This is in contrast to colorectal villous adenomas in which the villi seldom branch.

The degree of dysplasia varies considerably within an adenoma and careful examination of several sections of resected lesions should be conducted to rule out small foci of malignancy. Similarly, when an adenoma is biopsied, several samples are essential in order to obtain accurate assessment. Gastric dysplasia is discussed fully on p. 169. It is conventionally divided into low grade and high grade, the latter being characterized by marked architectural distortion with branching of glands and papillary ingrowth into the gland lumen. Cytologically there is marked nuclear pleomorphism, frequent mitoses with abnormal forms, nuclear stratification involving the full thickness of the cytoplasm and loss of polarity.

The development of malignancy in gastric adenomas is defined by invasion of the lamina propria by neoplastic epithelium (in contrast to colorectal adenomas, where malignancy is defined by submucosal invasion). Sometimes this can be clearly identified as irregular jagged budding of neoplastic epithelium into the surrounding loose lamina propria, but at other times it can only be inferred from severe abnormalities of

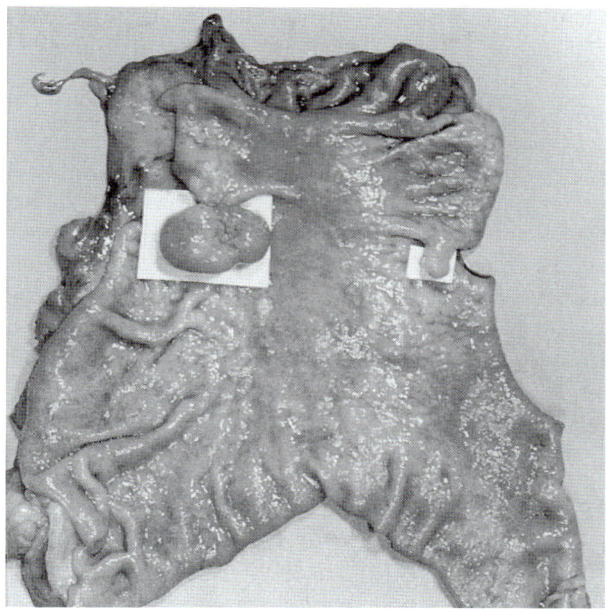

Fig. 14.1 Tubulovillous adenoma of stomach.

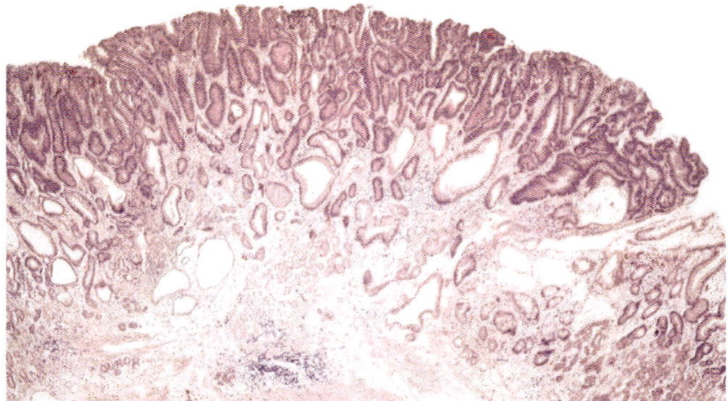

Fig. 14.2 Sessile tubulovillous adenoma. There is a two-layer structure. Hyperchromatic epithelium showing nuclear stratification and low-grade dysplasia occupies the superficial layer. Deep to this the glands are hyperplastic and dilated but not dysplastic.

architecture, such as a solid growth pattern or complex aggregation of back-to-back glands. Western pathologists usually demand the former to diagnose carcinoma while Japanese pathologists generally use the latter: this geographical difference in interpretation appears to contribute to the different reported frequencies in gastric cancer between East and West [11]. Estimates of the risk of malignant transformation in gastric adenomas are variable but two long-term follow-up studies indicated that carcinoma arose in 11 and 21% of adenomas, respectively [4,12]. Thus the risk is significant and sufficient to recommend complete excision of all adenomas to prevent progression to gastric cancer. Depressed adenomas appear to carry a similar risk to elevated lesions [6]. Features that have been associated with malignant transformation are increase in size, villiform architecture, sulphomucin secretion, a mixture of gastric and intestinal phenotypes and, most importantly, the presence of high-grade dysplasia. At molecular level, loss of heterozygosity at certain chromosomal regions is much less common in adenomas than in gastric carcinoma [13]. Overexpression of p53 gene protein is commoner in adenomas exhibiting an intestinal phenotype and in those with high-grade dysplasia [14].

Gastric adenoma and synchronous carcinoma coexist in a significant number of cases [12] indicating the need for careful examination of the surrounding mucosa during endoscopy or on examination of resected specimens.

Gastric adenomas in familial adenomatous polyposis (FAP) and Gardner's syndrome

While fundic gland polyps are the most common gastric lesions associated with FAP (see p. 217), adenomas also occur. They may affect a rather younger age group than in the general population [15] and are often small (less than 1 cm diameter). The antrum is the site predominantly affected and the lesions may be multiple. Their prevalence varies between series and appears to be considerably higher in Japanese series compared with the West where in most reports it is around 10% [10]. Duodenal adenomas are much more common. Most FAP-associated gastric adenomas have a tubular architecture [16,17] and the frequency with which they are found to have progressed to gastric cancer is generally low (<1%) in the West [17,18]. The corresponding figure in Japan is reported to be as high as 40% [19], but this difference is probably accounted for, at least in part, by the different criteria used for defining malignancy in adenomas between East and West (see above).

The association between gastric malignancy and Peutz–Jeghers syndrome is discussed on p. 169.

Malignant epithelial tumours

Adenocarcinoma

Gastric adenocarcinoma was said to be the commonest primary cancer in the world in 1980, with almost 670 000 new cases in that year [20]. By 1990, it had been overtaken by carcinoma of the lung, partly because of the rising incidence of lung cancer, but also because gastric cancer is one of the tumours whose frequency is falling worldwide [20,21]. It is generally a disease of the middle-aged and elderly, with a peak incidence in patients over 65 years [22]. Men are more often affected than women in a ratio of around 1.6 : 1 [20], and this is particularly so for adenocarcinoma arising at the cardia [23,24].

Epidemiology

There is considerable variation in the incidence of stomach cancer between countries. The highest recorded rate is in Japan, followed by Andean areas of Central and South America, Portugal, China, tropical Africa and Eastern Europe. Incidence rates are low in the USA, Canada, Australia and the Middle East while north and west Europe lie somewhere in between [22]. Even within countries there is marked variation between regions [25,26] and between socioeconomic groups, the disease being commoner in the lower social strata [27].

The overall incidence of gastric carcinoma appears to be declining in frequency in almost all countries, although this is not the case for carcinoma of the cardia and the gastro-oesophageal junction (see below). The rate of decline varies between and within countries. In the USA the drop in incidence rates has been quite sharp [28] while in Great Britain there has been a slower decline since the mid-1950s [29]. In the West Midlands region of England, age-standardized incidence rates decreased by 20% over a 20-year period from 1962 [23]. A similar decline has been noted in nearby Oxfordshire [30]. This trend continued nationwide, as reflected by a fall in mortality from gastric cancer in England and Wales between 1984 and 1994 from over 10 000 to approximately 7500 per annum [31]. In Finland the age-adjusted incidence in males fell from 65.4 to 21.4 per 100 000 between 1953 and 1985, with a similar decrease among females [32]. Here it was found that the reduction was largely in tumours of so-called intestinal type (see below), while the frequency of diffuse-type cancers remained steady.

The frequency of cancer arising at the cardia of the stomach has shown the opposite trend in Europe and the USA over the past 25 years [23,33–36]. In Great Britain the proportion of gastric adenocarcinoma arising at the cardia increased from approximately 13% in the early 1960s to over 20% in 1980 [23]. In the Netherlands cardial tumours constituted 26% of all gastric cancers by the end of the 1980s [35] and some studies indicate that, in contrast to 30–40 years ago, carcinoma of the corpus and cardia is now almost as common as carcinoma arising in the antrum [30,37]. In Connecticut, USA, the incidence rate of carcinoma of the cardia is reported to have trebled between 1964 and 1989 in males, with an even higher increase in females [38]. This is of particular concern because stage for stage, cardiac carcinomas carry a worse prognosis than those arising in other parts of the stomach [29,35]. Carcinoma of the gastric cardia shows a consistently higher male : female ratio than that of cancers arising in the more distal stomach [23,39]. There is also an association with hiatus hernia and chronic reflux symptoms [40], although the latter are more strongly associated with adenocarcinoma of the lower oesophagus [41]. Indeed, adenocarcinoma of the gastric cardia appears to share more in common epidemiologically with lower oesophageal adenocarcinoma than distal gastric cancer. Both tumours are increasing in incidence, show male predominance and have similar aetiological and clinicopathological features. The prevalence of *p53* mutations and DNA content abnormalities are also similar [42] and they have an equally poor prognosis.

Uncertainty frequently arises regarding the precise site of origin of tumours around the lower oesophagus, gastro-oesophageal junction and cardia, and Siewert *et al.* [43] have recently proposed a classification as follows: type I carcinomas arise in the distal third of the oesophagus, usually in a segment of Barrett's metaplasia, and may or may not directly involve the gastro-oesophageal junction (GOJ); type II straddle the GOJ and appear to arise at the true junction of the stomach and oesophagus; and type III are cardiac gastric cancers that have grown proximally to invade the GOJ. The cytokeratin expression profile of tumours arising in this location may also facilitate more accurate designation. Metaplastic columnar epithelium in Barrett's oesophagus shows a different distribution of CK7 and CK20 from that of intestinal metaplasia in the proximal stomach [44,45]. There is some evidence that this is reflected in the adenocarcinomas that arise from the two sites: 90% of oesophageal adenocarcinomas are reported to have a CK7 positive/CK20 negative profile while those arising in proximal stomach have a more variable profile and only around 20% are CK7 positive/CK20 negative [46].

Gastric carcinoma in young patients

Less than 5% of gastric cancers occur under the age of 35 years, after which age-specific incidence rates rise steeply [47–49]. The characteristics of the disease in the young differ from the overall pattern. The male : female ratio is approximately equal or shows female predominance [48], the tumours are usually poorly differentiated, diffuse-type or infiltrative carcinomas [47,49,50], and the prognosis is generally poor. Some are hereditary tumours in individuals with germline mutations of the E-cadherin gene [51].

Aetiology and pathogenesis

Gastric carcinogenesis is a multistep and multifactorial process that in many cases appears to involve a progression from normal mucosa through chronic gastritis, atrophic gastritis and intestinal metaplasia to dysplasia and carcinoma [52]. A number of precancerous conditions have been recognized such as atrophic gastritis and intestinal metaplasia due to *Helicobacter pylori* infection or autoimmunity, gastric ulcers, gastric polyps, previous gastric surgery and Menetrier's disease [53,54], and there are putative associations with environmental agents such as dietary constituents and the formation of carcinogenic N-nitroso compounds within the stomach. In a minority of cases there is good evidence for an inherited disposition. Each of these will now be discussed in some detail.

Chronic gastritis and intestinal metaplasia

The relationship between chronic gastritis, and in particular atrophic gastritis with intestinal metaplasia, and gastric cancer has been intensively studied and evidence for a true association comes from several sources. Epidemiologically, the prevalence of chronic atrophic gastritis within populations correlates closely with the incidence and death rate from gastric cancer [55,56] and in follow-up studies atrophic gastritis has been shown to precede the development of malignancy [57,58]. Conditions that predispose to gastric cancer, such as pernicious anaemia and the postoperative stomach, are frequently characterized by the presence of extensive atrophic gastritis and intestinal metaplasia, and it may be that the cancer risk is higher with severe atrophic gastritis of the antrum than with that of the body of the stomach. The observed increase in cell proliferation [59,60] and DNA aneuploidy [61] in chronic atrophic gastritis are potentially important factors in gastric carcinogenesis.

Nearly half a century ago, Morson showed that many gastric carcinomas arise from areas of intestinal metaplasia, and that these tumours often show an 'intestinal' phenotype morphologically [62]. This observation has been repeatedly corroborated by many other groups [63,64]. Atrophic gastritis with accompanying metaplasia is associated with increased prevalence of gastric cancer and with increased risk of developing cancer within 10 years [65], and the association with 'intestinal' as opposed to 'diffuse'-type tumours holds true for early adenocarcinomas [66], and for those arising at the gastric cardia [67]. Geographical studies have shown a strong correlation between the prevalence of intestinal metaplasia and the incidence of gastric cancer [68], and its particular importance in the context of chronic gastritis is indicated by the finding that gastric cancer is not particularly common in *H. pylori*-infected subjects unless they have concurrent intestinal metaplasia [69–71]. Because of the heterogeneous nature of intestinal metaplasia, interest has focused on the significance of the different variants (see p. 115) with respect to gastric carcinogenesis. While all three types are associated with gastric cancer, it is type III intestinal metaplasia, which is the least common and is characterized by the presence of columnar mucous cells containing sulphomucins, that is most closely associated, especially with the intestinal type of adenocarcinoma [72,73]. Despite this, type III metaplasia is not considered a sufficiently sensitive or specific marker for its routine use to be recommended in selecting individuals for gastric cancer surveillance [74,75].

Helicobacter pylori infection and gastric cancer

Because of the close association between *H. pylori* infection and development of chronic gastritis, atrophic gastritis and intestinal metaplasia, the possibility arises that *H. pylori* infection may itself be an important contributing factor to gastric cancer. A considerable body of evidence now exists indicating that this is the case. In a study of early gastric cancer *H. pylori* infection was found in all cases of diffuse carcinoma and around 80% of intestinal-type tumours [66]. Large prospective epidemiological investigations have indicated a consistent association between *H. pylori* seropositivity and an increased risk of gastric cancer [76,77] and a major study involving 13 countries with widely differing gastric cancer incidence and mortality rates showed a significant correlation between *H. pylori* infection and the incidence of gastric cancer and indicated an approximately sixfold risk [78]. Data from three other prospective studies carried out in different countries were used to calculate that the odds ratio for developing gastric cancer in patients with serological evidence of *H. pylori* infection in comparison with *H. pylori*-negative controls is 3.8 [79]. Similar results were obtained from a Swedish study, which also concluded that, in contrast to cancer of the more distal stomach, there is no association between cancer of the gastric cardia and *H. pylori* infection [80]. Such was the evidence from these and other studies that in 1994 *H. pylori* was designated a carcinogen by the International Agency for Research on Cancer [81]. However, not all studies have been confirmatory and the relationship is undoubtedly complex. No association between the seroprevalence of *H. pylori* and gastric cancer could be found in an area of low gastric cancer incidence in Germany [82], and another study from Poland found that *H. pylori* seroprevalence rates were lower in patients with gastric cancer than in patients with lung or colonic malignancy [83]. Furthermore, not all areas with a high prevalence of *H. pylori* infection have high rates of carcinoma. For example, in tropical Africa, where infection is exceedingly common and acquired at an early age, gastric carcinoma is relatively uncommon, possibly because of a low prevalence of intestinal metaplasia [84]. Moreover, duodenal ulcer patients in Western populations, in whom *H. pylori* infection is almost universal, have a generally low risk of gastric cancer [85]. Additional factors, so far incompletely defined, must also be involved [68,86].

As has been mentioned earlier, there is evidence from a number of studies that it is *H. pylori*-infected individuals who develop gastritis with atrophy and intestinal metaplasia that are at particular risk of gastric cancer [69,87]. In some of these the organism is no longer demonstrable in the stomach [88] although this may be due to extensive metaplasia or the fact that the bacteria sometimes assume the coccoid form, rather than the more familiar curved or S-shaped appearance, in resection specimens that have not been fixed promptly. The development of severe gastritis with atrophy and intestinal metaplasia is particularly associated with infection by CagA-positive strains of the bacillus [89,90] (see p. 112) and these strains have been associated with increased risk of gastric cancer in some studies [91], but not in others [92]. The issue is not just one of bacterial virulence, however, and other host factors that appear to govern the distribution of *H. pylori* gastritis within the stomach, its influence on acid output, and whether atrophy and metaplasia follow, probably further influence the carcinogenic process. Thus patients who develop hypochlorhydria and have predominantly corpus or pangastritis [93] with patchy but widespread atrophy and intestinal metaplasia involving both corpus and antrum may be the ones that are at particular risk of gastric carcinoma [94–96]. The importance of the host response has been elegantly demonstrated by the recent observation that certain polymorphisms in the interleukin-1 (IL-1) gene cluster on chromosome 2q are associated with an increased incidence of hypochlorhydria, atrophic gastritis and gastric carcinoma. The susceptible loci are associated with enhanced expression of the cytokine IL-1β in the presence of *H. pylori* infection. IL-1β is a potent inhibitor of gastric acid secretion and overexpression results in more widespread colonization of the gastric mucosa by *H. pylori* with resultant pangastritis and more extensive atrophic gastritis and subsequently an increased risk of carcinoma [97]. IL-1β is also an important enhancer of the host inflammatory response to infection capable of inducing expression of other proinflammatory cytokine genes. At least one of these, tumour necrosis factor alpha (TNF-α), also inhibits gastric acid secretion. Polymorphisms of the TNF-α gene may also determine gastric acid secretion in chronic *H. pylori* infection and hence the extent of atrophic gastritis and establishment of a gastric cancer phenotype [98].

There are a number of reviews of the putative sequence of atrophic gastritis, intestinal metaplasia, dysplasia and carcinoma resulting from *H. pylori* infection, and of pathogenetic mechanisms whereby the infection could act as an initiator or a promoter in gastric carcinogenesis [99–101]. These mechanisms include the following.

1 *Increased epithelial cell proliferation with a resultant increased risk of stable mutations*. Studies on gastric mucosal epithelial cell proliferation measured by a variety of different methods have produced consistent evidence of a hyperproliferative state in *H. pylori*-associated chronic gastritis, which is often reversed following eradication of the organism [59,102–105]. It is accompanied by an expansion of the proliferative zone in the gastric pits towards the gastric lumen and it has been suggested that this might increase the exposure of cells in the S-phase of the cell cycle to luminal carcinogens [106]. Increased proliferation also occurs in intestinal metaplasia [59,104,107], when it appears to extend to differentiated cell lineages, including goblet cells and Paneth cells that do not normally proliferate. This implies a certain degree of cell cycle deregulation with an enhanced likelihood of mutation [108], and there are reports [104] of DNA aneuploidy, oncogene expression and *p53* mutation in *H. pylori*-associated chronic gastritis and intestinal metaplasia without morphological evidence of dysplasia or carcinoma.

2 *Bacterial overgrowth with increased potential to generate intraluminal carcinogens*. Long-term *H. pylori* infection of the gastric body mucosa with atrophy and intestinal metaplasia leads to hypochlorhydria which facilitates overgrowth of bacteria within the lumen that convert ingested nitrate to nitrite and increase the potential to further generate carcinogenic N-nitroso compounds [109]. Increased excretion of nitrosoproline, an indicator of endogenous nitrosation, has been reported in patients with intestinal metaplasia and gastric dysplasia [110] although other workers have failed to find increased N-nitrosamines in the gastric juice of patients with gastric cancer precursor lesions [111].

3 *Increased free radicals*. The long-standing active inflammation associated with gastric *H. pylori* infection leads to production of potentially carcinogenic highly reactive oxygen metabolites by activated phagocytes, especially neutrophils [100,112,113]. In addition, bacterial lipopolysaccharide and cytokines released from inflammatory cells stimulate the release of nitric oxide which may combine with oxygen-derived free radicals to form highly reactive oxidants that damage DNA and cause mutations in human cells *in vitro* [114, 115].

4 *Reduced gastric antioxidant levels*. The cancer-protective effect of fresh fruit and vegetables and of antioxidants, vitamins C and E in particular, by preventing the formation of potentially carcinogenic N-nitroso compounds and scavenging oxygen-derived free radicals, is discussed below. Infection with *H. pylori* is associated with reduced levels of ascorbic acid, a component of vitamin C, in gastric juice [116–118] and a reduction in levels of vitamin E (α-tocopherol) in gastric corpus mucosa [119] although the reasons for this are unclear.

So far, molecular studies have failed to cast light on the mechanism of *H. pylori*-associated gastric carcinogenesis. In a series of early gastric cancers the profile of molecular alterations in those associated with *H. pylori* infection did not differ from those with no evidence of infection [120]. Any effect of *H. pylori* eradication on the growth of gastric cancer is also unknown, although a small study from Japan has claimed a beneficial effect [121]. This study also indicated some regression of intestinal metaplasia following bacterial eradication, in contrast to two prospective studies that failed to find any such effect [122,123].

While there is considerable evidence to implicate *H. pylori* infection in the pathogenesis of carcinoma of the stomach generally, it has been suggested that the infection may have a protective effect against Barrett's oesophagus and adenocarcinoma of the distal oesophagus and gastric cardia. The frequency of these tumours has been increasing at an alarming rate, especially among white males in developed countries, and this appears to have coincided with a falling incidence of *H. pylori* infection during the same period [124]. Since *H. pylori* pangastritis is associated with atrophic gastritis and hypochlorhydria, it has been hypothesized that reduced *H. pylori* infection in a population will be associated with a generally higher gastric acid output that might promote gastro-oesophageal reflux, Barrett's oesophagus and eventually adenocarcinoma of the oesophagogastric junction. Eradication of *H. pylori* in duodenal ulcer patients has indeed been shown to provoke reflux oesophagitis [125], and *H. pylori*-negative patients with symptoms of gastro-oesophageal reflux are reported to have more severe reflux disease and a higher prevalence of Barrett's oesophagus [126]. Infection with the more virulent CagA-positive strains of the organism has also been found to carry a reduced risk of adenocarcinoma of the oesophagus and gastric cardia [127]. While further evidence is needed, it has been suggested that eradication of *H. pylori*, while beneficial in reducing the risk of peptic ulcer and carcinoma of the distal stomach, may actually increase the risk of adenocarcinoma of the proximal stomach and oesophagus [128].

Diet

Dietary factors are potentially important in gastric cancer as ingested food is in contact with gastric mucosa for some considerable time. Intraluminal and intramucosal synthesis of carcinogens and excessive salt intake have been considered relevant in carcinogenesis whereas consumption of fresh fruit and vegetables, with their constituent antioxidants, are thought to have a protective effect [22,52,129].

The role of N-nitrosamines, a potent group of carcinogens, in the pathogenesis of gastric cancer has been particularly emphasized [130]. Their synthesis within the gastric lumen through the interaction of nitrites and secondary amines or amides is theoretically plausible and Correa *et al.* postulated that in the presence of extensive intestinal metaplasia, when the pH within the gastric lumen rises, bacteria proliferate and facilitate conversion of nitrates to nitrites within the stomach [131]. Nitrosable compounds occur naturally in many foods such as fish, meat and fava beans [132,133], and epidemiological studies suggest an increased risk of gastric cancer with consumption of smoked, cured and salted foods [129, 134]. Fava beans [133] and salted fish [135] have been shown to contain mutagenic compounds after nitrosation *in vitro*. Formation of N-nitroso compounds is reduced in the presence of ascorbate or α-tocopherol [136]. There is, however, no clear-cut correlation between levels of dietary nitrate or nitrite and the risk of gastric cancer [137,138].

Studies from various parts of the world repeatedly indicate that increased consumption of salt or salted foods is also associated with increased gastric cancer risk [139–141]. A high salt intake is believed to act as an irritant to the gastric mucosa, to cause inflammation and atrophic gastritis, and to increase mucal epithelial cell proliferation [52,142].

In contrast, there is consistent evidence that consumption of fresh fruit and vegetables gives some protection against development of cancer [143–147]. Relevant components of these foods include vitamin C, vitamin E and carotenoids [129], and pooled data from several case-control nutritional studies indicate that vitamin C (ascorbate) intake in particular is inversely related to the relative risk of gastric cancer [22]. Dietary supplementation with vitamins C, E and A has been reported to diminish the risk of gastric cancer [148]. Vitamins C and E inhibit the formation of N-nitroso compounds [149] and scavenge oxygen-derived free radicals but it is uncertain whether these represent the primary mechanisms of their protective effect.

Smoking

Evidence of a causative effect of smoking in gastric cancer is unclear. Some studies indicate that tobacco smokers are at increased risk [144,150] while others have found no such association or even a reduction in risk [151,152]. Hansson *et al.* found that both cigarette and pipe smokers were at considerably increased risk but that this risk could be offset to a large extent by high fruit and vegetable consumption [153].

Autoimmune gastritis and pernicious anaemia

It was recognized in the 1950s that pernicious anaemia was associated with an increased risk of gastric carcinoma [154,155] and this is now considered to be around three times that of the general population [155–157]. This is not surprising in view of the fact that the condition is characterized by an autoimmune chronic gastritis of the corpus that is often accompanied by marked atrophy, intestinal metaplasia, and hypo- or achlorhydria (see p. 117, Chapter 12) [158]. Atrophic changes in autoimmune gastritis tend to increase in severity and extent at about the age of 50 [159]. There is also an increased incidence of mucosal polyps in pernicious anaemia, and a proportion of these show adenomatous dysplasia of the glandular epithelium [160]. However, the majority are small carcinoid tumours that arise as a result of the proliferative effect of long-standing hypergastrinaemia on gastric fundic enterochromaffin-like (ECL) cells (see p. 183) [161,162].

Gastric polyps and cancer

Gastric epithelial polyps may be classified as hyperplastic or adenomatous, the former being much commoner. As has been described at the beginning of this chapter, adenomatous polyps represent localized areas of dysplasia in which malignant transformation is well recognized. The risk of this happening is directly related to the size of the lesion and the grade of dysplasia and is commoner in lesions with a tubulovillous or villous configuration [8,163,164], and it is generally regarded as sufficient to recommend endoscopic resection of all gastric adenomas if this is feasible.

The commoner hyperplastic polyps are discussed in Chapter 16 (p. 214) and consist of foveolar and pyloric-type glands lined mainly by normal gastric epithelium, although foci of intestinal metaplasia may also be present [165]. While the risk of malignancy arising in such lesions is much less than in adenomatous polyps, it is not negligible [163]. Dysplasia has been reported on close examination in 4% of small hyperplastic polyps (<1 cm diameter) and in 19% of those greater than 3 cm in diameter [165,166], and intramucosal carcinoma may be found in up to 2%, especially in lesions that are greater than 2 cm in diameter and that occur in elderly patients [164,166].

There is also evidence of some increase in the incidence of carcinoma arising elsewhere in the stomach in patients with multiple hyperplastic gastric polyps [163,164]. As such polyps

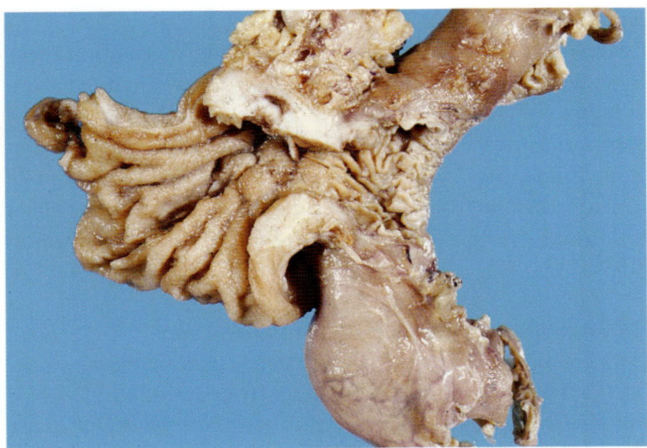

Fig. 14.3 Carcinoma arising at a gastroenterostomy stoma. The gastric 'stump' is seen at the left and the tumour is predominantly on the gastric side of the anastomosis.

are associated with atrophic gastritis and extensive intestinal metaplasia in the surrounding mucosa this association is perhaps not unexpected.

The operated stomach and cancer

The relative risk of adenocarcinoma arising in the gastric stump of patients who have undergone previous gastric surgery (Fig. 14.3) is increased compared to the general population [167–169]. This risk increases with time following the initial operation and while some studies have observed an effect after an interval of 10–12 years [170], it becomes more definite after 20 years [171]. It appears to be higher in females and following Billroth II gastrectomy, and a meta-analysis of 22 studies found that most of the increased risk applies to patients undergoing surgery for gastric ulcer while those operated on for duodenal ulcer are less susceptible [172].

The occurrence of bile reflux or reactive gastritis in postgastrectomy gastric stumps [173], discussed in Chapter 12 (p. 119), may well promote gastric carcinogenesis in this situation. It is often associated with intestinal metaplasia, whose prevalence increases with higher concentrations of bile in the gastric juice [174]. The likely importance of duodenogastric reflux in development of malignancy in the postoperative stomach is supported by experimental studies which indicate that in rats, gastric stump cancer develops quite frequently following Billroth II anastomosis. This is accompanied by elongation of the proliferative zone within the gastric mucosa and increased cell cycle time [175]. A high frequency of epithelial dysplasia was also reported in human gastric stump biopsies in the late 1970s [176,177], but much of this may represent florid regenerative atypia that is now recognized to occur in reactive gastritis and examples of genuine high-grade dysplasia are probably less frequent than previously reported. Another factor that may predispose to the development of stump cancer is the occurrence of single or multiple polyps, mainly hyperplastic in type, close to the stoma [178,179].

Hypertrophic gastropathy and gastritis, including Menetrier's disease

While it has been suggested that the incidence of carcinoma complicating Menetrier's disease is 8–10% [180,181], controversies surrounding the diagnosis of this condition (see Chapter 16, p. 221) make it difficult to assess the evidence properly. In some cases a finding of thickened gastric folds at endoscopy or on radiological examination at the time of diagnosis of gastric cancer has been attributed to Menetrier's disease but histological confirmation has been lacking and it is equally possible that an infiltrating carcinoma has given rise to the appearances secondarily. Nevertheless, there are case reports of early gastric cancer occurring synchronously with histologically proven Menetrier's disease [182,183].

Peptic ulcer disease

It has been widely accepted for some time that chronic duodenal ulcer is not associated with increased risk of gastric cancer and indeed there is some evidence that the risk is reduced [85,184,185]. The association between chronic gastric ulcer and cancer is less clear. Undoubtedly some early reports, in which histology was not carried out, failed to identify early ulcerating gastric cancers and thus exaggerated the supposed incidence of malignant transformation in benign ulcers. A more recent prospective study based on flexible endoscopy and histology failed to demonstrate any increased incidence of gastric carcinoma in patients treated medically for chronic gastric ulcer and followed for 5 years [186], and a large autopsy study demonstrated a lower than expected incidence of cancer in patients whose stomachs showed evidence of active or healed gastric ulcer [185]. However these findings are not supported by a study involving very large numbers of Swedish patients with gastric ulcer who did not undergo surgery and who were followed over an average of 9 years [85]. This showed the incidence of gastric cancer in such patients to be almost double the expected rate. The increased risk applied to patients with ulcers in the body of the stomach rather than prepyloric ulcers and was greater in women. Clearly, the debate regarding cancer risk in chronic gastric ulcer continues but it would seem premature to conclude that gastric ulcers proximal to the prepyloric area have no malignant potential.

Genetic predisposition

There is evidence of familial clustering in gastric cancer and around 8% of stomach cancers show evidence of a familial component. First-degree relatives of affected patients are almost three times as likely to develop the disease as the general population [187]. This may be partly attributable to *H. pylori* infection being commoner in families, and the potential role of IL-1 gene polymorphisms affecting this has already been discussed above [97,98]. However, there is now good evidence that germline truncating mutations in the gene for E-cadherin (CDH-1), a calcium-dependent cell adhesion protein, are responsible for a rare autosomal dominant inherited form of gastric carcinoma in young persons. This condition is highly penetrant and characterized by multiple tumours of diffuse or signet ring cell histological type that do not arise in a background of intestinal metaplasia [188]. Affected family members can be identified by mutation-specific genetic testing and offered prophylactic gastrectomy [189].

It is well known that the risk of malignancy in familial adenomatous polyposis (FAP) is not confined to the large intestine. The upper gastrointestinal tract is also at risk. Although in the West carcinoma is most common around the ampulla of Vater and the remainder of the duodenum, a small increased risk of gastric cancer exists [18]. In Korea patients with FAP are considered to have a sevenfold risk of gastric cancer in comparison with the general population [190]. Patients with hereditary non-polyposis colorectal cancer (HNPCC) (see Chapter 38), which results from germline mutation of one of the DNA mismatch repair genes *hMLH1*, *hMSH2*, *hMSH6*, *hPMS1* and *hPMS2*, also have an increased frequency of gastric cancers that are characterized by microsatellite instability. The tumours arise at an earlier age than sporadic neoplasms, most are of intestinal type histologically, but coincidental *H. pylori* infection of the background mucosa is relatively uncommon [191].

Peutz–Jeghers syndrome (PJS) is a rare inherited polyposis syndrome caused by mutation of the *LKB1/STK11* gene on chromosome 19p [192]. Hamartomatous polyps are found mainly in the small intestine but less frequently in colon, rectum and stomach. There is an increased risk of malignancy in PJS, frequently involving extragastrointestinal sites, but risk of gastric carcinoma is also increased, when it may occur at a relatively young age [193,194].

Gastric dysplasia

Dysplasia may be defined as unequivocal neoplastic transformation in the epithelium without invasion into the lamina propria [195]. The histological features are cellular atypia, abnormal differentiation and disorganized glandular architecture. These may occur in areas of intestinal metaplasia or in non-metaplastic mucosa. The difficulties in recognizing and categorizing these changes are reflected in various different classifications of gastric dysplasia [54,196–198]. Furthermore, inflammatory or regenerative changes within gastric mucosal epithelium can be mistaken for dysplasia, especially in reactive gastritis and at the edge of a benign ulcer or in the postoperative stomach. Here the distinction between regenerative changes and low-grade or mild dysplasia is especially difficult and is reflected in the wide observer variation that has been reported in the diagnosis of dysplasia [199]. In one study 15 out of 23 cases originally diagnosed as mild or low-grade dysplasia were reclassified as gastritis with regenerative atypia, and a further case as carcinoma, following review by specialist gastrointestinal pathologists [200]. High-grade or severe dysplasia is recognized more reproducibly, but since this diagnosis is often used as an indication for major surgery, it is recommended that it is confirmed by a second experienced pathologist [195] or by a second set of biopsies from the same area [200] before resection is carried out. As discussed above (p. 163) there are also major interpretative differences between Japanese and Western pathologists in the criteria used to define carcinoma occurring in the context of dysplasia, such that a significant proportion of cases diagnosed as dysplasia in the West are considered to be adenocarcinoma by Japanese workers [201].

Gastric dysplasia may be classified into metaplastic (arising in areas of intestinal metaplasia) and non-metaplastic or foveolar (arising in non-metaplastic epithelium) [54,198,202]. Like colonic dysplasia, gastric dysplasia is now usually graded as low grade or high grade [7]. The basic histological criteria are as follows [54,197,198].

1 Disorganized mucosal architecture manifested by irregularity of glands, back-to-back gland formation, budding and branching of glands, and papillary ingrowth into the gland lumen and on the surface. In general architectural disorganization is minimal in low-grade dysplasia and increases in higher grade lesions; it is also less prominent in dysplasia arising in non-metaplastic mucosa [202].

2 Cytological atypia characterized by nuclear pleomorphism, hyperchromasia, and increase in nuclear size and in nuclear : cytoplasmic ratio. Nuclear stratification is also common, especially in metaplastic dysplasia, but is not invariable [196,202]. In low-grade dysplasia the nuclei are confined to the basal part of the epithelium (Fig. 14.4) while in high-grade dysplasia nuclear stratification involves the full thickness of the epithelium. Loss of nuclear polarity (the long axis of nuclei lying at varying angles to or parallel to the basement membrane rather than perpendicular) is a feature of high-grade dysplasia (Fig. 14.5), as are vesicular nuclei and irregular clumping of nuclear chromatin with frequent mitoses [203]. It should be noted that increased mitotic activity *per se* is not pathognomonic of dysplasia as it is frequently seen in regenerating epithelium.

3 Abnormal differentiation characterized in metaplastic epithelium by progressive loss or reduction in the number of goblet cells and Paneth cells and poor development of brush border with increasing severity of dysplasia. In addition there may be expression of colon-type sulphomucins. In dysplasia there may be loss or reduction of mucin together with abnormal expression of sulphomucin and inappropriate antigens such as Lewis and sialylated Lewis antigen (CA 19-9) [198].

As stated previously gastric dysplasia is now categorized as low grade or high grade as there is better interobserver agreement than with a three-tier system of mild, moderate and severe. Management of the lesion, i.e. surveillance or excision, can be more easily based on a two-tier system [200,203].

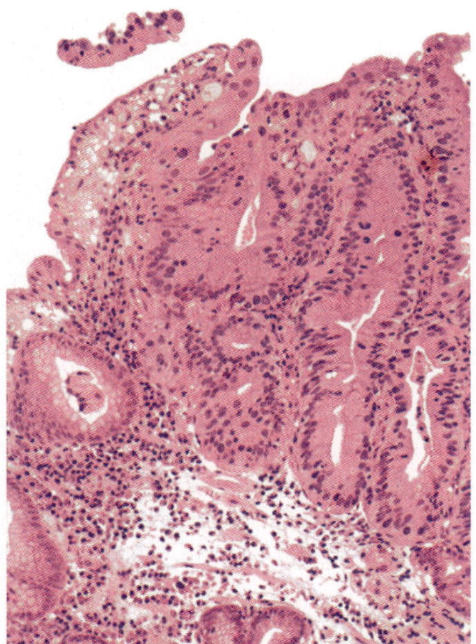

Fig. 14.4 Low-grade dysplasia showing hyperchromatism and mild stratification of nuclei, lack of surface maturation, but little architectural disorganization.

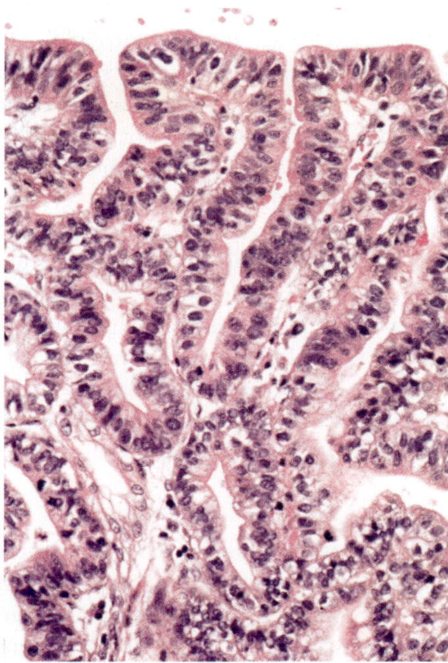

Fig. 14.5 High-grade dysplasia showing architectural and cytological atypia with nuclear stratification and loss of polarity.

Nevertheless, it is often useful to include a category of 'indefinitive for dysplasia', similar to that adopted for dysplasia in chronic inflammatory bowel disease [204] to indicate uncertainty and that early repeat biopsy may be required.

Table 14.1 Gastric dysplasia and related lesions: the Vienna classification.

1 Negative for neoplasia/dysplasia
2 Indefinite for neoplasia/dysplasia
3 Non-invasive neoplasia low grade (low-grade adenoma/dysplasia)
4 Non-invasive neoplasia high grade
  4.1 High-grade adenoma/dysplasia
  4.2 Non-invasive carcinoma (carcinoma *in situ*)
  4.3 Suspicious for invasive carcinoma
5 Invasive neoplasia
  5.1 Intramucosal carcinoma
  5.2 Submucosal carcinoma or beyond

In an attempt to standardize histopathological diagnosis and to allow valid comparisons between different centres, particularly between Japan and the West, the Vienna classification has recently been developed [205]. It is shown in Table 14.1 and incorporates five categories. This classification has been validated to some extent by a multinational panel of recognized experts in histological interpretation of gastric precancerous and cancerous lesions.

Gastric epithelial dysplasia has been most clearly characterized in adenomas, as described at the beginning of this chapter, but similar (and indeed commoner) histological changes in flat mucosa correspond to the metaplastic (or adenomatous) form of dysplasia [200,206]. The lesions consist of deeply stained tubular glands lined by epithelium composed of tall columnar cells crowded together. Small amounts of mucin, usually sulphated, may be present at the apex of the cell, and Paneth cells and goblet cells may also be seen. With increasing degrees of dysplasia the nuclei become oval or rounded, vary in size and are often not so deeply stained and contain prominent nucleoli. Nuclear stratification develops with loss of polarity in high-grade dysplasia. Increased mitotic figures are present and there is minimal or no mucin secretion. Along with these cytological changes there is increasing architectural disorganization with irregular glands, back-to-back arrangement of glands and micropapillary budding of cells within glands (Fig. 14.5). Carcinoma is diagnosed when dysplastic cells have penetrated the basal membrane of glands and invaded the lamina propria.

Dysplastic change within non-metaplastic mucosa may be more subtle. It is frequently very focal and can occur without architectural disorganization in the mucosa. Diagnosis depends on cytological features such as cellular and nuclear pleomorphism, enlarged vesicular hypochromatic nuclei or, in severe dysplasia, markedly anaplastic cells with hyperchromatic nuclei and loss of polarity [202]. This type of dysplasia is frequently associated with the development of diffuse-type gastric cancer.

The clinical significance and management of dysplasia depends to some extent on the grade. Many studies have shown that high-grade dysplasia frequently coexists with [207], or progresses to [206,208], invasive adenocarcinoma. Lansdown *et al.* [200] found that 85% of patients with high-grade dysplasia developed cancer within 15 months and 60% of those who underwent immediate gastrectomy were found to have concomitant gastric cancer. The diagnosis is therefore an indication for extirpation of the lesion by whatever means is most appropriate for the patient under consideration, provided that it is corroborated by a second experienced pathologist. If the lesion is small (<30 mm), not ulcerated, and well demarcated then endoscopic mucosal resection can be considered [209] but this must be followed by careful histological evaluation to confirm complete resection and exclude submucosal or lymphovascular invasion by carcinoma. Other patients with high-grade dysplasia may best be treated by more radical surgery from the outset. The best management of low-grade dysplasia is more uncertain, because apparent regression occurs in a significant proportion of patients followed up [206]. If there is a raised or demarcated lesion, then endoscopic mucosal resection as for high-grade dysplasia is probably indicated. However, for low-grade dysplasia in flat mucosa without a discrete endoscopic lesion, further multiple biopsies should be taken immediately to exclude a coexisting 'worse' lesion (such as high-grade dysplasia or carcinoma, which is found in about 15% of cases [207]), followed by regular endoscopic follow-up with multiple biopsies. Progression of dysplasia to a more severe grade or to early gastric cancer is said to be more likely in males, in older patients and in those with more extensive atrophic gastritis of the surrounding gastric mucosa [210].

Macroscopic features and topography of gastric adenocarcinoma

Carcinomas of the distal stomach are most common in the prepyloric region, in the pyloric antrum and on the lesser curvature; they are less common in the gastric body. Tumours arising at the cardia in the region of the oesophagogastric junction (OGJ), whose frequency is increasing (see above), are generally smaller than those of the distal stomach (Fig. 14.6), but this belies their aggressive nature.

Grossly, gastric cancers may be ulcerating, nodular, fungating or infiltrative in type. Ulcerated tumours occur most frequently in the cardia, antrum or region of the lesser curve. They differ from benign gastric ulcers in that they have an irregular margin with raised edges and the surrounding tissue is firm and appears thickened, uneven and indurated. The ulcer has a necrotic, shaggy and often nodular base. Mucosal folds radiating from the ulcer crater do not have a regular appearance as seen with benign ulcers and frequently show club-like thickening and fusion. Malignant ulcers tend to be larger than their benign counterparts. However, a significant proportion of malignant ulcers lack these appearances and endoscopic appearance alone is not a sufficiently reliable guide to diagnosis of malignancy [211]. Because of this it is particularly important that all ulcerated lesions seen at endoscopy, even when appearing to be healing, should be systematically and adequately biopsied.

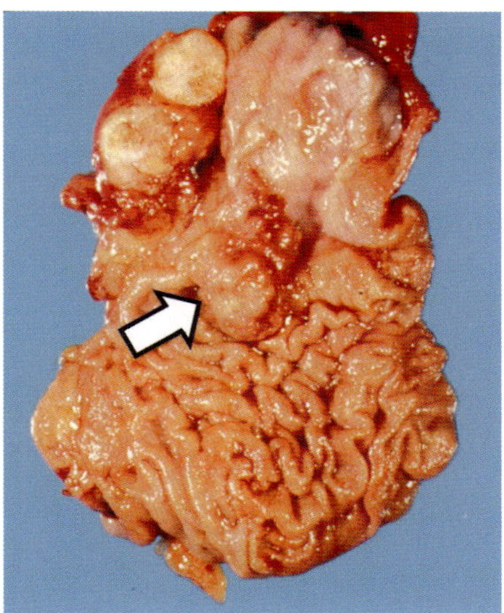

Fig. 14.6 Carcinoma arising at the gastro-oesophageal junction (arrow). There are also several enlarged para-oesophageal nodes containing metastases (top left of image).

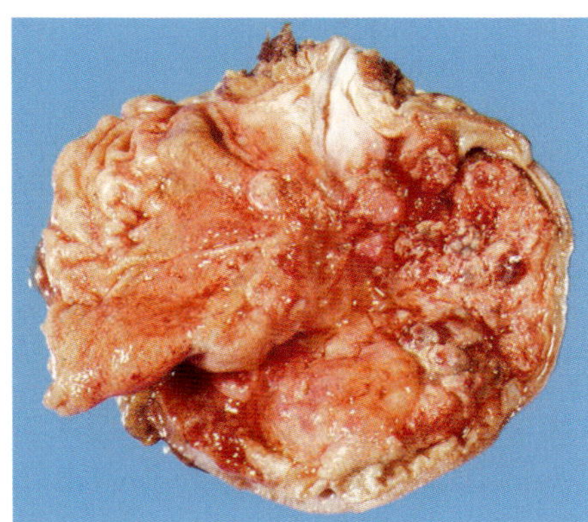

Fig. 14.7 Large fungating polypoid carcinoma occupying the posterior wall of the gastric corpus. The lower oesophagus is top centre.

Polypoid, fungating and nodular tumours typically consist of friable masses which project from a broad base into the cavity of the stomach. They tend to occur in the body of the stomach (Fig. 14.7), in the region of the greater curvature, posterior wall or fundus, and at the time of diagnosis are usually large when surface ulceration and bleeding may be prominent features.

Infiltrative cancers may spread superficially in the mucosa and submucosa giving rise to plaque-like lesions with flattening of the rugal folds and an opaque appearance of the mucosa.

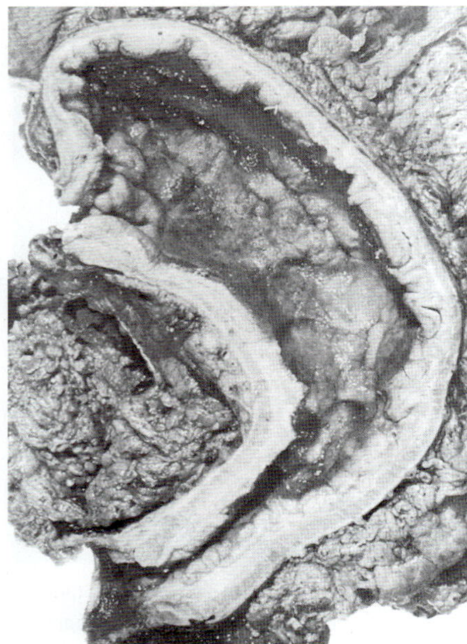

Fig. 14.8 Typical linitis plastica pattern of carcinoma.

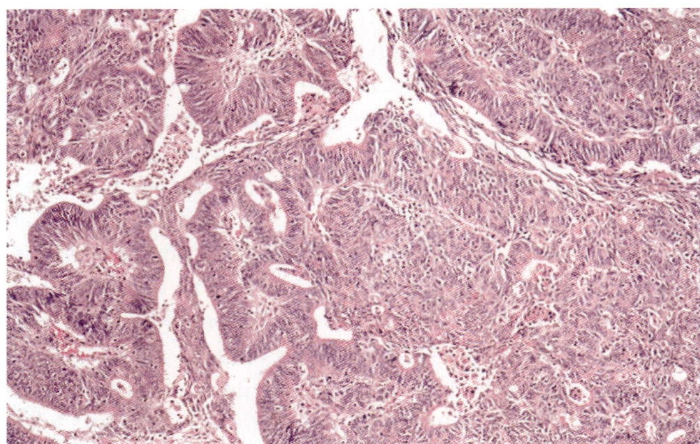

Fig. 14.9 Intestinal type of gastric adenocarcinoma showing a mixed tubular and papillary pattern on the right and left, respectively.

Superficial ulceration may supervene. More frequently infiltration involves the entire thickness of the stomach wall, usually over a limited area in the region of the pylorus but rarely extensively to produce the so-called linitis plastica or 'leather bottle' stomach (Fig. 14.8). In these cases the wall is markedly thickened and assumes a stiff consistency due to an extensive fibrotic response to tumour cells in the submucosa, muscle coats and subserosa which converts part or all of the stomach into a thick narrow tube. There is usually no visible localized growth.

Many gastric carcinomas, irrespective of type, secrete considerable amounts of mucin which gives the tumour or parts of it a gelatinous appearance to the naked eye. These are sometimes called mucinous or colloid carcinomas.

Microscopic appearances

Despite important differences in the aetiology, epidemiology and incidence of adenocarcinoma of the distal stomach compared with that of the cardia and OGJ, the microscopic appearances of these tumours are similar. The histological classification of gastric adenocarcinoma is made difficult because there are frequently marked differences in structure and/or differentiation, not only between separate carcinomas, but also within individual tumours. Nevertheless several histological classifications exist, some of which are widely used, and these will be considered.

World Health Organization (WHO) classification

This divides adenocarcinoma of the stomach into papillary, tubular, mucinous and signet ring types, the typing of any particular tumour being based on its predominant component [1]. Papillary adenocarcinomas are composed of pointed or blunt finger-like epithelial processes with fibrous cores. Some tubule formation may be present but the papillary pattern predominates, particularly in cystic structures. Typically this tumour grows as a polypoid mass into the lumen of the stomach. Tubular adenocarcinomas consist of branching glands embedded in or surrounded by a fibrous stroma. Mucinous carcinomas (mucoid or colloid carcinomas) contain large amounts of extracellular mucin in more than 50% of the tumour. In some such tumours the cells form glands lined by columnar mucus-secreting mucosa (well differentiated type). In others there are disaggregated ribbons or clusters of cells which appear to be floating in lakes of mucin (poorly differentiated type). Signet ring carcinomas do not form tubules. They are composed largely of mucin-containing signet ring cells but also contain cells with no mucin and cells with eosinophilic granular cytoplasm containing neutral mucin. Tumour cells are often accompanied by fibrous stroma and tend to infiltrate diffusely throughout muscularis propria and the serosal surface of the stomach. Tumours composed predominantly of signet ring cells are more common in younger patients and in the distal stomach [39]. All of the above types, with the exception of signet ring carcinoma, may be graded as well, moderately or poorly differentiated.

The Lauren classification

The Lauren classification [212] divides gastric carcinoma into intestinal and diffuse types. In general, intestinal-type tumours have a glandular pattern usually accompanied by papillary formations or solid components (Fig. 14.9). The glandular epithelium consists of large pleomorphic cells with large hyperchromatic nuclei often with numerous mitoses. They are usually fairly well polarized columnar cells, sometimes with a prominent brush border and goblet cells. Mucin

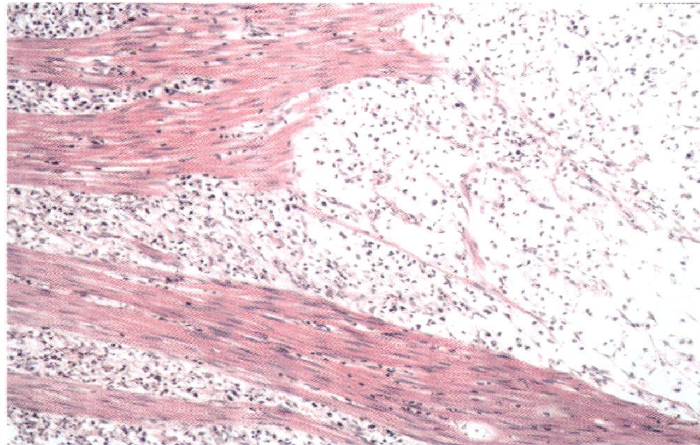

Fig. 14.10 Diffuse adenocarcinoma showing signet ring cells infiltrating the muscularis propria.

secretion is variable and occurs either focally in the cytoplasm of scattered cells or extracellularly in the lumina of neoplastic glands. By contrast, diffuse-type carcinomas are predominantly composed of poorly cohesive widely infiltrating small tumour cells with indistinct cytoplasm and regular, only faintly hyperchromatic though often pyknotic nuclei without many mitoses. Gland formation is inconspicuous, except sometimes in the superficial part of the tumour. Mucin secretion is common and widespread throughout the tumour. Signet ring cells are common and there may be extracellular mucin in the stroma (Fig. 14.10). Connective tissue proliferation is more marked and inflammatory cell infiltration less prominent than in intestinal cancers.

Of the 1344 tumours initially described by Lauren, 53% were intestinal, 33% diffuse and the remainder unclassified. The latter included tumours containing equal proportions of intestinal and diffuse types or ones that were undifferentiated with a solid growth pattern, composed of sheets of cells. In general, intestinal-type tumours are commoner in the elderly and in males while in the diffuse type the sex ratio is approximately equal and the mean age is younger. The overall falling incidence of gastric cancer appears to result from a reduction in intestinal-type tumours, and the frequency of diffuse tumours remains constant. The latter type is characteristic of the relatively rare cases of gastric carcinoma that occur in patients under 40 years of age [47,50], and of the tumours seen in inherited gastric cancer due to germline E-cadherin mutation. Recently, a very well differentiated variant of intestinal-type carcinoma has been described arising in association with complete (type I) intestinal metaplasia [213]. It arises mainly in the body of the stomach and is easily missed on endoscopy and biopsy because the histological features of malignancy are subtle and the intramucosal element closely resembles regenerative change within intestinal metaplasia. Cytological atypia is mild but the tumour glands show architectural distortion with branching and tortuosity.

The classification of Ming [214]

This divides tumours into an expanding type (67%) and an infiltrative type (33%). The expanding type has a pushing edge and forms discrete tumour nodules. It is twice as common in males, and tumour cells are surrounded by small amounts of fibrous tissue with a variable inflammatory cell response. It is very often accompanied by intestinal metaplasia in the adjacent mucosa. This compares roughly to the intestinal type of Lauren. The infiltrative type is ill defined and contains widely infiltrative tumour cells with poor inflammatory cell response and collagenous stroma. Accompanying intestinal metaplasia is less common. This type is equally common in males and females and while both types occur predominantly in patients over 50 years of age, infiltrative carcinoma is more common under the age of 50.

Classification of Mulligan and Rember [215]

This classifies gastric carcinoma into mucus cell type, intestinal type and pylorocardiac gland type. It is only the latter variant that distinguishes this classification from that of Lauren and, as the name suggests, it occurs predominantly in the cardia or pylorus. Pylorocardiac carcinomas are well demarcated exophytic tumours, frequently with surface ulceration. These tumours are commoner in men and are characterized microscopically by varying-sized glands lined by stratified or singly orientated cylindrical cells that often show striking vacuolation or clear cell change and stain brilliantly with the periodic acid–Schiff (PAS) reaction.

The Goseki classification

The Goseki classification attempts to encompass undifferentiated carcinomas as well as the more common types. It is based on tumour histology and includes four grades based on tubular differentiation and intracellular mucin production [216]. Group I consists of well differentiated tubules with poor intracellular mucin production; group II consists of well differentiated tubules and plentiful intracellular mucin; group III has poorly differentiated tubules and poor intracellular mucin; and group IV tumours are made up of poorly differentiated tubules and plentiful intracellular mucin.

Carneiro classification

Carneiro has proposed a 'new' classification that is also based on four histological types [217]. These include glandular and isolated cell carcinomas that are roughly equivalent to the intestinal and diffuse carcinomas of the Lauren classification, a solid variety composed of sheets, trabeculae or islands of undifferentiated cells with no glandular formation, and a mixed type that consists of a mixture of glandular and isolated cell types. Glandular tumours were commonest in the Portuguese population studied, followed by mixed, solid and isolated cell types in descending order.

Relative merits of the different classifications

To be of maximum benefit a histological classification of tumours should fulfil three criteria:

1 it should be easy to apply by different pathologists and be reproducible;

2 it should help in the assessment of the prognosis of the different types of tumour; and

3 it should relate to the histogenesis and if possible the aetiology of the several tumour types.

None of the current classifications satisfies all these criteria. Although the WHO and Lauren classifications are widely used they do not appear to be of much prognostic value. Nonetheless, the WHO classification is of undoubted value as a standard descriptive classification in routine work and serves as a base for achieving international uniformity [218]. The Lauren classification has been widely used in epidemiological investigations. Most studies in this context indicate that the proportion of intestinal-type cancers is greater in areas of high gastric cancer incidence and that the incidence of this type is decreasing. The diffuse type occurs in younger people and is equally common in women as in men. The incidence of this type appears to be unchanged. One drawback of both classifications is that many carcinomas are heterogenous and contain a variety of tumour patterns, and assessment of the predominant component is difficult.

Some reports indicate that the Ming classification is of prognostic value in that expanding tumours have considerably better prognosis than similarly advanced carcinomas of the infiltrative type [219,220]. Others make claims of prognostic value for the Goseki classification such that mucus-rich tumours (Goseki types II and IV) have a worse prognosis than tumours with sparse mucus (types I and III) [221] and others have found it to be highly reproducible [222]. The proponents of the Carneiro classification found that mixed-type tumours, which formed 38.5% of the cases studied, had a much worse prognosis than the other three types and multivariate analysis showed the classification to have independent prognostic significance that was second only to the TNM stage. Further evaluation of this system by other groups is clearly warranted.

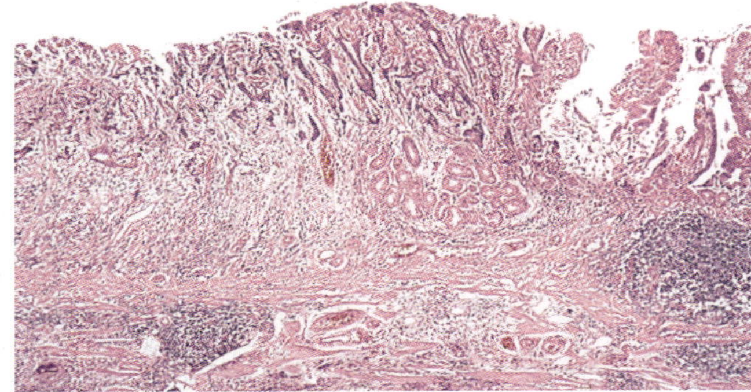

Fig. 14.11 Intramucosal early gastric carcinoma. Tumour cells occupy the superficial mucosa. There is underlying inflammation which extends into the muscularis mucosae with lymphoid aggregate formation.

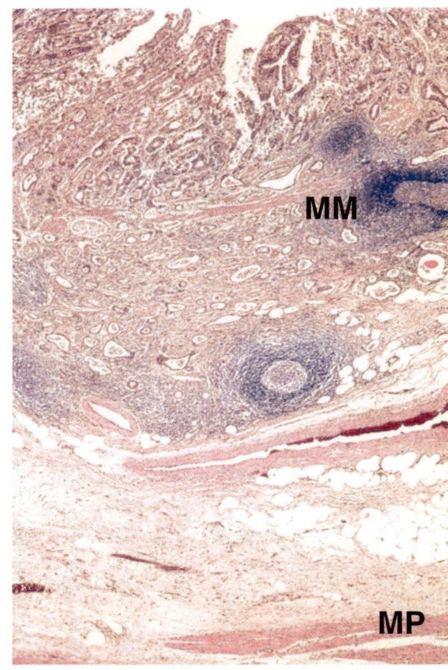

Fig. 14.12 Early gastric carcinoma. Tumour cells are present within the submucosa (arrow) but have not infiltrated the muscularis propria. MM, muscularis mucosa; MP, muscularis propria.

Early gastric cancer

Early gastric cancer (EGC) is defined as a carcinoma which is limited to the mucosa or the mucosa and submucosa only, irrespective of whether or not metastasis to lymph nodes has occurred. It can be subdivided therefore after histological examination into two groups, intramucosal (Fig. 14.11) and submucosal carcinoma (Fig. 14.12), both with potential for lymph node metastases. The term 'early' is not meant to imply a stage in the genesis of the cancer but is used to mean gastric cancer which can be cured [223]. Study of these cancers has shown that some may remain confined to the superficial layers for several years, although expanding laterally to a considerable degree, whereas others penetrate the gastric wall rapidly and can then invade into the submucosa when they are of the order of only 3–5 mm in diameter [224,225].

Cases of early gastric cancer as defined above have been reported for many years from several countries under a variety of terms such as superficial spreading carcinoma [226], surface carcinoma [227] and *cancer gastrique au début* [228]. However, it was as a result of a screening programme in Japan in the early 1960s that increasing numbers of early gastric cancers were detected.

The clinical characteristics of EGC differ from those of ad-

Table 14.2 Macroscopic classification of early gastric carcinoma.

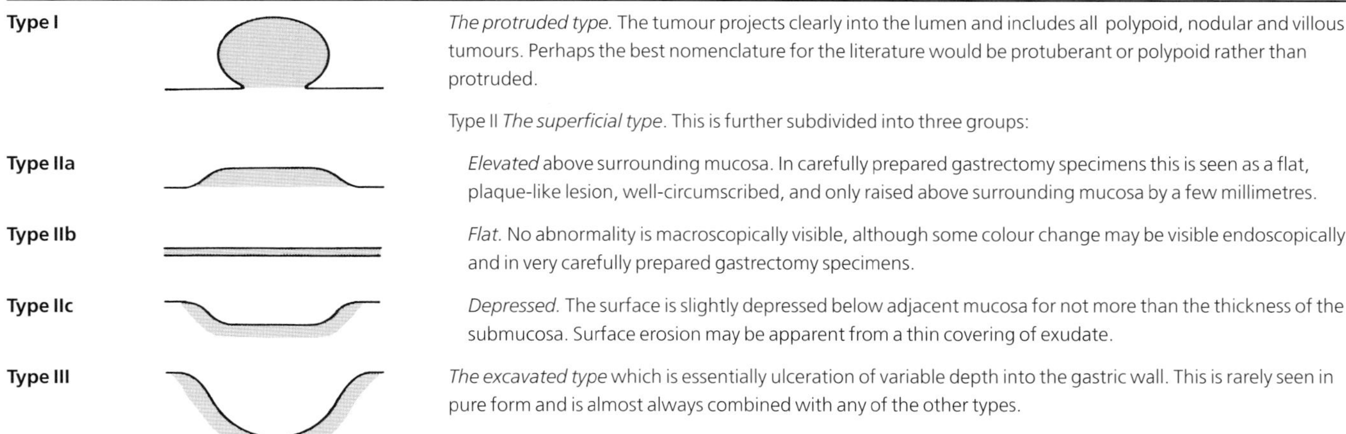

Type I	*The protruded type.* The tumour projects clearly into the lumen and includes all polypoid, nodular and villous tumours. Perhaps the best nomenclature for the literature would be protuberant or polypoid rather than protruded.
	Type II *The superficial type.* This is further subdivided into three groups:
Type IIa	*Elevated* above surrounding mucosa. In carefully prepared gastrectomy specimens this is seen as a flat, plaque-like lesion, well-circumscribed, and only raised above surrounding mucosa by a few millimetres.
Type IIb	*Flat.* No abnormality is macroscopically visible, although some colour change may be visible endoscopically and in very carefully prepared gastrectomy specimens.
Type IIc	*Depressed.* The surface is slightly depressed below adjacent mucosa for not more than the thickness of the submucosa. Surface erosion may be apparent from a thin covering of exudate.
Type III	*The excavated type* which is essentially ulceration of variable depth into the gastric wall. This is rarely seen in pure form and is almost always combined with any of the other types.

vanced gastric carcinoma. The mean age at presentation is somewhat lower [229] and the duration of symptoms, which resemble those of benign gastric ulcer more than advanced carcinoma, is generally longer [229,230]. Weight loss is infrequent. There is evidence that careful investigation with endoscopy and biopsy of patients aged over 40 years presenting for the first time with dyspeptic symptoms substantially increases the proportion of cases of gastric cancer diagnosed at an early stage [231].

Although the proportion of cases of gastric cancer that are diagnosed as EGC has increased over the past 30 years [232], the condition is still relatively rare in the UK and accounts for less than 20% of all cases of gastric cancer. In contrast, in Japan, EGC constitutes a higher proportion of resected gastric cancers [230,233,234]. This is undoubtedly related to the population gastric cancer screening that has taken place in Japan since the early 1960s, although differences in histological interpretation between Western and Japanese pathologists already referred to above (p. 163) also play a part: most cases interpreted by Western observers as high-grade dysplasia are regarded as carcinoma by Japanese pathologists [201].

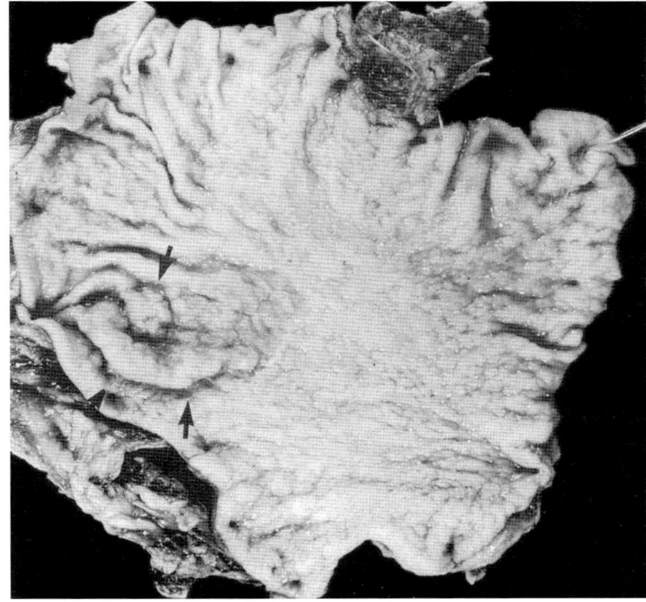

Fig. 14.13 Superficial elevated (IIa) type of early gastric cancer (arrowed).

Macroscopic features and classification

On the basis of macroscopic appearances at endoscopy and in gastrectomy specimens, early gastric cancers were classified by the Japanese Gastroenterological Endoscopic Society into three main types and three subtypes (Table 14.2). Combinations of types are commoner than single types and all possible combinations of the five varieties have been documented. When describing a particular lesion the dominant macroscopic feature is placed first, e.g. III + IIc, IIc + III, IIa + IIc. Whereas there is good correlation between the endoscopic recognition of early gastric cancer by an experienced observer and its subsequent confirmation as such on microscopical examination of the resected specimen, it should be remembered that a similar appearance can result from early and advanced cancers in fixed specimens. In some cases EGC may be very difficult to detect even in resected specimens (Figs 14.13 & 14.14), especially flat (type IIb) lesions and so-called minute cancers. Thus careful inspection of the specimen by an experienced pathologist and adequate sampling for histology is essential. Depressed and ulcerated lesions (types IIc and III) are more common than elevated lesions (types I and IIa) [233,235,236].

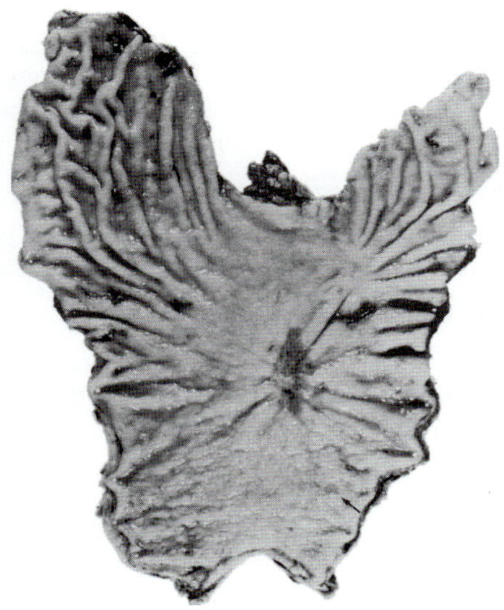

Fig. 14.14 Superficial depressed (IIc) type of early gastric cancer.

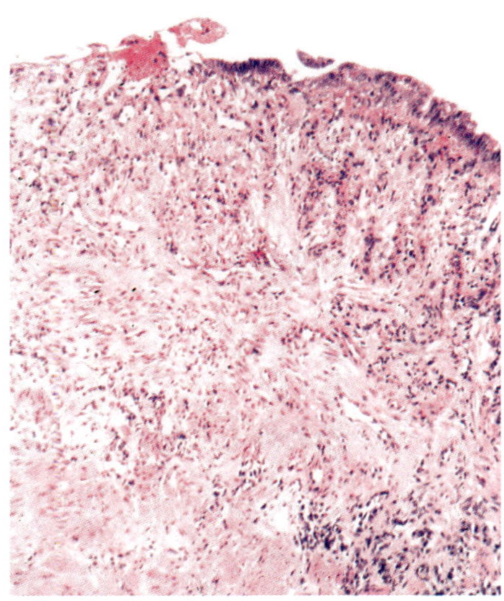

Fig. 14.15 Biopsy from a gastric erosion simulating carcinoma.

Some clinicians have found the above classification cumbersome and have suggested that the division of EGC into excavated and protruded forms is just as informative [237]. However, there is no doubt that the Japanese classification has resulted in a much more careful appraisal of the gastric mucosa by endoscopists looking for the variable, and often extremely subtle, appearances of EGC and this has resulted in an increasing proportion of such cancers being diagnosed in countries outside Japan.

EGC is located mainly in the corpus and antrum of the stomach; the cardia is involved in relatively few cases [229,233,236]. Lesions are multifocal in up to 14% of cases [238] and foci of dysplasia may also be present in adjacent mucosa. For this reason the pathologist should inspect the mucosal surface of resected specimens carefully and take multiple blocks in order to ensure that resection margins are not involved by synchronous carcinoma or dysplasia. The majority of ECG lesions are less than 4 cm in diameter, although occasionally they may extend up to 8 cm in diameter or more [233,239]. A small proportion of tumours are 5 mm in diameter or less. These are classified as minute cancers [238] and tend to be flat lesions [240] and are thus difficult to detect on endoscopy.

Histology

The microscopic appearances of EGC are similar to those of advanced carcinoma. Using the Lauren classification [212] the majority are intestinal carcinomas and approximately one-third are diffuse; mixed tumours are rare [238]. Using the WHO classification [1] most cases are tubular or signet ring cell in type. Elevated lesions (types I and IIa) are usually well differentiated and of intestinal type [233,235,241], while flat lesions (type IIb) and the majority of depressed or ulcerated tumours are poorly differentiated and composed of either intestinal or diffuse patterns.

The diagnosis of carcinoma from biopsies taken from a lesion suspected of being an early gastric cancer may not be straightforward. The presence of small numbers of differentiated or signet ring cells in the lamina propria can easily be missed and their detection may be facilitated if stains for mucin are routinely employed [242]. By the same token, muciphages and the finely vacuolated cells of a gastric xanthelasma, a benign lesion (see Chapter 16, p. 219), may be mistaken for cells of a diffuse carcinoma. Careful attention to nuclear morphology and the use of immunohistochemical epithelial and macrophage markers help to avoid this.

Carcinoma also has to be distinguished from regenerating epithelium, which may show nuclear pleomorphism, hyperchromatism and increased mitotic activity, and resemble tubular or intestinal-type carcinoma. Features that favour benign reactive atypia include homogeneous basophilia of the nuclei (even though they may be pleomorphic), small uniform nucleoli, maturation of the cells towards the luminal surface, and a gradual transition with the adjacent epithelium. On the other hand, neoplasia is favoured when there is irregular nuclear pleomorphism, the nucleoli are large and irregular, there is no surface maturation and the interface with the adjacent epithelium is abrupt. Diagnostic difficulties in biopsies from ulcers or erosions have been highlighted by Isaacson [243] who described two types of histological lesion. In the first, regenerating epithelium deep to an erosion but embedded in inflammatory exudate of granulation tissue may closely resemble adenocarcinoma, especially on frozen section (Fig. 14.15). In the other, bizarre non-epithelial spindle cells, of endothelial or myofibroblastic type, may simulate undifferentiated carcinoma (Fig. 13.2, p. 142). Careful assessment of nuclear chromatin, mitotic activity and the use of immunocytochemical markers and mucin stains are useful in avoiding erroneous diagnosis. For example, we have found widespread and strong nuclear immunoreactivity for p53 protein (as opposed to weak or focal staining of a proportion of the abnormal epithelial cells), if present, to be a useful pointer towards neoplasia, although it only occurs in less than 50% of definite cancers. In difficult cases pathologists should liaise with the endoscopist and discuss the histological appearances in the light of the clinical history and the endoscopic features. They should always be alert to the possibility of overdiagnosing carcinoma, and it is in the patient's interests to err on the side of caution and request repeat biopsies rather than precipitate unnecessary gastrectomy.

The distinction between severe degrees of adenomatous dysplasia and well differentiated tubular carcinoma, especially in type I and IIa early gastric cancers, can be virtually impossible in biopsy material. Indeed, there is good evidence that a proportion of type I and IIa EGCs result from malignant change in an adenoma [244] and the problem of diagnosing invasive malignancy has been discussed earlier in this chapter. Fortunately, the distinction is usually academic because the clinical management of both high-grade dysplasia and early gastric cancer is similar, and depends much more on the location, size and configuration of the lesion in question and on the patient's physical condition than on whether subtle invasion of the lamina propria can be confirmed.

Careful histological assessment of submucosal invasion with multiple sampling is important in resected EGCs because it correlates with the likelihood of lymph node metastasis [245]. Submucosal invasion occurs in about 50% of all EGCs, a figure that varies remarkably little between series from different parts of the world [238], and is least common in flat (type IIb) lesions [246]. Lymph node metastasis occurs in 10–20% of all cases of early gastric cancer [233,236,238,245] and, apart from being associated with the depth of submucosal invasion, it correlates with increasing tumour diameter [238,239,245,247]. Accordingly, endoscopic mucosal resection alone is only recommended for well or moderately differentiated tumours that are not ulcerated, are less than 30 mm in diameter, and in which subsequent histological examination confirms no submucosal invasion, no lymphovascular invasion and complete local excision [209].

Prognosis

A recent study of the natural history of untreated EGC has indicated a 63% cumulative 5-year risk of progression to advanced cancer [248]. On the other hand, the prognosis of surgically treated EGC is excellent. Five-year survival rates of greater than 90% have been regularly reported from Japan and indeed, some studies indicate that the long-term outlook for operated cases differs little from that of comparable subjects in the remainder of the population [249,250], or of those with benign gastric ulcer [229]. In Western populations reported recurrence rates are a little higher, between 5 and 15% [238]. Not unexpectedly, mucosal EGCs have a better prognosis than submucosal EGCs and patients with lymph node metastases have 10-year survival rates that are approximately 10–20% lower than those without [251–253]. Old age also appears to have an adverse effect on survival in EGC and, somewhat paradoxically, a number of studies have suggested that raised (types I or IIa) EGCs that are well or moderately differentiated and of intestinal type are more aggressive than depressed or ulcerated (types IIc or III) poorly differentiated tumours of diffuse type [230].

A significant incidence of recurrent or metachronous gastric cancers in patients treated for EGC has been noted in several papers. In the West this is reported to occur in between 5 and 15% of cases [236,238,252] and long-term endoscopic follow-up of patients treated for early gastric cancer is therefore to be recommended.

Spread of gastric carcinoma

Direct spread

Gastric carcinomas are highly infiltrative tumours and in resection specimens the majority have extended through the muscularis propria into the subserosa. According to the site of the primary growth, penetration of the serosa may result in direct spread to pancreas, liver, spleen, transverse colon and omentum, and often leads to early transperitoneal dissemination. Adhesions between the primary growth and neighbouring structures, particularly transverse colon, are common and tumour cells grow along them to reach the diaphgram or abdominal wall. Tumours at the cardiac end of the stomach infiltrate within the wall into the lower end of the oesophagus and at the distal end microscopic extension into the duodenum is not uncommon [254]. Widespread direct spread is particularly common in signet ring carcinomas and diffuse carcinomas that frequently show extensive lateral spread within the stomach wall and on the serosal surface, well beyond the macroscopically visible tumour. Intramural permeation of small lymphovascular vessels is widespread. There are reports of cases of linitis plastica which have extended along the wall of large segments of the intestinal tract producing an induration rather like that found in the stomach itself [255]. More commonly, secondary carcinoma of gastric origin in the small or large intestine presents as multiple strictures. Cancer cells are found in tissue spaces and lymphatics, and it is possible that peristalsis has played a part in their onward propulsion.

Macroscopical observation and palpation cannot be relied upon to define the margins of either early or advanced gastric cancer at operation, especially in the case of diffuse cancer, and frozen section examination of resected margins, particularly where the margin of excision is less than 4 cm, is desirable to ensure complete removal.

Lymphatic spread

Lymph node metastases were previously reported to be present in 90% of gastric carcinomas at autopsy and in 70% of surgical resections [256]. The latter figure may be rather less now as more lesions are diagnosed at the stage of early gastric cancer. The incidence of lymph node metastases increases with increasing depth of tumour invasion into the stomach wall [257] and occurs with equal frequency regardless of the histological type of the primary tumour. Their distribution varies according to the location of the tumour. Involvement of nodes along the lesser and greater curves is common and extension to the next zone, namely nodes along the left gastric, common hepatic and coeliac arteries, is often seen. More distant lymphatic spread may involve para-aortic and mesenteric nodes. Tumours of the midportion of the stomach may give rise to metastases in pancreatic and splenic nodes and lesions high in the stomach can metastasize to mediastinal lymph nodes. Spread by way of the thoracic duct to the left supraclavicular nodes (nodes of Troisier and of Virchow), although well recognized clinically, is not common. It is important for the surgeon to remove, and the pathologist to examine, all nodes, however small, since even the smallest apparently uninvolved node may contain secondary growth and there is good evidence that prognosis depends on the number of nodes involved.

Haematogenous spread

Spread via the bloodstream occurs from invasion of tributaries of the portal venous system and may occur even in the absence of lymph node involvement. Metastases can occur in almost any organ but are most commonly seen in the liver, followed by lung, peritoneum, adrenal glands, skin and ovaries; the latter are also involved by transperitoneal spread. The distribution of metastases is dictated to some extent by the histological tumour type. Intestinal-type carcinomas are likely to give rise to liver metastases by haematogenous spread while diffuse carcinomas are more likely to involve the peritoneum. Diffuse tumours tend to disseminate more widely, infiltrating lungs more extensively than the nodular metastases associated with intestinal-type tumours and involving unusual sites such as kidney, spleen, uterus and meninges more often [258,259]. Peritoneal involvement is more common in younger patients. In carcinomas showing unusual metastatic distribution, i.e. intestinal-type tumours involving peritoneum or diffuse tumours involving liver, the primary often shows a mixed histological pattern [260].

Transperitoneal spread

Secondary deposits of tumour from carcinoma of the stomach are common in omentum, peritoneum and mesentery but are rare over the spleen. Secondary ovarian deposits are well known as one form of Krukenberg's tumour, but in our view bloodstream spread is at least as likely as transperitoneal in their genesis. Krukenberg tumours are more frequently associated with diffuse primary carcinomas than the intestinal type.

Staging and prognosis of advanced gastric cancer

The prognosis of gastric cancer is closely related to the tumour stage at diagnosis. The TNM staging system [261], summarized in Table 14.3 and widely used in Western countries, is the best available predictor of outcome [262] and is recommended. The 'N' component has recently been modified to take into account the strong prognostic significance of the number of lymph nodes involved by tumour [263] and it can be seen that allocation of the correct 'N' stage requires at least 15 lymph nodes to be examined. The onus is on the pathologist to provide accurate staging of gastric carcinoma by careful examination of surgical resection specimens. Useful guidance on the gross examination of the resected stomach and completion of a clinically relevant report is available [264, 265].

Unfortunately, the TNM system is not applied worldwide (the Japanese, for example, have their own system [266]), and this makes international comparison of clinical studies difficult. However, the overall prognosis of advanced gastric carcinoma appears to vary from country to country with Japan having the best results with an overall 5-year survival rate of

Table 14.3 Pathological TNM staging of gastric carcinoma.

T—Primary tumour	
pT1	Tumour invades lamina propria or submucosa
pT2	Tumour invades muscularis propria or subserosa
pT3	Tumour penetrates serosa (visceral peritoneum) without invasion of adjacent structures
pT4	Tumour invades adjacent structures
N—Regional lymph nodes	
pN0	No regional lymph node metastasis
pN1	Metastasis in 1–6 regional lymph nodes
pN2	Metastasis in 7–15 regional lymph nodes
pN3	Metastasis in more than 15 regional lymph nodes
*M—Distant metastasis**	
M0	No distant metastasis
M1	Distant metastasis present

*Pathological staging cannot usually comment on the presence or absence of distant metastasis, unless biopsies of distant organs have been submitted for histological examination.

50% or better [267]. This can be explained at least partly by the aggressive Japanese surgical approach to treatment with extensive and meticulous lymph node dissection, although the employment of similar approaches in the West (so-called D2 gastrectomy) has not produced a corresponding benefit. In the non-screened populations of the West the prognosis of advanced gastric cancer is generally poor [29,268,269], and more than 75% of cases have such advanced disease at presentation that only palliative surgery is possible. Even for patients undergoing 'curative' gastrectomy the overall 5-year survival is generally 20–30% [270]. Mucinous carcinoma is associated with a worse prognosis than the other common histological types [271].

The outlook in carcinoma of the cardia is, if anything, worse than that for gastric carcinoma as a whole with 5-year survival rates in operable cases under 20% [272,273]. The median survival in all cases of carcinoma of the cardia, operable or otherwise, is in the region of only 7 months [274,275].

In resectable cases complete removal of tumour with good margins of clearance is important. Involvement of resection margins heralds early recurrence and death [268]. Apart from this, the depth of tumour invasion, the number of lymph nodes involved [276,277] and postoperative complications are important independent prognostic factors. The relatively good prognosis of early gastric cancer (pT1) tumours is discussed on p. 177 but pT2 tumours confined to the muscularis propria (so-called 'PM gastric cancer') also have considerably better 5-year survival rates than those showing serosal invasion [270].

Molecular aspects of gastric carcinoma

Huge advances have been made in our understanding of the molecular mechanisms underlying gastric carcinogenesis since the last edition of this book was published. They encompass identification of genetic lesions that range from gross structural chromosomal abnormalities to point mutations, defects of DNA repair, abnormalities of protein expression, and many others. They will be briefly reviewed here.

Chromosomal rearrangements

Cytogenetic studies of gastric adenocarcinoma have reported complex karyotypes with numerous numerical and/or structural abnormalities [278–280]. The most frequently documented include additional copies of chromosomes 7, 8, 9 and 12 [278,279,281] and the loss of the Y chromosome [278,282]. Loss of Y chromosome has also been reported in cell lines from both intestinal and diffuse types of gastric cancer [283]. A wide range of structural abnormalities have been described, but to date no non-random chromosomal abnormality has been consistently associated with gastric adenocarcinoma.

DNA aneuploidy

DNA aneuploidy has been reported in approximately 40–50% of gastric carcinomas including early gastric cancers [284–286]. Aneuploidy is significantly more common in adenocarcinomas of the cardia in comparison with those of body and antrum [42,287,288]. One study reported aneuploidy in 56% of adenocarcinomas arising in the cardia compared with 27% of those arising in the antrum [289]. Somewhat surprisingly, aneuploidy is commoner in intestinal-type adenocarcinoma than in the more aggressive diffuse type [285,286,288], but several studies conclude that aneuploid tumours are significantly associated with both lymph node and distant metastases and lower survival rates in comparison with diploid cancers [285,288,290–292].

Oncogene activation

Activation of several oncogenes has been implicated in gastric carcinoma including epidermal growth factor receptor (EGFR) [293] and *erb B-2* [294]. K-*ras* mutation is uncommon [295], while amplification or overexpression of c-*met* is reported in about 50% of tumours [296]. Amplification or overexpression of K-*sam* (particularly in diffuse-type cancers) [297], c-*myc* [298], the heparin-binding secretory transforming growth factor (HSTF-1 or *hst-1*) [299], and *bcl-2* [300] have also been reported.

Loss of heterozygosity

Loss of heterozygosity studies have identified a large number of regions of allelic loss in gastric adenocarcinoma. These include chromosomes 1q, 2q, 3p, 4p, 4q, 5q, 6p, 7q, 11p, 11q, 12q, 13q, 14q, 17p, 18q and 21q [301–308].

Inactivation of tumour suppressor genes

Adenomatous polyposis coli (APC)

This gene lies on chromosome 5q21. Allelic loss on 5q has been reported in 30–59% of gastric adenocarcinomas [302,304,307,308,] and *APC* gene mutations in 7–21% [309,310]. The *APC* gene product and E-cadherin exist in equilibrium with β-catenin, an intracytoplasmic protein whose function appears to be involved in organization of tissue architecture and polarity [311]. Mutation of *APC* appears to disturb the equilibrium between these molecules and the resulting increased levels of cytoplasmic β-catenin may act as a transcriptional factor through binding with the Tcf-Lef family [312]. Mutations of the β-catenin gene itself may have a similar effect, and these have also been reported in a significant proportion of gastric cancers [313].

p53

The *p53* gene is situated on chromosome 17p13. A substantial proportion of gastric adenocarcinomas demonstrate 17p allelic loss [302,314], especially those arising at the cardia [42]. Mutation of the *p53* gene was identified in approximately 25% of gastric carcinomas arising from all regions apart from the cardia, and this correlated well with demonstration of p53 protein overexpression by immunohistochemistry in these tumours [315]. Carcinomas of the cardia showed mutation of *p53* in a considerably higher proportion of cases than carcinoma of the body or antrum [42,316] and these tumours demonstrate a similar *p53* mutational spectrum to adenocarcinomas of the lower oesophagus, indicating that they may share a common aetiological basis and consistent with the fact that they show similar clinical and epidemiological features. Immunohistochemical studies have also indicated higher incidence of p53 protein overexpression in tumours of the cardia [317]. Overall the prevalence of p53 immunoreactivity in advanced gastric carcinoma is of the order of 50–60% [318–320].

Alterations of the *p53* gene have also been demonstrated in precancerous lesions of the stomach. Shiao *et al.* identified abnormalities in almost 60% of cases of dysplasia adjacent to adenocarcinomas [321] and similar results have been obtained by other groups [66]. More controversial was Shiao *et al.*'s finding of p53 abnormalities in almost 40% of cases of intestinal metaplasia, which has not been confirmed in other studies [66,322].

In established carcinomas *p53* gene mutation and overexpression of gene protein is more common in intestinal-type carcinomas than in diffuse tumours [66,315,319,323]. Some studies based on immunohistochemistry indicate that p53 protein overexpression is associated with shortened survival [324,325] but others, including a study of over 400 cases, failed to confirm this [319,323].

E-cadherin

In the past decade there has been considerable interest in the influence of cell adhesion molecules in the development and progression of tumours. The subject is highly complicated due to the large number of adhesion molecules and the huge potential they have for interacting and forming multimolecular complexes with, for example, epidermal growth factor receptor and APC and β-catenin [326,327], but one molecule that has assumed great importance recently is E-cadherin [326,328]. E-cadherin is expressed by epithelial cells and is a transmembrane protein which plays an important role in maintenance of intercellular connections, cell polarity and mucosal architecture. It is linked to the actin cytoskeleton within the cell by forming complexes with β- and γ-catenins which in turn are linked to actin microfilaments by binding to α-catenin. E-cadherin-mediated cell-to-cell adhesion may be destabilized by disturbed function or availability of either E-cadherin or the catenins and by alterations in other molecules such as APC gene protein which also form complexes with catenins. Germline mutations of the E-cadherin gene (*CDH-1*) resulting in a truncated gene product have been identified in New Zealand families showing high incidence of early-onset gastric carcinoma [188]. The associated cancers are of diffuse type and are highly aggressive. This finding has been confirmed by similar studies on European and Korean gastric cancer families [329,330]. While familial gastric cancer due to germline E-cadherin mutation is rare, the importance of E-cadherin abnormalities in sporadic gastric cancers of diffuse type has been shown by immunohistochemical studies that have demonstrated reduced E-cadherin expression in a high proportion of cases [331,332]. In contrast, intestinal carcinomas seldom show altered E-cadherin expression. This is supported by evidence of E-cadherin gene mutations in the majority of diffuse carcinomas and within the diffuse component of mixed carcinomas [333].

Microsatellite instability

Microsatellites are highly polymorphic short tandem-repeat DNA sequences. They are abundantly and evenly distributed throughout the genome and can be typed by PCR [334]. Microsatellite instability is manifest as alterations in the length of microsatellite alleles in tumour DNA as compared with matched normal DNA (see Chapter 38), and it results from abnormalities in DNA mismatch repair. Germline mutation in these mismatch repair genes results in widespread replication errors (RER+ phenotype) throughout the cancer cell genome and has been identified as the genetic basis of hereditary non-polyposis colorectal carcinoma (HNPCC) [335]. In HNPCC-associated carcinoma RER+ is indicated by detection of microsatellite instability at the majority of loci analysed and occasionally gastric cancers, usually of intestinal type, occur in this inherited background [191].

Microsatellite instability also occurs in up to a third of sporadic gastric cancers, but the mismatch repair defect in such cases is nearly always due to epigenetic silencing of DNA repair genes by promoter hypermethylation rather than somatic mutation [336]. Tumours showing this microsatellite instability occur mainly in the body and antrum [315,316,337,338], and it is rare in tumours of the cardia [339]. About a quarter of intestinal-type tumours are affected, but only a very small proportion of diffuse cancers [340]. Some reports indicate that the RER+ phenotype may be associated with rather better prognosis [315,337,338]; interestingly they seldom show coincident *p53* mutation [315,316]. Indeed there appears to be a reciprocal relationship between microsatellite instability and p53 abnormality between the two main anatomical forms of gastric cancer, cardiac tumours being generally RER negative and p53 positive while distal tumours often show the reverse.

Unusual variants of gastric carcinoma

Squamous cell and adenosquamous carcinoma

A pure squamous carcinoma at the cardia is likely to be of pri-

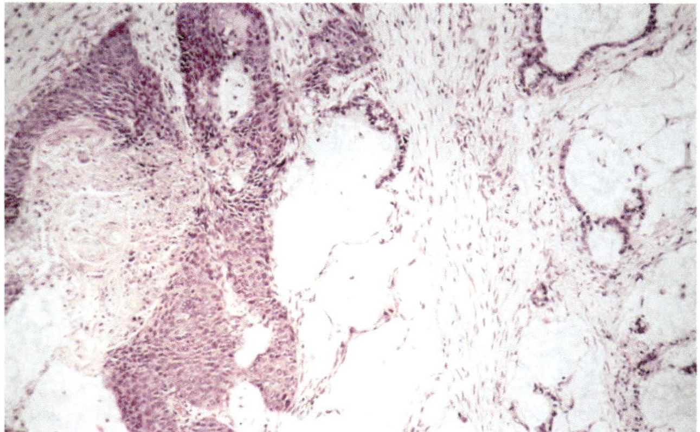

Fig. 14.16 Adenosquamous carcinoma. A focus of squamous cells producing keratin is present (left) while most of the tumour consists of mucinous adenocarcinoma (right).

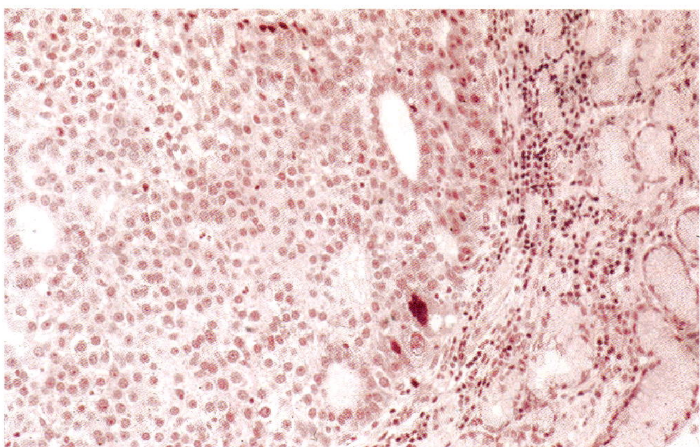

Fig. 14.17 Hepatoid gastric carcinoma showing uniform tumour cells (left) arising in gastric mucosa (right). Immunohistochemistry was positive for alpha-fetoprotein and there was extensive permeation of submucosal vessels by tumour.

mary oesophageal origin, but gastric squamous cell carcinoma does occur although it is rare [341,342] and a glandular component is often present when such tumours are extensively sampled following resection [343]. They have been described as a complication of gastric involvement in tertiary syphilis [344], after ingestion of corrosive acids [345], and following long-term cyclophosphamide therapy [346].

The histological diagnosis of primary adenosquamous carcinoma requires a squamous component characterized by keratin pearl formation and intercellular bridges in addition to the glandular element (Fig. 14.16) [10,347]. Such tumours are rare and occur most often in the antrum. Most examples are advanced carcinomas at the time of diagnosis but occasional cases of early gastric cancer of this type have been reported [348]. The squamous component consists of a very variable proportion of these tumours. Abrupt transition between squamous and glandular elements may occur or there may be intermingling of squamous foci within tumour glands [347,349]. Lymphovascular permeation by tumour cells is common and the prognosis of adenosquamous carcinoma is poor [341,347,348]. Ultrastructural demonstration of a tumour cell type showing evidence of both squamous and adenomatous differentiation supports the suggestion that this type of carcinoma arises from a multipotential common stem cell [350]. Metastases usually contain both glandular and squamous components but in some instances only one component may be present.

Hepatoid adenocarcinoma

A small number of gastric adenocarcinomas contain foci of tumour cells resembling hepatocellular carcinoma, usually interspersed with the common intestinal type of adenocarcinoma. These tumours may produce large amounts of alpha-fetoprotein (AFP) which is present in high levels in the serum and can be demonstrated by immunohistochemistry within the tumour [351]. AFP production is not invariable in such tumours, however, and conversely occasional intestinal-type adenocarcinomas without hepatoid features may demonstrate AFP production [352]. Hepatoid adenocarcinoma usually occurs in patients over the age of 50. Although occasional examples are detected at the stage of early gastric cancer [352,353], most are bulky polypoid tumours with ulceration and areas of necrosis and haemorrhage. The antrum is the most common site of origin followed by gastric fundus and occasionally the cardia [352].

Histologically these tumours may be heterogeneous. The characteristic hepatoid features consist of cells with eosinophilic or clear cytoplasm resembling those of hepatocellular carcinoma arranged in trabecular, sheeted or glandular patterns (Fig. 14.17). These may contain PAS–diastase-resistant hyaline globules [352,354] and occasionally secrete bile. Positivity for AFP on immunohistochemistry can be demonstrated usually, but not invariably, and overexpression of *p53* has been described [354]. These hepatoid foci are intermingled with intestinal-type adenocarcinoma, often showing a papillary pattern, and less differentiated areas may be seen containing bizarre giant cells and spindle cells [351,354]. A characteristic of these hepatoid carcinomas is extensive infiltration of venules within the gastric wall; this is reflected in the high incidence of liver metastases and a poorer prognosis even than conventional gastric adenocarcinoma [351,353,355].

Choriocarcinoma and adenocarcinoma

A number of gastric tumours have been described in which areas of choriocarcinoma containing syncytio- and cytotrophoblast occur, usually in association with poorly differentiated adenocarcinoma and with no evidence of primary choriocarcinoma elsewhere in the body. Immunohistochemical evidence of human chorionic gonadotrophin (HCG) expression within trophoblastic areas has been shown [356–358] and markedly elevated levels of circulating HCG are often present [356,359]. In occasional cases other germ cell tumour-like elements such as embryonal carcinoma may coexist. Gastric choriocarcinoma is rare and affects both sexes. In keeping with trophoblastic tumours arising elsewhere, the tumour often contains widespread areas of haemorrhagic necrosis that can be seen with the naked eye. Metastasis to the liver and lung are common and the prognosis is poor, typically with survival of a matter of months following diagnosis [357,360].

Medullary carcinoma with lymphoid stroma

This variant of gastric carcinoma has been described under several synonyms, such as gastric carcinoma with lymphoid stroma [361], undifferentiated gastric carcinoma with intense lymphocytic infiltrate, and lymphoepithelioma-like carcinoma [362]. Such tumours are reported to constitute around 4% of gastric carcinomas in the Far East but are less common in the West, and they display certain distinctive gross and histological characteristics [361,363]. On gross appearance they are usually ulcerated with a well circumscribed edge, and necrosis or haemorrhage are notably absent. Histologically the tumours usually have a well demarcated 'pushing' rather than an infiltrating margin and they are composed of poorly differentiated carcinoma cells infiltrated by a dense mixed infiltrate composed mainly of lymphocytes but also containing plasma cells, neutrophils and eosinophils (Fig. 14.18a). This infiltrate may be so intense that a diagnosis of gastric lymphoma is seriously considered. Lymphoid follicles may also be present. The tumour cells proper, which can be confirmed by immunostaining for epithelial markers, are generally large with eosinophilic cytoplasm but they show little cellular pleomorphism and low mitotic activity. They are arranged in nests, trabeculae or ill-defined tubules and well differentiated areas are rare.

The tumours occur predominantly in the antrum or body of the stomach and the age at presentation is slightly younger than conventional gastric carcinoma. Males are affected more often than females and the lesions may be diagnosed at both early and advanced stages [361,363], The prognosis is rather better than is usual in gastric carcinoma [363], possibly as a result of the brisk host immunological reaction to the tumour.

The other notable feature of this type of gastric carcinoma is its strong association with Epstein–Barr virus (EBV) infection that can be demonstrated in tumour cells by *in situ* hybridization (Fig. 14.18b) or PCR [362,364,365]. The nature of the association is so far unclear, and despite the ability of EBV-expressed proteins to bind with and stabilize p53 protein in some other EBV-related tumour types (raising the possibility of a direct role for the virus in oncogenesis), p53 immunoreactivity is less common in EBV-associated gastric carcinomas than in EBV-negative carcinomas [320,365]. Although much less prevalent, EBV genomic sequences have also been identified in up to 16% of conventional gastric carcinomas, raising the possibility that EBV infection may contribute to gastric carcinogenesis more generally [320,366].

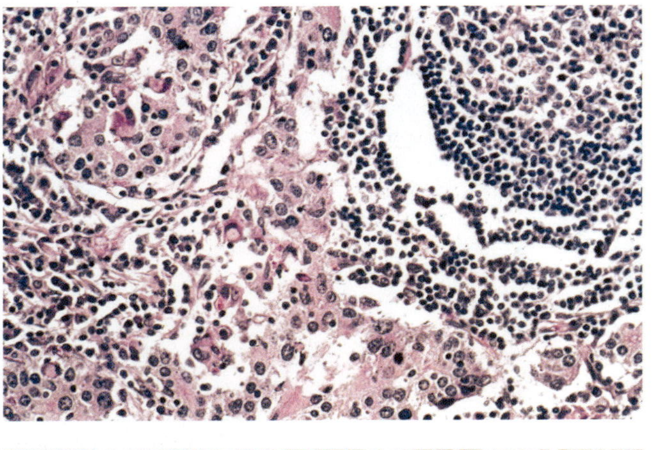
(a)

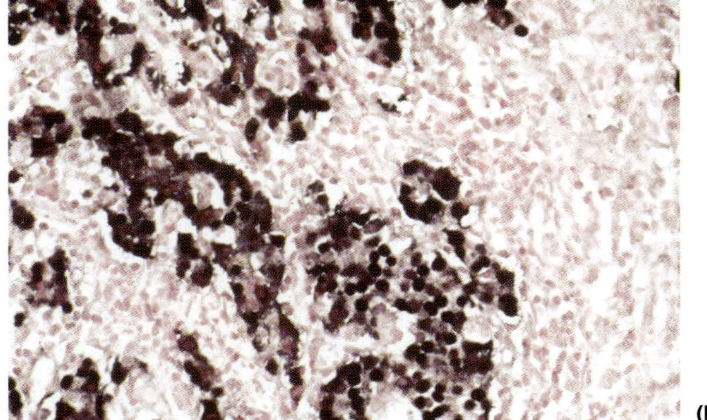
(b)

Fig. 14.18 (a) Medullary carcinoma with lymphoid stroma. The tumour is composed of undifferentiated cells with prominent lymphoid stroma. (b) Epstein–Barr virus DNA within tumour cells but not in lymphoid stroma. *In situ* hybridization.

Small cell carcinoma

This tumour is considered on p. 185 in the section on endocrine cell tumours.

Parietal cell carcinoma

These tumours are exceedingly rare. They present in a similar manner to adenocarcinoma and are bulky lesions involving both gastric body and antrum [367]. Histologically they have an expanding rather than infiltrating growth pattern and are composed of sheets of cells that may contain small gland-like clefts. The tumour cells resemble acid-secreting parietal cells in that they have eosinophilic granular cytoplasm and stain positively with PTAH (phosphotungstic acid haematoxylin) and Luxol fast blue. Electron microscopy shows them to have surface microvilli and numerous mitochondria in the cytoplasm. Lymph node metastases occur but are not extensive.

Endocrine cell tumours (carcinoid tumours, neuroendocrine tumours, neuroendocrine carcinomas)

These tumours, often referred to as carcinoid tumours when distinctive morphological patterns are seen microscopically, are not common in the stomach. While some increase has been reported in recent years as a result of more widespread use of endoscopy, they constitute less than 1% of all gastric tumours [368,369] and only some 3–5% of all gastrointestinal carcinoids [370,371]. They are a little commoner in females and the average age at diagnosis is slightly lower than that of non-carcinoid tumours [371].

Carcinoid tumours are neoplasms showing endocrine cell differentiation that is usually appropriate to their site of origin. The normal stomach contains a range of endocrine cells, including somatostatin (D) cells, gastrin (G) cells, X cells and P cells [372], but the great majority of gastric carcinoids arise from the ECL cells of the gastric body that normally secrete histamine. Endocrine neoplasms are generally recognized by their histological pattern; their cytoplasmic argentaffinity or argyrophilia; immunopositivity for cytosolic (neurone-specific enolase (NSE), protein gene product (PGP) 9.5 or CD56), vesicle (synaptophysin) or secretory granule (chromogranin) markers; immunohistochemistry or *in situ* hybridization for specific peptide hormones; or their electron microscopic features. Most carcinoids arising in the stomach are argyrophilic with the Grimelius technique and show immunopositivity for chromogranin A and synaptophysin, and these techniques are sufficient to confirm a diagnosis in the majority of cases. Difficulties only arise with poorly differentiated tumours that may only express NSE and/or PGP 9.5, neither of which is entirely specific for endocrine cell differentiation, and in such instances it may be necessary to utilize electron microscopy to look for intracytoplasmic membrane-bound secretory granules.

Over the past 10–15 years, considerable progress has been made in understanding the various types of gastric carcinoid tumours, their pathogenesis and precursor lesions, and the differing behaviour patterns of each type [373] and classification into three subtypes has been proposed [374,375]. These subtypes are:

1 tumours associated with chronic atrophic gastritis;
2 tumours associated with the Zollinger–Ellison syndrome—these occur almost always in patients with multiple endocrine neoplasia type I (MEN type I); and
3 sporadic tumours.

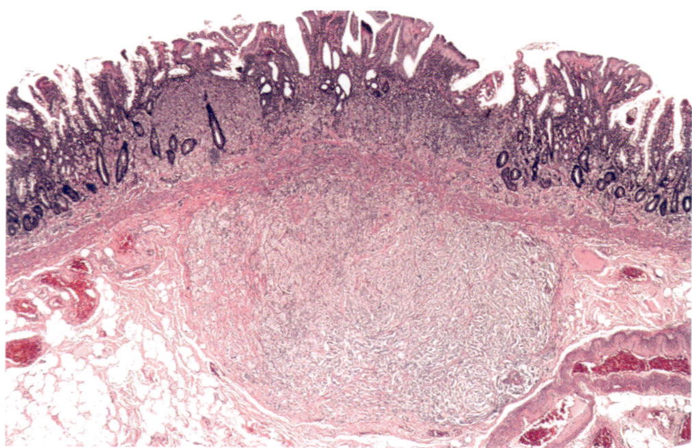

Fig. 14.19 A small neuroendocrine (carcinoid) tumour arising in the corpus of the stomach in association with severe atrophic gastritis and intestinal metaplasia.

Carcinoids associated with chronic atrophic gastritis are the commonest type and are more common in females. They are found in the corpus of the stomach or at the antral/corpus junction [376] and are frequently multiple. They present as small nodular polypoid swellings within the gastric mucosa that are usually less than 1 cm and virtually never greater than 2 cm in diameter and are usually confined to the mucosa and/or the submucosa [372,373] (Fig. 14.19). They are composed of small uniform cells arranged in nests, ribbons and/or a microglandular pattern. Mitotic activity is very low and tumour necrosis is not seen.

The adjacent mucosa shows features of chronic atrophic gastritis and intestinal metaplasia throughout the corpus of the stomach (type A chronic gastritis) that is frequently of the autoimmune type and associated with pernicious anaemia. Concomitant autoimmune conditions such as hypothyroidism are not uncommon. Within the severely atrophic gastric mucosa there is particular loss of parietal and chief cells and hyperplasia or dysplasia of neuroendocrine cells within the fundic mucosa [376]. The antral mucosa in contrast shows little atrophy, but immunohistochemistry may reveal hyperplasia of gastrin-containing G cells.

Carcinoid tumours of this type are not aggressive. Larger lesions (those measuring >2 cm but sometimes tumours of 1–2 cm) occasionally metastasize to local lymph nodes or (very rarely) spread to the liver, but they are virtually never fatal [377,378]. Indeed, there are well recorded examples of tumours undergoing spontaneous regression [379]. Accordingly, the only treatment required in most cases is local removal of visible lesions, followed by endoscopic follow-up and extirpation of any new lesions as they arise. Only exceptionally, if the tumours are unusually large or numerous, should gastrectomy be considered.

The pathogenesis of these carcinoid tumours is now well understood. They are proliferations of enterochromaffin-like

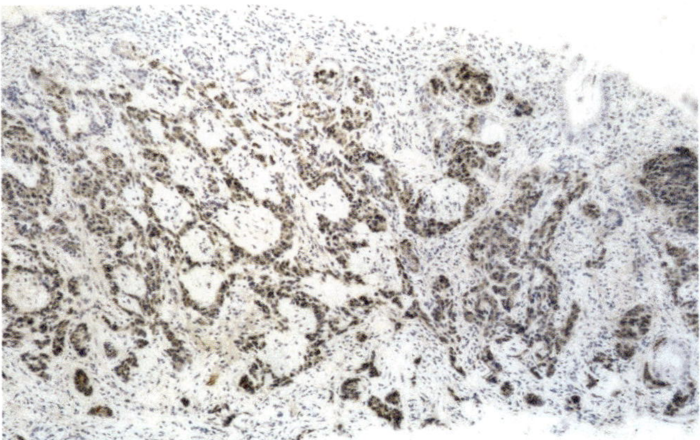

Fig. 14.20 Extensive neuroendocrine cell hyperplasia within and beneath the gastric mucosa in autoimmune gastritis. Chromogranin.

cells (ECL cells), consequent upon the trophic effect of hypergastrinaemia that is itself caused by the hypo- or achlorhydria that results from severe atrophic gastritis [368,375,380,381]. The hypergastrinaemia initially induces hyperplasia of intraglandular ECL cells that is first linear, i.e. forming chains of contiguous endocrine cells that are confined within the gland basement membrane, and then 'nodular', when small micronodular aggregates of cells escape into the lamina propria just above the muscularis mucosae. This is difficult to detect on routine haematoxylin and eosin (H&E) stain and immunohistochemistry is useful (Fig. 14.20). When these nodules measure 150–500 µm in size the term endocrine cell dysplasia is sometimes used [382]. Their further enlargement gives rise to proper carcinoids, which then acquire the capacity for invasion into and through the muscularis mucosae (Fig. 14.19). The tumours can often be induced to regress by blocking the hypergastrinaemic effect with somatostatin analogues or by removing the gastrin source with surgical antrectomy, though these approaches are seldom necessary in practice because of the tumours' innocent natural history.

ECL cell hyperplasia secondary to hypergastrinaemia may also occur in patients receiving long-term treatment with proton pump inhibitors, especially if there is concomitant *H. pylori* infection [383,384]. However, there is no evidence that this progresses to carcinoid tumours in humans.

Carcinoid tumours associated with the Zollinger–Ellison syndrome are rare and accounted for only 6% of gastric neuroendocrine tumours in one series [377]. They mostly occur in patients with multiple endocrine neoplasia (MEN) type 1, an autosomal dominantly inherited syndrome characterized by tumours of pituitary, pancreatic islets and parathyroids that is caused by germline mutation of the *MEN1* gene on chromosome 11q13 [385]. The gastric carcinoids that accompany the Zollinger–Ellison syndrome are also ECL cell proliferations that are induced by hypergastrinaemia. In most cases the gastrin-producing tumour arises in the duodenum or in the pancreas [370] and is accompanied by very high levels of circulating gastrin. It appears that the background germline defect of MEN-I is important for the tumours to develop. Patients with sporadic gastrinomas develop diffuse ECL cell hyperplasia within the corpus of the stomach but progression to overt carcinoids is unusual [386]. Allelic loss at the *MEN1* gene locus has been demonstrated in gastric carcinoid tumours occurring in MEN-I, suggesting that the gene behaves as a classical tumour suppressor gene in this scenario [387].

Zollinger–Ellison syndrome-associated gastric carcinoid tumours are similar to those associated with atrophic gastritis in that they are frequently multiple, usually less than 1 cm in diameter and confined to the mucosa or submucosa, and they are accompanied by ECL-cell hyperplasia in the surrounding mucosa [377]. In general they also have a good prognosis. However, in some instances, when they are larger (>2 cm) and show atypical histological features such as nuclear pleomorphism and prominent mitoses, they are aggressive and are associated with a poor prognosis [388,389].

Sporadic gastric carcinoids which arise in the absence of any background gastric pathology or hypergastrinaemia differ in several ways from subtypes 1 and 2. They are commoner in males and are usually solitary lesions [377]. They also tend to be larger and more deeply invasive, often ulcerating or reaching the serosa of the stomach and mimicking conventional gastric carcinomas macroscopically, and they are more likely to have atypical histological features and to behave aggressively [376,377]. Sporadic tumours measuring greater than 2 cm in diameter showing blood vessel invasion and deep infiltration of the stomach wall metastasized in over 60% of cases and around 50% had liver metastases [374]. Although most are non-functioning and show evidence of ECL cell differentiation, rare functional metastasizing tumours giving rise to the carcinoid syndrome or gastrin hypersecretion are recorded [374].

Sporadic gastric carcinoids may be subdivided histologically into well differentiated and poorly differentiated varieties [372]. Well differentiated tumours are composed of small uniform cells with a variety of patterns typical of neuroendocrine tumours, including islands or nests, anastomosing ribbons and, less often, rosettes or a microglandular pattern. A mixture of such patterns within each tumour is often seen. There is little cellular pleomorphism and mitotic activity is low (Fig. 14.21). Tumour necrosis is rare and there is a loose connective tissue stroma which is frequently hyalinized. Criteria have been proposed for dividing well differentiated gastric carcinoids into benign, borderline and low-grade malignant varieties. Benign tumours are less than 1 cm in diameter, confined to the mucosa or submucosa, show no evidence of angioinvasion, and are non-functioning. Borderline lesions comprise similar tumours that measure 1–2 cm and any tumour up to 2 cm with angioinvasion. Low-grade malignant tumours cor-

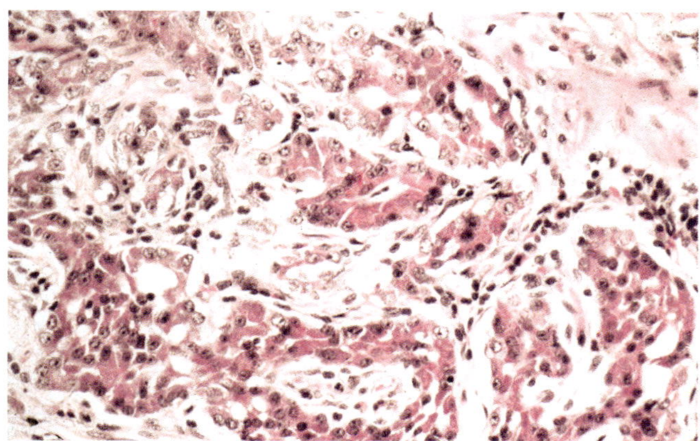

Fig. 14.21 Well differentiated carcinoid tumour composed of uniform cells showing insular and ribbon pattern.

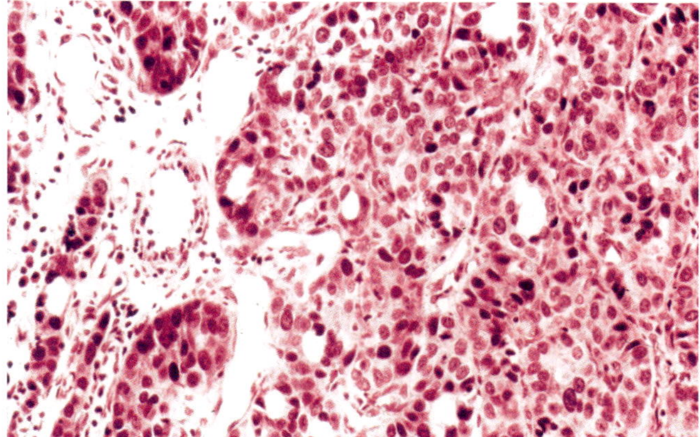

Fig. 14.22 Poorly differentiated carcinoid tumour resembling carcinoma and showing considerable pleomorphism and mitotic activity.

respond to any well differentiated tumour that is functioning, measures more than 2 cm in diameter, or invades beyond the submucosa [389].

Poorly differentiated or atypical carcinoids are all high-grade malignant tumours that show much more cellular pleomorphism and a variable spectrum of histology ranging from obvious carcinoid-like nesting to poorly differentiated tumours resembling small cell (oat cell) carcinoma [390] that may be found in different areas of the same lesion. Mitotic figures are frequent and widespread and may be abnormal. The classical neuroendocrine tumour patterns are less obvious and the tumour may simply be composed of sheets of cells. Most importantly, tumour necrosis is present, and may be prominent. These features are often accompanied by blood vessel invasion and deep infiltration of the stomach wall. Macroscopically they are generally larger than well differentiated carcinoid tumours and are commoner in the proximal stomach than in the antrum.

Tumours at the more undifferentiated end of the spectrum of atypical carcinoids are sometimes called neuroendocrine carcinomas and can be easily mistaken for poorly differentiated adenocarcinomas (Fig. 14.22). Small cell and large cell variants have been described [391] and both are highly aggressive tumours with a mean survival time of 12 months [374,391].

Small cell neuroendocrine cell carcinomas of the stomach are histologically similar to small cell lung carcinomas with solid organoid or trabecular patterns and small tumour cells with round or fusiform nuclei, little cytoplasm and finely granular nuclear chromatin but few nucleoli. Occasional rosettes are present and there may be peripheral palisading. In most cases the tumour cells are pleomorphic and rather larger than the classic oat cell type [392,393], and the main differential diagnosis is poorly differentiated adenocarcinoma and malignant lymphoma. Large cell neuroendocrine carcinomas have organoid, trabecular or pseudoglandular patterns. The tumour cells are large with eosinophilic cytoplasm, coarse nuclear chromatin and frequent nucleoli. Mitotic figures, apoptotic cells and necrosis are common in both small cell and large cell varieties and it is not uncommon to find scattered mucous cells or even areas of frank adenocarcinoma, indicating bidirectional differentiation. Immunocytochemistry is useful in reaching the diagnosis as most cases show positivity for chromogranin, neurone-specific enolase, synaptophysin or PGP 9.5 [391]. Electron microscopy shows intracytoplasmic dense-core secretory granules within tumour cells, although these may be scanty. Hormonal or paraneoplastic syndromes which may accompany pulmonary small cell carcinoma are seldom apparent in gastric tumours.

Composite tumours (adenoendocrine cell carcinomas)

These are defined as tumours showing both glandular and endocrine differentiation, in which the latter component accounts for at least one-third [394]: smaller numbers of scattered endocrine cells are not uncommon in conventional gastric adenocarcinomas [395]. Composite tumours are uncommon and generally composed of mixtures of adenocarcinoma and atypical carcinoid/neuroendocrine carcinoma. The glandular component may vary from well differentiated to a diffuse signet ring cell carcinoma [394], and in most cases the clinical behaviour is aggressive. Nevertheless, Caruso *et al.* [396] have reported a more differentiated case arising in a background of atrophic gastritis of the corpus with multiple gastric carcinoids.

Secondary carcinoma in the stomach

Carcinoma of the colon and of the pancreas uncommonly extends into the stomach by direct contiguous spread, invading the serosa and ulcerating the mucosa. Haematogenous metastatic spread from more distant primaries is commoner and possibly underestimated, and may present clinically with

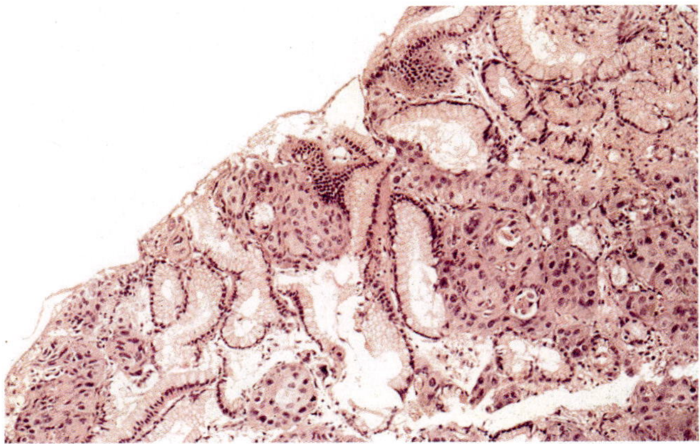

Fig. 14.23 Metastatic bronchial carcinoma infiltrating gastric mucosa. Tumour cells appear to grow within contours of mucosal glands.

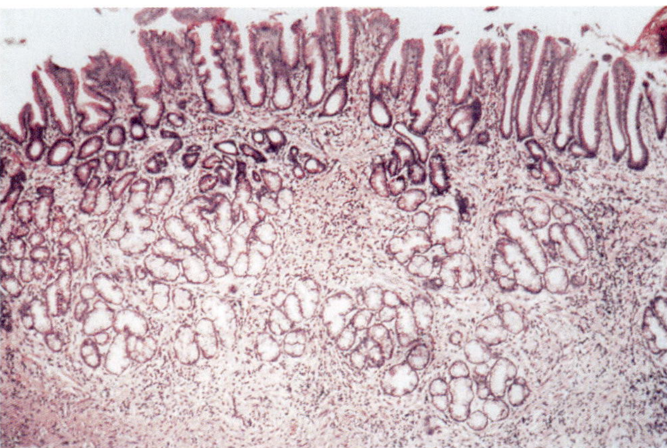

Fig. 14.24 Metastatic lobular carcinoma from breast showing very subtle infiltration of gastric mucosa.

any of the features of primary gastric cancer [397,398]. Metastatic deposits in the stomach are rare but may be single or multiple and appear as raised, volcano-like lesions with central ulceration. The most common primary tumours are carcinomas of the bronchus, breast and oesophagus, and malignant melanoma [10,398]. The correct diagnosis is greatly facilitated if the pathologist is informed of the clinical circumstances and the existence of extragastric malignancy, but sadly this is not always the case. Lewin and Appelman [10] describe an unusual pattern of infiltration of gastric mucosa by secondary carcinoma whereby tumour cells form nests and appear to grow within the contours of mucosal glands. Similar histological features are illustrated in Fig. 14.23.

The propensity of lobular carcinoma of breast to infiltrate widely and to involve the gastrointestinal tract is well known. The interval between diagnosis of the primary breast tumour and presentation of gastric metastases is considerable and averages around 6 years [399]. Infiltration of the stomach may simulate linitis plastica due to diffuse primary gastric carcinoma [400] and it is often impossible to make the distinction between these two tumours on the basis of histology alone (Fig. 14.24). Contrary to popular belief, the use of immunohistochemistry to detect oestrogen or progesterone receptors is of no value, because both steroid receptors are expressed in a significant proportion of primary gastric carcinomas.

References

1 Watanabe H, Jass JR, Sobin LH *et al*. *Histological typing of oesophageal and gastric tumours*. WHO International Histological Classification of Tumours. Berlin: Springer-Verlag, 1990.

2 Ming S-C, Goldman H. Gastric polyps: a histogenetic classification and the relation to carcinoma. *Cancer*, 1965; 18: 721.

3 Ito H, Hata J, Yokozaki H *et al*. Tubular adenoma of the human stomach. *Cancer*, 1986; 58: 2264.

4 Kolodziejczyk P, Yao T, Oya M *et al*. Long-term follow-up study of patients with gastric adenomas with malignant transformation. *Cancer*, 1994; 74: 2896.

5 Ming S-C. The classification and significance of gastric polyps. In: Yardley JH, Morson BC, Abell MR, eds. *The Gastrointestinal Tract*. Baltimore: Williams & Wilkins, 1977: 149.

6 Ito H, Yasui W, Yoshida K *et al*. Depressed tubular adenoma of the stomach: pathological and immunohistochemical features. *Histopathology*, 1990; 17: 419.

7 Goldstein NS, Lewin KJ. Gastric epithelial dysplasia and adenomas: historical review and histological evidence for grading. *Hum Pathol*, 1997; 28: 127.

8 Nakamura T, Nakano G-I. Histopathological classification and malignant change in gastric polyps. *J Clin Pathol*, 1985; 38: 754.

9 Morson BC. Gastric polyps composed of intestinal epithelium. *Br J Cancer*, 1955; 9: 550.

10 Lewin KJ, Appelman HD. *Tumors of the esophagus and stomach*. Atlas of Tumour Pathology, Fascicle 18. Washington: AFIP, 1996: 233.

11 Schlemper RJ, Itabashi M, Kato Y *et al*. Differences in diagnostic criteria for gastric carcinoma between Japanese and Western pathologists. *Lancet*, 1997; 349: 1725.

12 Kamiya T, Morishita T, Asakura H *et al*. Long-term follow-up study on gastric adenoma and its relation to gastric protruded carcinoma. *Cancer*, 1982; 50: 2496.

13 Tamura G, Sakata K, Nishizuka S *et al*. Allelotype of adenoma and differentiated adenocarcinoma of the stomach. *J Pathol*, 1996; 180: 371.

14 Kushima R, Muller W, Stolte M, Borchard F. Differential p53 protein expression in stomach adenomas of gastric and intestinal phenotypes: possible sequences of p53 alteration in stomach carcinogenesis. *Virchows Arch*, 1996; 428: 223.

15 Iida M, Yao T, Itoh H. Natural history of gastric adenomas in patients with familial adenomatous coli/Gardner's syndrome. *Cancer*, 1988; 61: 605.

16 Domizio P, Talbot IC, Spigelman AD *et al*. Upper gastrointestinal pathology in familial adenomatous polyposis: results from a prospective study of 102 patients. *J Clin Pathol*, 1990; 43: 738.

17 Sarre RG, Frost AG, Jagelman DG *et al*. Gastric and duodenal polyps in familial adenomatous polyposis: a prospective study of the nature and prevalence of upper gastrointestinal polyps. *Gut*, 1987; 28: 306.

18 Jagelman DG, Decosse JJ, Bussey HJR *et al*. Upper gastrointestinal cancer in familial adenomatous polyposis. *Lancet*, 1988; 1: 1149.

19 Watanabe H, Enjoji M, Yao T, Ohsato K. Gastric lesions in familial adenomatosis coli: their incidence and histologic analysis. *Hum Pathol*, 1978; 9: 269.

20 Parkin DM, Läärä E, Muir CS. Estimates of the worldwide frequency of 16 major cancers in 1980. *Int J Cancer*, 1988; 41: 184.

21 Pisani P, Parkin DM, Bray F, Ferlay J. Estimates of the worldwide mortality from 25 cancers in 1990. *Int J Cancer*, 1999; 83: 18.

22 Neugut AI, Hayek M, Howe G. Epidemiology of gastric cancer. *Semin Oncol*, 1996; 23: 281.

23 Powell J, McConkey CC. Increasing incidence of adenocarcinoma of the gastric cardia and adjacent sites. *Br J Cancer*, 1990; 62: 440.

24 Antonioli DA, Cady B. Changing aspects of gastric adenocarcinoma (letter). *N Engl J Med*, 1984; 310: 1538.

25 Guang-Wei X. Gastric cancer in China: a review. *J R Soc Med*, 1981; 74: 210.

26 Decarli LA, Vecchia C, Cislaghi C *et al*. Descriptive epidemiology of gastric cancer in Italy. *Cancer*, 1986; 58: 2560.

27 Weinberg GB, Kuller LH, Stehr PA. A case controlled study of stomach cancer in a coal mining region of Pennsylvania. *Cancer*, 1985; 56: 703.

28 *National Cancer Institute Annual Cancer Statistics Review 1973–91*. Bethesda MD: DHSS, 1994. DHSS Publications No. NIH 94: 2789.

29 Allum WH, Powell DJ, McConkey CC, Fielding JWL. Gastric cancer: a 25-year review. *Br J Surg*, 1989; 76: 535.

30 Rios-Castellani E, Sitas F, Shepherd NA, Jewell DP. Changing patterns of gastric cancer in Oxfordshire. *Gut*, 1992; 33: 1312.

31 Population and Health Monitor. DH2 85/3, DH2 96/1. Office for National Statistics.

32 Lauren PA, Nevalainen TJ. Epidemiology of intestinal and diffuse types of gastric carcinoma. *Cancer*, 1993; 71: 2926.

33 Blot WJ, Deves SS, Kneller RW, Fraumeni JF Jr. Rising incidence of adenocarcinoma of the oesophagus and gastric cardia. *JAMA*, 1991; 265: 1287.

34 Kalish RJ, Clancy PE, Orringer MB, Appelman HD. Clinical, epidemiologic and morphologic comparison between adenocarcinomas arising in Barrett's oesophageal mucosa and in the gastric cardia. *Gastroenterology*, 1984; 86: 461.

35 Craanen ME, Dekker W, Blok P *et al*. Time trends in gastric cancer: changing patterns of type and location. *Am J Gastroenterol*, 1992; 87: 572.

36 Dolan K, Sutton R, Walker SJ *et al*. New classification of oesophageal and gastric carcinoma derived from changing patterns in epidemiology. *Br J Cancer*, 1999; 80: 834.

37 Breaux JR, Bringaze W, Chappuis C, Cohn I. Adenocarcinoma of the stomach: a review of 35 years and 1710 cases. *World J Surg*, 1990; 14: 580.

38 Zheng T, Mayne ST, Holford TR *et al*. The time trend and age-period-cohort effects on incidence of adenocarcinoma of the stomach in Connecticut from 1955 to 1989. *Cancer*, 1993; 72: 330.

39 Wang HH, Antonioli DA, Goldman H. Comparative features of oesophageal and gastric adenocarcinoma. *Hum Pathol*, 1986; 17: 482.

40 MacDonald WC, MacDonald JB. Adenocarcinoma of the oesophagus and / or gastric cardia. *Cancer*, 1987; 60: 1094.

41 Lagergren J, Bergstrom M, Lindgen A, Nyren O. Symptomatic gastroesophageal reflux as a risk factor for esophageal adenocarcinoma. *N Engl J Med*, 1999; 340: 825.

42 Gleeson CM, Sloan JM, McManus DT *et al*. Comparison of p53 and DNA content abnormalities in adenocarcinoma of the oesophagus and gastric cardia. *Br J Cancer*, 1998; 77: 277.

43 Siewert RJ, Feith M, Werner M, Stein HJ. Adenocarcinoma of the esophagogastric junction: results of surgical therapy based on anatomical / topographic classification in 1,002 consecutive patients. *Ann Surg*, 2000; 232: 353.

44 Ormsby AH, Goldblum JR, Rice TW *et al*. Cytokeratin subsets can reliably distinguish Barrett's esophagus from intestinal metaplasia of the stomach. *Hum Pathol*, 1999; 30: 288.

45 Couvelard A, Cauvin J-M, Goldfain D *et al*. Cytokeratin immunoreactivity of intestinal metaplasia at normal oesophagogastric junction indicates its aetiology. *Gut*, 2001; 49: 761.

46 Ormsby AH, Goldblum JR, Rice TW *et al*. The utility of cytokeratin subsets in distinguishing Barrett's-related oesophageal adenocarcinoma from gastric adenocarcinoma. *Histopathology*, 2001; 38: 307.

47 Matley PJ, Dent DM, Madden MV, Price SK. Gastric carcinoma in young adults. *Ann Surg*, 1988; 208: 593.

48 Tamura PY, Curtis C. Carcinoma of the stomach in the young adult. *Cancer*, 1960; 13: 379.

49 Tso PL, Bringaze WL, Dauterive AH *et al*. Gastric carcinoma in the young. *Cancer*, 1987; 59: 1362.

50 Rugge M, Busatto G, Cassaro M *et al*. Patients younger than 40 years with gastric carcinoma. *Cancer*, 1999; 85: 2506.

51 Huntsman DG, Carneiro F, Lewis FR *et al*. Early gastric cancer in young, asymptomatic carriers of germ-line E-cadherin mutations. *N Engl J Med*, 2001; 344: 1904.

52 Correa P. Human gastric carcinogenesis. A multistep and multifactorial process. *Cancer Res*, 1992; 52: 6735.

53 Fenoglio-Preiser CM, Noffsinger AE, Belli J, Stemmermann GN. Pathologic and phenotypic features of gastric cancer. *Semin Oncol*, 1996; 23: 292.

54 Morson BC, Sobin LH, Grundmann E *et al*. Precancerous conditions and epithelial dysplasia in the stomach. *J Clin Pathol*, 1980; 33: 711.

55 Imai T, Kubo T, Watanabe H. Chronic gastritis in Japanese with reference to high incidence of gastric carcinoma. *J Natl Cancer Inst*, 1971; 47: 179.

56 Correa P, Cullo C, Duque E. Carcinoma and intestinal metaplasia of the stomach in Colombian migrants. *J Natl Cancer Inst*, 1970; 44: 297.

57 Siurala M, Varis K, Wiljasalo M. Studies of patients with atrophic gastritis: a 10–15 year follow-up. *Scand J Gastroenterol*, 1966; 1: 40.

58 Walker IR, Strickland RG, Ungar B, MacKay IR. Simple atrophic gastritis and gastric carcinoma. *Gut*, 1971; 12: 906.

59 Cahill RJ, Kilgallon C, Beattie S *et al*. Gastric epithelial cell kinetics in the progression from normal mucosa to gastric carcinoma. *Gut*, 1996; 38: 177.

60 Filipe MI, Mendes R, Lane DP, Morris RW. Assessment of proliferating cell nuclear antigen expression in precursor types of gastric carcinoma using the PC-10 antibody to PCNA. *Histopathology*, 1993; 22: 349.

61 Weiss H, Gütz H-J, Schröter J, Wildner GP. DNA distribution in chronic gastritis. *Scand J Gastroenterol*, 1989; 24: 643.

62 Morson BC. Carcinoma arising from areas of intestinal metaplasia in the gastric mucosa. *Br J Cancer*, 1955; 9: 377.
63 Nakamura K, Sugano H, Takagi K. Carcinoma of the stomach in incipient phase: its histogenesis and histological appearances. *Gann*, 1968; 59: 251.
64 Sipponen P, Kekki M, Siurala M. Atrophic chronic gastritis and intestinal metaplasia in gastric carcinoma. Comparison with a representative population sample. *Cancer*, 1983; 52: 1062.
65 Sipponen P, Kekki M, Haapakoski J *et al*. Gastric cancer risk in chronic atrophic gastritis: statistical calculations of cross-sectional data. *Int J Cancer*, 1985; 35: 173.
66 Solcia E, Fiocca R, Luinetti O *et al*. Intestinal and diffuse gastric cancers arise in a different background of *Helicobacter pylori* gastritis through different gene involvement. *Am J Surg Pathol*, 1996; 20 (Suppl 1): S8.
67 Ruol A, Parenti A, Zaninotto G *et al*. Intestinal metaplasia is the probable common precursor of adenocarcinoma in Barrett's oesophagus and adenocarcinoma of the gastric cardia. *Cancer*, 2000; 88: 2520.
68 Valle J, Sipponen P, Pajares JM. Geographical variations in *Helicobacter pylori* gastritis and gastric cancer. *Curr Opin Gastroenterol*, 1997; 13 (Suppl 1): 35.
69 Prabhu SR, Amrapurkar AD, Amrapurkar DN. Role of *Helicobacter pylori* in gastric carcinoma. *Natl Med J India*, 1995; 8: 58.
70 Genta RM, Gürer IE, Graham DY. Geographical pathological of *Helicobacter pylori* infection: is there more than one gastritis? *Ann Med*, 1995; 27: 595.
71 Asaka M, Kato M, Kudo M *et al*. Atrophic changes of gastric mucosa are caused by *Helicobacter pylori* infection rather than ageing. *Helicobacter*, 1996; 1: 52.
72 Jass JR. Role of intestinal metaplasia in the histogenesis of gastric carcinoma. *J Clin Pathol*, 1980; 33: 801.
73 Filipe MI, Munoz M, Matko J *et al*. Intestinal metaplasia types and the risk of gastric cancer: a cohort study in Slovenia. *Int J Cancer*, 1994; 54: 324.
74 Ectors N, Dixon MF. The prognostic value of sulphomucin positive intestinal metaplasia in the development of gastric cancer. *Histopathology*, 1986; 10: 1271.
75 Antonioli D. Precursors of gastric carcinoma. *Hum Pathol*, 1994; 25: 994.
76 Forman D, Newell DG, Fullerton F *et al*. Association between infection with *Helicobacter pylori* and risk of gastric cancer: evidence from a prospective investigation. *Br Med J*, 1991; 302: 1302.
77 Parsonnett J, Friedman GD, Vandersteen DP *et al*. *Helicobacter pylori* infection and the risk of gastric carcinoma. *N Engl J Med*, 1991; 325: 1127.
78 The Eurogast Study Group. An international association between *Helicobacter pylori* infection and gastric cancer. *Lancet*, 1993; 341: 1359.
79 Forman D. *H. pylori* infection and gastric carcinogenesis. *Eur J Gastroenterol Hepatol*, 1992; 4 (Suppl 2): S31.
80 Siman JH, Forsgren A, Berglund G, Floren C-H. Association between *Helicobacter pylori* and gastric carcinoma in the city of Malmo, Sweden. *Scand J Gastroenterol*, 1997; 32: 1215.
81 Chronic infection with *H. pylori*. In: *IARC Working Group on the Evaluation of Carcinogenic Risks to Humans. Schistosomes, Liver Flukes and Helicobacter pylori*. IARC Monographs on the Evaluation of Carcinogenic Risks to Humans, 61. Leon, France: International Agency for Research on Cancer, 1994: 177.
82 Rudi J, Müller M, von Herbay A *et al*. Lack of association of *Helicobacter pylori* sero-prevalence and gastric cancer in a population with low gastric cancer incidence. *Scand J Gastroenterol*, 1995; 30: 958.
83 Muszynski J, Dzierzanowska D, Sieminska J *et al*. Is *Helicobacter pylori* infection a real risk factor for gastric carcinoma? *Scand J Gastroenterol*, 1995; 30: 647.
84 Holcombe C. *Helicobacter pylori*: the African enigma. *Gut*, 1992; 33: 429.
85 Hansson L-E, Nyrén O, Hsing AW. The risk of stomach cancer in patients with gastric or duodenal ulcer disease. *N Engl J Med*, 1996; 335: 242.
86 Parsonnet J. *Helicobacter pylori* in the stomach—a paradox unmasked. *N Engl J Med*, 1996; 335: 278.
87 Hu PJ, Li YY, Lin HL. Gastric atrophy and regional variation in upper gastrointestinal disease. *Am J Gastroenterol*, 1995; 90: 1102.
88 Sipponnen P, Kosunen TU, Valle J *et al*. *Helicobacter pylori* infection and chronic gastritis in gastric cancer. *J Clin Pathol*, 1992; 45: 319.
89 Crabtree JE, Taylor JD, Wyatt JI. Mucosal IgA recognition of *Helicobacter pylori* 120 kDa protein, peptic ulceration and gastric pathology. *Lancet*, 1991; 338: 332.
90 Warburton VJ, Everett S, Mapstone NP *et al*. Clinical and histological association of CagA and VacA genotypes in *Helicobacter pylori* gastritis. *J Clin Pathol*, 1998; 51: 55.
91 Parsonnet J, Friedman GD, Orentreich N, Vogelman H. Risk for gastric cancer in people with Cag A positive or Cag A negative *H. pylori* infection. *Gut*, 1997; 40: 297.
92 Mitchell HM, Hazell SE, Hu PJ. Serological response to specific *Helicobacter pylori* antigens: antibody against Cag A protein is not predictive of gastric cancer in a developing country. *Am J Gastroenterol*, 1996; 91: 1785.
93 El-Omar EM, Oien K, El-Najumi A *et al*. *Helicobacter pylori* infection and chronic gastric acid hyposecretion. *Gastroenterology*, 1997; 113: 15.
94 Warburton VJ, Everett S, Mapstone NP *et al*. Clinical and histological association of Cag A + Vac A genotypes in *Helicobacter pylori* gastritis. *J Clin Pathol*, 1998; 51: 55.
95 Lee A, Dixon MF, Danon SJ *et al*. Local acid production and *Helicobacter pylori*; a unifying hypothesis of gastro-duodenal disease. *Eur J Gastroenterol Hepatol*, 1995; 7: 461.
96 Sipponen P, Kekki M, Seppala K, Siurala M. The relationship between chronic gastritis and gastric acid secretion. *Aliment Pharmacol Ther*, 1996; 10 (Suppl 1): 103.
97 El-Omar EM, Carrington M, Wong-Ho Chow *et al*. Interleukin-1 polymorphisms associated with increased risk of gastric cancer. *Nature*, 2000; 404: 398.
98 El-Omar EM. The importance of interleukin 1β in *Helicobacter pylori* associated disease. *Gut*, 2001; 48: 743.
99 O'Connor HJ. *Helicobacter pylori* and gastric cancer: a review and hypothesis. *Eur J Gastroenterol Hepatol*, 1992; 4: 103.
100 Goldstone AR, Quirke P, Dixon MF. *Helicobacter infection* and gastric cancer. *J Pathol*, 1996; 179: 129.
101 Correa P. *H. pylori* and gastric carcinogenesis. *Am J Surg Pathol*, 1995; 19 (Suppl 1): S37.
102 Lynch DAF, Mapstone NP, Clarke AMT *et al*. Cell proliferation in *Helicobacter pylori*-associated gastritis and the effect of eradication therapy. *Gut*, 1995; 36: 346.
103 Brenes F, Ruiz B, Correa P *et al*. *Helicobacter pylori* causes hyper-

proliferation of the gastric epithelium. Pre and post eradication indices of proliferating cell nuclear antigen. *Am J Gastroenterol*, 1993; 88: 1870.

104 Nardone G, Staibano S, Rocco A *et al*. Effect of *Helicobacter* pylori infection and its eradication on cell proliferation, DNA status and oncogene expression in patients with chronic gastritis. *Gut*, 1999; 44: 789.

105 Havard TJ, Sarsfield P, Wotherspoon AC, Steer HW. Increased gastric epithelial cell proliferation in *Helicobacter pylori*-associated follicular gastritis. *J Clin Pathol*, 1996; 49: 68.

106 Sorbye H, Svånes K. Gastric mucosal protection against penetration of carcinogens into the mucosa. *Scand J Gastroenterol*, 1995; 30: 929.

107 Wong W-M, Wright NA. Cell proliferation in gastro-intestinal mucosa. *J Clin Pathol*, 1999; 52: 321.

108 Wong W-M, Stamp GWH, Elia G *et al*. Proliferative populations in intestinal metaplasia: evidence of deregulation in Paneth and goblet cells but not endocrine cells. *J Pathol*, 2000; 190: 107.

109 Keefer LK, Roller PP. N-nitrosation by nitrite ion in neutral and basal medium. *Science*, 1973; 181: 1245.

110 Tilwell WG, Glogowski S, Xu HX *et al*. Urinary excretion of nitrate, N-nitrosoproline, 3-methyladenine and 7-methylguanine in a Colombian population at high risk for gastric cancer. *Cancer Res*, 1991; 51: 190.

111 Sobala GM, Pignatelli B, Schorah CJ *et al*. Levels of nitrite, nitrate, N-nitroso compounds, ascorbic acid and total bile acids in gastric juice of patients with and without precancerous lesions of the stomach. *Carcinogenesis*, 1991; 12: 193.

112 Davies GR, Symmons NJ, Stevens TRJ *et al*. *Helicobacter pylori* stimulates antral mucosal reactive oxygen metabolite production in vivo. *Gut*, 1994; 35: 179.

113 Phull PS, Green CJ, Jacyna MR. A radical view of stomach: the role of oxygen-derived free radicals and anti-oxidants in gastroduodenal disease. *Eur J Gastroenterol Hepatol*, 1995; 7: 265.

114 Nguyen T, Brunson D, Crespi CL *et al*. DNA damage and mutation in human cells exposed to nitric oxide in vitro. *Proc Natl Acad Sci USA*, 1992; 89: 3030.

115 Esumi H, Tannenbaum SR. US–Japan co-operative cancer research program. Seminar on nitric oxide synthase and carcinogenesis. *Cancer Res*, 1994; 54: 297.

116 Rathbone BJ, Johnson AW, Wyatt JI *et al*. Ascorbic acid: a factor concentrated in human gastric juice. *Clin Sci*, 1989; 76: 237.

117 Sobala GM, Crabtree JE, Dixon MF *et al*. Acute *Helicobacter pylori* infection: clinical features, local and systemic immune response, gastric mucosal histology and gastric juice ascorbic acid concentration. *Gut*, 1991; 32: 1415.

118 O'Connor HJ, Schorah CJ, Habibzedah N *et al*. Vitamin C in the human stomach: relation to gastric pH, gastroduodenal disease and possible sources. *Gut*, 1989; 30: 436.

119 Phull PS, Price AB, Thorniley MS *et al*. Vitamin E concentrations in the human stomach and duodenum—correlation with *H. pylori* infection. *Gut*, 1996; 39: 31.

120 Blok P, Craanen ME, Offerhaus J *et al*. Molecular alterations in early gastric carcinomas. No apparent correlation with *H. pylori* status. *Am J Clin Pathol*, 1999; 111: 241.

121 Uemura N, Mukai T, Okamoto S *et al*. *Helicobacter pylori* eradication inhibits the growth of intestinal type of gastric carcinoma in initial stage. *Gastroenterology*, 1997; 110: A282 (abstract).

122 Van der Hulst RWM, Van der Ende A, Dekker FW *et al*. Effect of *Helicobacter pylori* eradication on gastritis in relation to cag A: a prospective one year follow-up study. *Gastroenterology*, 1997; 113: 25.

123 Tepes B, Kavcic B, Zaletel LK *et al*. Two to four-year histological follow-up of gastric mucosa after *Helicobacter pylori* eradication. *J Pathol*, 1999; 188: 24.

124 Parsonnet J. The incidence of *Helicobacter pylori* infection. *Aliment Pharmacol Ther*, 1995; 9 (Suppl 2): 45.

125 Labenz J, Blum AL, Bayerdorffer E *et al*. Curing *Helicobacter pylori* infection in patients with duodenal ulcer may provoke reflux esophagitis. *Gastroenterology*, 1997; 112: 1442.

126 Schenk BE, Kuipers EJ, Klinkenberg-Knol EC *et al*. *Helicobacter pylori* and the efficacy of omeprazole therapy for gastro-oesophageal reflux disease. *Am J Gastroenterol*, 1999; 94: 884.

127 Chow W-H, Blaser MJ, Blot WJ *et al*. An inverse relation between cag-A positive strains of *Helicobacter pylori* infection and risk of oesophageal adenocarcinoma. *Cancer Res*, 1998; 58: 588.

128 Blaser MJ. *Helicobacter pylori* and gastric diseases. *Br Med J*, 1998; 316: 1507.

129 Kono S, Hirohata T. Nutrition and stomach cancer. *Cancer Causes and Control*, 1996; 7: 41.

130 Hill MJ, Hawksworth G, Tattersall G. Bacteria, nitrosamines and cancer of the stomach. *Br J Cancer*, 1973; 28: 562.

131 Correa P, Haenszel W, Cuello C *et al*. A model for gastric cancer epidemiology. *Lancet*, 1975; 2: 58.

132 Weisburger JH, Marquardt H, Hirota N *et al*. Induction of the glandular stomach in rats by extract of nitrite-treated fish. *J Natl Cancer Inst*, 1980; 64: 163.

133 Yang D, Tannenbaum SR, Buchi G, Lee GC. 4-chloro-6-methoxyindole is the precursor of a potent mutagen that forms during nitrosation of the fava bean. *Carcinogenesis*, 1984; 5: 1219.

134 Committee on Diet and Health. *Implications for Reducing Chronic Disease Risk*. Washington DC: National Academic Press, 1989.

135 Marquardt H, Rufino R, Weisburger JH. On the aetiology of gastric cancer: mutageneticity of food extracts after incubation with nitrate. *Food Cosmet Toxicol*, 1977; 15: 97.

136 Bilzer T, Reifenberger G, Wechsler W. Chemical induction of brain tumours in rats by nitrosoureas. *Neurotoxicol Teratol*, 1989; 11: 551.

137 Forman D. Are nitrates a significant risk factor in human cancer? *Cancer Surv*, 1989; 8: 443.

138 Hansson LE, Nyren O, Bergström R *et al*. Nutrients and risk of gastric cancer. A population-based case-control study in Sweden. *Int J Cancer*, 1994; 57: 638.

139 Correa P. A human model for gastric carcinogenesis. *Cancer Res*, 1988; 48: 3554.

140 Grain S, Haughey B, Marshall J *et al*. Diet in the epidemiology of gastric cancer. *Nutr Cancer*, 1990; 13: 19.

141 Ramón JM, Serra L, Cerdó C, Oromi J. Dietary factors and gastric cancer risk: a case controlled study. *Cancer* ,1993; 71: 1731.

142 Ames BN, Gold LS. Too many rodent carcinogens: mitogenesis increases mutagenesis. *Science*, 1990; 249: 970.

143 Trichopoulos D, Ouranos G, Day NE *et al*. Diet and cancer of the stomach: a case controlled study in Greece. *Int J Cancer*, 1985; 36: 291.

144 Correa P, Fontham E, Pickle L *et al*. Dietary determinants of gastric cancer in South Louisana. *J Natl Cancer Inst*, 1985; 75: 645.

145 Demirer T, Icli F, Uzunalimoglu O, Kucuk O. Diet and stomach

cancer incidence. A case controlled study in Turkey. *Cancer*, 1990; 65: 2344.
146 Chyou P-H, Nomura A, Hankan J, Stemmermann GN. A case cohort study of diet and stomach cancer. *Cancer Res*, 1990; 50: 7501.
147 Haenszel W, Kurihara M, Segi M, Lee RKC. Stomach cancer among Japanese in Hawaii. *J Natl Canc Inst*, 1972; 49: 969.
148 Hansson L-E, Nyrén O, Bergstrom R *et al*. Nutrients and gastric cancer risk: a population based case control study in Sweden. *Int J Cancer*, 1994; 57: 638.
149 Mirvish SS. Effects of vitamins C and E on N-nitroso compound formation, carcinogenesis and cancer. *Cancer*, 1986; 58: 1842.
150 Kneller RW, McLaughlin JL, Bjelke E *et al*. A cohort study of stomach cancer in a high risk American population. *Cancer*, 1991; 68: 672.
151 Buiatti E, Palli D, Decarli A *et al*. A case controlled study of gastric cancer on diet in Italy. *Int J Cancer*, 1989; 44: 611.
152 Boeing H, Frentzel-Beyme R, Berger M *et al*. Case-control study on stomach cancer in Germany. *Int J Cancer*, 1991; 47: 858.
153 Hansson L-E, Baron J, Nyrén O *et al*. Tobacco, alcohol and the risk of gastric cancer. A population-based case control study in Sweden. *Int J Cancer*, 1994; 57: 26.
154 Magnus HA. A re-assessment of the gastric lesion in pernicious anaemia. *J Clin Pathol*, 1958; 11: 289.
155 Mosbech J, Videbaek A. Mortality and risk of gastric carcinoma among patients with pernicious anaemia. *Br Med J*, 1950; 2: 390.
156 Brinton LA, Gridley G, Hrubec Z *et al*. Cancer risk following pernicious anaemia. *Br J Cancer*, 1989; 59: 810.
157 Hsing AW, Hansson L-E, McLaughlin JK *et al*. Pernicious anaemia and subsequent cancer. A population-based cohort study. *Cancer*, 1993; 71: 745.
158 Toh B-H, van Driel IR, Gleeson PA. Pernicious anaemia. *N Engl J Med*, 1997; 337: 1441.
159 Kekki M, Varis K, Pohjanpalo H *et al*. Course of antrum and body gastritis in pernicious anaemia families. *Dig Dis Sci*, 1983; 28: 698.
160 Stockbrügger RW, Menon GG, Beilby JOW *et al*. Gastroscopic screening in 80 patients with pernicious anaemia. *Gut*, 1983; 24: 1141.
161 Borch K, Renvall H, Liedberg C. Gastric endocrine cell hyperplasia and carcinoid tumours in pernicious anaemia. *Gastroenterology*, 1985; 88: 638.
162 Sjöblom SM, Sipponen P, Järvinen H. Gastroscopic follow-up of pernicious anaemia patients. *Gut*, 1993; 34: 28.
163 Laxen F, Sipponen P, Ihamaki T *et al*. Gastric polyps: their morphological and endoscopical characteristics and relation to gastric carcinoma. *Acta Pathol Microbiol Immunol Scand* Sect A, 1982; 90: 221.
164 Orlowska J, Jarosz B, Pachlewski J, Butruk E. Malignant transformation of benign epithelial gastric polyps. *Am J Gastroenterol*, 1995; 90: 2152.
165 Hattori T. Morphological range of hyperplastic polyps and cancers arising in hyperplastic polyps of the stomach. *J Clin Pathol*, 1985; 38: 622.
166 Diabo M, Itabashi M, Hirota T. Malignant transformation of gastric hyperplastic polyps. *Am J Gastroenterol*, 1987; 82: 1016.
167 Stalsberg H, Taksdal S. Stomach cancer following gastric surgery for benign conditions. *Lancet*, 1971; 2: 1175.
168 Viste A, Bjornestad E, Opheim P *et al*. Risk of carcinoma following gastric operations for benign disease. *Lancet*, 1986; 2: 502.
169 Offerhaus GJA, Tersemette AC, Huibregste K *et al*. Mortality caused by stomach cancer after remote partial gastrectomy for benign condition: 40 years of follow-up of an Amsterdam cohort of 2633 post-gastrectomy patients. *Gut*, 1988; 29: 1588.
170 Watt PCH, Patterson CC, Kennedy TL. Late mortality after vagotomy and drainage for duodenal ulcer. *Br Med J*, 1984; 288: 1335.
171 Caygill CPJ, Hill MJ, Hall CN *et al*. Increased risk of cancer at multiple sites after gastric surgery for peptic ulcer. *Gut*, 1987; 28: 924.
172 Tersmette AC, Offerhaus JA, Tersmette KWF *et al*. Meta-analysis of the risk of gastric stump cancer: Detection of high risk patient subsets for stomach cancer after remote partial gastrectomy for benign conditions. *Cancer Res*, 1990; 50: 6486.
173 Dixon MF, O'Connor HJ, Axon ATR *et al*. Reflux gastritis: a distinct histopathological entity. *J Clin Pathol*, 1986; 39: 524.
174 Sobala GM, O'Connor HJ, Dewar EP *et al*. Bile reflux and intestinal metaplasia in gastric mucosa. *J Clin Pathol*, 1993; 46: 235.
175 Miwa K, Kamata T, Miyazaki I, Hattori T. Kinetic changes and experimental carcinogenesis after Billroth I and II gastrectomy. *Br J Surg*, 1993; 80: 893.
176 Savage A, Jones S. Histological appearances of the gastric mucosa 15–27 years after partial gastrectomy. *J Clin Pathol*, 1979; 32: 179.
177 Watt PCH, Sloan JM, Kennedy TL. Changes in gastric mucosa after vagotomy and gastrojejunostomy for duodenal ulcer. *Br Med J*, 1983; 287: 1407.
178 Stemmermann GN, Hayashi T. Hyperplastic polyps of the gastric mucosa adjacent to gastroenterostomy stomas. *Am J Clin Pathol*, 1979; 71: 341.
179 Janunger K-G, Domellof L. Gastric polyps and precancerous mucosal changes after partial gastrectomy. *Acta Chir Scand*, 1978; 144: 293.
180 Scharschmidt BF. The natural history of hypertrophic gastropathy (Menetrier's disease). *Am J Med*, 1977; 63: 644.
181 Chusid EL, Hirsch RL, Colcher H. Spectrum of hypertrophic gastropathy: giant rugal folds, polyposis and carcinoma of the stomach. Case report and review of the literature. *Arch Intern Med*, 1964; 114: 621.
182 Johnson MI, Spark JI, Ambrose MS, Wyatt JI. Early gastric cancer in a patient with Menetrier's disease, lymphocytic gastritis and *Helicobacter pylori*. *Eur J Gastroenterol Hepatol*, 1995; 7: 187.
183 Wood GM, Bates C, Brown RC, Losowsky MS. Intramucosal carcinoma of the gastric antrum complicating Menetrier's disease. *J Clin Pathol*, 1983; 36: 1071.
184 Fischer A, Clagett OT, McDonald JR. Coexistent duodenal ulcer and gastric malignancy. *Surgery*, 1947; 21: 168.
185 Hole DJ, Quigley EMM, Gillis CR, Watkinson G. Peptic ulcer and cancer. An examination of the relationship between chronic peptic ulcer and gastric cancer. *Scand J Gastroenterol*, 1987; 22: 17.
186 Rollag A, Jacobson CD. Gastric ulcer and risk of cancer. *Acta Med Scand*, 1984; 206: 105.
187 La Vecchia C, Negri E, Franceschi S, Gentile A. Family history and the risk of stomach and colorectal cancer. *Cancer*, 1992; 70: 50.
188 Guilford P, Hopkins J, Harraway J *et al*. E-cadherin germline mutations in familial gastric cancer. *Nature*, 1998; 392: 402.

189 Huntsman DG, Carneiro F, Lewis FR. *et al*. Early gastric cancer in young, asymptomatic carriers of germ-line E-cadherin mutations. *N Engl J Med*, 2001; 344: 1904.

190 Park J-G, Park KJ, Ahn Y-O *et al*. Risk of gastric cancer among Korean familial adenomatous polyposis patients. *Dis Colon Rectum*, 1992; 35: 996.

191 Aarnio M, Salovaara R, Aaltonen LA, Mecklin JP, Jarvinen HJ. Features of gastric cancer in hereditary non-polyposis colorectal cancer syndrome. *Int J Cancer*, 1997; 74: 1551.

192 McGarrity TJ, Kulin HE, Zaino RJ. Peutz–Jeghers syndrome. *Am J Gastroenterol*, 2000; 95: 596.

193 Giardello FM, Welsh SB, Hamilton SR *et al*. Increased risk of cancer in the Peutz–Jegher syndrome. *N Engl J Med*, 1987; 316: 511.

194 Utsunomyia J, Gocho H, Miyanaga T *et al*. Peutz–Jeghers syndrome; its natural course and management. *Johns Hopkins Med J*, 1975; 136: 71.

195 Weinstein WM, Goldstein NS. Gastric dysplasia and its management. *Gastroenterology*, 1994; 107: 1543.

196 Jass JR. A classification of gastric dysplasia. *Histopathology*, 1983; 7: 181.

197 Ming SC, Bajtai A, Correra P *et al*. Gastric dysplasia. Significance and pathologic criteria. *Cancer*, 1984; 54: 1794.

198 Sipponen P. Gastric dysplasia. In: Williams GT, ed. *Current Topics in Pathology*, Vol. 81. *Gastrointestinal Pathology*. New York: Springer-Verlag, 1990: 61.

199 Sloan JM, Allen DC, Hamilton PW, Watt PCH. The place of quantitation in diagnostic gastrointestinal pathology. In: Williams GT, ed. *Current Topics in Pathology*, Vol. 81. *Gastrointestinal Pathology*. New York: Springer-Verlag, 1990: 192.

200 Lansdown N, Quirke P, Dixon MF *et al*. High grade dysplasia of the gastric mucosa: a marker for gastric carcinoma. *Gut*, 1990; 31: 977.

201 Lauwers GY, Shimizu M, Correa P *et al*. Evaluation of gastric biopsies for neoplasia. Differences between Japanese and Western pathologists. *Am J Surg Pathol*, 1999; 23: 511.

202 Ghandur-Mnaymneh L, Paz J, Roldan E, Cassady J. Dysplasia of non-metaplastic gastric mucosa. *Am J Surg Pathol*, 1988; 12: 96.

203 Lewin KJ. Nomenclature problems of gastrointestinal epithelial neoplasia. *Am J Surg Pathol*, 1998; 22: 1043.

204 Riddell RH, Goldman H, Ransohoff DF *et al*. Dysplasia in inflammatory bowel disease. *Hum Pathol*, 1983; 14: 931.

205 Schlemper RJ, Riddell RH, Kato Y *et al*. The Vienna classification of gastrointestinal epithelial neoplasia. *Gut*, 2000; 47: 251.

206 Rugge M, Farinati F, Baffa R *et al*. Gastric epithelial dysplasia in the natural history of gastric cancer: a multicentre prospective follow-up study. *Gastroenterology*, 1994; 107: 1288.

207 de Dombal FT, Price AB, Williams GT *et al*. The British Society of Gastroenterology early gastric cancer/dysplasia survey: an interim report. *Gut*, 1990; 31: 115.

208 Coma del Corral MJ, Pardo-Mindan FJ, Razquin S, Ojeda C. Risk of cancer in patients with gastric dysplasia. *Cancer*, 1990; 65: 2078.

209 Ono H, Kondo H, Gotoda T. Endoscopic mucosal resection for treatment of early gastric cancer. *Gut*, 2001; 48: 225.

210 Rugge M, Leandro G, Faranati F *et al*. Gastric epithelial dysplasia. *Cancer*, 1995; 76: 376.

211 Dekker W, Tytgat GN. Diagnostic accuracy of fiber-endoscopy in the detection of upper intestinal malignancy. *Gastroenterology*, 1977; 73: 710.

212 Lauren P. The two histological main types of gastric carcinoma: diffuse and so-called intestinal-type carcinoma. *Acta Pathol Microbiol Scand*, 1965; 64: 31.

213 Endoh Y, Tamura T, Motoyama T. Well differentiated adenocarcinoma mimicking complete-type intestinal metaplasia in the stomach. *Hum Pathol*, 1999; 30: 826.

214 Ming SC. Gastric carcinoma: a pathobiological classification. *Cancer*, 1977; 39: 2475.

215 Mulligan RM. Histogenesis and biologic behaviour of gastric carcinoma. In: Sommers SC, ed. *Gastrointestinal and Hepatic Pathology Decennial 1966–75*. New York: Appleton-Century-Crofts, 1975: 31.

216 Goseki N, Takizawa T, Koike M. Differences in the mode of extension of gastric cancer classified by histological type: new histological classification of gastric carcinoma. *Gut*, 1992; 33: 606.

217 Carneiro F. Classification of gastric carcinoma. *Curr Diag Pathol*, 1997; 4: 51.

218 Pagnini CA, Rugge M. Gastric cancer: problems in histological diagnosis. *Histopathology*, 1982; 6: 391.

219 Shennib H, Lough J, Klein HW, Hampson LG. Gastric carcinoma: intestinal metaplasia and tumour growth pattern as indicators of prognosis. *Surgery*, 1986; 100: 774.

220 Roy P, Piard F, Dusserre-Guion L *et al*. Prognostic comparison of the pathological classification of gastric cancer: a population based study. *Histopathology*, 1998; 33: 304.

221 Martin IG, Dixon MF, Sue-Ling H *et al*. Goseki histological grading of gastric cancer is an important predictor of outcome. *Gut*, 1994; 35: 758.

222 Songun I, van de Velde CJH, Arends JW. Classification of gastric carcinoma using the Goseki system provides prognostic information additional to TNM staging. *Cancer*, 1999; 85: 2114.

223 Murakami T. Pathomorphological diagnosis: definition and growth classification of early gastric cancer. In: Murakami T, ed. *Early Cancer*. Gann Monograph on Cancer Research 11. Tokyo: University of Tokyo Press, 1971: 53.

224 Oohara T, Tohma H, Takezoe K *et al*. Minute gastric cancers less than 5 mm in diameter. *Cancer*, 1982; 50: 801.

225 Kodama Y, Inokuchi K, Soejimi K *et al*. Growth patterns and prognosis in early gastric carcinoma. Superficially spreading and penetrating growth types. *Cancer*, 1983; 51: 320.

226 Stout AP. Superficial spreading type of carcinoma of the stomach. *Arch Surg*, 1942; 44: 651.

227 Mason MK. Surface carcinoma of the stomach. *Gut*, 1965; 6: 185.

228 Gutmann RA. De quelques signes radiologiques au cancer gastrique au début. *Bull Soc Radiol Med France*, 1933; 21: 347.

229 Eckardt VF, Giessler W, Kanzler G *et al*. Clinical and morphological characteristics of early gastric cancer. A case control study. *Gastroenterology*, 1990; 98: 708.

230 Everett SM, Axon ATR. Early gastric cancer: disease or pseudo-disease? *Lancet*, 1998; 351: 1350.

231 Hallissey MT, Allum WH, Jewkes AJ *et al*. Early detection of gastric cancer. *Br Med J*, 1990; 301: 513.

232 Sue-Ling HM, Johnston D, Martin IG *et al*. Gastric cancer: a curable disease in Britain. *Br Med J*, 1993; 307: 591.

233 Ohta H, Noguchi Y, Takagi K *et al*. Early gastric carcinoma with special reference to macroscopic classification. *Cancer*, 1987; 60: 1099.

234 Ikdea Y, Haraguchi Y, Mori M *et al*. Gastric cancer in a general hospital in Japan. *Semin Surg Oncol*, 1994; 10: 150.

235 Johansen A. *Early Gastric Cancer. A Contribution to the Pathology and to Gastric Cancer Histogenesis*. Copenhagen: Poul Petri, 1981.

236 Gardiner KR, Wilkinson AJ, Sloan JM. Early gastric cancer: a report of 30 cases. *J R Coll Surg Edinb*, 1990; 35: 237.

237 Hermanek P, Rosch W. Critical evaluation of the Japanese 'early gastric cancer' classification. *Endoscopy*, 1973; 5: 220.

238 Everett SM, Axon ATR. Early gastric cancer in Europe. *Gut*, 1997; 41: 142.

239 Kurihara N, Kubota T, Otani Y *et al*. Lymph node metastases of early gastric cancer with submucosal invasion. *Br J Surg*, 1998; 85: 835.

240 Mori M, Enjoji M, Sugimachi K. Histopathological features of minute and small human gastric adenocarcinomas. *Arch Pathol Lab Med*, 1989; 113: 926.

241 Nagayo T, Yokoyama H. Recent changes in the morphology of gastric cancer in Japan. *Int J Cancer*, 1978; 21: 407.

242 Yamashina M. A variant of early gastric carcinoma. Histologic and histochemical studies of early signet ring cell carcinomas discovered beneath preserved surface epithelium. *Cancer*, 1986; 58: 1333.

243 Isaacson P. Biopsy appearances easily mistaken for malignancy in gastrointestinal endoscopy. *Histopathology*, 1982; 6: 377.

244 Johansen A. Elevated early gastric carcinoma. Differential diagnosis as regards adenomatous polyps. *Pathol Res Pract*, 1979; 164: 316.

245 Yasuda K, Shiraishi N, Suematsu T *et al*. Rate of detection of lymph node metastases is correlated with the depth of submucosal invasion in early stage gastric carcinoma. *Cancer*, 1999; 85: 2119.

246 Fukutomi H, Sakita T. Analysis of early gastric cancer cases collected from major hospitals and institutes in Japan. *Jpn J Clin Oncol*, 1984; 14: 169.

247 Ishigami S, Hokita S, Natsugoe S *et al*. Carcinomatous infiltration into the submucosa as a predictor of lymph node involvement in early gastric cancer. *World J Surg*, 1998; 22: 1056.

248 Tsukuma H, Oshima A, Narahara H, Morii T. Natural history of early gastric cancer: a non-concurrent longterm follow-up study. *Gut*, 2000; 47: 618.

249 Yamazaki H, Oshima A, Murakami R *et al*. A long-term follow-up study of patients with gastric cancer detected by mass screening. *Cancer*, 1989; 63: 613.

250 Sue-Ling HM, Martin I, Griffith J *et al*. Early gastric cancer: 46 cases treated in one surgical department. *Gut*, 1992; 33: 1318.

251 Seto Y, Nagawa H, Muto T. Impact of lymph node metastasis on survival with early gastric cancer. *World J Surg*, 1997; 21: 186.

252 Guadagni S, Reed PI, Johnston BJ *et al*. Early gastric cancer: follow-up after gastrectomy in 159 patients. *Br J Surg*, 1993; 80: 325.

253 Pacelli F, Doglietto GB, Alfieri S *et al*. Survival in early gastric cancer: multivariate analysis in 72 consecutive cases. *Hepatogastroenterology*, 1999; 46: 1223.

254 Zinninger MM, Collins WT. Extension of carcinoma of the stomach into the duodenum and oesophagus. *Ann Surg*, 1949; 130: 557.

255 Fernet P, Azar HA, Stout AP. Intramural (tubal) spread of linitis plastica along the alimentary tract. *Gastroenterology*, 1965; 48: 419.

256 Stout AP. Pathology of carcinoma of the stomach. *Arch Surg*, 1943; 46: 807.

257 Maruyama K, Gunven P, Okabayashi K *et al*. Lymph node metastases of gastric cancer. *Ann Surg*, 1989; 210: 596.

258 Duarte I, Llanos O. Pattern of metastases in intestinal and diffuse types of carcinoma of the stomach. *Hum Pathol*, 1981; 12: 237.

259 Esaki Y, Hirayama R, Hirokawa K. A comparison of patterns of metastasis in gastric cancer by histological type and age. *Cancer*, 1990; 65: 2086.

260 Mori M, Sakaguchi H, Akazawa K *et al*. Correlation between metastatic site, histological type and serum tumour markers of gastric carcinoma. *Hum Pathol*, 1995; 26: 504.

261 Sobin LH, Wittekind CH. *TNM Classification of Malignant Tumours*, 5th edn. UICC. New York: John Wiley, 1997.

262 Setälä LP, Kosma V-M, Marin S *et al*. Prognostic factors in gastric cancer: the value of vascular invasion, mitotic rate and lymphoplasmacytic infiltration. *Br J Cancer*, 1996; 74: 766.

263 Wu CW, Hsieh MC, Lo SS *et al*. Relation of number of positive lymph nodes to the prognosis of patients with primary gastric adenocarcinoma. *Gut*, 1996; 38: 525.

264 Scott N, Quirke P, Dixon MF. Gross examination of the stomach. *J Clin Pathol*, 1992; 45: 952.

265 Dixon MF. *Minimum Dataset for Gastric Cancer Histopathology Reports*. London: Royal College of Pathologists, 2000.

266 Japanese Research Society for Gastric Cancer. *Japanese Classification of Gastric Carcinoma*. Tokyo: Kanehara & Co, 1995.

267 Noguchi Y, Imada T, Matsumoto A *et al*. Radical surgery for gastric cancer. *Cancer*, 1989; 64: 2053.

268 Bizer LS. Adenocarcinoma of the stomach. Current results of treatment. *Cancer*, 1983; 51: 743.

269 Lawrence W Jr, Menck HR, Steele GD Jr, Winchester DP. The National Cancer Data Base Report on Gastric Cancer. *Cancer*, 1995; 75: 1734.

270 Harrison JC, Dean PJ, Van Der Zwaag R *et al*. Adenocarcinoma of the stomach with invasion limited to the muscularis propria. *Hum Pathol*, 1991; 22: 111.

271 Wu C-Y, Yeh H-Z, Shih RT-P, Chen G-H. A clinicopathologic study of mucinous gastric carcinoma including multivariate analysis. *Cancer*, 1998; 83: 1312.

272 Jakl R, Miholic J, Koller R *et al*. Prognostic factors in adenocarcinoma of the cardia. *Am J Surg*, 1995; 169: 316.

273 Graham AJ, Finley RJ, Clifton JC *et al*. Surgical management of adenocarcinoma of the cardia. *Am J Surg*, 1998; 175: 418.

274 Bowrey DJ, Clark GW, Rees BI *et al*. Outcome of oesophagogastric carcinoma in young patients. *Postgrad Med J*, 1999; 75: 22.

275 Lardenoye JE, Kappetein AH, Lagaay MB *et al*. Survival of proximal third carcinoma. *J Surg Oncol*, 1998; 68: 183.

276 Fujii K, Isozaki H, Okajima K *et al*. Clinical evaluation of lymph node metastases in gastric cancer defined by the fifth edition of the TNM classification in comparison with the Japanese system. *Br J Surg*, 1999; 86: 685.

277 Siewert JR, Böttcher K, Stein HJ, Roder JD. Relevant prognostic factors in gastric cancer. *Ann Surg*, 1998; 228: 449.

278 Ochi H, Douglass J, Sandberg AA. Cytogenetic studies in primary gastric cancer. *Cancer Genet Cytogenet*, 1986; 22: 295.

279 Ferti-Passantonopoulou AD, Panani AD, Vlachos JD, Raptis SA. Common cytogenetic findings in gastric cancer. *Cancer Genet Cytogenet*, 1987; 24: 63.

280 Seruca R, Castedo S, Correia C *et al*. Cytogenetic findings in 11 gastric carcinomas. *Cancer Genet Cytogenet*, 1993; 68: 42.

281 Panani AD, Ferti A, Malliaros S, Raptis S. Cytogenetic study of 11 gastric adenocarcinomas. *Cancer Genet Cytogenet*, 1995; 81: 169.

282 Castedo S, Correia C, Gomes P *et al*. Loss of Y-chromosome in gastric carcinoma. Fact or artefact? *Cancer Genet Cytogenet*, 1992; 61: 39.

283 Ming PL, Yuan ZA, Baffa R *et al*. Molecular and cytogenetic characteristics of two cell lines derived from biologically distinct gastric carcinomas. *Am J Hum Genet*, 1992; 51A: 278.

284 Korenaga D, Haraguchi M, Okamura T *et al*. DNA ploidy and tumour invasion in human gastric cancer. *Arch Surg*, 1989; 124: 314.

285 Wyatt JI, Quirke P, Ward DC *et al*. Comparison of histological and flow cytometric parameters in prediction of prognosis in gastric cancer. *J Pathol*, 1989; 158: 195.

286 Brito MI, Filipe MJ, Williams GT *et al*. DNA ploidy in early gastric cancer (T1): a flow cytometric study of 100 European cases. *Gut*, 1993; 34: 230.

287 Nanus DM, Kelsen DP, Niedzwiecki D *et al*. Flow cytometry as a predictive indicator in patients with operable gastric cancer. *J Clin Oncol*, 1989; 7: 1105.

288 Johnson H, Belluco C, Masood S *et al*. The value of flow cytometric analysis in patients with gastric cancer. *Arch Surg*, 1993; 128: 314.

289 Flejou J-F, Muzeau F, Potet F *et al*. Over-expression of the p53 tumour suppressor gene product in esophageal and gastric carcinomas. *Pathol Res Pract*, 1994; 190: 1141.

290 Baba H, Korenaga D, Okamura T *et al*. Prognostic significance of DNA content with special reference to age in gastric cancer. *Cancer*, 1989; 63: 1768.

291 Rugge M, Sonego F, Panozzo M *et al*. Pathology and ploidy in the prognosis of gastric cancer with no extranodal metastases. *Cancer*, 1994; 73: 1127.

292 D'Agnano I, D'Angelo C, Savarese A *et al*. DNA ploidy, proliferative index and epidermal growth factor receptor: expression and prognosis in patients with gastric cancers. *Lab Invest*, 1995; 72: 432.

293 Lemoine NR, Jain S, Silverstre F *et al*. Amplification and over-expression of the EGF receptor and the c-*ERB* B-2 proto-oncogenes in human stomach cancer. *Br J Cancer*, 1991; 64: 79.

294 Ranzani GN, Pellegata NS, Previderz C *et al*. Heterogenous proto-oncogene amplification correlates with tumour progression and presence of metastases in gastric cancer patients. *Cancer Res*, 1990; 50: 7811.

295 Lin S-Y, Chen P-H, Wang C-K *et al*. Mutation analysis of K-*ras* oncogenes in gastroenterologic cancers by the amplified created restriction sites method. *Am J Clin Pathol*, 1993; 100: 686.

296 Ponzetto C, Giordano S, Peverali F *et al*. c-*met* is amplified but not mutated in a cell line with an activated *met* tyrosine kinase. *Oncogene*, 1991; 6: 553.

297 Hattori Y, Odagiri H, Nakatani H *et al*. K-*sam*, an amplified gene in stomach cancer, is a member of the heparin binding growth factor receptor genes. *Proc Natl Acad Sci USA*, 1990; 87: 5983.

298 Shibuya M, Yokota J, Ueyami Y. Amplification and expression of a cellular oncogene (c-*myc*) in human gastric adenocarcinoma cells. *Mol Cell Biol*, 1985; 5: 414.

299 Yoshida MC, Wada M, Satoh H *et al*. Human HST-1 (HSTF-1) gene maps to chromosome band 11q13 and co-amplifies with the INT2 gene in human cancer. *Proc Natl Acad Sci USA*, 1988; 85: 4861.

300 Saegusa M, Takano Y, Okayasu I. Bcl-2 expression and its associated cell kinetics in human gastric carcinomas and intestinal metaplasia. *J Cancer Res Clin Oncol*, 1995; 121: 357.

301 Motomura K, Nishisho I, Takai S-I *et al*. Loss of alleles at loci on chromosome 13 in human primary gastric cancers. *Genomics*, 1988; 2: 180.

302 Sano T, Tsujino P, Yoshida K *et al*. Frequent loss of heterozygosity on chromosomes 1q, 5q and 17p in human gastric carcinomas. *Cancer Res*, 1991; 51: 2926.

303 Uchino S, Tsuda H, Noguchi M *et al*. Frequent loss of heterozygosity at the DCC locus in gastric cancer. *Cancer Res*, 1992; 52: 3099.

304 Ranzani GN, Renault B, Pellegata NS *et al*. Loss of heterozygosity and K-*ras* gene mutations in gastric cancer. *Hum Genet*, 1993; 92: 244.

305 Rhyu M-G, Park W-S, Jung Y-J *et al*. Allelic deletions of MCC/APC and p53 are frequent late events in human gastric carcinogenesis. *Gastroenterology*, 1994; 106: 1584.

306 Schneider BG, Pulitzer DR, Brown RD *et al*. Allelic imbalance in gastric cancer: an affected site on chromosome arm 3p. *Genes Chromosomes Cancer*, 1995; 13: 263.

307 Tamura G, Sakata K, Nishizuka S *et al*. Allelotype of adenoma and differentiated adenocarcinoma of the stomach. *J Pathol*, 1996; 180: 371.

308 Gleeson CM, Sloan JM, McGuigan JA *et al*. Allelotype analysis of adencarcinoma of the gastric cardia. *Br J Cancer*, 1997; 76: 1455.

309 Horii A, Nakatsuru S, Miyoshi Y. The APC gene, responsible for familial adenomatous polyposis, is mutated in human gastric cancer. *Cancer Res*, 1992; 52: 3231.

310 Nakatsura S, Yanagisawa A, Ichii S *et al*. Somatic mutation of the APC gene in gastric cancer: frequent mutations in very well differentiated adenocarcinoma and signet ring cell carcinoma. *Hum Mol Genet*, 1992; 1: 559.

311 Ilyas M, Tomlinson IPM. The interactions of APC, E-cadherin and β-catenin in tumour development and progression. *J Pathol*, 1997; 182: 128.

312 Morin PJ, Sparks AB, Korinek V *et al*. Activation of β-catenin-Tcf signalling in colon cancer by mutations in β-catenin or APC. *Science*, 1997; 275: 1787.

313 Park WS, Oh RH Park R *et al*. Frequent somatic mutations of the β-catenin gene in intestinal-type gastric cancer. *Cancer Res*, 1999; 59: 4257.

314 Seruca R, Castedo S, Correia C *et al*. Cytogenetic findings in 11 gastric carcinomas. *Cancer Genet Cytogenet*, 1993; 68: 42.

315 Luinetti O, Fiocca R, Villani L *et al*. Genetic pattern, histological structure and cellular phenotype in early and advanced gastric cancers: evidence for structure-related genetic subsets and for loss of glandular structure during progression of some tumours. *Hum Pathol*, 1998; 29: 702.

316 Strickler JG, Zheng J, Shu Q *et al*. p53 mutations and microsatellite instability in sporadic gastric cancer: When guardians fail. *Cancer Res*, 1994; 54: 4750.

317 Flejou J-F, Muzeau F, Potet F *et al*. Over-expression of the p53 tumour-suppressor gene product in oesophageal and gastric carcinomas. *Pathol Res Pract*, 1994; 190: 1141.

318 Gulley ML, Pulitzer DR, Eagan PA, Schneider BG. Epstein–Barr infection is an early event in gastric carcinogenesis and is independent of bcl-2 expression and p53 accumulation. *Hum Pathol*, 1996; 27: 20.

319 Gabbert HE, Muller W, Schneiders A *et al*. The relationship of p53 expression to the prognosis of 418 patients with gastric carcinoma. *Cancer*, 1995; 76: 720.

320 Chapel F, Fabiani B, Davi F *et al*. Epstein–Barr virus and gastric carcinoma in Western patients: comparison of pathological parameters and p53 expression in EB-positive and negative tumours. *Histopathology*, 2000; 36: 252.

321 Shiao Y-H, Rugge M, Correa P *et al*. p53 alteration in gastric precancerous lesions. *Am J Pathol*, 1994; 144: 511.

322 Blok P, Craanen ME, Offerhaus GJ *et al*. Molecular alterations in early gastric carcinomas. *Am J Clin Pathol*, 1999; 111: 241.

323 Hurlimann J, Saraga EP. Expression of p53 protein in gastric carcinomas. *Am J Surg Pathol*, 1994; 18: 1247.

324 Martin HM, Filipe MI, Morris RW *et al*. p53 expression and prognosis in gastric carcinoma. *Int J Cancer*, 1992; 50: 859.

325 Joypaul BV, Hopwood D, Newman EL *et al*. The prognostic significance of the accumulation of p53 tumour-suppressor gene protein in gastric adenocarcinoma. *Br J Cancer*, 1994; 69: 943.

326 Wijnhoven BPL, Pignatelli M. E-cadherin-catenin: more than a sticky molecular complex. *Lancet*, 1999; 354: 356.

327 Ilyas M, Tomlinson IMP. The interactions of APC, E-cadherin and β-catenin in tumour development and progression. *J Pathol*, 1997; 182: 128.

328 Jawhari A, Farthing M, Pignatelli M. The importance of the E-cadherin-catenin complex in the maintenance of intestinal epithelial homeostasis is more than intercellular glue? *Gut*, 1997; 41: 581.

329 Gayther SA, Gorringe KL, Ramus SJ *et al*. Identification of germ-line E-cadherin mutations in gastric cancer families of European origin. *Cancer Res*, 1998; 58: 4086.

330 Yoon KA, Ku JL, Yang HK *et al*. Germ-line mutations of E-cadherin gene in Korean familial gastric cancer patients. *J Hum Genet*, 1999; 44: 177.

331 Blok P, Craanen ME, Dekker W, Tytgat GN. Loss of E-cadherin expression in early gastric cancer. *Histopathology*, 1999; 34: 410.

332 Shun CT, Wu MS, Lin JT *et al*. An immunohistochemical study of E-cadherin expression with correlations to clinicopathological features in gastric cancer. *Hepatogastroenterology*, 1998; 45: 944.

333 Machado JC, Soares P, Carneiro F *et al*. E-cadherin gene mutations provide a genetic basis for the phenotypic diagnosis of mixed gastric carcinomas. *Lab Invest*, 1999; 79: 459.

334 Weber JL, May PE. Abundant class of human DNA polymorphisms which can be typed using the polymerase chain reaction. *Am J Hum Genet*, 1989; 44: 388.

335 Aaltonen LA, Peltomaki P, Leach FS *et al*. Clues to the pathogenesis of familial colorectal cancer. *Science*, 1993; 260: 812.

336 Fleisher AS, Esteller M, Wang S *et al*. Hypermethylation of the hMLH1 gene promoter in human gastric cancers with microsatellite instability. *Cancer Res*, 1999; 59: 1090.

337 Seruca R, Santos NR, David L *et al*. Sporadic gastric carcinomas with microsatellite instability display a particular clinicopathologic profile. *Int J Cancer*, 1995; 64: 32.

338 dos Santos NR, Seruca R, Constancia M *et al*. Microsatellite instability at multiple loci in gastric carcinoma: clinicopathologic implications and prognosis. *Gastroenterology*, 1996; 110: 38.

339 Gleeson CM, Sloan JM, McGuigan JA *et al*. Widespread microsatellite instability occurs infrequently in adenocarcinoma of the gastric cardia. *Oncogene*, 1996; 12: 1653.

340 Buonsanti G, Calistri D, Padovan L *et al*. Microsatellite instability in intestinal- and diffuse-type gastric carcinoma. *J Pathol*, 1997; 182: 167.

341 Boswell JT, Helwig EB. Squamous cell carcinoma and adenoacanthoma of the stomach. *Cancer*, 1965; 18: 181.

342 Bonnheim DC, Sarac OK, Fett W. Primary squamous cell carcinoma of the stomach. *Am J Gastroenterol*, 1985; 80: 91.

343 Mori M, Iwashita A, Enjoji M. Squamous cell carcinoma of the stomach: Report of three cases. *Am J Gastroenterol*, 1986; 81: 339.

344 Vaughan WP, Straus FH, Paloyan D. Squamous carcinoma of the stomach after luetic linitis plastica. *Gastroenterology*, 1977; 72: 945.

345 Eaton H, Tennekoon GE. Squamous carcinoma of the stomach following corrosive acid burns. *Br J Surg*, 1972; 59: 382.

346 McLoughlin GA, Cave-Bigley DJ, Tagore V, Kirkham N. Cyclophosphamide and pure squamous cell carcinoma of the stomach. *Br Med J*, 1980; 280: 524.

347 Mori T, Iwashita A, Enjoji M. Adenosquamous carcinoma of the stomach. A clinicopathologic analysis of 28 cases. *Cancer*, 1986; 57: 333.

348 Yoshida K, Manabe T, Tsunoda T *et al*. Early gastric cancer of adenosquamous carcinoma type: Report of a case and review of the literature. *Jpn J Clin Oncol*, 1996; 26: 252.

349 Donald KJ. Adenocarcinoma of the pyloric antrum with extensive squamous differentiation. *J Clin Pathol*, 1967; 20: 136.

350 Mori M, Fukuda T, Enjoji M. Adenosquamous carcinoma of the stomach. Histogenetic and ultrastructural studies. *Gastroenterology*, 1987; 92: 1078.

351 Ishikura H, Kirimoto K, Shamoto M *et al*. Hepatoid adenocarcinoma of the stomach. *Cancer*, 1986; 58: 119.

352 Nagai E, Ueyama T, Yao T, Tsuneyoshi M. Hepatoid adenocarcinoma of the stomach. *Cancer*, 1993; 72: 1827.

353 Chang Y-C, Nagasue N, Kohno H *et al*. Clinicopathologic features and long term results of alpha-feto protein-producing gastric cancer. *Am J Gastroenterol*, 1990; 85: 1480.

354 Petrella T, Montagnon J, Roignot P *et al*. Alpha-fetoprotein-producing gastric adenocarcinoma. *Histopathology*, 1995; 26: 171.

355 Iskikura H, Kishimoto T, Andachi H. Gastrointestinal hepatoid adenocarcinoma: venous permeation and mimicry of hepatocellular carcinoma, a report of four cases. *Histopathology*, 1997; 31: 47.

356 Smith FR, Barkin JS, Hensley G. Choriocarcinoma of the stomach. *Am J Gastroenterol*, 1980; 73: 45.

357 Saigo PE, Sternberg SS, Brigati DJ *et al*. Primary gastric choriocarcinoma. An immunohistological study. *Am J Surg Pathol*, 1981; 5: 333.

358 Yonezawa S, Maruyama I, Tanaka S *et al*. Immunohistochemical localisation of thrombomodulin in chorionic diseases of the uterus and choriocarcinoma of the stomach. *Cancer*, 1988; 62: 569.

359 Krulewski T, Cohen LB. Choriocarcinoma of the stomach: pathogenesis and clinical characteristics. *Am J Gastroenterol*, 1988; 83: 1172.

360 Jindrak K, Bochetto JF, Alpert LI. Primary gastric choriocarcinoma. Case report with review of world literature. *Hum Pathol*, 1976; 7: 595.

361 Watanabe H, Enjoji M, Imai T. Gastric carcinoma with lymphoid stroma. *Cancer*, 1976; 38: 232.

362 Shibata D, Tokunaga M, Uemura Y *et al*. Association of Epstein–Barr virus with undifferentiated gastric carcinomas with intense lymphoid infiltration. *Am J Pathol*, 1991; 139: 469.

363 Minamoto T, Mai M, Watanabe K *et al*. Medullary carcinoma with lymphocytic infiltration of the stomach. *Cancer*, 1990; 66: 945.

364 Wang HH, Wu MS, Shun CT *et al*. Lymphoepithelioma-like carcinoma of the stomach: a subset of gastric carcinoma with distinct clinicopathological features and a high prevalence of Epstein–Barr virus infection. *Hepatogastroenterology*, 1999; 46:214.

365 Chang MS, Kim WH, Kim CW, Kim YI. Epstein–Barr virus in gastric carcinomas with lymphoid stroma. *Histopathology*, 2000; 37: 309.

366 Shibata D, Weiss LM. Epstein–Barr virus-associated gastric adenocarcinoma. *Am J Pathol*, 1992; 140: 769.

367 Capella C, Frigerio B, Cornaggio M. Gastric parietal cell carcinoma—a newly recognised entity: light microscopic and ultrastructural features. *Histopathology*, 1984; 8: 813.

368 Creutzfeldt W. The achlorhydria–carcinoid sequence. Role of gastrin. *Digestion*, 1988; 39: 61.

369 Modlin IM, Sandor A, Tang LH *et al*. A forty year analysis of 265 gastric carcinoids. *Am J Gastroenterol*, 1997; 92: 633.

370 Watson RGP, Johnston CF, Sloan JM *et al*. The frequency of gastrointestinal endocrine tumours in a well defined population—Northern Ireland 1970–1985. *Q J Med New Series*, 1989; 72: 647.

371 Modlin IM, Sandor A. An analysis of 8305 cases of carcinoid tumour. *Cancer*, 1997; 79: 813.

372 Rindi G. Clinicopathologic aspects of gastric neuroendocrine tumours. *Am J Surg Pathol*, 1995; Suppl 1: S20.

373 Gough DB, Thompson GB, Crotty TB *et al*. Diverse clinical and pathologic features of gastric carcinoid and the relevance of hypergastrinaemia. *World J Surg*, 1994; 18: 473.

374 Rindi G, Luinetti O, Cornaggia M *et al*. Three subtypes of gastric argyrophil carcinoid and the gastric neuroendocrine carcinoma: a clinicopathologic study. *Gastroenterology*, 1993; 104: 994.

375 Gilligan CJ, Lawton GP, Tang LH *et al*. Gastric carcinoid tumours: the biology and therapy of an enigmatic and controversial lesion. *Am J Gastroenterol*, 1995; 90: 338.

376 Bordi C, Yu J-Y, Baggi MT *et al*. Gastric carcinoids and their precursor lesions. *Cancer*, 1991; 67: 663.

377 Rindi G, Bordi C, Rappel S *et al*. Gastric carcinoids and neuroendocrine carcinomas: pathogenesis, pathology and behaviour. *World J Surg*, 1996; 20: 168.

378 Davies MG, O'Dowd G, McEntee GP, Hennessy TPJ. Primary gastric carcinoids. A view on management. *Br J Surg*, 1990; 77: 1013.

379 Harvey RF. Spontaneous resolution of multifocal gastric enterochromaffin-like cell carcinoid tumours. *Lancet*, 1988; i: 821.

380 Bordi C, D'Adda T, Azzoni C *et al*. Hypergastrinaemia and gastric enterochromaffin-like cells. *Am J Surg Pathol*, 1995; 19 (Suppl 1): S8.

381 Sjoblom S-M, Sipponen P, Karonen S-L, Jarvinen HJ. Mucosal argyrophil cells in pernicious anaemia and upper gastrointestinal carcinoid tumours. *J Clin Pathol*, 1989; 42: 371.

382 Solcia E, Bordi C, Creutzfeldt W *et al*. Histopathological classification of non antral gastric endocrine growths in man. *Digestion*, 1988; 41: 185.

383 Lamberts R, Creutzfeldt W, Strüber HG *et al*. Long term omeprazole therapy in paptic ulcer disease: gastrin, endocrine cell growth and gastritis. *Gastroenterology*, 1993; 104: 1356.

384 Eissele R, Brunner G, Simon B *et al*. Gastric mucosa during treatment with lansoprazole: *Helicobacter pylori* is a risk factor for argyrophil cell hyperplasia. *Gastroenterology*, 1997; 112: 707.

385 Kulke MH, Mayer RJ. Carcinoid tumours. *N Engl J Med*, 1999; 340: 858.

386 Feurle GE. Argryophil cell hyperplasia and a carcinoid tumour in the stomach of a patient with sporadic Zollinger–Ellison syndrome. *Gut*, 1994; 35: 275.

387 Cadiot G, Laurent-Puig P, Thuille B *et al*. Is the multiple endocrine neoplasia type-I gene a suppressor for fundic argyrophil tumours in the Zollinger–Ellison syndrome? *Gastroenterology*, 1993; 105: 579.

388 Bordi C, Falchetti A, Azzoni C *et al*. Aggressive forms of gastric neuroendocrine tumours in multiple endocrine neoplasia type I. *Am J Surg Pathol*, 1997; 21: 1075.

389 Klöppel G, Heitz Ph U, Capella C, Solcia E. The spectrum and classification of gastric and duodenal neuroendocrine tumours. *Curr Diag Pathol*, 1995; 2: 10.

390 Sweeney EC, McDonnell L. Atypical gastric carcinoids. *Histopathology*, 1980; 4: 215.

391 Matsui K, Jin XM, Kitagawa M, Miwa A. Clinicopathologic features of neuroendocrine carcinomas of the stomach. *Arch Pathol Lab Med*, 1998; 122: 1010.

392 Matsui K, Kitagawa M, Miwa A *et al*. Small cell carcinoma of the stomach: a clinicopathological study of 17 cases. *Am J Gastroenterol*, 1991; 86: 1167.

393 Chejfec G, Gould VE. Malignant gastric neuroendocrinomas. *Hum Pathol*, 1977; 8: 433.

394 Yang GCH, Rotterdam H. Mixed (composite) glandular-endocrine cell carcinoma of the stomach. *Am J Surg Pathol*, 1991; 15: 592.

395 Bonar SF, Sweeney EC. The prevalence, prognostic significance and hormonal content of endocrine cells in gastric cancer. *Histopathology*, 1986; 10: 53.

396 Caruso ML, Pilato FP, D'Adda T *et al*. Composite carcinoid–adenocarcinoma of the stomach associated with multiple gastric carcinoids and nonantral gastric atrophy. *Cancer*, 1989; 64: 1534.

397 Menuck LS, Amberg JR. Metastatic disease involving the stomach. *Am J Dig Dis*, 1975; 20: 903.

398 Green LK. Haematogenous metastases to the stomach. A review of 67 cases. *Cancer*, 1990; 65: 1596.

399 Schwarz RE, Klimstra DS, Turnbull AD. Metastatic breast cancer masquerading as gastrointestinal primary. *Am J Gastroenterol*, 1998; 93: 111.

400 Cormier WJ, Gaffey TA, Welch JM *et al*. Linitis plastica caused by metastatic lobular carcinoma of the breast. *Mayo Clin Proc*, 1980; 55: 747.

15 Non-epithelial tumours of the stomach

Although the overall incidence of non-epithelial tumours of the stomach is low compared with epithelial tumours, the stomach is the commonest site, in the gut, for both primary malignant lymphoma and gastrointestinal stromal tumours (GISTs). Furthermore, there is evidence that primary gastric lymphoma is increasing in prevalence in Western communities [1].

Tumours of lymphoid tissue

Definition

Defining what constitutes a benign lymphoid proliferation and a malignant lymphoma in the gastrointestinal tract is fraught with difficulties because many apparently benign lesions represent malignant lymphoma when molecular analysis is undertaken: on the other hand many low-grade lymphomas of the stomach are characterized by an indolent behaviour. There are also difficulties in strictly defining what constitutes a primary gastrointestinal lymphoma. Lymphoma in the gastrointestinal tract is most commonly due to secondary involvement from nodal disease: in one study in which gastroscopy was performed at the time of diagnosis of primary nodal lymphoma, 25% of cases showed evidence of gastric involvement [2]. It is eminently clear that strict criteria for the definition of primary gastrointestinal lymphoma are required. The original and well promulgated criteria, developed by Dawson, Cornes and Morson [3], required that the lymphoma be restricted to the gut with only local lymph node involvement. More recently these criteria have been considered too strict and would exclude lesions of undoubted primary gastrointestinal origin [4]. Most would now suggest that an appropriate working definition for primary gastrointestinal lymphoma would be when the tumour presents with the bulk of the disease in the gastrointestinal tract [5]. At the same time, it is important to recognize that, whilst most gastrointestinal lymphomas do have their place in standard lymphoma classifications, they represent a different spectrum of lymphoma subtypes. When considering a lymphoma to be primary in the gut, all attention should be paid to the lymphoma subtype, ensuring that it does represent one of the particular subtypes characteristic of the gut.

Incidence and distribution

The gastrointestinal tract is the commonest site for extranodal malignant lymphoma. In Western populations, it accounts for 30–50% of extranodal disease [6,7]. Primary gastrointestinal lymphoma accounts for between 4% and 18% of all non-Hodgkin's lymphomas [7]. Hodgkin's disease is vanishingly rare as a primary tumour in the gut, and the great majority of these tumours represent non-Hodgkin's lymphoma. There is considerable worldwide variation in the incidence of gastrointestinal lymphoma, with the highest incidence in the Mediterranean and Middle East due to a marked increase in incidence of immunoproliferative small intestinal disease (IPSID). Furthermore there are considerable regional variations, possibly in turn related to variations in *Helicobacter* colonization. In north-eastern Italy, the incidence of gastric lymphoma is more than 10 times higher than that in England and Wales [8]. In Western communities, the stomach accounts for 60% of all primary gastrointestinal lymphomas whilst 30% occur in the small intestine [6]. Oesophageal and colorectal primary lymphoma are distinctly rare, with the latter only accounting for between 5% and 10% of these tumours.

Staging of gastrointestinal lymphoma

There is relatively little agreement on the most appropriate staging system for gastrointestinal lymphoma. In some sites, notably the small and large bowel, simple staging systems such as a modified Dukes system have been utilized [9,10]. However, it is generally accepted that modifications of the Ann Arbor system, notably the Musshoff modification [11], are probably the most applicable. This system combines information on involvement of the wall of the gut (stage I_E) with local lymph node involvement (stage II_{1E}), regional lymph nodes (stage II_{2E}), thoracic lymph nodes (stage III) and splenic involvement (stage III_S). Stage IV refers to dissemination to bone marrow and non-lymphoid viscera. In recent larger studies of prognosis, this staging system provides useful information concerning treatment and prognosis although, more recently, modifications to the Musshoff system have been proposed [12].

Mucosa-associated lymphoid tissue (MALT)

Because the majority of primary lymphomas of the stomach arise from mucosa-associated lymphoid tissue (MALT), it is appropriate to consider this concept here. MALT was first conceptualized by Isaacson and Wright [13] who noted that many primary gastrointestinal malignant lymphomas recapitulated the histomorphological features of lymphoid aggregates in the gut, particularly Peyer's patches and other lymphoid tissue represented by MALT. Thus the MALT lymphomas are characterized by neoplastic marginal zone cells, with a centrocyte-like morphology (Fig. 15.1) (formerly termed centrocyte-like cells) [14] often around reactive germinal centres. There is a marked polymorphism to many of these tumours with evidence of plasma cell differentiation and blast cell transformation. Two characteristic features of the neoplastic marginal zone cells, once again recapitulating physiological MALT, is their ability to infiltrate epithelium, producing the characteristic lymphoepithelial lesions (LELs), in a similar way to the physiological involvement of dome epithelium seen in Peyer's patches (Fig. 15.1) [4]. Furthermore the neoplastic marginal zone cells also involve and infiltrate the germinal centre. Eventually both these structures, in MALT-type lymphoma, become overrun by the neoplastic lymphoid cells.

Such a concept of marginal zone lymphoma arising in lymphoid tissue is easy to comprehend in the intestine but less so in the stomach, which is usually devoid of any lymphoid tissue. However there is now compelling evidence that the importation of lymphoid tissue, primarily by chronic active gastritis induced by *Helicobacter pylori*, provides the seed bed for MALT lymphoma in the stomach. The links between chronic *H. pylori* infection and primary gastric lymphoma are

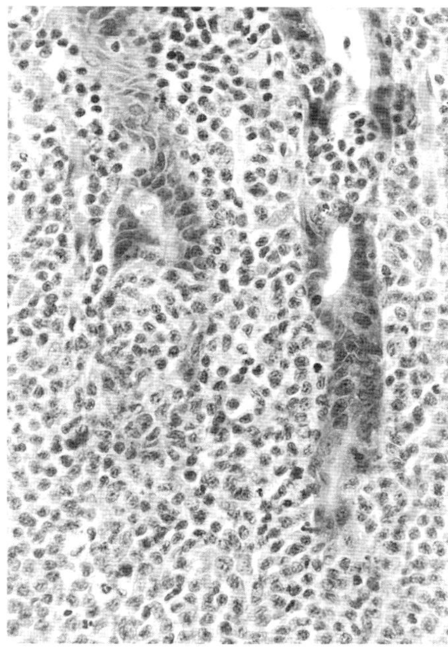

Fig. 15.1 A low-grade primary B-cell lymphoma of the stomach. Although the cell population is polymorphic, the predominant cell is the intermediate-sized lymphoid cell with centrocyte-like morphology. These cells are seen invading the crypt epithelium and destroying it, to produce lymphoepithelial lesions.

extremely strong and may account for an increasing prevalence of gastric lymphoma in recent years [1].

The classification of primary gastrointestinal lymphomas

From the previous discussion, it can be seen that nodal lymphoma classifications, such as the updated Kiel [15] and the Working Formulation [16], both of which were developed prior to the wide acceptance of the MALT concept, may not be entirely appropriate for classifying primary gastrointestinal lymphomas. The REAL classification, which combines both European and American concepts of lymphoma classification, is now widely promulgated and used: it does incorporate all those lymphomas that are commonly seen as primary lymphomas of the gut [17]. However, some reorganization of the REAL classification is appropriate to reflect the fact that the commoner lymphomas in the gut are certainly not those that are common in nodal disease. Furthermore, Hodgkin's disease is exquisitely rare as a primary tumour of the gut. Table 15.1 represents a reasonable classification of primary gastrointestinal lymphomas based on a reworking of the REAL classification.

It is appropriate to consider the low- and high-grade MALT lymphomas together as there is good evidence that transformation from low- to high-grade MALT-type lymphoma occurs: in many high-grade tumours, areas representing

Table 15.1 The classification of primary gastrointestinal lymphomas.

B cell
MALT-type lymphoma (marginal zone lymphoma)
Low grade
High grade
Immunoproliferative small intestinal disease (IPSID)
Low grade
High grade
Mantle cell lymphoma (malignant lymphomatous polyposis)
Burkitt-type lymphoma
Types corresponding to nodal equivalents
Follicular lymphoma
Other lymphomas
Immunodeficiency-related lymphoproliferative disease
Post-transplant immunoproliferative disease
High-grade lymphoma complicating AIDS
Congenital immunodeficiency lymphoproliferative disease
T cell
Enteropathy-associated T-cell lymphoma
Other T-cell lymphomas not associated with enteropathy

low-grade lymphoma can be readily identified. Current available information suggests that there are close parallels between low-grade and high-grade MALT-type lymphoma and that these should be considered part of the same spectrum. In a similar way, immunoproliferative small intestinal disease (IPSID), a comparatively common lymphoma in Mediterranean and Middle Eastern communities, is a MALT-type lymphoma (usually of the small bowel) characterized by a relatively indolent early natural history and by production of abnormal immunoglobulin heavy chains. Mantle cell lymphoma, which presents clinically as multifocal intestinal disease known as lymphomatous polyposis but may also involve the stomach, and Burkitt-type lymphoma, are also important primary lymphomas of the gut. Of the lymphomas more commonly associated with nodal disease, follicular lymphoma is probably the commonest in the gut and is most readily seen in the terminal ileum. The gastrointestinal tract is a relatively common site for immunodeficiency-associated lymphoproliferative disease. T-cell lymphomas are much less common than their B-cell counterparts in the gut. In the stomach and colorectum, they are described but are distinctly unusual. In the small bowel, they constitute about 40% of primary lymphomas at this site [10], largely because of their strong association with coeliac disease [4].

Benign lymphoid proliferations

It is notoriously difficult, often, to differentiate florid but benign lymphoid hyperplasia in the stomach from malignant lymphoma on morphological grounds alone. This accounts for the development of the term 'pseudolymphoma'. As immunohistochemistry and molecular studies can now convincingly differentiate, in most cases, between reactive states and low-grade lymphoma, we believe it is no longer appropriate to use this term. However, it is important to recognize that florid lymphoid hyperplasia does occur in the stomach. As already indicated, the stomach is devoid of lymphoid tissue in its normal state and the presence of lymphoid tissue demands its importation into the stomach by various pathophysiological mechanisms. This is usually due to infection with *H. pylori*. Chronic and severe infection of the stomach results in chronic active gastritis and the production of lymphoid follicles with germinal centres. These may have prominent marginal zones and, on occasion, some marginal zone cells are seen to infiltrate the juxtaposed glands creating small lymphoepithelial lesions [4]. These are specifically located adjacent to the lymphoid follicle: this *H. pylori*-related chronic follicular gastritis lacks the sheet-like morphology of MALT-type lymphoma and the lymphoepithelial lesions are geographically restricted within the mucosa. These features help to differentiate chronic follicular gastritis from low-grade MALT-type lymphoma, although on occasion this distinction may be difficult and may demand either further biopsies or even molecular analysis.

Chronic peptic ulcer of the stomach may be associated with lymphoid follicular hyperplasia. This may also be a reflection of concurrent *H. pylori* infection although often the lymphoid hyperplasia extends deeply into the submucosa. Differentiation from malignant lymphoma is relatively easy as the other features of peptic ulceration, including scarring of the muscularis propria, are present and the lymphoid follicles show normal cellular relationships and lack a marginal zone [4]. It should be noted that primary follicular lymphoma does occur in the stomach but is an extremely rare neoplasm: most cases represent secondary involvement of the stomach.

Primary low-grade MALT lymphoma

These indolent tumours of the stomach are the most common lymphoma in the gut, although their true incidence is difficult to define as many of these lesions have been previously regarded as 'pseudolymphomas'. They account, in most series, for at least half of all primary gastric lymphomas [18]. There is evidence of an increasing incidence [1]. There is strong evidence of a powerful relationship between *H. pylori* gastritis and these lymphomas [19]. Indeed some have suggested that these lymphomas only occur in a milieu of *H. pylori* gastritis. Although other diseases, notably autoimmune disease, can cause importation of lymphoid tissue, it would seem that the great majority of lymphomas do occur on a basis of *H. pylori* infection. This is supported by epidemiological [20], cell biological [21] and therapeutic studies [22], the latter demonstrating that treatment of *H. pylori* infection can lead to regression of the lymphoma.

Clinical features

As would be expected in a tumour that requires chronic inflammatory activity induced by *H. pylori*, the peak incidence of gastric low-grade MALT lymphoma is in the sixth and seventh decades. Men are more commonly affected than women but with a less marked sex inequality (approximately 1.5 : 1) than is seen in gastric carcinoma. Symptoms are non-specific with non-ulcer dyspepsia being the most common presentation. Nausea and vomiting also occur. Systemic symptoms, including weight loss, may presage more advanced disease, a relatively uncommon feature.

Endoscopic and macroscopic features

The antrum is the most common site for primary low-grade MALT lymphoma but any part of the stomach can be involved. The mucosa involved by this lymphoma is often relatively flat but has a somewhat infiltrated appearance: often the endoscopist demonstrates relatively subtle features such as nodulation, rugal fold thickening and/or non-specific 'gastritis' (Fig. 15.2). By the same token, macroscopic examination by the pathologist at the time of resection may be relatively unrewarding, with a flat, somewhat firm and infiltrated lesion being the only demonstrable abnormality. Deep infiltration, mass formation and ulceration (Figs 15.3 & 15.4) do all occur but they are usually not a substantial feature of this disease. One particular property of low-grade MALT lymphoma of the stomach is multifocality (Fig. 15.4). Whilst there may be a predominant lesion, small foci of lymphoma can often be demonstrated remote from the main mass. Mapping techniques on cases in which gastrectomy has been performed have demonstrated multifocal disease, often with lymphoma foci only demonstrable microscopically [23]. This multifocality is of importance in those cases treated by surgery. No demonstrable tumour at resection lines, in a partial gastrectomy specimen, does not guarantee complete excision. The diagnosis of low-grade MALT lymphoma of the stomach demands extensive biopsy mapping at the time of endoscopy to detect such multifocality. If surgery is contemplated, the multifocality may well be an indication for total gastrectomy.

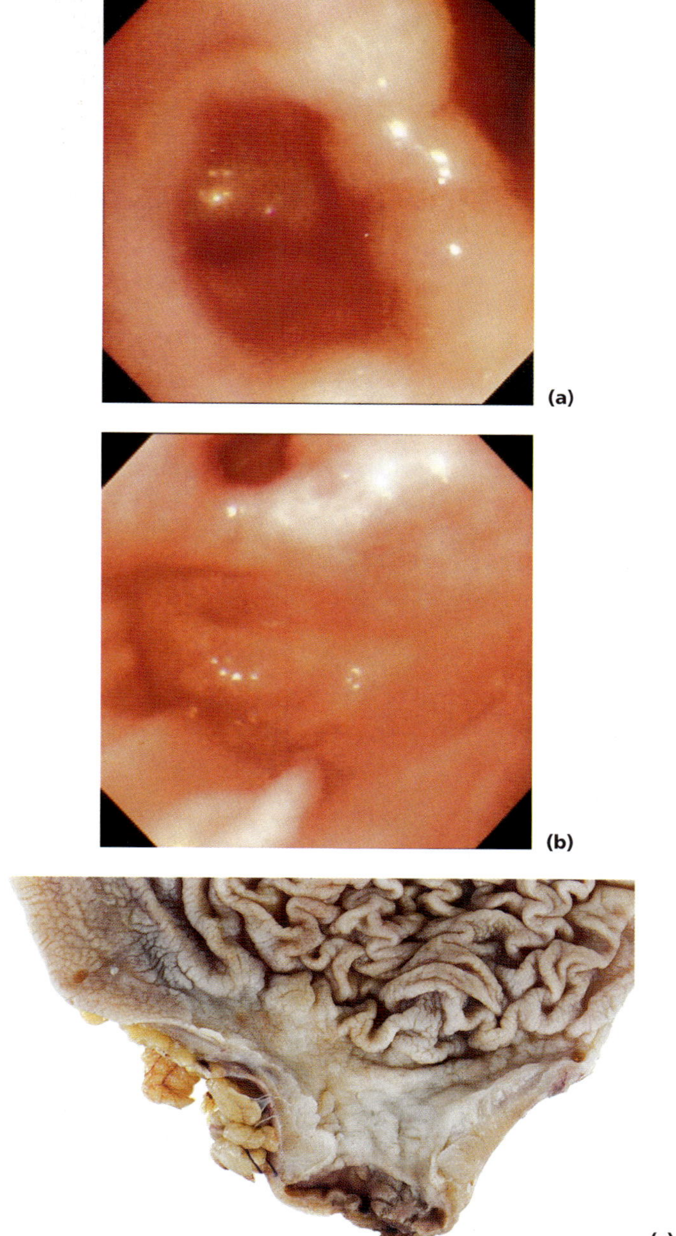

Fig. 15.2 Primary low-grade B-cell lymphoma of the stomach treated by antibiotic therapy. (a) The endoscopic appearances of the lymphoma: there is thickening of the rugae and a deep penetrating ulcer (centrally). (b) After antibiotic treatment for *Helicobacter pylori*, there is gross regression of the lesion with a relatively superficial ulcer remaining. The pylorus is seen above. (c) After resection, only a small residuum of lymphoma was demonstrated in the scarred area seen in the gastrectomy specimen.

Microscopic features

The histopathology of low-grade MALT lymphoma closely recapitulates the physiological appearances of gut lymphoid tissue such as in Peyer's patches (Fig. 15.5). Reactive lymphoid follicles with germinal centres are a prominent feature: interspersed between these are sheets of neoplastic marginal zone cells [24]. These cells have small to intermediate-sized nuclei that show prominent cleaving with moderate amounts of cytoplasm. The proportion of cells with these features varies. In some lymphomas there is a relative monotonous population of these cells whilst in others there is much more polymorphism, with many of the neoplastic cells resembling small lymphocytes and some showing monocytoid features [4]. Cells with plasmacytoid features are also present in 30% of cases and can be so predominant that the lymphomatous infil-

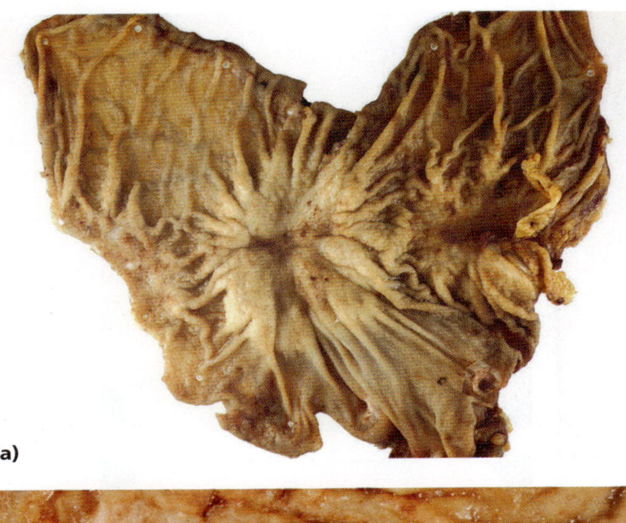

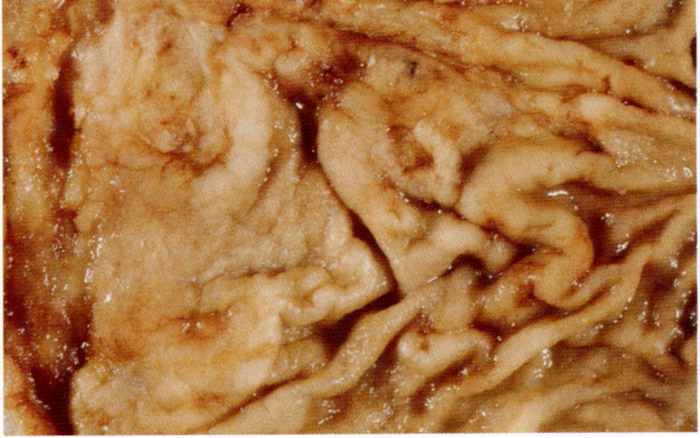

Fig. 15.3 Two cases of primary low-grade B-cell lymphoma of the stomach. (a) A total gastrectomy specimen showing a central tumour with heaped-up mucosa, which is largely intact, although there is central ulceration. (b) A higher-power view of another case shows the typical thickening of the rugae, which appear pale and infiltrated.

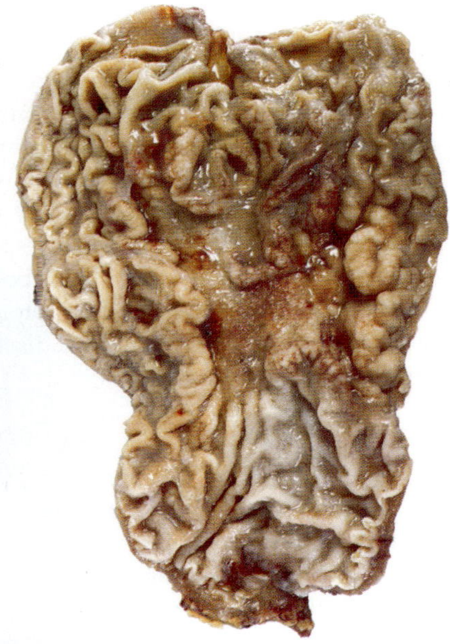

Fig. 15.4 A total gastrectomy specimen showing multicentric ulcerating lesions. Multicentricity is a typical feature of primary B-cell lymphoma of the stomach, one that usually means that total gastrectomy is the appropriate surgical procedure for this disease.

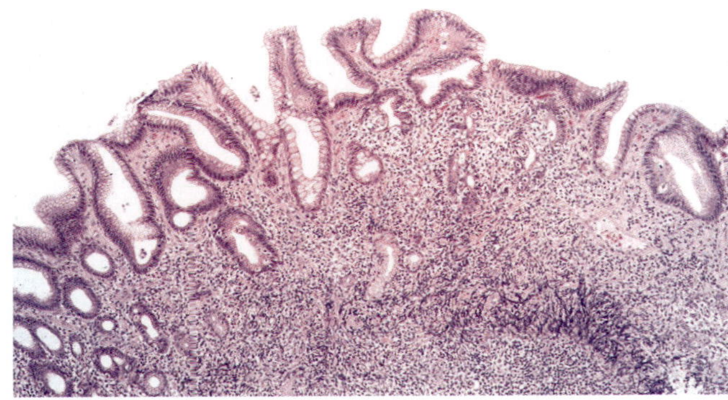

Fig. 15.5 Low-grade B-cell lymphoma of the stomach. The lamina propria is filled with lymphoid cells, which have partly destroyed a lymphoid follicle (lower right).

trate can be overlooked. These plasma cells characteristically have much intracytoplasmic immunoglobulin, which may be so pronounced that the nucleus becomes pushed to one side and the cell resembles the signet ring cells of diffuse-type gastric adenocarcinoma [25].

Within the infiltrate there are usually transformed cells present and these have a morphology similar to that of follicle centre cell blasts (centroblasts). These transformed cells are present in varying proportions and are usually diffusely admixed with the smaller lymphoid cells. Non-neoplastic reactive cells are also a distinctive feature of these lymphomas: small T lymphocytes, histiocytes and eosinophils are usually demonstrable, although only the former are usually present in substantial numbers. The neoplastic marginal zone cells, or centrocyte-like cells [14], have the ability to involve and infiltrate the gastrointestinal epithelium and this, once again, reproduces the physiology of marginal zone cells in lymphoid follicles (Figs 15.1 & 15.6). This infiltration creates the highly distinctive lymphoepithelial lesions, in which centrocyte-like cells displace and destroy the epithelium (Fig. 15.6) [26]. Characteristically the epithelium shows a striking eosinophilic change in the cytoplasm indicative of destruction [27]. These features allow the differentiation of true lymphoepithelial lesions from the reactive involvement of the epithelium seen in chronic follicular gastritis. Lymphoepithelial lesions are highlighted by cytokeratin immunohistochemistry that serves to demonstrate the destruction of epithelial structures. The reactive lymphoid follicles and germinal centres are such a composite part of the lymphoma and they produce a further highly characteristic feature of the disease [24]. The margins of the germinal centres become infiltrated and obscured by the

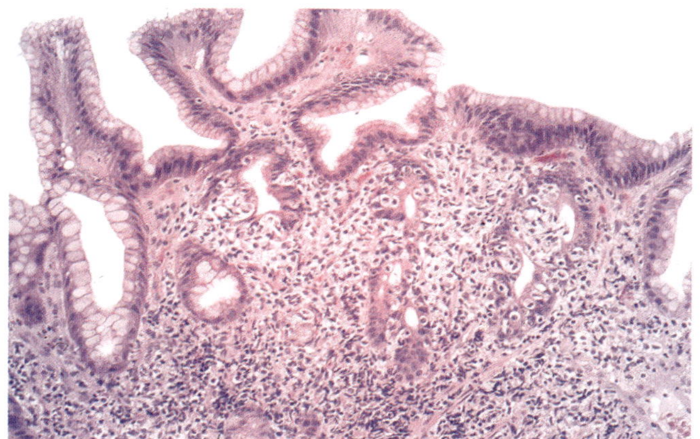

Fig. 15.6 Higher-power view of the low-grade B-cell lymphoma of the stomach shown in Fig. 15.5. Lymphoepithelial lesions are well seen centrally and at right.

neoplastic cells, producing a moth-eaten appearance in the germinal centre. Eventually the lymphoid follicle becomes completely overrun and destroyed by the lymphoma. This colonization of reactive lymphoid follicles produces the nodularity characteristic of low-grade MALT lymphoma.

Spread

The majority of these lymphomas are restricted to the gastric wall at the time of presentation [28]. The tumour predominantly involves the mucosa and submucosa but may spread into the muscularis propria and less commonly into the subserosa. Most cases are therefore stage I_E [29]. Local lymph node involvement (stage II_E) occurs in a minority of cases. Initially involved lymph nodes show enlargement of marginal zones, followed by interfollicular expansion and ultimately complete ablation of the normal architecture. Most of the histopathological features of the primary tumour, namely colonization of follicles, polymorphism, plasma cell differentiation and monocytoid differentiation, can be seen in lymph node involvement. Distant spread of this disease is distinctly uncommon. Spread to the spleen, particularly the marginal zone, is perhaps the commonest manifestation of distant spread whereas involvement of the small bowel, bone marrow and liver have been observed [27].

Immunohistochemistry and molecular pathology

Low-grade MALT lymphoma shows the immunophenotype of marginal zone cells and the tumour cells express CD20, CD21, CD35 and occasionally CD43. Light chain restriction is usually demonstrable and cytokeratin immunohistochemistry is also useful to demonstrate the epithelial destruction associated with lymphoepithelial lesions [27]. The molecular abnormalities that characterize this lymphoma include B-cell monoclonality [30], monoclonal rearrangement of the *IgH* gene demonstrable by PCR methodology [30,31], replication error phenotype [27] and trisomy 3 [32–34]. *p53* and *bcl-2* overexpression and gene mutation are features of high-grade transformation [27].

Treatment and prognosis

Although many reports suggest that gastrectomy with or without adjuvant therapy is the most appropriate treatment of primary gastric lymphoma [35–39], many of these series are biased towards high-grade lymphoma and do not include many cases of low-grade disease. There is now compelling evidence that low-grade lymphoma will regress in response to antibiotic therapy for *H. pylori* (Fig. 15.2) [40,41]: regression has been demonstrated by imaging and molecular methodology [42]. It would now appear undeniable that initial treatment of low-grade malignant lymphoma of the stomach should be antibiotic therapy assuming that appropriate imaging (particularly endoluminal ultrasound) is available to survey the wall of the stomach. Some cases do not respond to antibiotic therapy and these may benefit from local radiotherapy [43]. Chemotherapy may also be of benefit for advanced cases [44]. Stage is the most important determinant of long-term prognosis [45]. In general, low-grade MALT-type lymphoma is of early stage and has an excellent long-term prognosis when confined to the mucosa and submucosa [42,46]. It would also appear that tumour size is important [42].

Despite the evidence that *H. pylori* eradication therapy may lead to regression of low-grade MALT lymphoma of the stomach, it is uncertain whether all cases will show regression, whether those cases that show complete remission will stay in remission and, worryingly, whether eradication of the low-grade neoplastic clone may allow the expansion of a more aggressive high-grade neoplastic clone. More recent evidence would suggest that *H. pylori* eradication therapy leads to tumour regression in between 60% and 92% of cases [19]. With this in mind, the appropriate management of this tumour would be to treat *H. pylori* and survey the stomach, particularly with PCR-based clonality analysis, which has been suggested as a useful adjunct to histological surveillance [47]. Surveillance should also involve adequate imaging, perhaps most usefully by endoluminal ultrasound. At the same time, assessment of the stomach should include multiple biopsies to look for multifocality and to fully assess the stomach, at the time of diagnosis. If there is early relapse despite this treatment, then surgery and/or radiotherapy and chemotherapy should be considered. The value of surgery for this disease remains uncertain and should always be carefully considered [48]. In terms of prognosis, only very occasional surveys report survival rates with cases restricted for low-grade lymphoma and with specific treatment protocols. The series of Cogliatti is perhaps most relevant: they report a 91% 5-year survival rate and a 75% 10-year survival rate for low-grade primary gastric lymphoma [35].

There is evidence that *Helicobacter* colonization may disappear as lymphomas become more advanced [49]. It would also appear that the growth of lymphoma is sustained by *H. pylori* [50]. Further substantiating the relationship between *H. pylori* and lymphoma, there are now published cases of the synchronous and metachronous coexistence of primary malignant lymphoma and adenocarcinoma in the stomach [32].

Whilst the currently available literature would indicate that low-grade MALT lymphoma is the commonest form of lymphoma in the stomach, that it responds favourably to *Helicobacter* treatment and that it has an excellent prognosis, some caution is appropriate. Many of these reports derive from tertiary referral centres and it has been intimated that, in secondary referral centres, the spectrum of gastric lymphoma may well be different and that many patients will have bulk disease and indeed many will have high-grade lymphomas [51]. It may be that these patient groups respond poorly to *H. pylori* eradication therapy and may benefit from more aggressive treatment regimens.

High-grade B-cell lymphoma

In many large series of primary gastric lymphoma, high-grade tumours outnumber low-grade tumours [29,35–37,44]. It has been argued that this may not be a true reflection as many cases of low-grade lymphoma, in the time frame concerned, may have been regarded as pseudolymphoma [4]. A further problem is the lack of a clear definition of what constitutes high-grade MALT-type malignant lymphoma. Certainly a predominance of blast cells would fulfil the criteria for high-grade tumours but there remain cases where the blast cells are prominent but not predominant. In practice, the distinction is usually fairly obvious, particularly when allied to the endoscopic, macroscopic and staging features. A practical histological definition would be that a high-grade malignant lymphoma demonstrates sheets of transformed blast cells, whether accompanied by a low-grade cellular component or not (Fig. 15.7) [27]. Whether all diffuse large B-cell lymphomas (when classified as such in the REAL system) [17] represent high-grade MALT lymphoma when primary in the stomach is uncertain and controversial. As many are associated with typical low-grade components and as there is good evidence that most high-grade lymphomas are associated with *H. pylori* infection [20], it seems reasonable to consider all of these tumours as high-grade MALT lymphomas if histological, immunohistochemical and molecular features are compatible.

Clinical features

The median age range of high-grade tumours is slightly higher than for low-grade tumours, at 65 years. A male predominance is also seen. High-grade lymphomas are associated with more systemic symptoms and common presentations include abdominal pain, weight loss and gastrointestinal bleeding.

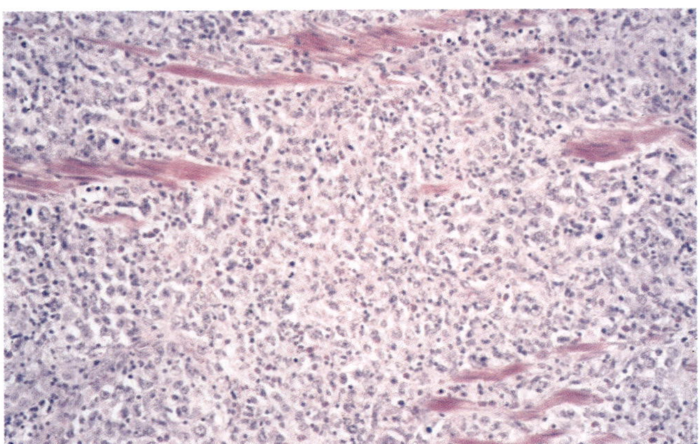

Fig. 15.7 High-grade B-cell lymphoma of the stomach showing sheets of transformed cells destroying muscularis propria.

Endoscopic and macroscopic features

High-grade lymphoma is usually, but not exclusively, associated with a mass lesion in the stomach. The antrum is the commonest site but no part of the stomach is immune. Mass lesions are likely to show ulceration but occasionally more diffuse infiltration with an intact mucosa is seen. Unlike low-grade tumours, local lymph node involvement is common and at least 50% of tumours will be at least stage II_E [35,37].

Microscopic features

High-grade MALT lymphoma, by definition, demonstrates sheets of transformed cells (Fig. 15.7). These have a morphology similar to centroblasts although nucleoli are often less conspicuous [4]. Lymphoepithelial lesions are formed by the transformed cells but they are less conspicuous than in low-grade disease. Equally, lymphoid follicles may be present but these are often destroyed, along with any low-grade component, by the high-grade neoplasm.

Many high-grade tumours will demonstrate a focal low-grade component suggesting transformation from such a lesion. A characteristic feature is that the tumour cells infiltrate between glands with little evidence of glandular destruction. This is a useful diagnostic feature as it helps to differentiate high-grade malignant lymphoma from poorly differentiated, diffuse-type adenocarcinoma and in particular the carcinoma variant, possibly linked to Epstein–Barr virus (EBV) infection, known as lymphoepithelioma-like carcinoma [52]. Whilst transformed cells, like centroblasts, usually predominate, occasional cases show large, bizarre and often multinucleated cells.

Immunohistochemistry and molecular pathology

The transformed cells of high-grade MALT lymphoma often contain plentiful intracytoplasmic immunoglobulin, usually

IgM [53]. Tumour cells express CD20 but often lack other distinguishing lymphocytic markers. Transformed high-grade lymphoma demonstrates the same immunoglobulin gene rearrangement as its low-grade component, strengthening the view that these tumours do represent MALT-type lymphoma [54]. c-*myc* mutation is a characteristic feature of these tumours [27], as are *p53* overexpression and gene mutation [55,56] and *bcl*-6 hypermutation and gene rearrangement [57,58].

Spread, treatment and prognosis

There is no doubt that high-grade lymphomas show a more advanced stage, case for case, than their low-grade counterparts and that their prognosis is worse [29,35,43,59]. However, it is clear that even high-grade lymphoma has a relatively good prognosis compared to lymphoma arising at other sites and compared to gastric adenocarcinoma. For instance, 5-year survival rates of 73% (for transformed high-grade disease) and 56% for primary high-grade lymphoma seem representative [35]. Treatment is primarily surgical [29] but there is evidence that adjuvant therapy, both radiotherapy and chemotherapy, can enhance survival rates [43,59].

Other primary lymphomas

Once lymphoid tissue has been imported into the stomach, either by *H. pylori* infection or by autoimmune pathology, there is no theoretical reason why any type of lymphoma should not arise there. In practice, MALT-type lymphomas undoubtedly predominate, notwithstanding the uncertainties in classification of some primary high-grade lymphomas. Why it is that common nodal lymphomas, such as follicular lymphoma, are so unusual in the stomach is entirely unknown. There are reports of other lymphoma subtypes arising in the stomach. Primary T-cell lymphoma has been described, particularly associated with human T-lymphotropic virus-1 (HTLV-1) infection [60,61], which appears to worsen their already poor prognosis [60]. Epitheliotropism is a characteristic feature of primary T-cell lymphoma of the stomach and can potentially mimic lymphoepithelial lesions of primary low-grade MALT lymphoma [62]. Most T-cell lymphomas show a helper–inducer phenotype although occasional examples of suppressor–cytotoxic phenotype occur [63]. Primary T-cell lymphomas may show a pronounced eosinophilia, which may partially obscure the neoplastic cells [64,65]. Primary Hodgkin's disease of the stomach is vanishingly rare and suggested cases should be treated with extreme scepticism. Many may represent either T-cell lymphoma or CD30-positive anaplastic (Ki-1) large cell lymphoma which is well recognized in the stomach [66–68].

Mantle cell lymphoma may involve the stomach as lymphomatous polyposis. This tumour tends to present with small and large bowel involvement and is further considered on pp. 382 and 613. Lymphoproliferative disease and frank lymphoma may complicate immunodeficiency. In the stomach, post-transplant lymphoproliferative disease and high-grade lymphoma complicating AIDS both occur [69–71]; these subjects are more fully dealt with on pp. 379 and 614.

Secondary lymphomatous and leukaemic involvement

Secondary involvement of the stomach by lymphoma is common in clinical and autopsy practice [2]. High-grade tumours are more likely and may be difficult to differentiate from primary high-grade MALT-type lymphomas. The distinctive features of primary MALT lymphoma, lymphoepithelial lesions, low-grade component and typical immunohistochemical and molecular phenotype, may be helpful differentiating features. Acute myeloblastic leukaemia may present as a myeloblastic sarcoma in the stomach [72] and may mimic primary lymphoma or even myeloma because the cells have plasmacytoid features (Fig. 15.8). Chloroacetate esterase demonstration (Fig. 15.8) and lysozyme immunohistochemistry are useful

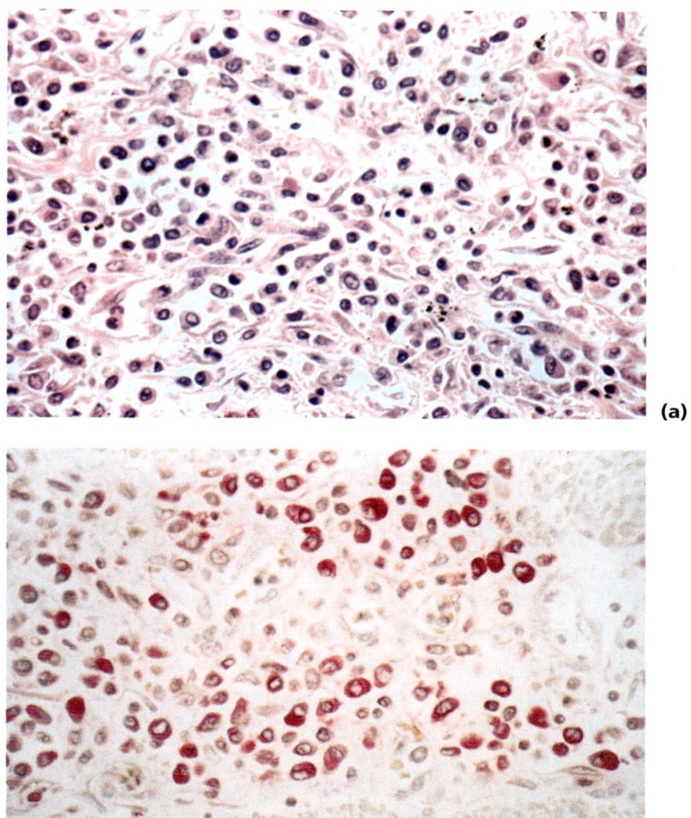

Fig. 15.8 A myeloblastic sarcoma of the stomach. (a) The cytology may mislead the unwary into making a diagnosis of lymphoma or plasmacytoma. (b) Chloroacetate esterase histochemistry shows striking positivity in this case.

diagnostic tests. Chronic leukaemia, both myeloid and lymphocytic, may involve the stomach: such involvement inevitably indicates advanced disease.

Gastrointestinal stromal tumours

Few tumours produce such consternation and confusion amongst clinicians and pathologists as gastrointestinal stromal tumours (GISTs). This is because they represent a morphologically heterogeneous group of tumours with diagnostic conundra and poorly defined management strategies: above all, it is notoriously difficult to predict their likely behaviour. No other tumour in the gut has undergone such rapid redefinition as stromal tumours: in the previous edition of this book, published only a decade ago, the term GIST does not appear, and most mesenchymal tumours with a spindle cell morphology occurring in the gut were regarded as smooth muscle tumours such as leiomyoma, leiomyoblastoma and leiomyosarcoma. This redefinition has been prompted by the advent of immunohistochemistry, the availability of markers such as CD34 and CD117 (c-kit) and molecular analysis. Much of the following discussion is appropriate to tumours of the small intestine and colon, but it is appropriate to initiate a general discussion on the definition and histogenesis of GISTs here.

Definition and histogenesis of GISTs

Tumours with the typical morphology of mesenchymal tumours elsewhere in the body, such as nerve sheath tumours and leiomyomas, are found in the gut but they are in a striking minority. For instance, tumours with unequivocal smooth muscle differentiation are most commonly seen in the oesophagus and rectum. It is surprising, considering the amount of muscularis present throughout the gut, that unequivocal evidence of smooth muscle derivation is lacking in the largest group of stromal tumours. This, and the presence of positivity for markers not indicative of a smooth muscle origin, has led to the concept of gastrointestinal stromal tumours. These tumours make up the great majority of spindle cell and epithelioid cell tumours of the stomach and small intestine. Whilst it is accepted that GIST is an umbrella term and tumours with more specific histogenesis may be incorporated into this category, we believe that the concept of GIST is clinically and histogenetically useful and would recommend its usage for the majority of mesenchymal tumours of the stomach, small intestine and colon. This stance is strongly supported by recent immunohistochemical and molecular evidence [73,74].

GISTs were formerly largely regarded as leiomyomas and leiomyosarcomas based on morphological appearances [75,76]. Because of difficulties in predicting their behaviour, a term for borderline tumours of 'stromal tumour of uncertain malignant potential' (STUMP) was introduced [77]. Subsequently immunohistochemical and ultrastructural studies showed that true evidence of smooth muscle differentiation was infrequent in gastric and small intestinal stromal tumours: desmin expression was unusual [78] and well developed myofilaments scanty [74]. Even in benign tumours, evidence of smooth muscle differentiation was often scanty or incomplete [79,80]. It was largely on this basis that the term GIST was introduced. Many have subsequently struggled with the concept because they perceive that, like in the uterus, the predominant connective tissue of the gastrointestinal tract is smooth muscle and that most tumours should, one would have thought, arise from these cells [81–83].

More recent immunohistochemical evidence has helped to reaffirm the concept of GISTs as a separate entity with specific histogenesis. Within the last decade, it has been appreciated that many GISTs (approximately 60%) express CD34, the myeloid progenitor cell antigen, a marker not expressed in smooth muscle cells [73,84–86]. Subsequently it has been demonstrated that the majority of GISTs express c-kit (CD117), a tyrosine kinase receptor of the immunoglobulin supergene family [73,74]. This antigen is widely expressed in haemopoietic stem cells, mast cells, melanocytes, various ductal epithelia and elsewhere [74]. Expression is also characteristic of the gut pacemaker cell, the interstitial cell of Cajal [87,88].

It is now apparent that between 68% and 90% of GISTs show strong expression for c-kit [73,86,89,90] whilst a gain-of-function mutation in the c-kit gene appears to be a novel and specific feature of GISTs [89]. Whether or not most GISTs do indeed derive from interstitial cells of Cajal, these studies have important implications as c-kit (CD117) is undoubtedly a diagnostically useful immunohistochemical marker [74] and c-kit mutation appears to have important prognostic implications, being associated with larger tumours with adverse prognosis in two recent large series [91,92]. It is also notable that a rare hereditary condition characterized by multiple GISTs (Fig. 15.9) is associated with a germline mutation of the c-kit gene,

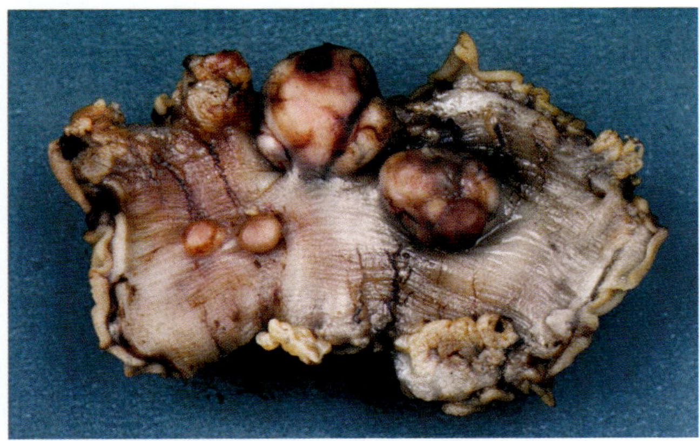

Fig. 15.9 Multiple subserosal gastrointestinal stromal tumours (GISTs) in a subserosal distribution in the stomach. Multiplicity of GISTs may indicate a hereditary syndrome.

the mutation being in a similar locus to that occurring in sporadic GISTs [89].

Because of the immunohistochemical and molecular evidence, it has been recommended that the term GIST should be replaced by 'gastrointestinal pacemaker cell tumour' (GI-PACT) [73]. We, and others [74], believe that this is premature. The term GIST is becoming widely accepted and promulgated and does not imply a specific cell of origin. Whilst there is evidence that many GISTs do indeed demonstrate similar phenotypes to interstitial cells of Cajal or pacemaker cells, it may be that GISTs arise from stem cells which are common to both interstitial cells of Cajal and other mesenchymal tissues [93]. Further evidence is required before the exact relationship between GISTs, pacemaker cells and other gastrointestinal cells of mesenchymal origin is fully understood.

GISTs in the stomach

The stomach is the commonest site for GISTs, accounting for about 60% of all cases [93]. Many GISTs in the stomach show some epithelioid features: hence the former designations of leiomyoblastoma and epithelioid leiomyoma [94,95]. One characteristic of GISTs (in general) is that many tumour subtypes show site specificity and this is apparent in the stomach as epithelioid features are relatively common and yet rare at other sites [96]. The second most common morphological phenotype of GISTs in the stomach is the cellular spindle cell tumour with a prominent palisading morphology and intracellular perinuclear vacuoles: this tumour is also unusual elsewhere in the gut [96]. Clinically significant GISTs remain an unusual tumour and this, together with the fact that most authors, in large series, combine gastric and intestinal GISTs, means that clinically, diagnostically and prognostically useful data specific to gastric GISTs are relatively lacking. It should also be appreciated that small, often subserosal, GISTs, sometimes multiple, are conversely commonplace in the stomach (Fig. 15.10), especially in autopsy practice (occurring in up to 50% of patients) [96], and this may introduce further bias into series of gastric GISTs.

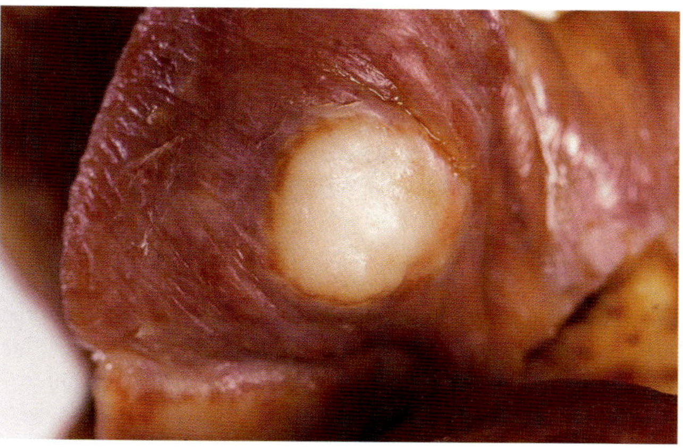

Fig. 15.10 A small subserosal gastrointestinal stromal tumour of the stomach. These are commonplace in autopsy (and even surgical) practice and such small subserosal lesions are invariably benign.

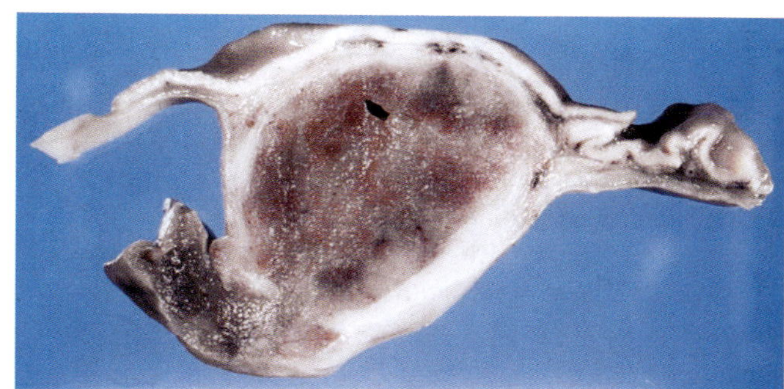

Fig. 15.11 The cut surface of a gastrointestinal stromal tumour of the stomach. It is intramural, grey in colour and granular in texture without whorling. Although circumscribed, it does not appear encapsulated.

Clinical, endoscopic and macroscopic features

GISTs occur mainly in the adult population with a median age of 60. The sex incidence is approximately equal. They are most commonly found in the fundus of the stomach and at this site are often asymptomatic unless the tumour is large. Presentation is largely dependent on size, site and associated ulceration. Small fundic tumours are usually discovered incidentally whilst small tumours of the pylorus can present with obstructive symptoms. Ulceration of a GIST results in bleeding and/or abdominal pain, common presenting features. A frankly malignant GIST may present with systemic symptoms, most notably weight loss.

The macroscopic features of gastric GISTs are more characteristic. They usually present as single intramural tumours (Fig. 15.11). An endophytic tumour is more likely to show ulceration, often with a central crater being the basis of the ulceration. Ulceration occurs in otherwise entirely benign tumours and does not necessarily presage malignancy. Some GISTs have a predominant extramural component and may only be attached to the stomach by a thin isthmus. Furthermore, some tumours may have both endophytic and exophytic aspects producing a dumb-bell shape with a narrow waist at the muscularis propria of the stomach. Frankly malignant tumours still appear predominantly expansile and only rarely is there frank infiltration into adjacent tissues.

The cut surface of a gastric GIST is characteristically grey in colour without the whorling pattern typical of leiomyomas at other sites, such as the uterus (Fig. 15.11). Instead the surface appears granular or rubbery. They are circumscribed but not encapsulated (Fig. 15.11). Coursing blood vessels may appear prominent. Malignant GISTs tend to be whiter in colour because of increased cellularity and are more likely to show areas of haemorrhage, necrosis and myxoid degeneration. Nevertheless none of these latter features are specific to malignant tumours and larger but benign GISTs may all show these changes as a result of mechanical forces.

Microscopic features

Despite recent studies of GISTs suggesting relative homogeneity relating to immunohistochemistry and molecular evidence, histologically gastric GISTs are strikingly heterogeneous. GISTs are primarily sited within the submucosa (Fig. 15.12) and muscularis propria, although predominant subserosal involvement is a feature of exophytic GISTs. The relationship with the gastric muscularis propria is a notable feature of GISTs. Often the muscularis appears hypertrophic with muscle bundles present within the tumour and forming muscular septa that may divide the tumour into lobules. The muscularis is often hyalinized. These features mean that very seldom is there a sudden transition from normal muscularis to the GIST [96].

The tumour cells of gastric GISTs are predominantly spindle celled (Fig. 15.13). They have oval often blunt-ended nuclei with abundant eosinophilic cytoplasm. Hyalinization, myxoid degeneration, haemorrhage and even necrosis may all occur in varying proportions in otherwise benign tumours. Features suggestive of a smooth muscle differentiation such as perinuclear vacuoles may be present but should not invite a diagnosis of leiomyoma in the absence of immunohistochemical evidence.

In line with the general acceptance that site-specific features are characteristic in GISTs, gastric GISTs show two predominant morphological phenotypes that are comparatively specific to the stomach. The relative incidence of these tumours is uncertain but it seems likely that they occur with approximately equal incidence and account for the majority of gastric GISTs. The 'cellular spindled cell stromal tumour' of the stomach is characterized by fascicles of spindle cells, often with pronounced palisades and, seemingly relatively specifically, a perinuclear vacuole, which indents the end of the nucleus [96]. Hyalinization and myxoid degeneration are both commonplace. The nuclei tend to be monotonous and uniform, although occasionally large forms may occur. The mitotic activity is low and these tumours usually behave in a benign fashion. Indeed, they account for many of the small tumours discovered incidentally in the stomach.

Epithelioid GISTs make up the majority of the remaining gastric GISTs. Whilst most occur in the fundus, these are the commonest GISTs in the antrum. It should be appreciated that few tumours are comprised entirely of epithelioid cells: most tumours in this category show varying amounts of spindle cell and epithelioid cell foci. These tumours account for those previously known as leiomyoblastoma and bizarre smooth muscle tumour [96]. The characteristic morphological features are rounded cells with prominent cleared cytoplasm although there is often condensation of the cytoplasm close to the nucleus (Fig. 15.14). The tumour cells are arranged in sheets or packets, rather than fascicles (Fig. 15.14), and tend to be orientated in a perivascular pattern. On frozen section, the clearing of the cytoplasm is not seen, indicating that it is an artefact of fixation [97]. As with other gastric GISTs, hyalinization and myxoid degeneration are common. Epithelioid GISTs are more likely to be multinodular than other types. Cellular pleomorphism is a characteristic of the tumour with large bizarre

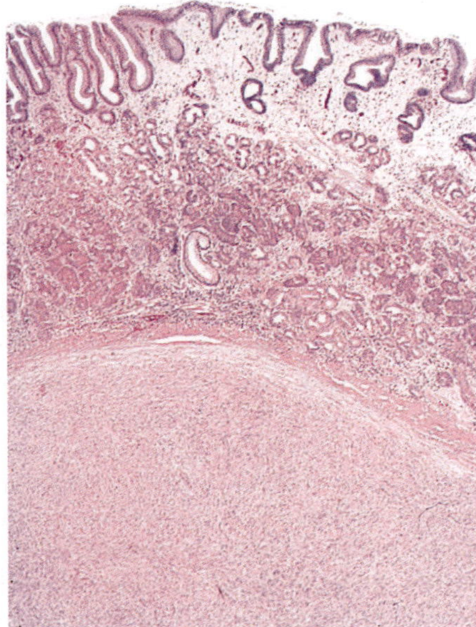

Fig. 15.12 Low-power histology of a gastrointestinal stromal tumour of the stomach. It is primarily sited in the submucosa and shows a spindle cell morphology.

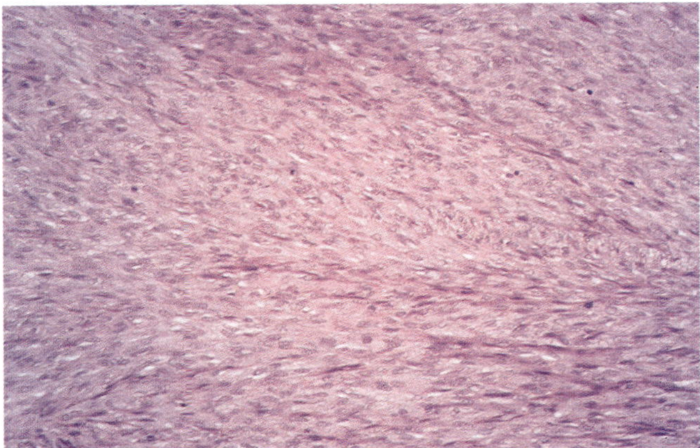

Fig. 15.13 High-power histology of a gastrointestinal stromal tumour of the stomach. The tumour cells are spindle celled with oval often blunt-ended nuclei with abundant eosinophilic cytoplasm.

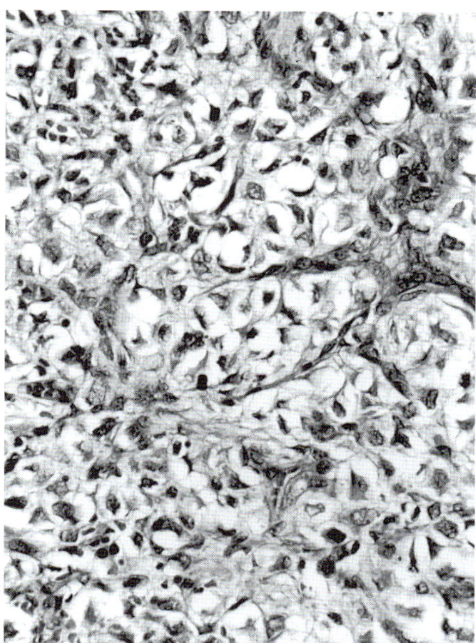

Fig. 15.14 An epithelioid gastrointestinal stromal tumour of the stomach. There is pronounced cytoplasmic clearing and the tumour cells are arranged in packets rather than fascicles.

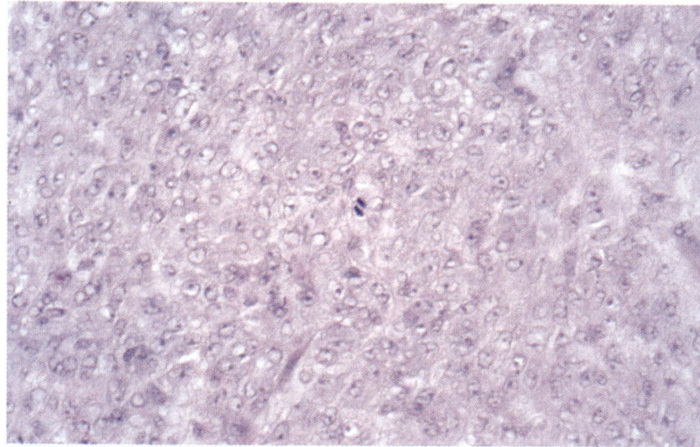

Fig. 15.15 A malignant gastrointestinal stromal tumour of the stomach. There is gross nuclear pleomorphism and the tumour showed numerous mitoses.

nuclei often present. This, *per se*, does not indicate likely malignancy. In fact, on the contrary, such features are more likely to be seen in benign tumours [96]. Malignant epithelioid GISTs tend to have smaller cells with less vacuolated cytoplasm. They are inclined to have more monotonous nuclei: cells appear clustered with an alveolar pattern often prominent. Malignancy in epithelioid GISTs is judged by the same criteria applied to other GISTs, most notably proliferative indices, tumour size and infiltrative pattern. They share the immunophenotype of other GISTs with a distinct lack of any evidence of smooth muscle differentiation [95].

Epithelioid tumours, because of their morphology and perivascular organization, can mimic other tumours. Endocrine cell tumours, haemangiopericytoma, glomus tumour, granular cell tumour and oncocytoma are all differential diagnoses to consider. In addition, epithelioid GISTs may show a striking morphological resemblance to gastrointestinal autonomic nerve tumour (GANT); indeed, given recent immunohistochemical evidence that GANTs express CD117, it is likely that there is overlap between these tumours. Indeed it is quite possible that many malignant epithelioid GISTs actually represent GANTs.

A further subtype of gastric GIST is the frankly malignant spindle cell sarcoma. These tumours lack epithelioid differentiation and demonstrate nuclear pleomorphism and high mitotic indices (Fig. 15.15). As their name implies, they are predominantly spindle celled and share some of the microscopic features of soft tissue sarcomas. However these tumours usually express markers of GISTs, such as CD117 and CD34, and are best considered malignant gastric GISTs. Unlike malignant epithelioid GISTs, which have an intermediate prognosis, with a median survival time of about 6 years, spindle cell sarcomas have an appreciably worse prognosis with a median survival of only about 1 year [96].

Immunohistochemistry and molecular pathology

It is largely the result of immunohistochemistry and molecular analysis that has allowed the reworking of our understanding of these enigmatic tumours and has allowed the general acceptance of the term GIST. The great majority of GISTs will show diffuse and strong staining for vimentin [86]. The relatively consistent expression (in more than 70% of cases) of CD117/c-kit is perhaps the most defining feature of GISTs and has promoted the view that many of these tumours derive not from smooth muscle but from stem cells related to pacemaker cells/interstitial cells of Cajal [73,86,90,91,98]. CD34 is also a useful marker of this tumour: about 70% of tumours will be positive [73,84–86,98,99]. Smooth muscle actin (SMA) is expressed often focally in GISTs; somewhere between 25% and 40% of GISTs will show some expression for SMA [84,85,99]. It would appear that gastric GISTs are less likely to express actin than their small intestinal equivalents [100]. Desmin expression is extremely rare in classical GISTs, despite the fact that this intermediate filament is usually expressed by the smooth muscle of the gut. Some GISTs will show focal expression for S-100 but this usually represents entrapped nerve fibres or antigen-presenting cells within the tumour. Diffuse strong staining for S-100 is most unusual and should suggest that the tumour is truly of neural origin. As schwannomas do occur in the stomach and share the palisaded morphology of cellular spindled cell stromal tumour of the stomach, it is likely that immunohistochemistry, for S-100 on the one hand and CD117 and CD34 on the other, will provide the primary method for differentiating these tumours.

Sixty per cent of GISTs will show mutation of the c-kit gene and this is more likely to occur in GISTs with metastatic potential [91,92]. The gain-of-function mutation of the c-kit gene appears to be specific for GISTs [89].

Prognostic indicators

GISTs are notoriously difficult to predict as far as biological behaviour and metastatic potential are concerned. There is no doubt that larger GISTs are more likely to be malignant and that the smaller, often subserosal, spindled cell stromal tumours are almost universally benign. Any GIST of the stomach over 6 cm in diameter, especially if it has epithelioid morphology, should be considered potentially malignant [96]. Size has undoubted univariate and multivariate prognostic implication but it is a weak prognostic parameter in comparison to proliferative indices [98,101]. Some studies have suggested that nuclear grade is a prognostic determinant [98,102] but some caution is appropriate here. Epithelioid GISTs are more likely to be benign when they show bizarre nuclei and malignant when they demonstrate nuclear monotony. Nevertheless a combination of nuclear grade assessment and mitotic activity (see below) is prognostically useful [103].

There is a gradual move toward regarding GISTs not as specifically benign or malignant, but as low risk, intermediate risk and high risk for recurrence and metastasis. We believe this assessment is best made by analysis of the morphological features (to determine whether the tumour fits into one of the more specific categories already described) and the proliferation activity. Assessment of mitotic index is the time-honoured method for the latter and is the parameter most easily and usefully assessed in clinical practice. The criteria for malignancy risk given by Newman *et al.* [103] remain clinically applicable and are reproduced in Table 15.2.

One important consideration concerning GISTs is that the malignancy risk, as determined by proliferative indices, is much higher than it is for the equivalent mitotic index for stromal tumours at other sites, most notably the myometrium. Leiomyosarcoma of the myometrium generally requires at least 15 mitoses/30 hpf whereas the equivalent figure for high-risk GIST is 5 mitoses/30 hpf [96]. Given the predictive applicability of mitotic indices for GISTs, it is not surprising that other proliferative markers such as Ki-67 and its analogues and proliferative cell nuclear antigen (PCNA) also show prognostic utility [98,101,104–107]. Studies have demonstrated that ploidy [101,108–110] and telomerase activity [111] also correlate with prognosis.

Table 15.2 Recurrence/metastatic risk of GISTs according to mitotic index and cell type.

Low risk	Spindle cell	0–2 mitoses/30 hpf
	Epithelioid cell	0–1 mitoses/30 hpf
Intermediate risk	Spindle cell with no atypia	3–4 mitoses/30 hpf
	Spindle cell with nuclear atypia	2–3 mitoses/30 hpf
	Epithelioid cell	1–2 mitoses/30 hpf
High risk	Spindle cell with no atypia	> 5 mitoses/30 hpf
	Spindle cell with nuclear atypia	> 3 mitoses/30 hpf
	Epithelioid cell	> 2 mitoses/30 hpf

hpf, high-power field.

Other GIST subtypes in the stomach

Gastrointestinal autonomic nerve tumour (GANT), first identified as a malignant stromal tumour of the small bowel known as plexosarcoma [112], does occur in the stomach but less often than in the small intestine [113]. The interested reader is referred to the 'GIST' section of the small intestine (see p. 384) for a full account of these tumours. GANTs, whether in the stomach or small bowel, are characterized by uniform positivity for CD117, large size, high mitotic rates and often a highly aggressive behaviour [113–115]. In the stomach, their main differential diagnosis is epithelioid GIST. In a recent series, all GANTs in a paediatric population occurred in the stomach and all four occurred in female children [116]. Gastrointestinal stromal tumours with skeinoid fibres appear to be a GIST subtype also more specific to the small bowel [82]. The specificity of skeinoid fibres to spindle cell tumours of the small bowel has been questioned by ultrastructural evidence that skein-like fibrillary material is demonstrable in all GANTs [117].

A form of (usually malignant) epithelioid GIST occurs, predominantly in young women, as part of a triad comprising these tumours, extra-adrenal paraganglioma and pulmonary chondroma, known as Carney's triad [118,119]. These tumours are characteristically multifocal in the stomach and they may show some features of GANTs [120].

Tumours of adipose tissue

Gastric lipomas are rare, unlike their colonic counterparts, and usually only come to attention because of haemorrhage due to ulceration [121,122]. They are usually single, relatively large and often project into the lumen. They are microscopically composed of lobulated adipose tissue (Fig. 15.16). Liposarcomas of the stomach are described [123] but are excessively rare: it is uncertain whether reported cases are truly liposarcomas or alternatively epithelioid GISTs [96].

Vascular tumours

True haemangiomas are described [124,125], but are very unusual in the stomach compared with the small and large bowel

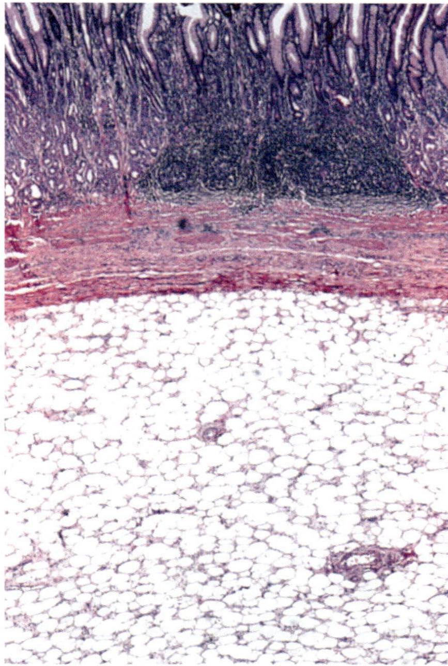

Fig. 15.16 A lipoma of the stomach. The tumour is submucosal and composed of lobules of normal-appearing adipose tissue.

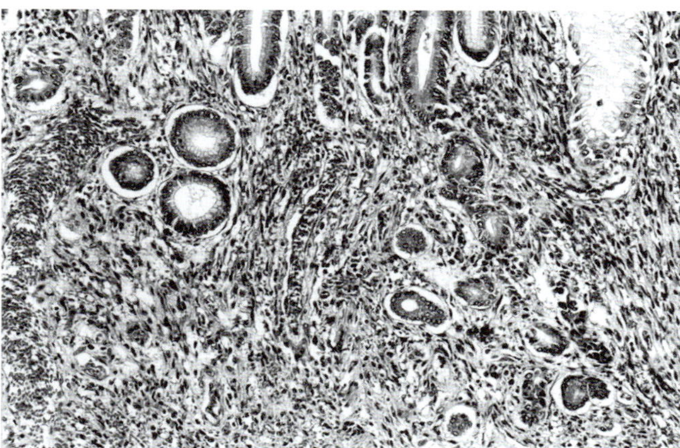

Fig. 15.17 Gastric involvement by Kaposi's sarcoma. The lamina propria is infiltrated by a tumour composed of bundles of spindle cells, thin-walled vessels and extravasated red blood cells.

[126], although vascular malformations such as submucosal arteriolar aneurysm/arteriovenous malformation of Dieulafoy are not uncommon and telangiectasias also occur in the stomach. For a general discussion of haemangiomas in the gastrointestinal tract, the reader is referred to p. 386. Haemangiopericytoma is described in the stomach [127] but some of these cases may represent GISTs with a prominent vascular component.

The stomach is a site of predilection for Kaposi's sarcoma (KS), arising in the context of AIDS [128] and now convincingly linked to human herpes virus 8 (HHV8) infection [129]. KS involvement of the stomach is almost exclusive to homosexuals with AIDS [128]. The disease is usually multifocal and up to 20% of homosexual patients with advanced immune paresis as a result of AIDS will show KS involvement of the gut [130]. The endoscopic appearances range from multiple purple maculopapular lesions to larger nodular and polypoid tumours [128,131]. Gastric lesions of KS are usually submucosal and superficial biopsies of the gastric mucosa may not detect the tumour. Histologically, KS is characterized by pleomorphic spindle cells with clefts in which erythrocytes are entrapped (Fig. 15.17). The tumour cells often demonstrate intracytoplasmic hyaline droplets. Whilst the presence of gastric KS indicates advanced immunosuppression, the prognosis is not usually further adversely influenced by the presence of gastric KS [128].

Nerve sheath tumours of the stomach

Older reports of neurilemmoma (schwannoma) in the stomach may well represent GISTs in that these tumours lack capsulation and definite evidence of nerve sheath differentiation [96]. Despite the resemblance of neurilemmoma to benign spindle cell stromal tumour of the stomach, there are reports of classical neurilemmoma in the post-GIST era in the stomach [132,133]. Rigid diagnostic criteria for neurilemmoma ensure that these tumours are distinctly rare and most benign palisaded spindle cell tumours probably represent GISTs [96]. Solitary neurofibroma also occurs in the stomach but gastric neurofibromas are more likely to be seen in von Recklinghausen's disease [134]. Confusingly, gastric GISTs are also seen in multiple neurofibromatosis although there may be considerable overlap between these tumour types in this syndrome [134,135]. As in the colon (see p. 619), polypoid and diffuse ganglioneuromatosis may occur sporadically or more often as part of von Recklinghausen's disease or multiple endocrine adenomatosis (MEA) type IIb [136,137].

Other mesenchymal tumours

Granular cell tumours of the gut are found most commonly in the oesophagus but they are occasionally described in the stomach [138]. They show the typical features of these tumours seen elsewhere: the intracytoplasmic granules are PAS positive and the cells stain with S-100 protein. Glomus tumours, in the gut, are almost always sited in the stomach [139,140]. The reason for the predilection of glomus tumours for the stomach is entirely unknown. They are particularly

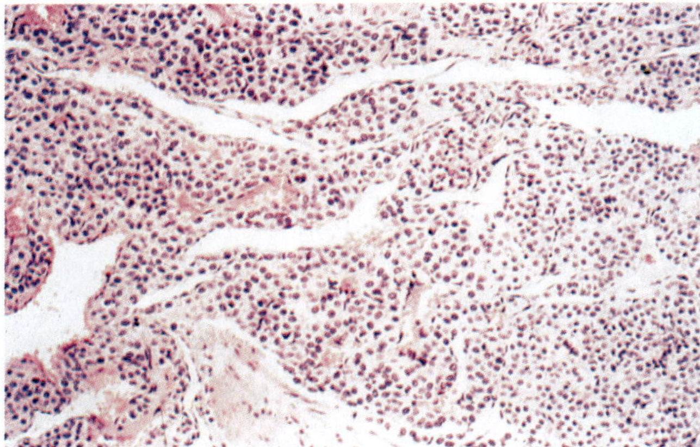

Fig. 15.18 A glomus tumour of the stomach. These are rare lesions but they do show similar morphology to the much more common skin glomus tumours.

found in the antrum and pylorus [139]. Glomus tumours are usually small and show features similar to those seen at other sites (Fig. 15.18), especially the skin. There is a unique report of a massive gastric glomus tumour filling the abdominal cavity, present for 20 years and apparently benign [141].

References

1 Severson RK, Davis S. Increasing incidence of primary gastric lymphoma. *Cancer*, 1990; 66: 1283.

2 Fischbach W, Kestel W, Kirchner T, Mossner J, Wilms K. Malignant lymphomas of the upper gastrointestinal tract. Results of a prospective study in 103 patients. *Cancer*, 1992; 70: 1075.

3 Dawson I, Cornes JS, Morson BC. Primary malignant lymphoid tumours of the gastrointestinal tract. *Br J Surg*, 1961; 49: 80.

4 Isaacson PG, Norton AJ. Malignant lymphoma of the gastrointestinal tract. In: *Extranodal Lymphomas*. Edinburgh: Churchill Livingstone, 1994: 15.

5 Isaacson PG. Gastrointestinal lymphoma. *Hum Pathol*, 1994; 25: 1020.

6 Freeman C, Berg JW, Cutler SJ. Occurrence and prognosis of extranodal lymphomas. *Cancer*, 1972; 29: 252.

7 Otter R, Bieger R, Kluin PM, Hermans J, Willemze R. Primary gastrointestinal non-Hodgkin's lymphoma in a population-based registry. *Br J Cancer*, 1989; 60: 745.

8 Doglioni C, Wotherspoon AC, Moschini A, de Boni M, Isaacson PG. High incidence of primary gastric lymphoma in northeastern Italy. *Lancet*, 1992; 339: 834.

9 Shepherd NA, Hall PA, Coates PJ, Levison DA. Primary malignant lymphoma of the colon and rectum. A histopathological and immunohistochemical analysis of 45 cases with clinicopathological correlations. *Histopathology*, 1988; 12: 235.

10 Domizio P, Owen RA, Shepherd NA, Talbot IC, Norton AJ. Primary lymphoma of the small intestine. A clinicopathological study of 119 cases. *Am J Surg Pathol*, 1993; 17: 429.

11 Musshoff K. Clinical staging classification of non-Hodgkin's lymphomas. *Strahlentherapie*, 1977; 153: 218.

12 Rohatiner A, d'Amore F, Coiffier B *et al*. Report on a workshop convened to discuss the pathological and staging classifications of gastrointestinal tract lymphoma. *Ann Oncol*, 1994; 5: 397.

13 Isaacson P, Wright DH. Extranodal malignant lymphoma arising from mucosa-associated lymphoid tissue. *Cancer*, 1984; 53: 2515.

14 Myhre MJ, Isaacson PG. Primary B-cell gastric lymphoma—a reassessment of its histogenesis. *J Pathol*, 1987; 152: 1.

15 Stansfeld AG, Diebold J, Noel H *et al*. Updated Kiel classification for lymphomas. *Lancet*, 1988; 1: 292.

16 Anonymous. National Cancer Institute sponsored study of classifications of non-Hodgkin's lymphomas: summary and description of a working formulation for clinical usage. The Non-Hodgkin's Lymphoma Pathologic Classification Project. *Cancer*, 1982; 49: 2112.

17 Harris NL, Jaffe ES, Stein H *et al*. A revised European-American classification of lymphoid neoplasms: a proposal from the International Lymphoma Study Group. *Blood*, 1994; 84: 1361.

18 Isaacson PG. Primary gastric lymphoma. *Br J Biomed Sci*, 1995; 52: 291.

19 Wotherspoon AC. Gastric lymphoma of mucosa-associated lymphoid tissue and *Helicobacter pylori*. *Annu Rev Med*, 1998; 49: 289.

20 Parsonnet J, Friedman GD, Vandersteen DP *et al*. *Helicobacter pylori* infection and the risk of gastric carcinoma. *N Engl J Med*, 1991; 325: 1127.

21 Hussell T, Isaacson PG, Crabtree JE, Spencer J. The response of cells from low-grade B-cell gastric lymphomas of mucosa-associated lymphoid tissue to *Helicobacter pylori*. *Lancet*, 1993; 342: 571.

22 Wotherspoon AC, Ortiz HC, Falzon MR, Isaacson PG. *Helicobacter pylori*-associated gastritis and primary B-cell gastric lymphoma. *Lancet*, 1991; 338: 1175.

23 Wotherspoon AC, Doglioni C, Isaacson PG. Low-grade gastric B-cell lymphoma of mucosa-associated lymphoid tissue (MALT): a multifocal disease. *Histopathology*, 1992; 20: 29.

24 Isaacson PG, Wotherspoon AC, Diss T, Pan LX. Follicular colonization in B-cell lymphoma of mucosa-associated lymphoid tissue. *Am J Surg Pathol*, 1991; 15: 819.

25 Zamboni G, Franzin G, Scarpa A *et al*. Carcinoma-like signet-ring cells in gastric mucosa-associated lymphoid tissue (MALT) lymphoma. *Am J Surg Pathol*, 1996; 20: 588.

26 Papadaki L, Wotherspoon AC, Isaacson PG. The lymphoepithelial lesion of gastric low-grade B-cell lymphoma of mucosa-associated lymphoid tissue (MALT): an ultrastructural study. *Histopathology*, 1992; 21: 415.

27 Isaacson PG. Lymphoproliferative disorders of the gastrointestinal tract. In: Ming S, Goldman H, eds. *Pathology of the Gastrointestinal Tract*. Baltimore: Williams & Wilkins, 1998: 339.

28 Eidt S, Stolte M, Fischer R. Factors influencing lymph node infiltration in primary gastric malignant lymphoma of the mucosa-associated lymphoid tissue. *Pathol Res Pract*, 1994; 190: 1077.

29 Radaszkiewicz T, Dragosics B, Bauer P. Gastrointestinal malignant lymphomas of the mucosa-associated lymphoid tissue: factors relevant to prognosis. *Gastroenterology*, 1992; 102: 1628.

30 Sanchez L, Algara P, Villuendas R *et al*. B-cell clonal detection in gastric low-grade lymphomas and regional lymph nodes: an immunohistologic and molecular study. *Am J Gastroenterol*, 1993; 88: 413.

31 Ono H, Kondo H, Saito D *et al*. Rapid diagnosis of gastric malignant lymphoma from biopsy specimens: detection of im-

munoglobulin heavy chain rearrangement by polymerase chain reaction. *Jpn J Cancer Res*, 1993; 84: 813.

32 Wotherspoon AC, Isaacson PG. Synchronous adenocarcinoma and low grade B-cell lymphoma of mucosa associated lymphoid tissue (MALT) of the stomach. *Histopathology*, 1995; 27: 325.

33 Zhang Y, Cheung AN, Chan AC *et al*. Detection of trisomy 3 in primary gastric B-cell lymphoma by using chromosome *in situ* hybridization on paraffin sections. *Am J Clin Pathol*, 1998; 110: 347.

34 Hoeve MA, Gisbertz IA, Schouten HC *et al*. Gastric low-grade MALT lymphoma, high-grade MALT lymphoma and diffuse large B cell lymphoma show different frequencies of trisomy. *Leukemia*, 1999; 13: 799.

35 Cogliatti SB, Schmid U, Schumacher U *et al*. Primary B-cell gastric lymphoma: a clinicopathological study of 145 patients. *Gastroenterology*, 1991; 101: 1159.

36 Cirillo M, Federico M, Curci G, Tamborrino E, Piccinini L, Silingardi V. Primary gastrointestinal lymphoma: a clinicopathological study of 58 cases. *Haematologica*, 1992; 77: 156.

37 Zinzani PL, Frezza G, Bendandi M *et al*. Primary gastric lymphoma: a clinical and therapeutic evaluation of 82 patients. *Leuk Lymphoma*, 1995; 19: 461.

38 Takenaka T, Maruyama K, Kinoshita T *et al*. A prospective study of surgery and adjuvant chemotherapy for primary gastric lymphoma stage II. *Br J Cancer*, 1997; 76: 1484.

39 Kodera Y, Yamamura Y, Nakamura S *et al*. The role of radical gastrectomy with systematic lymphadenectomy for the diagnosis and treatment of primary gastric lymphoma. *Ann Surg*, 1998; 227: 45.

40 Wotherspoon AC, Doglioni C, Diss TC *et al*. Regression of primary low-grade B-cell gastric lymphoma of mucosa-associated lymphoid tissue type after eradication of *Helicobacter pylori*. *Lancet*, 1993; 342: 575.

41 Eidt S, Lorenzen J, Ortmann M. Depth of infiltration of primary gastric B-cell lymphomas—correlations with proliferation, apoptosis and expression of p53 and bcl-2. *Pathol Res Pract*, 1996; 192: 925.

42 Bayerdorffer E, Neubauer A, Rudolph B *et al*. Regression of primary gastric lymphoma of mucosa-associated lymphoid tissue type after cure of *Helicobacter pylori* infection. MALT Lymphoma Study Group. *Lancet*, 1995; 345: 1591.

43 Fung CY, Grossbard ML, Linggood RM *et al*. Mucosa-associated lymphoid tissue lymphoma of the stomach: long term outcome after local treatment. *Cancer*, 1999; 85: 9.

44 Liang R, Todd D, Chan TK *et al*. Prognostic factors for primary gastrointestinal lymphoma. *Hematol Oncol*, 1995; 13: 153.

45 Sanchez BF, Garcia-Marcilla JA, Alonso JD *et al*. Prognostic factors in primary gastrointestinal non-Hodgkin's lymphoma: a multivariate analysis of 76 cases. *Eur J Surg*, 1998; 164: 385.

46 Kath R, Donhuijsen K, Hayungs J, Albrecht K, Seeber S, Hoffken K. Primary gastric non-Hodgkin's lymphoma: a clinicopathological study of 41 patients. *J Cancer Res Clin Oncol*, 1995; 121: 51.

47 Aiello A, Giardini R, Tondini C *et al*. PCR-based clonality analysis: a reliable method for the diagnosis and follow-up monitoring of conservatively treated gastric B-cell MALT lymphomas? *Histopathology*, 1999; 34: 326.

48 Koch P, Grothaus PB, Hiddemann W *et al*. Primary lymphoma of the stomach: three-year results of a prospective multicenter study. The German Multicenter Study Group on GI-NHL. *Ann Oncol*, 1997; 8 (Suppl 1): 85.

49 Nakamura S, Yao T, Aoyagi K, Iida M, Fujishima M, Tsuneyoshi M. *Helicobacter pylori* and primary gastric lymphoma. A histopathologic and immunohistochemical analysis of 237 patients. *Cancer*, 1997; 79: 3.

50 Cammarota G, Tursi A, Papa A *et al*. The growth of primary low-grade B-cell gastric lymphoma is sustained by *Helicobacter pylori*. *Scand J Gastroenterol*, 1997; 32: 285.

51 Muller AF, Maloney A, Jenkins D *et al*. Primary gastric lymphoma in clinical practice 1973–1992. *Gut*, 1995; 36: 679.

52 Shibata D, Tokunaga M, Uemura Y, Sato E, Tanaka S, Weiss LM. Association of Epstein–Barr virus with undifferentiated gastric carcinomas with intense lymphoid infiltration. Lymphoepithelioma-like carcinoma. *Am J Pathol*, 1991; 139: 469.

53 Isaacson PG. Gastrointestinal lymphomas of T- and B-cell types. *Mod Pathol*, 1999; 12: 151.

54 Montalban C, Manzanal A, Castrillo JM, Escribano L, Bellas C. Low grade gastric B-cell MALT lymphoma progressing into high grade lymphoma. Clonal identity of the two stages of the tumour, unusual bone involvement and leukemic dissemination. *Histopathology*, 1995; 27: 89.

55 Gisbertz IA, Schouten HC, Bot FJ, Arends JW. Proliferation and apoptosis in primary gastric B-cell non-Hodgkin's lymphoma. *Histopathology*, 1997; 30: 152.

56 Dogusoy G, Karayel FA, Gocener S, Goksel S. Histopathologic features and expression of Bcl-2 and p53 proteins in primary gastric lymphomas. *Pathol Oncol Res*, 1999; 5: 36.

57 Liang R, Chan WP, Kwong YL *et al*. Bcl-6 gene hypermutations in diffuse large B-cell lymphoma of primary gastric origin. *Br J Haematol*, 1997; 99: 668.

58 Liang R, Chan WP, Kwong YL, Xu WS, Srivastava G, Ho FC. High incidence of BCL-6 gene rearrangement in diffuse large B-cell lymphoma of primary gastric origin. *Cancer Genet Cytogenet*, 1997; 97: 114.

59 Salvagno L, Soraru M, Busetto M *et al*. Gastric non-Hodgkin's lymphoma: analysis of 252 patients from a multicenter study. *Tumori*, 1999; 85: 113.

60 Horie R, Yatomi Y, Wakabayashi T *et al*. Primary gastric T-cell lymphomas: report of two cases and a review of the literature. *Jpn J Clin Oncol*, 1999; 29: 171.

61 Itatsu T, Miwa H, Ohkura R *et al*. Primary gastric T-cell lymphoma accompanied by HTLV-I, HBV and *H. pylori* infection. *Dig Dis Sci*, 1999; 44: 1823.

62 Foss HD, Schmitt GA, Daum S *et al*. Origin of primary gastric T-cell lymphomas from intraepithelial T-lymphocytes: report of two cases. *Histopathology*, 1999; 34: 9.

63 Banerjee D, Walton JC, Jory TA, Crukley C, Meek M. Primary gastric T-cell lymphoma of suppressor-cytotoxic (CD8+) phenotype: discordant expression of T-cell receptor subunit beta F1, CD7, and CD3 antigens. *Hum Pathol*, 1990; 21: 872.

64 Shepherd NA, Blackshaw AJ, Hall PA *et al*. Malignant lymphoma with eosinophilia of the gastrointestinal tract. *Histopathology*, 1987; 11: 115.

65 Shimada HM, Fukayama M, Hayashi Y *et al*. Primary gastric T-cell lymphoma with and without human T-lymphotropic virus type 1. *Cancer*, 1997; 80: 292.

66 Mori N, Yatabe Y, Oka K *et al*. Primary gastric Ki-1 positive anaplastic large cell lymphoma: a report of two cases. *Pathol Int*, 1994; 44: 164.

67 Paulli M, Rosso R, Kindl S *et al*. Primary gastric CD30 (Ki-1)-positive large cell non-Hodgkin's lymphomas. A clinicopathologic analysis of six cases. *Cancer*, 1994; 73: 541.
68 Nakamura S, Aoyagi K, Ohkuni A *et al*. Rapidly growing primary gastric CD30 (Ki-1)-positive anaplastic large cell lymphoma. *Dig Dis Sci*, 1998; 43: 300.
69 Levine AM. AIDS-associated malignant lymphoma. *Med Clin N Am*, 1992; 76: 253.
70 Craig FE, Gulley ML, Banks PM. Posttransplantation lymphoproliferative disorders. *Am J Clin Pathol*, 1993; 99: 265.
71 Nalesnik MA. Clinical and pathological features of post-transplant lymphoproliferative disorders (PTLD). *Semin Immunopathol*, 1998; 20: 325.
72 Brugo EA, Marshall RB, Riberi AM, Pautasso OE. Preleukemic granulocytic sarcomas of the gastrointestinal tract. Report of two cases. *Am J Clin Pathol*, 1977; 68: 616.
73 Kindblom LG, Remotti HE, Aldenborg F, Meis-Kindblom JM. Gastrointestinal pacemaker cell tumor (GIPACT): gastrointestinal stromal tumors show phenotypic characteristics of the interstitial cells of Cajal. *Am J Pathol*, 1998; 152: 1259.
74 Chan JK. Mesenchymal tumors of the gastrointestinal tract: a paradise for acronyms (STUMP, GIST, GANT, and now GIPACT), implication of c-kit in genesis, and yet another of the many emerging roles of the interstitial cell of Cajal in the pathogenesis of gastrointestinal diseases? *Adv Anat Pathol*, 1999; 6: 19.
75 Evans HL. Smooth muscle tumors of the gastrointestinal tract. A study of 56 cases followed for a minimum of 10 years. *Cancer*, 1985; 56: 2242.
76 Appelman HD. Smooth muscle tumors of the gastrointestinal tract. What we know now that Stout didn't know. *Am J Surg Pathol*, 1986; 10 (Suppl 1): 83.
77 Appelman HD. Mesenchymal tumors of the gut: historical perspectives, new approaches, new results, and does it make any difference? In: Goldman H, Appelman HD, Kaufman N, eds. *Gastrointestinal Pathology*. Baltimore: Williams & Wilkins, 1990: 220.
78 Evans DJ, Lampert IA, Jacobs M. Intermediate filaments in smooth muscle tumours. *J Clin Pathol*, 1983; 36: 57.
79 Hjermstad BM, Sobin LH, Helwig EB. Stromal tumors of the gastrointestinal tract: myogenic or neurogenic?. *Am J Surg Pathol*, 1987; 11: 383.
80 Pike AM, Lloyd RV, Appelman HD. Cell markers in gastrointestinal stromal tumors. *Hum Pathol*, 1988; 19: 830.
81 Saul SH, Rast ML, Brooks JJ. The immunohistochemistry of gastrointestinal stromal tumors. Evidence supporting an origin from smooth muscle. *Am J Surg Pathol*, 1987; 11: 464.
82 Ueyama T, Guo KJ, Hashimoto H, Daimaru Y, Enjoji M. A clinicopathologic and immunohistochemical study of gastrointestinal stromal tumors. *Cancer*, 1992; 69: 947.
83 Ma CK, Amin MB, Kintanar E, Linden MD, Zarbo RJ. Immunohistologic characterization of gastrointestinal stromal tumors: a study of 82 cases compared with 11 cases of leiomyomas. *Mod Pathol*, 1993; 6: 139.
84 van de Rijn M, Hendrickson MR, Rouse RV. CD34 expression by gastrointestinal tract stromal tumors. *Hum Pathol*, 1994; 25: 766.
85 Miettinen M, Virolainen M, Maarit SR. Gastrointestinal stromal tumors—value of CD34 antigen in their identification and separation from true leiomyomas and schwannomas. *Am J Surg Pathol*, 1995; 19: 207.
86 Sircar K, Hewlett BR, Huizinga JD, Chorneyko K, Berezin I, Riddell RH. Interstitial cells of Cajal as precursors of gastrointestinal stromal tumors. *Am J Surg Pathol*, 1999; 23: 377.
87 Huizinga JD, Thuneberg L, Kluppel M *et al*. W/kit gene required for interstitial cells of Cajal and for intestinal pacemaker activity. *Nature*, 1995; 373: 347.
88 Yarden Y, Kuang WJ, Yang-Feng T *et al*. Human proto-oncogene c-kit: a new cell surface receptor tyrosine kinase for an unidentified ligand. *EMBO J*, 1987; 6: 3341.
89 Nakahara M, Isozaki K, Hirota S *et al*. A novel gain-of-function mutation of c-kit gene in gastrointestinal stromal tumors. *Gastroenterology*, 1998; 115: 1090.
90 Sarlomo RM, Kovatich AJ, Barusevicius A, Miettinen M. CD117: a sensitive marker for gastrointestinal stromal tumors that is more specific than CD34. *Mod Pathol*, 1998; 11: 728.
91 Taniguchi M, Nishida T, Hirota S *et al*. Effect of c-kit mutation on prognosis of gastrointestinal stromal tumors. *Cancer Res*, 1999; 59: 4297.
92 Lasota J, Jasinski M, Sarlomo RM, Miettinen M. Mutations in exon 11 of c-Kit occur preferentially in malignant versus benign gastrointestinal stromal tumors and do not occur in leiomyomas or leiomyosarcomas. *Am J Pathol*, 1999; 154: 53.
93 Miettinen M, Sarlomo-Rikala M, Lasota J. Gastrointestinal stromal tumors: recent advances in understanding of their biology. *Hum Pathol*, 1999; 30: 1213.
94 Appelman H, Helwig EB. Cellular leiomyomas of the stomach in 49 patients. *Arch Pathol Lab Med*, 1977; 101: 373.
95 Knapp RH, Wick MR, Goellner JR. Leiomyoblastomas and their relationship to other smooth-muscle tumors of the gastrointestinal tract. An electron-microscopic study. *Am J Surg Pathol*, 1984; 8: 449.
96 Appelman HD. Mesenchymal tumors of the gastrointestinal tract. In: Ming S, Goldman H, eds. *Pathology of the Gastrointestinal Tract*. Baltimore: Williams & Wilkins, 1998: 361.
97 Cornog JL. The ultrastructure of leiomyoblastoma. With comments on the light microscopic morphology. *Arch Pathol Lab Med*, 1969; 87: 404.
98 Seidal T, Edvardsson H. Expression of c-kit (CD117) and Ki67 provides information about the possible cell of origin and clinical course of gastrointestinal stromal tumours. *Histopathology*, 1999; 34: 416.
99 Monihan JM, Carr NJ, Sobin LH. CD34 immunoexpression in stromal tumours of the gastrointestinal tract and in mesenteric fibromatoses. *Histopathology*, 1994; 25: 469.
100 Franquemont DW, Frierson HF Jr. Muscle differentiation and clinicopathologic features of gastrointestinal stromal tumors. *Am J Surg Pathol*, 1992; 16: 947.
101 Rudolph P, Gloeckner K, Parwaresch R, Harms D, Schmidt D. Immunophenotype, proliferation, DNA ploidy, and biological behavior of gastrointestinal stromal tumors: a multivariate clinicopathologic study. *Hum Pathol*, 1998; 29: 791.
102 Rudolph P, Bonichon F, Gloeckner K *et al*. Comparative analysis of prognostic indicators for sarcomas of the soft parts and the viscerae. *Verh Dtsch Ges Pathol*, 1998; 82: 246.
103 Newman PL, Wadden C, Fletcher CD. Gastrointestinal stromal tumours: correlation of immunophenotype with clinicopathological features. *J Pathol*, 1991; 164: 107.
104 Amin MB, Ma CK, Linden MD, Kubus JJ, Zarbo RJ. Prognostic value of proliferating cell nuclear antigen index in gastric stro-

mal tumors. Correlation with mitotic count and clinical outcome. *Am J Clin Pathol*, 1993; 100: 428.

105 Sbaschnig RJ, Cunningham RE, Sobin LH, O'Leary TJ. Proliferating-cell nuclear antigen immunocytochemistry in the evaluation of gastrointestinal smooth-muscle tumors. *Mod Pathol*, 1994; 7: 780.

106 Franquemont DW, Frierson HF Jr. Proliferating cell nuclear antigen immunoreactivity and prognosis of gastrointestinal stromal tumors. *Mod Pathol*, 1995; 8: 473.

107 Emory TS, O'Leary TJ. Prognosis and surveillance of gastrointestinal stromal/smooth muscle tumors. *Ann Chir Gynaecol*, 1998; 87: 306.

108 el Naggar AK, Ro JY, McLemore D, Garnsey L, Ordonez N, MacKay B. Gastrointestinal stromal tumors: DNA flow-cytometric study of 58 patients with at least five years of follow-up. *Mod Pathol*, 1989; 2: 511.

109 Cooper PN, Quirke P, Hardy GJ, Dixon MF. A flow cytometric, clinical, and histological study of stromal neoplasms of the gastrointestinal tract. *Am J Surg Pathol*, 1992; 16: 163.

110 Tsushima K, Rainwater LM, Goellner JR, van Heerden JA, Lieber MM. Leiomyosarcomas and benign smooth muscle tumors of the stomach: nuclear DNA patterns studied by flow cytometry. *Mayo Clin Proc*, 1987; 62: 275.

111 Sakurai S, Fukayama M, Kaizaki Y *et al*. Telomerase activity in gastrointestinal stromal tumors. *Cancer*, 1998; 83: 2060.

112 Herrera GA, Pinto DM, Grizzle WE, Han SG. Malignant small bowel neoplasm of enteric plexus derivation (plexosarcoma). Light and electron microscopic study confirming the origin of the neoplasm. *Dig Dis Sci*, 1984; 29: 275.

113 Lauwers GY, Erlandson RA, Casper ES, Brennan MF, Woodruff JM. Gastrointestinal autonomic nerve tumors. A clinicopathological, immunohistochemical, and ultrastructural study of 12 cases. *Am J Surg Pathol*, 1993; 17: 887.

114 Shanks JH, Harris M, Banerjee SS, Eyden BP. Gastrointestinal autonomic nerve tumours: a report of nine cases. *Histopathology*, 1996; 29: 111.

115 Tornoczky T, Kalman E, Hegedus G *et al*. High mitotic index associated with poor prognosis in gastrointestinal autonomic nerve tumour. *Histopathology*, 1999; 35: 121.

116 Kerr JZ, Hicks MJ, Nuchtern JG *et al*. Gastrointestinal autonomic nerve tumors in the pediatric population: a report of four cases and a review of the literature. *Cancer*, 1999; 85: 220.

117 Ojanguren I, Ariza A, Navas-Palacios JJ. Gastrointestinal autonomic nerve tumor: further observations regarding an ultrastructural and immunohistochemical analysis of six cases. *Hum Pathol*, 1996; 27: 1311.

118 Carney JA. The triad of gastric epithelioid leiomyosarcoma, functioning extra-adrenal paraganglioma, and pulmonary chondroma. *Cancer*, 1979; 43: 374.

119 Carney JA. The triad of gastric epithelioid leiomyosarcoma, pulmonary chondroma, and functioning extra-adrenal paraganglioma: a five-year review. *Medicine*, 1983; 62: 159.

120 Tortella BJ, Matthews JB, Antonioli DA, Dvorak AM, Silen W. Gastric autonomic nerve (GAN) tumor and extra-adrenal paraganglioma in Carney's triad. A common origin. *Ann Surg*, 1987; 205: 221.

121 Bijlani RS, Kulkarni VM, Shahani RB, Shah HK, Dalvi A, Samsi AB. Gastric lipoma presenting as obstruction and hematemesis. *J Postgrad Med*, 1993; 39: 42.

122 Alberti D, Grazioli L, Orizio P *et al*. Asymptomatic giant gastric lipoma: What to do? *Am J Gastroenterol*, 1999; 94: 3634.

123 Seki K, Hasegawa T, Konegawa R, Hizawa K, Sano T. Primary liposarcoma of the stomach: a case report and a review of the literature. *Jpn J Clin Oncol*, 1998; 28: 284.

124 Smith JW, Jensen DM. Gastrointestinal angiomas. Source of recurrent bleeding. *Postgrad Med*, 1987; 82: 171.

125 Wan YL, Eng HL, Lee TY, Tsai CC, Chen SM, Chou FF. Computed tomography of an exophytic gastric hemangioma with torsion and intratumoral hemorrhage. *Clin Imaging*, 1993; 17: 210.

126 Oswalt CE, Kasal NG. Gastric hemangioma in a 15-year-old girl. *Texas Med*, 1983; 79: 37.

127 Vauclin P, Thau FF. A case of gastric haemangiopericytoma. *Mem Acad Chir*, 1966; 92: 368.

128 Parente F, Cernuschi M, Orlando G, Rizzardini G, Lazzarin A, Bianchi PG. Kaposi's sarcoma and AIDS: frequency of gastrointestinal involvement and its effect on survival. A prospective study in a heterogeneous population. *Scand J Gastroenterol*, 1991; 26: 1007.

129 Strickler HD, Goedert JJ, Bethke FR *et al*. Human herpes virus 8 cellular immune responses in homosexual men. *J Infect Dis*, 1999; 180: 1682.

130 Friedman SL. Kaposi's sarcoma and lymphoma of the gut in AIDS. *Baillières Clin Gastroenterol*, 1990; 4: 455.

131 Weprin L, Zollinger R, Clausen K, Thomas FB. Kaposi's sarcoma: endoscopic observations of gastric and colon involvement. *J Clin Gastroenterol*, 1982; 4: 357.

132 Sarlomo RM, Miettinen M. Gastric schwannoma—a clinicopathological analysis of six cases. *Histopathology*, 1995; 27: 355.

133 Prevot S, Bienvenu L, Vaillant JC, Saint-Maur PP. Benign schwannoma of the digestive tract: a clinicopathologic and immunohistochemical study of five cases, including a case of esophageal tumor. *Am J Surg Pathol*, 1999; 23: 431.

134 Fuller CE, Williams GT. Gastrointestinal manifestations of type 1 neurofibromatosis (von Recklinghausen's disease). *Histopathology*, 1991; 19: 1.

135 Schaldenbrand JD, Appelman HD. Solitary solid stromal gastrointestinal tumors in von Recklinghausen's disease with minimal smooth muscle differentiation. *Hum Pathol*, 1984; 15: 229.

136 Carney JA, Go VL, Sizemore GW, Hayles AB. Alimentary-tract ganglioneuromatosis. A major component of the syndrome of multiple endocrine neoplasia, type 2b. *N Engl J Med*, 1976; 295: 1287.

137 Shekitka KM, Sobin LH. Ganglioneuromas of the gastrointestinal tract. Relation to Von Recklinghausen disease and other multiple tumor syndromes. *Am J Surg Pathol*, 1994; 18: 250.

138 Johnston J, Helwig EB. Granular cell tumors of the gastrointestinal tract and perianal region: a study of 74 cases. *Dig Dis Sci*, 1981; 26: 807.

139 Appelman HD, Helwig EB. Glomus tumors of the stomach. *Cancer*, 1969; 23: 203.

140 Almagro UA, Schulte WJ, Norback DH, Turcotte JK. Glomus tumor of the stomach. Histologic and ultrastructural features. *Am J Clin Pathol*, 1981; 75: 415.

141 Warner KE, Haidak GL. Massive glomus tumor of the stomach: 20-year follow-up and autopsy findings. *Am J Gastroenterol*, 1984; 79: 253.

16 Tumour-like lesions of the stomach

Tumour-like lesions in the stomach present macroscopically either as focal lesions or as a more diffuse involvement of the lining of the stomach. They will be considered here under the two general headings of gastric polyps and thickened gastric folds. It is appreciated that the distinction between the two is blurred in a few patients with polyposis syndromes where multiple confluent polyps can result in a picture of grossly hypertrophied and nodular gastric folds.

Gastric polyps

The clinical term 'polyp' describes any focal lesion that projects above the surface of the surrounding mucosa, and when used alone gives no indication of its nature. Gastric polyps are found in only about 0.4% of autopsies [1] but have been present in up to 5% of routine endoscopies, although many of them are small [2,3]. Although a polypoid appearance can result from unaffected islands of mucosa occurring in a diffusely atrophic stomach (these are more appropriately termed pseudopolyps) [4], in common usage the term implies a substantive process occurring in the mucosa or less commonly submucosa.

The classification of gastric mucosal polyps is a matter of debate but, from a clinical point of view, the most important distinction is between the neoplastic and non-neoplastic groups. Neoplastic polyps, in practice predominantly adenomas, polypoid carcinomas and carcinoid tumours, are considered elsewhere (see Chapter 14). Non-neoplastic polyps can be considered under three headings—hyperplastic, hamartomatous and a miscellaneous group that includes epithelial and non-epithelial types.

Hyperplastic (regenerative) polyps

These are the commonest type of gastric polyp, constituting from 50 to 90% of the total [5–7]. They are smooth surfaced or only slightly lobulated, oval or hemispherical in shape, and rarely greater than 1.5 cm in diameter. Their surface is often eroded. The majority are sessile but larger polyps may be pedunculated. They can be single or multiple and may occur anywhere in the stomach, although most commonly in the antrum (Fig. 16.1). When multiple, they may be widely scattered or confined to one area, sometimes being concentrated at the junction of the body and antral mucosa.

Histologically, they consist of markedly hyperplastic and elongated foveolae in which intraluminal infolding and apparent branching [8] is frequent and cystic dilatation almost invariable in the deeper parts of the polyp (Fig. 16.2). The lining cells consist of a single layer of regularly arranged hypertrophied foveolar epithelium containing abundant neutral mucin. In some areas the cells may be cuboidal with granular eosinophilic cytoplasm [9,10]. Small groups of pyloric-type glands are present beneath the proliferating foveolae and connect with some of them. Parietal and chief cells are uncommon even when the polyp occurs in the body mucosa. Intestinal metaplasia can occur but is rarely a conspicuous feature and, when present, usually focal and of incomplete type [10]. Bundles of smooth muscle fibres growing into the polyp from the muscularis mucosae are frequently seen and the lamina propria is variably oedematous and infiltrated by plasma cells and lymphocytes. Lymphoid aggregates with germinal centres can sometimes be present. At sites of erosion there is a fibrinopurulent exudate associated with the presence of numerous acute inflammatory cells and proliferated capillaries in the subjacent tissues. In such areas, bizarre-appearing, pleomorphic cells with hyperchromatic nuclei and prominent nucleoli may be seen scattered or in small groups in the stroma. Some of them show mitoses. These are regenerative and not malignant cells [11], and have been described in inflammatory polyps and ulcers at other sites of the gastrointestinal tract [12]. They stain strongly for vimentin and in some cases for muscle-specific actin, and negatively for epithelial and lymphoid markers, suggesting that they are reactive fibroblasts or myofibroblasts [13]. The mucosa adjacent to a hyperplastic polyp usually shows similar, though less marked, changes of hypertrophy and hyperplasia of the foveolar cells, and mild to moderate inflammation with or without focal intestinal metaplasia and cyst formation, so that there is no clear demarcation between the two.

Because of their histological features, and the fact that they can develop at the site of, or bordering, ulcers and erosions

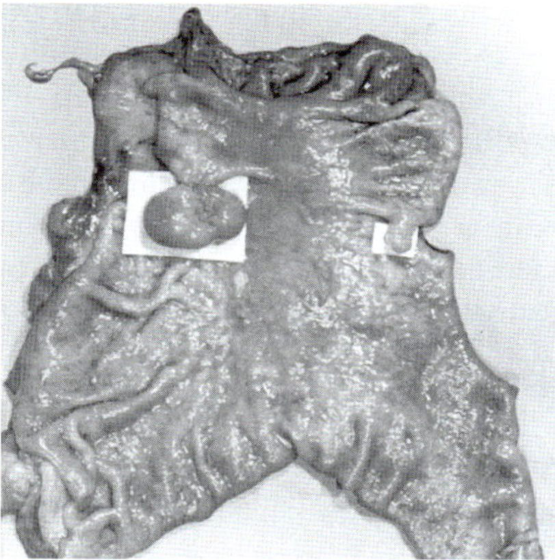

Fig. 16.1 Two hyperplastic polyps in the gastric antrum.

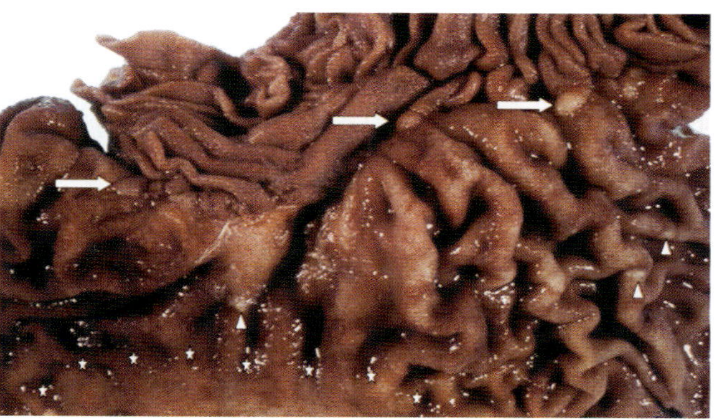

Fig. 16.3 Several hyperplastic polyps (arrowed) are present at the junction of stomach and small intestine (stomal polypoid hypertrophic gastritis) in this operated stomach specimen. Part of an ill-defined carcinoma (asterisks) and several xanthelasmas (arrowheads) are also present.

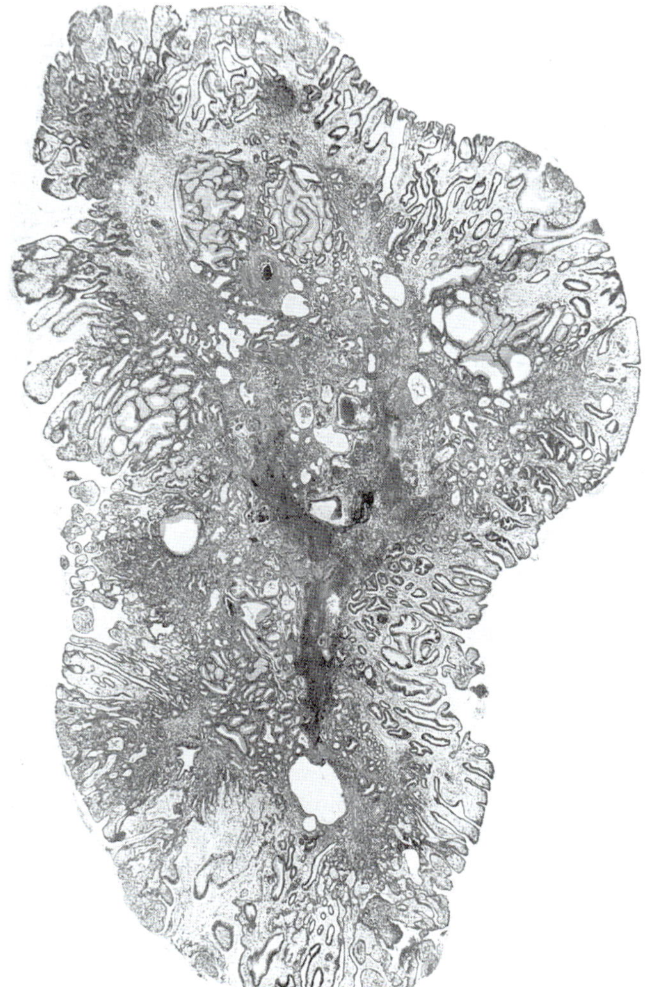

Fig. 16.2 Hyperplastic polyp. The surface is composed of elongated crypts lined by foveolar epithelium with some cystic change. Beneath this there is a mixture of gastric glands, collagen fibres and smooth muscle. There is no epithelial atypia and inflammatory changes are minimal.

[14], it seems that these polyps arise on the basis of excessive regeneration following mucosal damage—hence their alternative name of regenerative polyps. *Helicobacter pylori* organisms are usually associated with these polyps [15], although a causal role is speculative [16]. However, in a recent randomized controlled study, eradication therapy resulted in disappearance of hyperplastic polyps in a majority [17]. Both spontaneous regression [3,18] and the appearance of new polyps [3,19] have been observed on follow-up.

Hyperplastic polyps may also occur at, or close to, the stoma of operated stomachs (Fig. 16.3), where they have been reported in about 10% of cases at long-term follow-up [20,21]. They may be single or multiple, discrete or confluent, and occur along the line of the anastomosis on the gastric side. Not uncommonly they have been associated with submucosal cysts (one form of so-called gastritis cystica profunda—see also Menetrier's disease, p. 221) lined by columnar or flattened mucous cells, but occasionally by parietal and chief cells, and accompanied by irregularly arranged smooth muscle and collagen fibres [22–25]. The terms gastritis cystica polyposa [22] and stomal polypoid hypertrophic gastritis [26] have been used to describe this lesion, and its pathogenesis has been related to inflammation following biliary reflux, mucosal prolapse, ischaemia and the effects of surgery including the presence of suture material [25,27].

A distinctive feature of a minority of hyperplastic polyps has been a concentric infolding of the papillary surface epithelium (Fig. 16.4), which macroscopically corresponds to a central dimple. These polyps, which have been separately categorized by Nakamura [7,28], are usually multiple and arranged in a band in the distal fundic mucosa adjacent to the pyloric antrum (Fig. 16.5). They probably result from overexuberant healing of gastric erosions. Another classification separates those polyps with foveolar hyperplasia only and which tend to be small, from larger polyps in which there is in addition stromal and glandular hyperplasia, and which are re-

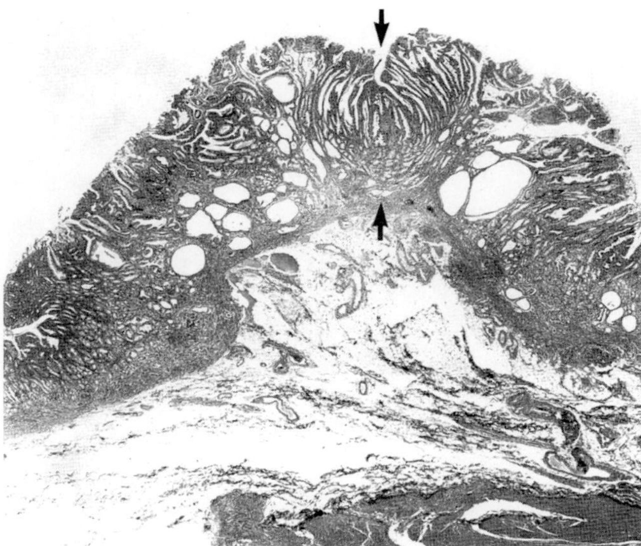

Fig. 16.4 Hyperplastic polyp showing 'onion skin' infolding of papillary surface epithelium in the centre of the polyp (arrowed).

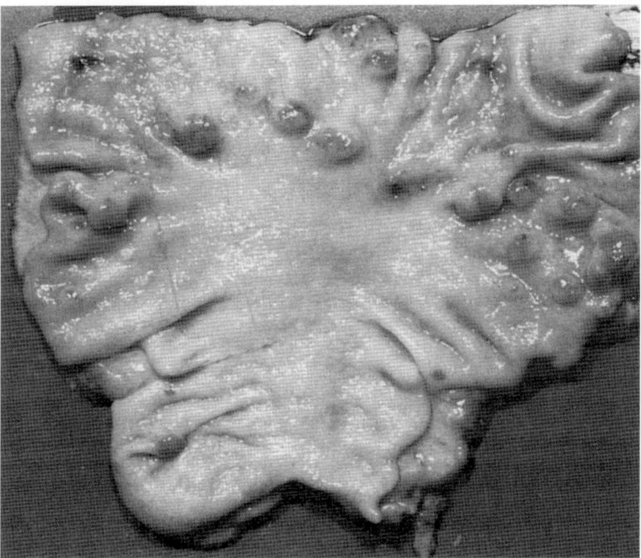

Fig. 16.5 Multiple hyperplastic polyps with a band-like arrangement at the junction of gastric antrum and body.

ferred to as hyperplasiogenous polyps [29]. The essential change, however, in all of them appears similar, varying only in degree. Although there is general agreement that the malignant potential of hyperplastic polyps is low, examples of epithelial dysplasia and malignant change are being increasingly reported [7,10,30–33]. In one large series, focal carcinoma was identified in 1.3% of hyperplastic polyps, although this rose to 2.1% when those polyps showing foveolar hyperplasia only were excluded. This compared to a malignancy rate of 7.4% in adenomas [34]. p53 overexpression has been identified in focal areas of dysplasia in hyperplastic gastric polyps [35]. A recent case report identified the same activating point mutation in codon 12 of the K-*ras* oncogene in three independent hyperplastic polyps with focal high-grade dysplasia and, in one of them, intramucosal carcinoma [36]. On the other hand, these polyps are often associated with an independent carcinoma elsewhere in the stomach, being found in 10% of cases of advanced gastric cancer and 18% of early gastric carcinomas in one report [2].

Hamartomatous polyps

Peutz-Jeghers polyps

Endoscopy has shown that polyps with a characteristic histological appearance are present in the stomach in nearly half of those individuals with Peutz–Jeghers syndrome [37]. In this site they are lobulated, rarely pedunculated, and mostly number less than 10. Although usually found incidentally, gastric polyps may bleed and there is a low but definite risk of malignant change [38,39], so that regular endoscopy with removal of any polyps present has been recommended in the management of patients with this rare autosomal dominant disorder [40]. In addition there appears to be an excess of tumours at a number of other extraintestinal sites including bilateral breast cancer, pancreatic cancer, ovarian sex cord tumours, adenoma malignum of the cervix and feminizing Sertoli cell tumours in the testis of prepubertal boys [41–44]. The genetic basis of this condition is a germline mutation affecting the serine/threonine kinase 11 (*LKB1/STK11*) gene on the short arm of chromosome 19 [45–47]. Histologically, the characteristic feature is the tree-like branching of the muscularis mucosae with overlying mucosa being of normal or hyperplastic antral or fundal type depending on the site of the polyp. As well as the typical polyp, hyperplastic polyps may also occur in this condition.

Juvenile polyps

As the name suggests, juvenile polyps occur predominantly in children and adolescents, and when solitary or few in number mostly affect the large bowel, particularly the lower rectum. When numerous, the upper gastrointestinal tract is frequently involved. Familial and non-familial cases of juvenile polyposis have been described. Rarely, multiple polyps of this type have been restricted to the stomach [48,49]. Multiple gastric polyps have resulted in chronic and severe loss of blood and protein [48,50].

Characteristically, the polyps are round and smooth surfaced and may show evidence of haemorrhage. In the stomach they have been more numerous in the antrum or restricted to that site [51] and larger lesions have been pedunculated. Microscopic examination shows cystically dilated glands lined by foveolar epithelium lying in an abundant oedematous lamina propria infiltrated by variable numbers of inflammatory cells. The smooth surface of the polyp may be focally eroded. Rarely, foci of cartilaginous or osseous metaplasia are present in the stroma. Fibres of the muscularis mucosae are absent from the polyp. In some cases of juvenile polyposis, the gastric lesions have been indistinguishable histologically from hyperplastic polyps [51].

The malignant potential of juvenile polyps is low, although there are reports describing areas of epithelial dysplasia and even of invasive carcinoma in polyps of the large bowel in cases of juvenile polyposis [51–56] (see p. 629). There are also occasional reports of this sequence occurring in the stomach [49,57]. Recently, the genetic basis of juvenile polyposis syndrome has been elucidated, with defects localized to the *PTEN* gene on chromosome 10q and the *SMAD4* gene on chromosome 18q [58,59]. In a recent study, deletion or mutation of a tumour suppressor gene mapping to the long arm of chromosome 10 was identified in non-epithelial cells in the lamina propria of a majority of juvenile polyps by fluorescent *in situ* hybridization, raising the possibility that the primary defect occurs in a stromal cell which induces secondary epithelial abnormalities [60].

Cowden's disease (multiple hamartoma syndrome)

In this rare condition, which has also been linked to germline mutation of the *PTEN* gene, gastric polyps may be present as one element of a more generalized gastrointestinal polyposis, and associated with a range of extraintestinal manifestations including multiple hamartomas, cutaneous trichilemmomas, macrocephaly, ataxias, and breast and thyroid tumours. Histology of the gastric polyps has described foveolar hyperplasia, along with more basal, cystically dilated glands that contained papillary infoldings. Intermingled smooth muscle fibres may be present and sometimes the cysts extend into the submucosa. In other cases, with more complex lesions, there has been a resemblance to Peutz–Jeghers polyps [61–63].

Miscellaneous polyps

Fundic gland polyps (fundic glandular cysts)

This polyp, first described by Elster in 1976 [64], has been observed in up to 1.9% of routine gastroscopies when carefully looked for [65,66]. The majority of cases have been in middle-aged women, and no specific association with other primary gastric diseases has been noted. However, along with adenomas and hyperplastic polyps [67,68], fundic gland polyps have been reported in the stomachs of patients with familial adenomatous polyposis (FAP) [69–71]. Indeed, it is the commonest type of gastric polyp in this setting with a reported prevalence of 26–73% [72,73] and a slight male predominance [74]. Fundic gland polyps are also more common in individuals with the hereditary flat adenoma syndrome [75]. While

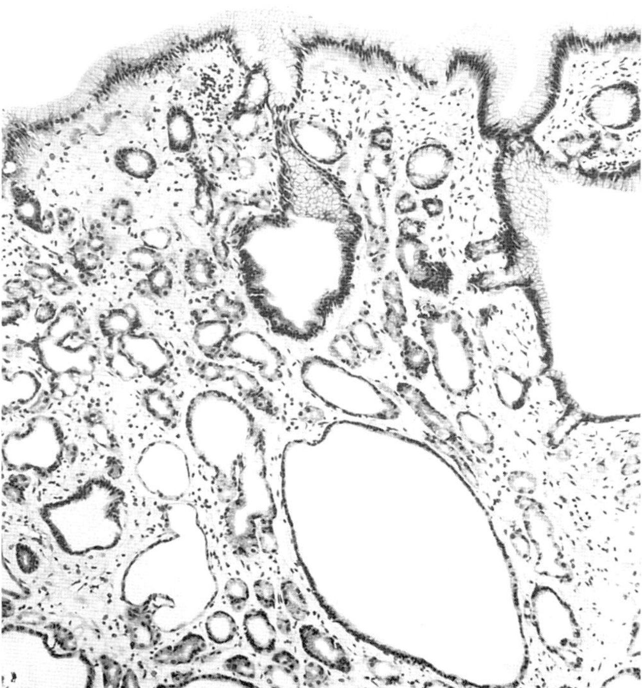

Fig. 16.6 Fundic gland polyp. Cystic change in body glands. The flattened epithelium of the cysts includes parietal and chief cells.

the great majority of patients with fundic gland polyps have no other gastrointestinal problem, formal examination of the large bowel has shown an increased frequency of epithelial neoplasms [76]. Whether individuals who are found to have multiple fundic gland polyps should undergo screening for colorectal neoplasia is controversial, but a case could be made for this in young subjects.

Occasionally single, but often numbering in the order of 15–30, fundic gland polyps appear endoscopically as clusters of small, mostly sessile lesions (up to about 5 mm in diameter) with a glassy transparent appearance. They are restricted to the body and fundus of the stomach, within the acid-secreting area [77]. One case has also been described in heterotopic gastric body mucosa in the duodenal bulb [78]. Histologically, microcysts are present at different levels of the gastric glands admixed with normal glands (Fig. 16.6). Disordered glandular architecture with budding and tortuosity is a conspicuous feature [79]. The cysts are often interconnected and are lined by mucin-secreting cells, rather atrophic parietal cells and some chief cells, although the latter are not obvious. There is usually no associated inflammation. There is a low prevalence of associated *H. pylori* infection [80].

The histogenesis of this type of polyp is unclear. Whilst generally regarded as hamartomatous, this seems unlikely in view of its predominantly epithelial composition, without an associated proliferated connective tissue element, as occurs with other hamartomatous lesions of the gastrointestinal tract.

Follow-up has shown that the number and size of polyps tend to remain unchanged, but in some cases spontaneous disappearance over a period of several months or a few years has been observed, particularly after colectomy in patients with FAP [69,81]. There have been recent reports of an association with long-term proton pump inhibitor treatment [82,83], which has also been accompanied by parietal cell enlargement and hyperplasia [84,85]. This association has recently been questioned [86].

Whilst these polyps were previously regarded as innocuous, there are several reports in the recent literature of dysplasia, predominantly low grade, of foveolar and surface epithelium and occurring in up to 25% of fundic gland polyps associated with FAP [73,87,88]. In addition, a few cases of gastric adenocarcinoma have been reported in this setting [89,90], two of which involved a brother and sister from a large kindred with attenuated FAP [91,92].

Cronkhite–Canada syndrome

In this rare disorder, of unknown aetiology and without any familial tendency, there is generalized gastrointestinal polyposis associated with skin pigmentary changes including hyperpigmentation and white patchy vitiligo, alopecia and atrophy of the nails [93]. There have been approximately 80 cases reported in the literature [94]. The major symptom is watery diarrhoea which can precede [95,96] or follow the ectodermal changes [97] and which can give rise to marked electrolyte disturbances and hypoproteinaemia. Unlike most cases of intestinal polyposis the majority of patients have been middle-aged or elderly.

Endoscopically, the polyps have a glistening, glassy appearance due to the presence of mucous cysts and may be sessile or finger-like or result in irregular, polypoid, nodular folds resembling the appearances seen, for example, with a diffusely infiltrating malignant lymphoma. Histologically, there is intense oedema of the lamina propria, usually associated with an increased cellularity, and elongation and tortuosity of the foveolae with marked cystic change in the pits and glands (Fig. 16.7). Cysts may rupture and result in inflammation and the presence of muciphages in the lamina propria. The histological appearances are not specific and may be indistinguishable from those of juvenile and hyperplastic polyps [98,99].

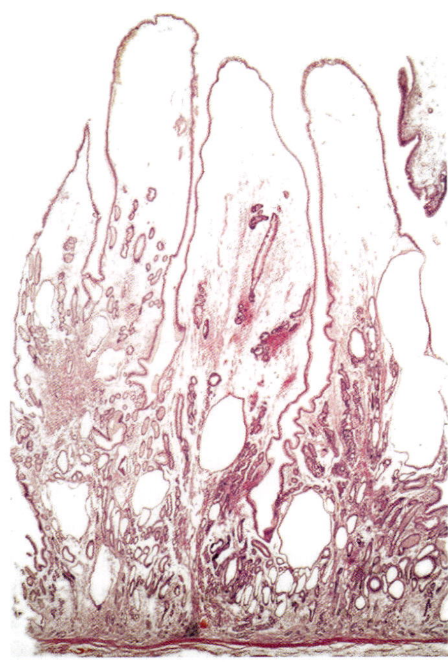

Fig. 16.7 Cronkhite–Canada syndrome. Finger-like polyps with marked elongation of foveolae and cystic change associated with oedema of the lamina propria.

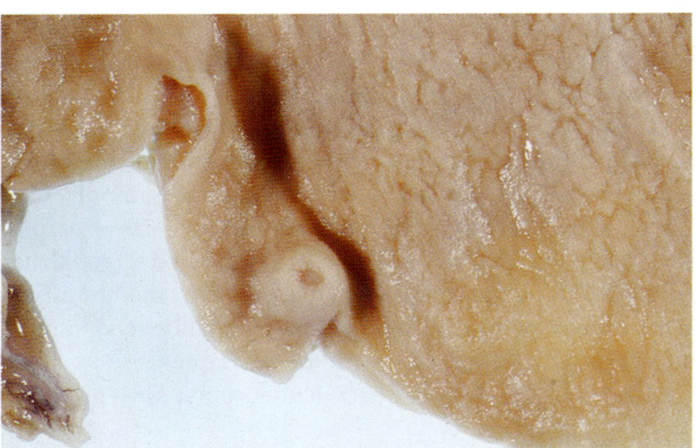

Fig. 16.8 Heterotopic pancreas. A sessile polyp with a central dimple is present in the gastric antrum.

Heterotopic pancreatic tissue ('adenomyoma', 'myoepithelial hamartoma')

Heterotopic pancreatic tissue in the stomach and duodenum is a congenital abnormality thought to result from separation of fragments from the main mass of the pancreas during rotation of the foregut. At endoscopy, the usual appearance of this uncommon lesion is indistinguishable from many other submucosal masses, namely a hemispherical sessile polyp, of variable size, anything from a few millimetres to several centimetres in diameter. A distinctive feature of some has been the presence of an opening, visible as a dimple on the surface (Fig. 16.8). They are invariably single and the majority occur within 3–4 cm of either side of the pylorus [100].

Histological examination shows pancreatic acini and ducts, in which cystic change is common, present in the submucosa. Sectioning may disclose ducts leading to the lumen. Islets of Langerhans are present in approximately one-third of cases (Fig. 16.9) [101]. This pancreatic tissue may be accompanied by bundles of hypertrophied smooth muscle surrounding ducts lined by tall columnar or cuboidal epithelium along with col-

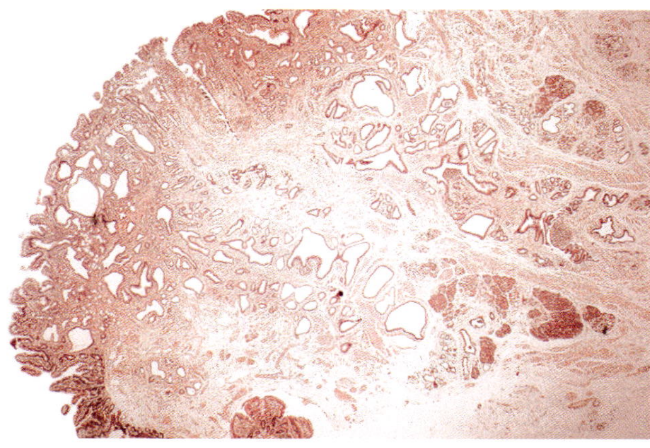

Fig. 16.9 Heterotopic pancreas. In this example from the duodenopyloric junction, dilated ducts, some associated with smooth muscle fibres, extend to the surface from the submucosa. Pancreatic acinar tissue is seen to the right.

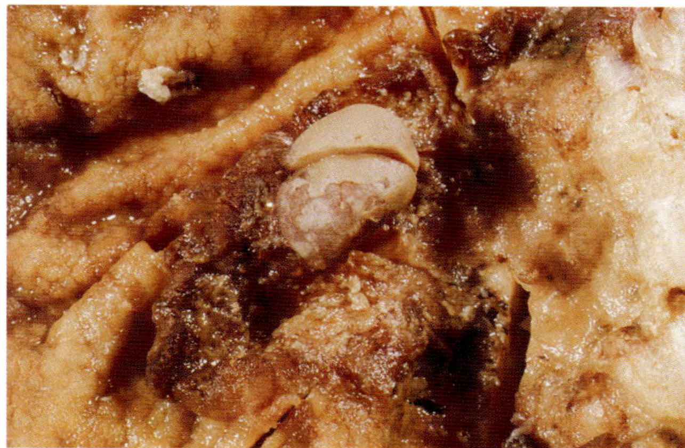

Fig. 16.10 A focally eroded inflammatory fibroid polyp is present at the margin of an ulcerated gastric cancer.

lections of Brunner's glands. The latter elements without pancreatic tissue may be found alone, when the term 'adenomyoma' or 'myoepithelial hamartoma' have been applied (see Fig. 11.2, p. 100). Larger lesions near the pylorus produce symptoms of gastric outlet obstruction, and ulceration and bleeding may occur. Lesions near the ampulla can cause obstruction of the common bile duct [102]. Multiple cysts up to 3 cm in diameter in the submucosa and muscularis propria of the duodenal and gastric wall accounted for obstructive symptoms necessitating surgery in one report of 10 patients, all of whom were young or middle-aged white males [103]. The large majority of these lesions, however, are incidental findings, either at endoscopy or at postmortem [104]. Very rare cases of malignancy in heterotopic pancreas have also been described [105,106].

Cases of true gastric gland heterotopia are very uncommon. They have usually manifested as intramural cysts [107], in one case associated with a dense lymphoid stroma [108].

Gastric inflammatory fibroid polyps

The stomach is the commonest site in the gastrointestinal tract for this uncommon lesion, which has also been called eosinophil granuloma, gastric fibroma with eosinophil infiltration, gastric submucosal granuloma, polypoid eosinophilic gastritis and inflammatory pseudotumour. In the majority of cases a single, smooth-surfaced oval polyp with a short pedicle which often shows surface erosion has been present in the pyloric antrum or prepyloric region of the stomach. Most examples are less than 3 cm in diameter and associated with episodic abdominal pain, although gastric outlet obstruction has been recorded with larger lesions. They most commonly occur in adults with a median age of 60 years and show a slight male preponderance, though cases have been reported in children [109].

Histologically, inflammatory fibroid polyps consist of non-encapsulated, extremely vascular and usually loose connective tissue, centred on the submucosa, infiltrated by variable numbers of eosinophils, plasma cells, basophils, lymphocytes and histiocytes. The latter two cell types may form aggregates, but true granuloma formation is rare. Blood vessels range from capillaries to larger thin- or thick-walled channels that are often surrounded by a zone of loose connective tissue containing palisaded fibroblasts with plump, spindle-shaped nuclei, giving a characteristic whorled or onion-skin pattern. These lesions have been misdiagnosed as haemangiopericytomas [110]. When small in size they have been amenable to endoscopic removal [111,112].

The precise nature and aetiology of inflammatory fibroid polyps is unknown, but they are not generally regarded as true neoplasms. Occasional cases have arisen at the edge of a peptic ulcer [113] or carcinoma (Fig. 16.10), and a jejunal polyp has been described following mucosal damage after a saline emetic [114], suggesting an over-reactive healing process. There is a report of multiple and recurrent fibroid polyps occurring in the stomach and ileum of three generations of a family [115]. A proposed neurogenic origin [116] appears unlikely and is not substantiated by ultrastructural examination [117]. The suggestion that inflammatory fibroid polyps may be a localized variant of eosinophilic gastroenteritis [118] has been convincingly refuted [119]. Ultrastructural studies have suggested that the spindle cells have fibroblastic and myofibroblastic features [120], while a detailed immunohistochemical study showed that they stained for CD34 but not for other endothelial and smooth muscle markers, suggesting a reactive proliferation of perivascular fibroblastic cells [121].

Xanthelasma

Gastric xanthelasmas, also known as lipid islands, have been noted at endoscopy in 0.4–6.3% of non-operated patients

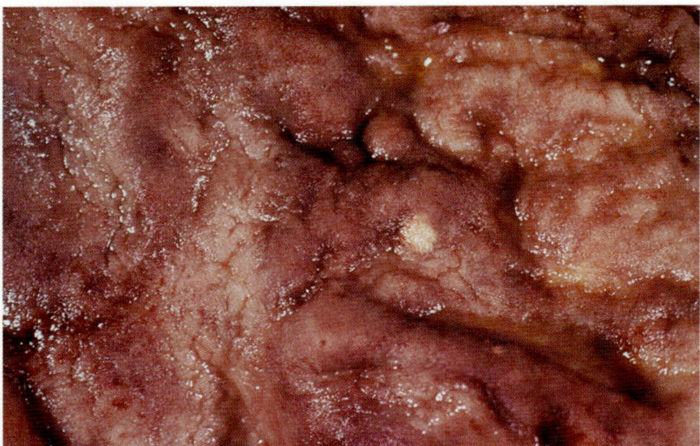

Fig. 16.11 Gastric xanthelasma. This 2-mm creamy-yellow macule was one of several in this operated stomach specimen.

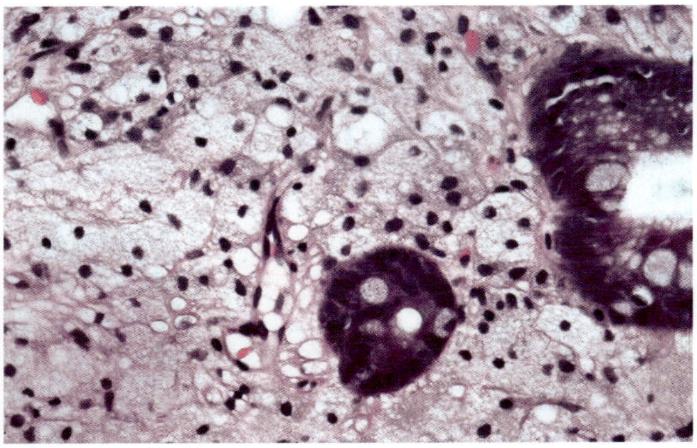

Fig. 16.12 Xanthelasma. Macrophages with foamy cytoplasm and small round nuclei are present between gastric glands.

[122,123], but their prevalence is higher in patients with a gastric stump, increasing with length of follow-up. Thus in one series, 60% of patients had lesions 23 years after Billroth II resection [122].

Macroscopically, they appear as yellow or orange, clearly demarcated macules (Fig. 16.11) with a somewhat irregular outline, mostly 1–2 mm in diameter and rarely exceeding 5 mm, which occur preferentially in the antrum and related to the lesser curve in non-operated subjects, and close to the stoma, on the posterior wall or along the greater curvature in operated patients. Larger lesions may be nodular and protrude above the surface [124]. Xanthelasmas may be single or multiple but rarely exceed 10 in number.

Histologically, a focal group of foam cells is present in the lamina propria, predominantly in the superficial parts of the mucosa. Individual cells are polygonal or rounded with distinct cell outlines and 10–30 μm in diameter. The cytoplasm has a distinctive mesh-like network with vacuoles from one to several microns in diameter, outlined by remnants of fine eosinophilic cytoplasm. The nucleus is small, round or oval, and central or slightly eccentric. No mitoses or atypia are present (Fig. 16.12). Inflammatory cells are scanty or absent, although adjacent mucosa often shows gastritis, sometimes with atrophy and intestinal metaplasia.

The most important distinction in practice is from infiltrating carcinoma of signet ring and other mucin-secreting varieties [125], particularly in the setting of the postoperative stomach where there is an increased risk of malignancy. Indeed, there are case reports of their simultaneous occurrence [126]. Apart from the distinctive endoscopic appearances and the cytological features described above, the use of a periodic acid–Schiff/alcian blue (PAS/AB) stain is very helpful in differentiating the two. Carcinoma cells will stain strongly because of their content of either PAS- or alcian blue-positive mucin (not infrequently a mixture), whereas foam cells are unstained or only faintly PAS positive. Foam cells are also sudanophilic. Focal collections of mucin-containing macrophages (muciphages) are extremely uncommon in gastric biopsy material and are easily distinguished from carcinoma cells by their low nuclear : cytoplasmic ratio and the bland appearance of their centrally located and pyknotic-appearing nuclei. Immunohistochemical staining for cytokeratins can also be used to distinguish the lesions.

The pathogenesis of xanthelasma is unclear. Chemical analysis has shown the presence of cholesterol in all, and of neutral fat in one-third [127]. A recent study has also identified oxidized low-density lipoprotein [128]. The association with chronic gastritis and intestinal metaplasia and their frequency in the operated stomach suggests that biliary reflux is an important aetiological factor. Ultrastructural and immunohistochemical studies have shown that the foam cells are mostly macrophages with smaller numbers of lipid-containing smooth muscle cells, plasma cells, pericytes, fibroblasts and Schwann cells [128–130].

Other polyps

Plasma cell granuloma is a localized inflammatory condition of unknown cause that can mimic a tumour at endoscopy. Histologically, it consists of large numbers of mature plasma cells, but small numbers of lymphocytes and other inflammatory cells are seen as well. Intra- or extracellular hyaline globules of immunoglobulin are often prominent. The polyclonal immunoglobulin pattern demonstrable immunohistochemically confirms the reactive nature of this lesion [131–133] and distinguishes it from plasmacytoma and from malignant lymphoma with plasmacytoid differentiation. Some cases have occurred in association with gastric carcinoma [134].

Tumour-like masses of amyloid may occur in the stomach as part of systemic amyloidosis [135] or as a primary lesion [136]. One case of multiple gastric polyps in a patient with familial amyloid polyneuropathy has recently been described [137].

Localized amyloid has also been associated with a primary gastric lymphoma [138].

Thickened gastric folds

Enlarged or thickened gastric folds on radiological examination or at endoscopy occur in a variety of disorders and may be associated with a nodular or polypoid appearance of the mucosa. *État mamelonné* is an uncommon variation of the normal where the gastric rugae are thickened and have a fine cobblestone appearance. Pathological conditions resulting in thickened gastric folds include infections due to tuberculosis, syphilis and fungi such as *Candida* and *Histoplasma*, Crohn's disease, eosinophilic gastroenteritis, lymphangiectasia, amyloid deposits, and malignant infiltrations by carcinoma or lymphoma. Gastric varices may also result in this appearance, as do certain types of polyposis when very extensive. Two other conditions that give rise to giant folds, which characteristically are restricted to the body mucosa, are the Zollinger–Ellison syndrome and Menetrier's disease. In the former, there is marked thickening of the body mucosa due to glandular hyperplasia as a result of gastrin-stimulated proliferation of parietal cells. This condition is considered in detail in Chapter 13 (p. 154).

Menetrier's disease

Since the original description in 1888 of what Menetrier called *'polyadenomes en nappe'* [139], approximately 400 cases have been reported of this enigmatic disorder. Clinically it occurs more commonly in middle-aged males than females, but has been described in children [140]. The common clinical symptoms are epigastric pain, which is often food related, weight loss, vomiting and diarrhoea. Occasionally presentation is with haematemesis or melaena. Acid secretion studies show that the majority of patients have hypo- or achlorhydria [141] and there is a non-selective loss of plasma proteins into the gastric lumen, often resulting in a low serum albumin and sometimes associated with peripheral oedema.

Macroscopically, it is characterized by enormous thickening of gastric folds that may additionally have a nodular or polypoid appearance. Body mucosa is affected, particularly along the greater curve [142], with or without antral sparing [143]. Localized forms (one case described by Menetrier in his original paper) have also been reported [144]. The mucosal folds are enormously enlarged, varying from 1 to 3 cm in height with an appearance typically resembling cerebral convolutions (Fig. 16.13). At endoscopy superficial erosions may be present and large amounts of viscous mucus coat the enlarged folds. The latter are not effaced after maximal air insufflation. Differential diagnosis must be made from *état mamelonné*, which is a variation of normal (see above), and from the increased parietal cell mass sometimes seen in patients with duodenal ulcer [145]. In both these situations the enlargement is usually far less marked.

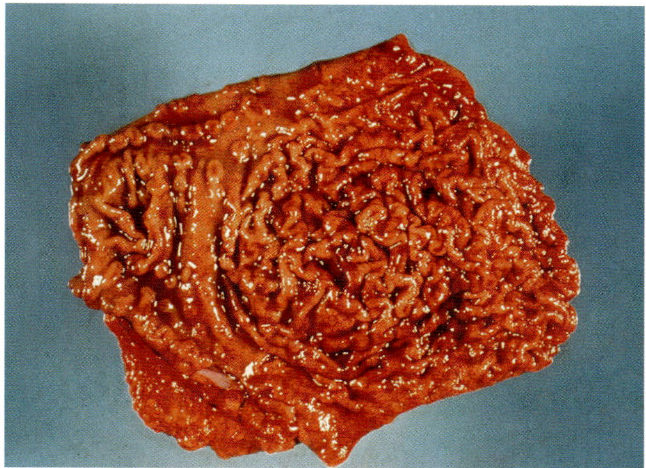

Fig. 16.13 Menetrier's disease. There is marked thickening and tortuosity of mucosal ridges involving the fundus and body and sparing the antrum. Compare with the pattern seen in Zollinger–Ellison syndrome, Fig. 13.11.

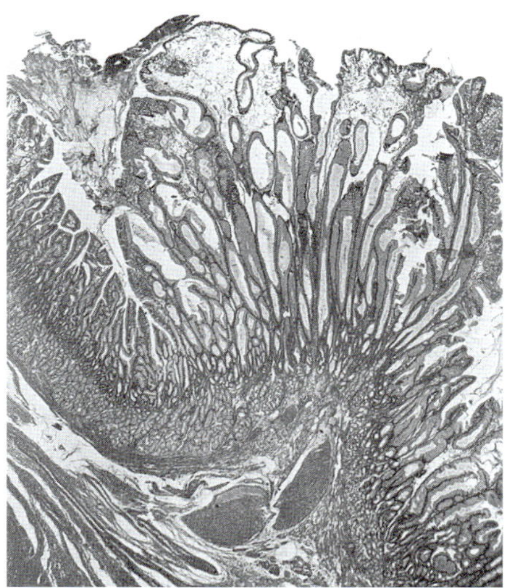

Fig. 16.14 Menetrier's disease. There is marked elongation and some tortuosity of gastric pits.

Microscopically, there is marked thickening of the mucosa as a result of extreme elongation and tortuosity of the gastric pits, which often have a somewhat corkscrew appearance, and, to a lesser extent, of elongation of the glands (Fig. 16.14). This is most prominent in the apical regions of the gastric folds, and between the folds the mucosa may be of normal thickness. The body glands may contain a relatively normal distribution of specialized cells but usually there is a variable replacement by mucin-secreting cells. Cysts lined by similar epithelium often develop, most commonly in the basal portion of the glan-

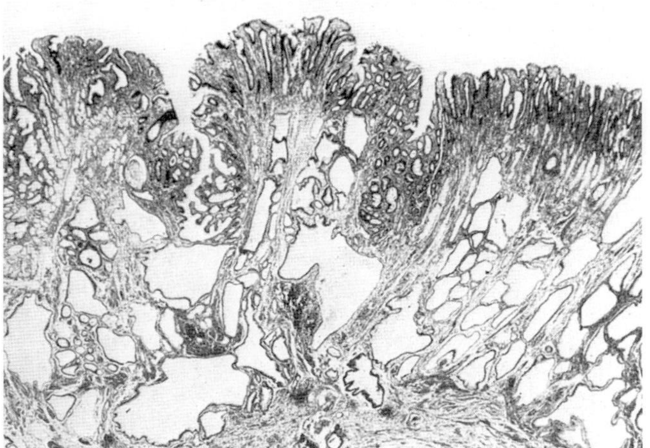

Fig. 16.15 Menetrier's disease. There is conspicuous cystic dilatation of glands in the deeper part of the mucosa.

dular layer (Fig. 16.15) but sometimes higher. These cysts may penetrate the muscularis mucosae, resulting in one type of so-called gastritis cystica profunda (see also p. 215). Inflammation is usually not a conspicuous feature but polymorphs may be present in the lamina propria and within the lumen of glands. Lymphoid follicles can be prominent. There is often considerable oedema, particularly in the superficial part of the mucosa. Thickening and fragmentation of the muscularis mucosae occurs and prolongations of this smooth muscle extend between the glands and may reach the surface. Intestinal metaplasia is unusual. Because of the enormous thickening of the mucosa it is obvious that normal-sized biopsies will only contain hyperplastic surface and foveolar epithelium which, although consistent with a diagnosis of Menetrier's disease, can also result from other disorders associated with thickened gastric folds (see above). Thus a full-thickness mucosal biopsy, obtained either at laparotomy or by an electrosurgical snare at endoscopy [146], is essential to make the diagnosis.

The nature of Menetrier's disease and its aetiology is almost certainly multifactorial. Cases reported in children have been of a self-limited illness, and the presence of a peripheral eosinophilia in some has suggested the possibility of an allergic reaction in this age group [147,148]. In others there has been an association with acute cytomegalovirus infection [149–151]. *H. pylori* infection may result in thickening of gastric rugae seen at endoscopy or radiologically [152,153]. The natural history of the disease in adults has been unclear since in the past the majority of cases in the literature have had a gastric resection soon after diagnosis. Occasional examples of spontaneous remission have been reported in which protein loss from the stomach has stopped, and this has been accompanied by histological transition to an atrophic gastritis [154,155]. A role for growth factors to explain the abnormal proliferation of the gastric mucosa has received support from a study showing enhanced immunostaining for transforming growth factor alpha (TGF-α) in the gastric mucosa of four patients with Menetrier's disease. A transgenic mouse model in which TGF-α was overproduced showed a number of features characteristic of the disease in humans including foveolar hyperplasia, cystic glandular dilatation and reduced basal and histamine-stimulated rates of acid production [156].

The identification of lymphocytic gastritis in seven patients described as having Menetrier's disease [157,158] led to a re-evaluation of 23 cases previously diagnosed as Menetrier's disease at the Mayo Clinic between 1950 and 1991 [159]. As a result of this study two distinct histological entities (with similar clinical and macroscopic features) were delineated, namely massive foveolar hyperplasia (MFH) with little inflammation (10 cases) and hypertrophic lymphocytic gastritis (HLG) in which there was severe, usually diffuse, mucosal inflammation and a striking increase in intraepithelial lymphocytes (13 cases). Although the height of the mucosal folds in MFH and HLG was comparable, statistical analysis showed that patients with MFH had a thicker mucosa, higher foveolar to gland ratios, minimal inflammation and greater mucosal oedema compared to HLG. The authors concluded that the term Menetrier's disease should be restricted to those with the histological picture of MFH and that the others represented one end of the pathological spectrum of lymphocytic gastritis (see also p. 120). In another report, an association was found between giant gastric folds in the fundus and corpus and heavy colonization with *H. pylori* in some 90% of patients studied [160]. There have been several reports where eradication of *H. pylori* has resulted in resolution of enlarged gastric folds and of hypoproteinaemia [161–164], although in some this took several months. In one report increased production of interleukin-1-beta (IL-1β) and hepatocyte growth factor fell concomitantly with foveolar thickness and fold width on antibacterial treatment [165].

A major point of controversy, dating from the original paper, has related to the cancer risk in Menetrier's disease [166]. In several cases the finding of thickened gastric folds at endoscopy, or after radiological examination at the time of diagnosis of gastric cancer, has been attributed to Menetrier's disease, but adequate histological confirmation has been lacking and it is more likely that an infiltrating carcinoma has given rise to this appearance secondarily. As well as this, gastric resection soon after the diagnosis of Menetrier's disease has been the usual method of treatment in the past, so that in these instances any possible cancer risk could not be assessed. In a few cases, however, gastric cancer has been detected several years after the diagnosis of Menetrier's disease [166–168]. Because of this, it would seem advisable to advocate regular endoscopic follow-up with gastric biopsy in the increasing proportion of patients who are managed medically.

In summary, Menetrier's disease, always a rare condition, and one subject to varying clinical and pathological diagnostic criteria in the literature, is likely to be even less commonly reported in the future as a result of an appreciation that identical gross morphological and clinical features, namely thickened folds predominantly involving the body of the stomach and accompanying hypoproteinaemia, can result from other conditions, particularly lymphocytic and *H. pylori*-associated gastritis.

References

1 Plachta A, Speer FD. Gastric polyps and their relationship to carcinoma of the stomach. *Am J Gastroenterol*, 1957; 28: 160.
2 Rosch W. Epidemiology, pathogenesis, diagnosis and treatment of benign gastric tumours. *Front Gastrointest Res*, 1980; 6: 167.
3 Laxen F, Sipponen P, Ihamaki T, Hakkiluoto A, Dortscheva Z. Gastric polyps: their morphological and endoscopical characteristics and relation to gastric carcinoma. *Acta Pathol Microbiol Immunol Scand (A)*, 1982; 90: 221.
4 Ikeda T, Senoue I, Hara M, Tsutsumi Y, Harasawa S, Miwa T. Gastric pseudopolyposis: a new clinical manifestation of type A gastritis. *Am J Gastroenterol*, 1985; 80: 82.
5 Ming S-C, Goldman H. Gastric polyps: a histogenetic classification and its relation to carcinoma. *Cancer*, 1965; 18: 721.
6 Tomasulo J. Gastric polyps: histologic types and their relationship to gastric carcinoma. *Cancer*, 1971; 27: 1346.
7 Nakamura T, Nakano G-I. Histopathological classification and malignant change in gastric polyps. *J Clin Pathol*, 1985; 38: 754.
8 Muller-Lissner SA, Wiebecke B. Investigations on hyperplasiogenous gastric polyps by partial reconstruction. *Pathol Res Pract*, 1982; 174: 368.
9 Muto TR, Oota K. Polypogenesis of gastric mucosa. *Gann*, 1970; 61: 435.
10 Hattori T. Morphological range of hyperplastic polyps and carcinomas arising in hyperplastic polyps of the stomach. *J Clin Pathol*, 1985; 38: 622.
11 Dirschmid K, Walser J, Hugel H. Pseudomalignant erosion in hyperplastic gastric polyps. *Cancer*, 1984; 54: 2290.
12 Isaacson P. Biopsy appearances easily mistaken for malignancy in gastrointestinal endoscopy. *Histopathology*, 1982; 6: 377.
13 Shekitka KM, Helwig EB. Deceptive bizarre stromal cells in polyps and ulcers of the gastrointestinal tract. *Cancer*, 1991; 67: 2111.
14 Mori K, Shinya H, Wolff WI. Polypoid reparative mucosal proliferation at the site of a healed gastric ulcer: sequential gastroscopic, radiological and histological observation. *Gastroenterology*, 1971; 61: 523.
15 Saito Y, Ohkusa T, Endo S, Okayasu I. Detection of *Helicobacter pylori* in gastric hyperplastic polyps: comparison between foveolar and fundic polyps. *Eur J Gastroenterol Hepatol*, 1992; 4 (Suppl 1): 589.
16 Veereman-Wauters G, Ferrell L, Ostroff JW, Hayman MB. Hyperplastic gastric polyps associated with persistent *Helicobacter pylori* infection and active gastritis. *Am J Gastroenterol*, 1990; 85: 1395.
17 Ohkusa T, Takashimizu I, Fujiki K *et al*. Disappearance of hyperplastic polyps in the stomach after eradication of *Helicobacter pylori*. A randomized, controlled trial. *Ann Intern Med*, 1998; 129: 712.
18 Mizuno H, Kobayashi S, Kasugai T. Endoscopic follow-up of gastric polyps. *Gastrointest Endosc*, 1975; 21: 112.
19 Joffe N, Goldman H, Antonioli DA. Recurring hyperplastic gastric polyps following subtotal gastrectomy. *Am J Roentgenol*, 1978; 130: 301.
20 Janunger K-G, Domellof L. Gastric polyps and precancerous mucosal changes after partial gastrectomy. *Acta Chir Scand*, 1978; 144: 293.
21 Savage A, Jones S. Histological appearances of the gastric mucosa 15–27 years after partial gastrectomy. *J Clin Pathol*, 1979; 32: 179.
22 Littler ER, Gleibermann E. Gastritis cystica polyposa. (Gastric mucosal prolapse at gastroenterostomy site, with cystic and infiltrative epithelial hyperplasia.) *Cancer*, 1972; 29: 205.
23 Chakravorty RC, Schatzki PF. Gastric cystic polyposis. *Dig Dis*, 1975; 20: 981.
24 Stemmermann GN, Hayashi T. Hyperplastic polyps of the gastric mucosa adjacent to gastroenterostomy stomas. *Am J Clin Pathol*, 1979; 71: 341.
25 Franzin G, Novelli P. Gastritis cystica profunda. *Histopathology*, 1981; 5: 535.
26 Koga S, Watanabe H, Enjoji M. Stomal polypoid hypertrophic gastritis. A polypoid gastric lesion at gastroenterostomy site. *Cancer*, 1979; 43: 647.
27 Griffel B, Engleberg M, Reiss R. Multiple polypoid cystic gastritis in old gastroenteric stoma. *Arch Pathol*, 1974; 97: 316.
28 Nakamura T. Pathologische Einteilung der Magenpolypen mit specifischer Betrachtung ihrer malignen Entartung. *Der Chirurg*, 1970; 41: 122.
29 Elster K. A new approach to the classification of gastric polyps. *Endoscopy*, 1974; 6: 44.
30 Kozuka S, Masamoto K, Suzuki S *et al*. Histogenetic types and size of polypoid lesions in the stomach, with special reference to cancerous change. *Gann*, 1977; 68: 267.
31 Remmele W, Kolb EF. Malignant transformation of hyperplasiogenic polyps of the stomach. *Endoscopy*, 1978; 10: 63.
32 Daibo M, Itabashi M, Hirota T. Malignant transformation of gastric hyperplastic polyps. *Am J Gastroenterol*, 1987; 82: 1016.
33 Carneiro F, David L, Seruca R *et al*. Hyperplastic polyposis and diffuse carcinoma of the stomach. A study of a family. *Cancer*, 1993; 72: 323.
34 Orlowska J, Jarosz D, Pachlewski J, Butruk E. Malignant transformation of benign epithelial gastric polyps. *Am J Gastroenterol*, 1995; 90: 2152.
35 Lauwers GY, Wahl SJ, Melamed J, Rojas-Corona RR. p53 expression in precancerous gastric lesions: an immunohistochemical study of Pab 1801 monoclonal antibody on adenomatous and hyperplastic gastric polyps. *Am J Gastroenterol*, 1993; 88: 1916.
36 Dijkhuizen SMM, Entius MM, Clement MJ *et al*. Multiple hyperplastic polyps in the stomach: evidence for clonality and neoplastic potential. *Gastroenterology*, 1997; 112: 561.
37 Utsunomiya J, Gocho H, Miyanaga T *et al*. Peutz–Jeghers syndrome: its natural course and management. *Johns Hopkins Med J*, 1975; 136: 71.
38 Dodds WJ, Schulte WJ, Hensley GT, Hogan WJ. Peutz–Jeghers syndrome and gastrointestinal malignancy. *Am J Roentgenol*, 1972; 115: 374.
39 Cochet B, Carrel J, Desbaillets L, Widgren S. Peutz–Jeghers syn-

drome associated with gastrointestinal carcinoma. Report of two cases in a family. *Gut*, 1979; 20: 169.

40 Williams CB, Goldblatt M, Delaney PV. 'Top and tail endoscopy' and follow-up in Peutz–Jeghers syndrome. *Endoscopy*, 1982; 14: 82.

41 Giardiello FM, Welsh SB, Hamilton SR *et al*. Increased risk of cancer in the Peutz–Jeghers syndrome. *N Engl J Med*, 1987; 316: 1511.

42 Spigelman AD, Murday V, Phillips RKS. Cancer and the Peutz–Jeghers syndrome. *Gut*, 1989; 30: 1588.

43 Hizawa K, Iida M, Matsumoto T *et al*. Cancer in Peutz–Jeghers syndrome. *Cancer*, 1993; 72: 2777.

44 Tomlinson I, Houlston R. Peutz–Jeghers syndrome. *J Med Genet*, 1997; 34: 1007.

45 Hemminki A, Tomlinson I, Markie D *et al*. Localization of a susceptibility locus for Peutz–Jeghers syndrome to 19p using comparative genomic hybridization and targeted linkage analysis. *Nat Genet*, 1997; 15: 87.

46 Jenne DE, Reimann H, Nezu J *et al*. Peutz–Jeghers syndrome is caused by mutations in a novel serine threonine kinase. *Nat Genet*, 1998; 18: 38.

47 Wang Z-J, Ellis I, Zauber P *et al*. Allelic imbalance at the *LKB1 (STK11)* locus in tumours from patients with Peutz–Jeghers' syndrome provides evidence for a hamartoma–(adenoma)–carcinoma sequence. *J Pathol*, 1999; 188: 9.

48 Watanabe A, Nagashima H, Motoi M, Ogawa K. Familial juvenile polyposis of the stomach. *Gastroenterology*, 1979; 77: 148.

49 Hizawa K, Iida M, Yao T, Aoyagi K, Fujishima M. Juvenile polyposis of the stomach: clinicopathological features and its malignant potential. *J Clin Pathol*, 1997; 50: 771.

50 Ruymann FB. Juvenile polyps with cachexia. Report of an infant and comparison with Cronkhite–Canada syndrome in adults. *Gastroenterology*, 1969; 57: 431.

51 Goodman ZD, Yardley JH, Milligan FD. Pathogenesis of colonic polyps in multiple juvenile polyposis. Report of a case associated with gastric polyps and carcinoma of the rectum. *Cancer*, 1979; 43: 1906.

52 Stemper TJ, Kent TH, Summers RW. Juvenile polyposis and gastrointestinal carcinoma. A study of a kindred. *Ann Intern Med*, 1975; 83: 639.

53 Beacham CH, Shields HM, Raffensperger EC, Enterline HT. Juvenile and adenomatous gastrointestinal polyposis. *Dig Dis*, 1978; 23: 1137.

54 Grigioni WF, Alampi G, Martinelli G, Piccaluga A. Atypical juvenile polyposis. *Histopathology*, 1981; 5: 361.

55 Jarvinen H, Franssila KO. Familial juvenile polyposis coli: increased risk of colorectal cancer. *Gut*, 1984; 25: 792.

56 Jass JR, Williams CB, Bussey HJR, Morson BC. Juvenile polyposis: a precancerous condition. *Histopathology*, 1988; 13: 619.

57 Sassatelli R, Bertoni G, Serra L *et al*. Generalized juvenile polyposis with mixed pattern and gastric cancer. *Gastroenterology*, 1993; 104: 910.

58 Wang Z-J, Taylor F, Churchman M, Norbury G, Tomlinson I. Genetic pathways of colorectal carcinogenesis rarely involve the PTEN and LKB1 genes outside the inherited hamartoma syndromes. *Am J Pathol*, 1998; 153: 363.

59 Howe JR, Roth S, Ringold JC *et al*. Mutations in the SMAD4/DPC4 gene in juvenile polyposis. *Science*, 1998; 180: 1086.

60 Jacoby RF, Schlack S, Cole CE, Skarbek M, Harris C, Meisner LF. A juvenile polyposis tumor suppressor locus at 10q22 is deleted from nonepithelial cells in the lamina propria. *Gastroenterology*, 1997; 112: 1398.

61 Weinstock JV, Kawanishi H. Gastrointestinal polyposis with orocutaneous hamartomas (Cowden's disease). *Gastroenterology*, 1978; 74: 890.

62 Hauser H, Ody B, Plojoux O, Wettstein P. Radiological findings in multiple hamartoma syndrome (Cowden's disease). A report of three cases. *Radiology*, 1980; 137: 317.

63 Gorensek M, Matko I, Skralovnik A, Rode M, Satler J, Jutersek A. Disseminated hereditary gastrointestinal polyposis with orocutaneous hamartomatosis (Cowden's disease). *Endoscopy*, 1984; 16: 59.

64 Elster K. Histologic classification of gastric polyps. In: Morson BC, ed. *Pathology of the Gastro-Intestinal Tract. Current Topics in Pathology 63*. Berlin: Springer-Verlag, 1976: 77.

65 Sipponen P, Laxen F, Seppala K. Cystic 'hamartomatous' gastric polyps: a disorder of oxyntic glands. *Histopathology*, 1983; 7: 729.

66 Kinoshita Y, Tojo M, Yano T *et al*. Incidence of fundic gland polyps in patients without familial adenomatous polyposis. *Gastrointest Endosc*, 1993; 39: 161.

67 Utsunomiya J, Maki T, Iwama T *et al*. Gastric lesion of familial polyposis coli. *Cancer*, 1974; 34: 745.

68 Ranzi T, Castagnone D, Velio P *et al*. Gastric and duodenal polyps in familial polyposis coli. *Gut*, 1981; 22: 363.

69 Watanabe H, Enjoji M, Yao T, Ohsato K. Gastric lesions in familial adenomatosis coli. Their incidence and histological analysis. *Hum Pathol*, 1978; 9: 269.

70 Eichenberger P, Hammer B, Gloor F *et al*. Gardner's syndrome with glandular cysts of the fundic mucosa. *Endoscopy*, 1980; 12: 63.

71 Burt RW, Berenson MM, Lee RG *et al*. Upper gastrointestinal polyps in Gardner's syndrome. *Gastroenterology*, 1984; 86: 295.

72 Sarre RG, Frost AG, Jagelman DG *et al*. Gastric and duodenal polyps in familial adenomatous polyposis: a prospective study of the nature and prevalence of upper gastrointestinal polyps. *Gut*, 1987; 28: 306.

73 Domizio P, Talbot IC, Spigelman AD *et al*. Upper gastrointestinal pathology in familial adenomatous polyposis: results from a prospective study of 102 patients. *J Clin Pathol*, 1990; 43: 738.

74 Iida M, Yao T, Watanabe H *et al*. Fundic gland polyposis in patients without familial adenomatous coli: its incidence and clinical features. *Gastroenterology*, 1984; 86: 1437.

75 Lynch HT, Smyrk TC, Lanspa SJ *et al*. Upper gastrointestinal manifestations in families with hereditary flat adenoma syndrome. *Cancer*, 1993; 71: 2709.

76 Eidt S, Stolte M. Gastric glandular cysts. Investigations into their genesis and relationship to colorectal epithelial tumors. *Z Gastroenterol*, 1989; 27: 212.

77 Tatsuta M, Okuda S, Tamura H, Taniguchi H. Polyps in the acid-secreting area of the stomach. *Gastrointest Endosc*, 1981; 27: 145.

78 Elster K, Eidt H, Ottenjann R *et al*. Drusenkorperzysten, eine polypoide Läsion der Magenschleimhaut. *Deutsche Med Wochenshr*, 1977; 102: 183.

79 Lee RG, Burt RW. The histopathology of fundic gland polyps of the stomach. *Am J Clin Pathol*, 1986; 86: 498.

80 Sakai N, Tatsuta M, Hirasawa R *et al*. Low prevalence of

Helicobacter pylori infection in patients with hamartomatous fundic polyps. *Dig Dis Sci*, 1998; 43: 766.

81 Iida M, Yao T, Watanabe H *et al.* Natural history of fundic gland polyposis in patients with familial adenomatosis coli/Gardner's syndrome. *Gastroenterology*, 1985; 89: 1021.

82 El-Zimaity HMT, Jackson FW, Graham DY. Fundic gland polyps developing during omeprazole therapy. *Am J Gastroenterol*, 1997; 92: 1858.

83 Choudry U, Boyce HW Jr, Coppola D. Proton-pump inhibitor-associated gastric polyps: a retrospective analysis of their frequency, and endoscopic, histological and ultrastructural characteristics. *Am J Clin Pathol*, 1998; 110: 615.

84 Stolte M, Bethke B, Ruhl G, Ritter M. Omeprazole-induced pseudohypertrophy of gastric parietal cells. *Z Gastroenterol*, 1992; 30: 134.

85 Declich P, Ambrosiani L, Prada A *et al.* Fundic metaplasia with parietal cell hyperplasia of the antrum: a lesion possibly associated with long term use of omeprazole (letter). *Am J Gastroenterol*, 1999; 94: 2317.

86 Vieth M, Stolte M. Fundic gland polyps are not induced by proton pump inhibitor therapy. *Am J Clin Pathol*, 2001; 116: 716.

87 Odze RD, Quinn PS, Terrault NA *et al.* Advanced gastroduodenal polyposis with ras mutations in a patient with familial adenomatous polyposis. *Hum Pathol*, 1993; 24: 442.

88 Wu T-T, Kornacki S, Rashid A, Yardley JH, Hamilton SR. Dysplasia and dysregulation of proliferation in foveolar and surface epithelia of fundic gland polyps from patients with familial adenomatous polyposis. *Am J Surg Pathol*, 1998; 22: 293.

89 Coffey RJ Jr, Knight CD Jr, van Heerden JA *et al.* Gastric adenocarcinoma complicating Gardner's syndrome in a North American woman. *Gastroenterology*, 1985; 88: 1263.

90 Goodman AJ, Dundas SAC, Scholfield JH, Johnson BF. Gastric carcinoma and familial adenomatous polyposis (FAP). *Int J Colorectal Dis*, 1988; 3: 201.

91 Zwick A, Munir M, Ryan CK *et al.* Gastric adenocarcinoma and dysplasia in fundic gland polyps of a patient with attenuated adenomatous polyposis coli. *Gastroenterology*, 1997; 113: 659.

92 Hofgartner WT, Thorp M, Ramus MW *et al.* Gastric adenocarcinoma associated with fundic gland polyps in a patient with attenuated familial adenomatous polyposis. *Am J Gastroenterol*, 1999; 94: 2275.

93 Cronkhite LW Jr, Canada WJ. Generalized gastrointestinal polyposis. An unusual syndrome of polyposis, pigmentation, alopecia and onychotrophia. *N Engl J Med*, 1955; 252: 1011.

94 Ikeda K, Sannohe Y, Murayama H. A case of Cronkhite–Canada syndrome developing after hemi-colectomy. *Endoscopy*, 1981; 13: 251.

95 Johnstone MM, Vosburgh JW, Wiens AT, Walsh GC. Gastrointestinal polyposis associated with alopecia, pigmentation and atrophy of the fingernails and toenails. *Ann Intern Med*, 1962; 56: 935.

96 Jarnum S, Jensen H. Diffuse gastrointestinal polyposis with ectodermal changes. A case with severe malabsorption and enteric loss of plasma proteins and electrolytes. *Gastroenterology*, 1966; 50: 107.

97 Ali M, Weinstein J, Biempica L *et al.* Cronkhite–Canada syndrome: report of a case with bacteriologic, immunologic, and electron microscopic studies. *Gastroenterology*, 1980; 79: 731.

98 Kindbloom L, Angervall L, Santesson B, Selander S. Cronkhite–Canada syndrome. *Cancer*, 1977; 39: 2651.

99 Burke AP, Sobin LH. The pathology of Cronkhite-Canada polyps. A comparison to juvenile polyposis. *Am J Surg Pathol*, 1989; 13: 940.

100 Zarling EJ. Gastric adenomyoma with coincidental pancreatic rest: a case report. *Gastrointest Endosc*, 1981; 27: 175.

101 Nickels J, Laasonen EM. Pancreatic heterotopia. *Scand J Gastroenterol*, 1970; 5: 639.

102 Bill K, Belber JP, Carson JW. Adenomyoma (pancreatic heterotopia) of the duodenum producing common bile duct obstruction. *Gastrointest Endosc*, 1982; 28: 182.

103 Fléjou J-F, Potet F, Mollas G, Bernardes P, Amouyal PF, Fékété F. Cystic dystrophy of the gastric and duodenal wall developing in heterotopic pancreas: an unrecognized entity. *Gut*, 1993; 34: 343.

104 Lai ECS, Tompkins RK. Heterotopic pancreas. Review of a 26 year experience. *Am J Surg*, 1986; 151: 697.

105 Goldfarb WB, Bennett D, Monafo W. Carcinoma in heterotopic gastric pancreas. *Ann Surg*, 1963; 158: 56.

106 Hickman DM, Frey CF, Carson JW. Adenocarcinoma arising in gastric heterotopic pancreas. *West J Med*, 1981; 135: 57.

107 Gensler S, Seidenberg B, Rifkin H *et al.* Ciliated lined intramural cyst of the stomach: case report and suggested embryogenesis. *Ann Surg*, 1966; 163: 954.

108 Delvaux S, Ectors N, Geboes K, Desmet V. Gastric gland heterotopia with extensive lymphoid stroma: a gastric lymphoepithelial cyst. *Am J Gastroenterol*, 1996; 91: 599.

109 Schroeder BA, Wells RG, Sty JR. Inflammatory fibroid polyp of the stomach in a child. *Pediatr Radiol*, 1987; 17: 71.

110 Helwig EB, Ranier A. Inflammatory fibroid polyps of the stomach. *Am J Pathol*, 1952; 28: 535.

111 Tada S, Iida M, Yao T *et al.* Endoscopic removal of inflammatory fibroid polyps of the stomach. *Am J Gastroenterol*, 1991; 86: 1247.

112 Matsushita M, Hajiro K, Okazaki K, Takakuwa H. Endoscopic features of gastric inflammatory fibroid polyps. *Am J Gastroenterol*, 1996; 91: 1595.

113 Vanek J. Gastric submucosal granuloma with eosinophilic infiltration. *Am J Pathol*, 1949; 25: 397.

114 Calam J, Krasner N, Haqqani M. Extensive gastrointestinal damage following a saline emetic. *Dig Dis Sci*, 1982; 27: 936.

115 Allibone RO, Nanson JK, Anthony PP. Multiple and recurrent inflammatory fibroid polyps in a Devon family ('Devon polyposis syndrome'). An update. *Gut*, 1992; 33: 1004.

116 Goldman RL, Friedman NB. Neurogenic nature of so-called inflammatory fibroid polyps of the stomach. *Cancer*, 1967; 20: 134.

117 Williams RM. An ultrastructural study of a jejunal inflammatory fibroid polyp. *Histopathology*, 1981; 5: 193.

118 Ureles AL, Alschibaja T, Lodico D, Stabins SJ. Idiopathic eosinophilic infiltration of the gastrointestinal tract, diffuse and circumscribed. *Am J Med*, 1961; 30: 899.

119 Johnstone JM, Morson BC. Inflammatory fibroid polyp of the gastrointestinal tract. *Histopathology*, 1978; 2: 349.

120 Widgren S, Pizzolato GP. Inflammatory fibroid polyp of the gastrointestinal tract: possible origin in myofibroblasts? A study of twelve cases. *Ann Pathol*, 1987; 7: 184.

121 Wille P, Borchard F. Fibroid polyps of gastrointestinal tract are inflammatory-reactive proliferations of CD34-positive perivascular cells. *Histopathology*, 1998; 32: 498.

122 Domellöf L, Eriksson S, Helander HF, Janunger K-G. Lipid islands in the gastric mucosa after resection for benign ulcer disease. *Gastroenterology*, 1977; 72: 14.
123 Terruzzi V, Minoli G, Butti GC, Rossini A. Gastric lipid islands in the gastric stump and in non-operated stomach. *Endoscopy*, 1980; 12: 58.
124 McCaffery TD Jr. Xanthomas of the stomach. *Gastrointest Endosc*, 1975; 21: 167.
125 Heilmann K. Lipid islands in gastric mucosa. *Beitr Pathol*, 1973; 149: 411.
126 Ludvikova M, Michal M, Datkova D. Gastric xanthelasma associated with diffuse signet ring carcinoma. A potential diagnostic problem. *Histopathology*, 1994; 25: 581.
127 Kimura K, Hiramoto T, Buncher CR. Gastric xanthelasma. *Arch Pathol*, 1969; 87: 110.
128 Kaiserling E, Heinle H, Itabe H, Takano T, Remmele W. Lipid islands in human gastric mucosa: morphological and immunohistochemical findings. *Gastroenterology*, 1996; 110: 369.
129 Takebayashi S. Fine structure of xanthelasma of the stomach. *Acta Pathol Jpn*, 1970; 20: 357.
130 Boger A, Hort W. The importance of smooth muscle cells in the development of foam cells in the gastric mucosa. An electron microscopic study. *Virchows Arch Pathol Anat*, 1977; 372: 287.
131 Soga J, Saito K, Suzuki N, Sakai T. Plasma cell granuloma of the stomach. A report of a case and review of the literature. *Cancer*, 1970; 25: 618.
132 Isaacson P, Buchanan R, Mepham BL. Plasma cell granuloma of the stomach. *Hum Pathol*, 1978; 9: 355.
133 Domenichini E, Martiarena HM, Rubio H. Gastric plasma cell granuloma (report of a case). *Endoscopy*, 1982; 14: 148.
134 Tada T, Wakabayashi T, Kishimoto H. Plasma cell granuloma of the stomach. A report of a case associated with gastric cancer. *Cancer*, 1984; 54: 541.
135 Jensen K, Raynor S, Rose SG *et al*. Amyloid tumors of the gastrointestinal tract: a report of two cases and review of the literature. *Am J Gastroenterol*, 1985; 80: 784.
136 Bjornsson S, Johansson JH, Sigurjonsson F. Localised primary amyloidosis of the stomach presenting with gastric haemorrhage. *Acta Med Scand*, 1987; 221: 115.
137 Greaney TV, Nolan N. Malone DE. Multiple gastric polyps in familial amyloid polyneuropathy. *Abdom Imaging*, 1999; 24: 220.
138 Goteri G, Ranaldi R, Pileri SA, Bearzi I. Localized amyloidosis and gastrointestinal lymphoma: a rare association. *Histopathology*, 1998; 32: 348.
139 Menetrier P. Des polyadénomes gastriques et de leurs rapports avec le cancer de l'estomac. *Arch Physiol Norm Pathol*, 1888; 1: 32.
140 Burns B, Gay B. Ménétrier's disease of the stomach in children. *Am J Roentgenol*, 1968; 103: 300.
141 Scharschmidt BF. The natural history of hypertrophic gastropathy (Ménétrier's disease). Report of a case with 16 year follow-up and review of 120 cases from the literature. *Am J Med*, 1977; 63: 644.
142 Kenney FD, Dockerty MB, Waugh JM. Giant hypertrophy of gastric mucosa. A clinical and pathological study. *Cancer*, 1954; 7: 671.
143 Olmsted WW, Cooper PH, Madewell JE. Involvement of the gastric antrum in Ménétrier's disease. *Am J Roentgenol*, 1976; 126: 524.
144 Stamm B. Localized hyperplastic gastropathy of the mucous cell- and mixed cell-type (localized Menetrier's disease): a report of 11 patients. *Am J Surg Pathol*, 1997; 21: 1334.
145 Stempien SJ, Dagradi AE, Riengold IM *et al*. Hypertrophic hypersecretory gastropathy. *Am J Dig Dis*, 1964; 9: 417.
146 Bjork JT, Geenen JE, Soergel KH *et al*. Endoscopic evaluation of large gastric folds. A comparison of biopsy techniques. *Gastrointest Endosc*, 1977; 24: 22.
147 Chouraqui JP, Roy CC, Brochu P *et al*. Ménétrier's disease in children: report of a patient and review of sixteen other cases. *Gastroenterology*, 1981; 80: 1042.
148 Fishbein M, Kirschner BS, Gonzales-Valina R. Ménétrier's disease associated with formula protein allergy and small intestinal injury in an infant. *Gastroenterology*, 1992; 103: 1664.
149 Coad NAG, Shah KJ. Ménétrier's disease in childhood associated with cytomegalovirus infection: a case report and review of the literature. *Br J Radiol*, 1986; 59: 615.
150 Kovacs AAS, Churchill MA, Wood D, Mascola L, Zaia JA. Molecular and epidemiologic evaluations of a cluster of cases of Menetrier's disease associated with cytomegalovirus. *Pediatr Infect Dis J*, 1993; 12: 1011.
151 Eisenstat DDR, Griffiths AM, Cutz E, Petric M, Drumm B. Acute cytomegalovirus infection in a child with Menetrier's disease. *Gastroenterology*, 1995; 109: 592.
152 Morrison S, Dahms BB, Hoffenberg E, Czinn SJ. Enlarged gastric folds in association with *Campylobacter pylori* gastritis. *Radiology*, 1989; 171: 819.
153 Chaloupka JC, Gay BB, Caplan D. Campylobacter gastritis simulating Ménétrier's disease by upper gastrointestinal radiography. *Pediatr Radiol*, 1990; 20: 200.
154 Frank BW, Kern F Jr. Menetrier's disease. Spontaneous metamorphosis of giant hypertrophy of the gastric mucosa to atrophic gastritis. *Gastroenterology*, 1967; 53: 953.
155 Berenson MM, Sanella J, Freston JW. Menetrier's disease. Serial morphological, secretory, and serological observations. *Gastroenterology*, 1976; 70: 257.
156 Dempsey PJ, Goldenring JR, Soroka CJ *et al*. Possible role of transforming growth factor α in the pathogenesis of Ménétrier's disease: supportive evidence from humans and transgenic mice. *Gastroenterology*, 1992; 103: 1950.
157 Hayot J, Bogomoletz WV, Jouret A, Mainget P. Menetrier's disease with lymphocytic gastritis: an unusual association with possible pathogenic implications. *Hum Pathol*, 1991; 22: 379.
158 Mosnier JF, Fléjou JF, Amouyal G *et al*. Hypertrophic gastropathy with gastric adenocarcinoma: Menetrier's disease and lymphocytic gastritis? *Gut*, 1991; 32: 1565.
159 Wolfsen HC, Carpenter HA, Talley NJ. Menetrier's disease: a form of hypertrophic gastropathy or gastritis? *Gastroenterology*, 1993; 104: 1310.
160 Stolte M, Batz C, Eidt S. Giant fold gastritis—a special form of *Helicobacter pylori* associated gastritis. *Z Gastroenterol*, 1993; 31: 289.
161 Bayerdorffer E, Ritter MM, Hatz R *et al*. Healing of protein losing hypertrophic gastropathy by eradication of *Helicobacter pylori*. Is *Helicobacter pylori* a pathogenic factor in Menetrier's disease? *Gut*, 1994; 35: 701.
162 Avunduk C, Navab F, Hampf F, Coughlin B. Prevalence of *Helicobacter pylori* infection in patients with large gastric folds: evaluation and follow-up with endoscopic ultrasound before and after antimicrobial therapy. *Am J Gastroenterol*, 1995; 90: 1969.

163 Kawasaki M, Hizawa K, Aoyagi K, Nakamura S, Fujishima M. Menetrier's disease associated with *Helicobacter pylori* infection: resolution of enlarged gastric folds and hypoproteinemia after antibacterial treatment. *Am J Gastroenterol*, 1997; 92: 1909.
164 Kaneko T, Akamatsu T, Gotoh A *et al*. Remission of Menetrier's disease after a prolonged period with therapeutic eradication of *Helicobacter pylori*. *Am J Gastroenterol*, 1999; 94: 272.
165 Yasunaga Y, Shinomura Y, Kanayama S *et al*. Increased production of interleukin 1β and hepatocyte growth factor may contribute to foveolar hyperplasia in enlarged fold gastritis. *Gut*, 1996; 39: 787.
166 Chusid EL, Hirsch RL, Colcher H. Spectrum of hypertrophic gastropathy. Giant rugal folds, polyposis and carcinoma of the stomach—case report and review of the literature. *Arch Intern Med*, 1964; 114: 621.
167 van Loewenthal M, Steinitz H, Friedlander E. Gastritis hypertrophica gigantea und Magenkarzinom. *Gastroenterologia*, 1960; 93: 133.
168 Wood GM, Bates C, Brown RC, Losowsky MS. Intramucosal carcinoma of the gastric antrum complicating Ménétrier's disease. *J Clin Pathol*, 1983; 36: 1071.

17 Miscellaneous conditions of the stomach

Acute gastric dilatation

Acute spontaneous gastric dilatation is rare in humans [1] (occurring more commonly in fur seals, macaques, cats and horses). It occurs mainly in patients with respiratory problems or with paralytic ileus. It may also be seen in eating disorders [2], including anorexia nervosa in association with superior mesenteric artery syndrome [3], and postoperatively. Other associations include diabetes mellitus [4] especially in diabetic ketoacidosis [5], drugs [6], Duchenne muscular dystrophy [7] and Prader–Willi syndrome. It has also been reported following insertion of a percutaneous endoscopic gastrostomy (PEG) feeding tube [8,9], or after injection sclerotherapy of oesophageal varices [10]. Acute gastric dilatation may also be seen following severe trauma [11]. Gastric rupture is unusual, but when it occurs it may be fatal. The dilatation is due to gas and the onset is usually rapid, leading to regurgitation of small amounts of fluid, shock and collapse.

Motility disorders

Adult pyloric obstruction

The gastric outlet in adults may be narrowed due to a number of causes. A congenital diaphragm comprised of mucosa, submucosa and muscularis mucosae has been described at the pyloric ring [12,13]. This has a distinct similarity to a gastric diaphragm described in a patient taking non-steroidal anti-inflammatory drugs [14], which resembled diaphragm disease elsewhere in the gastrointestinal tract (see p. 298) [15]. The commonest form of adult pyloric stenosis is in fact hypertrophic stenosis due to previous prepyloric or duodenal ulceration [16–19], tumour or extrinsic adhesions. It may occasionally be due to eosinophilic gastroenteritis, when the circular muscle is fibrosed and not hypertrophic.

The rare primary adult hypertrophic pyloric stenosis is associated with total or segmental hypertrophy of the circular muscle coat without obvious disease [20–25]. A few cases appear to represent persistent infantile pyloric stenosis and it is occasionally familial. The macroscopic appearance is of an enlarged pylorus, similar to that seen in infancy (see p. 100). Microscopically there may be a uniform or segmental muscular hypertrophy, sometimes with fibrosis but no mucosal inflammation.

Gastric motility disorders associated with neuromuscular disorders

Gastroparesis may complicate several generalized neuromuscular disorders. Patients with Duchenne muscular dystrophy, mitochondrial myopathies and the syndrome of polyneuropathy, ophthalmoplegia and leukoencephalopathy (so-called POLYP syndrome) [26] and patients with oculogastrointestinal muscular dystrophy are included in this group, along with progressive muscular dystrophy. The appearances seen in the stomach in progressive muscular dystrophy are similar to those seen in the oesophagus and small bowel [27].

Patients with Friedreich's ataxia may have repetitive uncoordinated gastric contractions, as may be seen throughout the gastrointestinal tract. The myenteric plexus will usually show a reduction in neurone numbers and the presence of eosinophilic nuclear inclusions, similar to those seen in the rest of the nervous system in these patients. Dystrophia myotonica may produce delayed gastric emptying, and in this autosomal dominant inherited condition the gastrointestinal effects may precede the more classical systemic features. The nerves appear normal, but there is smooth muscle atrophy with fatty replacement and fibrosis. Surviving smooth muscle fibres may appear pleomorphic, oedematous and hypereosinophilic with nuclear pyknosis and perinuclear vacuolation.

Postviral gastroparesis

Gastric outlet obstruction has been reported to follow viral illnesses in previously healthy young to middle-aged people. These cases are not well characterized, since the histology has not been studied and the nature of the precipitating viral infection is not always known [28]. However, this remains an unusual but important differential diagnosis in gastric outlet obstruction in the young and middle-aged.

Familial visceral myopathies

There are several different types of familial visceral myopathy, all of which are uncommon. They are inherited and are characterized by the histological findings of degeneration, thinning and fibrous replacement of the smooth muscle of the gastrointestinal tract. Some of these also involve the smooth muscle of the bladder. Although the histological features are similar in these different disorders, the pattern of involvement of the organs and the inheritance may differ between the conditions. Schuffler has subdivided them into types I to IV, type I showing autosomal dominant inheritance and the remainder autosomal recessive [29]. Type I does not involve the stomach. Its effects are seen in the oesophagus, duodenum, colon and bladder. Type II is associated with gastric and jejunoileal dilatation and the presence of multiple diverticula in the small bowel. The duodenum is usually spared. Ptosis and ophthalmoplegia also occur in this variety. Type III results in marked dilatation of the whole of the gastrointestinal tract [30]. In Type IV there is gastroparesis and a narrow small intestine without diverticula. The histological features in all of these forms of visceral myopathy include marked vacuolar degeneration with a characteristic honeycomb appearance of the longitudinal muscle and hypertrophy of the circular muscle coat. The smooth muscle cells are reported to include spheroidal inclusions that are grey on haematoxylin and eosin staining and PAS positive, but the authors have observed similar inclusions in isolation or in very small numbers in patients without visceral myopathy.

Non-familial visceral myopathies

These conditions may occur sporadically without obvious inheritance. Patients may present at all ages with pseudo-obstruction involving the whole gastrointestinal tract. Unlike the inherited conditions, the sporadic varieties may show an inflammatory infiltrate in the smooth muscle layers.

Systemic sclerosis

Involvement of the gastrointestinal tract is common in systemic sclerosis. It most commonly affects the oesophagus [31] (see p. 32) where it may result in severe dysmotility and regurgitation, sometimes with fatal inhalation of gastro-oesophageal contents, but other sites in the gut, including the stomach, may be affected.

Motility disorders in patients with malignancy

Tumour-associated gastric paresis may be associated with the general effects of neoplasia or with therapy—radiation and chemotherapy [32–34]. Local effects of vagal infiltration may be contributory, as may stiffness of the gastric wall from tumour infiltration. Gastroparesis may also be seen in patients with brain stem or posterior fossa tumours, and in paraneoplastic neuropathy in association with small cell carcinoma of the lung.

Gastric volvulus

Gastric volvulus may affect patients at any age. It may present acutely [35] or chronically [36]. Acute presentation is with haemorrhage and ischaemia and infarction. Chronic volvulus presents with recurrent pain and vomiting and sometimes with haematemesis. Gastric volvulus has been subdivided anatomically. Approximately two-thirds of cases have organoaxial volvulus, in which there is volvulus around the long axis of the lesser curve of the stomach. The stomach effectively turns upside down. There is therefore obstruction at the proximal and distal ends of the stomach. Rotation is more commonly anterior in direction in these cases. The second type is mesenteroaxial volvulus, in which the stomach twists around a line from the middle of the greater curve to the porta hepatis. In some instances the stomach may also twist around the gastrohepatic omentum to result in torsion rather than volvulus.

Amyloid

Gastric amyloid (Fig. 17.1) may occur in isolation or as part of generalized amyloidosis [37]. It may present with bleeding and may be seen to infiltrate the whole gastric wall to give a rigid, indistensible and non-collapsible stomach that resembles the leather bottle stomach of diffuse gastric carcinoma. The causes, associations and diagnostic techniques are the same as those elsewhere in the intestine and will be discussed fully in Chapter 41 (see p. 634).

Gastric bezoars

A bezoar is a mass of foreign material in the stomach or intestine [38,39]. In young people and psychiatric patients, trichobezoars consisting of balls or mats of swallowed hair

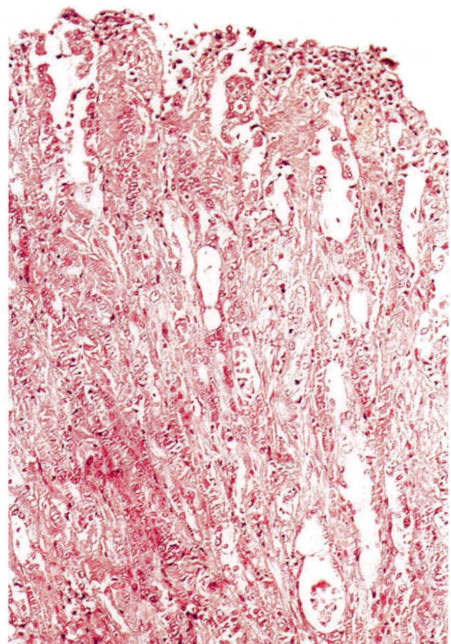

Fig. 17.1 Gastric amyloidosis. The lamina propria of the mucosa is largely replaced by amyloid, which compresses the gastric glands. There is inflammation and erosion of the surface epithelium that is probably due to secondary ischaemia.

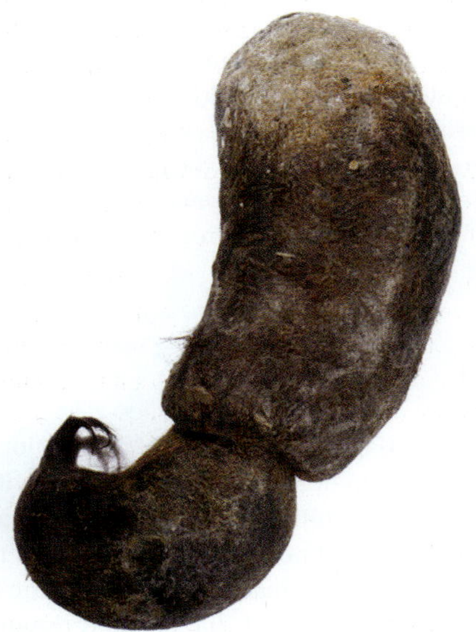

Fig. 17.2 A huge gastric trichobezoar that filled and expanded the lumen of the stomach.

are the most common (Fig. 17.2) [40]. Rapunzel's syndrome refers to the extension of the hair mass through the pylorus into the duodenum, like the mane of hair associated with the Grimm's fairy tale character [41]. In adults, phytobezoars composed of indigestible vegetable matter (often persimmon) are the rule. These are usually cylindrical, ovoid or spheroid with a smooth, bossed or pitted surface. They may be dark brown, green or black, and friable or calcified. Combined bezoars (trichophytobezoars) may sometimes occur. Occasionally unusual substances may be eaten by psychiatric patients and form bezoars. Identification of these has been aided by use of several analytical techniques including X-ray energy spectroscopy [42].

Gastric hyalinization

A small number of thickened stomachs that resemble linitis plastica have been described as incidental findings at autopsy [43,44]. There is marked thickening of the submucosa and the muscle coats of the fundus in the presence of a normal pylorus. Submucosal collagen is increased, whilst the blood vessels are normal. Some patients have received antimetabolic drugs or irradiation, but in others the cause remains obscure. The condition may be distinguished from systemic sclerosis by the absence of appropriate clinical or serological features or involvement of some other part of the gut, and the fact that changes in the muscle coat are relatively minor.

Pseudolipomatosis

A single case of gastric pseudolipomatosis has been identified in the literature. Whether or not its origin is the same as that in the colorectum is unclear [45].

Pseudoxanthoma elasticum

Pseudoxanthoma elasticum is a rare, but recognized cause of gastric bleeding that may occasionally require gastrectomy for treatment [46]. Endoscopically, there are usually yellow submucosal nodules resembling xanthomas in the skin [47–49] and histology shows degenerative changes in gastric submucosal arterioles with elastic lamina degeneration and dystrophic calcification. Angiography, which may demonstrate angiomatous malformation, aneurysmal dilatation and narrowing or occlusion of visceral arteries, can aid the diagnosis. The stomach is not usually affected in isolation in pseudoxanthoma elasticum, and such patients will usually have a characteristic papular rash and retinal angioid streaks to confirm the diagnosis [50].

Graft-versus-host disease

Graft-versus-host disease is a complication of allogenic bone marrow transplantation or transfusion, particularly in immunocompromised patients [51]. It may occur in acute or

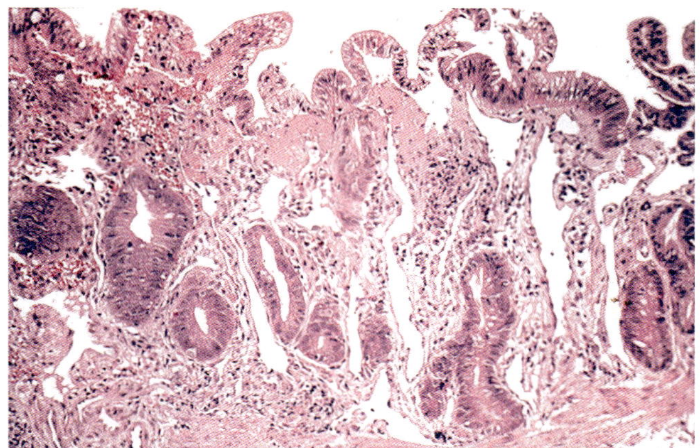

Fig. 17.3 Angiodysplasia of the stomach. Numerous dilated intramucosal vascular spaces are seen, many containing fibrin thrombus. The presence of such thrombi correlates with recent bleeding.

chronic forms. The acute phase occurs 2–10 weeks after bone marrow transplantation, usually with skin rash and gastrointestinal symptoms of nausea, vomiting, abdominal pain and diarrhoea. Endoscopically, the stomach may be congested with erosions [52] and sometimes there may be prominent vascular ectasia [53]. The cardinal histological feature is apoptosis, located especially in the mucous neck cells of the gastric foveolae, associated with granular debris within the glands and varying degrees of gland loss [54]. An acute inflammatory reaction may be seen, and here a careful search for cytomegalovirus inclusions is vital because this is an important differential diagnosis (see p. 125). Other potential mimics are herpes simplex gastritis and human immunodeficiency virus (HIV)-related changes [55]. Graft-versus-host changes may also coexist with other forms of pre-existing gastritis such as that induced by *Helicobacter pylori*.

The histological diagnosis of acute graft-versus-host disease also needs caution in the immediate post-transplant period (before 20 days post transplant), since some of the pre-bone marrow transplant chemotherapy conditioning regimes may produce similar histological changes. It must also be remembered that the changes of graft-versus-host disease may be subtle, are characteristically focal, and often require a diligent search over many sections from the biopsy. It seems that gastric and duodenal biopsies are more sensitive than rectal biopsies for diagnosing gastrointestinal graft-versus-host disease, even when diarrhoea is the predominant symptom: a rectal biopsy will yield the diagnosis in about a half of cases, whereas combined gastric and duodenal biopsies will be diagnostic in more than 90% [54]. Opportunistic infections may also complicate graft-versus-host disease and there is a single report of pseudomembranous gastritis due to *Aspergillus* in a patient with graft-versus-host disease [56].

Chronic graft-versus-host disease is seen between 3 and 13 months after bone marrow transplant in approximately one-third of patients [52]. Some of the clinical features may resemble systemic sclerosis [57]. The histological changes are not specific or diagnostic but glandular atrophy is often prominent.

Vascular disorders

Angiodysplasia

Angiodysplasia may be isolated to the stomach but is more commonly part of a generalized gastrointestinal angiodysplasia. The lesions are comprised of dilated submucosal vessels with perforating vessels going through the muscularis mucosae into the mucosa (Fig. 17.3) [58,59]. These lesions may be associated with long-term haemodialysis or renal failure [60,61], or with von Willebrand's disease [62]. Occasionally they are part of the infantile haemorrhagic angiodysplasia syndrome [63]. How and when angiodysplastic lesions bleed is not clear. It is possible that coexistent pathologies may predispose to bleeding. These include atrophic gastritis, aortic stenosis [64,65] and mitral valve disease [66].

Dieulafoy's disease

The lesions of Dieulafoy are small and likely to be underestimated in some patients when a source of considerable gastric haemorrhage is being sought [67]. Over 100 cases are recorded and reviewed in the literature [68]. The first account of such a lesion was by Gallard in 1884 [69], some 14 years before that of Dieulafoy [67]. The presentation is with massive, occasionally recurrent, sometimes fatal, gastric haemorrhage. Most patients are in the fifth decade and men are affected twice as commonly as women [68]. The lesions are difficult to detect endoscopically because of their site in the fundus: most are situated within 6 cm of the cardia. Microscopically, there is an unusually large, tortuous and aneurysmal artery in the base of a small well circumscribed ulcer 2–5 mm in diameter. The surrounding gastric mucosa is quite normal [70]. This abnormal vessel is thought to represent a congenital calibre persistent submucosal artery [71].

References

1 Todd SR, Marshall GT, Tyroch AH. Acute gastric dilatation revisited. *Am Surg*, 2000; 66: 709.

2 Adson DE, Mitchell JE, Trenkner SW. The superior mesenteric artery syndrome and acute gastric dilatation in eating disorders: a report of two cases and a review of the literature. *Int J Eat Disord*, 1997; 21: 103.

3 Stheneur C, Rey C, Pariente D, Alvin P. Acute gastric dilatation with superior mesenteric artery syndrome in a young girl with anorexia nervosa. *Arch Pediatr*, 1995; 2: 973.

4 Nagai T, Yokoo M, Tomizawa T, Mori M. Acute gastric dilatation accompanied by diabetes mellitus. *Intern Med*, 2001; 40: 320.

5 Magee MF, Bhatt BA. Management of decompensated diabetes. Diabetic ketoacidosis and hyperglycaemic hyperosmolar syndrome. *Crit Care Clin*, 2001; 17: 75.
6 Sarici SU, Yurdatok M, Unal S. Acute gastric dilatation complicating the use of mydriatics in a preterm newborn. *Pediatr Radiol*, 2001; 31: 581.
7 Bensen ES, Jaffe KM, Tarr PI. Acute gastric dilatation in Duchenne muscular dystrophy: a case report and review of the literature. *Arch Phys Med Rehabil*, 1996; 77: 512.
8 Vautier G, Scott BB. Early acute gastric dilatation following percutaneous endoscopic gastrostomy. *Gastrointest Endosc*, 1995; 42: 189.
9 Ghosh S, Eastwood MA, Palmer KR. Acute gastric dilatation—a delayed complication of percutaneous endoscopic gastrostomy. *Gut*, 1993; 34: 859.
10 Sabanathan K, Dean J, Carr-Locke D, Pohl JE. Acute gastric dilatation after injection sclerotherapy. *Lancet*, 1984; i: 1240.
11 Cogbill TH, Bintz M, Johnson JA, Strutt PJ. Acute gastric dilatation after trauma. *J Trauma*, 1987; 27: 1113.
12 Chamberlain D, Addison NV. Adult pyloric obstruction due to a mucosal diaphragm. Report on 2 cases. *Br Med J*, 1959; ii: 1381.
13 Spencer SS. Adult pyloric obstruction due to a mucosal diaphragm. *Med J Aust*, 1961; 1: 816.
14 Warren BF, Shepherd NA. Iatrogenic pathology of the gastrointestinal tract. In: Kirkham N, Hall P, eds. *Progress in Pathology*. Edinburgh: Churchill Livingstone, 1995: 31.
15 Lang J, Price AB, Levi AJ, Burke M, Gumpel JM, Bjarnason I. Diaphragm like disease of the small intestine induced by non steroidal anti-inflammatory drugs. *J Clin Pathol*, 1988; 41: 516.
16 Ger R. Postoperative extrinsic pyloric stenosis. *Br Med J*, 1964; ii: 294.
17 Balint JA, Spence MP. Pyloric stenosis. *Br Med J*, 1959; i: 890.
18 Howe CT, Spence MP. Pyloric stenosis in adults. *Postgrad Med J*, 1960; 36: 743.
19 Knoght CD. Hypertrophic pyloric stenosis in the adult. *Ann Surg*, 1961; 153: 899.
20 McLaughlin RT, Madding GF. Primary pyloric hypertrophy in the adult. *Ann Surg*, 1962; 104: 874.
21 Christiansen KH, Grantham A. Idiopathic hypertrophic pyloric stenosis in the adult. *Arch Surg*, 1962; 85: 207.
22 Wellman KF, Kagan A, Fang H. Hypertrophic pyloric stenosis in adults. *Gastroenterology*, 1964; 46: 601.
23 Hiebert BW, Farris JM. Hypertrophic pyloric stenosis in adults. *Am Surg*, 1961; 32: 712.
24 Woo-Ming M. Familial relationship between adult and infantile hypertrophic pyloric stenosis. *Br Med J*, 1961; i: 476.
25 Raia A, Curti P, DeAlmeida AC, Fry W. The pathogenesis of hypertrophic pyloric stenosis of the pylorus in the newborn and the adult. *Surg Gynecol Obstet*, 1956; 102: 705.
26 Simon LT, Dikram S, Horoupian DS *et al*. Polyneuropathy, opthalmoplegia, leukoencephalopathy and intestinal pseudo-obstruction: POLYP *syndrome*. *Ann Neurol*, 1990; 28: 349.
27 Bevans M. Changes in the musculature of the gastrointestinal tract and the myocardium in progressive muscular dystrophy. *Arch Pathol*, 1945; 40: 225.
28 Oh JJ, Kim OH. Gastroparesis after a presumed viral illness: clinical and laboratory features and natural history. *Mayo Clin Proc* 1990; 65: 636.
29 Schuffler MD, Pope CE. Studies of idiopathic intestinal pseudo-obstruction 2. Hereditary hollow visceral myopathy: family studies. *Gastroenterology*, 1977; 73: 339.
30 Fenoglio-Preisser CM, Noffsinger AE, Stemmermann GN, Lantz PE, Listrom MB, Rilke FO. *Gastrointestinal Pathology: An Atlas and Text*. New York: Lippincott-Raven, 1999: 622.
31 Sjogren R. Gastrointestinal motility disorders in scleroderma. *Arthritis Rheum*, 1994; 37: 1265.
32 Shivshanker K, Bennett RW, Haynie TP. Tumour associated gastroparesis; correction with metoclopramide. *Am J Surg*, 1983; 145: 221.
33 Layer P, Demol P, Hotz J, Goebell H. Gastroparesis after radiation. *Dis Dis Sci*, 1986; 31: 1377.
34 Choe AI, Ziessman HA, Fleischer DE. Tumor associated gastroparesis with esophageal carcinoma. Use of intravenous metoclopramide during radionuclide gastric emptying studies to predict clinical response. *Dig Dis Sci*, 1989; 34: 1132.
35 Miller D, Pasquale M, Seneca R, Hodin E. Gastric volvulus in the pediatric population. *Arch Surg*, 1991; 126: 1146.
36 Patel NM. Chronic gastric volvulus: report of a case and review of the literature. *Am J Gastroenterol*, 1985; 80: 170.
37 Usui M, Matsuda S, Suzuki H, Hirata K, Ogura Y, Shiraishi T. Gastric amyloidosis with massive bleeding requiring emergency surgery. *J Gastroenterol*, 2000; 35: 924.
38 De Bakey M. Bezoars and concretions. *Surgery*, 1938; 4: 934.
39 De Bakey M, Ochsner A. Bezoars and concretions. *Surgery*, 1938; 5: 132.
40 Singh A, Khanna RC, Jolly SS. Three unusual cases of trichobezoar. *Gastroenterology*, 1961; 40: 441.
41 Schiller KFR, Cockel R, Hunt RH, Warren BF. *Atlas of Gastrointestinal Endoscopy and Related Pathology*. Oxford: Blackwell Science, 2001: 195.
42 Levison DA, Crocker PR, Boxall TA, Randall KJ. Coconut matting bezoar identified by a combined analytical approach. *J Clin Pathol*, 1986; 39: 172.
43 Smith JC, Bolande RP. Radiation and drug induced hyalinisation of the stomach. *Arch Pathol*, 1965; 79: 310.
44 Smith JC. Gastric hyalinisation without irradiation. *Arch Pathol*, 1966; 81: 42.
45 Stebbing J, Wyatt JI. Gastric pseudolipomatosis. *Histopathology*, 1998; 33: 394.
46 Morgan AA. Recurrent gastrointestinal haemorrhage: an unusual cause. *Am J Gastroenterol*, 1982; 77: 925.
47 Costopanagiotou E, Spyrou S, Farantos C, Kostopanagiotou G, Smymiotis V. An unusual cause of massive gastric bleeding in a young patient. *Am J Gastroenterol*, 2000; 95: 2400.
48 Spinzi G, Strocchi E, Imperiali G, Sangiovanni A, Terruzzi V, Minoli G. Pseudoxanthoma elasticum: a rare cause of gastrointestinal bleeding. *Am J Gastroenterol*, 1996; 91: 1631.
49 Kundrotas L, Novak J, Kremzier J, Meenaghan M, Hassett J. Gastric bleeding in pseudoxanthoma elasticum. *Am J Gastroenterol*, 1988; 83: 868.
50 Belli A, Cawthorne S. Visceral angiographic findings in pseudoxanthoma elasticum. *Br J Radiol*, 1988; 61: 368.
51 Snover DC, Weisdorf SA, Vercellotti GM *et al*. A histopathologic study of gastric and small intestinal graft-versus-host disease following allogenic bone marrow transplantation. *Hum Pathol*, 1985; 16: 387.
52 McDonald GB, Shulman HM, Sullivan KM, Spencer GD. Intesti-

nal and hepatic complications of human bone marrow transplantation. *Part I. Gastroenterology*, 1986; 90: 460.
53 Marmaduke DP, Greenson JK, Cunningham I, Herderick EE, Cornhill JF. Gastric vascular ectosia in patients undergoing bone marrow transplantation. *Am J Clin Pathol*, 1994; 102: 708.
54 Snover DC. Graft versus host disease of the gastrointestinal tract. *Am J Surg Pathol*, 1991; 14 (Suppl 1): 101.
55 Washington K, Bentley RC, Green A, Olson J, Treem WR, Krigman HR. Graft versus host disease: a blinded histologic study. *Am J Surg Pathol*, 1997; 21: 1037.
56 Yong S, Attal H, Chedjfec G. Pseudomembranous gastritis: a novel complication of *Aspergillus* infection in a patient with a bone marrow transplant and graft versus host disease. *Arch Pathol Lab Med*, 2000; 124: 619.
57 Shulman HM, Sullivan KM, Weiden PI *et al*. Chronic graft versus host syndrome in man. A long term clinicopathologic study of 20 Seattle patients. *Am J Med*, 1980; 69: 204.
58 Warren BF, Davies JD. Vascular disorders of the oesophagus. In: Whitehead R, ed. *Gastrointestinal and Oesophageal Pathology*. Edinburgh: Churchill Livingstone, 1995: 662.
59 Hunt RH. Angiodysplasia of the colon. In: Salmon, PR ed. *Gastrointestinal Endoscopy. Advances in Diagnosis and Therapy*. London: Chapman & Hall, 1984: 1997.
60 Cunningham JT. Gastric telangiectasia in chronic haemodialysis patients: a report of six cases. *Gastroenterology*, 1981; 81: 1131.
61 Dave PB, Romeu J, Antonelli A, Eiser AR. Gastrointestinal telangiectasias: a source of bleeding in patients receiving hemodialysis. *Arch Intern Med*, 1984; 144: 1781.
62 Duray PH, Marcal JM, LiVolsi VA, Fisher R, Scholmacher C, Brand MH. Gastrointestinal angiodysplasia: a possible component of Von Willebrand's disease. *Hum Pathol*, 1984; 15: 539.
63 Odell JM, Haas JE, Tapper D, Nugent D. Infantile haemorrhagic angiodysplasia. *Pediatr Pathol*, 1987; 7: 629.
64 Cairns HS, Rees H, Bevan G. Iron deficiency anaemia, gastritis and antral vascular malformation. *J Roy Soc Med*, 1986; 79: 46.
65 Stamp GWH, Palmer K, Misiewicz JJ. Antral hypertrophic gastritis: a rare cause of iron deficiency. *J Clin Pathol*, 1985; 38: 390.
66 Ponsot P, Theodore C, Julien PE *et al*. Gastric angiodysplasias and Rendu–Osler's disease. *Gastroenterol Clin Biol*, 1983; 7: 321.
67 Dieulafoy G. Exulceratio simplex: l'intervention surgicale dans les hématemèses foudroyantes consecutives à l'exulcération simple de l'estomac. *Bull Acad Med*, 1898; 49: 49.
68 Veldhuyzen van Zanten SJO, Bartelsman JFWM, Schipper MEI, Tytgat GNJ. Recurrent massive haematemesis from Dieulafoy malformations: a review of 101 cases. *Gut*, 1986; 27: 213.
69 Gallard T. Aneurysmes miliares de l'estomac, donnant lieu à des hématemèses mortelles. *Bull Soc Med Hop Paris*, 1884; 1: 84.
70 Mortensen NJ McC, Mountford RA, Davies JD, Jeans WD. Dieulafoy's disease: a distinctive arteriovenous malformation causing massive gastric haemorrhage. *Br J Surg*, 1983; 70: 76.
71 Miko TL, Thomazy VA. The calibre persistent artery of the stomach: a unifying approach to gastric aneurysm, Dieulafoy's lesion and submucosal arterial malformation. *Hum Pathol*, 1988; 19: 914.

PART

4 Small intestine

18 Normal small intestine

For an organ from which portions are so frequently resected with potentially damaging results, surprisingly little is known about the length of the small bowel and its variation in normal people. Measurements taken at autopsy and on operation specimens suggest adult lengths of between 300 and 900 cm with a mean just greater than 600 cm [1], but others taken endosopically during life give a much lower figure of about 280 cm [2], presumably due to tone in the longitudinal muscle coat. In infants and young children the length is from three to seven times the crown–heel length [3] and a prospective autopsy study of fetuses and infants of gestational age 19–40 weeks reports that the overall length for infants of 19–27 weeks' gestation is 142 ± 22 cm, increasing to 304 ± 44 cm by 35 weeks' gestation [4]. These figures may be important in resections for neonatal intestinal obstruction.

The duodenum, which is almost entirely retroperitoneal and was so named because it was supposed to be 12 fingers in breadth, has a fairly constant length of 20 cm. Its first, second and third parts are fixed and extend from the pylorus, at first upwards and backwards, then downwards on the right side from the 2nd to the 4th lumbar vertebrae, then across the 4th vertebra forming a C-shaped organ which embraces the head of the pancreas; the pancreatic and bile ducts open into its second part, usually through a common orifice on the ampulla of Vater but sometimes separately. The fourth part is short, unfixed, becomes invested in a mesentery and continues as the jejunum.

There is no visible line of division between the duodenum and jejunum or between jejunum and ileum; both are supported by a common mesentery arising from a relatively narrow origin between the left side of the second lumbar vertebra and the right sacroiliac joint. Traditionally the jejunum represents the proximal 40% and the ileum the distal 60%. Some guide as to the level of a resected specimen can be obtained by naked-eye inspection of the mucosal surface. In the duodenum this shows crescentic folds about 3 mm thick and up to 9 mm deep which extend a little over halfway round the circumference of the bowel. They begin in the second part, are most conspicuous in the third and fourth parts and gradually diminish in the jejunum to disappear in the ileum. They are not obliterated by distension and presumably increase the absorptive area.

The so-called ileocaecal valve is not a true valve but a sphincter [5]. In humans there is a web of muscle extending from the circular layer of the muscularis propria into the submucosa, towards the muscularis mucosae. The muscle layers are not appreciably thickened but the last 0.5–1.0 cm contracts after the administration of acetylcholine or adrenaline, which suggests a true sphincteric mechanism.

The duodenum is supplied by the superior pancreaticoduodenal branch of the gastroduodenal artery; its fourth part and the remainder of the small bowel are supplied by the superior mesenteric artery which forms numerous arcades in the mesentery, allowing a wide collateral circulation. The venous drainage is to the portal system. The microcirculation within the mucosa has been described in detail in relation to countercurrent effects [6]. Capillaries and lymphatic lacteals traverse the villi and can be difficult to distinguish from one another, except after a fatty meal when the latter are dilated and contain fatty globules. Duodenal lymphatics drain to portal and pyloric lymph nodes, jejunal and ileal lymphatics into haphazardly arranged nodes in the mesentery and thence to the superior mesenteric group, while lymphatics from the terminal ileum drain to ileocaecal nodes. The innervation of the small bowel is described on p. 245.

Physiology

The small bowel has digestive, absorptive, secretory and immunological functions. Much of the physiology is outside the scope of this book but some aspects of digestion and absorption can be investigated using biopsy material with appropriate histochemical and immunocytochemical techniques, and a brief account of relevant features is appended. Good recent general reviews are available [7–17].

Protein digestion and absorption

Protein is derived from exogenous (70–100 g/day) and endogenous (30–200 g/day) sources [7,11]. When exogenous it is often linked to fat or carbohydrate moieties; endogenous protein is mainly derived from the breakdown and shedding of degenerate cells. It is denatured within the lumen to oligopeptides which are then hydrolysed to amino acids by peptidases situated on the brush borders of mucosal enterocytes; small amounts of unhydrolysed protein, including, in neonates, maternal antibody derived from breast milk [2] can be absorbed unchanged. Experimental studies suggest that longer-chain peptides are hydrolysed at brush border level [18] by a number of different aminopeptidases. Aminopeptidases are readily demonstrable histochemically and immunocytochemically [19] (see also Chapter 2) and it may be possible, by using appropriate substrates, to differentiate between aminopeptidases, endopeptidases and glutamyl-aminotransferases [20].

In any disorder with mucosal flattening and increased cell turnover, protein malnutrition may occur because fewer enterocytes are present for absorption of dietary protein and because the increased cell turnover itself increases the amount of endogenous protein lost.

Fat digestion and absorption

Nearly all dietary fat is water-insoluble triglyceride. This is emulsified and hydrolysed in the small intestinal lumen by the combined action of bile salts and lipases, first to di- and then to monoglycerides, free fatty acids and glycerol [9]. The resulting micelles are transferred across the surface membrane of enterocytes and resynthesized to triglyceride within the cell. An isolated rabbit enterocyte model system has been used to demonstrate that apo-β-48 is utilized in this process [21]. The various lipases involved are not readily demonstrated histochemically and the only worthwhile investigation is a simple stain for neutral fat that may be useful in such conditions as suspected α-β-lipoproteinaemia.

Carbohydrate digestion and absorption

Carbohydrates are ingested as polysaccharides, oligo- or disaccharides, all of which are broken down to monosaccharides for absorption [10]. Much of the breakdown takes place on the enterocyte brush border by saccharidases and absorption takes place against a concentration gradient.

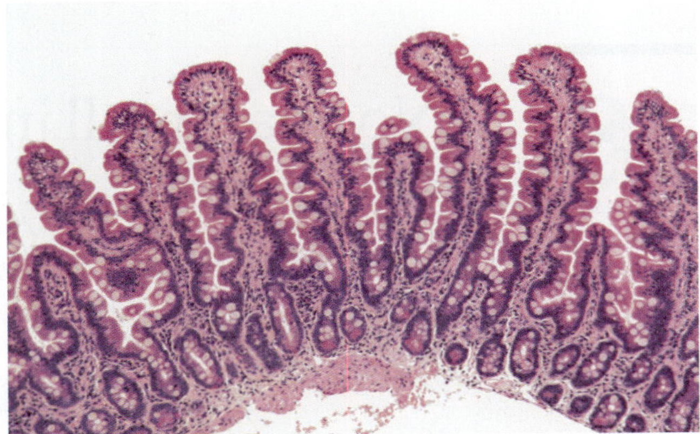

Fig. 18.1 Histology of biopsy of mucosa from the distal duodenum. This sample does not include Brunner's glands and is indistinguishable from the jejunal mucosa. Note the 'sawtooth' indentations along the sides of the villi.

Microscopic anatomy

Small bowel mucosa is readily sampled blind from the jejunum by capsule biopsy or from the duodenum under direct endoscopic vision. The advantages and disadvantages of each method as regards the interpretation of the biopsy obtained are discussed below.

Microscopy

Knowledge of the histopathology of small bowel mucosa has been revolutionized by the application of such techniques as plastic embedding, thin sectioning, electron microscopy, morphometry and quantification with automated equipment, histochemistry, immunocytochemistry and tissue and organ culture. However, examination of haematoxylin and eosin (H&E)-stained paraffin sections remains the mainstay of diagnostic practice.

Mucosa

The normal human small bowel mucosa consists of a basal layer varying from 120 to 270 μm thick, from which villi project into the lumen. Between the villi, crypts extend down into the basal layer and often reach the muscularis mucosae. The epithelium covering the villi arises from and is continuous with that lining the crypts (Figs 18.1 & 18.2).

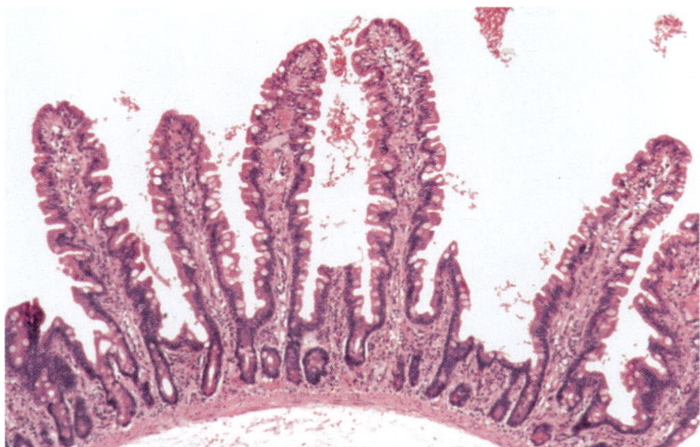

Fig. 18.2 Histology of normal ileal mucosal biopsy. The villi are longer than those in the duodenal and jejunal mucosa and the 'sawtooth' indentations are less conspicuous.

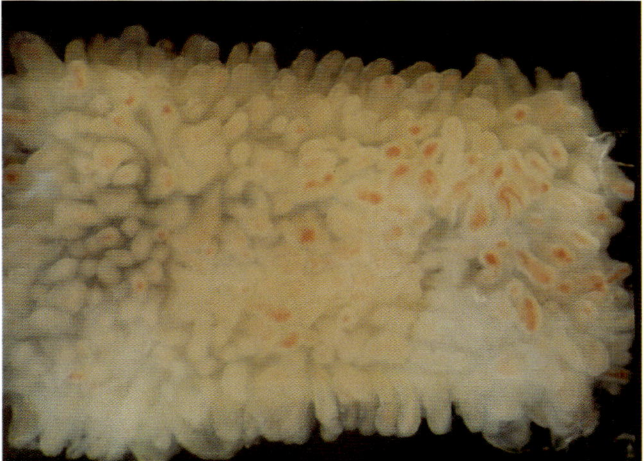

Fig. 18.3 Normal jejunal villi as seen by dissecting microscopy. Although most of the villi are truly finger-shaped, a few leaf forms are present.

Villi

There are between 10 and 40 villi/mm^2 of mucosa.

Dissecting microscopy

There is good evidence that the morphology of duodenal and jejunal mucosa differs from race to race, though these differences are probably more the result of environment and diet than genetically determined. In Caucasians, villi from different regions of the gut have a characteristic appearance [22–24]. The majority project luminally as finger-like processes; in children, the villi are shorter [26a]. In the duodenum and upper jejunum an appreciable number are leaf-like or spade-shaped and in the duodenum occasional ridges or convolutions are normal and are more frequent in tropical countries [25–27]

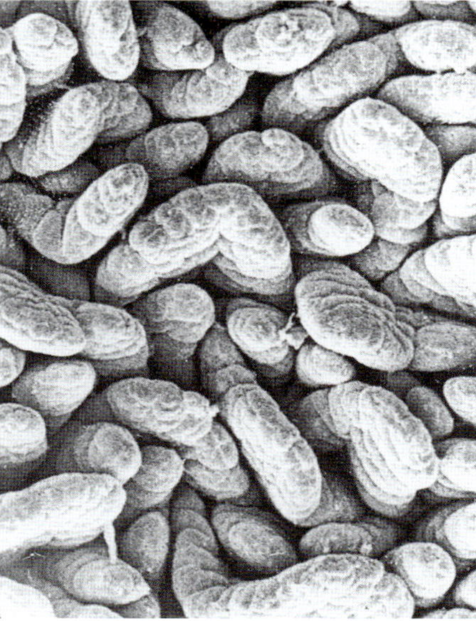

Fig. 18.4 Scanning electron micrograph of normal small bowel. Both finger- and spade-shaped villi are present.

(Fig. 18.3). There is probably a normal ratio of three crypts to each villus, and small intervillous ridges link adjacent villi. A central vascular arcade can often be seen in the lamina propria. The presence of fairly numerous leaf and spade forms in the upper part of the small bowel is not reliable evidence of gluten-induced enteropathy. It is our experience that when there is doubt as to whether or not a minor degree of change is present under the dissecting microscope the histology is likely to be within normal limits.

Scanning electron microscopic appearances

The appearances of villi under the scanning electron microscope are now well documented [28–31] and illustrated (Fig. 18.4). They are of great interest and beauty but are not further described here because they add little to diagnosis and the equipment needed is not widely available.

Conventional microscopy

When assessed on conventionally processed material from adults, jejunal villi vary in height from 320 to 570 μm and in width from 85 to 140 μm. They are responsible for 60–75% of the total mucosal thickness [32]. Microdissection techniques on alcohol- and acetic acid-fixed material give values for height as great as 500–1100 μm [33] but the values here quoted still hold good for conventionally handled biopsies. They are supported by morphometric analyses using computer-aided microscopy [34]. Villi are longest in the distal duodenum and proximal jejunum, gradually shortening to more stubby finger-like forms in the mid-small bowel [35] but again be-

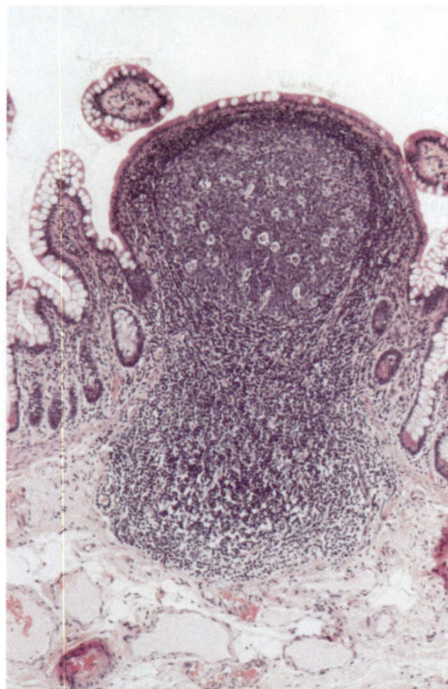

Fig. 18.5 The epithelium overlying small intestinal mucosal lymphoid follicles is thin and flat rather than forming villi.

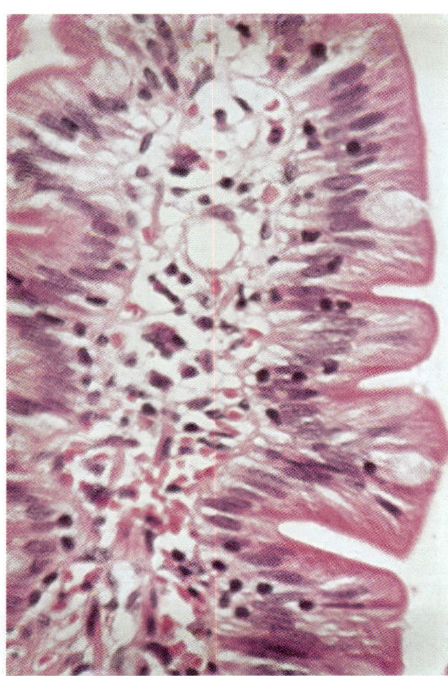

Fig. 18.6 A single normal villus in histological section. Enterocytes with distinguishable brush borders, goblet cells and intraepithelial lymphocytes are clearly visible.

come elongated in the distal ileum. Quantitative studies in children show that their villi are slightly smaller [36].

In the duodenum and upper jejunum of Caucasians a number of villi are broad and leaf- or spade-shaped; these forms are more numerous in apparently normal Asiatic, African and Afro-Caribbean adults in whom finger-shaped villi are often scanty, though they are present in fetuses and in children [27,37]. It has been suggested that the shape of villi is governed by the rate of epithelial cell turnover, a high turnover rate being associated with tall finger-like villi [38]. In the duodenum and upper jejunum there is commonly some villous branching and the branches may reunite to form bridges; this can also occur in the ileum and, contrary to some workers, we have seen it as often in adults as in children. In the ileum villi over lymphoid aggregates are often absent or poorly formed (Fig. 18.5) and this should be remembered in assessing material from this region. We have found certain features of value in assessing the level of a biopsy. Biopsies from duodenum and upper jejunum show a 'sawtooth' appearance of the sides of the villi which is less prominent in the ileum (Figs 18.1 & 18.2). The ileal villi are longer and less straight so that it is common to see the villous tips in tangential section; also, the more proximal the biopsy the fewer the goblet cells present in villous epithelium.

Because a number of disease processes are, in their early stages, characterized only by minor variations from normal, some of which are quantitative rather than qualitative, a number of workers have routinely measured one or more of such factors as villous height and breadth, the height of the basal layer, the number of mitoses in the crypt zone, the ratio of absorptive to goblet cells and their absolute numbers, the villous surface area, the numbers of plasma cells synthesizing immunoglobulin A (IgA), IgG and IgM, and the numbers of intraepithelial lymphocytes and macrophages.

Accurate measurements may be helpful in determining minor degrees of variation in villous size that can be significant [39,40]. However, there is a limit to the value of such precision and there is also some evidence that the villi in those capsular biopsies that include muscularis mucosae appear longer and thinner than those lacking a basal layer of supporting muscle, perhaps because the muscle prevents the biopsy 'spreading out'.

The cells covering villi are basically of two types. Enterocytes or absorptive cells predominate over goblet cells at the tips of the villi in a ratio of about 8:1. In 5-μm sections they appear to become less numerous as one approaches the crypt zone; this may be illusory as in semithin (0.5-μm) sections they appear numerous but crowded together. They are tall columnar cells with oval, basally situated reticular nuclei, eosinophilic cytoplasm and a microvillous brush border which can often be seen under the light microscope, especially in cryostat sections (Fig. 18.6).

Specialized techniques give information about enterocyte function. Microvilli are regularly arranged, vary in height from 1.3 μm at the tips to 0.7 μm just above the crypt zone and project at right angles to the surface (Fig. 18.7). Each microvillus is from 0.1 to 0.2 μm wide and has a fine filamentous core

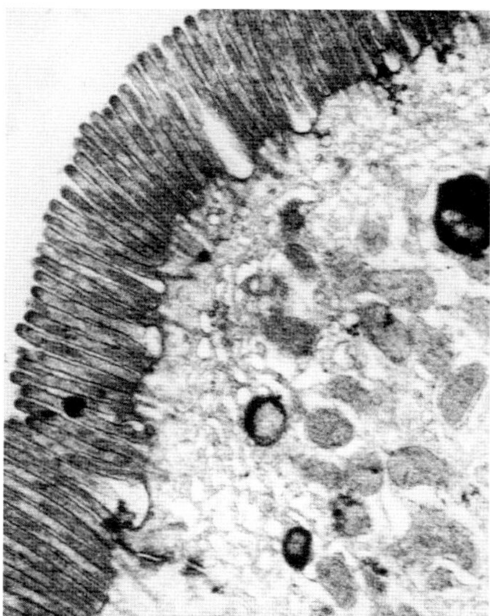

Fig. 18.7 Electron micrograph showing normal microvilli on surface enterocytes.

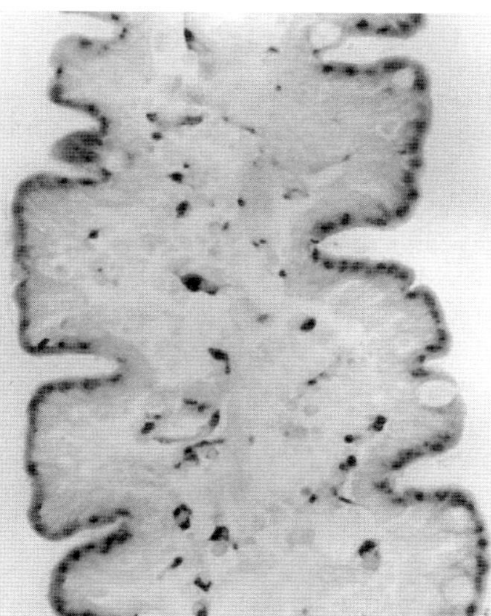

Fig. 18.8 Acid phosphatase in jejunal mucosa. The enzyme is intracellular and mainly confined to lysozomes; the unstained brush border is clearly visible. Macrophages within the lamina propria also stain (naphthol pararosanilin technique).

with an outer trilaminar membrane from which fine filaments radiate out to form a fuzzy surface coat [31,41–44]. This surface 'fuzz' throughout the small bowel contains acid mucosubstances that stain faintly with alcian blue at pH 0.5. Within it are brush border enzymes, including alkaline phosphatase, aminopeptidases (Fig. 18.8) and saccharidases which are demonstrable using histochemical or biochemical assay techniques [45–54] Enterokinase is present in the duodenum and upper jejunum only [55]. Other important substances demonstrable in the brush border include carcinoembryonic antigen [56,57]. The enterocytes themselves contain lysozyme [58], α_1-antitrypsin [59] localized mainly in crypt and lower villous epithelium, apolipoproteins A1, A4 and B [60] mainly at the villous tips, some antigens, including the common acute lymphoblastic leukaemia antigen [61,62], secretory component [63], oxidoreductive enzymes in mitochondria, acid phosphatase in digestive sacs and lysosomes (Fig. 18.8) and possibly alkaline phosphatase in non-brush border form. The role of some of these proteins, HLA-DR antigens and the modification of surface enterocytes to form M cells is discussed on p. 244.

Crypt zone

The cells which clothe the villi and those which form the basal layer are generated and regenerated from the crypt proliferative zone (Fig. 18.9) situated between the crypt base and the villous compartment [64–66]. Three or four crypts open into a common vestibule and a number of vestibules coalesce to form a basin around each villus, the basins intercommunicating to form intervillous spaces [67]. The crypt stem cells give rise to all types of epithelial cell. They migrate upward to cover the villi, differentiating and maturing as they do so, to form enterocytes, M (membranous) cells, oligomucous cells and goblet cells, which are shed off from the villous tips as effete in 2–4 days. They also migrate downward to form the cells of the basal layer (see below) which explains the thickening of this

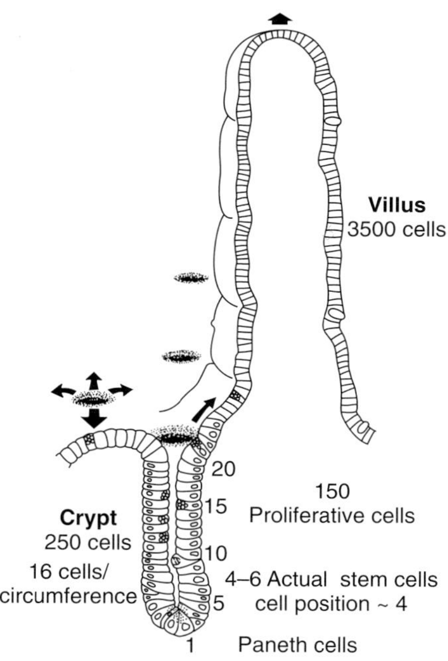

Fig. 18.9 Diagram of the three-dimensional architecture of the small intestine, showing the numbers assigned to each cell position and the hierarchy of cells from the cells at the base of the crypt to the villous tip (after [158]).

layer seen in many instances of mucosal flattening associated with increased crypt zone proliferation.

Investigation of crypt cell dynamics has been assisted by mapping of the cells with numbered positions, as proposed by Potten and colleagues [157, 157a]. The model crypt consists of 20 annuli of cells from the base to the top of the crypt (Fig. 18.9). The average number of epithelial cells in each annulus is 16. Studies in mice show that there are 4–6 stem cells in each crypt, situated above the base at position four. These are relatively undifferentiated, proliferative cells which divide, apparently asymmetrically, to both maintain their own numbers and simultaneously generate more differentiated transit cells which migrate upwards to reach the base of the villi [158]. Three-dimensional reconstruction studies in a mouse chimeric model [68a] have revealed that the columns of cells migrating upwards from the crypts to replenish the surface of the villi remain in tight cohorts with little deviation or mixing. Cells from each crypt feed to more than one villus.

Basal layer

Four types of cell are found in the lower crypt zone throughout the small intestine (Fig. 18.10). There are oligomucous and goblet cells immediately beneath the generative zone, Paneth cells and endocrine cells. Paneth cells are found towards the base of the crypts throughout the small bowel and in the appendix; a few are present in the right colon. They are not found in the normal stomach though they can be seen in intestinal metaplasia, nor in the normal transverse or left-sided large bowel, though they can be present in inflammatory bowel disease [68]. They are derived from crypt cells and have a life span of about 30 days [69]. Mature cells are large and flask-shaped and contain acidophil supranuclear cytoplasmic granules that readily disintegrate and autolyse. They stain with phloxine-tartrazine [70] and fluoresce after staining with eosin; the granules contain lysozyme [71] and the cells themselves also contain IgA and IgG [72]. Paneth cells may contribute to the maintenance of crypt epithelial integrity by inhibiting apoptosis of crypt epithelial cells. They express CD95L (fas ligand) but are CD95 (fas) negative, suggesting that they themselves are protected from fas-mediated apoptosis in an analogous way to cells in the brain and eye [72a]. Paneth cell granules are highly cationically charged which accounts for their staining properties and perhaps also for some of their biological activity in stabilizing the environment of the crypt base. Paneth cells have also been shown to contain the natural antibiotics known as defensins, possibly for protection of the adjacent stem cells from attack by microbes [72b]. Endocrine cells are described below.

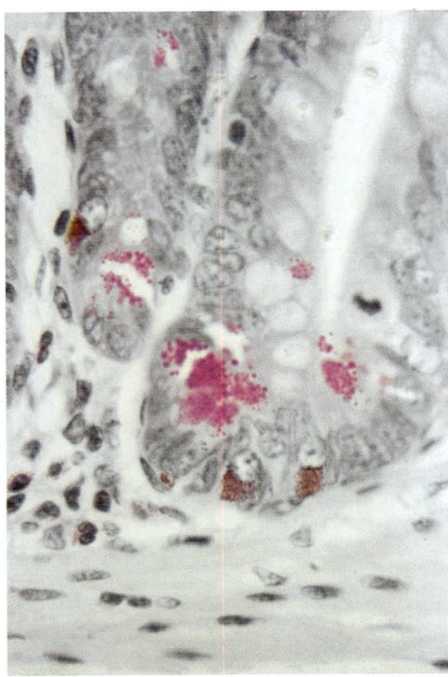

Fig. 18.10 The cell types at the crypt base in normal small intestinal mucosa. The absorptive columnar cells and goblet cells are stained with haematoxylin but the bright red supranuclear granules belong to Paneth cells and the brown infranuclear granules are within the enterochromaffin (EC) cells (Kultschitsky cells). The latter are argyrophyllic and argentaffin and have large 'open' nuclei (phloxine tartrazine and silver impregnation toned with gold chloride, haematoxylin counterstain).

The diffuse endocrine system of the gut

The concept of a diffuse endocrine system in the gut has been widely surveyed in modern literature [66,73–75]. It is a family of enteroendocrine epithelial cells originating from the crypt zone [76,77] and scattered throughout the mucosa, though most numerous in the bases of the glands [64,74,78]. It should not be confused with the peptidergic intercalating neurones that are part of the autonomic nervous system of the gut and, as such, are derived from the neural crest. These are discussed further under 'The innervation of the small intestine' on p. 245. The endocrine cells of epithelial origin vary from columnar to triangular in shape, with a broad base resting on the basement membrane. After conventional formaldehyde fixation small subnuclear acidophilic granules can occasionally be seen in their cytoplasm between the nucleus and the basal aspect of the cell. The cells tend to lie towards the base of the crypts in the basal layer or in Brunner's glands and are rare on the sides of the villi (Fig. 18.10). Those cells whose apex reaches the lumen possess modified microvilli and are classified as 'open' cells. Other, less conspicuous, flattened cells, from which slender processes extend along the basement membrane, are known as 'closed' cells [79].

Enteroendocrine cells can be identified immunohistochemically, using antibody to chromogranin [79a] or synaptophysin [79b] or by using more traditional semispecific histochemical screening techniques such as lead haemotoxylin and argy-

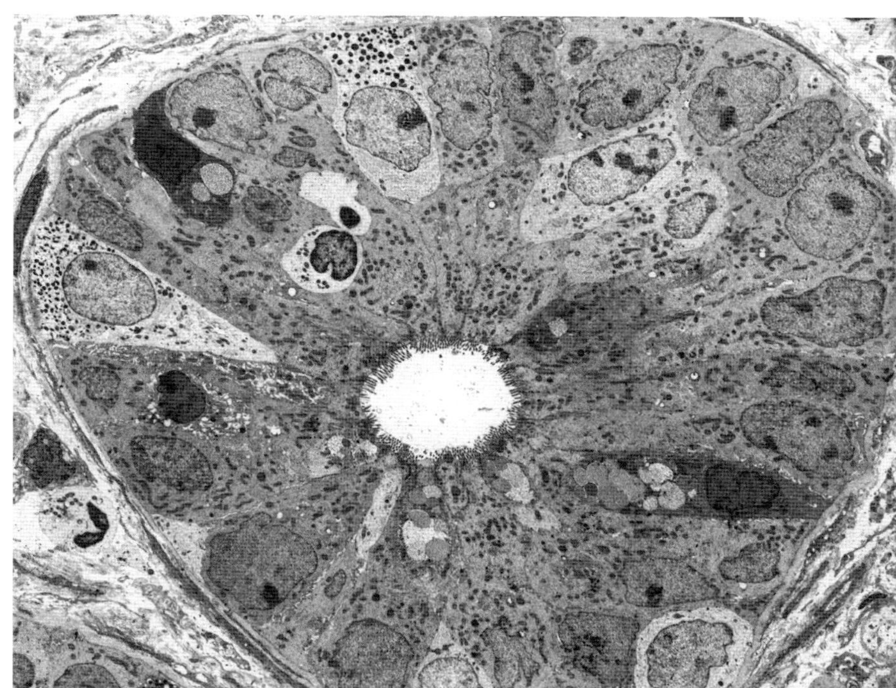

Fig. 18.11 Low-power electron micrograph of lower end of a crypt, cut transversely. The basally situated granules of two endocrine cells are well shown.

rophil methods (see Chapter 2). After aldehyde fixation, staining by an argentaffin technique, or the diazo reaction, or by means of aldehyde-induced fluorescence, identifies cells containing 5-hydroxytryptamine (5-HT). So-called 'neurone-specific' enolase [80] (which is not in fact specific for neurones) can be useful as a marker for diffuse endocrine cells.

By the use of specific antisera or monoclonal antibodies to identify the secretory products by radioimmunoassay [81,82], immunohistochemistry and ultrastructural examination of the size, shape and appearance of individual granules [83] (Figs 18.11–18.13) the distribution of different subgroups of endocrine cells has been mapped along the gastrointestinal tract [84]. Cells with granules containing serotonin (5-HT), vasoactive intestinal peptide (VIP), enkephalins, bombesin (gastrin-releasing peptide) and somatostatin are diffusely distributed throughout the gut. Cholecystokinin (pancreatozymin), secretin, gastric inhibitory peptide (GIP) and motilin-containing cells are found mainly in the upper small intestine and, in addition, there are gastrin-containing cells in the proximal duodenum. Neurotensin is most prominent in the distal ileum and proximal colon. However, antibodies detect only about six amino acid residues of any polypeptide [85] and polypeptide hormones exist in precursor pre and pro forms in which the antigenic elements of the active form may be buried; conversely fragments of active peptide hormone too small to be physiologically effective but containing the appropriate antigenic determinant may be detected and regarded as representing active hormone. Endocrine cell tumours do not therefore always exactly correspond in hormone profile with the neighbouring normal cells.

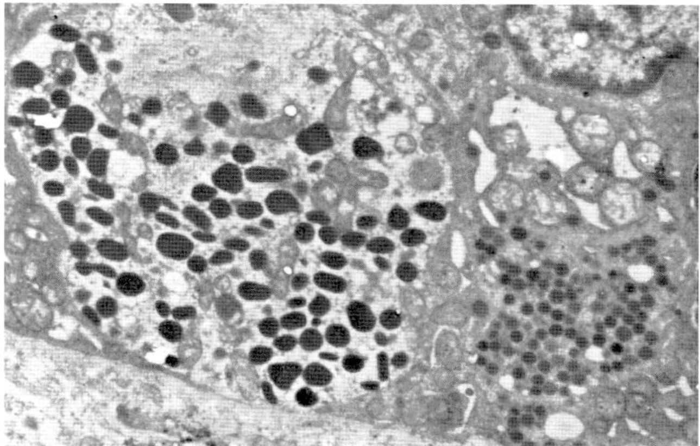

Fig. 18.12 Electron micrograph of duodenum showing a 5HT-secreting cell with characteristic dense pleomorphic granules on the left and a second endocrine cell, probably a secretin-containing cell, with small round granules of varying density on the right.

The lamina propria

Each villus has a central connective tissue core which is continuous with the lamina propria of the basal layer and contains arterioles, venules, capillaries, lymphatics, smooth muscle and a variety of other cells (Fig. 18.6). Full details of the microcirculation are available [6,86]. Estimation of lymphatic diameter may be important since protein-losing enteropathy can be associated with lymphangiectasia, but we know of only one study, which gives the normal diameter as varying from 16 to

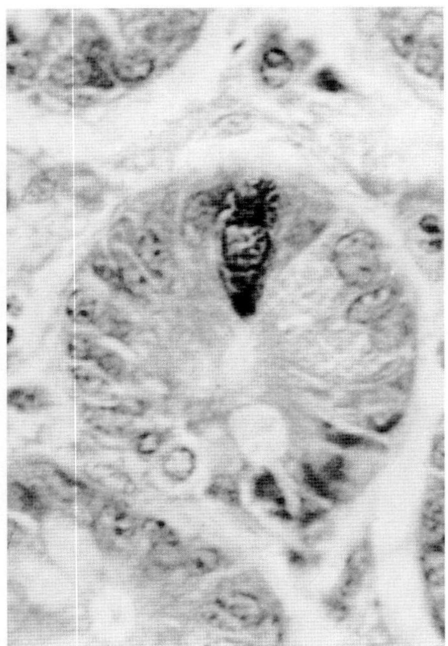

Fig. 18.13 Enteroglucagon-containing cell in ileal crypt (immunoperoxidase).

64 μm [87]. A mesenchymal cell layer immediately beneath epithelial cells (the so-called pericryptal fibroblastic sheath) has been described [88], homologous to that in the colon (p. 439). The cells forming it are of smooth muscle rather than fibroblastic nature; it may play a part in regulating and maintaining normal absorption and secretion. The lamina propria also normally contains mast cells, plasma cells, lymphocytes and eosinophils [89]; the last-named may be increased in type 1 allergic reactions to ingested protein [90].

The gut-associated lymphoid tissue

Perhaps more than any other part of the body, the digestive tract is exposed to antigenic material in the form of microorganisms and ingested food. This continually reaches the small bowel from birth onward. It is the unique function of the small and large bowel to avoid constant inappropriate inflammatory reaction by recognizing which antigens to tolerate. The response depends on free access between the immune system and antigenic material and some knowledge of its working is essential for the proper interpretation of small bowel biopsies [91–93].

A specialized *lymphoepithelium* overlies Peyer's patches and probably solitary follicles also (Fig. 18.5). It contains M cells [94] which histologically resemble flattened enterocytes and ultrastructurally have modified microvilli or microfolds (from which the cells derive their name) and lack a terminal web [95,96]. They transfer many antigens to the underlying tissue, probably by pinocytosis. Some of the lymphoepithelial cells also possess HLA-DR-like antigens and are able to function as antigen-presenting cells [97–99]. More conventional antigen-presenting cells, homologous to dendritic cells and Langerhans cells at other sites, are the macrophage-like cells with dendritic processes (dendritic cells), situated between the base of the M cells and the underlying lymphoid tissue. These cells also possess HLA-DR antigens [100], are rich in ATPase and express S100 protein [100a] and CDIA [100b]. Morphologically similar are phagocytic effector cells, which contain acid phosphatase and are S100 negative. It seems probable that particular HLA antigens play a role in gastrointestinal disease [101] and that most of the foreign antigenic material enters via the M cells or enterocytes and is phagocytosed by dendritic macrophages for immune presentation [102].

In the duodenum and jejunum the lymphoid tissue is localized in scattered follicles of lymphocytes, 0.6–3.0 mm in diameter, in the mucosa and submucosa, which may or may not contain germinal centres. In the lower ileum these aggregate to form Peyer's patches, up to 12 × 20 mm in size, and germinal centres are more usual (Fig. 18.5). Both B and T lymphocytes are present, the B cells around germinal follicles and T cells in interfollicular zones; both types are also scattered diffusely in the lamina propria [103]. Most B cells have IgA or IgM surface antibody. They appear to be involved in a continuous circular migratory cycle from epithelium to mesenteric nodes and thence via the thoracic duct and bloodstream either back to the intestinal epithelium or to other secretory epithelia such as bronchial [104]. The T cells predominantly express CD4 [105] and include helper [106], suppressor, killer and null cells [107,108].

Plasma cells synthesizing IgA, IgM and IgG are present in a ratio of approximately 20 : 10 : 1 [109,110]. IgA is synthesized in its 11S dimeric form together with J chain which forms a clasp between the two monomers and acts as a site of attachment for secretory piece which is formed on the basal surface of enterocytes [111]. The complex is transported across the enterocyte to its luminal surface where it becomes attached to the mucocalyx and forms a protective 'paint' which binds and agglutinates microbial and food antigens and prevents microorganisms from attaching themselves to the mucosa. IgM is treated in a similar fashion which explains why patients with isolated IgA deficiency do not necessarily develop immune deficiency syndromes in relation to the gut. There are few IgG-synthesizing cells in the normal gut, reflecting the need for immune protection (by IgA and IgM) without lytic destruction of mucosal tissue.

A regular feature of the villous epithelium, which shows significant changes in a number of diseases including gluten-induced enteropathy, is the presence between individual enterocytes of round cells of which the majority are T lymphocytes of CD8 (suppressor) type; a minority are macrophages. The receptors on many of the T cells are made up of gamma and delta chains. These (γ-δ cells probably serve to damp down immune responses [112,113]. In total they average about one to every 10 enterocytes, although they can number up to 40% of the enterocytes in normal small bowel mucosa; their numbers appear raised in many conditions associated with mucosal flattening though this rise is likely to be relative rather than absolute. These cells seem to have a dual role, being concerned with both immune regulation and protection of the mucosa from infectious agents. Good reviews are available [114–116].

Immunoglobulins, their light and heavy chain components, J chain, secretory piece, C3 complement factors, B cells, subgroups of T cells and HLA antigens can be identified immunocytochemically. Unfortunately, in paraffin sections of formalin-fixed tissue, there is a tendency for specific cell surface immunoglobulins to be masked by the large pool of heterogeneous immunoglobulins normally present in the interstitial fluid.

The muscularis mucosae

This coat consists of a narrow band of smooth muscle fibres running mainly longitudinally, though some circular fibres are present. In the duodenum, where it lies on the luminal side of Brunner's glands, it is not always distinct.

Brunner's glands

These glands are a morphological continuation of antral-type mucosa into the submucosa of the duodenum (Fig. 18.14). They extend beneath the muscularis mucosae from the pylorus, which they often infiltrate in advancing age, to the inferior duodenal papilla and sometimes into the upper jejunum [117,118]. Their number is variable and decreases with age. They consist of ramifying tubules which drain by way of ducts which empty into the lumen either part way up the crypts or in between the villi [119]. The cells are microscopically and ultrastructurally of one type [120] resembling the mucous cells of antral glands and they stain only faintly with stains for acid mucosubstances. Brunner's glands are functionally homologous with the glands of 'pyloric metaplasia'/ulcer-associated cell lineage [159] and their cells express the trefoil peptides PS2 and human spasmolytic polypeptide 1 (HSP-1), proteins which are concerned with epithelial cell motility in the healing process, indicating that a physiological role of Brunner's glands is maintenance of the integrity of the mucosa in the comparatively hostile acid environment of the proximal duodenum.

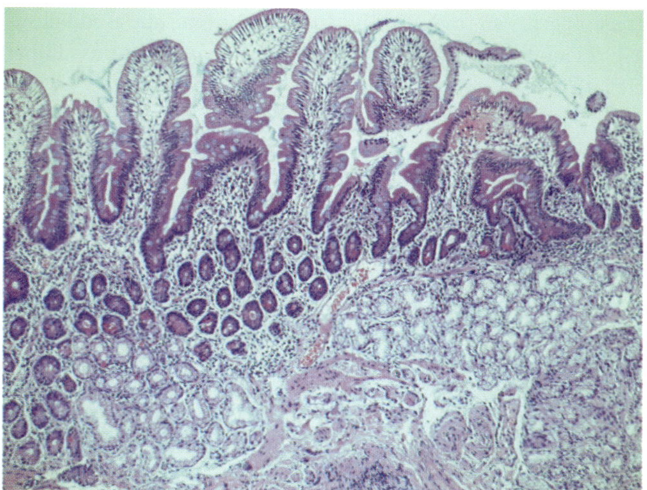

Fig. 18.14 Normal mucosa from the proximal duodenum, with Brunner's glands. These resemble gastric antral glands and lie deep to the muscularis mucosae which intermingles with them.

The submucosa

The small intestinal submucosa is composed of loose, moderately vascular connective tissue in which lie blood vessels, lymphatics and an autonomic nerve plexus (see below). Aggregates of lymphocytes without a follicular pattern, solitary lymphoid follicles and Peyer's patches, already described, lie astride the muscularis mucosae and project down into the submucous layer.

The muscle coats

Continuous inner circular and outer longitudinal smooth muscle coats are present throughout the small bowel; there is no taenia formation. A myenteric plexus (see below) is present between the two muscle coats.

The innervation of the small intestine

In recent years great advances have been made in our understanding of the nervous control of the gut [121–124]. As immunocytochemical techniques have become available for identifying neurotransmitters the large degree of autonomy possessed by the enteric nervous system has become appreciated, a separate non-cholinergic co-ordinating component has been recognized and rational explanation for a number of disorders previously considered as of undetermined origin is now possible.

The enteric nervous system has extrinsic sympathetic and parasympathetic components and its intrinsic components are peptidergic [125]. The sympathetic nerves are adrenergic, inhibitory and usually argyrophilic and derived from branches of the coeliac and superior mesenteric ganglia which in turn receive efferent fibres from T4–T8 and L1–L2. The parasympathetic nerves are cholinergic, excitatory and usually unstained in silver preparations; they come from the vagus via the coeliac axis. Both silver and acetylcholine esterase (AChE) techniques have limitations that are not always appreciated. Most if not all adrenergic fibres are argyrophilic, but not all argyrophilic fibres or ganglion cells are necessarily adrenergic. Histochemically demonstrable AChE is present in all cholinergic fibres and neurones synthesizing ACh, but has also been demonstrated, at least in the kidney, in fibres that are not cholinergic [126]. The neurotransmitters of the peptidergic nerves include 5-HT and related indolamines [127], neuropeptides [125,128] including VIP, substance P [129], encephalin, bombesin, somatostatin, neurotensin and motilin [130].

The myenteric (Auerbach's) plexus lies between the longitudinal and circular muscle coats, resting on the former; its ganglion cells are found in small groups and are of a number of types. The submucosal (Meissner's) plexus lies, as its name suggests, in the submucosa; its ganglion cells are found singly and in it also a number of types are present. Experimental studies in quail chick chimeras [131] have shown that the intrinsic gut innervation is of neural crest origin. Future ganglion cells specifically migrate to the gut and arrest in the sites designated for myenteric or submucosal plexuses. Their ultimate function and the substance they will synthesize may in part be regulated by local environmental factors, though differentiating enteric neuroblasts appear to express cholinergic properties soon after migration and may develop them at the neural crest stage. Adrenergic properties may be related to the induction of cells at the later neural tube or notochordal stage. There is also some evidence that a switch of synthesis from one transmitter to another can be brought about by local influences in the developing gut, though where and at what stage the programming of ganglion cells to synthesize other (peptide) transmitters takes place is not yet known. What is established is that there is a variety of ganglion cells in myenteric and submucosal plexuses synthesizing a variety of possible neurotransmitters.

Ganglion cells cannot readily be classified in terms of what they synthesize on a histological or ultrastructural basis [132,133] though attempts have been made to do so [132]. They are surrounded by a tightly packed mass of axons, dendrites and glial cells as well as the interstitial cells of Cajal, without connective tissue; there are numerous contacts between nerve endings and cell bodies or cell processes. It may prove easier to classify axonal types on the basis of their contained vesicles. Sympathetic nerves do not supply muscle directly; multiaxonal, multifibrillar fibres surround other ganglia in both plexuses [134,135] and exert an inhibitory influence. Some of the ganglia thus surrounded are cholinergic and their fibres directly supply muscle including muscularis mucosae [136] and possibly the smooth muscle fibres present in individual villi. Some adrenergic fibres do reach the lamina propria [137]. In addition there is, in both plexuses, an extensive intermediate plexus of ganglion cells, axons and neurofibrils synthesizing and containing neuropeptides [138–141], ATPase and 5-HT which acts as a complex regulatory controlling mechanism for motor and perhaps sensory activity. It has become evident that inhibition of smooth muscle contraction in the gut is mediated by local release of nitric oxide [141a]. Nitric oxide is released immediately after its local synthesis by nitric oxide synthase (NOS). Inhibition of NOS may have a physiological role in mediating smooth muscle contraction in some circumstances, such as in the fasting state [142].

The interstitial cells of Cajal, which form an inconspicuous meshwork around the myenteric plexus and throughout the muscle layers of the bowel [142a], are stainable by the antibody to C-kit (stem cell factor, CD117). These cells, like the myocytes, are of mesenchymal origin [143] and seem to communicate directly with the myocytes through their gap junctions [143a] and with tiny sites of contact on varicosities on autonomic neurones [144]. They play a crucial role as pacemaker of the gastrointestinal tract [144a], apparently acting as facilitators of synthesis of nitric oxide [145,146]. They are necessary for propagation of the slow waves that are the essential element of peristalsis [147].

In summary it appears that there is a largely autonomous enteric nervous system, with the interstitial cells of Cajal acting as pacemakers and with an extrinsic cholinergic parasympathetic excitatory component that acts directly through nerve endings in muscle. Co-ordination seems to be through a complex intercalating system, mediated by neuropeptides. An extrinsic adrenergic sympathetic inhibitory component probably acts indirectly on this rather than directly on muscle. The precise physiological role of variations in nitric oxide in inducing relaxation remains to be elucidated but the interstitial cells of Cajal seem to have a central role in this function. The interest for the practising pathologist lies in the linking of a recognizable pattern of neuronal or axonal damage or defect with an identifiable clinical disorder [148–150]. Further discussion is given under individual conditions, and good clinical reviews of gut motility and its disorders are available [151,152].

The serosa

The small bowel serosa consists of a thin layer of connective and adipose tissue containing blood vessels and lymphatics but no lymphoid follicles or aggregates. The peritoneum is formed by a layer of flattened mesothelial cells resting on a well developed elastic membrane.

The luminal content

It is possible to measure the pH of different regions of the bowel using a telemetering device [153] but we do not know the relevance of altered pH to histological appearances.

Bacteriological studies are now well established. The normal small bowel contains spaces (also known as niches or habitats) formed partly by the concentric folds and also by mucosal surfaces and crypts. These spaces are normally colonized permanently by indigenous organisms that are strict or facultative anaerobes, predominantly bacteroides. They are more readily cultured from the ileum than from the upper reaches of the intestine [154–156]. In addition, particularly in the duodenum and upper jejunum, there is a variable non-indigenous and non-permanent flora of ingested bacteria, mainly aerobes and facultative anaerobes. This ingested population cannot normally permanently colonize the spaces already occupied by the indigenous anaerobes, but alterations in conditions within the bowel producing stagnant loop syndromes or small bowel bacterial 'contamination' can produce changes in ecology potentially damaging to the mucosa.

References

1 Underhill BML. Intestinal length in man. *Br Med J*, 1955; ii: 1243.

2 Hirsch J, Ahrens EH, Blankenhorn DH. Measurement of human intestinal length *in vivo*. *Gastroenterology*, 1956; 31: 274.

3 Reiquam CW, Allen RP, Akers DR. Normal and abnormal small bowel lengths. An analysis of 389 autopsy cases in infants and children. *Am J Dis Child*, 1965; 109: 447.

4 Touloukian RJ, Walker-Smith GJ. Normal intestinal length in pre-term infants. *J Pediatr Surg*, 1983; 18: 720.

5 Gazet JC, Jarrett RJ. The ileocaeco-colic sphincter. Studies *in vitro* in man, monkey cat and dog. *Br J Surg*, 1964; 51: 368.

6 Granger DN, Barrowman JA. Microcirculation of the alimentary tract, II. Pathophysiology of oedema. *Gastroenterology*, 1983; 84: 1035.

7 Lucas M. Physiology of the small intestine. *Curr Opin Gastroenterol*, 1985; 1: 203.

8 Clark ML. Small intestinal pathophysiology. *Curr Opin Gastroenterol*, 1985; 1: 212.

9 Glickman RM. Fat absorption and malabsorption. *Clin Gastroenterol*, 1983; 12: 323.

10 Ravich WJ, Bayless TM. Carbohydrate absorption and malabsorption. *Clin Gastroenterol*, 1983; 12: 335.

11 Freeman HJ, Sleisenger MH, Kim YS. Human protein digestion and absorption; normal mechanisms and protein–energy malnutrition. *Clin Gastroenterol*, 1983; 12: 357.

12 Turvill JL, Farthing MJG. Water and electrolyte absorption and secretion. *Curr Opin Gastroenterol*, 1996; 12: 129–33.

13 Turvill JL, Farthing MG. Water and electrolyte secretion in the small intestine. *Curr Opin Gastroenterol*, 1997; 13: 94.

14 Turvill JL, Farthing MG. Water and electrolyte secretion in the small intestine. *Curr Opin Gastroenterol*, 1998; 14: 94.

15 Turvill JL, Farthing MJG. Water and electrolyte absorption and secretion in the small intestine. *Curr Opin Gastroenterol*, 1999; 15: 108–12.

16 Kumar NS, Nutting DF, Mansbach CM. Nutrient absorption and malabsorption. *Curr Opin Gastroenterol*, 1997; 13: 99.

17 Kumar NS, Nutting DF, St Hilaire RJ, Mansbach CM. Nutrient absorption. *Curr Opin Gastroenterol*, 1998; 14: 99.

18 Nicholson JA, Peters TJ. Subcellular distribution of di- and tripeptidase activity in human jejunum. *Clin Sci Mol Med*, 1977; 52: 168.

19 Feracci H, Bernadac A, Gorvel JP, Maroux S. Localization by immunofluorescence and histochemical labelling of aminopeptidase N in relation to its biosynthesis in rabbit and pig enterocytes. *Gastroenterology*, 1982; 82: 317.

20 Lojda Z. The histochemical demonstration of brush border endopeptidase. *Histochemistry*, 1979; 64: 205.

21 Cartwright IJ, Higgins JA. Isolated rabbit enterocytes as a model cell system for investigations of chylomicron assembly and secretion. *J Lipid Res*, 1999; 40: 1357–65.

22 Holmes R, Hourihane DO'B, Booth CC. Dissecting microscope appearances of jejunal biopsy specimens from patients with 'idiopathic steatorrhoea'. *Lancet*, 1961; i: 81.

23 Holmes R, Hourihane DO'B, Booth CC. The mucosa of the small intestine. *Postgrad Med J*, 1961; 37: 717.

24 Brackenbury W, Stewart JS. Macroscopic appearances of mucosal biopsies from the small intestine. *Med Biol Illust*, 1963; 13: 220.

25 Bennett MK, Sachdev CK, Jewell DP, Anand BS. Jejunal mucosal morphology in healthy North Indian subjects. *J Clin Pathol*, 1985; 38: 368.

26 Cook GC, Kajubi SK, Lee FD. Jejunal morphology of the African in Uganda. *J Pathol*, 1969; 98: 157.

26a Penna FJ, Hill ID, Kingston D, Robertson K, Slavin G, Shiner M. Jejunal mucosal morphemetry in children with and without gut symptoms and in normal adults. *J Clin Pathol*, 1981; 34: 386.

27 Baker SJ. Geographical variations in the morphology of the small intestinal mucosa in apparently healthy individuals. *Pathol Microbiol*, 1973; 39: 222.

28 Toner PG, Carr KE. The use of scanning electron microscopy in the study of the intestinal villi. *J Pathol*, 1969; 97: 611.

29 Toner PG, Carr KE, Ferguson A, Mackay C. Scanning and transmission electron microscopic studies of human intestinal mucosa. *Gut*, 1970; II: 471.

30 Millington PF, Critchley DR, Tovell PWA, Pearson R. Scanning electron microscopy of intestinal microvilli. *J Microscopy*, 1969; 89: 339.

31 Carr KE, Toner PG. *Cell Structure. An Introduction to Biomedical Electron Microscopy*, 3rd edn. Edinburgh: Churchill Livingstone, 1982.

32 Shiner M, Doniach I. Histopathologic studies in steatorrhoea. In: *Proceedings of the World Congress of Gastroenterology, Washington*. Baltimore: Williams & Wilkins, 1958: 586.

33 Ferguson A, Sutherland A, MacDonald TT, Allan F. Technique for microdissection and measurement in biopsies of human small intestine. *J Clin Pathol*, 1977; 30: 1068.

34 Slavin G, Sowter C, Robertson K, McDermott S, Paton K. Measurement in jejunal biopsies by computer-aided microscopy. *J Clin Pathol*, 1980; 33: 254.

35 Williams PL, ed. *Gray's Anatomy*, 38th edn. Edinburgh: Churchill Livingstone, 1995: 1765.

36 de Peyer E, France NE, Philips AD, Walker-Smith JA. Quantitative evaluation of small intestinal morphology in childhood. *Acta Paediatr Belg*, 1978; 31: 173.

37 Baker SJ, Ignatius M, Mathan VI, Vaish SK, Chako CC. In: Wolstenholme GEW, ed. *Intestinal Biopsy*. Ciba Foundation Study Group no. 19. London: J & A Churchill, 1962: 84.

38 Creamer B. Variations in small intestinal villous shape and mucosal dynamics. *Br Med J*, 1964; ii: 1371.

39 Corazza GR, Frazzoni M, Dixon MF, Gasbarrini G. Quantitative assessment of the mucosal architecture of jejunal biopsy specimens; a comparison between linear measurement, stereology and computer-aided microscopy. *J Clin Pathol*, 1985; 38: 765.

40 Corazza GR, Bonvicini F, Frazzoni M, Gatto M, Gasbarrini G. Observer variation in assessment of jejunal biopsy specimens. A comparison between subjective criteria and morphometric measurement. *Gastroenterology*, 1982; 83: 1217.

41 Sinclair TS, Jones DA, Kumar PJ, Phillips AD. The microvillus in adult jejunal mucosa—an electron microscopic study. *Histopathology*, 1984; 8: 739.

42 Trier JS, Rubin CE. Electron microscopy of the small intestine: a review. *Gastroenterology*, 1965; 49: 574.

43 Trier JS. The surface coat of gastrointestinal epithelial cells. *Gastroenterology*, 1969; 56: 618.

44 Dobbins WO III. Morphologic and functional correlates of intestinal brush borders. *Am J Med Sci*, 1969; 258: 150.

46 Mason DY, Piris J. Immunohistochemistry and the gastrointestinal tract. In: Wright R, ed. *Recent Advances in Gastrointestinal Pathology*. London: WB Saunders, 1980: 3.

47 Lojda Z. The application of enzyme histochemistry in diagnostic pathology. In: Stoward PJ, Polak JM, eds. *Histochemistry; the Widening Horizons*. Chichester: John Wiley, 1981: 205.

48 Lev R, Griffiths WC. Colonic and small intestinal alkaline phosphatase. A histochemical and biochemical study. *Gastroenterology*, 1982; 82: 1427.

49 Shields HM, Bair FA, Bates ML, Yedlin ST, Alpers DH. Localization of immunoreactive alkaline phosphatase in the rat small intestine at the light microscopic level by immunocytochemistry. *Gastroenterology*, 1982; 82: 39.

50 Keane R, O'Grady JG, Shiel J *et al*. Intestinal lactase, sucrase and alkaline phosphatase in relation to age, sex and site of intestinal biopsy in 477 Irish subjects. *J Clin Pathol*, 1983; 36: 74.

51 Triadou N, Bataille J, Schmitz J. Longitudinal study of the human intestinal brush border membrane proteins; distribution of the main disaccharidases and peptidases. *Gastroenterology*, 1983; 85: 1326.

52 Lojda Z. Indigogenic methods for glycosidases I. An improved method for β-D glucosidase and its application to localisation studies of intestinal and renal enzymes. *Histochemie*, 1970; 22: 347.

53 Lojda Z. Indigogenic methods for glycosidases II. An improved method for β-D galactosidase and its application to localisation studies of the enzymes in the intestine and in other tissues. *Histochemie*, 1970; 23: 266.

54 Nordstrom C, Dahlquist A, Josefsson L. Quantitative determination of enzymes in different parts of the villi and crypts of rat small intestine. Comparison of alkaline phosphatase, disaccharidases and dipeptidases. *J Histochem Cytochem*, 1967; 15: 713.

55 Hermon-Taylor J, Perrin J, Grant DAW, Appleyard A, Bupel M, Magee AI. Immunofluorescent localization of enterokinase in human small intestine. *Gut*, 1977; 18: 259.

56 Isaacson P, Judd MA. Immunohistochemistry of carcinoembryonic antigen in the small intestine. *Cancer*, 1978; 42: 1554.

57 Goldenberg DM, Sharkey RM, Primus FJ. Immunocytochemical detection of carcinoembryonic antigen in conventional histopathology specimens. *Cancer*, 1978; 42: 1546.

58 Montero C, Erlandsen SL. Immunocytochemical and histochemical studies on intestinal epithelial cells producing both lysozyme and mucosubstance. *Anat Rec*, 1978; 190: 127.

59 Geboes K, Ray MB, Rutgeerts P, Callea F, Desniet VJ, VanTrappen G. Morphological identification of alpha-1-antitrypsin in the human small intestine. *Histopathology*, 1982; 6: 55.

60 Green PHR, Lefkowitch JH, Clickman RM, Riley JW, Quinet E, Blum CR. Apolipoprotein localization and quantitation in the human intestine. *Gastroenterology*, 1982; 83: 1223.

61 Trejeloziewicz LK, Malizia G, Oakes J, Losowsky MS, Janossy G. Expression of the common acute lymphoblastic leukaemia antigen (CALLA gp. 100) in the brush border of normal jejunum and jejunum of patients with coeliac disease. *J Clin Pathol*, 1985; 38: 1002.

62 Hershberg R, Eghtesady R, Sydora B *et al*. Expression of the thymus leukemia antigen in mouse intestinal epithelium. *Proc Natl Acad Sci USA*, 1990; 87: 9727.

63 Brown WR. Relationships between immunoglobulins and the intestinal epithelium. *Gastroenterology*, 1978; 75: 129.

64 MacDonald WC, Trier JS, Everett NB. Cell proliferation and migration in the stomach, duodenum and rectum of man: radioautographic studies. *Gastroenterology*, 1964; 46: 405.

65 Lipkin M. Proliferation and differentiation of gastrointestinal cells. *Physiol Rev*, 1973; 53: 811.

66 Bjerknes M, Cheng H. The stem-cell zone of the small intestinal epithelium. III. Evidence from columnar, enteroendocrine and mucous cells in the adult mouse. *Am J Anat*, 1981; 160: 77.

67 Cocco AE, Dohrmann MJ, Hendrix TR. Reconstruction of normal jejunal biopsies: three dimensional histology. *Gastroenterology*, 1966; 51: 24.

68 Sandow MJ, Whitehead R. The Paneth cell. *Gut*, 1979; 20: 420.

68a Wilson TJ, Ponder BA, Wright NA. Use of a mouse chimaeric model to study cell migration patterns in the small intestinal epithelium. *Cell Tissue Kinetics*, 1985; 18: 333.

69 Bjerknes M, Cheng H. The stem-cell zone of the small intestinal epithelium. I. Evidence from Paneth cells in the adult mouse. *Am J Anat*, 1981; 160: 51.

70 Lewin K. The Paneth cell in disease. *Gut*, 1969; 10: 804.

71 Peeters T, Van Trappen G. The Paneth cell: a source of intestinal lysozyme. *Gut*, 1975; 16: 553.

72 Rodning CB, Wilson ID, Erlandsen SL. Immunoglobulins within small intestinal Paneth cells. *Lancet*, 1976; i: 984.

72a Porter EM, Liu L, Oren A, Anton PA, Ganz T. Localization of human intestinal defensin 5 in Paneth cell granules. *Infect Immun*, 1997; 65: 2389.

72b Moller P, Walczak H, Reidl S, Strater J, Krammer PH. Paneth cells express high levels of CD95 ligand transcripts: a unique property among gastrointestinal epithelia. *Am J Pathol*, 1996; 149: 9.

73 Dawson IMP. Visualisation of the diffuse endocrine system. *J Clin Pathol*, 1979; 33 (Suppl): 8A.

74 Dawson IMP. Diffuse endocrine and neuroendocrine tumours. In: Anthony PP, MacSween RMN, eds. *Recent Advances in Histopathology*. Edinburgh: Churchill Livingstone. 1984, 12: 111.

75 Sjolund K, Sanden G, Hakanson R, Sundler F. Endocrine cells in human intestine; an immunocytochemical study. *Gastroenterology*, 1983; 85: 1120.

76 Novelli MR, Williamson JA, Tomlinson IP *et al*. Polyclonal origin of colonic adenomas in an XO/XY patient with FAP. *Science*, 1996; 272: 1187.
77 Andrew A, Kramer B, Rawdon BB. The origin of gut and pancreatic neuroendocrine (APUD) cells—the last word? *J Pathol*, 1998; 186: 117.
78 Sidhu GS. The endodermal origin of digestive and respiratory tract APUD cells. *Am J Pathol*, 1979; 96: 5.
79 Sjolund K, Sanden G, Hakanson R, Sundler F. Endocrine cells in human intestine: an immunocytochemical study. *Gastroenterology*, 1983; 85: 1120.
79a Facer R, Bishop AE, Lloyd RV, Wilson BS, Hennessy RJ, Polak JM. Chromogranin: a newly recognized marker for endocrine cells of the human gastrointestinal tract. *Gastroenterology*, 1985; 89: 1366.
79b Buffa R, Rindi G, Sessa F *et al*. Synaptophysin immunoreactivity and small clear vesicles in neuroendocrine cells and related tumours. *Mol Cell Probes*, 1987; 1: 367.
80 Bishop AE, Polak JM, Facer P, Ferry G-L, Marangos PJ, Pearse AGE. Neuronspecific enolase: a common marker for the endocrine cells and innervation of the gut and pancreas. *Gastroenterology*, 1982; 83: 902.
81 Bryant MG, Bloom SR. Distribution of the gut hormones in the primate intestinal tract. *Gut*, 1979; 20: 653.
82 Bryant MC, Bloom SR, Polak JM *et al*. Measurement of gut hormonal peptides in biopsies from human stomach and proximal small intestine. *Gut*, 1983; 24: 114.
83 Solcia E *et al*. Lausanne 1977 classification of gastroenteropancreatic endocrine cells. In: Bloom SR, ed. *Gut Hormones*. Edinburgh: Churchill Livingstone, 1978: 42.
84 Bloom SR. Gut hormones. *Curr Opin Gastroenterol*, 1986; 2: 816.
85 Irvine GB, Murphy RF. Multiple forms of gastroenteropancreatic hormones. *Gut*, 1981; 22: 1048.
86 Lundgren O. The circulation of the small bowel mucosa. *Gut*, 1974; 15: 1005.
87 Bank S, Fisher G, Marks IN, Groll A. The lymphatics of the intestinal mucosa. A clinical and experimental study. *Ant J Dig Dis*, 1967; 12: 619.
88 Parker FG, Barnes EN, Kaye GI. The pericryptal fibroblast sheath. IV. Replication, migration and differentiation of the subepithelial fibroblasts of the crypt and villus of the rabbit jejunum. *Gastroenterology*, 1974; 67: 607.
89 Brandborg LL. The lamina propria: orphan of the gut. *Gastroenterology*, 1969; 57: 191.
90 Perdue MH, Chung M, Gall DG. Effect of intestinal anaphylaxis on gut function in the rat. *Gastroenterology*, 1984; 86: 391.
91 Bienenstock J. The physiology of the local immune response. In: Asquith P, ed. *Immunology of the Gastrointestinal Tract*. Edinburgh: Churchill Livingstone, 1979: 3.
92 Doe WF, Hapel AJ. Intestinal immunity and malabsorption. *Clin Gastroenterol*, 1983; 12: 415.
93 Marsh MN. *Immunopathology of the Small Intestine*. Chichester: John Wiley, 1987.
94 Owen RL, Jones AL. Epithelial cell specialisation within human Peyer's patches: an ultrastructural study of intestinal lymphoid follicles. *Gastroenterology*, 1974; 66: 189.
95 Bhalla DK, Owen RL. Cell renewal and migration in lymphoid follicles of Peyer's patches and cecum: an autoradiographic study in mice. *Gastroenterology*, 1982; 82: 232.
96 Bye WH, Allan CH, Trier JS. Structure, distribution and origin of M cells in Peyer's patches of mouse ileum. *Gastroenterology*, 1984; 86: 789.
97 Scott H, Sothern BG, Brandtzaeg P, Thorsby E. HLA-DR-like antigens on the epithelium of the human small intestine. *Scand J Immunol*, 1980; 12: 77.
98 Spencer J, Finn T, Isaacson PC. Expression of HLA-DR antigen on epithelium associated with lymphoid tissue in the human gastrointestinal tract. *Gut*, 1986; 27: 153.
99 Ernst PB, Song F, Klimpel GR *et al*. Regulation of the mucosal immune response. [Review] [90 references] *Am J Trop Med Hyg*, 1999; 60: 2.
100 Golder JP, Doe WF. Isolation and preliminary characterization of human intestinal macrophages. *Gastroenterology*, 1983; 84: 795.
101 Rossen RD. HLA and disease: a postulated role for HLA in gastrointestinal diseases. *Gastroenterology*, 1980; 78: 1629.
102 Mowat AM, Viney JL. The anatomical basis of intestinal immunity. *Immunol Rev*, 1997; 156: 145.
103 Arnaud-Battandier F. Lymphoid population of the gut. *Rec Adv Gastroenterol Clin Biol*, 1984; 8: 632.
104 Brandtzaeg P, Farstad IN, Haraldsen G, Jahnsen FL. Cellular and molecular mechanisms for induction of mucosal immunity. [Review] [57 references] *Dev Biol Stand*, 1998; 92: 93.
105 MacDonald TT, Pender SL. Lamina propria T cells. [Review] [68 references] *Chem Immunol*, 1998; 71: 103.
106 Clancy R, Cripps A, Chipchase H. Regulation of human gut lymphocytes by T lymphocytes. *Gut*, 1984; 25: 47.
107 Cerf-Bensussan N, Guy-Grand D, Griscolli C. Intra-epithelial lymphocytes of human gut: isolation, characterisation and study of killer activity. *Gut*, 1985; 26: 81.
108 Nanno M, Kanamori Y, Saito H, Kawaguchi-Miyashita M, Shimada S, Ishikawa H. Intestinal intraepithelial T lymphocytes. Our T cell horizons are expanding. *Immunol Res*, 1998; 18: 41.
109 Kingston D, Pearson JR, Penna FJ. Plasma cell counts of human jejunal biopsy specimens examined by immunofluorescence and immunoperoxidase techniques; a comparative study. *J Clin Pathol*, 1981; 34: 381.
110 Husband AJ, Gowans JLN. The origin and antigen dependent distribution of IgA-containing cells in the intestine. *J Exp Med*, 1978; 148: 1146.
111 Brandtzaeg P, Prydz H. Direct evidence for an integrated function of J-chain and secretory component in epithelial transport of immunoglobulins. *Nature*, 1984; 311: 71.
112 Selby WS, Janossy G, Jewell DP. Immunohistological characterization of intraepithelial lymphocytes of the human gastrointestinal tract. *Gut*, 1981; 22: 169.
113 Greenwood JH, Austin LL, Dobbins WO III. In vitro characterization of human intestinal intraepithelial lymphocytes. *Gastroenterology*, 1983; 85: 1023.
114 Dobbins WO. Human intestinal intraepithelial lymphocytes. *Gut*, 1986; 27: 972.
115 Mestecky J. The common mucosal immune system and current strategies for induction of immune response in external secretions. *J Clin Immunol*, 1987; 7: 265.
116 Takahashi I, Kiyono H. Gamma delta T cells: bodyguards and/or sleepers in the gut. *Chem Immunol*, 1998; 71: 77.

117 Landboe-Christensen E. The duodenal glands of Brunner in man, their distribution and quantity. *Acta Pathol Microbiol Scand Suppl*, 1944; 52A.
118 Grossman MI. The glands of Brunner. *Physiol Rev*, 1958; 38: 675.
119 Treasure T. The ducts of Brunner's glands. *Anatomy*, 1978; 127: 299.
120 Leeson T, Leeson CR. The fine structure of Brunner's glands in man. *J Anat*, 1968; 103: 263.
121 Gershon MD, Erde SM. The nervous system of the gut. *Gastroenterol Suppl*, 1981; 80: 1571.
122 Smith B. *The Neuropathology of the Alimentary Tract*. London: Edward Arnold, 1972.
123 Burnstock G. Studies of autonomic nerves in the gut—past, present and future. *Scand J Gastroenterol* (Suppl), 1982; 17: 135.
124 Polak JM, Bloom SR, Wright NA, Daly MJ, eds. Autonomic nerves of the gut. *Scand J Gastroenterol* (Suppl 71), 1982; 1.
125 Bishop AE, Ferri GL, Probert L, Bloom SR, Polak JM. Peptidergic nerves. *Scand J Gastroenterol* (Suppl), 1982; 17: 43.
126 Barajas L, Wong P. Demonstration of acetylcholin-esterase in the adrenergic nerves of the renal glomerular arterioles. *J Ultrastruct Res*, 1975; 53: 244.
127 Gershon MD. Serotinergic neurotransmission in the gut. *Scand J Gastroenterol* (Suppl), 1982; 17: 27.
128 Polak JM, Bloom SR. Peptidergic nerves of the gastrointestinal tract. *Invest Cell Pathol*, 1978; 1: 301.
129 Llewellyn-Smith IJ, Furness JB, Murphy R, O'Brien PE, Costa M. Substance-P-containing cells in the human small intestine. Distribution, ultrastructure and characterization of the immuno-reactive peptide. *Gastroenterology*, 1984; 86: 421.
130 Furness JB *et al*. Detection and characterisation of neurotransmitters, particularly peptides, in the gastrointestinal tract. *Scand J Gastroenterol* (Suppl), 1982; 17: 61.
131 Cochard P, Le Douarin NM. Development of the intrinsic innervation of the gut. *Scand J Gastroenterol* (Suppl), 1982; 17: 1.
132 Cook RD, Burnstock G. The ultrastructure of Auerbach's plexus in the guinea pig. *J Neurocytol*, 1976; 5: 171.
133 Gabella G. On the ultrastructure of the enteric nerve ganglia. *Scand J Gastroenterol* (Suppl), 1982; 17: 15.
134 Furness JB, Costa M. The adrenergic innervation of the gastrointestinal tract. *Ergeb Physiol*, 1979; 69: 1.
135 Llewellyn-Srnith IJ, Furness JB, O'Brien PE, Costa M. Noradrenergic nerves in human small intestine. Distribution and ultrastructure. *Gastroenterology*, 1984; 87: 513.
136 Angel F, Schmalz PF, Morgan KG, Go VLW, Szurszewski JH. Innervation of the muscularis mucosae in the canine stomach and colon. *Scand J Gastroenterol* (Suppl), 1982; 17: 71.
137 Ahlman H, Lundberg J, Dahlstrom A, Kerwenter J. A possible vagal adrenergic release of serotonin from enterochromaffin cells in the cat. *Acta Physiol Scand*, 1976; 98: 366.
138 Ferri GL, Botti PL, Vezzadini P, Biliotti G, Bloom SR, Polak JM. Peptide-containing innervation of the human intestinal mucosa. An immunocytochemical study on wholemount preparations. *Histochemistry*, 1982; 76: 413.
139 Ferri GL, Adrian TE, Ghatei MA *et al*. Tissue localization and relative distribution of regulatory peptides in separated layers from human bowel. *Gastroenterology*, 1983; 84: 777.
140 Ferri GL, Botti P, Biliotti G *et al*. VIP-, substance P, and metencephalin-immunoreactive innervation of the human gastroduodenal mucosa and Brunner's glands. *Gut*, 1984; 25: 948.
141 Llewellyn-Smith IJ, Furness JB, Murphy R, O'Brien PE, Costa M. Substance P-containing nerves in the human small intestine. Distribution, ultrastructure and characterization of the immunoreactive peptide. *Gastroenterology*, 1984; 86: 421.
141a Lamas S, Perez-Sala D, Moncada S. Nitric oxide: from discovery to the clinic. *Trends Pharmacol Sci*, 1998; 19: 436.
142 Russo A, Fraser R, Adachi K, Horowitz M, Boeckxstaens G. Evidence that nitric oxide mechanisms regulate small intestinal motility in humans. *Gut*, 1999; 44: 72.
142a Hagger R, Finlayson C, Jeffrey I, Kumar D. Role of the interstitial cells of Cajal in the control of gut motility. *Br J Surg*, 1997; 84: 445.
143 Young HM, Ciampoli D, Southwell BR, Newgreen DF. Origin of interstitial cells of Cajal in the mouse intestine. *Dev Biol (Orlando)*, 1996; 180: 97.
143a Sanders KM. A case for interstitial cells of Cajal as pacemakers and mediators of neurotransmission in the gastrointestinal tract. [Review] [154 references] *Gastroenterology*, 1996; 111: 492.
144 Thuneberg L. Interstitial dells of Cajal: intestinal pacemaker cells? *Adv Anat Embryol Cell Biol*, 1982; 71: 1.
144a Rumessen JJ, Thuneberg L. Pacemaker cells in the gastrointestinal tract: interstitial cells of Cajal. *Scand J Gastroenterol Suppl* 1996; 216: 82.
145 Publicover NG, Hammond EM, Sanders KM. Amplification of nitric oxide signaling by interstitial cells isolated from canine colon. *Proc Natl Acad Sci USA*, 1993; 90: 2087.
146 Vannucchi MG. Receptors in interstitial cells of Cajal: identification and possible physiological roles. *Microsc Res Tech*, 1999; 47: 325.
147 Thomsen L, Robinson TL, Lee JC *et al*. Interstitial cells of Cajal generate a rhythmic pacemaker current. *Nat Med*, 1998; 4: 848.
148 Smith B. The neuropathology of pseudo-obstruction of the intestine. *Scand J Gastroenterol* (Suppl), 1982; 17: 103.
149 Riemann JF, Schmidt H. Ultrastructural changes in the gut autonomic nervous system following laxative abuse and in other conditions. *Scand J Gastroenterol* (Suppl), 1982; 17: 111.
150 Cohen S. Clinical aspects of autonomic nerve dysfunction of the gut. *Scand J Gastroenterol* (Suppl), 1982; 17: 125.
151 Kellow JE, Borody TJ, Phillips SP, Tucker RL, Haddad AC. Human interdigestive motility: variations in pattern from esophagus to colon. *Gastroenterology*, 1986; 91: 386.
152 Vantrappen G, Janssens J, Coremans G, Jian R. Gastrointestinal motility disorders. *Dig Dis Sci*, 1986; 31 (Suppl 9).
153 Kitagawa K, Nishigori A, Murata N, Nishimoto K, Takada H. Radiotelemetry of the pH of the gastrointestinal tract by glass electrode. *Gastroenterology*, 1966; 51: 368.
154 Savage DC. Microbial ecology of the gastrointestinal tract. *Ann Rev Microbiol*, 1977; 31: 107.
155 Simon GL, Gorbach SL. Intestinal flora in health and disease. *Gastroenterology*, 1984; 86: 174.
156 Justesen T, Nielsen OH, Jacobsen IE, Lave J, Rasmussen SN. The normal cultivable microflora in upper jejunal fluid in healthy adults. *Scand J Gastroenterol*, 1984; 19: 279.
157 Potten CS, Hendry H. The microcolony assay in mouse small intestine. In: Potten CS, Hendry JH, eds. *Cell Clones: Manual of Cell Techniques*. Edinburgh: Churchill Livingstone, 1985: 50.
157a Potten CS, Booth C, Pritchard DM. The intestinal epithelial stem cell: The mucosal governor. *Int J Exp Pathol* 1997; 78: 219.

158 Potten CS. Stem cells in the gastrointestinal epithelium: numbers, characteristics and death. *Phil Trans R Soc Biol Sci*, 1998; 353: 821.
159 Hanby AM, Poulsom R, Elia G, Singh S, Longcroft JM, Wright NA. The expression of the trefoil peptides pS2 and human spasmolytic polypeptide (hSP) in 'gastric metaplasia' of the proximal duodenum: implications for the nature of 'gastric metaplasia'. *J Pathol* 1993; 169: 355.

19 Normal embryology and fetal development; developmental abnormalities of the small intestine

An extensive study of 8390 childhood autopsies has shown that particular anomalies in the gastrointestinal tract, including Meckel's diverticulum, atresias, Hirschsprung's disease and pyloric stenosis, are commonly associated with other anomalies elsewhere [1]. The majority of serious developmental abnormalities reveal themselves at birth or during early childhood [2,3] and present as obstructions with perforation and peritonitis as likely complications. Those that are less severe and the majority of hamartomas present later with less dramatic symptoms, though intussusception is relatively more common. To understand many of the developmental anomalies in the small bowel it is necessary to review briefly its development and rotation [4–6].

Normal development

Some pathologists are unfamiliar with the relationship between gestational age and embryo length. Because there are individual differences in development between fetuses, and it is not always possible to know the exact date of fertilization, especially when this has to be deduced from the date of the last menstrual period, Table 19.1 gives a rough approximation only of this relationship.

In the 1.5–3-mm stage (4th week) the head and somites appear. The notochord develops and mesoderm grows into the embryonic disc and separates ectoderm from endoderm except at the *buccopharyngeal membrane* anteriorly and at the *cloacal membrane* posteriorly. The head and tail now curve ventrally and the *cloacal membrane* comes to lie on the ventral surface. Failure of the mesodermal ingrowth may result in non-separation of neural and gut elements and so to those duplications associated with defects of spinal cord and vertebrae. By this stage the former yolk sac, seen in longitudinal section, is shaped somewhat like a mushroom; its anterior limb lies between the developing central nervous system and the heart, where it forms the primitive foregut, while the posterior limb lies in the tail fold and forms the primitive hindgut. The central portion, which will form the midgut, is in free communication through a wide opening, the vitellointestinal duct, with the remains of the yolk sac, which is now outside the embryo (Fig. 19.1). As the embryo grows the body becomes bounded by definitive folds which form the ventral body wall and narrow the broad body stalk, which will later form the umbilical cord, and which, between the 23-mm and 60-mm stages, will contain the midgut in a physiological hernia.

The foregut is at first short and lies in close apposition to the developing vertebrae, from which it becomes suspended by a short dorsal mesentery. It has its own arterial blood supply from the coeliac axis, and from it develop the oesophagus, stomach, first part of duodenum, trachea and respiratory system. The dorsal wall of the stomach grows relatively more rapidly than the ventral, producing the greater curve; the stomach rotates to the left causing a slight left deviation of the lower oesophagus and a slight deviation of the duodenum to the right. The oesophageal and duodenal mesenteries are later absorbed and these organs become anchored to the posterior thoracic and abdominal walls.

The hindgut is suspended by a similar mesentery and is supplied by the inferior mesenteric artery; from it develop the descending and sigmoid colons and the rectum.

The midgut is supplied by the superior mesenteric artery and from it develop the third and fourth parts of the duodenum, the jejunum, ileum, caecum, appendix and ascending and transverse colons. At the 5–12-mm stage it begins to lengthen and become tubular, at first growing away from the vertebral axis in the sagittal plane and later becoming coiled, which induces a marked development of the dorsal mesentery

Table 19.1 Approximate relationship between fetal age and embryo length.

Age after fertilization (days)	Embryo length (mm)
22	1.5–2.0
25	2.5–3.5
30	6.0–7.5
35	12–15
40	20–23
45	24–28
50	29–34
55	35–41
60	42–50
70	53–67
84	80–95
98	110–130
112	130–150
126	155–180
140 (20 weeks)	175–205

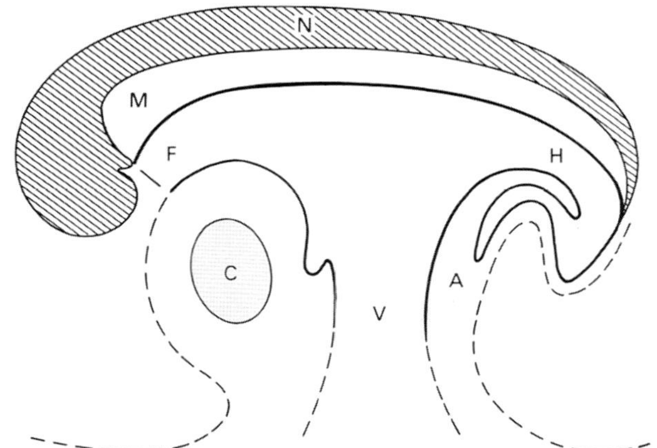

Fig. 19.1 The figure shows the normal development of the gut. A, allantoic diverticulum; C, developing heart; F, foregut; H, hindgut; M, mesodermal ingrowth; N, neural tube; V, vitellointestinal duct.

in which the superior mesenteric artery runs. By the 14–23-mm stage, due to lack of intra-abdominal space caused partly by the rapid growth of the liver and also by the marked elongation of the gut itself, the midgut is extruded into the umbilical cord as a physiological hernia; the caecum develops on its caudal limb and the vitellointestinal duct lies at its apex. Further growth in a purely sagittal plane now becomes impossible and rotation begins. It is completed as the bowel returns to the abdominal cavity at the 50–60-mm stage. This process may be divided into phases which are most easily followed by taking a piece of flexible rubber tubing, marking it into cranial and caudal loops and using it as a model.

Phase 1

The cranial (ventral) loop of bowel rotates to the fetal right and caudally. The caudal (dorsal) loop, on which lies the caecum, is correspondingly displaced upwards and to the fetal left through 90° (this is an anticlockwise rotation around the superior mesenteric artery when the embryo is viewed from the front). It takes place between the 6th and 10th weeks.

Phase 2

This takes place at the end of phase 1, at about the 10th week, when there is room for the bowel to return to the abdominal cavity. The cranial (ventral) loop of small bowel re-enters first and passes to the fetal right of the superior mesenteric artery; it then rotates through a further 180° making a total rotation of 270°. The caecum, which returns last, has a similar rotation and comes to lie to the fetal right of the umbilicus and in front of the small bowel. The future transverse colon lies across the abdomen in front of the superior mesenteric artery and the mesenteric attachment, though it is no longer thought that its further growth is responsible for pushing the caecum down into the right iliac fossa [7]. The descending colon is displaced to the left and comes to lie in the left loin. When rotation is complete the small intestine is approximately six times as long as the large.

Phase 3

This is a phase of fixation. The mesenteries of the caecum, ascending and descending colons shorten and become absorbed, leaving those parts of the large bowel also attached to the posterior abdominal wall. The transverse and sigmoid colons retain a full mesentery.

Mucosal development

A number of studies are available on the mucosal development of human fetuses [6,8–15]. At the 10–20-mm stage the small bowel is lined by a layer of cubical cells, two to four cells thick around a central lumen [16]. These cells proliferate and some become vacuolated (Fig. 19.2). The duodenum can appear occluded for a time but there is probably never occlusion below this level. The structural development of the small intestinal mucosa appears to be determined by the expression of products of so-called homeobox, or *HOX* genes [16a], particularly *Cdx-1* and *Cdx-2*. Contact of the epithelial cells with their environment causes up-regulation of growth factors TGF-α, TGF-β, EGF and HGF, which stimulate cell proliferation. Tissue organization is brought about by differential apoptosis by up-regulation of the *bcl-2/bax* family of genes, triggered by contact with mesenchymal elements, together with differential stimulation of motility of the cells by differential expression of motilins such as the trefoil peptides [17]. Rudimentary microvilli appear on the luminal cells at the 35–40-mm stage [11,12] and this is followed by villus formation which becomes complete by the 80–90-mm stage

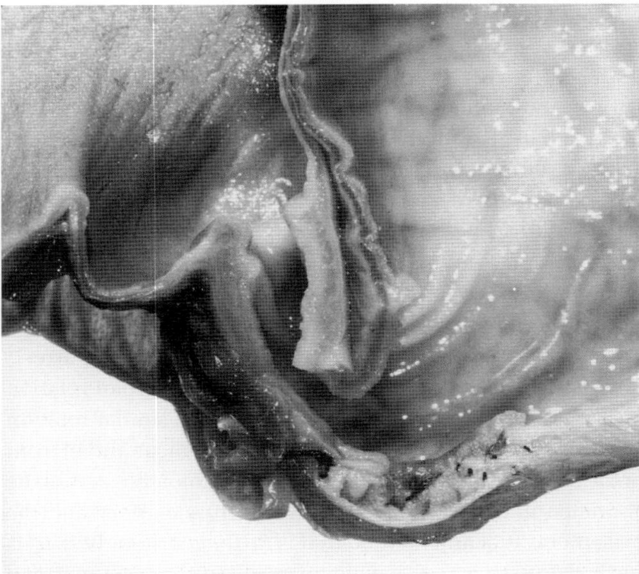

Fig. 19.2 Severe duodenal stenosis with narrowing of the lumen over a length of about 1 cm. The duodenum on the right is dilated because of the stenosis.

[13,15], somewhat earlier in the jejunum than in the ileum. Some workers have considered that villi are produced by the vacuolation and breakdown of intervening cells [16] but our own studies and those of others [8] do not support that view. Surface enterocytes differentiate on the developing villi and alkaline phosphatase, aminopeptidases, adenosine triphosphatase and succinate dehydrogenase become demonstrable histochemically as early as the 25-mm stage [8,10] and are followed by lactase and other disaccharidases [14,15], at first in equal concentrations throughout the bowel but later showing regional differences with higher concentrations of sucrase and lactase in the jejunum. Mucin granules and goblet cells appear at the same time. Crypts are formed by budlike down-growths into the surrounding mesenchyme at the 50–60-mm stage [13,15]. Endocrine cells containing gastrin, secretin, motilin, gastric inhibitory peptide (GIP), vasoactive intestinal polypeptide (VIP), enteroglucagon and somatostatin have been recognized as early as the 40–45-mm stage [18,19] and are said to have an adult distribution by 175–205 mm. Paneth cells have been present in our own material by 110–130 mm.

Lymphoid follicles first appear in the mucosa at 110–150 mm and recognizable Peyer's patches by 175–205 mm [20]. Cells which may be membranous (M) cells have been described at 130–150 mm [13].

The circular muscle coat appears first in the duodenum at the 30-mm stage and extends distally throughout the small bowel; the longitudinal coat follows at the 60–75-mm stage and the muscularis mucosae much later at about 20 weeks. An intramuscular ganglionic plexus is present at 35–40 mm and a submucosal plexus at 60 mm [21]; neurotensin and VIP can be demonstrated at the 80–90 mm stage.

The myenteric plexus appears to be fully formed in the 60 mm fetus but there is doubt about the functionality of the innervation before birth, at least in dogs [21a].

Malformations

Our knowledge of the development of the human small intestine has advanced greatly, largely due to the availability of suitable material for study following the legalization of abortions. There has not as yet been a corresponding advance in the understanding of many human bowel malformations.

Comparatively few congenital anomalies in the bowel are genetically inherited; examples are mucoviscidosis and anomalies associated with certain chromosomal trisomies [5]. A good, though now somewhat dated review is available [2]. Very few are linked with known environmental factors such as maternal rubella. There is, however, considerable evidence that many are associated with interference with the blood supply at critical periods in development between the 3rd and 8th weeks, although we do not know the primary causative factor for the interruption. A small study which compared children with congenital anomalies of the mesentery with normal children, using postmortem arteriography, showed a significant number of vascular aberrations in the affected children [22].

Malpositions

Malrotation and malfixation

Minor degrees of malrotation and, more commonly, malfixation are not uncommon [2,3,23] but the more severe forms are rare [24–28]. Their importance lies in their secondary effects, particularly volvulus and obstruction. The recognized types are described below.

Reversed rotation

In phase 1 (see p. 253) the ventral and dorsal loops rotate to the fetal left through 90° instead of to the fetal right. The caecum still comes to lie in the right iliac fossa, but the small bowel is now ventral (superficial) to the transverse colon, which often passes through an aperture in the small bowel mesentery. The caecum and ascending colon may retain a mesentery and fail to become fixed [28,29].

Failure of the small bowel to rotate fully

This is a failure in phase 2, following a normal phase 1. As the small bowel returns to the abdomen it remains on the right side without rotation. The caecum also fails to rotate, retains its mesentery and lies either in the left iliac fossa or in the midline; the ascending colon also retains its mesentery and lies just to the left of the midline behind the greater curve of the stomach; a shortened loop of transverse colon connects it to a normally situated descending colon. The whole bowel from duodenum to splenic flexure is unanchored and is supported by a single mesentery with a very narrow base, prone to volvulus. Symptoms of appendicitis can be central or left sided [25,28,30,31].

Other rotational anomalies
After a normal phase 1 the caecum may undergo normal rotation but retain a mesentery, while the small bowel does not rotate further [30] or undergoes reverse rotation, in which case the caecum will come to lie in the pyloric region [32,33].

Anomalies of fixation
After normal rotation the caecum initially lies over the right kidney. It may become fixed here or, conversely, delay in absorption of the mesentery may result in a pelvic caecum or a mobile ascending colon. Abnormal peritoneal bands may be found between caecum or ascending colon and the posterior abdominal wall; they are clinically important because they often cross and compress the duodenum [26,34].

Consequences of failures of rotation or fixation

There may be an unusually long mesentery extending from duodenum to splenic flexure and arising from an abnormally narrow base. Volvulus leading to duodenal obstruction and formation of varices with haemorrhage due to involvement of superior mesenteric vessels can occur [35]. Duodenal obstruction can result from direct pressure of a malrotated caecum or from abnormal peritoneal bands. These result from imperfect mesenteric absorption and can also act as potential sacs for internal hernias. Such bands often coexist with volvulus and must always be looked for. It should be remembered that the above abnormalities may not be present in isolation. Even after apparently adequate surgical correction of a malrotation, persisting pseudo-obstruction frequently occurs [36]. This may be due to other congenital mechanical anomalies or to defective intrinsic innervation.

Situs inversus and Kartagener's syndrome

Some form of situs inversus occurs once in every 1400 births [37]. It may be complete, when thoracic and abdominal organs are both involved, but more commonly involves the abdominal viscera only. When complete it can be associated with bronchiectasis and abnormal nasal sinuses—Kartagener's syndrome. Reversals of position can cause difficulties in diagnosis but do not directly predispose to pathological complications.

Omphalocoele (exomphalos) and related defects

Omphalocoele and exomphalos are commonly used as synonyms and will not be separated here.

A physiological hernial sac composed of amnion is normally present from the 10–60-mm stage and becomes obliterated after the bowel returns to the body cavity (see p. 253). The most common form of omphalocoele results from a persistence of this sac, which usually contains a variable length of ileum, the caecum and part of the ascending colon, usually unrotated [38–40]. Liver, spleen and stomach can also be found in it. The sac may persist because its neck becomes abnormally narrowed, because the bowel adheres to it before the end of the 10th week, or because of undue enlargement of the liver, all of which hinder the normal return of the bowel.

Other defects include herniation of the bowel into the umbilical cord through an umbilical ring which has failed to close and non-formation of the fetal part of the umbilical cord because of defective condensation of mesenchyme around the attachment of the cord to the embryo. This condition is allied to complete eventration, in which a large sac forms which occupies much of the abdominal wall above and below the umbilicus and contains gut and other abdominal viscera. These defects, which resemble omphalocoeles clinically and in their appearance, are not due to the persistence of a physiological hernia; they must also be distinguished from upper and lower abdominal and paraumbilical hernias which are associated with malformations of the abdominal wall, are covered by skin and lined by peritoneum and are not of primary umbilical origin. Cases are also described in which, in the absence of hernia or exomphalos, the bowel is surrounded by an adherent sac or encapsulation of peritoneum thought to be derived from the primitive peritoneum lining the physiological hernial sac which has become adherent some time in the 20–60-mm stage [41,42]. This condition is distinct from that of abdominal cocooning. The association of abdominal muscle defects with malformations of the gut is well recognized [43].

Maldevelopment

Aplasia and agenesis

Complete absence of the small bowel is not, to our knowledge, recorded. The term aplasia is used in the literature in two ways: either to describe a short but otherwise normal small bowel in adults [44] or children [45]; or to indicate a solid cord of tissue of variable length, without a lumen [46–48]. The latter is probably more correctly considered as an acquired atresia due to interference with the blood supply (see below).

Atresias and stenoses

We use the term *atresia*, which means 'non-perforated', to describe a congenital anomaly which can involve any part of the gut and in which there is complete discontinuity of the lumen over a variable length of bowel. We use the term *stenosis* to indicate a narrowing of the lumen without complete obliteration. About 60% of all cases presenting as stenoses and a higher proportion with duodenal obstruction result from extrinsic causes such as peritoneal bands or an annular pancreas [49].

The incidence of intrinsic atresias and stenoses together varies in different series from 1 in 2000 to 1 in 6000 live births [50]. Sex incidence is equal and there is rarely any evidence of a familial predisposition [51]. Atresias are more common than stenoses and may be single or multiple. They are often associated with mesenteric defects. Sixty per cent occur in the ileum, 40% in duodenum or upper jejunum, where they often give rise to maternal hydramnios [52]. There is an association with a single umbilical artery and with Down's syndrome [53]. Stenoses are more common in the duodenum than elsewhere, and are usually single [54]; occasional multiple stenoses are accompanied by malrotation. They are important since the malrotation may be diagnosed and corrected, and the stenosis missed [55].

There are three main types of atresia [56,57].

Type 1. An imperforate septum, covered on both sides by mucosa and often with smooth muscle in the septal wall, stretches across an otherwise continuous bowel.

Type 2. A variable length of bowel is replaced by a thin cord of fibromuscular tissue; there may or may not be an associated defect in the mesentery.

Type 3. Two blind ends of bowel are separated by a gap with a corresponding mesenteric defect.

These types may coexist and any may be single or multiple. Recently a variety has been described with a segmental absence of muscle coats but with normal ganglion cells [58].

There are two main types of stenosis.

Type 1. A septum identical to that seen in type 1 atresia is present, but with a central perforation of variable size.

Type 2. The lumen of the bowel is uniformly narrowed over a variable length but all the coats are more or less normally formed.

Studies on the histology of atresias and stenoses are few. Mucosal ulceration with replacement of the lamina propria by granulation tissue containing haemosiderin-filled macrophages has been described [59,60], a finding which supports the suggestion that an interruption of blood supply is causative. The mucosa may regenerate simple crypts, but not villi, and the muscularis mucosae and submucosa often show distortion with fibrosis. In complete atresia the bowel proximally is dilated and can become gangrenous, while distally it is collapsed and small. When stenoses are multiple the intervening normal segments are usually dilated (Fig. 19.2).

There have been numerous theories as to the cause of atresias and stenoses [5,61]. Suggestions that developing epithelial cells normally occlude the lumen at one stage of development and fail to break down [62], or that at some stage epithelial proliferation fails to keep pace with longitudinal growth [63] appear to be excluded by the finding of bile, squames and lanugo hairs distal to atretic segments, indicating that atresia developed after the 20-mm stage [64] and that a lumen was originally present and subsequently became occluded. The currently accepted explanation, supported by experimental evidence from the ligature of mesenteric vessels in dogs [56,65] and sheep [66], is that local interruption of the blood supply occurs, due either to intrauterine intussusception [67] or to splanchnic shunting of blood in intrapartum asphyxia [60]. In stenoses involving long segments of bowel Hirschsprung's disease must always be excluded.

Idiopathic dilatation of small bowel

Idiopathic segmental dilatation of the small bowel is described [68] but its aetiology remains undetermined; ganglion cells appear to be normal. Occasional cases of unexplained megaduodenum are also recorded [69].

Duplications, diverticula and cysts

In few fields in pathology has so much speculative literature been written based on so little concrete evidence as on the nature and genesis of these lesions; we refer the reader to the few valuable general surveys in the field [70–76].

Duplications

We define a *duplication* as the complete or partial doubling of a variable length of small bowel. The anomaly is always congenital. The duplicated segment may possess its own independent mesentery, but is more commonly included in the mesentery of the normal bowel. It may communicate with the normal bowel at either or both ends or not at all, when it may be regarded as a cyst (see below). It is normally lined by intestinal epithelium and usually possesses a submucosa and an inner circular muscle coat. The longitudinal muscle coat is frequently incomplete [77] but a myenteric plexus is usually present. Gastric epithelial heterotopia is common [78]. Examples of triplication have been recorded [79].

Diverticula

We define a *diverticulum* as an outpouching of mucosa into or through the muscle coats. It can be congenital or acquired. Congenital diverticula are often outpouchings of the full-thickness bowel wall including muscle coats. Those of foregut origin arise in the duodenum; they may be small and localized; when large they may either pass upward behind the stomach through a separate opening in the diaphragm to enter the right thoracic cavity where they are often attached to a defective thoracic vertebra [80], or penetrate the pancreas along the line of fusion between its ventral and dorsal components [81]. The majority, which are of midgut origin, and vary in size from small to the so-called giant diverticula, are not associated with vertebral anomalies. In all varieties, heterotopic gastric mucosa is extremely common. The majority, which are of midgut origin, and vary in size from small to the so-called giant diverticula, are not associated with vertebral anomalies. Multiple jejunal diverticula are notable but are often only discovered incidentally during investigation for other conditions. They are typically wide-necked and, unlike Meckel's diverticula, tend to lie close to the mesentery of the small bowel (Fig. 19.3).

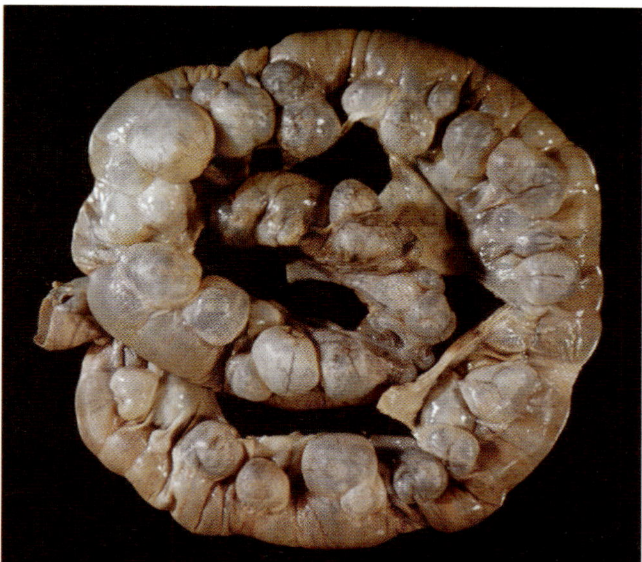

Fig. 19.3 Multiple jejunal diverticula.

Cysts

Enterogenous cysts are common. They are found incorporated into the bowel wall, lying on its serosal aspect or in the mesentery, posterior mediastinum or pelvis, detached and separate from the tract.

Those cysts that lie within the bowel wall can be submucosal, intramuscular or subserosal in position and may secondarily invaginate into the lumen producing symptoms and signs of obstruction, especially in the duodenum or at the ileocaecal valve. Those that are detached are usually surrounded by smooth muscle and, if they are of foregut origin, may be associated with anomalies of spinal cord and vertebrae. All types of cyst have a mucosal lining of alimentary-type epithelium which may be more primitive than the normal; ciliated cells are not uncommon.

Rarely cysts, fistulae, sinus tracks or diverticula lined by alimentary-type epithelium and often surrounded by smooth muscle are found either beneath the skin which covers the dorsal vetebral spines or opening onto it. There is always an associated vertebral defect, sometimes with local duplication of the spinal cord. It is clear that endoderm giving rise to bowel has failed to separate from ectoderm giving rise to skin and spinal cord and that mesoderm has failed to grow inward to form normal vertebrae. Cysts containing alimentary epithelium described in the spinal cord [82] are of similar origin.

Complications

These are not numerous. Diverticula can be associated with stagnant loop syndromes, disturbed bowel ecology and signs of malabsorption; intussception, intraluminal obstruction, infarction [83], perforation and haemorrhage have all been described.

Causative factors

Many earlier theories must now be discarded, including imperfect luminal recanalization and the outgrowth of epithelium through the bowel wall [84].

Many diverticula and cysts of foregut and hindgut origin are associated with vertebral anomalies or Klippel–Feil syndrome [70,72,74]; midgut anomalies do not have this association but are otherwise similar. It seems logical to consider one embryological concept to explain them all. In the 2–4-mm embryo the endoderm, which forms the roof of the yolk sac and is destined to give rise to the future fore- and hindgut, is in contact with the ectoderm, which forms the floor of the amniotic sac and will give rise to the neural crest and tube (see Fig. 19.1). The two communicate through the neurenteric canal. This canal normally closes and the notochord grows forward to become intercalated with the endoderm and to separate it from the ectoderm. Mesoderm grows inward to surround the notochord and form the future vertebrae and surrounding muscle; this separates the ectoderm and endoderm still further. At the same time the midgut develops from the yolk sac and thus has no relationship to the ectoderm. Failure of separation of ectoderm from endoderm at this early stage would explain the formation of diverticula and cysts of the fore- and hindgut and their association with spinal cord abnormalities; failure of mesoderm to grow inwards would explain the vertebral anomalies [70,72,74,85,86], and the development of the midgut from the yolk sac which is unrelated to the ectoderm provides the reason for the non-association of neural and vertebral anomalies with midgut anomalies.

That the development of diverticula may also be linked to genetic defects is suggested by their infrequent but significant association with Marfan's syndrome [87].

Duodenocolic fistulae

Examples are described of fistulae between the third part of the duodenum and the transverse colon which are thought to have developed at the time of physiological herniation [88].

Anomalies of the vitellointestinal duct

This duct, also known as the omphalomesenteric duct, links the developing midgut to the yolk sac. It is normally obliterated and disappears at about the 7-mm stage though its distal end can be recognized as a fibrous strand in most umbilical cords at birth. Remnants of it persist in a number of individuals.

Meckel's diverticulum

Meckel's diverticulum is the persisting proximal part of the vitellointestinal duct. It is present equally in males and females in 1–4% of the population but causes symptoms much

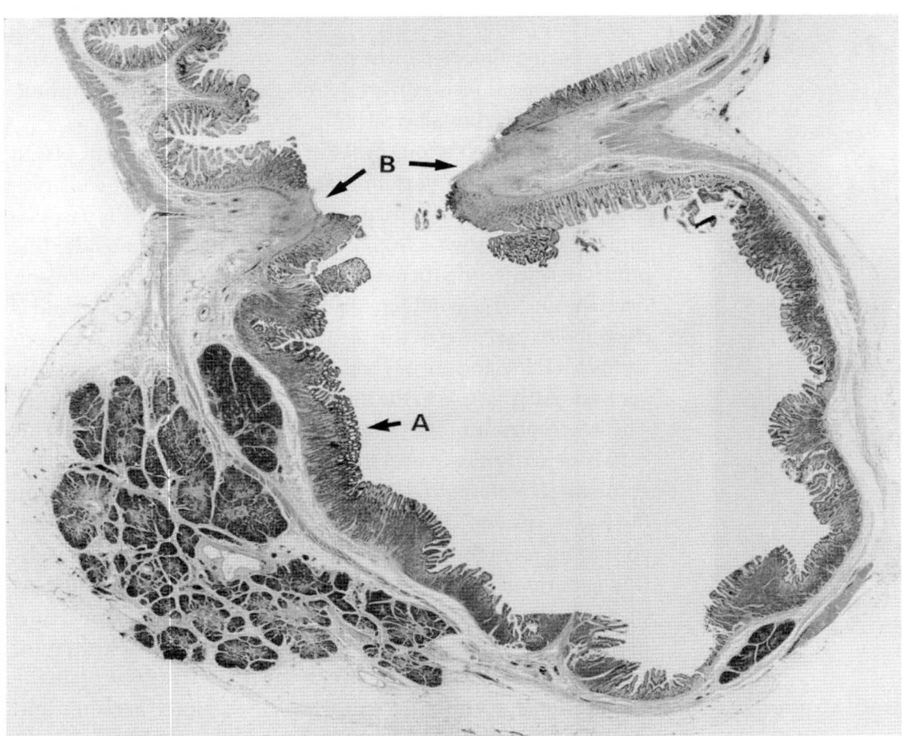

Fig. 19.4 Meckel's diverticulum lined partly by gastric body-type mucosa (arrowed A). There is pancreatic tissue in the wall and peptic ulceration is present at the junction of the diverticulum with the small intestine (arrowed B).

more commonly in men [89,90]. It lies on the antimesenteric border of the ileum, some 30 cm from the ileocaecal valve in infants and some 90 cm from it in adults. It varies from 2 to 8 cm in length and usually possesses a narrow lumen which is patent throughout, though the opening into the bowel is occasionally valvular or occluded. The tip is usually free but may be attached to the umbilicus by the remains of the vitellointestinal duct, which can be fibrous or have a wholly or partially patent lumen.

The lining mucosa is small intestinal, though patches of heterotopic gastric epithelium-containing pepsinogen or acid-secreting cells are common. Large intestinal-type epithelium is rare. Pancreatic tissue is frequently present in the wall [89] (Fig. 19.4).

Symptoms occur in about 20% of individuals and are numerous and diverse [91]. Acid secretion may lead to peptic ulceration with haemorrhage and perforation either in the diverticulum itself or in the adjacent ileum. A cord which anchors the diverticulum to the umbilicus can give rise to volvulus or obstruction. The diverticulum may invaginate or act as the starting point for an intussception [92]; it may herniate into an internal sac or be perforated by a foreign body [93] and enteroliths may form in it, pass out and obstruct the ileum [94]. It may become inflamed and adhesions may form. Occasional cases of eversion of a Meckel's diverticulum have been reportedly mistaken for a polyp of the ileal mucosa. Tumours, usually leiomyomas or endocrine cell tumours, are rare [95–98]. Endometriosis and regional enteritis involving the diverticulum have both been described [99].

Complete or partial patency of the vitellointestinal duct

The duct may remain patent throughout, giving rise to an umbilical fistula; segments may remain patent producing cysts; or the umbilical end may remain patent producing a sinus which may contain pancreatic tissue in its wall and may be lined by intestinal or gastric epithelium [100]. The mucosal lining sometimes undergoes hyperplasia, producing one form of umbilical polyp.

The intestinal lesions of cystic fibrosis (mucoviscidosis)

An analysis of babies with neonatal intestinal obstruction shows that about 15% have a thick putty-like mass of meconium in the terminal ileum which adheres to the mucosa and resists onward propulsion by peristalsis [101], a condition usually described as meconium ileus. The majority of patients have or will develop other stigmata of cystic fibrosis [102]. Conversely, although only some 10% of babies with cystic fibrosis present with meconium ileus at birth, many show suggestive mucosal changes on small intestinal or rectal biopsy [103–107]. In a small number the ileum perforates in the antenatal period and meconium peritonitis develops. A good general review of all the gastrointestinal manifestations of cystic fibrosis is available [108].

The disease is a generalized disorder of exocrine glands, including sweat glands, inherited as an autosomal recessive genetic condition. Either patients synthesize an abnormal glycoprotein which is more viscid than normal mucin or there is a variation of polymerization in normal mucin which increases its viscosity [102,109–112]. Some recent studies suggest that carcinoembryonic antigen and an α-glycoprotein (Mec 6) may also be reduced in concentration and that measurement of these may be a useful screening procedure [113]. Since the exocrine pancreas is also affected there is a theoretical possibility that lack of pancreatic enzymes may prevent breakdown of the thick meconium but the abnormality of the mucin itself is the most significant factor. Some patients have associated intestinal atresia, probably as a result of inspissated meconium producing ischaemic ulceration by pressure, followed by scarring, rather than as a separate anomaly [112,114].

In babies with meconium ileus the terminal ileum is enlarged and often congested; the small intestine proximally is dilated but the large intestine often appears empty and shrunken. The lower ileum is filled with greenish-grey meconium with the consistency of putty which adheres to the mucosal surface and is difficult to remove manually (Fig. 19.5); the bowel content above this meconium is usually fluid. Microscopic appearances are the same whether or not ileus is present though they vary in degree from patient to patient. There are streaks and pools of mucin between villi and within crypts which are often distended (Fig. 19.6). This mucin is predominantly acid non-sulphated (sialomucin) and does not differ histochemically from normal ileal mucin. Goblet cells are distended but not increased in number. Villus flattening is common, but this probably results from a secondary pressure effect. There may be evidence of previous meconium peritonitis.

Similar appearances are found in Brunner's glands and in rectal biopsies, though in the latter there is usually less mucin present on the mucosal surface. Muciphages, surprisingly, have not been a feature either in the lamina propria or in the submucosa. Histochemical studies on rectal biopsies have shown no quantitative differences from normal [115] and there are apparently no differences from normal controls in stereological studies [116]. Since both parents must carry the recessive gene concerned, one of us made (with informed consent) an unpublished study of rectal biopsies from a number of parents in an attempt to identify the carrier state; no diagnostic histological or histochemical changes were found.

Some patients with cystic fibrosis develop intestinal obstruction later in childhood [117,118] or even in adult life [119,120]—a condition termed meconium ileus equivalent or meconium plugging. They present with small intestinal obstruction, a palpable mass in the right iliac fossa and the presence of 'bubbly' intestinal contents on straight X-ray.

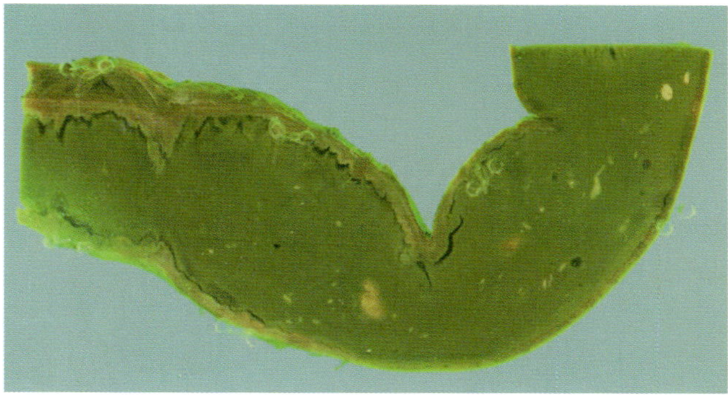

Fig. 19.5 Terminal ileum from a 4-day-old child who had cystic fibrosis with meconium ileus. The tenacious putty-like material is clearly shown.

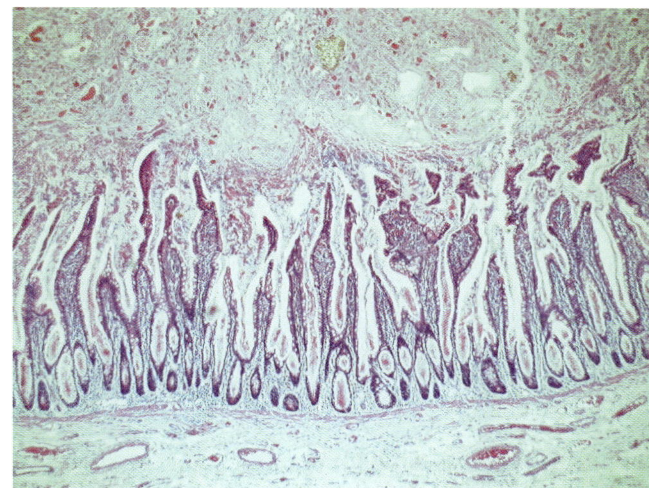

Fig. 19.6 Section from the terminal ileum of an infant with cystic fibrosis, showing inspissated mucin and debris in the crypts, between the villi and in the lumen.

Intussusception occurs with increased frequency [121]. The histology is similar to that already described.

Meconium plug syndrome

In a small number of babies who present with small intestinal obstruction, plugs of meconium are present but the mucosa is histologically normal and there are no other stigmata of cystic fibrosis [122]. If the viscid meconium is washed out, no sequelae usually follow. The cause of the plugging is uncertain. A similar syndrome may occur in the large intestine, sometimes in association with Hirschsprung's disease [123].

Fetal and neonatal peritonitis

Peritonitis in neonates and evidence of peritonitis *in utero* in stillbirths are rare but well recognized [124,125]. Both are related to perforation, usually in zones of distension proximal

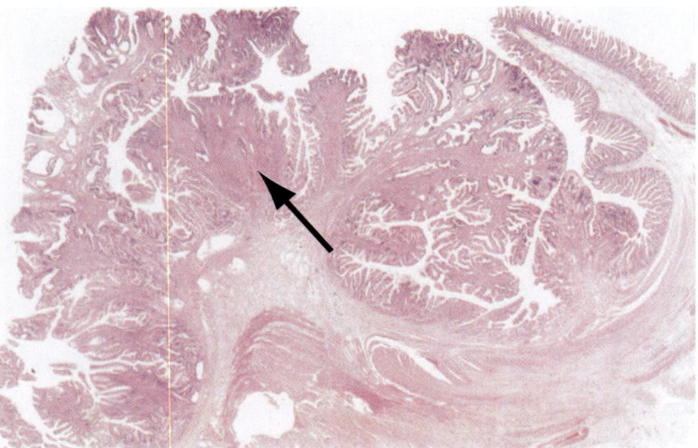

Fig. 19.7 Polypoid gastric heterotopia. Section of a polyp which was obstructing the jejunum. Much of the epithelium in the polyp is of gastric type and there is a focus of gastric body glands (arrowed).

to an obstruction, but sometimes without obvious cause. The peritonitis can be infective or sterile, due to irritation by meconium. In infections there is an acute inflammatory reaction with numerous pus cells and the site of perforation is usually obvious; in meconium peritonitis, which is often associated with cystic fibrosis, there is granulation tissue formation leading to fibrosis with formation of adhesions and the site of perforation may not be detectable. Swallowed fetal squames from the vernix caseosa can sometimes be seen in the reparative tissue.

Heterotopias and heteroplasias

Heterotopia is the presence of a particular type of tissue in a place where it is not normally found. Under the heterotopias we include the term *heteroplasia*, which some authors reserve for the anomalous differentiation of a developing tissue, as for example the development of gastric epithelium in a Meckel's diverticulum [126]. We separate both of these from metaplasia which we regard as a change of one type of fully developed tissue to another, usually as a result of inflammation or irritation. The pyloric gland metaplasia described in a number of inflammatory disorders including Crohn's disease [127] falls into this group.

There are a number of useful reviews of what are probably true heterotopias in the small intestine [126,128–133]. The heterotopic epithelium is nearly always gastric, either of body or antral type, or pancreatic. In rats it has been shown that underexpression of CDX-2 protein, as a result of haplodeletion of the gene, inhibits small intestinal differentiation and causes a shift of phenotype to a more proximal type of mucosa [134]. Heterotopic gastric mucosa has rarely been described in the normal small bowel [135,136]. We have seen a case of polypoid gastric heterotopia of the jejunum (Fig. 19.7). Heterotopic gastric mucosa is not uncommon in Meckel's diverticula (Fig. 19.4) or in other persisting parts of the vitellointestinal duct and in duplications, diverticula and cysts. A number of pathologists now consider that full-thickness body-type mucosa, seen as small nodules in the first part of the duodenum, may represent a true heterotopia rather than metaplasia [131–133]; the immunocytochemical demonstration of cells synthesizing gastrin may be helpful in deciding whether pyloric-type mucosa is heterotopic or metaplastic [137]. Examples of gastric-type epithelium seen in the duodenum in association with gastric ulcer, Zollinger–Ellison syndrome and hyperacidity are almost certainly metaplastic [138].

Heterotopic pancreatic tissue is most common in the duodenum, where it lies in submucosa or muscle coats and projects into the lumen as elevations which occasionally become pedunculated [139,140]. These are most common around the ampulla of Vater and microscopically consist of normal pancreatic tissue in which islets are often present. They may form the origin of at least some duodenal islet cell neoplasms. Heterotopic pancreas is also found in Meckel's diverticulum (Fig. 19.4).

Hamartomas

Hamartomas are not primarily neoplastic lesions, though some have neoplastic potential. They are primarily malformations of epithelial or of connective tissue. They tend, however, to resemble neoplasms both clinically and in their gross appearance and have to be distinguished from them, usually on microscopical grounds. For this reason they are discussed in Chapters 25 and 26 (see p. 448).

Aganglionosis of small bowel

In about 5% of patients with Hirschsprung's disease the aganglionic segment extends proximally to involve the small intestine [141]. These patients present with intestinal obstruction without evidence of megacolon and the diagnosis must be considered in all babies with neonatal obstruction for which no mechanical cause can be found. In this form of the disease a full-thickness small intestinal biopsy is essential. Ganglion cells are absent in both plexuses but nerve trunks do not always show hypertrophy and palisading, and acetylcholinesterase techniques for thickened nerves in mucosa are therefore not reliable. Patients have been described in whom both ganglion cells and nerve trunks were absent [142]; this is probably a developmental anomaly related to Hirchsprung's disease but may have resulted from temporary ischaemia during the normal phases of bowel rotation with selective damage to ganglion cells [143]. In some patients with the very rare condition of total aganglionosis of small bowel [144–146] the disorder may be inherited as an autosomal recessive characteristic.

Under the name *adynamic ileus with dilatation* occasional patients are described with persistent non-motility of small and large bowel resembling pseudo-Hirschsprung's disease in which ganglion cells were normal [147]. The defect here may be in the central nervous system and the condition may be related to that of idiopathic dilatation described on p. 256.

References

1 Evans PR, Polani N. Congenital malformations in a post-mortem series. *Teratology*, 1980; 22: 207.

2 Santulli TV, Amoury RA. Congenital anomalies of the gastrointestinal tract. *Pediatr Clin North Am*, 1967; 14: 21.

3 Silverberg M, Davidson M. Paediatric gastroenterology. A review. *Gastroenterology*, 1970; 58: 229.

4 Crelin ES. Development of gastrointestinal tract. *Ciba Clin Symp*, 1961; 13: 67.

5 Louw JH. The pathogenesis of congenital abnormalities of the digestive tract. *S Afr Med J*, 1967; 2: 1057.

6 Grand RJ, Watkins JB, Torti FM. Development of the human gastrointestinal tract. A review. *Gastroenterology*, 1976; 70: 790.

7 Fitzgerald MJT, Nolan JP, O'Neill MN. The formation of the ascending colon. *Irish J Med Sci*, 1971; 140: 258.

8 Jirasek JE, Uher J, Koldovsky O. A histochemical analysis of the development of the small intestine of human fetuses. *Acta Histochem*, 1965; 22: 33.

9 Garbarsch C. Histochemical studies on the early development of the human small intestine. *Acta Anat*, 1969; 72: 357.

10 Lev R, Siegel HI, Bartman J. Histochemical studies of developing human fetal small intestine. *Histochemie*, 1972; 29: 103.

11 Kelley R. An ultrastructural and cytochemical study of developing small intestine in man. *J Embryol Exper Morph*, 1973; 29: 411.

12 Varkonyi T, Gergely G, Varro V. The ultrastructure of the small intestinal mucosa in the developing human fetus. *Scand J Gastroenterol*, 1974; 9: 495.

13 Moxey PC, Trier JS. Specialised cell types in the human fetal small intestine. *Anat Rec*, 1978; 191: 269.

14 Triadou N, Bataille J, Schmitz J. Longitudinal study of the human intestinal brush border membrane proteins; distribution of the main disaccharidases and peptidases. *Gastroenterology*, 1983; 85: 1326.

15 Lacroix B, Kedinger M, Simon-Assmann P, Haffen K. Early organogenesis of human small intestine; scanning electron microscopy and brush border enzymology. *Gut*, 1984; 25: 925.

16 Johnson FP. The development of the mucus membrane of the stomach and small intestine in the human embryo. *Am J Anat*, 1910; 10: 521.

16a Walters JR, Howard A, Rumble HE, Prathalingam SR, Shaw-Smith CJ, Lagon S. Differences in expression of homeobox transcription factors in proximal and distal human small intestine. *Gastroenterology* 1997; 113: 472.

17 Scarlet YV, Brenner DA. Molecular and cellular biology of the small intestine. *Curr Opin Gastroenterology* 1998; 14: 90.

18 Bryant MG, Buchan ANJ, Gregor M, Ghatei MA, Polak JM, Bloom SR. Development of intestinal regulatory peptides in the human fetus. *Gastroenterology*, 1982; 83: 47.

19 Koldovsky O. Longitudinal specialization of the small intestine; developmental aspects. *Gastroenterology*, 1983; 85: 1436.

20 Cornes JS. Number, size and distribution of Peyer's patches in the human small intestine. *Gut*, 1965; 6: 225.

21 Read JB, Burnstock G. The development of adrenergic innervation and chromaffin cells in human fetal gut. *Dev Biol*, 1970; 22: 513.

21a Daniel EE, Wang YF. Control systems of gastrointestinal motility are immature at birth in dogs. *Neurogastroenterology and Motility* 1999; 11: 375.

22 Jimenez FA, Reiner L. Arteriographic findings in congenital abnormalities of the mesentery and intestines. *Surg Gynecol Obstet*, 1961; 113: 346.

23 Wang C, Welch CE. Anomalies of intestinal rotation in adolescents and adults. *Surgery*, 1963; 54: 839.

24 Frazer JE, Robbins RH. On the factors concerned in causing rotation of the intestine in man. *J Anat*, 1915; 50: 75.

25 Dott NM. Anomalies of intestinal rotation: their embryology and surgical aspects: with report of 5 cases. *Br J Surg*, 1923; II: 251.

26 McIntosh R, Donovan EJ. Disturbances of rotation of the intestinal tract. *Am J Dis Child*, 1939; 57: 116.

27 Bremer JL. *Congenital Anomalies of the Viscera: Their Embryological Basis*, Chapter 4. Cambridge, Massachusetts: Harvard University Press, 1957.

28 Söderlund S. Anomalies of midgut rotation and fixation. *Acta Paediatr (Stockh) Suppl*, 1962; 135: 225.

29 Glasgow EF. Unsuspected malrotation of gut in an adult male. *Lancet*, 1962; i: 621.

30 Rixford E. Failure of primary rotation of the intestine (left-sided colon) in relation to intestinal obstruction. *Ann Surg*, 1920; 72: 114.

31 Thorlakson PHT, Monie IW, Thorlakson TK. Anomalous peritoneal encapsulation of the small intestine. A report of 3 cases. *Br J Surg*, 1953; 40: 490.

32 Denzer BS. Congenital duodenal obstruction, malrotation of the intestine: report of case. *Am J Dis Child*, 1922; 24: 534.

33 Eggers C. Non rotation of the large intestine. *Ann Surg*, 1922; 75: 757.

34 Waugh GE. The morbid consequences of a mobile ascending colon with a record of 180 operations. *Br J Surg*, 1920; 7: 343.

35 Park RW, Watkins JB. Mesenteric vascular occlusion and varices complicating midgut malrotation. *Gastroenterology*, 1979; 77: 565.

36 Devane SP, Coombes R, Smith VV *et al*. Persistent gastrointestinal symptoms after correction of malrotation. *Arch Dis Child*, 1992; 67: 218.

37 Brown NM, Smith AN. Kartagener's syndrome with fibrocystic disease. *Br Med J*, 1960; ii: 725.

38 Soper RT, Green EW. Omphalocoele. *Surg Gynecol Obstet*, 1961; 113: 501.

39 Eckstein HB. Exomphalos. A review of 100 cases. *Br J Surg*, 1963; 50: 405.

40 Wyburn GM. Congenital defects of the anterior abdominal wall. *Br J Surg*, 1953; 40: 553.

41 Lewin K, McCarthy LJ. Peritoneal encapsulation of the small intestine. *Gastroenterology*, 1970; 59: 270.

42 Sieck JO, Cowgill R, Larkworthy W. Peritoneal encapsulation and abdominal cocoon. Case reports and a review of the literature. *Gastroenterology*, 1983; 84: 1597.

43 Silverman FN, Huang N. Congenital absence of the abdominal muscles associated with malformation of the genito-urinary and alimentary tracts: report of cases and review of literature. *Am J Dis Child*, 1950; 80: 91.

44 Raeburn C, Brafield AJ. A short small intestine associated with fibrosis of the liver. *Lancet*, 1956; i: 884.
45 Hamilton JR, Reilly BJ, Morecki R. Short small intestine associated with malrotation: a newly described congenital cause of intestinal malabsorption. *Gastroenterology*, 1969; 56: 124.
46 Miller MM, Amir-Jahed AK. Total intestinal atresia. *Surgery*, 1963; 55: 737.
47 Okmian LG, Kövamees A. Jejunal atresia with intestinal aplasia. *Acta Paediatr (Stockh)*, 1964; 53: 65.
48 Bennington JL, Haber SL. The embryologic significance of an undifferentiated intestinal tract. *J Pediatr*, 1964; 64: 735.
49 Forshall I. Duodenal obstruction in newborn with description of 4 cases. *Br J Surg*, 1947; 35: 58.
50 Moore TC, Stokes GE. Congenital stenosis and atresia of the small intestine. *Surg Gynecol Obstet*, 1953; 97: 719.
51 Mishalany HG, Najjar FB. Familial jejunal atresia: three cases in one family. *J Pediatr*, 1968; 73: 753.
52 Lloyd JR, Clatworthy HW Jr. Hydramnios as an aid to the early diagnosis of congenital obstruction of the alimentary tract. A study of the maternal and foetal factors. *Pediatrics*, 1958; 21: 903.
53 Bodian M, White LLR, Carter CO, Louw JH. Congenital duodenal obstruction and mongolism. *Br Med J*, 1952; i: 77.
54 Ehrenpreis T, Sandblom P. Duodenal atresia and stenosis. *Acta Paediatr (Stockh)*, 1949; 38: 109.
55 Knutrud O, Eek S. Combined intrinsic duodenal obstruction and malrotation. *Acta Chir Scand*, 1960; 119: 506.
56 Louw JH. Congenital intestinal atresia and stenosis in the newborn. *Ann R Coll Surg*, 1959; 25: 209.
57 Willis RA. *The Borderland of Embryology and Pathology*, 2nd edn. London: Butterworths, 1962: 187.
58 Alvarez SP, Greco MA, Geneiser NB. Small intestinal atresia and segmental absence of muscle coats. *Hum Pathol*, 1982; 13: 948.
59 Louw JH. Congenital intestinal atresia and severe stenosis in the new born. *S Afr J Clin Sci*, 1952; 3: 109.
60 De Sa DJ. Congenital stenosis and atresia of the jejunum and ileum. *J Clin Pathol*, 1972; 25: 1063.
61 O'Neill JF, Anderson K, Bradshaw HH, Lawson RB, Hightower F. Congenital atresia of small intestine in newborn. *Am J Dis Child*, 1948; 75: 214.
62 Feggetter S. Congenital intestinal atresia. *Br J Surg*, 1955; 42: 378.
63 Morison JE. *Foetal and Neonatal Pathology*, 2nd edn. London: Butterworths, 1963.
64 Santulli TV, Blanc WA. Congenital atresia of the intestine. Pathogenesis and treatment. *Ann Surg*, 1961; 154: 939.
65 Louw JH, Barnard CN. Congenital intestinal atresia: observations on its origin. *Lancet*, 1955; ii: 1065.
66 Abrams JS. Experimental intestinal atresia. *Surgery*, 1968; 64: 185.
67 Parkkulainen KV. Intrauterine intussusception as a cause of intestinal atresia. *Surgery*, 1958; 44: 1106.
68 Sjölin S, Thoren L. Segmental dilatation of the small intestine. *Arch Dis Child*, 1962; 37: 422.
69 Hillemand P, Cherigic E, Hillemand B, Mirande JL. Les megagrêles chroniques. *Arch Mal Appar Dig*, 1961; 50: 5.
70 Fallon M, Gordon ARG, Lendrum AC. Mediastinal cysts of foregut origin: association with vertebral abnormalities. *Br J Surg*, 1953; 41: 520.
71 McLetchie NGB, Purves JK, Saunders RL De CH. The genesis of gastric and certain intestinal diverticula and enterogenous cysts. *Surg Gynecol Obstet*, 1954; 99: 135.
72 Rhaney K, Barclay GPT. Enterogenous cysts and congenital diverticula of the alimentary canal with abnormalities of the vertebral column and spinal cord. *J Pathol Bacteriol*, 1959; 77: 457.
73 Smith JR. Accessory enteric formations. A classification and nomenclature. *Arch Dis Child*, 1960; 35: 87.
74 Bentley JRF, Smith JR. Developmental posterior enteric remnants and spinal malformations. *Arch Dis Child*, 1960; 35: 76.
75 Anderson MC, Silverman WW, Shields TW. Duplications of the alimentary tract in the adult. *Arch Surg*, 1962; 85: 94.
76 Avni F, Kalifa G, Sauvegrain J. Gastric and duodenal duplications in infants and children. *Ann Radiol*, 1980; 23: 195.
77 Gross RE, Holcomb GW Jr, Farber S. Duplications of the alimentary tract. *Pediatrics*, 1952; 9: 449.
78 Duffy G, Enriquez AA, Watson WC. Duplication of the ileum with heterotopic gastric mucosa, pseudomyxoma peritonei and non-rotation of the midgut. *Gastroenterology*, 1974; 67: 341.
79 Basu R, Forshall I, Rickham PP. Duplications of the alimentary tract. *Br J Surg*, 1966; 47: 477.
80 Goldberg HM, Johnson TP. Posterior abdominothoracic enteric duplication. *Br J Surg*, 1963; 50: 445.
81 Suda K, Mizuguchi K, Matsumoto M. A histopathological study on the etiology of duodenal diverticulum related to the fusion of the pancreatic anlage. *Am J Gastroenterol*, 1983; 78: 335.
82 Harriman DGF. An intraspinal enterogenous cyst. *J Pathol Bacteriol*, 1958; 75: 413.
83 Fan ST, Lau WY, Pang SW. Infarction of a duodenal duplication cyst. *Am J Gastroenterol*, 1985; 80: 337.
84 Lewis FT, Thyng FW. The regular occurrence of intestinal diverticula in embryos of the pig, rabbit and man. *Am J Anat*, 1908; 7: 505.
85 Veeneklaas GMH. Pathogenesis of intrathoracic gastrogenic cysts. *Am J Dis Child*, 1952; 83: 500.
86 Abell MR. Mediastinal cysts. *Arch Pathol*, 1956; 61: 360.
87 Clunie GJA, Mason JM. Visceral diverticula and the Marfan syndrome. *Br J Surg*, 1962; 50: 51.
88 Torrance B, Jones C. Three cases of spontaneous duodeno colic fistula. *Gut*, 1972; 13: 627.
89 Söderland S. Meckel's diverticulum. A clinical and histologic study. *Acta Chir Scand Suppl*, 1959; 248.
90 Jackson RH, Bird AR. Meckel's diverticulum in childhood. *Br Med J*, 1961; ii: 1399.
91 Ker H. A muckle of Meckels. *Lancet*, 1962; i: 617.
92 McKenzie G, Gault EW, Wood IJ. Meckel's diverticulum: invagination causing recurrent ileal obstruction. *Aust N Z J Surg*, 1966; 35: 272.
93 Dowse JLA. Meckel's diverticulum. *Br J Surg*, 1961; 48: 392.
94 Bergland RL, Gump F, Price JB Jr. An unusual complication of Meckel's diverticulum seen in older patients. *Ann Surg*, 1963; 158: 6.
95 Doyle JL, Severance AO. Carcinoid tumours of Meckel's diverticulum. *Cancer*, 1966; 19: 1591.
96 Freeman GC. Adenocarcinoma in a Meckel's diverticulum with perforation. *Arch Surg*, 1957; 75: 158.
97 Jones EL, Thompson H, Williams JA. Argentaffin-cell tumour of Meckel's diverticulum. A report of 2 cases and review of the literature. *Br J Surg*, 1972; 59: 213.
98 Lie ST. Leiomyosarcoma of Meckel's diverticulum. *Br J Surg*, 1966; 53: 336.

99 Won KH. Endometriosis, mucocele and regional enteritis of Meckel's diverticulum. *Arch Surg*, 1969; 98: 209.
100 Nicholson GW. Gastric glands in the extroverted distal end of the vitelline duct. *J Pathol Bacteriol*, 1922; 25: 201.
101 Schwachman H, Pryles CV, Gross RE. Meconium ileus. Clinical study of 20 surviving patients. *Am J Dis Child*, 1956; 91: 223.
102 Di Sant'Agnese PA, Talamo RC. Pathogenesis and physiopathology of cystic fibrosis of the pancreas. *N Engl J Med*, 1967; 77: 1287, 1344, 1399.
103 Bodian M. *Fibrocystic Disease of the Pancreas: a Congenital Disorder of Mucus Production—Mucosis*. London: Heinemann, 1952.
104 Di Sant'Agnese PA, Lepore MJ. Involvement of abdominal organs in cystic fibrosis of the pancreas. *Gastroenterology*, 1961; 40: 64.
105 Thomaidis TS, Arey JB. The intestinal lesions in cystic fibrosis of the pancreas. *J Pediatr*, 1963; 63: 444.
106 Grossman H, Berdon WE, Baker DH. Gastrointestinal findings in cystic fibrosis. *Am J Roentgenol*, 1965; 97: 227.
107 Kopel FB. Gastrointestinal manifestations of cystic fibrosis. *Gastroenterology*, 1972; 62: 483.
108 Park RW, Grand RJ. Gastrointestinal manifestations of cystic fibrosis: a review. *Gastroenterology*, 1981; 81: 1143.
109 Green MN, Clarke JT, Schwachman H. Studies in cystic fibrosis of the pancreas; protein pattern in meconium ileus. *Pediatrics*, 1958; 21: 635.
110 Anderson C, Freeman F. A chemical study of mutin in fibrocystic disease of the pancreas. *Arch Dis Child*, 1956; 31: 31.
111 Di Sant'Agnese PA. Fibrocystic disease of the pancreas. A generalised disease of exocrine glands. *JAMA*, 1956; 160: 846.
112 Blanck C, Okmian L, Robbe H. Mucoviscidosis and intestinal atresia. A study of 4 cases in the same family. *Acta Paediatr (Stockh)*, 1965; 54: 557.
113 Ryley HC. Distribution of non-plasma protein components in meconium from healthy and cystic fibrosis neonates. *J Clin Pathol*, 1981; 34: 179.
114 Bernstein J, Vawter G, Harris GBC, Young V, Hillman LS. The occurrence of intestinal atresia in new born with meconium ileus. *Am J Dis Child*, 1960; 99: 804.
115 Johansen PG, Kay R. Histochemistry of the rectal mucosa in cystic fibrosis of the pancreas. *J Pathol*, 1969; 99: 299.
116 Hage E, Anderson U. Light and electron microscopical studies of rectal biopsies in cystic fibrosis. *Acta Pathol Microbiol Scand*, 1972; 80: 345.
117 Fanconi A. Postneonataler Kotileus bei cystischer Pancreasfibrose. *Helvt Paediat Acta*, 1960; 15: 566.
118 Cordonnier JK, Izant RJ Jr. Meconium ileus equivalent. *Surgery*, 1963; 54: 667.
119 Hunton DB, Long WK, Tsumagari HY. Meconium ileus equivalent: an adult complication of fibrocystic disease. *Gastroenterology*, 1966; 50: 99.
120 Hodgson WJB. Intestinal obstruction in an adult suffering from mucoviscidosis. *Br J Surg*, 1969; 56: 472.
121 Eggermont E, De Boeck K. Small intestinal abnormalities in cystic fibrosis patients. *Eur J Pediatr*, 1991; 150: 824.
122 Emery JC. Abnormalities in meconium of foetus and newborn. *Arch Dis Child*, 1957; 32: 17.
123 Swischuk LE. Meconium plug syndrome: a cause of neonatal intestinal obstruction. *Am J Roentgenol*, 1968; 103: 339.
124 Fonkalsrud EW, Ellis DG, Clatworthy HW Jr. Neonatal peritonitis. *J Pediatr Surg*, 1966; 1: 227.
125 Birtch AG, Coran AG, Cross RE. Neonatal peritonitis. *Surgery*, 1967; 61: 305.
126 Willis RA. Some unusual developmental heterotopias. *Br Med J*, 1968; ii: 267.
127 Lee FD. Pyloric metaplasia in the small intestine. *J Pathol Bacteriol*, 1964; 87: 267.
128 Taylor AL. Epithelial heterotopias of the alimentary tract. *J Pathol Bacteriol*, 1927; 30: 415.
129 Kimpton AR, Crane DR. Heterotopic gastric mucosa. *N Engl J Med*, 1938; 218: 627.
130 Kimpton AR, Crane DR. Heterotopic gastric mucosa and reduplication of the intestinal tract. *Am J Surg*, 1940; 49: 342.
131 Lessels AM, Martin DF. Heterotopic gastric mucosa in the duodenum. *J Clin Pathol*, 1982; 35: 591.
132 Spiller RC, Shousha S, Barrison IG. Heterotopic gastric tissue in the duodenum: a report of 8 cases. *Dig Dis Sci*, 1982; 27: 880.
133 Kundrotas LW, Camara DS, Meenaghan MA, Montes M, Wosick WF, Weiser MM. Heterotopic gastric mucosa: a case report. *Am J Gastroenterol*, 1985; 80: 253.
134 Beck F, Chawengsaksophak K, Waring Playford RJ, Furness JB. Reprogramming of intestinal differention and intercalary regeneration in Cdx2 mutant mice. *Proc Natl Acad Sci USA*, 1999; 96: 7381.
135 Gore I, Williams WJ. Adenomatous polyp of the jejunum composed of gastric mucosa. *Cancer*, 1953; 6: 164.
136 Nawaz K, Graham DY, Fechner RE, Eiband JM. Gastric heterotopia in the ileum with ulceration and bleeding. *Gastroenterology*, 1974; 66: 113.
137 Dayal Y, Wolfe HJ. Gastrin-producing cells in ectopic gastric mucosa of developmental and metaplastic origin. *Gastroenterology*, 1978; 75: 655.
138 James AH. Gastric epithelium in the duodenum. *Gut*, 1964; 5: 285.
139 Barbosa JJC, Dockerty MB, Waugh JM. Pancreatic heterotopia. *Surg Gynecol Obstet*, 1946; 82: 527.
140 Feldman M, Weinberg T. Aberrant pancreas: a cause of duodenal. syndrome. *JAMA*, 1952; 148: 893.
141 Walkor AW, Kempson RL, Ternberg JL. Aganglionosis of the small intestine. *Surgery*, 1966; 60: 449.
142 Boggs JD, Kidd JM. Congenital abnormalities of intestinal innervation: absence of innervation of jejunum, ileum and colon in siblings. *Pediatrics*, 1958; 21: 261.
143 Earlam RJ. A vascular cause for aganglionic bowel. A new hypothesis. *Am J Dig Dis*, 1972; 17: 255.
144 MacKinnon AE, Cohen SJ. Total intestinal aganglionosis; an autosomal recessive condition? *Arch Dis Child*, 1977; 52: 898.
145 Saperstein L, Pollack J, Beck AR. Total intestinal aganglionosis. *Mt Sitzai Med J*, 1980; 47: 72.
146 Descos B, Lachaux A, Louis D *et al*. Extended aganglionosis in siblings. *J Pediatr Gastroenterol Nutr*, 1984; 3: 641.
147 Ehrenpreis T, Bentley JFR, Nixon HH. Seminar on pseudo Hirschsprung's disease and related disorders. *Arch Dis Child*, 1966; 41: 143.

20 Muscular and mechanical disorders of the small intestine

Many of the mechanical disorders of the small bowel are associated with anomalies of rotation and mesenteric resorption, or abnormalities in development. The small bowel is, apart from the first three parts of the duodenum, entirely suspended from a mesentery which arises from a relatively narrow base, through which the superior mesenteric artery enters and the superior mesenteric vein drains. The bowel and mesentery are, within limits, freely mobile. Apart from congenital atresias and stenoses (see p. 255), the majority of purely mechanical effects in this group arise as the result of herniation of the bowel or torsion of the mesentery, for which there may or may not be a recognizable antecedent cause. They usually result in acute intestinal obstruction, with the risk of haemorrhagic infarction due to vascular obstruction. The principal conditions in each group are described below.

Intussusception

Intussusception is the telescopic invagination of a variable length of the bowel into the bowel immediately distal to it. Once initiated, the invaginated segment, called the intussusceptum, is propelled further distally by the peristaltic activity of the ensheathing outer bowel, or intussuscipiens (Fig. 20.1). The process is usually triggered by the presence of a 'mass' of poorly propagated material within the intestinal lumen. Most often this is either a bolus of firmly adherent ingested material or a polypoid lesion of the intestinal wall itself. The presence of this intraluminal mass gives rise to increased peristaltic activity which eventually succeeds in propelling the obstruction distally, taking with it the attached bowel wall. This initiates the intussusception, which is then self-perpetuated by further peristaltic activity which continues until it is terminated by stretching of the mesentery of the intussusceptum and the consequent complete intestinal obstruction. Although it is customary to regard intussusception as a distal propulsion of invaginated intestine, retrograde intussusceptions are recorded [1].

Intussusception occurs most commonly in childhood, with an incidence of between one to four cases per 1000 live births [2]. It is likely that the incidence is greater than this, because many intussusceptions could be self-correcting and never diagnosed. Males outnumber females by about 2 : 1, and this proportion rises with age of onset. The condition is rare in the neonatal period, becomes increasingly common from 3 to 6 months, and is infrequent after the age of 3 years [3]. Multiple or single intussusceptions are occasionally seen in the small bowel at necropsy on babies and children; they are rarely associated with antemortem obstructive symptoms or visible change in the bowel and are considered to be agonal, and of no clinical significance.

In most children intussusception occurs for no easily recognized reason [4–6], although occasional examples appear to be triggered by foreign bodies such as bezoars, Meckel's diverticula, rare intestinal tumours or Peutz–Jeghers polyps. Well nourished children are affected more commonly than the poorly nourished and the condition is said to occur more commonly in siblings than would be expected by chance [2]. Many children with 'idiopathic' intussusception often have mesenteric adenitis, sometimes associated with adenovirus infection [7,8]. Intussusception is a frequent cause of abdominal pain and melaena in Henoch–Schönlein purpura. Other cases have been associated with an excess intake of fluids [9]. Intussusception due to heterotopic pancreas in the small bowel has also been described [10]. There is an increased incidence of intussusception in cystic fibrosis [11], possibly related to the tenacious, adherent intestinal contents that are typical of this condition.

The usual site of intussusception in childhood is at the ileocaecal valve, and this is probably related to the abundant lym-

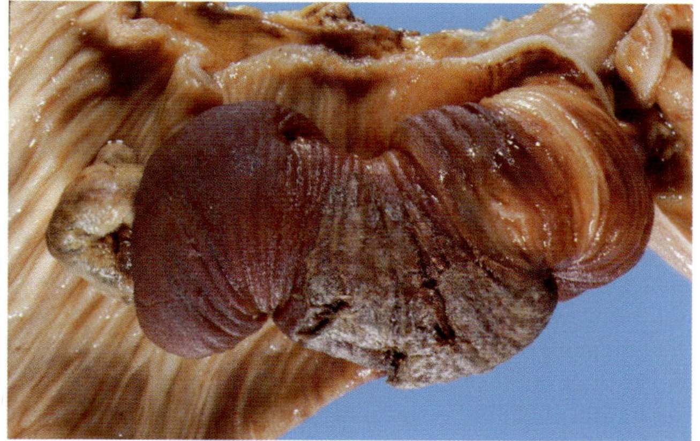
(a)

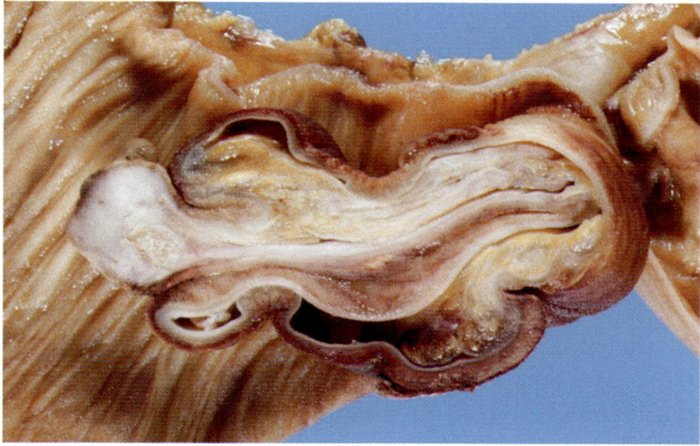
(b)

Fig. 20.1 (a) Intussusception in terminal ileum. (a) shows a necrotic nodular mass at the tip of a haemorrhagic intususceptum. This is seen on slicing (b) to be a discrete nodule and appears to be an everted Meckel's diverticulum.

phoid tissue at this site. Hyperplasia of this lymphoid tissue, possibly due to viral infection or antigenic stimulation from intestinal contents, results in its protrusion into the lumen of the terminal ileum, triggering the process of intussusception which then becomes self-perpetuating [12]; the leading point of the intussusceptum frequently reaches the transverse colon. Additional factors are probably involved, however, since the high frequency of childhood ileal lymphoid hyperplasia continues well beyond the age of 5 years, when the incidence of intussusception falls markedly. Childhood ileoileal intussusception is less common, and in our experience jejunal intussusceptions are rare unless there is a particular anatomical abnormality.

Intussusception in adults is rare, and although some cases are idiopathic [4,13], an organic cause is found in the vast majority. In contrast to childhood cases, adult intussusception is frequently chronic and recurrent. Among the more common causes are swallowed foreign bodies, polypoid epithelial tumours (especially Peutz–Jeghers polyps and carcinoids), tumours of connective tissue in the bowel wall (especially submucosal lipomas and so-called inflammatory fibroid polyps), metastatic tumours (especially malignant melanomas) [14,15], Meckel's diverticula (Fig. 20.1) and gastroenterostomy sites [16]. Intussusception in adults is less commonly ileocaecal than in children, and other varieties, including gastroduodenal intussusception, occur [17].

Early symptoms of intussusception are those of obstruction: if an appreciable length of mesentery is drawn into the ensheathing bowel the venous return may be occluded, and gangrene with perforation and peritonitis supervenes. On macroscopic examination of a longitudinally sectioned specimen three definite layers can be distinguished, namely the outermost investing *intussuscipiens* and the entering (inner) and returning (outer) layers of the invaginated *intussusceptum*. The intussusceptum itself is oedematous and engorged (it has been likened to a bloated phallus!) and if its vasculature has been severely compromised it may appear black from infarction. Microscopically the picture is one of developing haemorrhagic necrosis of both inner coats, often with acute inflammatory changes on the peritoneal surface. It is important to examine histologically the apex of the intussusceptum to exclude neoplasia.

Internal (intra-abdominal) hernia

Obstruction of bowel associated with internal hernia accounts for between 1 and 5% of all cases of intestinal obstruction [18,19]. The most common type is entrapment of a loop of intestine within a so-called paraduodenal hernia, where there is a protrusion of peritoneum beneath the inferior mesenteric vein and left colic artery [20]. Various other types occur, including those through the foramen of Winslow [21], and are well classified [22]. A small but important group are those in which bowel herniates through a mesenteric or omental defect [23,24]; the most common sites for these are in the terminal ileal region or the transverse mesocolon. The majority of internal hernias are developmental in origin, although some have been associated with trauma or previous abdominal surgery.

The complications of internal hernias occur in adults more commonly than children. They include strangulation of bowel with necrosis and gangrene, perforation with peritonitis, or incomplete small intestinal obstruction when part of the circumference of the bowel is involved as a so-called Richter's hernia.

Volvulus

Volvulus is defined as a twist of a loop of bowel to such a degree that obstruction occurs either to the lumen or to the blood supply, or to both. In the Western world it accounts for only a small proportion of all cases of small intestinal obstruction, without predilection for any special sex or age. Aetiological factors include a congenitally long mesentery with a narrow base, congenital omental and mesenteric bands, acquired inflammatory or postoperative adhesions, and possibly overloading of the small bowel due to a copious semifluid diet [25]. Nevertheless, in some parts of the world, notably Iran [26], India [27] and Zimbabwe [28], small intestinal volvulus is much commoner, possibly related to a high-residue diet. An interesting study from Afghanistan found that hospital admissions for small intestinal volvulus were much commoner during the religious period of Ramadan, a time of daylight fasting and the consumption of a single large, high-residue meal in the evening [29]. A related condition is intestinal knotting, in which two loops of bowel twist around each other. This too is more common in the Third World, especially in central Africa [30].

Symptoms of small intestinal volvulus are those of obstruction, often with disproportionate shock requiring early operation [31]. Findings in the resected bowel depend largely on whether there is partial or complete venous obstruction with or without arterial obstruction. The bowel involved is distended, and gas-producing organisms frequently proliferate. Haemorrhagic infarction and gangrene are common.

Chronic volvulus can lead to repeated episodes of relatively mild ischaemia with the formation of granulation tissue in the submucosa. There is patchy mucosal ulceration and dense fibrosis often extending into the mesenteric tissues, although the muscularis of the small intestine is relatively spared. A stricture is formed, the histology of which can be difficult to distinguish from ischaemic stricture due to other causes and from Crohn's disease.

Perforation and rupture

Small intestinal perforations in adults may follow ingestion of foreign bodies, peptic or other ulceration, acute or chronic inflammatory bowel disease, thinning and weakening of the bowel wall due to systemic sclerosis [32] or diverticula, or follow obstruction of the bowel lumen from a large number of causes. Meconium ileus is an additional cause in infancy while trauma, often of a blunt nature, may produce a single laceration on the antimesenteric surface of the ileum in both adults and children [33]. The usual consequence is peritonitis or local abscess formation, and shock is often a concomitant feature. Apparent spontaneous rupture of the small intestine has been recorded infrequently, sometimes following sudden muscular effort [34]. Many such cases have occurred in patients with hernia, suggesting a causal association.

Small intestinal obstruction

The mechanical causes of small intestinal obstruction are often divided into those situated within the lumen, those within the bowel wall, and extramural causes. The latter are nearly always diseases of the peritoneum, and include congenital mesenteric or omental bands, peritonitis and its consequences, peritoneal adhesions [35], and primary or secondary tumours of the peritoneal cavity. Intramural causes may similarly be congenital atresias, inflammatory conditions such as Crohn's disease, tuberculosis or drug-induced stenoses, ischaemic strictures, irradiation damage and polypoid or infiltrative neoplasms. They are described in other chapters.

The commonest luminal cause of mechanical small intestinal obstruction is a bolus of food, nearly always of fruit or vegetable origin [36,37]. Persimmon is the most common offender in America, but oranges, peaches, grapefruit, apples, raw figs, mushrooms and coconut have all been incriminated. Macaroni, sauerkraut, onion and tomato skins, potato skin and peanuts are among the vegetable foods reported as causing obstruction. Predisposing factors include false teeth, previous gastrectomy [38] and intestinal adhesions, but undoubtedly a greedy attitude to eating, accompanied by inadequate mastication and bolting of large amounts of food, is the most important single factor. Bolus obstruction due to food can lead to mucosal ulceration and perforation, with release of food into the submucosa, muscle coats and even the abdominal cavity to give rise to so-called food granulomas. Abscesses follow perforation of sharp objects, such as undigested peanuts and whole quarters of orange, into the mesenteric attachment of the gut. A variety of food bolus obstruction in neonates is called the milk curd syndrome. In this condition, which usually occurs during the 2nd week of life in babies fed with artificial milk products, impaction of thick milk curds in the terminal ileum produces acute intestinal obstruction [39].

Ingested therapeutic agents may also give rise to bolus obstruction. Barium sulphate used for radiological imaging is probably the most common offender but there are also reports of intestinal obstruction following the use of antacid gels [40]. Bezoars, concretions formed within the stomach from ingested hairs, vegetables or other materials (see p. 229), may also give rise to small intestinal obstruction after fragmentation, and in parts of the world where roundworm (*Ascaris lumbricoides*) infestation is endemic, a mass of worms may form an obstructing bolus [41].

Swallowed foreign bodies are not infrequently the cause of mechanical small intestinal obstruction, especially in children, the mentally ill and prisoners. The variety of articles involved is almost limitless but among the most common are dentures, bones, pins, coins, screws and nails. In fact the vast majority of swallowed objects which are able to negotiate the gastro-oesophageal junction will traverse the remainder of the alimentary tract with little difficulty, although potential sites of obstruction are the second part of the duodenum and the terminal ileum. Experimental studies suggest that soft, malleable objects are more dangerous than hard ones [42]. In recent years international drug smugglers have turned to the use of ingested balloons filled with illicit drugs for avoiding detection at customs points. Offenders place themselves in great personal danger, not only from intestinal obstruction but also from lethal drug overdose following rupture of the balloons [43].

Luminal obstruction of the small intestine may also be of 'endogenous' origin. Two varieties are well described: meconium ileus and gallstone ileus. Meconium ileus nearly always occurs in infants with cystic fibrosis (mucoviscidosis), in whom the abnormally viscid mucus secreted into the gut lumen makes meconium tenacious and liable to cause obstruction, notably at the mid- or terminal ileum [44]. The mucin hyperviscosity is due to decreased fluid and increased chloride ion secretion due to defective cystic fibrosis transmembrane conductance regulator (CFTR) [45]. Occasionally intestinal obstruction develops during fetal life, leading to intrauterine perforation and meconium peritonitis. A similar acute intestinal obstruction by viscid luminal contents may also occur in older children or even adults with cystic fibrosis. It is usually called 'meconium ileus equivalent' [46]. Gallstone ileus, on the other hand, is a disease of adults, and in most instances elderly women [47]. It is said to account for about 1–2% of all cases of adult small intestinal obstruction [48]. Patients obviously have underlying gallbladder disease and the obstructing gallstone, which is nearly always more than 2.5 cm in diameter, lodges in the terminal ileum. It usually reaches the small intestinal lumen through a cholecystoduodenal fistula although in rare instances a small stone passing down the biliary tree may grow within the intestinal lumen (a so-called enterolith) until it reaches obstructing proportions [49]. Since multiple gallstones are common in cholelithiasis, it is not infrequent for patients with gallstone ileus to have recurrent attacks of intestinal obstruction unless any additional stones are removed during surgery for the first attack [50]. We have also seen obstruction of the ileum in an elderly patient by huge enteroliths that had escaped from jejunal diverticula.

Intestinal pseudo-obstruction

Although many cases of small intestinal obstruction are caused by some recognizable mechanical obstructing lesion this is not always so. When no localized lesion is apparent the name intestinal pseudo-obstruction is given. The functional obstruction is due to a failure of intestinal propulsion, due to either disorders of intestinal smooth muscle, the innervation of the bowel, or both. Intestinal pseudo-obstruction may be divided into acute and chronic forms.

Acute intestinal pseudo-obstruction (paralytic ileus)

By far the commonest variety of small intestinal pseudo-obstruction is so-called paralytic (or adynamic) ileus [51]. This acute self-limiting condition is usually a complication of peritoneal irritation, from either acute peritonitis, trauma or abdominal surgery. Rarer causes are metabolic disturbances (especially hypokalaemia, uraemia, diabetic ketoacidosis and myxoedema), spinal injuries and the use of ganglion-blocking drugs. The clinical picture is one of acute small intestinal obstruction with abdominal distension, vomiting and absent bowel sounds. In most cases the whole of the small intestine is affected and on gross examination it is distended by gas and a watery brown faeculent fluid [52]. The wall is thin and often dusky in appearance.

The aetiology of the smooth muscle paralysis in ileus is poorly understood but is probably multifactorial. There is evidence that postoperative ileus is at least partly related to changes in autonomic nervous function, either from overstimulation of the splanchnic sympathetic system [53] or from damage to cholinergic fibres [54] due to surgical manipulation of the mesentery. Contributing factors may be electrolyte imbalance and the use of anaesthetic agents. Abnormalities of autonomic function are also important when ileus is associated with acute peritonitis, when toxins absorbed through the inflamed peritoneal membrane and anoxia due to vascular stasis contribute to the smooth muscle dysfunction.

Chronic intestinal pseudo-obstruction

Chronic intestinal pseudo-obstruction is manifested clinically by recurrent attacks of nausea, vomiting, abdominal pain and distension that vary greatly in their frequency, severity and duration [55]. These attacks are the result of acute or subacute functional obstruction of the small intestine but motility studies in the intervening 'asymptomatic' periods usually show an impaired propulsive capacity of the intestinal smooth muscle. In many cases they also show a more widespread abnormality of motor function of the whole alimentary tract than would be suspected from the clinical features, such that subclinical involvement of the oesophagus, colon and, less frequently, the stomach are quite common. Nevertheless localized functional obstruction in some patients leads to segmental dilatation of one part of the small intestine, resulting in so-called megaduodenum or megajejunum while in others it leads to the formation of intestinal diverticula [56]. The abnormality of propulsive action frequently predisposes to overgrowth of colonic-type microorganisms within the affected small bowel, leading to malabsorption. Sometimes this complication may even produce more clinical effects than the underlying motor disorder. Malabsorption may also lead to the accumulation of lipofuscin (ceroid) pigment within the smooth muscle coats of the intestine, giving the appearance of the so-called 'brown bowel syndrome' (Fig. 20.2). Whether this ceroid accumulation impairs smooth muscle function, aggravating the motility disturbance even further, is uncertain [56].

Chronic intestinal pseudo-obstruction may result from a

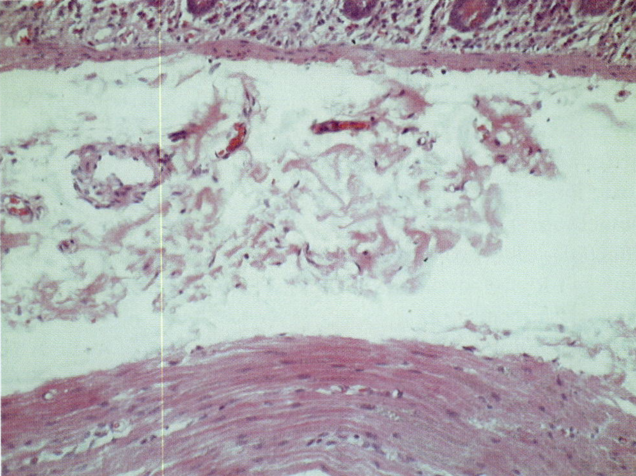

Fig. 20.2 Brown bowel syndrome. A full-thickness biopsy of the jejunum from a man of 60 being investigated for intractable malabsorption. He was found to have jejunal diverticular disease, and the serosal surface of the small bowel was brown at laparotomy. The brown granular ceroid pigment is concentrated in the perinuclear cytoplasm of the myocytes of the muscularis propria.

wide variety of disease processes [55,56], as is shown in Table 20.1. Involvement of the whole of the gastrointestinal tract is common, and sometimes there are similar disorders of motility in other organs, notably the urinary bladder.

Intestinal pseudo-obstruction may be due to smooth muscle disease or, more rarely, a neuropathy [57].

Disorders of intestinal smooth muscle

Both inherited and acquired disorders of intestinal smooth muscle may give rise to intestinal pseudo-obstruction. Familial visceral myopathy may be inherited as both autosomal dominant and autosomal recessive traits [56,58,59]. Generally speaking, the dominant form of the disease is often localized to the duodenum (although also affecting the oesophagus, colon and urinary bladder), while a more severe and widespread involvement of the small intestine is usual in the recessive type, sometimes with the development of intestinal diverticulosis [56]. In rare autosomal recessive variants extraintestinal involvement has included skeletal myopathy or ophthalmoplegia [60,61]. We have seen one patient with acquired visceral myopathy due to Epstein–Barr virus infection [62], and self-limiting or curable idiopathic (and presumably acquired) pseudo-obstruction due to enteric myositis has been described in a child [63].

When definite morphological abnormalities are evident, there can be vacuolar degeneration of the smooth muscle coats of the intestinal wall (Fig. 20.3), most marked in the muscularis propria but sometimes including the muscularis mucosae, with progressive replacement by fibrosis (Fig. 20.4) [56,58,59].

Table 20.1 Causes of chronic small intestinal pseudo-obstruction.

Smooth muscle disorders
Primary
  Inherited visceral myopathy:
    autosomal dominant
    autosomal recessive
  Sporadic visceral myopathy

Secondary
  Collagen diseases:
    scleroderma
    dermatomyositis
    mixed connective tissue disease
  Myotonic dystrophy
  Progressive muscular dystrophy
  Amyloidosis

Neurological disorders
Primary
  Inherited visceral neuropathy:
    autosomal recessive
    autosomal dominant
  Developmental disorders:
    aganglionosis
    hyperganglionosis (neuronal intestinal dysplasia)
  Sporadic visceral neuropathy

Secondary
  Inflammatory disorders:
    infective (Chagas' disease, cytomegalovirus)
    immunological (small cell carcinoma of bronchus)
  Crohn's disease
  Idiopathic (isolated 'plexitis')
  Metabolic disorders:
    diabetes mellitus
    hypothyroidism
  Drug-induced:
    psychotropic drugs (phenothiazines, tricyclic antidepressants, anticholinergic drugs)
    antineoplastic drugs (vinca alkaloids, daunorubicin)

The myenteric plexus is normal on both light and electron microscopy. Occasionally the clinical and pathological features of familial visceral myopathy are found without evidence of an inherited defect. The fundamental smooth muscle abnormality in most cases of visceral myopathy is unknown and, histologically, many of these cases are ill defined [64]. However, in one sporadic case, in which there was also external ophthalmoplegia, skeletal myopathy and peripheral neuropathy, a generalized defect of mitochondrial cytochrome-c-oxidase was established [65].

So-called 'secondary' smooth muscle disorders [55] leading to chronic intestinal pseudo-obstruction include those associated with the collagen diseases, especially systemic sclerosis and dermatomyositis [66], polymyositis [67], myotonic dystrophy, progressive muscular dystrophy [68] and muscle

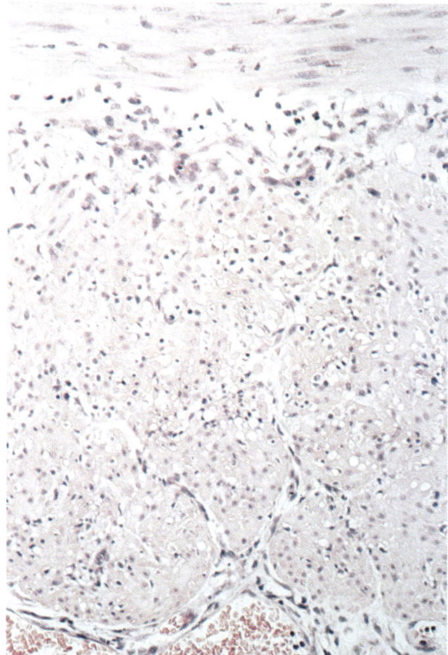

Fig. 20.3 Idiopathic hollow visceral myopathy. Section of the ileal muscularis propria from a patient with small intestinal pseudo-obstruction. The myocytes of the longitudinal muscle layer (lower three-quarters of field) are vacuolated.

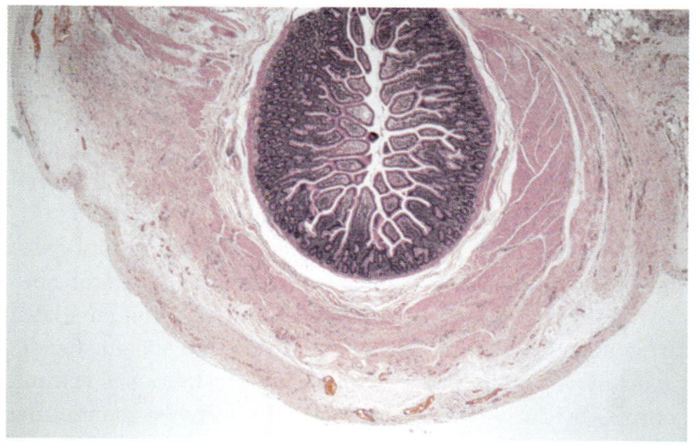

(a)

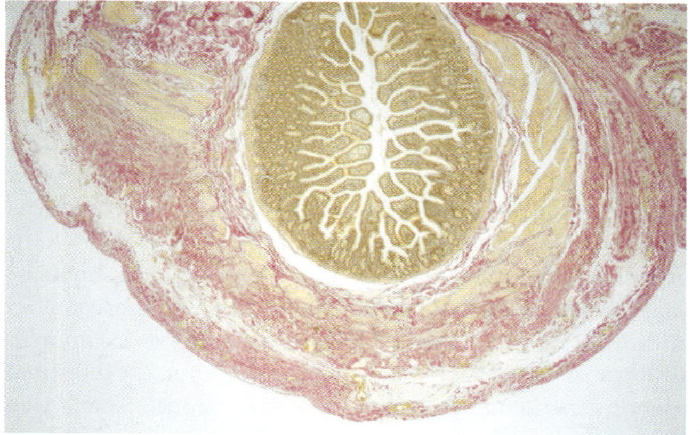

(b)

Fig. 20.4 (a,b) Small intestine from a child with visceral myopathy. The muscularis propria, particularly the longitudinal layer, shows patchy thinning and replacement by pale fibrous tissue, pale on H&E (a), red on van Giesen (b).

dysfunction from amyloid infiltration [69]. While the microscopic appearances of the latter lesion are characteristic, the changes in the other conditions are often far from distinct and may be difficult to distinguish from those of primary visceral myopathy [56]. We have not found that vacuolation of the smooth muscle cells [66] is particularly specific in distinguishing visceral myopathy from the changes of systemic sclerosis.

Neurological disorders

Abnormalities of visceral nervous innervation leading to chronic intestinal pseudo-obstruction have been recognized only recently, since special neuropathological techniques have been applied to the gastrointestinal tract [70]. They may be divided into the inherited familial visceral neuropathies, developmental disorders, and a number of acquired lesions.

Familial visceral neuropathies may be inherited as either autosomal dominant [71] or autosomal recessive [72] traits. Although genetic disorders, they rarely present with intestinal symptoms before adult life. The dominant form affects the small intestine almost exclusively, and on histological examination there is a degeneration of the argyrophilic neurones in the submucosal and myenteric plexuses with a consequent reduction in their numbers. Denervation of smooth muscle often leads to increased but uncoordinated peristalsis, and there may be work hypertrophy of the ileal smooth muscle coats [71]. Autosomal recessive visceral neuropathy usually affects the alimentary tract in a more widespread form, and frequently has extraintestinal manifestations [56]. A number of varieties have been described, including one which is associated with abnormalities of the central and peripheral nervous systems and which is characterized by the presence of intranuclear eosinophilic inclusions within the degenerating neurones [72], and another which is associated with mental retardation and calcification of the basal ganglia [73]. Isolated cases of chronic intestinal pseudo-obstruction with the features of neuronal degeneration seen in familial visceral neuropathy occur rarely without any apparent genetic predisposition [56]. Whether or not they are true sporadic cases is uncertain.

Developmental abnormalities of the innervation of the small intestine leading to motility disorders are similar to those that occur more commonly in the large intestine (see p. 447). Thus aganglionosis of the small intestine, which rarely may extend proximally up to the duodenum, represents proximal extension from total colonic involvement by Hirschsprung's disease [74] while hyperganglionosis of the small intestine, characterized by hyperplasia of the submucosal and myenteric plexuses with formation of giant ganglia, corresponds to neuronal colonic dysplasia [75]. Both conditions may present with functional small intestinal obstruction, usually in the neonatal period.

The major causes of acquired damage to the small intestinal neuronal innervation are infective agents, metabolic disturbances, drugs and, rarely, non-metastatic manifestations of malignant disease [55,56,76]. Granulomatous visceral neuropathy has been reported in association with non-small cell carcinoma of the lung [77].The lesions are not specific for the small bowel, and indeed the clinical manifestations of visceral neuropathy derive more commonly from involvement of the large intestine. For this reason the reader is referred to Chapter 35 (p. 461) where the lesions are discussed in some detail. Suffice it to say that chronic intestinal pseudo-obstruction may be found in diabetes mellitus and hypothyroidism [55] and that while inflammatory damage to the myenteric plexus of the small intestine is well recorded in Chagas' disease [78], it is also described rarely in cytomegalovirus infection [79] and in patients with oat cell carcinoma of the lung in whom it is thought to be immunologically mediated [56,76,80,81]. Axonal necrosis of enteric nerves has been reported in Crohn's disease [82] and this could lead to intestinal pseudo-obstruction, adding to the effect of the obstruction which is so common in Crohn's disease. There is a single case report of intestinal pseudo-obstruction in which there was idiopathic selective inflammatory destruction of axons in the myenteric plexus, with sparing of the neuronal bodies [83]. Its aetiology was not established. Drug-induced visceral neuropathy leading to functional obstruction of the small intestine is an uncommon side-effect of tricyclic antidepressants, phenothiazines, anticholinergic drugs and the vinca alkaloids [56,70]. They are probably chiefly responsible for the high frequency of intestinal motility disorders, including pseudo-obstruction of the small intestine, in psychiatric patients and those with Parkinson's disease [55].

References

1 Gough M. Multiple intussusception and intestinal perforation due to a bezoar. *Br J Surg*, 1960; 48: 222.

2 MacMahon B. Data on the etiology of acute intussusception in childhood. *Am J Hum Genet*, 1955; 7: 430.

3 Talwalker VC. Intussusception in the newborn. *Arch Dis Child*, 1962; 37: 203.

4 Smith IS, Gillespie C. Adult intussusception in Glasgow. *Br J Surg*, 1968; 55: 925.

5 Ein SH. Leading points in childhood intussusception. *J Pediatr Surg*, 1976; 11: 209.

6 Wayne E, Campbell J, Burrington J, Davis W. Management of 344 children with intussusception. *Radiology*, 1973; 107: 597.

7 Gardner PS, Knox EG, Court SDM, Green CA. Virus infection and intussusception in childhood. *Br Med J*, 1962; 2: 697.

8 Nicholas JL, Ingrand D, Fortier B, Briscout F. A one year virological survey of acute intussusception in childhood. *J Med Virol*, 1982; 9: 267.

9 Knox EC, Court SDM, Gardner PS. Aetiology of intussusception in children. *Br Med J*, 1962; 2: 692.

10 Abel R, Keen CE, Bingham JB *et al*. Heterotopic pancreas as lead point in intussusception: new variant of vitellointestinal tract malformation. *Pediatr Dev Pathol*, 1999; 2: 367.

11 Holsclaw D, Rocmans C, Shwachman H. Intussusception in patients with cystic fibrosis. *Pediatrics*, 1971; 48: 51.

12 Cornes JS, Dawson IMP. Papillary lymphoid hyperplasia at the ileocaecal valve as a cause of acute intussusception in infancy. *Arch Dis Child*, 1963; 38: 89.

13 Burke M. Intussusception in adults. *Ann R Coll Surg Engl*, 1977; 59: 150.

14 Das Gupta TK, Brasfield RD. Metastatic melanoma of the gastrointestinal tract. *Arch Surg*, 1964; 88: 969.

15 Fawaz F, Hill GJ. Adult intussusception due to metastatic tumors. *South Med J*, 1983; 76: 522.

16 Donhauser JH, Kelly RC. Intussusception in the adult. *Am J Surg*, 1950; 79: 673.

17 Riccabono XJ, Haskins RM. Gastroduodenal intussusception: report of 2 cases. *Gastroenterology*, 1970; 38: 995.

18 Mock CJ, Moock HE Jr. Strangulated internal hernia associated with trauma. *Arch Surg*, 1958; 77: 881.

19 Rooney JA, Carroll JP, Keeley JL. Internal hernias due to defects in the meso-appendix and mesentery of small bowel, and probable Ivemark syndrome. *Ann Surg*, 1963; 157: 254.

20 Willwerth BM, Zollinger RM, Izant R. Congenital mesocolic (paraduodenal) hernia. Embryological basis of repair. *Am J Surg*, 1974; 128: 358.

21 Cook JL. Bowel herniation through the foramen of Winslow. *Am Surg*, 1970; 36: 241.

22 Hansmann GH, Morton SA. Intraabdominal hernia. Report of a case and review of the literature. *Arch Surg*, 1939; 39: 973.

23 Janin Y, Stone AM, Wise I. Mesenteric hernia. *Surg Gynecol Obstet*, 1980; 150: 747.

24 Stewart JOR. Transepiploic hernia. *Br J Surg*, 1962; 49: 649.

25 Kerr WG, Kirkaldy-Willis WH. Volvulus of the small intestine. *Br Med J*, 1946; 1: 799.

26 Saidi F. The high incidence of intestinal volvulus in Iran. *Gut*, 1969; 10: 838.

27 Agarwal RL, Misra MK. Volvulus of the small intestine in northern India. *Am J Surg*, 1970; 120: 366.

28 Wapnick S. Treatment of intestinal volvulus. *Ann R Coll Surg*, 1973; 53: 57.

29 Duke JH, Yar MS. Primary small bowel volvulus. *Arch Surg*, 1977; 112: 685.

30 Shepherd J. The epidemiology and clinical presentation of sigmoid volvulus. *Br J Surg*, 1969; 56: 353.

31 Talbot CH. Volvulus of the small intestine in adults. *Gut*, 1960; 1: 76.

32 Ebert EC, Ruggiero FM, Seibold JR. Intestinal perforation. A common complication of scleroderma. *Dig Dis Sci*, 1997; 42: 549.

33 Evans JP. Traumatic rupture of the ileum. *Br J Surg*, 1973; 60: 119.

34 Mullins AEJ. Perforation of the small intestine by sudden muscular effort. *Br J Surg*, 1962; 50: 191.

35 Ellis H, Moran BJ, Thompson JN *et al*. Adhesion-related hospital readmissions after abdominal and pelvic surgery: a retrospective cohort study. *Lancet*, 1999; 353: 1476.

36 Norberg PB. Food as a cause of intestinal obstruction. *Am J Surg*, 1962; 104: 444.

37 Connelly HJ, Del Carmen BV. Intestinal obstruction due to food. *Am Surg*, 1969; 35: 820.

38 Koott H, Urca H. Intestinal obstruction after partial gastrectomy due to orange pith. *Arch Surg*, 1970; 100: 79.

39 Cook RCM, Rickham PP. Neonatal intestinal obstruction due to milk curds. *J Pediatr Surg*, 1969; 4: 599.

40 Brettschneider L, Monafo W, Osborne DP. Intestinal obstruction due to antacid gels. *Gastroenterology*, 1965; 49: 291.

41 Hhekwaba EN. Intestinal ascariasis and the acute abdomen in the tropics. *J Roy Coll Surg Edinb*, 1980; 25: 452.

42 Harjola P-T, Scheinin TM. Experimental observations on intestinal obstruction due to foreign bodies. *Acta Chir Scand*, 1963; 126: 144.

43 McCarroon MM, Wood JO. The cocaine body packer syndrome. *Diagnosis* and *treatment*. *JAMA*, 1983; 250: 1417.

44 Holsclaw OS, Eckstein HB, Nixon HH. Meconium ileus: a 20-year review of 109 cases. *Am J Dis Child*, 1965; 109: 101.

45 Eggermont E, De Boeck K. Small-intestinal abnormalities in cystic fibrosis patients. *Eur J Pediatr*, 1991; 150: 824.

46 Jeffrey I, Durrans O, Wells M, Fox H. The pathology of meconium ileus equivalent. *J Clin Pathol*, 1983; 36: 1292.

47 Brockis JC, Gilbert MC. Intestinal obstruction by gall stones. A record of 179 *cases*. *Br J Surg*, 1957; 44: 461.

48 Stitt RB, Heslin DJ, Currie DJ. Gallstone ileus. *Br J Surg*, 1967; 54: 673.

49 Newman JH. A case of gall-stone ileus in the absence of a biliary-enteric fistula. *Br J Surg*, 1972; 59: 573.

50 Rogers EA, Carter R. Recurrent gallstone ileus. *Am J Surg*, 1958; 96: 379.

51 Ellis H. *Intestinal obstruction*. New York: Appleton-Century Crofts, 1982.

52 Shields R. The absorption and secretion of fluid and electrolytes by the obstructed bowel. *Br J Surg*, 1965; 52: 774.

53 Smith J, Kelly KA, Weinshilboum RM. Pathophysiology of postoperative ileus. *Arch Surg*, 1977; 112: 203.

54 Davison JS. Selective damage to cholinergic nerves: possible cause of postoperative ileus. *Lancet*, 1979; i: 1288.

55 Faulk DL, Anuras S, Christensen J. Chronic intestinal pseudo-obstruction. *Gastroenterology*, 1978; 74: 922.

56 Knishnamurthy S, Schuffler MD. Pathology of neuromuscular disorders of the small intestine and colon. *Gastroenterology*, 1987; 93: 610.

57 Mann SD, Debinski HS, Kamm MA. Clinical characteristics of chronic idiopathic intestinal pseudo-obstruction in adults. *Gut*, 1997; 41: 675.

58 Mitros FA, Schuffler MD, Teja K, Aneiras S. Pathologic features of familial visceral myopathy. *Hum Pathol*, 1982; 13: 825.

59 Alstead EM, Murphy MN, Flanagan AM, Bishop AE, Hodgson HJF. Familial autonomic visceral myopathy, with degeneration of the muscularis mucosae. *J Clin Pathol*, 1988; 41: 424.

60 Anuras S, Mitros FA, Nowak TV *et al*. A familial visceral myopathy with external ophthalmoplegia and autosomal recessive transmission. *Gastroenterology*, 1983; 84: 346.

61 Ionasescu VV, Thompson HS, Aschenbrener C, Aneuras S. Late onset oculogastrointestinal muscular dystrophy. *Am J Med Genet*, 1984; 18: 781.

62 Debinski HS, Kamm MA, Talbot IC *et al*. DNA viruses in the pathogenesis of sporadic chronic idiopathic intestinal pseudo-obstruction. *Gut*, 1997; 41: 100.

63 Ginies JL, Francois H, Joseph MG *et al*. A curable cause of chronic idiopathic intestinal pseudo-obstruction in children: idiopathic myositis of the small intestine. *J Pediatr Gastroenterol Nutr*, 1996; 23: 426.

64 Ladabaum U, Hasler WL. Motility of the small intestine. *Curr Opin Gastroenterol*, 1999; 15: 125.

65 Barejoosi A, Creutzfeldt W, DiMauro S *et al*. Myo-, neuro-, gastrointestinal encephalopathy (MNGIE syndrome) due to partial deficiency of cytochrome-c-oxidase. *Acta Neuropathol (Berl)*, 1987; 74: 248.

66 Schuffler MD, Beegle RG. Progressive systemic sclerosis of the gastrointestinal tract and hereditary, hollow visceral mycopathy: two distinguishable disorders of intestinal smooth muscle. *Gastroenterology*, 1979; 77: 664.

67 Boardman P, Nolan DJ. Case report: Small intestinal pseudo-obstruction: an unusual manifestation of polymyositis. *Clin Radiol*, 1998; 53: 706.

68 Nowak TV, Ionasescu V, Anuras S. Gastrointestinal manifestations of the muscular dystrophies. *Gastroenterology*, 1982; 82: 800.

69 Tada S, Iida M, Yao T, Kitamoto T, Fujishima M. Intestinal pseudo-obstruction in patients with amyloidosis: clinicopathologic differences between chemical types of amyloid protein [see comments]. *Gut*, 1993; 34: 1412.

70 Smith B. *The Neuropathology of the Alimentary Tract*. Baltimore: Williams & Wilkins, 1972.

71 Mayer EA, Schuffler MD, Rotter JI, Hanna P, Mogard M. Familial visceral neuroopathy with autosomal dominant transmission. *Gastroenterology*, 1986; 91: 1528.

72 Schuffler MD, Bird TO, Sumi SM, Cook A. A familial neuronal disease presenting as intestinal pseudo-obstruction. *Gastroenterology*, 1978; 75: 889.

73 Cockel R, Hill FE, Rushton DI, Smith B, Hawkins CF. Familial steatorrhoea with calcification of the basal ganglia and mental retardation. *Q J Med*, 1973; 42: 771.

74 Ahmed S, Cohen SJ, Jacobs SI. Total intestinal aganglionosis presenting as duodenal obstruction. *Arch Dis Child*, 1971; 46: 868.

75 Scharli AF, Meier-Ruge W. Localized and disseminated forms of neuronal intestinal dysplasia mimicking Hirschsprung's disease. *J Pediatr Surg*, 1981; 16: 835.

76 Smith B. The neuropathology of pseudo-obstruction of the intestine. *Scand J Gastroenterol*, 1982; 17 (Suppl 71): 103.

77 Roberts PF, Stebbings WS, Kennedy HJ. Granulomatous visceral neuropathy of the colon with non-small cell lung carcinoma. *Histopathology*, 1997; 30: 588.

78 Martins-Campos JV, Tafuri WL. Chagas' enteropathy. *Gut*, 1973; 14: 910.

79 Sonsino F, Mouy R, Foucaud P *et al*. Intestinal pseudoobstruction related to cytomegalovirus infection of myenteric plexus. *N Engl J Med*, 1984; 311: 196.

80 Schuffler MD, Baird HW, Fleming CR *et al*. Intestinal pseudoobstruction as the presenting manifestation of small cell carcinoma of the lung: a paraneoplastic neuropathy of the gastrointestinal tract. *Arch Intern Med*, 1983; 98: 129.

81 Bell CE Jr, Seetharam S. Identification of the Schwann cell as a peripheral nervous system cell possessing a differentiation antigen expressed by a human lung tumor. *J Immunol*, 1977; 118: 826.

82 Dvorak AM, Silen W. Differentiation between Crohn's disease and other inflammatory conditions by electron microscopy. *Ann Surg*, 1085; 201: 53.

83 Krishnamurthy S, Schuffler MD, Belic L, Schweid A. An inflammatory axonopathy of the myenteric plexus causing rapidly progressive intestinal pseudoobstruction. *Gastroenterology*, 1986; 90: 754.

21 Inflammatory disorders of the small intestine

Inflammatory pathology of the small bowel is relatively common. This includes specific infections, usually either viral or bacterial, non-specific inflammatory pathology and chronic enteritis, most noticeably caused by chronic infection, inflammatory bowel diseases and drugs. Many enteritides are entirely non-specific in nature and the majority of patients recover without surgery or biopsy: often they are not even subjected to formal microbiological assessment. Thus these conditions do not often come to the attention of the histopathologist. Formerly the more chronic conditions and more severe acute pathological entities only came to the attention of pathologists when resection was performed. However, now that colonoscopic examination can regularly reach the terminal ileum, such ileoscopy is increasingly able to demonstrate many forms of enteritis [1]. Enteroscopy, performed via the upper gastrointestinal tract, may be used for the demonstration of inflammatory pathology but is more often indicated for obscure small intestinal bleeding [2].

Inflammation due to identifiable microorganisms

Viral gastroenteritis

Acute gastrointestinal infection is a major cause of morbidity throughout the world and viruses play a leading part in its aetiology [3]. Children are particularly prone whereas, in adults, viral gastroenteritis is often a relatively minor and self-limiting condition. In all age groups, viral gastroenteritis is characteristically associated with outbreaks and epidemics, although isolated viral gastroenteritis is also well recognized. The relationship between viral enteritis and acquired immune deficiency sydrome (AIDS) is less clear than for bacteria and other opportunistic infections occurring in AIDS. Nevertheless, evidence of viral infection can be detected in up to 10% of AIDS patients: the relationship between such viral presence and the production of symptoms such as diarrhoea is less certain [4].

A comprehensive analysis of the epidemiology and virology of the condition is beyond the scope of the current text, as the disease is so rarely the subject of histopathological assessment. This review will simply highlight those viruses of importance in the genesis of gastroenteritis and briefly review the morphological features associated with these infections.

Small round structured viruses (SRSVs) are a common cause of adult viral gastroenteritis, often after the ingestion of food [5], particularly shellfish [6]. Norwalk virus is perhaps the best known cause but several others including Hawaii, Mexico, Montgomery County, Grimsby and Southampton viruses are all well described [7,8]. These are now classified as caliciviruses [9]. The disease presents with a self-limiting diarrhoea, often accompanied by nausea, vomiting and abdominal pain after the ingestion of contaminated food and water. These viruses are particularly associated with outbreaks of diarrhoea in the UK and elsewhere [10]. Histological changes are seen in the jejunal mucosa, including villous blunting and irregularity and vacuolation of the surface enterocytes. There

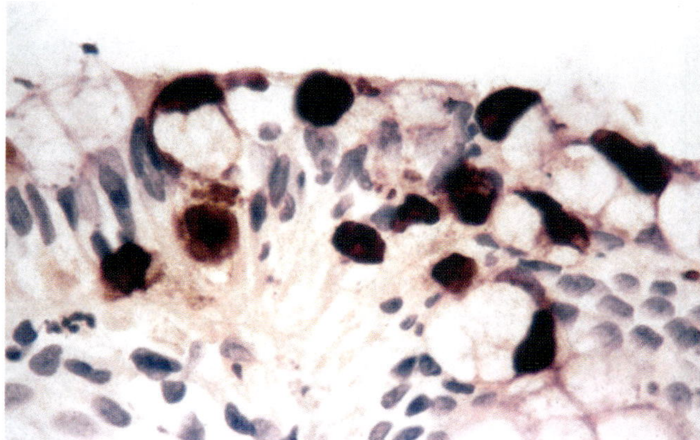

Fig. 21.1 Immunohistochemistry demonstrating adenovirus infection in the small intestinal mucosa.

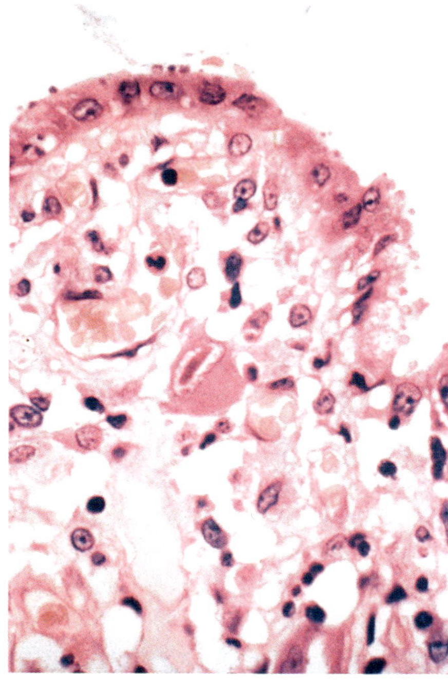

Fig. 21.2 Small intestinal mucosa in an AIDS patient. A classical cytomegalovirus inclusion is present centrally whilst the epithelial surface demonstrates innumerable adherent cryptosporidia.

are also modest inflammatory changes. The disease is particularly associated with outbreaks in hospitals and residential facilities for the elderly: in one study in the UK, 76% of the total number of infections occurred in these institutions [11]. Many of these viruses are also important causes of traveller's diarrhoea [12] and they also cause outbreaks of gastroenteritis in children and infants [13].

Rotaviruses are so called because of their wheel-like morphology on electron microscopic examination. They are the most common cause of infective gastroenteritis in infants and children [14,15]. Interestingly, neonates and adults are relatively immune from infection and usually have only a mild disease whilst infants up to the age of 1 year suffer more pronounced symptoms. Large outbreaks and epidemics are well recognized [16]. The morphological features are loss of absorptive cells with replacement by immature cuboidal cells, villous blunting and a lymphocytic infiltrate in the lamina propria [17]. Virus particles are present in the villi and crypts, demonstrable by electron microscopy [6]. Infection with rotavirus may increase the susceptibility of the intestine to other pathogens [18].

Adenoviruses are most commonly associated with respiratory infection but they also cause acute diarrhoea [19]. They are a cause of outbreaks of acute diarrhoea in children. However, it is important to realize that these DNA viruses can be detected in the stools of asymptomatic children. For the histopathologist, probably the most important associations are with lymphoid hyperplasia in the terminal ileum and subsequent intussusception in infants [20], and the common occurrence of the infection in AIDS diarrhoea. The inclusions are readily demonstrable by immunohistochemical techniques (Fig. 21.1) [21,22].

The *picornaviruses* (named because they are small and of RNA type) incorporate the *enteroviruses* (including polio, coxsackie A and B and echovirus), *astroviruses* and *coronaviruses*. Enteroviruses are well recognized as causing severe gastroenteritis in immunocompromised patients but they may also be found in asymptomatic carriers. Astroviruses are associated with gastroenteritis in children but produce only mild symptoms in adults [23,24]. Coronaviruses [25] are a cause of gastroenteritis in the tropics and in Asia but rarely in the UK and Europe, although they have been associated with necrotizing enterocolitis in infants [26].

Cytomegalovirus in the small intestine

Cytomegalovirus infection (CMV) is most likely to be seen in the small bowel in the context of profound immune suppression, especially with HIV infection and AIDS (Fig. 21.2) [27,28]. In the colon, it is seen in immunocompetent hosts, especially when associated with ulcerative colitis [29], but in the small intestine such infection is less commonly seen. There remains some doubt as to the primary pathogenicity of the virus and it may well be that it is nearly always an opportunistic infection, especially involving ulcers and other pathological situations where granulation tissue is a prominent feature [30]. The histological diagnosis depends on recognizing the characteristic intranuclear inclusions (Fig. 21.2): these are most commonly seen in endothelial cells within small capillary-type blood vessels [31]. They may also be seen in histiocytes and, less commonly, in epithelial cells. In the small bowel, CMV infection is often evident in otherwise nonspecific ulcers and, occasionally, in areas of perforation [28,32].

Whether it is the primary pathogen in this situation is often uncertain [33]. In the context of profound immunosuppression, especially AIDS, it is important to remember that CMV infection often coexists with evidence of other pathogens, especially atypical mycobacterial infection, giardiasis and other opportunistic infections (Fig. 21.2) [27]. In such situations, the CMV changes may be striking, often with evidence of a vasculitis [34].

HIV and AIDS in the small intestine

Chronic diarrhoea remains a considerable problem in AIDS, notwithstanding the success of antiviral therapy in controlling the disease and its complications [35]. There is now increasing evidence that infection by the virus itself causes both functional and morphological abnormalities in the small bowel, outside of the numerous opportunistic infections that complicate the disease [36]. The small bowel mucosa, whether in duodenal, jejunal or ileal biopsies, shows various morphological abnormalities, from complete normality to varying chronic inflammation in the lamina propria and partial villous atrophy [21]. Both crypt hyperplastic [37] and crypt hypoplastic atrophy patterns have been described [38]. Furthermore, HIV antigens and RNA are readily demonstrated in lamina propria inflammatory cells, histiocytes and intraepithelial lymphocytes (IELs) [39]. Enhanced apoptosis is a characteristic feature [40]. Such increased apoptotic activity is often closely associated with IELs and is typically prominent in crypt bases [40]. The features are similar to those seen in graft-versus-host disease, suggesting an early phase of cell-mediated immunity, cell–cell recognition [21]. Despite these changes, epithelial cells usually appear morphologically and morphometrically normal, despite the villous atrophy and inflammatory changes [38,41]. However there are functional abnormalities: β-glucosidase activity, for instance, is greatly reduced, indicating a profound functional immaturity in epithelial cells [36]. The powerful effect of combination therapy in AIDS on gastrointestinal symptoms and on morphological, immunological and virological abnormalities, in terms of decreased apoptotic activity, reduced viral RNA load, and raised intraluminal CD4 counts, suggests that the intestinal dysfunction seen in AIDS could well be a direct result of HIV infection [42].

Opportunistic infection of the small intestine has been extremely common in the small bowel in AIDS. Nevertheless histopathologists are called upon less often than previously to diagnose such opportunistic infections. This may relate to enhanced detection of these diseases by microbiological techniques, but also to a steady decline in the prevalence of some of these infections because of the success of combination therapy in AIDS [35,43]. Indeed, the effect of highly active antiretroviral therapy (HAART) has seen a marked decrease in opportunistic infection in AIDS, and has also decreased the incidence of Kaposi's sarcoma and the mortality from infectious disease in AIDS over the past few years [44–46].

Nevertheless, infectious diarrhoea remains a considerable problem and histopathological assessment of small bowel biopsies still provides valuable information. Viral, bacterial and protozoal infections are particularly common in AIDS and the pathologist must always be alert to the potential for multiple infections (Fig. 21.2) [22,47]. We have seen cases with no less than six separate infections, including Kaposi's sarcoma and systemic *Pneumocystis carinii* infection in a single section from a small intestinal resection specimen. Whilst individual infections are more comprehensively covered elsewhere in this chapter, because almost all of them also occur outside AIDS, it is appropriate to outline the infections likely to be detected histopathologically in AIDS. In the UK chronic diarrhoea in AIDS is most likely to be caused by cryptosporidiosis whilst microsporidiosis, CMV, adenovirus infection and giardiasis are also common [22,48]. It is important to emphasize that the spectrum of infections may be very different in other countries, especially tropical countries, with their very different spectrum of infectious disease in the gut and the less common usage of HAART [43]. CMV infection may be particularly associated with Kaposi's sarcoma, in the small bowel and elsewhere [27]. Most of these infections can be demonstrated by simple morphological and immunohistochemical methods, the latter especially important for viral infection, such as adenovirus and CMV [38]. Electron microscopic assessment is used less often, especially as microsporidiosis and cyclosporidiosis can now be recognized by light microscopic techniques (see below) [43,49].

Bacterial infection

Whilst bacterial infection specific and localized to the small bowel does occur, it is important to realize that, in acute bacterial infection, there is usually evidence of an enterocolitis. The primary presentation is with diarrhoea, with or without evidence of blood loss [50]. The pathology of such acute enteritides ranges from a superficial exudative inflammatory process, best characterized by shigellosis and *Escherichia coli* infection, to deeper penetrating inflammatory pathology, as seen in yersiniosis and amoebiasis [51]. The pathology is often caused by the elaboration of enterotoxins, and this is particularly the case with cholera, *Shigella* and *E. coli* [51]. These diseases are especially prone to epidemics and this is partly related to the small inoculum often required to produce infection. For instance, with some strains of *Shigella*, only about 100 bacteria are required to produce an acute enteritis [51]. Whilst such bacterial enteritides are extremely common worldwide, histopathologists seldom see evidence of such diseases in routine practice. Only occasionally will duodenal and proximal small bowel biopsies, on the one hand, and ileoscopic biopsies, on the other, demonstrate infectious enteritis [1]. It is much more common for pathologists to see evidence of such infections in colonic biopsy series [52]. Furthermore, resection of the small intestine is seldom performed for these diseases.

These enteritides are common in autopsy practice in the Third World but are not often seen at postmortem in the UK, Europe or North America.

Shigellosis, salmonellosis and *Campylobacter* infection

Shigella infection is extremely common worldwide. It afflicts about 20 million people each year and kills about three quarters of a million people every year [53]. It is the classical superficial enterocolitis and is caused by four species: *Shigella sonnei, dysenteriae, flexneri* and *boydii*. Evidence of infection starts, clinically, in the small bowel with fever and a secretory diarrhoea [50]. Subsequently, in the next few days, bacteria localize to the colon, causing a colitis with ulceration and erosions. Thus the symptoms of bloody diarrhoea, tenesmus and systemic symptoms supervene. Chronicity does occur but is rare. Shigellosis is particularly prevalent in children, especially undernourished children [54], and the disease exacerbates such undernourishment by its propensity to enteric protein loss [55]. Because of the predominant colonic involvement later in the disease's natural history, demonstration of the disease in small bowel biopsies is unusual.

Salmonella infection is the classical food-related enteritis. Infectious enteritis is most commonly caused by *Salmonella enteritidis* and its serotypes (*typhimurium, heidelberg* and *newport*). *S. choleraesuis* is the other important cause of enteritis [50]. Salmonellae cause an acute gastroenteritis, ileocolitis or colitis alone. For the most part the duration of the disease is short lived and self-limiting. Seldom is histopathological assessment required, except in longer duration enterocolitis [56]. In severe cases, the changes of an acute colitis may be prominent whilst the small bowel mucosa shows more subtle signs of a mucosal enteropathy [57]. Like shigellosis, salmonellosis causes epithelial damage, probably mediated by host inflammatory reactions, especially by production of tumour necrosis factor alpha (TNF-α) [58].

Campylobacter jejuni causes an infectious enterocolitis. It occurs in all age groups and results in a syndrome of acute abdominal pain, fever and an inflammatory enterocolitis, which ranges from a mild secretory diarrhoea through to a severe dysentery-like syndrome [51]. It is a relatively common cause of diarrhoea, being demonstrated in the stools of about 10% of Western patients with diarrhoea [51,59]. Campylobacter colitis has been studied pathologically but there is little data on the pathological features of the associated enteritis [59,60].

The enteric fevers: typhoid and paratyphoid

Caused by *Salmonella typhi*, the incidence of typhoid (enteric) fever has declined greatly in the Western world. The fall in its incidence and the great improvement in its prognosis are due to improved living conditions and sanitation and the introduction of effective antibiotic therapy, which have made the disease now much less important in Western communities. However typhoid epidemics still regularly occur in the Third World and typhoid remains a significant cause of mortality in these communities, mainly because of poor sanitation and living conditions. It is important to realize that other salmonella species, notably the three subtypes of *S. paratyphi*, but also *S. choleraesuis*, yersiniosis and *Campylobacter* infection can be clinically indistinguishable from classical enteric fever [61].

Salmonella typhi reaches the small intestine in food or drink contaminated by carriers or polluted by infected excreta. The organisms enter the bloodstream through the Peyer's patches without producing any local lesions, and may be isolated by blood culture during the first week or two of the illness. Septicaemia and the accompanying toxaemia are responsible for many of the characteristic clinical features of the disease, such as the eruptions of 'rose spots' in the skin, the peculiar type of continued fever and the clouded mental state. After multiplication in the bloodstream, the organisms are excreted by the liver into the bile and enter the gallbladder and intestinal contents in rapidly increasing numbers; they can be cultured from the faeces in an increasing proportion of cases as the disease progresses, the highest incidence of positive stool cultures occurring in the 3rd week of the illness. They are also excreted in the urine and cultures of urine may be of diagnostic value. Towards the end of the 1st week of the illness, specific agglutinating antibodies begin to appear in the patient's blood and the titre rises to its peak by the end of the 3rd week (the Widal reaction). Bacilli are reabsorbed through Peyer's patches in which some degree of local immunity has now developed, leading to a localized antigen–antibody reaction with ulceration and necrosis.

This immunological reaction results in the characteristic macroscopic and microscopic features of the disease. There are ulcers over Peyer's patches, particularly in a longitudinal orientation, with more circular ulcers over smaller lymphoid follicles (Fig. 21.3). Occasionally the large bowel is also involved [62] and in some the appendix is involved. Because of the marked inflammatory reaction and oedema, the ulcers are often raised above the surrounding mucosa, from which they are sharply demarcated. The base of the ulcer contains black necrotic material: healing begins with shedding of the slough. Healing is complete within a week or so of the subsidence of the acute manifestations of the illness and there is little fibrosis. This accounts for the low frequency of stenosis and strictures as a result of previous typhoid fever. Local lymph nodes are considerably enlarged, soft and hyperaemic at the height of the disease. Foci of necrosis sometimes form in their substance. Histologically, enteric fever shows hyperaemia and oedema in the early stages with proliferation of large, often deeply staining mononuclear cells, which are modified histiocytes (Fig. 21.3) [63]. Moderate numbers of lymphocytes and plasma cells are present but neutrophil polymorphs are strikingly rare, accounting for the typical neutropenia found in the blood. Later, focal necrosis develops in lymphoid tissue, the necrotic foci becoming confluent, and ulceration occurs. Large

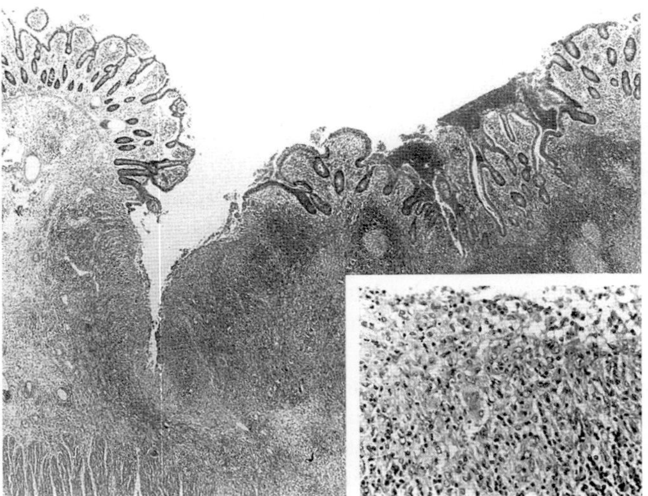

Fig. 21.3 Ulceration in typhoid fever. The insert demonstrates the paucity of acute inflamatory cells and the abundance of pale-staining mononuclear cells lining the ulcer floor.

numbers of typhoid bacilli are present in the intestinal lesions and in the regional lymph nodes.

Enteric fever is associated with significant complications. These include local complications of perforation of the ulcers and haemorrhage. Perforation occurs most frequently in the terminal ileum, in about 5–10% of cases, and it may be that many ulcers perforate or are close to perforation at the same time [64]. At operation, the small bowel is markedly friable. Perforation is a common cause of death from the disease [64,65]. Haemorrhage from the ulcers is the next most frequent complication and occurs at about the same stage in the course of the disease. Acute typhoid cholecystitis is another frequent complication. Other findings and complications in cases of typhoid include paralytic ileus, splenomegaly, myocarditis, multifocal necrosis in parenchymatous organs, particularly the liver, kidneys and bone marrow, and Zenker's degeneration of the abdominal muscle. Acute bronchitis, meningitis, nephritis, orchitis, arthritis and periosteitis due to the presence of the typhoid bacillus in the tissues concerned have all been described. Typhoid osteitis may remain in a state of low-grade activity for a very long period whilst patients may carry the organism, especially in the biliary tract, for many years [66].

Paratyphoid is usually a much less serious illness than typhoid. It is caused by three subtypes of *Salmonella paratyphi*, now named *S. paratyphi A*, *S. schottmulleri* (formerly *paratyphi B*) and *S. hirschfeldii* (formerly *paratyphi C*) [61]. Pathologically the lesions of paratyphoid resemble those of typhoid, but are confined to a smaller area of the terminal ileum. Ulceration is not such a marked feature, and serious complications, comparable with those of typhoid fever, are correspondingly rare.

Cholera

Worldwide, cholera is extremely common and is a major source of morbidity and mortality, especially in those areas associated with poor sanitation and an infected water supply [67]. It is caused by non-invasive toxogenic strains of *Vibrio cholerae* 0:1, and is endemic in southern Asia and parts of Africa. Seasonal outbreaks are particularly associated with areas of poor sanitation. Clinically the condition manifests with severe dehydration accompanied by the passing of enormous quantities of watery fluid flecked with mucus, known as 'rice-water stool'. Epidemics were once common in Europe but have not been seen since the 19th century.

There is not often cause to seek the histopathological features of cholera, as treatment is largely supportive and biopsy adds little to the management of the disease. Clinical and experimental studies have shown villous damage with necrosis of enterocytes, disruption of the underlying basement membrane and necrosis of lymphoid tissue [68]. In the lamina propria there is commonly an increase in numbers of lymphocytes and plasma cells but not of eosinophils or neutrophils [69]. The secretory diarrhoea is induced by the action of the cholera enterotoxin. This molecule has two important functioning moieties. The first, the beta subunit, is responsible for adhesion to the enterocyte surface while the second, the A unit, enters the cytoplasm and activates adenylate cyclase, which in turn increases intracellular cyclic AMP, stimulates secretion of water and electrolytes from the enterocyte and inhibits absorption [70].

Escherichia coli infection

Escherichia coli is responsible for a high proportion of cases of infective diarrhoea and is responsible for about 30–50% of cases of 'traveller's diarrhoea' in visitors to Africa, Asia and Latin America [51]. These are caused by enterotoxogenic *E. coli*. Some strains of such enterotoxogenic (or enterohaemorrhagic—EHEC) *E. coli* can cause much more severe dysentery-like syndromes due to toxin elaboration, notably a Shiga-like toxin (verocytotoxin) of two major forms, SLT I and SLT II [71]. Serogroup 0157:H7 is particularly associated with epidemics of *E. coli*-mediated enterocolitis and these infections often occur through food (particularly infected meat of bovine origin) and water vehicles [72]. This serogroup, in particular, causes severe complications, especially the haemolytic–uraemic syndrome, with an attendant 5–10% mortality [73]. Whilst the pathological changes in the colon are well described [74], the small bowel also shows significant pathology. The bacterium is able to target the lymphoid tissue of the small bowel and produces a characteristic attaching/effacing lesion on the epithelial surface, by which it instigates an immune reaction that exacerbates the pathological effects [72]. There is evidence that tumour necrosis factor alpha (TNF-α) is important in this immune reaction [75] and anti-TNF monoclonal antibody has successfully reversed the effects of the bacterium in experimental animals [76].

A second group of *E. coli* associated with infective enteritis comprises the enteroinvasive *E. coli*. Infections with these bacteria have much in common with shigellosis and, in microbiological analysis, may be mistaken for them [51]. As their name implies, they are capable of cell invasion [77]. These are primarily infections of the colon and are described more fully elsewhere (see p. 475). The third major group of *E. coli* comprises the enteropathogenic *E. coli*, which are mainly responsible for outbreaks of diarrhoea in infants and neonates. They do not invade cells and do not produce SLT I and SLT II toxins. They have the ability to adhere to, and colonize, the mucosa of the small and large bowel, and this is the major mode of pathogenicity. The production of adherence antigens, termed CFA (colonization factor antigen) in human disease, appears to be genetically encoded in transmissible plasmids [51].

Clostridial infections and pseudomembranous ileocolitis

Clostridia are part of the normal flora of the large intestine and are also found in the distal part of the small intestine. These are potentially pathogenic but probably only after mucosal damage with necrosis of underlying tissues has occurred. Following infarction of the bowel, secondary clostridial infection may occur and may contribute to the haemorrhagic and haemolytic appearances frequently seen in infarcts. In fact it is likely that many cases of 'primary clostridial infection' represent secondary effects with ischaemia as the predominant pathology. Nevertheless significant primary clostridial infection does occur in the small bowel, although the exact relationship between the bacterial infection and any ischaemic pathology present is often uncertain [78]. The two most common small bowel manifestations of clostridial infection are *Clostridium perfringens* food poisoning and *C. difficile*-mediated pseudomembranous enterocolitis.

Although *C. difficile*-mediated disease is primarily colonic, there also may be an accompanying ileitis [79]. This is particularly seen in severe pseudomembranous colitis, especially occurring in the immunosuppressed, when extension of the disease into the distal ileum is commonplace. It is also well recognized as a complication of previous surgery, both colonic and ileal [80–82]. The pathophysiology of the disease involves the alteration of gut flora, especially in the colon, by antibiotic therapy and the overgrowth of toxin-producing *C. difficile* [79]. The toxins may be cytotoxic (toxin B) or enterotoxic (toxins A and C) [83]. The macroscopic and microscopic features of pseudomembranous ileitis are identical to those in the large intestine (see p. 516).

Pig-bel (or enteritis necroticans) is a focal necrotizing and inflammatory disease of the small intestine, especially in poorly nourished children, and is a major cause of morbidity in the highlands of Papua New Guinea where it often follows local pig feasting (hence its name) [84]. It is found elsewhere [85,86] and has been described in a well nourished white vegetarian in the UK [87]. It seems to be a very similar disease to *Darmbrand* (meaning 'fire bowels'), a necrotizing small bowel disease, epidemic in Northern Germany after World War II [88]. Serosal congestion, necrosis, bowel wall thinning and ultimately perforation are the characteristic macroscopic findings of enteritis necroticans, especially occurring in the jejunum [78]. Histologically there is infarction of the mucosa that can be clearly demarcated by a line of inflammatory cells from viable areas [89]. Haemorrhagic infarction and necrosis can extend through the bowel wall. Thrombosis of small vessels may be present and occasionally gas cysts [85,89]. This describes the most severe acute pattern of disease but there is a complete clinical and pathological spectrum with some patients having more chronic disease and surviving without surgery [85]. Resolution occurs and a subsequent stricture can develop [78]. Both pig-bel and *Darmbrand* are the result of *C. perfringens* infection, usually type C, in the small bowel [51,78].

Staphylococcal enteritis

Staphylococcus aureus toxin is responsible for some cases of 'food poisoning' and there may be response to appropriate antibiotics. The organism's role in the production of enterocolitis remains more controversial. Cases of necrotizing enterocolitis, purported to be due to staphylococci, both *S. aureus* and *S. epidermidis*, are still described in infants, especially after antibiotic administration [90,91]. Methicillin-resistant *S. aureus* (MRSA) may be especially responsible for such necrotizing and ulcerating enteritis [91]. Typically transverse linear ulcers occur throughout the small bowel and these may result in perforation [91]. However, in the past staphylococcus had been implicated in the genesis of necrotizing enteritis in adults because of the presence of large numbers of cocci lining necrotic ulcers in the small bowel [92,93]. In many of these cases, it remained uncertain whether the coccal bacteria were a primary cause or a secondary effect of ischaemic ulceration and necrosis. As these organisms can be found in 30% of healthy persons and 90% of those on certain antibiotics with no evidence of diarrhoea [93], the role of staphylococcus in the cause of ulcerating enteritis in patients other than very young children remains uncertain. Many such cases may well represent antibiotic-associated enteritis and are probably caused by bacteria other than staphylococcus, such as clostridia and *E. coli*.

Yersiniosis

The genus *Yersinia* includes two human enteric pathogens, *Yersinia enterocolitica* and *Yersinia pseudotuberculosis*. Both are important causes of mesenteric adenitis with or without inflammation of the terminal ileum and appendix [94,95]. *Y. enterocolitica*, however, can also cause a colitis and in some

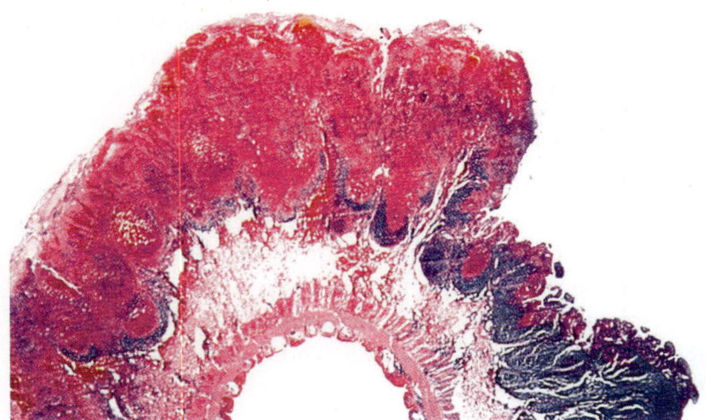

Fig. 21.4 A terminal ileal resection for acute-on-chronic yersiniosis. The thickening of the ileal wall is apparent, with ulceration of the mucosa over the hyperplastic lymphoid tissue.

countries, for instance Germany, Canada, New Zealand and Scandinavia, the organism can rival other bacteria described above as an important cause of acute enterocolitis [96,97]. It can cause an enteric fever-like syndrome with systemic illness, most usually in adults with significant comorbidity, especially chronic liver disease [98,99].

Epidemiological studies have shown that consumption of pork and contact with untreated sewage are important risk factors for yersinia infection [100,101]. Yersiniosis causing mesenteric adenitis is most common in children and young adults, especially boys [97,102]. Both *Y. enterocolitica* and *Y. pseudotuberculosis* cause a terminal ileitis and localized mesenteric adenitis, with thickening of the terminal ileum and local nodes being enlarged and matted together [94,103]. Involvement of the appendix is surprisingly uncommon, although when sequential serological samples were studied in a group of patients presenting with an acute abdomen, 31% of patients with proven *Y. pseudotuberculosis* were found to have appendicitis [104]. The clinical presentation of yersinia-related mesenteric adenitis may be indistinguishable from acute appendicitis. In terminal ileal acute yersiniosis (Fig. 21.4), the ileoscopic features may suggest Crohn's disease, especially as aphthoid ulceration, typically over lymphoid aggregates and Peyer's patches, is a characteristic feature [103]. The ulceration may be extensive and involve the adjacent caecum and, in fatal cases, it may involve the whole small and large intestine [94].

Yersiniosis is characterized by an acute-on-chronic histiocytic and granulomatous inflammation histologically, especially that caused by *Y. pseudotuberculosis* (Fig. 21.5). Granulomas are not such a conspicuous feature of *Y. enterocolitica* infection [1]. There appear to be four stages of disease: lymphoid hyperplasia, histiocytic hyperplasia, epithelioid granuloma formation and finally central granuloma necrosis (Fig. 21.5) [95]. These are best demonstrated in yersinial mesenteric adenitis. Firstly, there is a generalized reactive

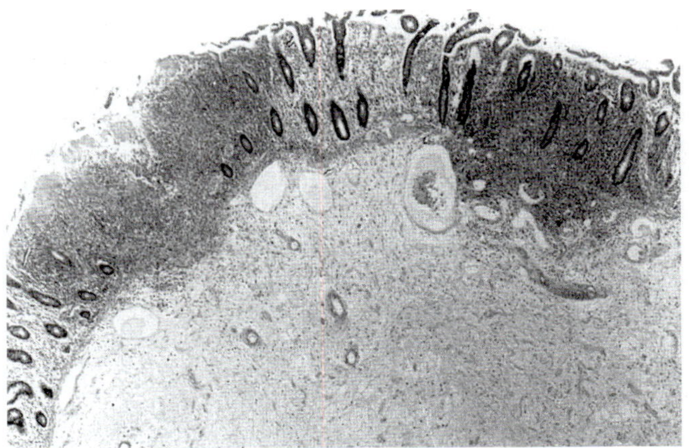

(a)

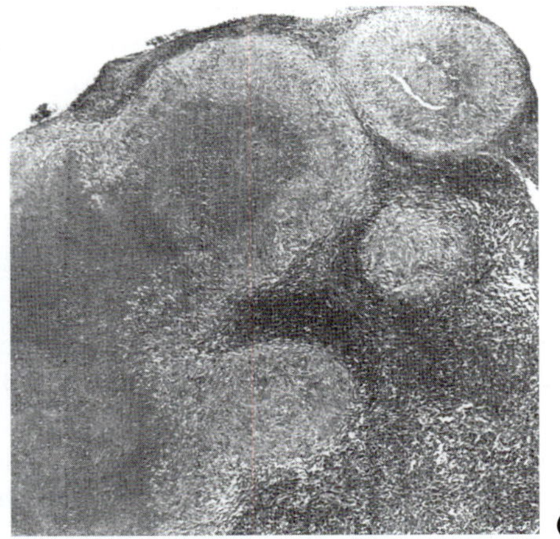

(b)

Fig. 21.5 (a) Yersinosis showing ulceration and necrosis of mucosal lymphoid follicles. (b) Mesentric lymph node in yersinia infection showing numerous granulomas with central necrosis surrounded by epitheloid cells.

hyperplasia with preservation of the normal architecture. Histiocytes are conspicuous and may produce a 'starry-sky' appearance. The formation of granulomas, often of geographical shapes and confluent, then supervenes. These often have a central necrotic zone infiltrated by polymorphs and forming a microabscess, surrounded by epithelioid cells and histiocytes (Fig. 21.5). This pattern of large geographical necrotizing granulomatosis is similar to that seen in other infective lymphadenitides, most notably cat scratch fever and lymphogranuloma venereum. Even giant cells of Langhans' type may be present. The granulomas are predominantly in paracortical zones, particularly in relation to lymphatic sinuses, and the surrounding capsule usually shows fibrous thickening. Colonies of Gram-negative organisms can be seen [103].

In the ileum and appendix, there is ulceration and focal chronic active inflammation, with or without necrotizing granulomas (Fig. 21.4). Evidence of granulomatous pathology is more likely in *Y. pseudotuberculosis* infection but is less likely to be seen in ileal biopsies than in involved mesenteric lymph nodes. When the disease is more pronounced, there may be evidence of deep ulceration and submucosal oedema, although involvement of the muscularis propria is unusual. Between 60 and 80% of cases of acute terminal ileitis are due to yersinia infection. When this is seen in ileal biopsies, especially in children and young adults and in the absence of clinical and radiological evidence of Crohn's disease, it is always advisable to suggest serology to confirm a diagnosis of yersiniosis as the histological features of ileal biopsies are often relatively non-specific [1].

Other bacterial causes of enteritis

Acute bacterial enteritis can be caused by *Klebsiella* infection [105], by *Pleisomonas* species and by *Aeromonas* species [106]. The latter bacterium is associated with increasing numbers of reports of acute enterocolitis, and infection has been related to the consumption of untreated water [107]. In children, it appears to be a relatively common cause of acute self-limiting diarrhoea [108] whilst in older adults, it may cause a more chronic enterocolitis [109].

Although strictly not an enteritis, in that it usually presents with an ileocaecal chronic inflammatory phlegmon, actinomycosis should always be considered in the differential diagnosis of chronic active inflammatory pathology affecting the terminal ileum and proximal colon, especially in women using an intrauterine contraceptive device. The disease can closely mimic Crohn's disease, both clinically and pathologically, and it may also, rarely, complicate Crohn's disease [110]. It is a cause of fistulation [111] and can also cause ileal strictures [112]. A Gram stain will reveal the causative filamentous Gram-positive bacilli, *Actinomyces israelii*, usually demonstrable in large colonies known as 'sulphur granules'.

Bacterial overgrowth in the small intestine

Bacterial overgrowth is increasingly recognized as a clinical syndrome, presenting with malabsorption, weight loss and diarrhoea [113] (see p. 337). It is primarily a disease of the elderly, in which case it is most often of unknown cause [114,115]. Nevertheless, small intestinal bacterial overgrowth is also caused by previous surgery, especially gastrectomy [116], small intestinal dysmotility [117], jejunal diverticulosis [118] and previous vagotomy [118]. Histopathology is not used as a primary diagnostic procedure in this disease as the changes are usually mild and non-specific and tend to undercall the severity of the functional abnormality of the small intestinal mucosa [119]. In fact breath testing for hydrogen is the preferred diagnostic modality. Nevertheless bacterial overgrowth does cause variable villous atrophy and minor chronic inflammatory changes in the mucosa and has the potential to mimic other causes of malabsorption [119,120]. Furthermore small intestinal bacterial overgrowth may cause elevated antigliadin antibody levels in small intestinal luminal secretions and has the potential therefore to cause overdiagnosis of coeliac disease [119].

Tuberculosis and other mycobacterial diseases

In Western pathological practice, intestinal tuberculosis remains rare, but there is no doubt that there has been a steady increase in the number of recorded cases in the last decade, in part related to increased immigration from countries where intestinal tuberculosis is endemic [121]. Furthermore AIDS has wrought a dramatic increase in systemic and localized tuberculosis in many parts of the world, and together they are a dangerous combination [121].

In one study in the UK, 84% of cases of intestinal tuberculosis were seen in immigrants, especially from the Asian subcontinent [122]. Within the immigrant Asian community the highest incidence of gastrointestinal involvement occurs in the years soon after arrival in the West. It is customary to divide intestinal tuberculosis into primary and secondary forms. In the first, ingested bacilli are believed to set up a primary reaction in the intestinal wall or mesenteric lymph nodes; in the second, the source is swallowed infected sputum from a primary lung lesion or a further oral dose of bacilli establishing a reinfection in an already sensitized individual. The latter used to be the commoner form but in more recent studies accounts for less than one half of all cases [122–124]. Intestinal tuberculosis is still more common in younger adults and somewhat commoner in females.

Acute intestinal tuberculosis usually presents as a severe enterocolitis (so-called dysenteric tuberculosis), especially in children. Free perforation leading to tuberculous peritonitis is a common complication of acute disease. The macroscopic appearances of intestinal tuberculosis vary considerably according to the acuteness and severity of the infection and the stage of disease. Areas of involvement, often multiple, are found with increasing frequency from the jejunum to the ileum, being particularly common in the terminal ileum and ileocaecal area [125,126]. This distribution follows the localization of lymphoid tissue in the small intestine. Ulcerative intestinal tuberculosis, as its name implies, presents as one or more annular circular or oval ulcers lying transversely, raised above the normal mucosa and usually producing a stricture (Fig. 21.6) [126,127]. It is a characteristic of intestinal tuberculosis that single ulcers are relatively large whilst multiple ulcers are usually much smaller [123,127]. The appearances of the cut surface of the affected bowel depend on the stage of the disease. In acute ulcerating tuberculosis, caseation is usually definable and there may be evidence of miliary tuberculosis on the peritoneal surface [123]. Regional lymph nodes are usually enlarged and show caseation on the cut surface [128]. Later-stage disease gives rise to dense fibrosis and strictures (Fig. 21.7) [126]. It is such strictures with bowel obstruction that predispose to perforation in chronic intestinal tuberculosis [129]. These chronic cases are also prone to fistulae and ileocaecal

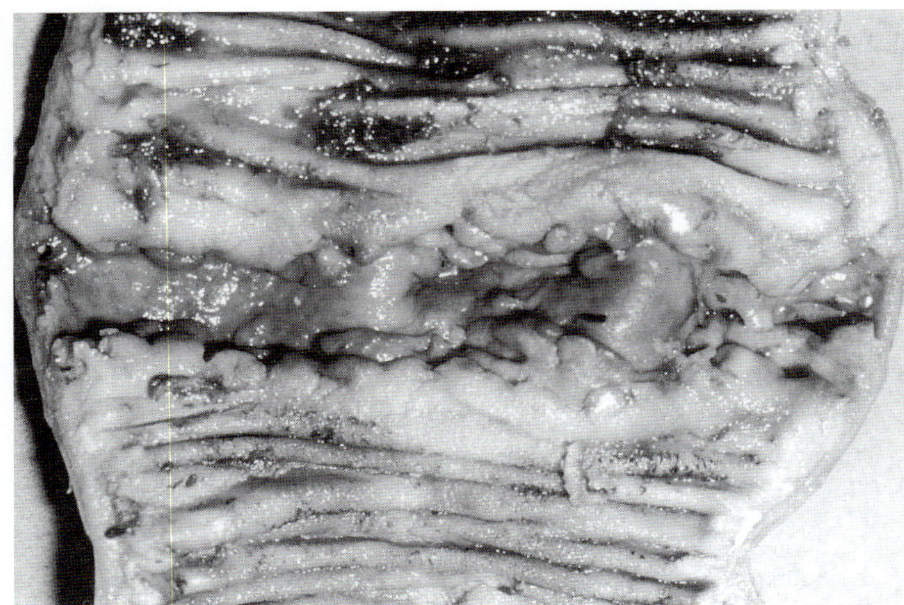

Fig. 21.6 Transverse ulceration of the ileum in tuberculosis.

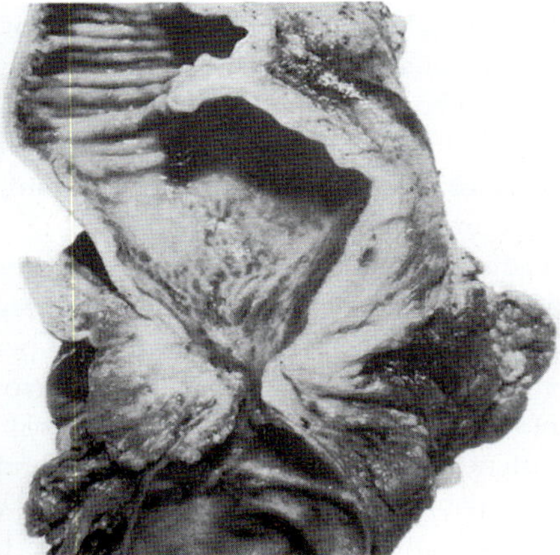

Fig. 21.7 Chronic intestinal tuberculosis with stricturing and fibrosis.

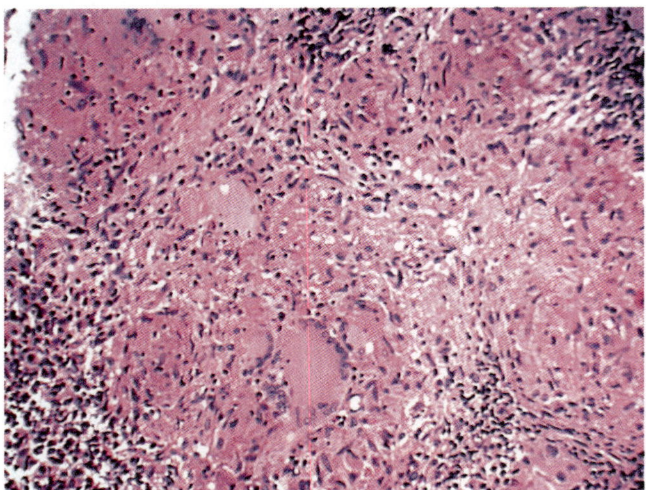

Fig. 21.8 Coalescent epithelioid cell granulomas in intestinal tuberculosis. Langhans' giant cells are present.

inflammatory masses, the pathological features combining to induce mimicry of Crohn's disease [130,131]. However, in countries where tuberculosis is endemic, notably India, tuberculosis is the commonest cause of small intestinal stricture [121].

The microscopic appearances of intestinal tuberculosis also vary with the stage of the disease. It is not appropriate to give a detailed description of the morphological features of intestinal tuberculosis because they do not differ significantly from those of tuberculosis elsewhere. Coalescent (Fig. 21.8) and caseating granulomas are seen in all layers of the bowel wall and in regional nodes, but are especially seen in Peyer's patches and lymphoid follicles [128]. In more chronic disease, caseation may not be a feature and the pathology is dominated by dense fibrosis with destruction of the normal tissues of the bowel wall, including the muscularis propria. In very chronic lesions, the granulomas become hyalinized and eventually disappear, leaving behind only small aggregates of lymphocytes, an excess of fibrous tissue and, sometimes, 'tombstones' of effete coalescent granulomas. Then, the appearances can closely mimic chronic or burnt-out Crohn's disease with the associated mucosal (ulcer-associated cell lineage) and connective tissue changes (including vascular, neural and muscular changes) [132]. The principal microscopic features that separate tuberculosis from Crohn's disease are a relative lack of fissuring, coalescence of granulomas with caseation, lack of submucosal oedema, the presence of small serosal tubercles and, clinically, the rarity of anal lesions [127]. Examination of regional lymph nodes is particularly important, as they can show better any evidence of former tuberculous infection. In our experience the regional lymph nodes nearly always contain granulomas in intestinal tuberculosis, while these are relatively infrequent in Crohn's disease.

Acid-fast bacilli can usually be found, on Ziehl–Neelsen (ZN) staining, in intestinal tuberculosis when there is caseous necrosis, although their detection may require a prolonged search. However, in chronic fibrosing and stricturing tuberculosis, demonstrable mycobacteria may be very scanty or absent. In this situation, it is imperative that ZN stains are performed on involved regional lymph nodes, as these are much more liable to harbour organisms.

Tuberculosis is a major problem in AIDS patients in places where TB is endemic such as Africa: it is a major determinant in death in up to 40% of AIDS patients there [133]. However, in Western countries, atypical mycobacteriosis, predominantly caused by *M. avium-intracellulare* (MAI) is more important. The small bowel is a site of predilection for this opportunistic infection and it appears that the gastrointestinal tract is an early, possibly primary, site of colonization [43,134]. The disease is a late manifestation in AIDS, usually occurring when the CD4 count falls below 100/dL [135]. In autopsy studies evidence of MAI infection is demonstrated in about 50% of cases but only about 10% of AIDS patients with diarrhoea will demonstrate the organism [135,136]. MAI infection causes a granulomatous reaction in which foamy macrophages predominate (Fig. 21.9). These are periodic acid–Schiff (PAS) positive and thus may closely mimic Whipple's disease [43,137]. Sometimes the changes are very subtle with just scanty collections of foamy histiocytes in the lamina propria. In known AIDS patients with any form of histiocytic infiltrate in small bowel biopsies, a ZN stain is imperative as this will demonstrate the (often large numbers of) mycobacteria and will help to refute a diagnosis of Whipple's disease (Fig. 21.10) [138]. The importance of a search, in such biopsies, for other infecting organisms in AIDS is once again emphasized: MAI infection is often coexistent with other infections, especially CMV and cryptosporidiosis [22].

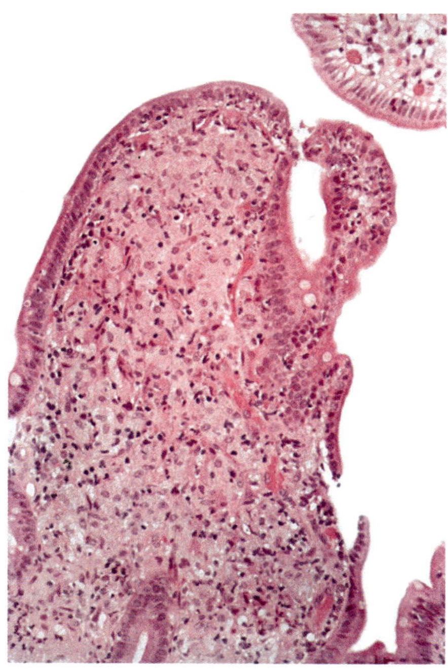

Fig. 21.9 The histology of small intestinal *M. avium-intracellulare* infection in AIDS. There is an ill-defined granulomatous infiltrate with numerous foamy macrophages.

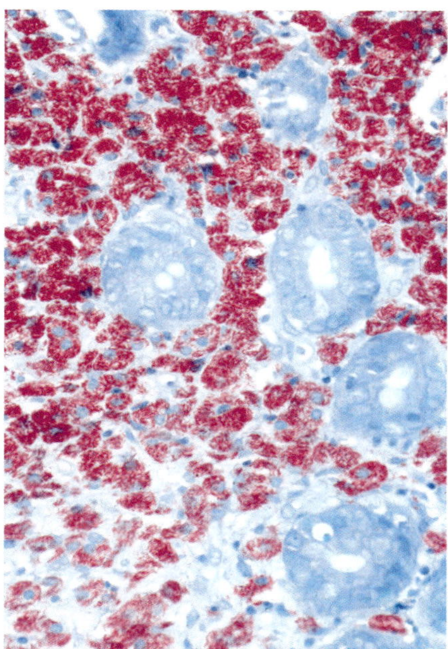

Fig. 21.10 A Ziehl–Neelsen stain of *M. avium-intracellulare* infection in AIDS demonstrates innumerable acid-fast bacilli.

Whipple's disease

Whipple's disease was first described in 1907 by George Hoyt Whipple, who christened the alternative title of 'intestinal lipodystrophy' in the mistaken belief that the disease was an abnormality of lipid metabolism [139]. It is now recognized as a multisystemic chronic disease of infective (indeed bacterial) aetiology. The disease mostly affects middle-aged men, with a male to female ratio of 8:1, who present with weight loss, malabsorption, diarrhoea, arthralgia and abdominal pain [140]. The disease has a propensity to systemic involvement, with lymphadenopathy and cardiac (especially endocarditis), pulmonary and central nervous system involvement all well described. Nevertheless, it primarily involves the intestines, particularly the small intestine, and the disease is most usually diagnosed by small bowel (either duodenal or jejunal) biopsy. The disease does involve the large intestine and rectal biopsies can also reveal the characteristic pathological appearances [141].

Whipple originally demonstrated rod-shaped structures within the cytoplasm of macrophages in the disease [139] but, for many years, the causative organism could not be identified. This was mainly due to its refusal to grow on recognized microbiological media. In fact it took the development of molecular biological techniques, specifically polymerase chain reaction (PCR) and sequencing, to allow the identification of the causative organism [142,143] as a specific actinomycete, and the genus *Tropheryma* (Greek for barrier to nourishment) *whippelii* proposed [143]. The bacillary nature of the organism had been previously identified as a Gram-positive rod and was

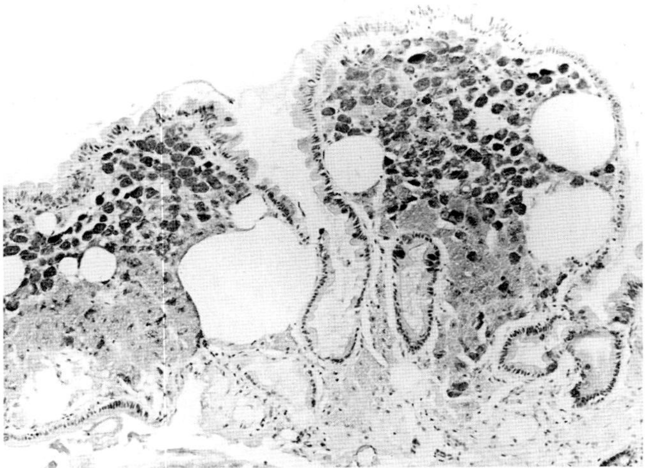

(a)

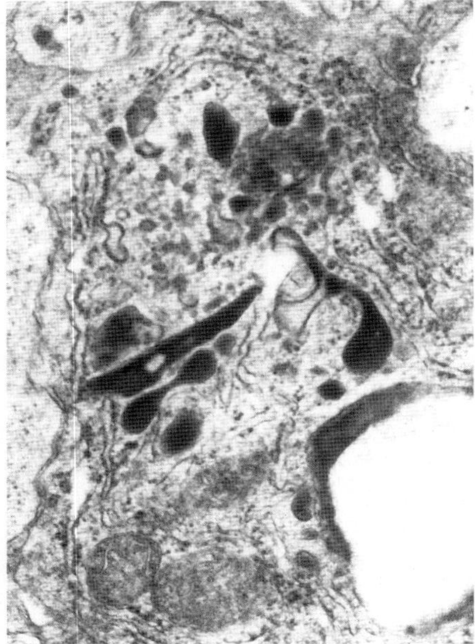

(b)

Fig. 21.11 Whipple's disease in a duodenal biopsy. (a) Section stained by PAS. The villi are expanded by PAS-positive macrophages and large vacuoles. (b) Electron microscopy shows the intracytoplasmic rod-shaped structures, now confirmed as bacteria.

shown to be present within the cytoplasm of affected histiocytes by electron microscopy (Fig. 21.11) [144,145]. That the disease is a primary infection of the gut caused by an environmental bacterium has been further supported by the demonstration of bacterial gene products in waste water supplies from sewerage works [146].

Whilst the disease can be now regarded as an infection caused by a Gram-positive actinomycete, it is clear that the disease is associated with profound immunological defects which allow the survival of the bacteria within macrophages, the build-up of which causes many of the deleterious effects of the disease [147]. The immunological defects in Whipple's disease are almost unique, with a diminution of immunocompetent B cells despite the massive histiocytic influx [148,149]. There are also abnormalities of T-cell function, with reduced CD4 : CD8 ratios, a shift towards mature T-cell populations, increased T-cell activation and decreased T-cell-mediated responses [150,151]. There are also abnormalities of histiocytic function, as would be expected from the pathological appearances, with evidence of reduced histiocytic phagocytic activity [151] and reduced macrophage production of interleukin-12, a cytokine with important cell-mediated immune response regulation [152,153]. However, none of these features provides definitive evidence of a primary immunological abnormality to explain a predilection to infection by *T. whippelii* in Whipple's disease patients. It still seems more logical to reason that the bacterial infection causes secondary immunological abnormalities, in susceptible individuals, which enhance the pathological effects of the infection [147,154].

The small bowel affected by Whipple's disease shows characteristic, and sometimes highly specific, macroscopic features. Erosions are common, but yellow plaques and pale yellow shaggy mucosa are considered highly suggestive of Whipple's disease [155]. At laparotomy, the affected small bowel serosa is lined by exudate and the intestine appears thickened, dilated and rigid. The mesentery is also thickened and there is lymphadenopathy. There may also be peritoneal plaques [156].

Histologically there is usually a degree of villous atrophy on examination of small bowel biopsies, whilst the lamina propria is greatly expanded by numerous pale-staining histiocytes. These contain abundant PAS-positive granular material, representing the intracellular bacilli (Fig. 21.11). Whilst the diagnosis remains primarily a pathological endeavour, PCR is now regarded as a useful confirmatory test [157]. Furthermore, cases are described where gastrointestinal symptomatology and intestinal involvement is minimal [158,159], or focal [160]. Such cases underpin the importance of PCR, either on duodenal biopsies or on other specimens: positive PCR results have been described on analysis of faeces, peripheral blood cells, lymph node biopsies and cerebrospinal fluid from patients with Whipple's disease [161–164]. More recently PCR for the *hsp65* gene has been proposed as a suitable target for *T. whippelii* detection [165].

The disease has demonstrated an excellent response to antibiotic therapy for many years. Whilst tetracycline has been the mainstay of treatment, relapse is well described [155] and many now use multiple antibiotic regimes. These have included penicillin and streptomycin and, more recently, trimethoprim and sulphamethoxazole, the latter being the recommended treatment now [166,167]. PCR has been advocated as an excellent means of assessing response to treatment and the diagnosis of relapse [168], not least because PAS-positive histiocytes may remain in the small intestinal mucosa for many years after treatment and thus histology may not be a useful means for diagnosing relapse [169]. Such relapses usually occur only a few years after treatment and are accompanied by a re-emergence of viable bacteria [167]. Some patients remain refractory to antibiotic treatment and may require both comprehensive antibiotic regimes and immunomodulatory therapy [170].

For the pathologist, Whipple's disease provides a striking pathological picture, enhanced by PAS histochemistry, electron microscopy and PCR analysis (Fig. 21.11). Nevertheless it is important to emphasize that other conditions may mimic Whipple's disease. Certainly the most important differential diagnosis is that of mycobacterial infection in AIDS, specifically that by MAI, in which numerous pale-staining histiocytes characteristically pack the distended lamina propria of the intestines [137]. A ZN stain is an important analysis in this situation as it does not stain *T. whippelii* [137]. Other histiocytic accumulations may also mimic Whipple's disease in rectal biopsies [171]. Occasionally aggregations of histiocytes in the small intestine may also resemble sarcoidosis, and even Crohn's disease, on biopsy [172].

Fungal infection

Fungal infection of the small intestine is rare: it is virtually never primary and usually occurs in the severely immunocompromised. In these patient groups, in the UK at least, candidiasis and aspergillosis are most commonly seen [173]. Candidiasis can occur in the small bowel in AIDS [174] and can result in perforation [175]. Macroscopically these fungal infections usually present with ulceration, irregular shaggy mucosal surfaces resembling pseudomembranous enterocolitis or inflammatory masses [173]. Histologically, *Candida* is usually detectable in the surface ulcer debris whilst *Aspergillus* is more likely to be demonstrated in and around submucosal blood vessels [173].

The association of ulceration with extensive fungal involvement of intramural blood vessels is also a feature of mucormycosis in the small bowel. This fungal infection, caused by *Mucor* and *Rhizopus* species, is once again only effectively seen in the immunosuppressed, particularly children [176,177], although it is curiously rare as a complication of AIDS [178]. The fungal hyphae are characteristically broad and irregular, rarely septate and show irregular branching: these features help to differentiate *Mucor* from *Aspergillus*.

Pneumocystis carinii can very rarely involve the small intestine. Although there remains some doubt about its phylogeny, evidence now favours the view that the organism is a fungus [179]. Involvement of the small intestine is, apparently, uniquely in the profoundly immunosuppressed, especially those with advanced AIDS: the bowel wall involvement can be transmural, which can lead to fatal perforation of the small bowel [180,181].

Histoplasmosis, caused by the dimorphic fungus *Histoplasma capsulatum*, involves the small intestine in its disseminated form [182]. In the latter case, it is usually associated with immunosuppression and is particularly common in AIDS patients [183]. Occasionally disseminated histoplasmosis can cause malabsorption as a result of small intestinal involvement [184]. The histological appearances vary according to the level of immunocompromise present: in advanced AIDS there may be little cellular reaction, extensive necrosis and numerous typical capsulate yeast forms of the fungus. Morphologically the fungus measures about 3 μm in diameter and resembles *Leishmania*. It is often weakly birefringent in polarized light and is well demonstrated with the PAS stain.

Protozoal infection

Several species of protozoa infect the small intestine primarily, causing diarrhoea and/or malabsorption. All are particularly associated with immunosuppression, especially AIDS, but it is increasingly realized that several species also cause enteropathy in the immunocompetent: this is particularly the case with cryptosporidiosis, microsporidiosis and cyclosporidiosis [185]. Giardiasis is the most commonly recognized protozoal infection of the small bowel in histopathological practice. Many of the other infections are more likely to be demonstrated by microbiological means: histopathologists are rarely asked to diagnose some of the more unusual protozoal infections, except in the context of advanced AIDS [38].

Giardiasis

Infection by *Giardia lamblia* (or *duodenalis*), a motile flagellate protozoan, is the most common small intestinal protozoal infection worldwide [186]. The disease usually presents with diarrhoea and it is curiously commoner in males than females [187]. There is pronounced variation in the clinical response to the infection, from an asymptomatic carrier state to debilitating chronic diarrhoea and malabsorption [186,188,189]. The infection is most often related to infected water supplies and epidemics are well described. Giardiasis is particularly associated with immunological deficiency, most notably with hypogammaglobulinaemia [190] and AIDS [22]. In these diseases, there is often evidence of extremely heavy colonization by the protozoan.

The mechanism by which giardiasis causes diarrhoea and malabsorption remains poorly understood; direct physical injury by the parasite, release of parasite products such as lectins and enzymes and mucosal inflammation due to cytokine release have all been postulated [186]. Nevertheless, whilst an increased intraepithelial T-cell infiltrate is on occasion demonstrated in small intestinal biopsies, there is little evidence of activation of cytotoxic T cells [191]. Ultimately, it is likely that the pathogenesis of giardiasis is multifactorial [192].

In biopsies, the parasites are usually demonstrated in clusters in the lumen, on or adjacent to the superficial epithelial surface (Fig. 21.12). They appear as sickle-shaped, slightly basophilic structures, often with a greyish nucleus. Flagella may be demonstrable at high power. A Giemsa preparation stains the organism well but, in normal or heavy infestation, such special stains are usually not required. Whilst varying degrees of villous atrophy, chronic inflammation in the lamina propria and modest intraepithelial lymphocytosis are all seen in duodenal biopsies with giardiasis, it is important to emphasize that in most cases (96% in one series) the duodenal mucosa appears normal [187]. Thus a search for the parasite should be undertaken in all duodenal biopsies in patients presenting with diarrhoea and malabsorption, whether the biopsies are morphologically normal or not [187]. Furthermore the protozoan may be detected in gastric, jejunal, ileal and colonic mucosa; these mucosae are also usually normal histologically [187]. The presence of giardiasis may presage immunocompromise and a search for other infecting organisms is especially important in AIDS and hypogammaglobulinaemia. Outside of these conditions, there is a strong positive association between giardiasis and gastric *Helicobacter* infection [187].

Coccidiosis

The gut coccidia represent a group of obligate intracellular protozoan parasites, four species of which are human pathogens: *Cryptosporidium*, *Cyclospora*, *Isospora* and *Sarcocystis*. The first three are especially associated with enteropathy and diarrhoea in AIDS, but it must be emphasized that all are increasingly recognized as causing diarrhoea, especially in epidemics and/or as traveller's diarrhoea, in the immunocompetent [185].

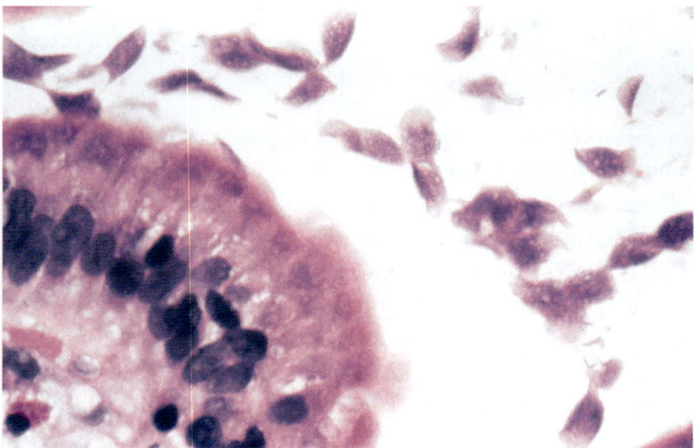

Fig. 21.12 A duodenal biopsy showing innumerable *Giardia lamblia* protozoa. They appear as clustered, sickle-shaped, slightly basophilic structures adjacent to the surface of the epithelium.

Cryptosporidiosis

Cryptosporidium parvum is the only type of this genus known to infect humans [193] although a murine cryptosporidium has been detected in otherwise healthy children [194]. The primary site of infection is the upper small bowel, although the disease is most often diagnosed microbiologically in stool samples. While a characteristic and prevalent feature in AIDS patients, cryptosporidiosis is increasingly associated with outbreaks of diarrhoea in the immunocompetent, especially due to contaminated water supplies, and it is also a cause of traveller's diarrhoea [51]. In the immunocompetent, the disease is self-limiting with the organisms spontaneously clearing after a few weeks as the cryptosporidia are, in this situation, minimally invasive mucosal pathogens [193].

In AIDS, cryptosporidiosis is the commonest cause of diarrhoea in the UK [22], occurring in about 21% of patients [195], and in about 15% of US patients [196]. In Haiti and in Africa up to 50% of AIDS patients are infected [21]. The small bowel mucosa shows strikingly variable changes that correlate with a highly variable clinical picture from minor symptoms, through a cholera-like acute enteritis, to chronic diarrhoea. The symptomatology and morphological changes also correlate with the oocyst concentration in the stool [197]. Whilst in most AIDS patients with cryptosporidiosis the small intestinal mucosa is normal, those with the most severe symptoms show pronounced villous atrophy with an intense neutrophilic infiltration [198]. Such severe cryptosporidial enteritis is often associated with coinfection, particularly with cytomegalovirus [199]. Extensive involvement of the small and large bowel with heavy oocyst load correlates with the most severe clinical features [199]. The pathogenesis of the enteritis remains poorly understood in both the immunocompetent and the immunocompromised [200]. In AIDS patients there may also be involvement of the stomach, biliary tract and, particularly, the colon [21].

The coccidian, in histological sections, is recognized by its proximity to the epithelial surface, being attached to the microvillous border of the epithelial cells of the small bowel (Figs 21.2 & 21.13) [21]. The organism becomes internalized within the cytoplasm by extension of the cytoplasm around it [201]. In AIDS, the organisms have been shown to enter the lamina propria and may also be found within the cytoplasm of M cells and macrophages [201]. The oocysts measure between 4.5 and 6 μm in diameter and are ZN negative in histological sections (although they are positive in modified ZN stains in stool samples). They are stained by Giemsa. Probably the most

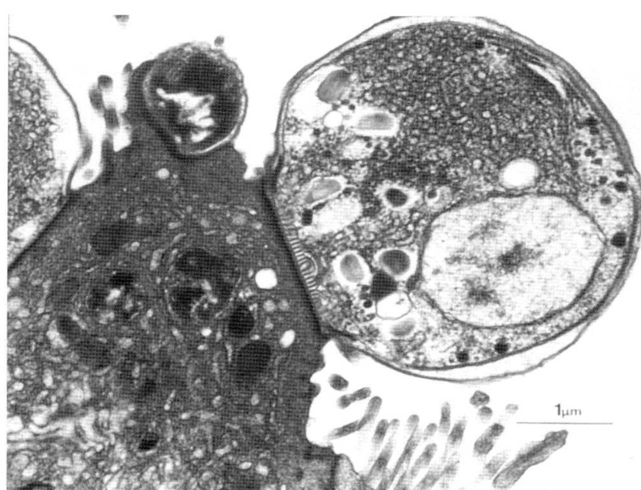

Fig. 21.13 Electron microscopy of a *Cryptosporidium parvum* coccidian. It is attached to the microvillous border of the epithelial cell of the duodenum.

useful special stains are mucin stains, which help to differentiate the organisms from blobs of mucin, the most likely confounding histopathological feature.

Isosporiasis

Like cryptosporidium, *Isospora belli* is an upper small bowel pathogen that is a relatively common cause of enteropathy in tropical countries. It is an unusual cause of diarrhoea in the immunocompetent in Western countries, although sporadic outbreaks are described in the USA [202]. It accounts for only about 2% of cases of chronic diarrhoea in AIDS patients in Western populations but up to 15–20% in countries such as Haiti and in Africa [21]. Unlike cryptosporidia, isospora organisms are internalized within the enterocyte cytoplasm, and are readily detected here by high-power light microscopy and by electron microscopy. Nevertheless the diagnosis is usually achieved microbiologically by examining stools with a modified ZN stain. In AIDS patients, it may cause severe diarrhoea and can, on occasion, become systemic [203].

Cyclosporidiosis

Cyclospora cayetanensis is increasingly recognized as cause of diarrhoea, especially in travellers to Nepal, the Caribbean and Central America [204–207]. Once again, this coccidian primarily involves the proximal small bowel and may be demonstrated in duodenal biopsies [208]. Heavy infection may cause inflammation and epithelial injury with villous blunting [209,210]. The infection results in a cyclical pattern of diarrhoea (hence the name), lasting 6–8 weeks [209], although this is more prolonged in the immunosuppressed, especially in AIDS [211]. It can be caused by infected water supplies [212] but, in the US at least, it is particularly associated with infected imported fruit, especially berries [213].

The diagnosis is usually achieved by parasitological examination of the stool [214]. In histological sections, the parasites are visible, with difficulty, within the cytoplasm of enterocytes, where 2–3-μm schizonts and the 5-μm elongated merozoites are visible at high power, with experience, especially in thick sections [215]. They are smaller than *Isospora* and not PAS positive [215]. Co-trimoxazole usually results in rapid relief of symptoms, although relapses occur, particularly in AIDS patients [209].

Sarcosporidiosis

Sarcocystis hominis is the least common of the human coccidial small intestinal infections, in Western countries at least [185]. It is only rarely associated with AIDS and then usually in tropical countries [185].

Microsporidiosis

These obligate intracellular parasites remain of uncertain phylogeny, although they are generally considered closely related to other coccidioses [216]. There are five genera, although just two species commonly involve the small bowel, especially in AIDS patients. These are *Enterocytozoon bieneusi* and *Septata intestinalis* [217–219]. Infection, causing diarrhoea, does occur in the immunocompetent, usually from infected water supplies [219], but the disease is most readily recognized by pathologists in the small intestinal epithelium of AIDS patients [43]. Sophisticated microbiological methods of diagnosis, including PCR, are now available and pathological examination is becoming less often required [216,220].

The pathological features of microsporidial infection are subtle and require experience to demonstrate: indeed the complex life cycle of the protozoon and the difficulties associated with the light microscopic demonstration of the disease make the diagnosis the realm of experts [43]: only a brief description of the major changes is appropriate here. Electron microscopic examination has been important for the understanding of the different stages of parasite development and thus for light microscopic diagnosis (Fig. 21.14) [43]. Furthermore semithin resin-embedded sections will demonstrate the parasite better than routine sections (Fig. 21.14). The duodenal mucosa often shows villous blunting and feathering of the surface epithelium at the tips of the villi. Three stages of the coccidian's life cycle can be recognized histologically. *E. bieneusi* shows meronts, sporonts and spores, the former two appearing as haematoxyphilic intracytoplasmic bodies (Fig. 21.14) and the latter as 1-μm diameter intracytoplasmic bodies. *S. intestinalis* is characterized by numerous intracytoplasmic spores separated by granular material (hence the name *Septata*) [43]. In some AIDS cases, *E. bieneusi* spores have been demonstrated within the lamina propria, although this is not commonly associated with systemic infection [221]. On the other hand, systemic dissemination is described in *S. intestinalis* infection [217].

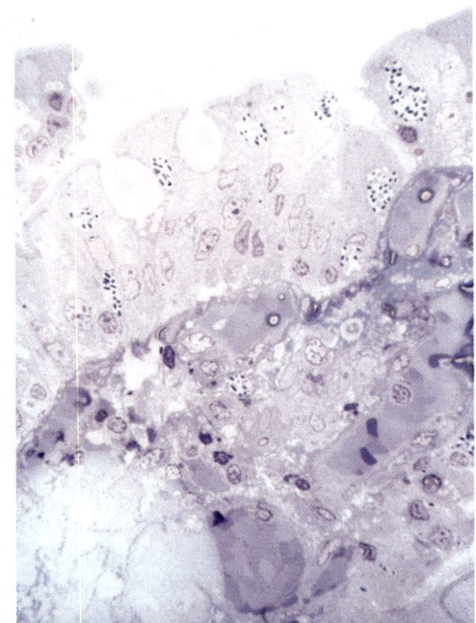

(a)

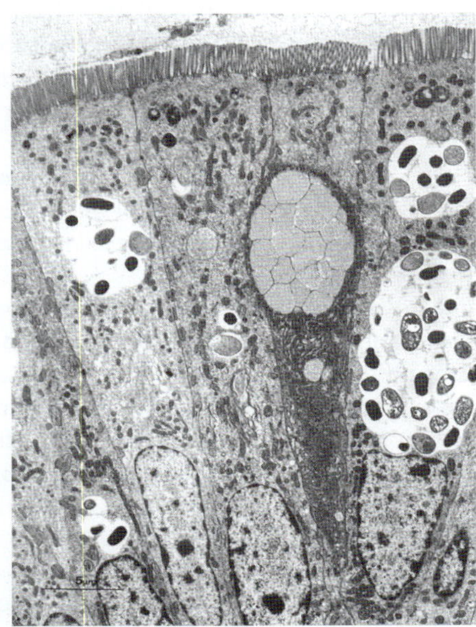

(b)

Fig. 21.14 Microsporidiosis in the small intestine. This is infection by *Enterocytozoon bieneusi* in an AIDS patient. (a) Semithin resin-embedded sections demonstrate the intracellular meronts and sporonts much better than routine sections. (b) Electron microscopy shows the numerous meronts and sporonts.

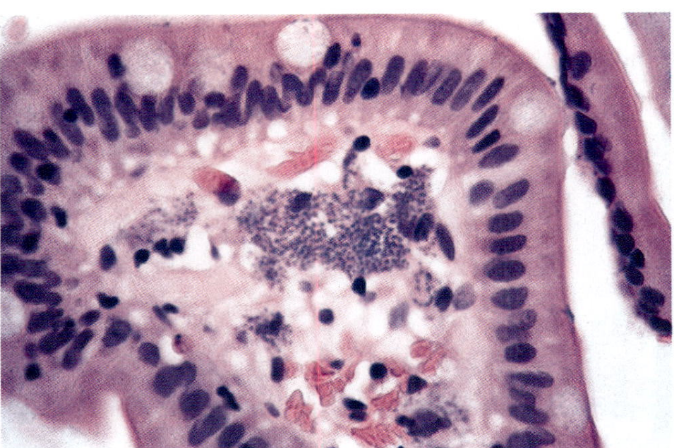

Fig. 21.15 *Leishmania donovani* infection in the duodenal mucosa of an AIDS patient. There are numerous Leishman–Donovan bodies within the cytoplasm of intralaminal macrophages.

Leishmaniasis

Visceral leishmaniasis can involve the small intestine but Western pathologists very rarely see the disease at this site. However, the spectrum of leishmanial infection has been changed dramatically by HIV/AIDS and there has been a European epidemic of visceral leishmaniasis in AIDS patients, despite the fact that the disease is not endemic [215, 222, 223]. HIV-associated visceral leishmaniasis presents with fever, diarrhoea and hepatosplenomegaly and is associated with a high mortality in those untreated [223]. Mucosal biopsies from the small bowel reveal innumerable histiocytes within the lamina propria packed by classical Leishman–Donovan bodies (Fig. 21.15), representing the amastigotes of *Leishmania donovani* [215]. Whilst techniques such as PCR have been successfully applied to the diagnosis of leishmaniasis [215], the diagnosis is usually very straightforward, once the possibility has been entertained, because of the number and characteristic morphology of the parasites. Special stains are not normally required.

Other protozoa

Amoebiasis, caused by *Entamoeba histolytica*, and the ciliate protozoan, *Balantidium coli*, can both involve the small intestine, especially the terminal ileum, and may be seen in ileoscopic biopsies. Nevertheless the colorectum is the primary site of infection and large intestinal biopsies are much more likely to detect these parasites. Similarly Chagas' disease, chronic infection with *Trypanosoma cruzi*, can involve the small intestine with enteromegaly, neuropathy, loss of myenteric ganglia and muscle hypertrophy of the small bowel [224]. However, it is doubtful whether small bowel disease ever occurs in the absence of more marked disease in the oesophagus and colon; clinical and pathological features are usually much more marked in these organs than in the small intestine.

Helminthic infection

A large number of helminthic infections can involve the small intestine. These commonly present with lassitude, abdominal pain, diarrhoea and anaemia, the latter a typical presentation of hookworms. The diagnosis of helminthic infection is usually made by microbiological investigation of the stool. Nevertheless some infections may be demonstrated in histological specimens, both duodenal and ileal biopsies, and in resection specimens. Strongyloidiasis and schistosomiasis are perhaps the most commonly encountered, although hookworm larvae and ascariasis may be demonstrated in biopsy specimens. Because these diseases are not often encountered in histopathological practice, the interested reader should consult specialist texts for more comprehensive descriptions of these helminths, their life cycles and their morphological and histopathological appearances [225–227].

Hookworms

Hookworm infestation is commonly caused by *Ankylostoma duodenale* in Southern Europe, Asia and the Middle East and by *Necator americanus* in Africa and the American continents, though mixed infections are common [225]. The disease infects around 1.3 billion people worldwide and about 100 million of these suffer profound long-term morbidity as a result of the infestation [228]. Patients with severe hookworm infestation present with anaemia due to profound blood loss from the small intestine. The blood loss, and subsequent anaemia, appear to be directly proportional to the number of adult worms in the bowel [229]. Most patients do not suffer from true malabsorption and probably have a normal small intestinal mucosa [230]. However, infestation in some has been associated with a malabsorption syndrome, with shortening and broadening of the villi, many of which have a club-shaped appearance; these morphological changes are said to revert to normal if the disease is successfully treated [231]. The worms have characteristic features seen in jejunal or duodenal fluid and are visible on the mucosa in biopsies [225].

Ascariasis

Ascaris lumbricoides is the most common and largest nematode infecting the human gastrointestinal tract [232]. The worms are ingested as ova in infected food or drink. Hatched larvae penetrate the intestinal mucosa and reach the lung via the portal system. Here they develop further before being coughed up and swallowed. The worms then develop in the small intestine and the adult worms, which may be up to 20 cm long, can inhabit any part of the small bowel. The geographical distribution of ascariasis is worldwide, although it is commoner in tropical countries [233]. The disease is usually asymptomatic but concentrations of the large worms in the small intestine can cause obstruction, volvulus and even appendicitis [234–236]. More sinister is the worm's ability to migrate into ducts, especially the pancreatic and biliary ducts, where the parasites are a recognized cause of pancreatitis, biliary obstruction and hepatic pathology [232,237].

Anisakiasis

Infection by the helminths *Anisakis* are increasingly recognized in the small intestine and, more particularly, in the stomach [238]. *Anisakis simplex* is most often implicated and this worm has been recognized as a cause of allergic gastroenteritis with or without anaphylaxis, eosinophilic gastroenteritis and intestinal obstruction [238–240]. The disease is particularly associated with the ingestion of raw fish and its gastric manifestations are most readily encountered in Japan [241].

Capillariasis

Infection with the small nematode, *Capillaria philippinensis*, is mainly restricted to south-eastern Asia, especially the Philippines and Thailand, although it is now well recognized in other parts of Asia and in Egypt [227,242]. The disease has also been described in patients from non-endemic areas [243]. A range of symptoms occur, depending on the parasite population, but severe infection produces diarrhoea, malabsorption with wasting, and sometimes death. The worm, 3–4 mm long, may be demonstrated embedded in jejunal mucosa. Humans are infected by ingestion of raw freshwater fish [242].

Schistosomiasis

Intestinal schistosomiasis is classically associated with infection with the trematode *Schistosoma mansoni*. However, less commonly *S. haematobium* can involve the intestines, as can *S. japonicum* in eastern Asia. However, in all forms of schistosomiasis, large bowel involvement is much commoner than small bowel pathology [244–246]. Small intestinal involvement by schistosomiasis can mimic Crohn's disease, with small bowel stricturing, or tuberculosis, with extensive transmural fibrosis and small white serosal nodules resembling milia, or alternatively present with malabsorption [244,247,248]. Schistosomal polyposis does not occur in the small bowel. Microscopically the ova with their characteristic morphology (see p. 485), especially their spines, are surrounded by a granulomatous reaction in which epithelioid cells, giant cells, lymphocytes and sometimes eosinophils predominate [225].

Strongyloidiasis

Strongyloides stercoralis is a small nematode that inhabits the upper small bowel. Its distribution is worldwide and its prevalence rate may reach up to 80% in lower socioeconomic groups of the developing countries [249]. Indigenous cases are well described in Western countries [250,251]. The helminth is almost unique in its ability to remain dormant in the small intestine for many years and reactivate, often with hyperinfestation, especially in immunocompromised hosts [249]. The disease is particularly seen in veterans of the Far Eastern cam-

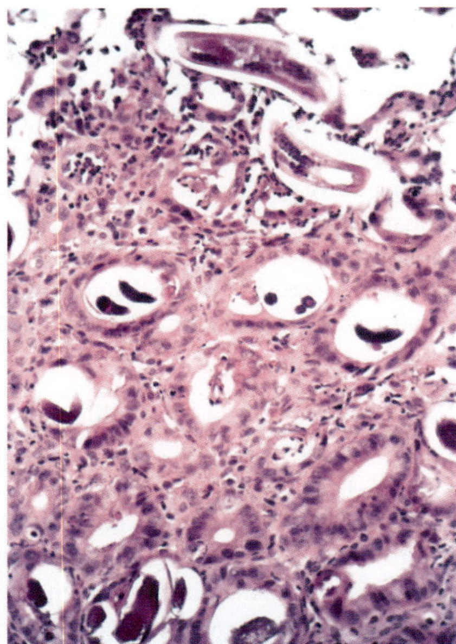

Fig. 21.16 Hyperinfestation of the duodenal mucosa with *Strongyloides stercoralis* larvae. They are characteristically seen within the lumina of crypts.

paign of World War II, who have been shown to be carrying the worm up to 40 years later [252,253].

Primary infection presents with abdominal pain and diarrhoea; around 90% of patients will demonstrate a peripheral eosinophilia. The worm is small, measuring 2–3 mm long, and the female is demonstrated in the crypts of the duodenal and jejunal mucosa (Fig. 21.16). The male nematode is seldom seen. Biopsy findings are variable but there may be villous atrophy that reverts to normal after therapy. Malabsorption is rare in the primary infection. Hyperinfection with strongyloidiasis is associated with immunocompromise, such as in patients treated for neoplastic disease or in AIDS. Perhaps surprisingly, *Strongyloides* hyperinfection has not been as common as might be expected in AIDS patients [249]. In hyperinfection, there is massive proliferation of rhabtidiform larvae of *S. stercoralis* and maturation to filariform larvae, which are demonstrable in large numbers embedded in the crypts of the small intestinal mucosa (Fig. 21.16). The filariform larvae can invade into the mucosa and soon become systemic, resulting in widespread dissemination. The disease is then rapidly fatal unless detected quickly and treated appropriately [249].

Other helminthic infestations of the small intestine

Many other helminths have life cycles that involve the small intestine and/or may present with symptoms and signs referable to the small bowel. These include *Toxocara canis*, *Trichuris trichuria*, *Trichinella spiralis*, *Angiostrongylus costaricensis*, fluke infections including *Clonorchis sinensis*, *Fasciola hepatica* and *Opisthorchis viverrini*, other trematodes and tapeworm infections. However seldom, if ever, do any of these infestations present to the histopathologist and a comprehensive account of their pathology is deemed beyond the scope of this book. The interested reader is referred to specialist texts [225,227,254,255].

Crohn's disease

Introduction

In 1932, Crohn, Ginzberg and Oppenheimer, from the USA, first described the condition of regional enteritis, the terminal ileal presentation of Crohn's disease [256]. Nevertheless, it is now generally accepted that the Scottish surgeon, Dalziel (pronounced 'Dee-ell') gave the first account of the disease, much earlier, in 1913 [257]. Until the 1960s it was believed that Crohn's disease only affected the small intestine. It was then that Lockhart-Mummery and Morson described involvement of the large intestine by Crohn's disease [258]. Subsequently it has become increasingly important to differentiate colorectal Crohn's disease from that other major form of chronic inflammatory bowel disease, ulcerative colitis. This distinction remains a major part of the gastrointestinal pathologist's workload.

It was also in the 1950s that anal and anorectal Crohn's disease were fully described [259]. Subsequently it became clear that Crohn's disease could involve any part of the gut, from mouth to anus, and that there could be extraintestinal manifestations of the disease, especially in the skin, eyes and joints [260–264]. Thus Crohn's disease is now accepted as a pangastrointestinal pathology with systemic manifestations. It remains an enigmatic condition, not least because it is still uncertain whether it represents one or several different diseases.

Epidemiology

The prevalence of Crohn's disease has been difficult to estimate because of inaccuracies in diagnosis, in particular the distinction between large intestinal Crohn's disease and ulcerative colitis. It is now clear, however, that the condition is becoming much more common, particularly in the UK, Scandinavia and other parts of northern Europe. The highest prevalence figures in Western countries are between 26 and 56 per 10 000 of the population [265,266]. The increase in incidence is particularly in large bowel disease [267,268]. There are two peaks of incidence, one in early adulthood and the other in the 60–70 age group. The disease is seen with increasing frequency in southern Europe, although much more rarely than in northern Europeans [269], but it remains rare in Africa, the Middle East, the Far East and South America. It is especially common in the white population of North America, South Africa, Australia and New Zealand. The incidence in Jewish populations is also particularly high. In epidemiological terms, there are many similarities between Crohn's disease and ulcerative colitis [265,269].

Aetiology and pathogenesis

Perhaps the greatest conundrum of Crohn's disease is its aetiology. Theories abound in an attempt to explain its multifocal involvement, its very protean clinical presentations, its epidemiology and its variable pathological features. It has to be admitted that its aetiology remains completely unknown at this time, although several theories currently hold sway and have been associated with intense media interest. Each one of the main theories concerning the aetiology will be considered separately, although it may well be that two, or more, of these theories are important in the genesis of the disease.

Genetic factors

There is increasing evidence for the involvement of specific gene loci in the predisposition to Crohn's disease [270]. Such genetic predisposition was initially suggested by family and twin studies. First-degree relatives of patients with Crohn's disease have an incidence of the disease of between 13 and 18% [271–273]. There is also a high concordance for the disease in monozygotic twins [274]. Now studies such as genomic scanning have confirmed this genetically determined predisposition.

Animal models and studies of different ethnic groups indicate the likelihood of a polygenic contribution to inflammatory bowel disease susceptibility [274]. It is also likely that certain of these multiple gene loci predispose to both ulcerative colitis and Crohn's disease, helping to explain the epidemiological and genetic overlaps between these two forms of inflammatory bowel disease [275,276]. Genomic screening has identified linkage for inflammatory bowel disease predisposition, both ulcerative colitis and Crohn's disease, initially to chromosome 16 [277] and then to chromosomes 12, 7 and 3 [273]. Linkages to chromosomes 12 and 16 have been confirmed by several other groups [274]. More recently, two groups working independently have established that variants of the *NOD2* gene on chromosome 16 predispose to Crohn's disease specifically [278,279], a finding made particularly interesting because the *NOD2* gene product is involved in controlling the inflammatory response to gut bacteria.

Environmental factors, including diet

Certain environmental risk factors, especially social factors and diet, are acknowledged, aided by the recognition that Crohn's disease is a relatively modern condition and most common in Western society. Smokers have an increased risk of Crohn's disease, both initially and with recurrence [280,281]. Furthermore the prevalence of the disease in Western communities suggests that a refined diet may be an important factor; patients with Crohn's disease have increased sugar consumption [282] and it has been suggested that other ingested compounds in a Western diet, such as Corn Flakes [283] and toothpaste [284], may be important in promoting the disease. None of these is in any way proven to be important [285]. Support for diet being important in the genesis of the disease is manifest by the amelioration of the disease by dietary manipulation. For instance, an elemental diet has been shown to considerably improve small intestinal Crohn's disease [286]. Whether this is a primary or secondary effect remains unknown; it may be that dietary components merely trigger an abnormal immunological reaction already at play.

Infective agents

There have been numerous studies attempting to link Crohn's disease to bacterial infection but none of these has been, by any means, conclusive [287–291]. The resemblance of the pathology of Crohn's disease to intestinal tuberculosis has led workers to seek a mycobacterial cause for Crohn's disease [292] and the causation of Crohn's disease by mycobacteria (especially *Mycobacterium avium* subspecies *paratuberculosus*) is strongly championed in some quarters [293]. However, many studies, particularly those using sophisticated molecular biological methodology, have been at best equivocal and probably favour the lack of a relationship between mycobacteria and Crohn's disease [294–300] and trials of antituberculous chemotherapy have shown no observable benefit. Current opinion holding sway is that mycobacteria are unlikely to be the cause of Crohn's disease but that continued research is required to finally lay this attractive but unsubstantiated theorem to rest [301,302].

There has been intense interest in the possibility of a relationship between the disease and the measles virus or its vaccine. Initial descriptions of the electron microscopic demonstration of measles-like virus in Crohn's tissue led some researchers to seek a relationship between measles exposure and the subsequent development of Crohn's disease, especially in pregnant women and in their offspring [303–306]. More recently the same authors have suggested that the measles vaccine, particularly when in combination as MMR (measles, mumps and rubella), may be responsible for Crohn's disease and also for the purported lymphoid follicular hyperplasia and 'inflammatory bowel disease' that these workers believe are characteristic lesions of autism [307,308]. Epidemiological evidence has failed to support any of these theories, but public concern over this issue in the UK has resulted in a worrying diminished uptake of the vaccine [309,310].

Immunopathology

The pathogenesis of Crohn's disease involves a complex interplay between those factors involved in the aetiology of the disease, whether genetic, environmental or possibly infective, and the immune system. As the immune system is primarily responsible for the inflammatory changes that are such an important component of the disease, it is clearly important to understand the immunological factors that are involved. The study of the immunopathology of Crohn's disease has been particularly hindered by the complex microenvironment of the intestines, especially the presence of innumerable food and bacterial antigens, and the complexity of the immune system. Thus the numerous studies that have been performed to assess the immunopathology of Crohn's disease remain difficult to interpret and are, at the current time, inconclusive. In this review it is intended to cover only very briefly the abnormalities described in the different parts of the immune system.

In Crohn's disease, there is a marked increase in total immunoglobulin production within the intestine mucosa, particularly IgG [311]. IgG2 predominates, an antibody produced in response to carbohydrate and bacterial antigens [312]. There is less evidence for autoantibody production in Crohn's disease compared with ulcerative colitis, for instance perinuclear antineutrophil cytoplasmic antibody (p-ANCA) being demonstrable less readily in Crohn's disease compared with ulcerative colitis [313]. In the lamina propria of the intestines in Crohn's disease, T cells are increased but with a relatively normal CD4/CD8 ratio [314]. However, the number of T cells with an activated phenotype, expressing interleukin (IL)-2 and transferrin receptor, is increased [315].

There is an increase in production of monocytes in patients with Crohn's disease, with increased recruitment into the intestinal wall as macrophages [316,317]. There are two main types of intestinal macrophages, mature tissue macrophages (RFD7 antibody positive) and interdigitating dendritic cells, which are antigen presenting and are found predominantly in organized lymphoid tissue. The distribution of these histiocytic subsets is grossly altered in Crohn's disease, especially with clustering of RFD7-positive cells in granulomas [318,319]. Crohn's disease is characterized by a florid neutrophil polymorph infiltrate and this produces superoxide radicals and nitric oxide which are thought to be important in the production of epithelial damage [320]. Furthermore it has been shown that the mucosa in Crohn's disease lacks antioxidant defences [321]. Eosinophils are also elevated in the mucosa of Crohn's disease: these secrete proteins such as eosinophilic basic protein and IL-5 that may enhance the mucosal damage [322].

Cytokine expression in Crohn's disease has been extensively studied as many of these proteins appear to have a major involvement in the initiation, propagation and recurrence of inflammation. There is increased production of the immunostimulatory cytokines, notably IL-1, from polymorphs, and levels of IL-6, both in peripheral blood and in tissues, and the proinflammatory tumour necrosis factor alpha (TNF-α) are increased [323–327]. Indeed, there has been some success in the treatment of Crohn's disease with chimeric monoclonal antibody to TNF-α [328,329]. Immunomodulatory cytokines have been less extensively studied: there appears to be overactivity of IL-2 in Crohn's disease whereas in ulcerative colitis there is reduced activity [330,331]. There is also evidence of increased activity of interferon-γ [332,333] and possible involvement of IL-4 in early recurrences of Crohn's disease [322].

Further evidence for the importance of immunological mechanisms in Crohn's disease has been sought from animal models. There are numerous gene knockout animal models that show intestinal inflammation, including IL-2- and IL-10-deficient mouse models [334,335]. Another mouse model has shown that intestinal inflammation can be produced when there are abnormalities of the epithelial cell junction complexes, notably N-cadherin expression, suggesting that altered epithelial permeability is an important, and possibly primary, abnormality in inflammatory bowel disease [336].

The very complex nature of the intestinal microenvironment and of the interactions of the immune system have ensured that our knowledge of the immunopathology of Crohn's disease remains strictly limited. The target for future research is the identification of the important immunostimulatory and immunomodulatory elements, enabling treatment by immunomodulation and molecular means against specific targets in the inflammatory process.

Macroscopic appearances

The classical macroscopic manifestations of small intestinal Crohn's disease are ulceration, strictures and fissuring, the latter manifesting as a cobblestoning pattern of the mucosa. The macroscopic features of ulceration in Crohn's disease are characteristic: the ulcers are serpiginous and discontinuous and in their earliest form present as small, aphthoid ulcers. They vary in size from tiny, pinpoint haemorrhagic lesions to small, clearly defined shallow ulcers with a white base, and are easily missed if the specimen is not carefully prepared and examined (Fig. 21.17). Evidence suggests that these early lesions may take several years to progress sufficiently to give rise to detectable clinical or radiological signs and serial studies have followed their progression through more extensive linear ulceration to stenosis, the latter developing after at least 3 years [337,338].

Small bowel strictures in Crohn's disease may be short or long, single or multiple. The classical single long segment 'hosepipe' stricture of the terminal ileum is the basis for the 'string sign of Kantor' seen radiologically (Fig. 21.18). Although classical of Crohn's disease, there is some evidence that such extensive stricturing terminal ileal disease is becoming less common [338]. This is possibly because it represents a more advanced form of the disease, less readily seen now because of the relative success of anti-inflammatory treatment

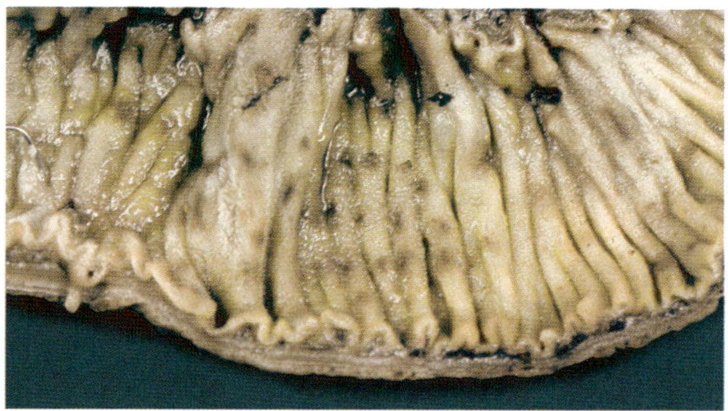

Fig. 21.17 Crohn's disease in the ileum. Numerous aphthous ulcers are seen in this segment, proximal to a terminal ileal stricture.

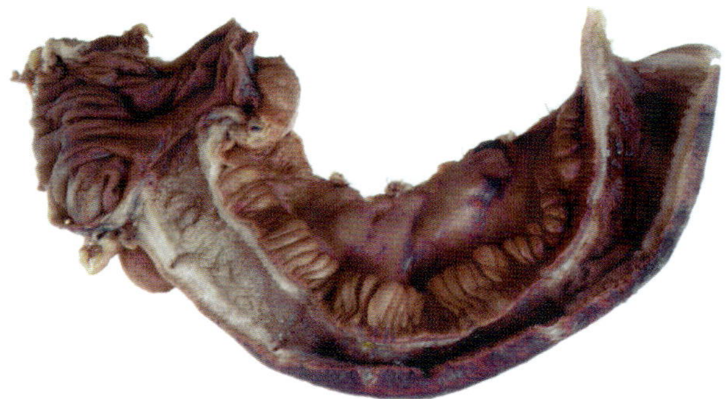

Fig. 21.18 A classical hosepipe-type stricture of the terminal ileum with extensive stricturing due to Crohn's disease.

regimes. In fact strictures can be seen in any part of the small bowel but are still more common in the ileum as a whole than in the jejunum (Fig. 21.19), and certainly much more common than in the duodenum.

The classical 'cobblestone' appearance of the mucosal surface of the small intestine in Crohn's disease is seen in only about a quarter of all cases. The cobblestones are formed as a result of intercommunicating crevices or fissures surrounding islands of surviving mucosa, raised up by the underlying inflammation and oedema (Fig. 21.20). Considerable oedema of the intestinal mucosa is often a useful sign of active disease. Fissuring is a very important sign of Crohn's disease and must be looked for carefully, at both the macroscopic and microscopic level of observation. Extensive fissuring and cobblestoning can progress to inflammatory polyp formation, although this feature is much less common than in the large bowel afflicted by chronic inflammatory bowel disease [339].

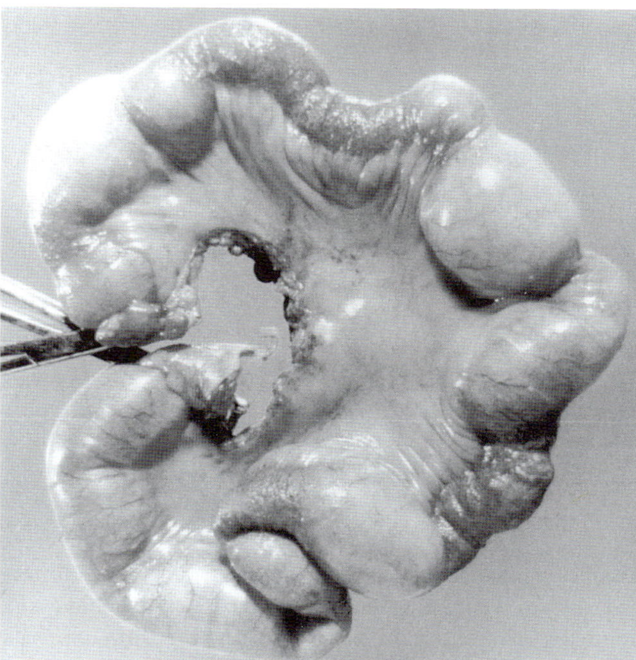

Fig. 21.19 Multiple short ileal strictures in Crohn's disease. The specimen was inflated with formalin which accentuates the features.

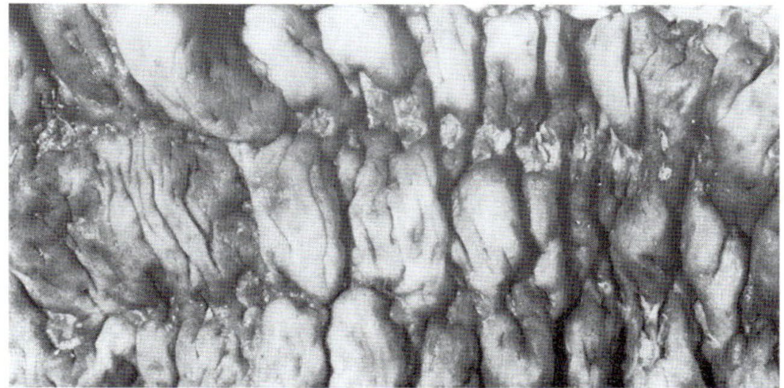

Fig. 21.20 Cobblestoning of the mucosa in Crohn's disease. Intercommunicating fissures (cleft-like ulcers) and crevices in the mucosa separate islets of more or less intact epithelium, which are raised up by submucosal oedema.

Whether Crohn's disease presents primarily as an ulcerative, stricturing or cobblestone form, or as a combination of these changes, it is nearly always a discontinuous pathology of gut. Multiple lesions are common and may be widely separated, but even in extensively diseased small or large intestine, there are nearly always small patches of intervening normal bowel (Fig. 21.19). Small intestinal Crohn's disease has been divided into three main types, depending on whether the disease is primarily perforating, ulcerating or fibrostenosing [340,341]. Whilst this subdivision was originally thought to be

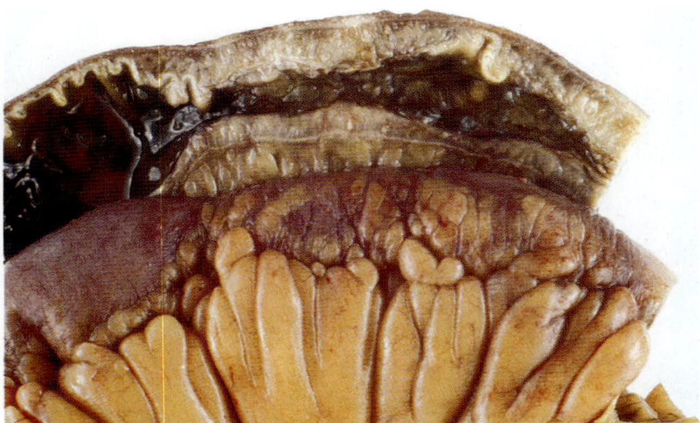

Fig. 21.21 A Crohn's stricture of the ileum. This demonstrates the marked thickening of the bowel wall. The serosal surface shows prominent fat wrapping, the extent of which correlates directly with the stricture.

of some predictive value in terms of recurrence and ultimate prognosis of Crohn's disease, more recent studies have cast doubt on its utility and have shown these three patterns cannot be regularly or usefully separated in terms of natural history or underlying pathological features [342,343].

In small bowel Crohn's disease, the bowel wall is usually considerably thickened and the inflammation is obviously transmural, sometimes with involvement of peri-intestinal fat and serosa by fibrosis and adhesions (Fig. 21.21). Often pathological examination of surgical specimens has concentrated on the mucosal aspect of the small bowel, once the specimen has been opened and pinned mucosal surface upwards. This is a pity, because the serosal surface provides useful macroscopic features pointing towards a diagnosis of Crohn's disease (Fig. 21.21). These serosal changes include the presence of tiny 'tubercles' which, when examined microscopically, are seen to be the sarcoid-like granulomas of Crohn's disease. Occasionally this may be a very prominent feature, resembling the appearance in tuberculosis [344]. Serosal congestion and fibrosis are both common, and deep fissures developing into internal fistulae may be demonstrable here. The connective tissue changes of Crohn's disease include neuronal, vascular, muscular, fibrosing and fat abnormalities. Fat wrapping, in which hyperplasia of the subserosal and mesenteric fat extends around the bowel wall to become circumferential on the antimesenteric aspect of the bowel, is a highly characteristic, and possibly pathognomonic, feature of small bowel Crohn's disease (Fig. 21.21) [345,346]. It correlates closely with activity of disease, most notably transmural inflammation, and is used by surgeons to gauge the extent of disease at the time of resection [345,346].

It should be emphasized that changes in the proximal small intestine, especially the duodenum, can be much more subtle. Whilst earlier studies have suggested that duodenal involvement is unusual, only occurring in about 2% of cases [347], it has become clear, from large-scale endoscopic and histopathological studies, that more subtle duodenal pathology is relatively commonplace, changes being demonstrable in about 25% of Crohn's disease patients [348,349].

In small intestinal Crohn's disease, the regional lymph nodes are often enlarged but in many cases they are quite normal histologically. It must be remembered that the ileocaecal lymph nodes in particular are normally relatively large and that the size of nodes varies with age. Mesenteric lymph nodes in Crohn's disease may contain non-caseating epithelioid granulomas, but only in a minority of cases. Consequently, biopsy of such nodes is not a sensitive method of making the diagnosis. However, it can be useful for distinguishing Crohn's disease from important mimics, notably tuberculosis and yersiniosis (see below).

Microscopic appearances

It cannot be overemphasized that small intestinal Crohn's disease exhibits a very variable microscopic pattern, and some of the more important histopathological features may be entirely absent in some cases. Only rarely are all the characteristic histological features present in a single specimen. The most characteristic microscopic features of the disease are its multifocal involvement and the triumvirate of focal ulceration (which is often fissuring and may result in fistula formation), transmural inflammation in the form of lymphoid aggregates and granulomas. These three features are generally regarded as the hallmarks of intestinal Crohn's disease. Although it is usually considered a granulomatous disease, it is important to recognize that granulomas may be completely absent in up to 50% of cases of small intestinal Crohn's disease [350]. Nevertheless, when present, especially in the small bowel, they are a very useful diagnostic pointer.

A granuloma is a circumscribed collection of epithelioid histiocytes, with or without giant cells, which are usually of the Langhans type. Granulomas, when present in Crohn's disease, may be found throughout the bowel wall, including the mucosa and superficial submucosa of duodenal and ileoscopic biopsies (Fig. 21.22). They are less common in the small bowel than in the large bowel and anal region [351], are less commonly seen in patients with a long clinical history [338,351,352], and are commoner in younger patients with a shorter duration of disease [338,350]. Their presence (or absence) does not influence recurrence rates or prognosis in small intestinal Crohn's disease [351,353–355]. Granulomas are often related to areas of ulceration and transmural inflammation but they may be seen in isolation away from areas of active disease [356]. They often have a close relationship to lymphatics, especially in the submucosa and subserosa of the small intestine [357], whilst a lower proportion are related to small blood vessels (Fig. 21.23) [358,359]. In about 25% of cases, the local lymph nodes in the small intestinal mesentery will contain similar granulomas but it is exceptional for granulomas to be present in lymph nodes and not in the bowel wall

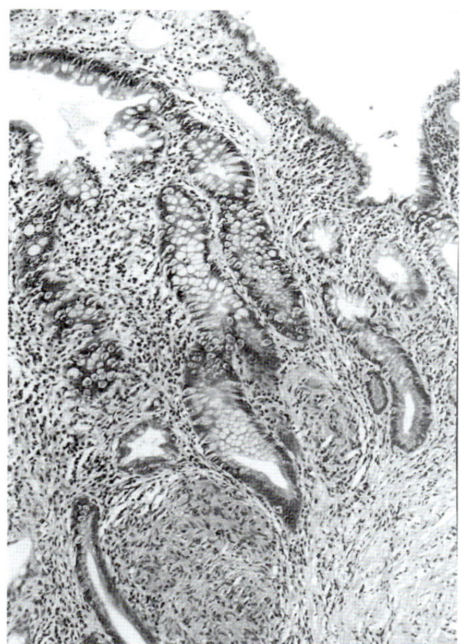

Fig. 21.22 An ileoscopic biopsy demonstrating two well formed epithelioid cell granulomas, basally situated in the mucosa.

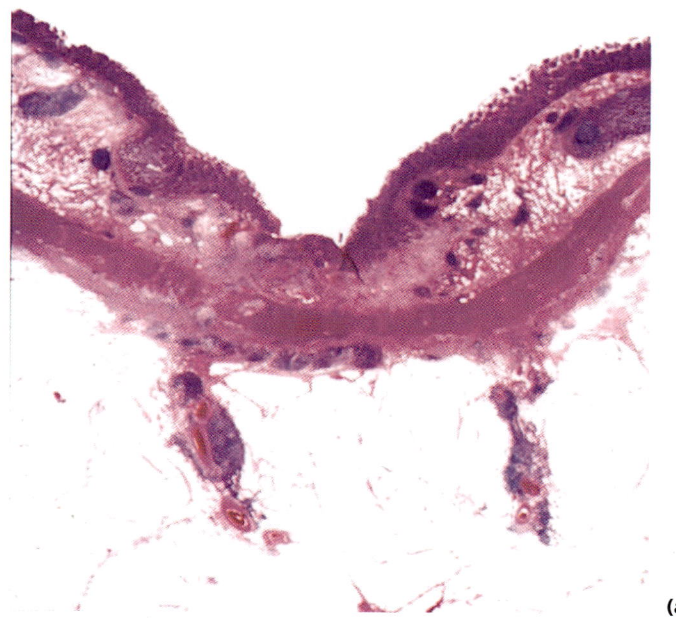

(a)

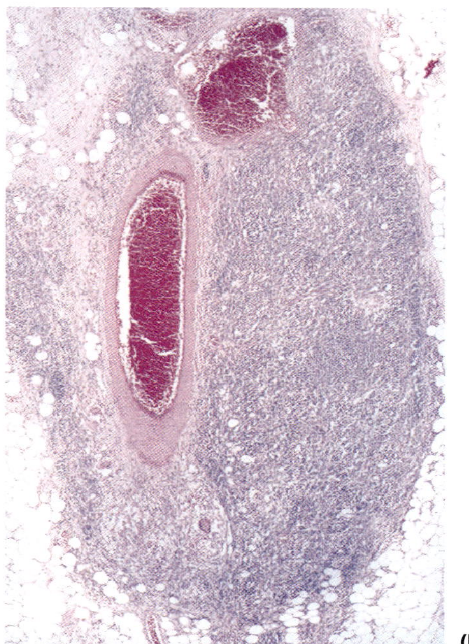

(b)

Fig. 21.23 (a) A wholemount section of jejunal Crohn's disease. The transmural inflammation is evident, with inflammation extending along two mesenteric blood vessel bundles. (b) A high-power view of one of the blood vessel bundles shows prominent chronic inflammation around a vein and artery with a single well formed granuloma (with giant cell) close to the arterial wall (below).

[52]. Nodes containing granulomas are no larger than those without [360].

Focal inflammation is a characteristic and highly prevalent feature of small intestinal Crohn's disease. It would appear that the earliest lesion in the disease is a zone of mucosal inflammation, often superficial to lymphoid aggregates and/or Peyer's patches, which then develops into the characteristic aphthoid ulcer (Fig. 21.24). It has been suggested that such early inflammatory changes are induced by damage to small capillaries [361] although there is no objective evidence to support this. Other mucosal changes may signify previous (or concurrent) ulceration, especially so-called pseudopyloric metaplasia. This lesion, which comprises glands of the 'ulcer-associated cell lineage' (UACL), secretes trefoil peptides and growth factors, notably epidermal growth factor (EGF), that may accelerate healing mechanisms subsequent to ulceration [362–364]. UACL is diagnostically useful but is not specific to Crohn's disease: it may be seen in any chronic inflammatory pathology of the small intestine where previous ulceration has occurred, although it is most often seen in Crohn's disease.

Whilst small aphthoid-type ulcers are a characteristic accompaniment of relatively early Crohn's disease, the subsequent more extensive ulceration often takes the form of longitudinally orientated or deep crevice-like fissures. These knife-like clefts, sometimes branching, extend deeply into the bowel wall and are the histological basis for the formation of fistulae. Usually lined by granulation tissue, they may demonstrate epithelioid histiocytes and giant cells in their walls. They are particularly useful for the diagnosis of Crohn's disease when granulomas are absent, but they are not pathognomonic; similar fissuring ulcers may sometimes occur in other small intestinal conditions including drug-induced ulceration, Behçet's disease and malignant lymphoma. Indeed, fissuring ulceration is also an especially prominent feature of 'ulcerative jejunitis', which represents early lymphomatous transformation in coeliac disease (see p. 382).

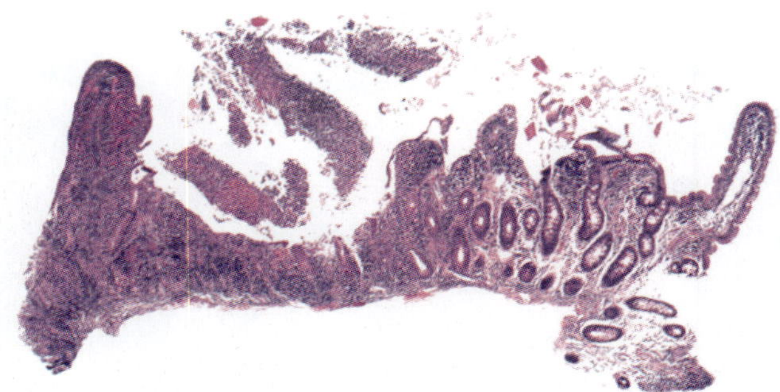

Fig. 21.24 An ileoscopic biopsy from a patient with Crohn's disease. It shows focal inflammation and an aphthous ulcer, distinctive features of the disease in ileoscopic biopsies.

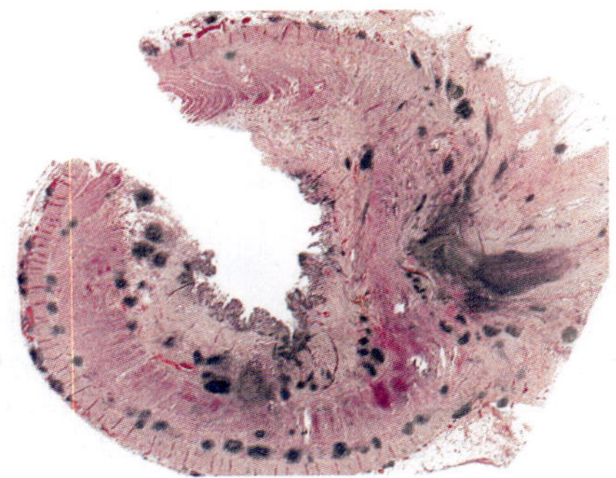

Fig. 21.25 A wholemount section of jejunal Crohn's disease. There is transmural inflammation in the form of lymphoid aggregates, forming the distinctive 'Crohn's rosary. The subserosal aspect of a fistula is discernible (right).

Even when granulomas and fissuring ulceration are absent, there remain distinctive histological features of Crohn's disease. Perhaps the most prevalent and diagnostically useful feature is transmural inflammation in the form of multiple lymphoid aggregates (Fig. 21.25). Often about the size of granulomas or somewhat larger, such well-formed lymphoid collections are scattered throughout the bowel wall but are particularly obvious in the submucosa and subserosa. In the latter, they are usually orientated in a line immediately adjacent to the outer aspect of the muscularis propria, forming the characteristic 'Crohn's rosary' which is readily identifiable in histological slides to the naked eye (Fig. 21.25). Associated with the transmural inflammation, there is gross bowel wall thickening, involving all the layers, with oedema and fibrosis being especially prominent in the submucosa. Lymphangiectasia is also a common feature, which is best appreciated in the submucosa and subserosa.

In more chronic disease, the 'connective tissue changes' of Crohn's disease become useful diagnostic features. The macroscopic changes of fat wrapping have already been described. Its microscopic basis is adipose cell hyperplasia, almost certainly related to chronic inflammation: the presence of fat wrapping correlates well with the degree of transmural chronic inflammation (Fig. 21.21) [345,346]. Indeed, it may be that the fat hyperplasia perpetuates the inflammation as hyperplastic fat has been shown to secrete TNF-α [365]. Histological changes in nerves in Crohn's disease may be pronounced with marked hyperplasia of nerve fibres, especially in the submucosal and myenteric plexuses and in the subserosal and mesenteric tissues [366]. It could be that the basis of this neuronal hyperplasia is inflammation-induced axonal necrosis, a feature that is readily identifiable at the electron microscopic level [366,367]. Fibrosis of the submucosa is another common feature. It may be accompanied by abnormalities of the musculature with splaying of the muscularis mucosae and distortion of the muscularis propria, while muscularization of the fibrotic submucosa is a common feature in chronic 'burnt-out' Crohn's disease [132].

Vascular abnormalities have received much recent attention because of the suggestion that the pathogenesis of Crohn's disease may include an arteritic and thus ischaemic element [358,368]. There is no doubt that remodelling of the wall of arterioles and arteries with medial atrophy is a feature of early and late disease [369], but how these changes relate to active inflammation is uncertain. Vasculitis, including a granulomatous vasculitis [359], is a striking feature of a small number of cases of Crohn's disease (Fig. 21.23) [370], more often seen in the early stages, but it is commoner to find a granulomatous phlebitis. Vascular abnormalities could explain the way that active disease, particularly ulceration, is sometimes concentrated at the mesenteric aspect of the small bowel [370,371]. The arteries here are end arteries and their stenosis or occlusion would lead to ulceration. Although the finding of a granulomatous vasculitis or arteritis can aid the diagnosis of Crohn's disease, it remains unproven, and in our view unlikely, that ischaemia is a major determinant of the pathogenesis of the disease, not least because the pathological features are usually so unlike those of ischaemic enteritis. Apart from granulomatous phlebitis, veins in Crohn's disease may show irregular thickening of the media as a result of hyperplasia of fibres, elastic and muscle tissue [372]. Finally, lymphatic changes include prominent lymphangiectasia. This feature, along with the submucosal oedema and the close relationship of lymphocytic aggregates and granulomas to intramural and extramural lymphatic channels, suggests that chronic lymphangitis and/or lymphatic obstruction may play a significant role in the pathogenesis of Crohn's disease.

Crohn's disease in the duodenum

There is increasing interest in gastroduodenal involvement in Crohn's disease, not least because minor abnormalities, easily detectable in mucosal biopsies at the time of upper gastrointestinal endoscopy, appear to be much more common than previously thought. These may provide substantial corroborative evidence for a diagnosis of Crohn's disease, especially when symptoms and signs are caused by more distal occult small intestinal disease that is poorly accessible to conventional diagnostic modalities. About 15% of patients with Crohn's disease will have histological changes in the duodenum, although gross involvement only affects about 2% of patients [347–349]. Focal active gastritis, in the absence of *Helicobacter pylori* involvement, is said to be characteristic of gastric Crohn's disease, and in a similar way, a focal polymorph infiltration with moderate chronic inflammation and villous architectural abnormalities in the duodenum provides relatively strong evidence for a diagnosis of Crohn's disease in the appropriate clinical setting [348]. Granulomas are clearly useful but are less commonly seen in the duodenum than in other parts of the intestines in Crohn's disease [349]. Micrograpulomas are more common, occurring in about a third of cases [373], and are particularly useful in subtyping chronic inflammatory bowel disease [374]. It should be stressed that duodenal Crohn's disease very often demonstrates abnormal histology in the presence of entirely normal endoscopic features [375].

Macroscopic involvement at the duodenum is characterized by three patterns of disease: duodenal stenosis, fistulation and ulcerating disease which often does not evolve into the other two types and often resolves [376]. Fistulae may involve the stomach, other parts of the small bowel or the abdominal skin [377]. Duodenal involvement may be complicated by common bile duct obstruction and pancreatitis [378]. Whilst duodenal involvement can result in severe pathology, it is emphasized that duodenal Crohn's disease is associated with less morbidity and less need for surgical intervention than more distal small bowel disease [347]. Only very rarely is neoplastic change described in duodenal Crohn's disease [379].

The diagnosis of Crohn's disease in ileoscopic biopsies

There is increasing usage of ileoscopic biopsies in the assessment of chronic inflammatory bowel disease at the time of colonoscopy [380]. Reaching the terminal ileum is now regarded as a prerequisite for adequate colonoscopy and the colonoscope can reach a considerable distance into the terminal ileum and so assess that part of the intestine most likely to be affected in Crohn's disease. Terminal ileal biopsies in chronic inflammatory bowel disease are most useful in two circumstances: the diagnosis of isolated terminal ileal disease and the differential diagnosis of obvious colonic chronic inflammatory bowel disease, both 'pancolitis' and left-sided disease [380].

Focal active inflammation and disturbed villous architecture are the most common histological features of terminal ileal Crohn's disease (Figs 21.24 & 21.26) [1,380]. Granulomas are less often demonstrated in terminal ileal mucosal biopsies than in the colonic biopsies [351] but are clearly of great diagnostic value when detected. Other useful pointers include isolated giant cells, an eosinophil infiltrate and the presence of the ulcer-associated cell lineage (pseudopyloric metaplasia) within the epithelium [380]. Isolated terminal ileal chronic inflammatory pathology, in a Western population, with some or all of these additional features, is most likely to represent Crohn's disease but caution is always advisable. In a younger age group, yersiniosis is a potential differential diagnosis while drugs, other infections, Behçet's disease and the small bowel manifestations of ulcerative colitis should also be considered [1].

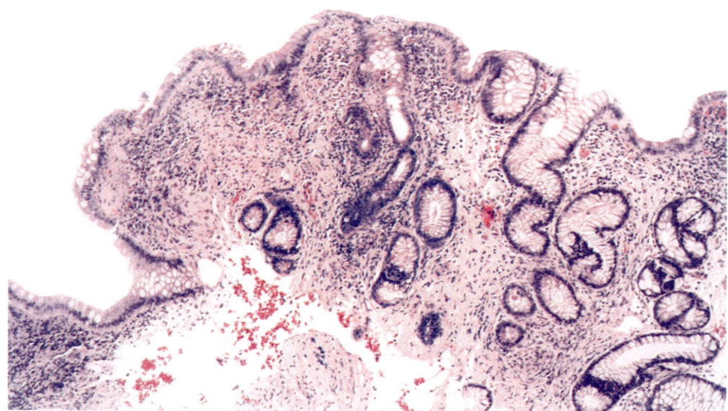

Fig. 21.26 An ileoscopic biopsy from a patient with Crohn's disease. Villous architectural abnormalities and focal inflammation, as seen here, are the two commonest histological abnormalities seen in ileoscopic biopsies in Crohn's disease.

Differential diagnosis

A discussion of the pathological differential diagnosis of small intestinal Crohn's disease depends critically on the specimens available. In biopsies of duodenum and ileum, the differential diagnosis is primarily non-specific duodenitis (see below), coeliac disease (see Chapter 22) and infective enteritis, including bacterial overgrowth, for the former, and infective enteritis, especially yersiniosis, tuberculosis, drug-induced pathology and small intestinal manifestations of ulcerative colitis for the latter.

Tuberculosis remains an important differential diagnosis of small intestinal Crohn's disease. It can show evidence of active necrotizing granulomatous pathology but also can appear effete and closely mimic (burnt-out) Crohn's disease. Histological features favouring a diagnosis of tuberculosis include the number, size and coalescence of granulomas and the presence of caseating necrosis [381]. Small granulomas, microgranulomas and focal inflammation with transmural inflammation in the form of lymphoid aggregates favour Crohn's disease [381]. In only about 50% of cases of tuberculosis will mycobacteria be detected by Ziehl–Neelsen staining [52]. Nodal granulomas may be seen in the absence of intramural granulomas in tuberculosis, unlike in Crohn's disease [52]. Other infective granulomatous conditions, including schistosomiasis, deep mycoses and larval infestations, are not often confused with Crohn's disease as the causative organisms are usually readily identifiable. Similarly viral enteritis, perhaps most notably caused by CMV, can be a source of confusion but the cytopathic viral effects are usually evident.

Apart from tuberculosis, yersiniosis is the most likely infective enteritis to be confused with Crohn's disease. The most useful differentiating features are the central suppurative necrosis with coalescent granulomatosis, the relative lack of transmural inflammation and the presence of suppurative granulomatosis in local lymph nodes, all of which favour yersiniosis [95]. Yersiniosis is characteristically a disease of children and young adults and tends to present more acutely than Crohn's disease. If there is any doubt, then yersinia serology should be recommended.

Ulceration and/or stricturing of the small intestine may be seen as a result of drugs (especially NSAIDs), Behçet's disease, ischaemia, vasculitis and malignant lymphoma [52]. These all remain important differential diagnoses of small intestinal Crohn's disease. Furthermore, so-called burnt-out Crohn's disease may lack the usual inflammatory pathology and may mimic various hamartomas, ganglioneuromatous pathology and effete tuberculosis [52]. Crohn's disease is an important differential diagnosis of a florid eosinophil infiltrate in the small intestine (see below).

Whilst granulomas are an important feature of Crohn's disease, it is important not to assume a diagnosis of Crohn's disease just because granulomas are present. In young children the autosomal recessive disorder, chronic granulomatous disease (CGD), may involve the small intestine although it is more usually seen in the colon [382,383]. In CGD, the granulomas contain lipid vacuoles and lipofuscin-like pigment. If there is any doubt, leucocyte bactericidal activity should be assessed, for this is normal in Crohn's disease [384]. In the pelvic ileal reservoir, granulomas are almost a normal phenomenon, being seen in the lymphoid aggregates of the ileal mucosa in patients with unequivocal ulcerative colitis and in those with familial adenomatous polyposis [385]. Barium granuloma may be present in the small bowel but these granulomas usually contain refractile crystals of barium sulphate [386]. Foreign body-type granulomas containing suture material may mimic Crohn's-type granulomas after previous surgery. Finally, it is possible for sarcoidosis to affect the small intestine but, in our experience, it is exceptional for sarcoidosis to mimic small intestinal Crohn's disease.

Natural history of Crohn's disease

Only about 10% of patients present with 'acute terminal ileitis', i.e. an acute illness subsequently progressing to characteristic small bowel Crohn's disease [387]. Indeed, most patients who present with such an acute ileitis will probably have an infective aetiology such as yersiniosis. Furthermore, as indicated above, the majority of patients with histological evidence of duodenal Crohn's disease will also not progress, in the duodenum at least, to classical disease. It is thus apparent that most patients with symptomatic small intestinal disease present insidiously with recurrent abdominal pain, signs of malabsorption, blood loss and/or change of bowel habit. Investigation, which may include duodenal and/or terminal ileal biopsies, may reveal evidence to support the diagnosis. However, especially in isolated small intestinal disease, the pathological diagnosis may only be attained at the time of surgical resection. Even then, the changes may not be specific and a guarded diagnosis of Crohn's disease may be appropriate.

It has already been indicated that granulomatous inflammation is more characteristic of early than of late small intestinal disease. Occasionally, however, resection is carried out in the more chronic phase of Crohn's disease and then the pathology may reveal the 'healed' or burnt-out phase of the disease. Ulceration may be absent and transmural inflammation minimal. The 'connective tissue changes' of Crohn's disease may predominate with dense fibrosis, muscularization, neuronal hyperplasia and vascular changes notable [132]. In this situation, the late effects of drug-induced enteritis and 'healed' tuberculosis are probably the most important differential diagnoses. In the chronic phase of Crohn's disease, granulomas are often converted into hyalinized tombstones in which Schaumann bodies may be particularly prominent: this feature is especially seen in Crohn's disease diverted from the faecal stream [388].

Through the years, there has been considerable debate concerning the extent of surgery required in intestinal Crohn's disease and the utility of pathological assessment in predicting recurrence of disease. Initially it was thought that surgery should attempt to remove all disease [389] but it is now clear that relative surgical conservatism (especially in the small bowel) should be practised, underpinning the importance of limited resections and stricturoplasty in the surgical management of small intestinal disease [390]. Endoscopic and histological studies of patients after previous resection have shown that most (72–84%) will demonstrate endoscopic lesions just proximal to the anastomosis [337,391,392]. In the great majority (approximately 90%) these lesions occur in the neoterminal ileum just proximal to an ileocolonic anastomosis. Such endoscopic lesions do not themselves predict proper anastomotic recurrence [393] and many affected patients will remain asymptomatic [394]. It appears that these changes are induced by exposure to intestinal contents in the first few days after surgery [395,396].

Since apparent endoscopic and histological changes at the anastomosis are seen in the majority of patients and do not predict recurrence, how important is it for the pathologist to assess resection margins in small intestinal resection specimens? This has become a time-honoured and time-expending task in many pathology laboratories. Whilst it was originally thought that the presence of the disease, whether determined by active inflammation or by the presence of granulomas, was of importance for the prediction of recurrence [389], it is now abundantly clear from numerous studies that the histological demonstration of disease at or close to margins is of no value in predicting recurrence [397–401]. Whilst the observed histological parameters were variable in these studies, none predicted recurrence. Thus pathological time can be more usefully spent in other directions; furthermore, unsurprisingly, it has been shown that frozen section is equally inexact in this regard and cannot be recommended [398]. These studies underpin current surgical practice which is increasingly conservative. Indeed, recurrence is also not influenced by the margin of disease-free bowel at the time of primary surgery [402].

In conclusion, pathologists have little role in predicting the natural history of small intestinal Crohn's disease. The distinction between fibrostenosing, perforating and ulcerating phenotypes of the disease is of little practical value and the pathological assessment of resection margins cannot be encouraged at this time. It is clear, however, that there are clinical factors that predict recurrence, perhaps most notably extensive anal disease [403] and smoking [281].

Complications

The complications of small intestinal Crohn's disease can be usefully considered as local or systemic. Subacute small intestinal obstruction is a common presentation of the disease relating to its stricturing nature whilst ulceration may cause haemorrhage. The latter usually presents with iron deficiency anaemia but, on occasion, it can be more dramatic. Perforation does occur but only in about 2% of cases [404,405]. Fissuring and fistulation may lead to intra-abdominal abscess formation, especially in the ileocaecal region. Fistulae are commonest, in the disease as a whole, in the terminal ileum: 10% of patients have clinically significant fistulae. Enteroenteric, enterocolic and enterocutaneous are the commonest types, although fistulae from the small bowel to the bladder and vagina are also occasionally seen. Extensive small bowel involvement may cause malabsorption, especially of vitamin B_{12}, although malabsorption may also be caused by fistulae, blind loops, strictures and surgical resection.

Neoplastic change in small intestinal Crohn's disease

Sporadic small intestinal epithelial malignancy is rare and the now well described association between small intestinal Crohn's disease and dysplasia and adenocarcinoma of the small bowel is undoubtedly real, although it is much less common than colorectal cancer occurring in the context of chronic inflammatory bowel disease [264,406,407]. The increased risk of small intestinal cancer in Crohn's disease is somewhere between six- and 20-fold [408]. About two-thirds of carcinomas occur in the ileum and one-third in the jejunum; neoplastic transformation of Crohn's disease is exceptionally rare in the duodenum [409]. The diagnosis is not usually apparent radiologically or at the time of surgery [410], and often neoplastic stricturing of the small bowel is only discovered at the time of histological assessment [411].

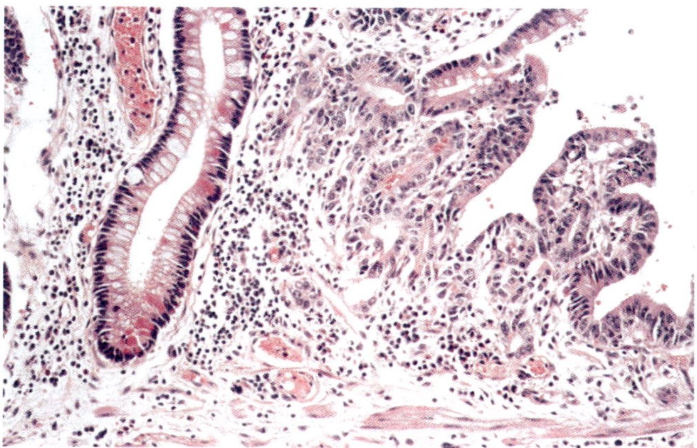

Fig. 21.27 Dysplasia in small intestinal Crohn's disease. The dysplasia (at right) contrasts with a prominent non-neoplastic ileal crypt (at left).

Most cases of adenocarcinoma in small intestinal Crohn's disease are associated with adjacent dysplasia, and there is evidence of a dysplasia–carcinoma sequence (Fig. 21.27) [412–414]. Neoplastic transformation is commoner in males and typically occurs in patients with extensive disease, evidence of both small and large intestinal involvement and a long history [406,414].

Because cancer in small intestinal Crohn's disease is usually 'occult', having not been demonstrated or even suspected by clinical, radiological or surgical means, it is important that the pathologist examines and samples diligently every resection specimen. In 70% of cases, he or she will be the first to identify small intestinal neoplasia in Crohn's disease and it is thus important that there is a high level of suspicion at the time of macroscopic evaluation [411]. Carcinomas in the small bowel are often flat and stricturing and indistinguishable from more 'ordinary' chronic strictures of Crohn's disease [411]. Many are advanced at diagnosis and it is reported that up to 60% are poorly differentiated [414]. Although much less common, there is some evidence of an increased incidence of small intestinal neuroendocrine tumours in ileal Crohn's disease [415] and rare associations with primary intestinal lymphoma are also recorded [416–418].

Systemic complications

A comprehensive review of the systemic effects of Crohn's disease is beyond the scope of this book and only a brief summary will be given here. Arthritis is a common accompaniment of Crohn's disease: there may be a migratory asymmetrical arthritis or there may be associated ankylosing spondylitis

[419–421]. Dermatological lesions include perianal inflammation and fistulation, ulceration around stomas, metastatic Crohn's disease of the skin, pyoderma gangrenosum, erythema nodosum and constitutional eczema [422–425]. About 10–15% of patients with Crohn's disease will develop ocular pathology, especially uveitis and episcleritis [419]. Abnormalities of liver function tests are common but severe hepatic pathology such as pericholangitis and primary sclerosing cholangitis are not so clearly associated with Crohn's disease as they are with ulcerative colitis [426].

Drug-induced enteropathy

Theoretically any number of drugs can induce pathology in the small bowel but drug-induced changes are less well described in the small bowel than in other parts of the gut (such as the stomach and large intestine) because of poor access by clinical investigative means, especially endoscopy. The most important drug-induced enteritides are undoubtedly those due to non-steroidal anti-inflammatory agents (NSAIDs), which produce a wide variety of pathological effects in the duodenum, jejunum and ileum [427,428]. Potassium chloride tablets, gold and chemotherapeutic agents have also received some attention because of their effects on the small bowel mucosa.

NSAIDs in the small intestine

NSAIDs are widely used, especially for chronic arthritis, and it is this patient group that is likely to suffer small intestinal complications of their therapy. Up to 65% of patients on long-term NSAIDs will develop small intestinal pathology [427] and about 10% show evidence of ulceration in autopsy studies [429]. Non-selective cyclooxygenase inhibitors, such as indomethacin, are much more likely to result in small intestinal damage than the more recently introduced specific (COX-2) inhibitor drugs [430]. In the duodenum, erosions and ulcers are common and NSAIDs are likely to increase, relatively, as a cause of duodenitis as *H. pylori*-related duodenitis and peptic ulcer disease become less common [431]. In the more distal small intestine, perforation, ulcers, stricturing and obscure bleeding are the most likely presentations of NSAID enteropathy [428,430,432].

The pathogenesis of mucosal pathology induced by NSAIDs is complex and multifactorial [433,434]. Specific biochemical effects and intracellular organelle damage may be initiating factors [433] but vascular pathology inducing decreased mucosal blood flow, impaired neutrophil function, defective mucosal defence mechanisms and prostaglandin inhibition are all further factors in inducing mucosal damage [433–436]. Increased mucosal permeability leads to protein loss whilst ulceration causes obscure haemorrhage, presenting as unexplained anaemia [437,438].

Mucosal biopsies from the proximal small intestine of patients on NSAIDs may demonstrate specific features, but often terminal ileal biopsies show non-specific changes and may be unrewarding. Increased epithelial apoptotic activity and mucosal eosinophilia are useful signs of NSAID enteropathy [439] and there may be intraepithelial lymphocytosis, although this is more often found in colonic mucosal biopsies. In resection specimens, performed because of NSAID therapy complications, the changes of ulceration and stricturing may be non-specific. However, NSAIDs should always be considered as a cause of 'non-specific ulceration' and perforation in the small intestine as these drugs are widely prescribed and are also now freely available without prescription (Fig. 21.28).

Although relatively rare, there is one distinctive pathological feature of chronic NSAID enteropathy. This is so-called diaphragm disease (Fig. 21.29) [440]. In this condition, which usually affects the ileum but is also now increasingly recognized more proximally in the small intestine and in the colon, patients present with subacute obstruction due to thin mucosa-lined septa that resemble a perforated diaphragm when seen *en face* (Fig. 21.29). They may be single but are usually multiple and they are increasingly recognized in small intestinal radiological studies [441]. It is particularly important for surgeons to know of their existence because their involvement of only the mucosa and submucosa means that the small bowel containing diaphragms may appear entirely normal externally. Diaphragms may be associated with ulcers but often the adjacent mucosa is entirely normal [440]. Their pathogenesis appears to relate to superficial circumferential ulceration, followed by submucosal fibrosis and a high degree of mucosal restitution. They show a close resemblance to the normal plicae circulares of the small bowel, but have addition-

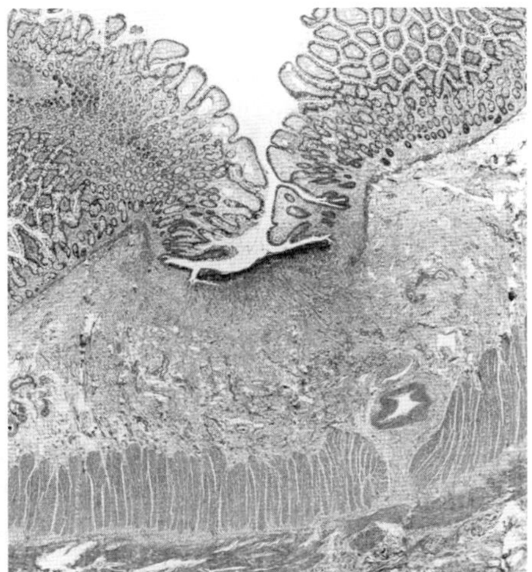

Fig. 21.28 A so-called solitary ulcer of the small intestine. Once other pathologies have been excluded, the diligent pathologist should seek an accurate drug history as many of these lesions are caused by drugs, especially non-steroidal anti-inflammatory drugs.

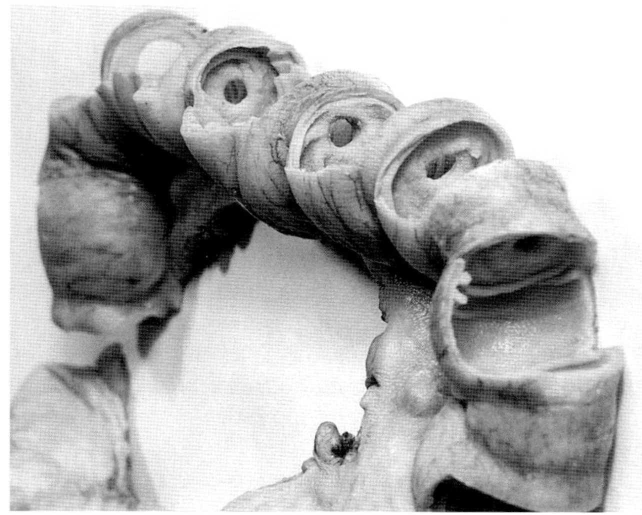

Fig. 21.29 The multiple 'diaphragms' compartmentalizing the ileum from a patient taking long-term non-steroidal anti-inflammatory drugs. Inflation of the unopened fresh specimen is important to display the lesions to the best advantage.

al characteristic features. Immediately adjacent to the stenotic lumen there is mucosal attenuation and ulceration, often with features of mucosal prolapse in the form of fibromuscular proliferation in the lamina propria in the adjacent intact mucosa (Fig. 21.30). There is a well defined area of underlying submucosal fibrosis, which is more prominent in broad-based lesions (Fig. 21.30) [440]. If suspected clinically, diaphragm disease can be diagnosed either radiologically and/or endoscopically and may be treated by enteroscopic means rather than having to resort to surgical resection.

Other drug-induced enteropathies

Enteric-coated potassium supplements and hydrochlorthiazide are both associated with small intestinal ulceration and haemorrhage [442]. Localized ischaemia is a likely mechanism (see p. 353). As a treatment for hyperkalaemia in uraemic patients, kayexalate (sodium polystyrene sulphonate in sorbitol) may be given by mouth, via a nasogastric tube, or by enema. This can cause localized ulceration and mucosal necrosis in any part of the gut, although small bowel inflammation is less commonly seen than in the colorectum [443]. The characteristic crystalline deposits of kayexalate, which usually have large, polygonal profiles with angulated contours and are refractile, basophilic, PAS and Ziehl–Neelsen positive, are identifiable in the bed of the small intestinal ulcers [443].

Patients treated for rheumatoid arthritis with gold therapy occasionally develop an eosinophilic enterocolitis. This usually occurs within 3 months of initiating therapy and the disease presents with diarrhoea, abdominal pain, fever and, sometimes, peripheral eosinophilia [444,445]. The small and large intestine may be involved with haemorrhagic, oedematous and thickened mucosa at endoscopy. Histopathologically, there is ulceration with diffuse inflammatory changes, including both chronic inflammation and a polymorph infiltrate with crypt abscesses. Eosinophils are often particularly prominent [444].

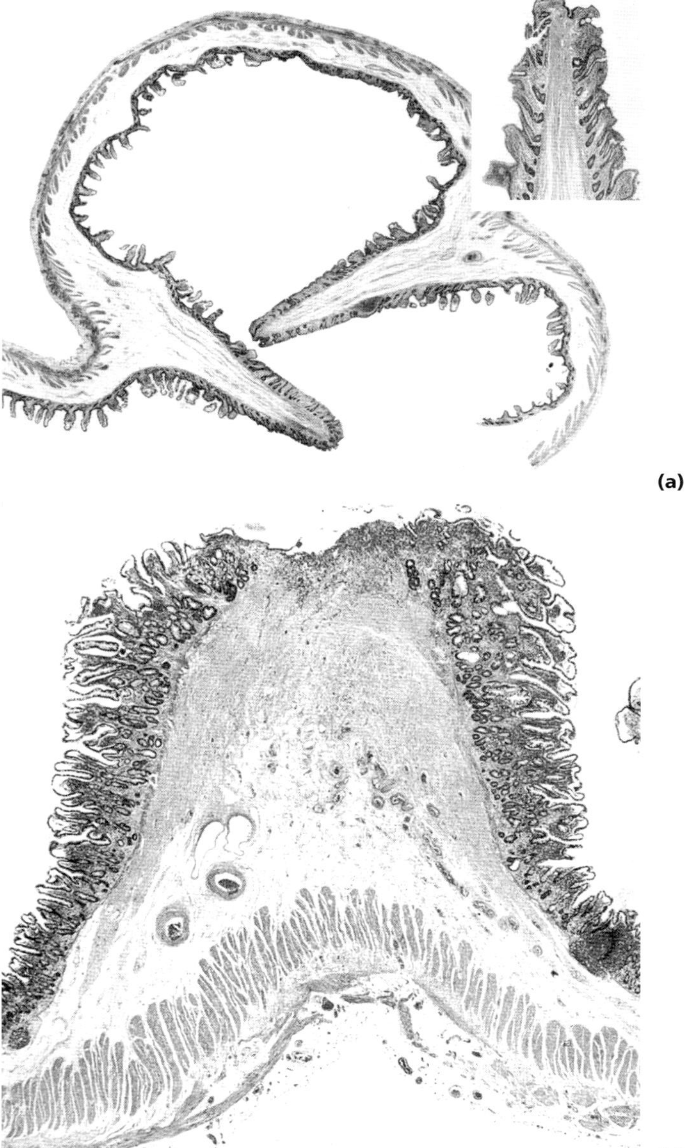

Fig. 21.30 (a) Microscopy of the 'diaphragms' in Fig. 21.29 shows a close resemblance to the plicae circulares. At higher power the insert demonstrates submucosal fibrosis at the tip and villous blunting. (b) Broader-based lesion in the same case as (a) showing an increased degree of submucosal fibrosis. There is now some resemblance to the pattern of microscopy in the potassium-induced ulceration.

Given the rapid cell turnover of the small intestinal mucosa, it is not surprising that chemotherapeutic agents may cause enteropathy. Cyclophosphamide, methotrexate and 5-

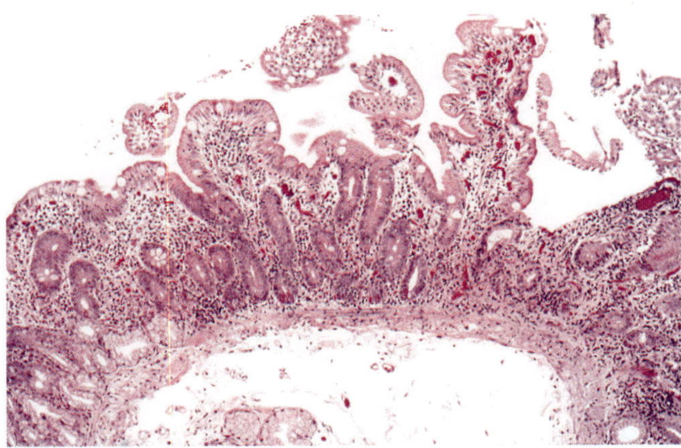

Fig. 21.31 A duodenal biopsy from a patient on 5-fluorouracil therapy for metastatic colorectal carcinoma. There is hypoplastic villous atrophy. Enhanced apoptotic activity was prominent in the crypt bases.

fluorouracil are the agents most associated with, and most widely studied in, drug-induced enteropathy [446–448]. Acute injury is induced by enhanced apoptotic activity, increased migration of crypt epithelial cells and reduced compensatory mitotic activity leading to a hypoplastic villous atrophy (Fig. 21.31) [447,448]. Chemotherapy-induced enteropathy may be exacerbated by radiotherapy [449], whilst there is some evidence that vitamin A treatment may lessen the effects of methotrexate enteropathy [450]. Successful chemotherapeutic ablation of primary tumours of the small intestine, notably malignant lymphoma, can have devastating consequences: perforation of the intestine can occur through the necrotic tumour and strictures can develop much later [451,452].

Miscellaneous inflammatory conditions of the small intestine

Numerous miscellaneous inflammatory conditions affect the small bowel. Some of these are relatively specific to certain parts of the small bowel, and there are interrelationships between some of these conditions and other better recognized enteritides. Initially it is appropriate to consider two pathological phenomena that not uncommonly present to the surgical pathologist and provide a taxing differential diagnosis, often requiring clinical, therapeutic and radiological correlation. These are ulceration and tissue eosinophilia of the small intestine.

Ulceration in the small bowel

Pathologists are occasionally asked to examine small intestinal resections, performed for penetrating ulceration and perforation. Such specimens are often a source of diagnostic difficulty, usually because entirely diagnostic histopathological features are absent (Fig. 21.28). The differential diagnosis of such penetrating small intestinal ulcers, which may be multiple, is broad, and it is intended to give a guide herewith to the salient pathological features and the appropriate additional clinical features to be sought. Perforating Crohn's disease is high on the list of differential diagnoses and transmural inflammation, granulomas and the connective tissue changes should be looked for. Some of these features may be less pronounced in the more chronic, fibrotic and burnt-out phases of the disease [132]. Rarely, Behçet's disease (see below) may show similar changes to Crohn's disease and the appropriate clinical setting should be investigated [453]. In young children, obscure ulceration may represent a distinct inherited disease, intractable ulcerating enterocolitis of infancy [454].

Small intestinal ulceration may be infective in origin. Diligent search for cytopathic effect of viruses, particularly CMV, may be rewarding. The pathological features of ulceration related to bacterial infection may be non-specific and microbiological investigation may be required. Especially in AIDS, protozoal infection may cause deep penetrating ulceration and perforation. Ischaemia, whether acute or subacute, causes ulceration and perforation. Nevertheless, the characteristic pathological features of ischaemia should be demonstrable in the adjacent small intestinal mucosa. Jejunal and ileal ulceration may be peptic in origin, especially in Zollinger–Ellison syndrome [455,456]. Peptic digestion of the ulcer bed and multiplicity of ulcers should prompt investigation of acid secretion and serum gastrin levels. Vascular pathology, including vasculitis, arteritis and irradiation enteritis, may all cause perforating ulceration in the small bowel. Ulcerative jejunitis, effectively representing an early stage of lymphoma in the small bowel, has been considered elsewhere (see p. 381). Suffice it to say that the features of lymphoma may be very subtle in ulcers of the jejunum and ileum, and evidence of lymphoid malignancy should be diligently sought by morphological, histochemical and, if necessary, molecular biological methodology.

Once all these avenues of investigation have been exhausted drugs should be strongly considered as the cause of small intestinal ulceration. NSAIDs are available without prescription and are a highly prevalent cause of small intestinal disease. Apart from diaphragm disease due to NSAIDs (see above) and eosinophilic enterocolitis due to gold therapy, the histopathology of drug-induced enteritis and ulceration may be relatively non-specific (Fig. 21.28). Enteric-coated potassium tablets [457] and NSAIDs [458] have a similar pathogenetic effect by causing localized mucosal ischaemia.

Despite comprehensive searching for evidence of drug ingestion, there will remain some cases of small intestinal ulceration that have to be regarded as primary idiopathic disease [459,460]. Despite regular ileoscopy during colonoscopy and the advent of enteroscopic methods, this small patient group remains enigmatic at present.

Eosinophilic infiltrates in the small intestine

Tissue eosinophilia of the small intestine is by no means a specific diagnosis and merely represents a histological pattern of inflammation [461]. It is described in a wide number of conditions: diagnoses for the pathologist to consider include drug-induced enteropathy, inflammatory bowel disease (in the small intestine alone, Crohn's disease is of course much more likely), malignant lymphoma, systemic disorders such as polyarteritis nodosa and Churg–Strauss syndrome, inflammatory fibroid polyp (see p. 397) and parasitic infection (see above) [461]. In the absence of evidence of these diseases, a diagnosis of eosinophilic gastroenteritis or enterocolitis should be considered.

Eosinophilic (gastro)enteritis

A wide variety of diagnostic criteria have been used for this condition and this has resulted in a lack of standards for its recognition and diagnosis [462,463]. Most commonly eosinophilic enteritis (or eosinophilic gastroenteritis in association with gastric involvement or enterocolitis if associated with large bowel involvement) presents with signs of small intestinal obstruction [464,465], although perforation, haemorrhage, protein-losing enteropathy and malabsorption are all presenting features [466–468]. There may be associated gastric involvement, especially prepyloric obstruction, and the disease may involve the entire gut [463,469]. Rarely, eosinophilic gastroenteritis may be the presentation of a systemic disorder such as connective tissue disease [470] or Churg–Strauss syndrome (allergic granulomatosis) [471].

Associated clinical features aid in the pathological diagnosis of eosinophilic enteritis. About 70% of patients have a history of allergic disorder, especially asthma, hay fever or drug sensitivity. Even more (up to 90%) have a peripheral eosinophilia [461,472,473]. This association with 'allergy' underpins the relative success of therapy such as corticosteroids and sodium cromoglycate in the treatment of the disorder [463,474]. It would seem logical that eosinophilic enteritis represents a localized allergic reaction to an intraluminal antigen. Indeed, some cases have been demonstrated to represent a reaction to parasites; the herring worm, *Eustoma rotundatum*, has been implicated in a small number of cases. However, more recent serological evidence has implicated anisakiasis as a cause in up to 40% of cases [238], particularly in association with gastric involvement in eosinophilic gastroenteritis [238,241]. Other parasites such as *Toxocara canis* have occasionally been implicated [475].

The diagnosis of eosinophilic enteritis is often only achieved at the time of small intestinal resection although duodenal, jejunal and ileal biopsies may occasionally be diagnostic. The involved small intestine shows thickening and oedema with luminal narrowing and a serosal reaction (Fig. 21.32), although there is variation according to what part of the gut wall is predominantly involved. Klein's classification [462] divides cases into mucosal/submucosal, muscular and subserosal [472,473]. The submucosal type, usually with secondary eosinophilic involvement in the overlying mucosa, is predominant, accounting for about 60% of cases (Fig. 21.32) [472]. The striking submucosal eosinophilic infiltrate, often with a distinct paucity of any other inflammatory cell types, is accompanied by oedema. Predominant involvement of the muscularis propria occurs in about 30% of cases, whilst subserosal eosinophilic enteritis is the rarest [472]. The number of eosinophils (up to 80 per high-power field) and their predominance over other inflammatory cells helps with the differentiation from other causes of eosinophilic infiltration [461].

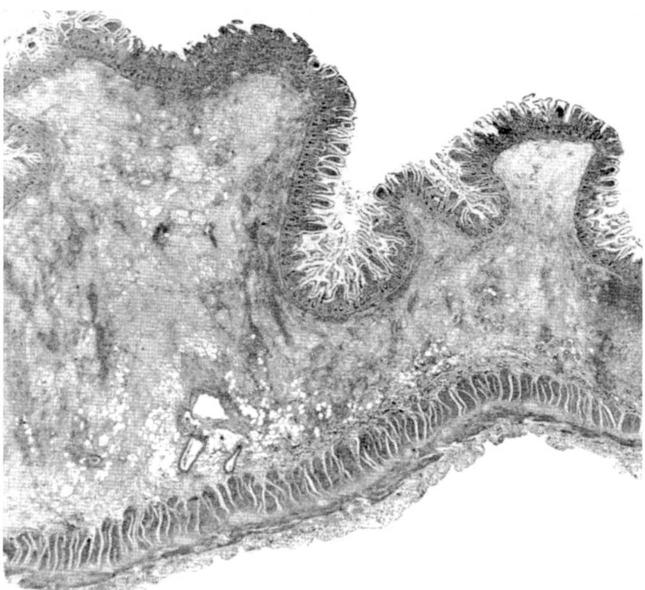

Fig. 21.32 Eosinophilic enteritis. Note the intact mucous membrane and the widening of the submucosa by oedema. There is diffuse infiltration by eosinophils.

In children, allergic or eosinophilic gastroenteritis tends to be a more specific and readily diagnosed condition [463] presenting with anaemia, malabsorption, protein-losing enteropathy, failure to thrive or asthma. Unlike in adults, it is relatively easily to determine the cause of the allergy, which is usually a dietary antigen. Cow's milk protein is most common [476,477]. Eosinophilic infiltration is only a feature of the immediate postchallenge period. At other times, and usually at the time of biopsy, villous atrophy is the predominant feature with a non-specific increase in chronic inflammatory cells in the lamina propria [476]. The diagnosis is often readily apparent clinically and it is only rarely that biopsies are taken except to exclude other conditions, most notably coeliac disease.

Radiation enteritis

Radiotherapy is increasingly given for abdominal and pelvic malignancies, and radiation enteritis continues to cause considerable morbidity and some mortality, despite attempts by radiotherapists (and surgeons at the time of cancer surgery) to minimize damage to the small bowel [478,479]. The severity of radiation enteritis is dependent on several factors, anatomical features, host mechanisms and the type of therapy being the most important [479]. The severity of acute radiation enteritis appears primarily to determine the severity of chronic disease: whilst the effects upon epithelial cell integrity and kinetics and on vascular epithelium are considerable, host defence responses to intraluminal antigens and pathogens are also of some importance [479].

Radiation enteritis is most likely to be demonstrated in parts of the small bowel that are fixed, thus allowing a constant maximal dose of radiotherapy to reach them. The duodenum, proximal jejunum and terminal ileum are therefore most likely to show maximal changes but small bowel fixed by adhesions after previous surgery, for instance, would also be subject to the maximum radiation dose and may exhibit marked radiation change [479,480].

Acute radiation enteritis shows predominant mucosal changes with epithelial stem cell damage leading to villous atrophy and crypt epithelial cell damage with widespread apoptosis [478]. This is accompanied by pronounced regenerative activity in the surviving crypts, which may show marked reactive cytological atypia that can trap the unwary pathologist into a diagnosis of dysplasia [481]. Perforation, adhesions and fistulation (enteroenteric, enterovesical and enterovaginal are the commonest) may all be an early complication of radiation enteritis [481,482].

The late effects of radiation enteritis may be seen months or even years (up to 30 years) after radiotherapy. Stricture and malabsorption are common presenting features [483], with fistula and perforation less common [481]. Even at this stage there may be mucosal ulceration whilst fibrosing strictures and fine serosal adhesions are the commonest macroscopic manifestations [478,481]. The submucosa is most affected with hyaline sclerosis, 'atypical' or stellate fibroblasts and vascular changes prominent (Fig. 21.33) [478,481]. Enteritis cystica profunda is also not uncommon [481]. The mucosa may be ulcerated, may show variable villous atrophic changes with chronic inflammation or may be relatively normal [478]. Telangiectasia is common and mucosal ectatic blood vessels may be a source of gastrointestinal haemorrhage [484]. Vascular changes, particularly in the submucosa and subserosa, include thickening of arteries and arterioles with hyaline fibrosis of the muscularis and foam cells in the intima (Fig. 21.33) [485]. The muscularis may be relatively normal or show hyalinizing fibrosis. Subserosal fibrosis and fibrous adhesions are usually present [481].

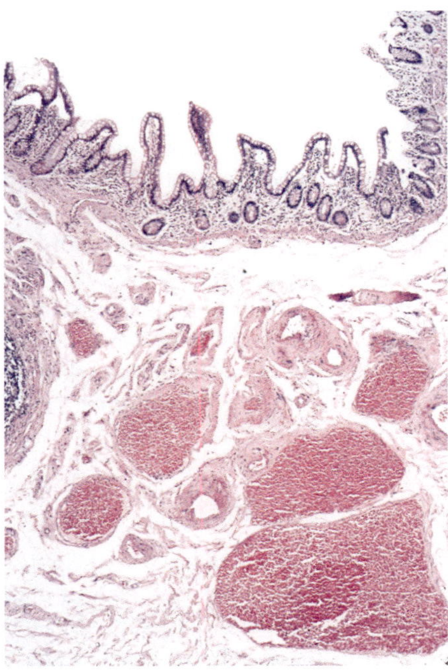

Fig. 21.33 Chronic radiation enteritis. This was from an area of stricture. The mucosa is intact but shows architectural distortion. There is gross hyaline thickening of submucosal blood vessels.

Behçet's disease

Behçet's disease is an idiopathic multisystem syndrome characterized by orogenital ulceration and ocular manifestations. It is a disease of young adults and is more severe in males. It has high prevalence rates in the Mediterranean basin, especially Turkey, from where the disease was originally described. Neurological involvement, either from direct parenchymal involvement of the brain or from major vascular involvement, is one of the most severe manifestations of the disease [486]. Pathologically the disease is characterized by a vasculitis that is usually lymphocytic and affects veins to a greater extent than arteries, although occasionally there may be more necrotizing inflammation with leucocytoclasis. Involvement of the gut is relatively unusual. In one series 5% of patients had significant gastrointestinal symptoms [487] whilst only about 1–2% of patients will have small intestinal involvement [488,489]. Distribution of the disease appears to be geography dependent, ileocaecal involvement being relatively more common in Japan [490]. The disease is described in children [491] and the differential diagnosis from Crohn's disease and other ulcerating diseases may be particularly difficult in this age group [454,491].

Whilst it is clear that the disease is primarily a vasculitis, the cause remains uncertain. Familial cases are well described [492] but no specific genetic abnormalities have been discovered. An association with CMV infection has been suggested [493]. Defective T-suppressor function has been described

[494] and this may possibly be related to Epstein–Barr virus [495]. More recently high levels of truncated actin have been described in polymorph neutrophils of patients with Behçet's disease and it has been suggested that this is a specific abnormality [496,497]. Furthermore, it is clear that the disease represents vasculitis targeting the vasa vasorum and other small blood vessels [498].

Small intestinal involvement is primarily in the terminal ileum [499] and lymphoid aggregates and Peyer's patches are a particular site of involvement [500]. Macroscopically the disease is characterized by penetrating ulcers, often with a flask-shaped morphology and perforation is a relatively common feature (Fig. 21.34) [499,501]. Adjacent to the larger ulcers, there are often smaller aphthoid ulcers. Fissuring and linear ulcers up to 5 cm long may also be present [490]. Behçet's disease is particularly characterized by adjacent macroscopically normal-appearing mucosa [502]. Histologically, the ulcers have non-specific appearances, although the flask-shaped morphology is rather characteristic. The adjacent ileal mucosa may appear almost entirely normal. A common feature is the presence of a lymphocytic vasculitis, often involving small veins and venules [453,502]. There may also be fibrinoid necrosis in involved veins and venules.

Perforation and massive gastrointestinal haemorrhage are the most severe complications of intestinal Behçet's disease [502]. As in Crohn's disease, inflammatory masses may involve the ileocaecal region [488]. Patients with involvement of the small bowel in Behçet's disease often come to surgery but this is complicated by high rates of recurrence of disease [489,499]. The vasculitis of Behçet's disease may be difficult to demonstrate histologically and the condition provides diagnostic challenges to the histopathologist. Indeed, there remains a considerable overlap between intestinal Behçet's disease and Crohn's disease [503]. A diagnosis of intestinal involvement by Behçet's disease requires the presence of the typical extraintestinal manifestations, along with pathology in keeping with the diagnosis. Recurrent oral ulceration is a prerequisite for the diagnosis, and additional features such as ocular involvement, arthritis, erythema nodosum and recurrent genital ulceration are very helpful corroborative features.

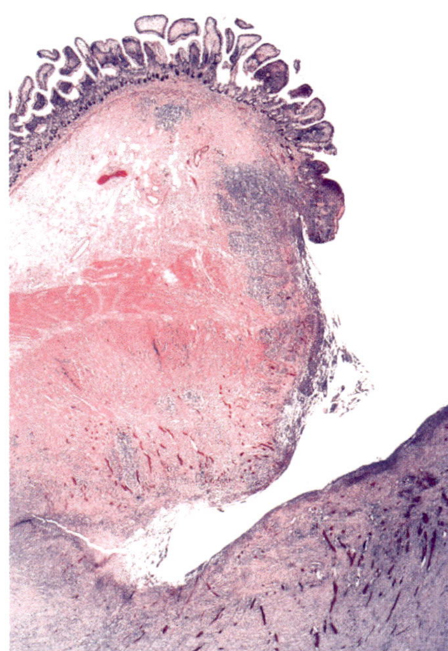

Fig. 21.34 Behçet's disease of the ileum. The edge of a deeply penetrating flask-shaped ulcer extending to the subserosa is well seen. There was evidence of a venulitis elsewhere.

Ileal reservoirs and pouchitis

Pelvic ileal reservoirs were first used for ulcerative colitis and familial adenomatous polyposis (FAP) [504] but more recently they have been used for other conditions, such as juvenile polyposis, necrotizing colitis and severe megacolon when total colectomy is necessary. Most pouches show a degree of mucosal chronic inflammation and villous architectural abnormality (Fig. 21.35) [505,506]. It is likely that these represent a response of the ileal mucosa to the altered environment and probably to stasis and changes in the bacterial flora of the ileum [505,507]. Studies of serial mucosal biopsies indicate that the changes in the ileal pouch mucosa occur soon after faecal stream exposure and, once present, the mucosa appears to reach a steady state in terms of inflammation, architectural abnormality, histochemistry and proliferation [508]. Such changes are probably the prerequisite for subsequent acute inflammatory changes that occur in pouchitis [506,509].

The chronic changes that are almost universal are particularly concentrated in the posterior and inferior parts of the pouch suggesting that contact with static faecal residue is a

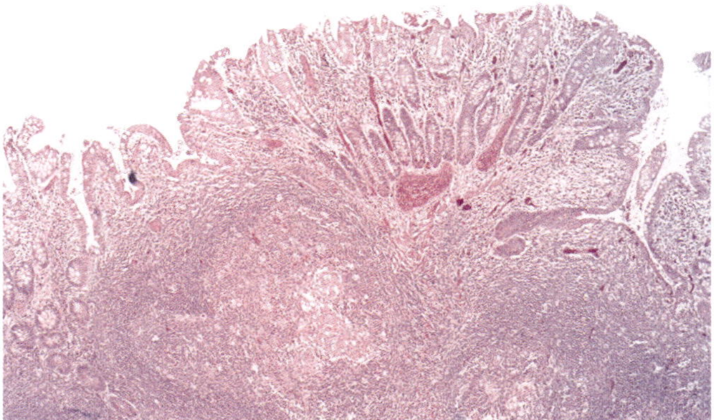

Fig. 21.35 A mucosal biopsy from a pelvic ileal reservoir. The biopsy shows villous atrophy and dense chronic inflammation. Within a germinal centre (below) is a small granulomatous focus. This is a common feature of pouch mucosa and should not be taken as evidence, necessarily, for a diagnosis of Crohn's disease.

major determinant [508]. Despite this, no consistent changes have been demonstrated in bacterial flora [510–512]. Those pouches with the more severe chronic changes are more likely to show so-called colonic phenotypic change in the mucosa, demonstrated by the acquisition of morphological, immunohistochemical, mucin histochemical, lectin histochemical and electron microscopic features of large bowel epithelium [508]. However, certain small intestinal characteristics [506] are retained and immunohistochemical evidence suggests that the mucosa does not undergo complete colonic metaplasia [508].

Pouchitis must not be equated simply with inflammation in the reservoir mucosa. The term pouchitis should be restricted to those patients with an acute-on-chronic, relapsing, inflammatory and ulcerating condition of the functioning reservoir with characteristic clinical, endoscopic and pathological features. Because of the confusion over terminology, many now consider the term chronic relapsing pouchitis to be more appropriate for this condition [388]. Symptomatology includes diarrhoea, often bloody, abdominal pain, urgency, discharge, bloating and systemic symptoms: thus the clinical features are not dissimilar to those of the main disease for which pouch surgery is performed, ulcerative colitis. Endoscopic examination in pouchitis patients reveals increased vascularity, contact bleeding and ulceration, typical features of active chronic inflammatory bowel disease.

Whilst it is important to realize that several conditions cause active inflammation in the reservoir, the pathological hallmarks of the disease pouchitis are acute inflammation and focal ulceration, occurring on a background of marked chronic inflammation and villous atrophy (Fig. 21.36) [505,513]. The overall histological appearances bear a close likeness to those of ulcerative colitis and are unlike those of Crohn's disease. Ulceration in pouchitis is usually superficial; deep ulceration with mucosal erosion is unusual and should raise suspicions of a more specific pathology such as Crohn's disease or ischaemic enteritis [508]. Pouchitis has been defined histopathologically by the presence of severe active inflammation and ulceration and a number of scoring systems are in existence for assessing disease activity [505]. Once these clinical, endoscopic and histopathological characteristics are present, the diagnosis is effectively established [514,515]. When so defined the prevalence of pouchitis usually varies between 10% and 20% of ulcerative colitis patients, although striking variation in prevalence rates continues to characterize the ileal reservoir literature [508].

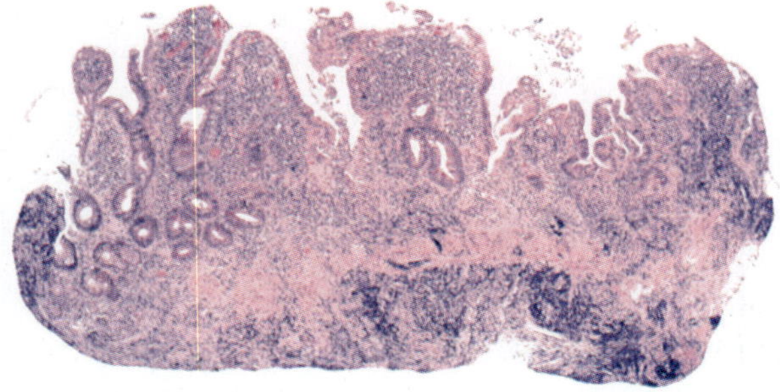

Fig. 21.36 Pouchitis in a pelvic ileal reservoir. There is villous atrophy, chronic inflammation and activity in the form of superficial erosions and disruptive crypt abscesses.

There is little doubt that once other pathologies that cause active inflammation in the pouch (such as Crohn's disease, infective enteritis, mucosal prolapse and mucosal ischaemia) are excluded, chronic relapsing pouchitis occurs specifically in a small subgroup of patients, almost universally with an original diagnosis of ulcerative colitis, who show more advanced chronic inflammatory and villous atrophic change [516,517]. If such patients can be identified at an early stage, then this does have major implications for their management and particularly surveillance.

Theories abound concerning possible pathogenetic mechanisms for pouchitis: these include stasis, bacterial changes, mucosal ischaemia, mucosal prolapse, mucolysis, Crohn's disease, mucosal pathology as a result of a lack of small intestinal nutrients and recurrent ulcerative colitis in a pouch with colonic phenotypic change [388]. Whilst it is clearly possible for Crohn's disease to involve the reservoir, particularly if the pouch was constructed on the basis of an erroneous initial diagnosis or alternatively deliberately in a Crohn's patient [518], there is no evidence to implicate Crohn's disease as the cause of chronic relapsing pouchitis [519,520]. Similarly there is no good evidence that mucosal ischaemia, stasis and/or bacterial changes or epithelial nutrient deficiency (specifically glutamine, in a suggested corollary with butyrate and diversion colitis; see p. 520) are the cause of pouchitis [388]. There is now much stronger evidence to implicate the resurgence of ulcerative colitis in metaplastic mucosa as the most likely cause of the disease [388].

There are interesting associations between an original diagnosis of ulcerative colitis and pouchitis. Most accept that pouchitis is essentially a disease of ulcerative colitis patients. Ulcerative colitis patients show more inflammatory change in their reservoirs than FAP patients [505,513] and there are intriguing connections between ulcerative colitis, extraintestinal manifestations and pouchitis [509,521,522]. Similarities in the immunopathology of pouchitis and ulcerative colitis have also been reported [388]. The most contentious facet of the ulcerative colitis theory is the extent or importance of colonic phenotypic change in the mucosa. As already indicated, current evidence would suggest that colonic metaplasia is not complete in the reservoir: it is this area of pouch mucosal pathophysiology that demands further research.

We are learning more about the pathology and management of chronic relapsing pouchitis but the pathogenesis and prognosis (particularly with regard to neoplastic risk) remain ill understood. Previously the neoplastic risk was thought to be largely theoretical [523], but of more concern is the description of patients with dysplasia in the ileal pouch, apparently supported by flow cytometric abnormalities, although this has only been well described from Huddinge in Sweden [517,524]. Very occasional cases of carcinomas arising in the pouch have been described [525–527]. There have also been descriptions of inflammation relating to remaining rectal cuff [528], and dysplasia and carcinoma have also been described here [529–531]. Potential neoplastic transformation would seem a powerful argument to ensure all reservoirs, particularly those with the most advanced adaptive changes, with pouchitis and with a remaining inflamed rectal cuff, are comprehensively surveyed by endoscopy and biopsy.

Kock's continent ileostomy is performed for the same indications as the pelvic ileal reservoir but the pouch is intra-abdominal and continuity is not restored. There was a vogue for this operation in the UK and Europe, especially Sweden, but in most places, the pelvic reservoir is now much preferred. Unlike the pelvic pouch, Kock's pouches appear to have a different natural history with lower rates of pouchitis: indeed after two decades, the mucosa appears relatively normal in the majority of patients [532]. Nevertheless occasionally cases of neoplasia are described [533].

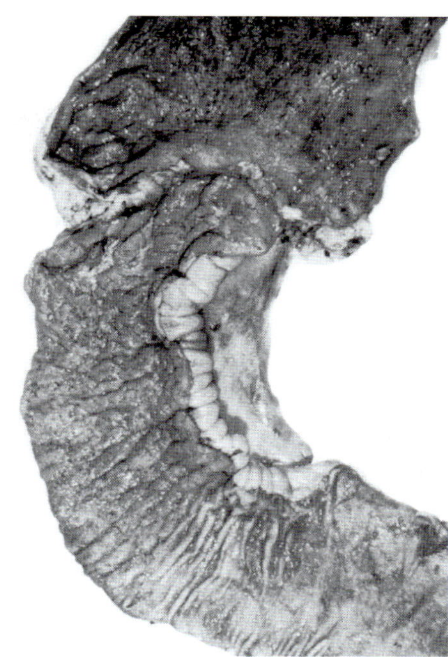

Fig. 21.37 Backwash ileitis associated with a dilated and incompetent ileocaecal valve in continuity with total involvement of the large bowel by ulcerative colitis.

Ulcerative colitis in the small intestine

An increasing number of inflammatory complications of ulcerative colitis are described in the small bowel. Clinically the most important are ileal reservoir inflammation and chronic relapsing pouchitis. Evidence of inflammation in the small bowel, associated with colorectal inflammatory bowel disease, should always raise suspicions for a diagnosis of Crohn's disease. Nonetheless pathologists are increasingly exposed to other enteritides associated with otherwise classical ulcerative colitis.

Backwash ileitis

Ten per cent of total colectomy specimens in ulcerative colitis will show inflammation in the terminal ileum [534]. The inflammation is usually confined to the terminal 10–15 cm of the ileum. Macroscopically the mucosa appears diffusely reddened and granular with erosions and ulcers often prominent (Fig. 21.37). In its milder form, the disease is superficial but deep ulceration may occur and inflammatory polyp formation is well described [534,535]. The ileocaecal valve is usually dilated, allowing the contents of the colon to enter the small intestine. Given the usual continuity of inflammatory pathology between the proximal colon and the terminal ileum and the incompetent ileocaecal valve, it is generally believed that backwash ileitis is not a primary enteritis but rather an effect upon ileal mucosa induced by the contents of the colon.

The histological hallmarks of backwash ileitis are villous atrophy, chronic active inflammation, ulceration and vascular ectasia (Fig. 21.38). There is diffuse chronic inflammation of the mucosa and crypt abscesses are often prominent. Deep ulceration may be fissuring. It is important to differentiate backwash ileitis from Crohn's disease. Discontinuity of disease, granulomas, transmural inflammation and connective tissue changes are all features that would make the pathologist highly suspicious for a diagnosis of Crohn's disease. On ileoscopic biopsy, the same features should be sought, although often only full clinical, radiological and endoscopic correlation will allow the biopsy appearances to be accurately diagnosed [380]. Late-stage backwash ileitis manifests as gross

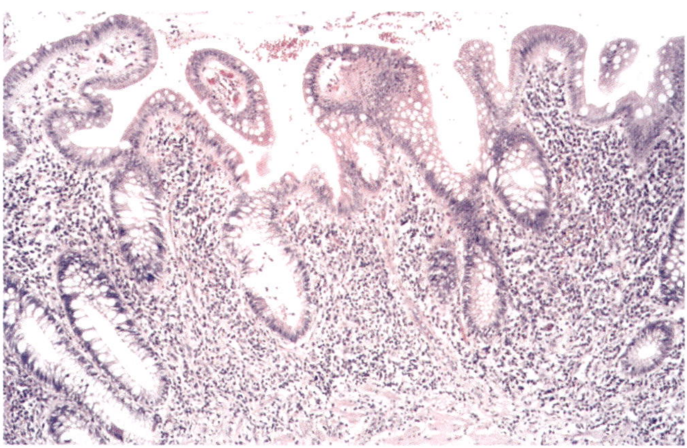

Fig. 21.38 The histology of backwash ileitis. There is villous atrophy, diffuse chronic inflammation and activity in the form of small crypt abscesses.

villous atrophy with epithelial regeneration, leading to a flattened mucosa which may closely resemble colonic mucosa. Evidence for true colonic metaplasia, due to the long-term presence of colonic contents, is currently lacking.

Backwash ileitis has relatively little clinical significance apart from its potential for a misdiagnosis as evidence of Crohn's disease. It is usually associated with severe pancolonic ulcerative colitis and the colonic complications of the disease are usually much more significant than those of the terminal ileum. Perforation of 'backwash ileitis' should raise suspicions for an alternative diagnosis. It remains controversial whether the presence of backwash ileitis predicts the subsequent onset of pouchitis in the pelvic ileal reservoir after proctocolectomy [536,537]. Given the current theories that the disease is a secondary phenomenon, it would seem more likely that the severity of the colonic disease (which itself determines the presence or absence of backwash ileitis) might predict subsequent pouchitis rather than the presence of backwash ileitis.

The duodenum and jejunum in ulcerative colitis

Evidence of inflammatory pathology in the proximal small bowel in putative ulcerative colitis would usually raise suspicions for an alternative diagnosis, such as Crohn's disease. However, the jejunal mucosa has been shown to harbour chronic inflammation in ulcerative colitis patients [538] and there may also be architectural disturbance [539]. Severe and often fatal panenteritis is also described in ulcerative colitis [540]. Diffuse duodenitis is a rare complication of ulcerative colitis [539,541]. Both before and after colectomy, there may rarely be varying degrees of chronic inflammation and villous architectural disturbance in the duodenal mucosa [539]. Such diffuse duodenitis is also described in children with ulcerative colitis [542]. These changes, in the jejunum and duodenum, may be the result of bacterial flora changes as a result of the colonic disease [541].

Postcolectomy small intestinal pathology in ulcerative colitis

Whilst pelvic ileal reservoir pathology is the most clinically important entity in this category (see above), further pathological changes are seen in the small intestinal mucosa as a result of colectomy and proctocolectomy for ulcerative colitis.

Ileorectal anastomosis

Until about 25 years ago, there was a vogue for ileorectal anastomosis in ulcerative colitis before it was appreciated that the rectum was an important site for carcinoma development in ulcerative colitis and before the advent of pelvic pouch surgery. The ileal mucosa proximal to an ileorectal anastomosis shows florid changes on biopsy not unlike those of backwash ileitis. There is villous architectural change, active inflammation and occasional erosions and ulceration [543]. Studies have shown that active inflammation and epithelial cell proliferation are prominent early after the operation but that the epithelial proliferation, in particular, returns to relative normality with time [543]. Eventually, as in backwash ileitis, the mucosa appears relatively atrophic. In this situation, it may well be difficult, on biopsy, to differentiate between ileal and rectal mucosa, both showing architectural distortion and the long-term effects of chronic ulcerative colitis.

Prestomal ileitis

Obstructive ileitis is now well recognized proximal to an obstructive lesion in the small bowel, but true prestomal ileitis is a condition specific to patients who have undergone total proctocolectomy and permanent ileostomy [544]. It is characterized by profuse watery ileostomy discharge with marked systemic symptoms [544]. Perforation is common. The macroscopic features are of deep linear ulceration with normal intervening mucosa (Fig. 21.39). The ulcers may be fissuring and thus there is some resemblance to Crohn's disease. However, the disease lacks the other pathological hallmarks of Crohn's disease such as granulomas, transmural inflammation and connective changes. The condition is fortunately rare as it has a high mortality. Despite its associations with ulcerative colitis, its pathogenesis remains unclear.

Ileostomy pathology

Various mechanical and ischaemic mechanisms are responsible for villous architectural changes and inflammation that

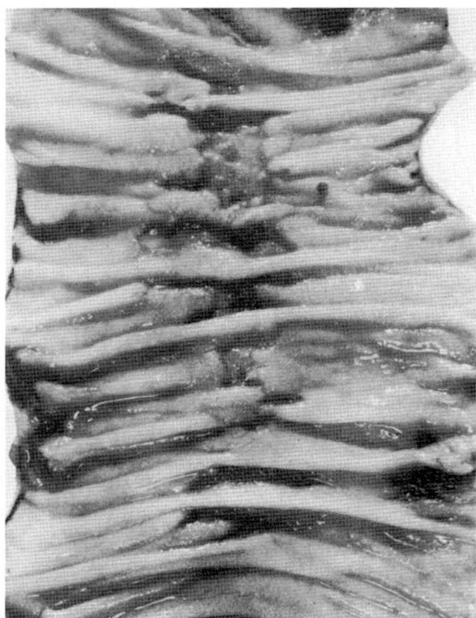

Fig. 21.39 Prestomal ileitis. The ulcers are linear, deep and very clear cut, and the intervening mucosa is normal.

are almost inevitable in the ileostomy mucosa regardless of the indication for ileostomy (Fig. 21.40). Furthermore, minor degrees of obstruction are commonplace and these may induce more pronounced inflammation, villous atrophy and ulceration. There may also be the changes of mucosal prolapse, well recognized in ileostomy mucosa as at other sites where mechanical forces are at play in the intestinal mucosa (Fig. 21.41) [545]. Obstructive ileitis and prestomal ileitis may be seen proximal to an ileostomy. Finally, dysplasia and carcinoma are well recognized at ileostomies, especially those performed for inflammatory bowel disease and familial adenomatous polyposis [546,547]. How important the inflammatory pathology of the stomal mucosa is in carcinogenesis is uncertain.

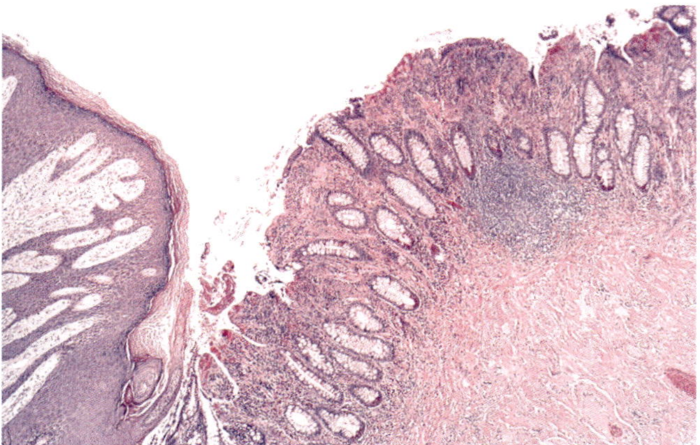

Fig. 21.40 Villous atrophy and chronic inflammation are very commonly seen in the ileal mucosa adjacent to an ileostomy. They should not be taken as evidence of Crohn's disease.

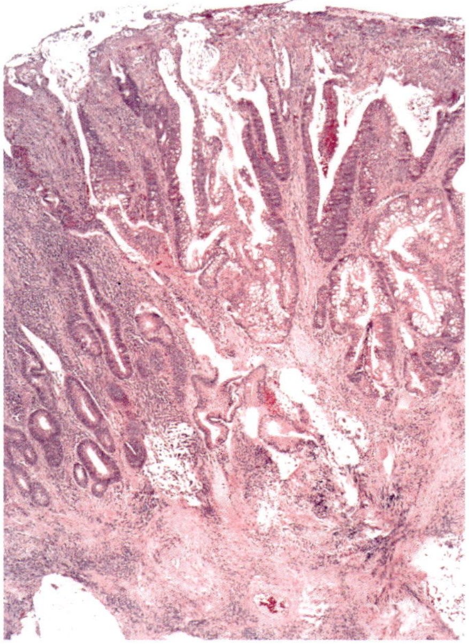

Fig. 21.41 Mucosal prolapse changes in the ileal mucosa of an ileostomy. The dramatic epithelial hyperplasia and the enteritis cystica profunda with mucin lakes can trick the unwary into a diagnosis of malignancy.

Ileal conduits

Ileal conduits are urinary reservoirs constructed after bladder resection for malignancy. Varying degrees of mucosal abnormality are described, including villous architectural changes and mucin depletion [548]. There is evidence of some increased malignancy risk, transitional cell carcinomas at the ureteroileal junction being most commonly described [549].

Obstructive ileitis

Obstructive colitis is now well recognized to have characteristic macroscopic and histopathological features [550]. We have seen several cases of 'obstructive ileitis' where similar macroscopic and histological changes have been observed in the small intestine, but the condition is relatively poorly documented in the literature [551]. As in the colon, there appears to be a vascular element to the pathogenesis with mural hypoperfusion and secondary localized ischaemia apparently accounting for relatively sharply localized ischaemic-type inflammation and ulceration, often adjacent to relatively normal-appearing mucosa [551]. We have seen several cases now, as described by others [552], in which obstructing carcinoid tumours of the small intestine have produced proximal ulceration and granulation tissue polyposis, presumably a consequence of obstruction and relative ischaemia due to compromise of blood supply. The latter is putatively induced by a combination of the mechanical effects of the obstructing tumour and vascular spread by small intestinal carcinoid, a feature that seems to predict the presence of associated granulation tissue polyposis.

Non-specific jejunitis

Isolated jejunitis often has relatively non-specific histological features but it occurs in several specific situations. So-called ulcerative jejunitis is now recognized to be a neoplastic complication of coeliac disease: there is good pathological and molecular evidence that most, if not all, of such cases represent early T-cell lymphoma complicating coeliac disease (see p. 381) [553,554]. Isolated jejunitis is rarely an early manifestation of systemic disorders such as Henoch–Schönlein purpura [555] and microscopic polyarteritis [556]. Severe necrotizing jejunitis is an uncommon condition that occurs in children; its potential causes are many, but often no cause is found [557]. The disease shows similarities to enteritis necroticans (see above) and may represent a bacterial overgrowth pathology [557,558]. Corrosive jejunitis due to the ingestion of acids may occur, but this is only likely after previous gastroenterostomy allows the undiluted acid to enter the jejunum [559].

Chronic 'non-specific' duodenitis

Inflammation of the duodenum is caused by a large number of pathogenic mechanisms with diverse clinical implications. For the purposes of this discussion, it will be divided into two main groups: inflammation maximal in the duodenal bulb and clearly associated with *Helicobacter pylori* infection, chronic active gastritis and peptic ulcer disease (variably called chronic non-specific duodenitis, chronic active duodenitis and, even, *H. pylori* bulbitis) [560–562]; and that due to other specific causes such as coeliac disease, Crohn's disease, drugs, Whipple's disease, parasitic infection and ulcerative colitis. To the practising pathologist, the differentiation between *H. pylori*-related duodenitis, coeliac disease and Crohn's disease is probably the most important. For an account of the pathology of individual causes of duodenitis, the reader should seek the appropriate sections elsewhere. This account will concentrate on the pathology of duodenitis associated with *H. pylori*, maximal in the bulb of the duodenum.

Macroscopically, especially on endoscopic examination, duodenitis may be manifest by mucosal swelling, erythema, erosions and petechial haemorrhages. These changes are particularly prominent adjacent to established peptic ulcer. However, it should be emphasized that there is often poor correlation between endoscopic and histopathological features; it is well recognized that the endoscopically normal duodenum will harbour inflammatory changes on biopsy [562]. However, those with detectable macroscopic features, especially erosions, are at significant risk for subsequent peptic ulcer disease in the duodenum [563].

The microscopic assessment of duodenitis has not been aided by a lack of uniformity and definition and by the fact that assessment of inflammation is particularly difficult in a mucosa with a considerable mononuclear cell presence in the physiological state [564]. Furthermore, the variation in villous architecture in the normal duodenal bulb is considerable, with leaf and clubbed forms common, and this underpins the importance of well orientated sections for histological assessment [564]. For these reasons, only gross abnormalities of mononuclear cell numbers and villous architecture can be regarded as reliable markers for duodenitis (Fig. 21.42) [565,566].

Neutrophil polymorph infiltration is a much more reliable indicator of duodenitis; this is seen in the lamina propria and in crypt and surface epithelium [566]. The polymorph infiltrate is often focal, emphasizing the importance of examining multiple levels. Surface and crypt epithelial changes are also of importance, with degenerative changes in the former and regenerative changes in the latter. Finally, active duodenitis is associated with gastric metaplasia (Fig. 21.42). Although this feature may be seen in duodenal Crohn's disease [564], and less commonly in coeliac disease [567], it is an important component of *H. pylori*-associated duodenitis and peptic ulcer disease (Fig. 21.43) [560,568]. There is increasing evidence of the importance and prevalence of gastric metaplasia in peptic ulcer disease and its strong association with active inflammation in the duodenal bulb [569]. *H. pylori* will not normally colonize small intestinal mucosa. Marshall and colleagues [570] first suggested that the organism could colonize antral-type mucosa in the duodenum bulb, but it was Wyatt and Dixon who popularized the view that gastric metaplasia is an important part of the pathogenesis of *H. pylori*-related duodenitis and duodenal peptic ulceration [571,572].

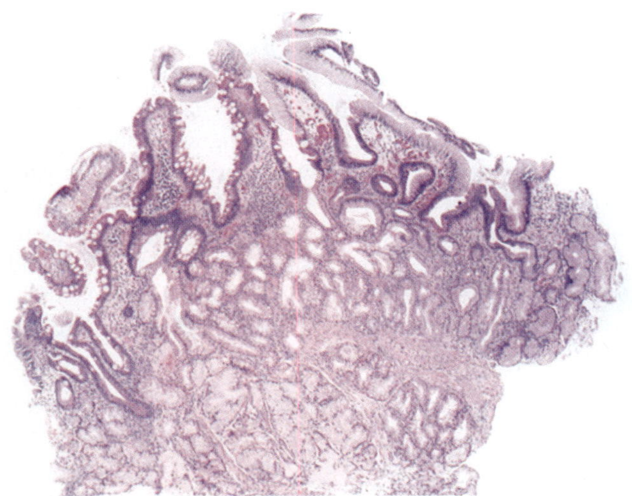

Fig. 21.42 A chronic duodenitis with minor abnormalities of crypt architecture. Gastric metaplasia is just discernible at this power. The pathology was *H. pylori* related.

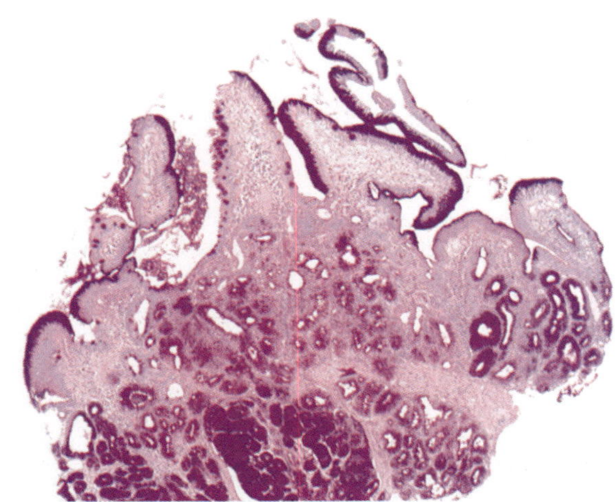

Fig. 21.43 A PAS stain serves to highlight the gastric metaplasia in the biopsy from Fig. 21.42. We believe that a PAS stain should be a routine procedure for duodenal biopsies.

More recently the evidence for *H. pylori*-induced, gastric metaplasia-associated duodenitis being the most common and important inflammatory pathology in the duodenal bulb has become more compelling [562]. Factors known to be important in the genesis of chronic active gastritis are also important in the duodenum. For instance, increased *H. pylori* pathogenicity, determined by CagA and vacuolating toxin positivity, is predictive of duodenitis and ulceration [560,562,573]. It should be emphasized, however, that *H. pylori* is much more difficult to demonstrate in duodenal mucosal biopsies than in gastric mucosal biopsies. They are usually scanty and in coccoid forms [562]. Initial studies suggested that only about 50% of inflamed duodenal biopsies will show identifiable *H. pylori* [572]. However, there is a much higher prevalence of specific IgA anti-*H. pylori* antibodies in the first part of the duodenum, providing firmer evidence of the association between the organism and 'bulbitis' [574]. From the practising histopathologist's viewpoint, these studies emphasize the importance of differentiating duodenitis of the duodenal bulb, almost uniquely associated with *H. pylori* infection and its gastric manifestations, from other chronic active duodenitides that are prevalent in the more distal duodenum and associated with other pathological mechanisms [562,575].

References

1 Cuvelier C, Demetter P, Mielants H, Veys EM, De Vos M. Interpretation of ileal biopsies: morphological features in normal and diseased mucosa. *Histopathology*, 2001; 38: 1.

2 O'Mahony S, Morris AJ, Straiton M, Murray L, Mackenzie JF. Push enteroscopy in the investigation of small-intestinal disease. *Q J Med*, 1996; 89: 685.

3 Blacklow NR, Greenberg HB. Viral gastroenteritis. *N Engl J Med*, 1991; 325: 252.

4 Kaljot KT, Ling JP, Gold JW *et al.* Prevalence of acute enteric viral pathogens in acquired immunodeficiency syndrome patients with diarrhea. *Gastroenterology*, 1989; 97: 1031.

5 Luthi TM, Wall PG, Evans HS, Adak GK, Caul EO. Outbreaks of foodborne viral gastroenteritis in England and Wales: 1992 to 1994. *Commun Dis Rep CDR Rev*, 1996; 6: R131.

6 Madeley CR. Viruses associated with acute diarrhoeal illness. In: Zuckerman AJ, Banatvala JE, Pattison JR, eds. *Principles and Practice of Clinical Virology*. Chichester: John Wiley & Sons, 1995: 189.

7 Caul EO. Viral gastroenteritis: small round structured viruses, caliciviruses and astroviruses. Part I. The clinical and diagnostic perspective. *J Clin Pathol*, 1996; 49: 874.

8 Hale AD, Crawford SE, Ciarlet M *et al.* Expression and self-assembly of Grimsby virus: antigenic distinction from Norwalk and Mexico viruses. *Clin Diagn Lab Immunol*, 1999; 6: 142.

9 Glass RI, Noel J, Ando T *et al.* The epidemiology of enteric caliciviruses from humans: a reassessment using new diagnostics. *J Infect Dis*, 2000; 181 (Suppl 2): S254.

10 Maguire AJ, Green J, Brown DW, Desselberger U, Gray JJ. Molecular epidemiology of outbreaks of gastroenteritis associated with small round-structured viruses in East Anglia, United Kingdom, during the 1996–1997 season. *J Clin Microbiol*, 1999; 37: 81.

11 Dedman D, Laurichesse H, Caul EO, Wall PG. Surveillance of small round structured virus (SRSV) infection in England and Wales, 1990–5. *Epidemiol Infect*, 1998; 121: 139.

12 Kapikian AZ. Overview of viral gastroenteritis. *Arch Virol Suppl*, 1996; 12: 7.

13 Nakata S, Honma S, Numata KK *et al.* Members of the family caliciviridae (Norwalk virus and Sapporo virus) are the most prevalent cause of gastroenteritis outbreaks among infants in Japan. *J Infect Dis*, 2000; 181: 2029.

14 Walker-Smith J. Rotavirus gastroenteritis. *Arch Dis Child*, 1978; 53: 355.

15 Lieberman JM. Rotavirus and other viral causes of gastroenteritis. *Pediatr Ann*, 1994; 23: 529.

16 Hrdy DB. Epidemiology of rotaviral infection in adults. *Rev Infect Dis*, 1987; 9: 461.

17 Davidson GP, Barnes GL. Structural and functional abnormalities of the small intestine in infants and young children with rotavirus enteritis. *Acta Paediatr Scand*, 1979; 68: 181.

18 Moreau MC, Corthier G, Muller MC, Dubos F, Raibaud P. Relationships between rotavirus diarrhea and intestinal microflora establishment in conventional and gnotobiotic mice. *J Clin Microbiol*, 1986; 23: 863.

19 Jeffries BC, Brandt CD, Kim HW, Rodriguez WJ, Arrobio JO, Parrott RH. Diarrhea-associated adenovirus from the respiratory tract. *J Infect Dis*, 1988; 157: 1275.

20 Nicolas JC, Ingrand D, Fortier B, Bricout F. A one-year virological survey of acute intussusception in childhood. *J Med Virol*, 1982; 9: 267.

21 Francis N. Light and electron microscopic appearances of pathological changes in HIV gut infection. *Baillieres Clin Gastroenterol*, 1990; 4: 495.

22 Blanshard C, Francis N, Gazzard BG. Investigation of chronic diarrhoea in acquired immunodeficiency syndrome. A prospective study of 155 patients. *Gut*, 1996; 39: 824.

23 Nazer H. Astrovirus gastroenteritis. *J Trop Pediatr*, 1985; 31: 67.

24 Glass RI, Noel J, Mitchell D *et al.* The changing epidemiology of astrovirus-associated gastroenteritis: a review. *Arch Virol Suppl*, 1996; 12: 287.

25 Macnaughton MR, Davies HA. Human enteric coronaviruses. Brief review. *Arch Virol*, 1981; 70: 301.

26 Rousset S, Moscovici O, Lebon P *et al.* Intestinal lesions containing coronavirus-like particles in neonatal necrotizing enterocolitis: an ultrastructural analysis. *Pediatrics*, 1984; 73: 218.

27 Francis ND, Boylston AW, Roberts AH, Parkin JM, Pinching AJ. Cytomegalovirus infection in gastrointestinal tracts of patients infected with HIV-1 or AIDS. *J Clin Pathol*, 1989; 42: 1055.

28 Cheung AN, Ng IO. Cytomegalovirus infection of the gastrointestinal tract in non-AIDS patients. *Am J Gastroenterol*, 1993; 88: 1882.

29 Cooper HS, Raffensperger EC, Jonas L, Fitts WT. Cytomegalovirus inclusions in patients with ulcerative colitis and toxic dilation requiring colonic resection. *Gastroenterology*, 1977; 72: 1253.

30 Goodman ZD, Boitnott JK, Yardley JH. Perforation of the colon associated with cytomegalovirus infection. *Dig Dis Sci*, 1979; 24: 376.

31 Sindre H, Haraldsen G, Beck S *et al.* Human intestinal endothelium shows high susceptibility to cytomegalovirus and altered

expression of adhesion molecules after infection. *Scand J Immunol*, 2000; 51: 354.

32 Genta RM, Bleyzer I, Cate TR, Tandon AK, Yoffe B. In situ hybridization and immunohistochemical analysis of cytomegalovirus-associated ileal perforation. *Gastroenterology*, 1993; 104: 1822.

33 Iwasaki T. Alimentary tract lesions in cytomegalovirus infection. *Acta Pathol Jpn*, 1987; 37: 549.

34 Shintaku M, Inoue N, Sasaki M, Izuno Y, Ueda Y, Ikehara S. Cytomegalovirus vasculitis accompanied by an exuberant fibroblastic reaction in the intestine of an AIDS patient. *Acta Pathol Jpn*, 1991; 41: 900.

35 Plosker GL, Noble S. Indinavir: a review of its use in the management of HIV infection. *Drugs*, 1999; 58: 1165.

36 Ullrich R, Zeitz M, Heise W, L'age M, Hoffken G, Riecken EO. Small intestinal structure and function in patients infected with human immunodeficiency virus (HIV): evidence for HIV-induced enteropathy. *Ann Intern Med*, 1989; 111: 15.

37 Batman PA, Miller AR, Forster SM, Harris JR, Pinching AJ, Griffin GE. Jejunal enteropathy associated with human immunodeficiency virus infection: quantitative histology. *J Clin Pathol*, 1989; 42: 275.

38 Francis N. Histopathology of the gut in the acquired immune deficiency syndrome. *Eur J Gastroenterol Hepatol*, 1992; 4: 449.

39 Fox CH, Kotler D, Tierney A, Wilson CS, Fauci AS. Detection of HIV-1 RNA in the lamina propria of patients with AIDS and gastrointestinal disease. *J Infect Dis*, 1989; 159: 467.

40 Kotler DP, Weaver SC, Terzakis JA. Ultrastructural features of epithelial cell degeneration in rectal crypts of patients with AIDS. *Am J Surg Pathol*, 1986; 10: 531.

41 Bjarnason I, Sharpstone DR, Francis N *et al*. Intestinal inflammation, ileal structure and function in HIV. *AIDS*, 1996; 10: 1385.

42 Kotler DP, Shimada T, Snow G *et al*. Effect of combination antiretroviral therapy upon rectal mucosal HIV RNA burden and mononuclear cell apoptosis. *AIDS*, 1998; 12: 597.

43 Francis N. Infectious complications of HIV disease: a selective review. *Curr Diag Pathol*, 1994; 1: 142.

44 Sepkowitz KA. Effect of HAART on natural history of AIDS-related opportunistic disorders. *Lancet*, 1998; 351: 228.

45 Bower M, Fox P, Fife K, Gill J, Nelson M, Gazzard B. Highly active anti-retroviral therapy (HAART) prolongs time to treatment failure in Kaposi's sarcoma. *AIDS*, 1999; 13: 2105.

46 Sansone GR, Frengley JD. Impact of HAART on causes of death of persons with late-stage AIDS. *J Urban Health*, 2000; 77: 166.

47 Laughon BE, Druckman DA, Vernon A *et al*. Prevalence of enteric pathogens in homosexual men with and without acquired immunodeficiency syndrome. *Gastroenterology*, 1988; 94: 984.

48 Connolly GM, Forbes A, Gazzard BG. Investigation of seemingly pathogen-negative diarrhoea in patients infected with HIV1. *Gut*, 1990; 31: 886.

49 Peacock CS, Blanshard C, Tovey DG, Ellis DS, Gazzard BG. Histological diagnosis of intestinal microsporidiosis in patients with AIDS. *J Clin Pathol*, 1991; 44: 558.

50 Surawicz CM. Diarrhea. In: Dale DC, Federman DD, eds. *Scientific American Medicine*. New York: WebMD Reference, 2000: III:1.

51 Guerrant RL, Lima AAM. Inflammatory enteritides. In: Mandell GL, Bennett JE, Dolin R, eds. *Principles and Practice of Infectious Diseases*. Philadelphia: Churchill Livingstone, 2000: 1126.

52 Shepherd NA. Pathological mimics of chronic inflammatory bowel disease. *J Clin Pathol*, 1991; 44: 726.

53 Lindberg AA, Pal T. Strategies for development of potential candidate *Shigella* vaccines. *Vaccine*, 1993; 11: 168.

54 Townes JM, Quick R, Gonzales OY *et al*. Etiology of bloody diarrhea in Bolivian children: implications for empiric therapy. Bolivian Dysentery Study Group. *J Infect Dis*, 1997; 175: 1527.

55 Bennish ML, Salam MA, Wahed MA. Enteric protein loss during shigellosis. *Am J Gastroenterol*, 1993; 88: 53.

56 Day DW, Mandal BK, Morson BC. The rectal biopsy appearances in *Salmonella* colitis. *Histopathology*, 1978; 2: 117.

57 Boyd JF. Pathology of the alimentary tract in *Salmonella typhimurium* food poisoning. *Gut*, 1985; 26: 935.

58 Arnold JW, Niesel DW, Annable CR *et al*. Tumor necrosis factor-alpha mediates the early pathology in *Salmonella* infection of the gastrointestinal tract. *Microb Pathog*, 1993; 14: 217.

59 Blaser MJ, Parsons RB, Wang WL. Acute colitis caused by *Campylobacter fetus* ss. *jejuni*. *Gastroenterology*, 1980; 78: 448.

60 Price AB, Jewkes J, Sanderson PJ. Acute diarrhoea: *Campylobacter colitis* and the role of rectal biopsy. *J Clin Pathol*, 1979; 32: 990.

61 Pearson RD, Guerrant RL. Enteric fever and other causes of abdominal symptoms with fever. In: Mandell GL, Bennett JE, Dolin R, eds. *Principles and Practice of Infectious Diseases*. Philadelphia: Churchill Livingstone, 2000: 1136.

62 Gonzalez A, Vargas V, Guarner L, Accarino A, Guardia J. Toxic megacolon in typhoid fever. *Arch Intern Med*, 1985; 145: 2120.

63 Chuttani HK, Jain K, Misra RC. Small bowel in typhoid fever. *Gut*, 1971; 12: 709.

64 Noorani MA, Sial I, Mal V. Typhoid perforation of small bowel: a study of 72 cases. *J R Coll Surg Edinb*, 1997; 42: 274.

65 Khanna AK, Misra MK. Typhoid perforation of the gut. *Postgrad Med J*, 1984; 60: 523.

66 Mandal BK. Typhoid and paratyphoid fever. *Clin Gastroenterol*, 1979; 8: 715.

67 Cook GC. Gastroenterological emergencies in the tropics. *Baillieres Clin Gastroenterol*, 1991; 5: 861.

68 Moyenuddin M, Weiss R, Wachsmuth IK, Ahearn DG. Non-toxigenic *Vibrio cholerae* O1 intestinal pathology in adult mice. *Zentralbl Bakteriol*, 1995; 283: 43.

69 Asakura H, Morita A, Morishita T *et al*. Pathologic findings from intestinal biopsy specimens in human cholera. *Am J Dig Dis*, 1973; 18: 271.

70 Rabbani GH. Cholera. *Clin Gastroenterol*, 1986; 15: 507.

71 O'Brien AD, Newland JW, Miller SF, Holmes RK, Smith HW, Formal SB. Shiga-like toxin-converting phages from *Escherichia coli* strains that cause hemorrhagic colitis or infantile diarrhea. *Science*, 1984; 226: 694.

72 Phillips AD, Navabpour S, Hicks S, Dougan G, Wallis T, Frankel G. Enterohaemorrhagic *Escherichia coli* 0157:H7 target Peyer's patches in humans and cause attaching / effacing lesions in both human and bovine intestine. *Gut*, 2000: 47: 377.

73 Richardson SE, Karmali MA, Becker LE, Smith CR. The histopathology of the hemolytic uremic syndrome associated with verocytotoxin-producing *Escherichia coli* infections. *Hum Pathol*, 1988; 19: 1102.

74 Murray KF, Patterson K. *Escherichia coli* 0157:H7-induced

hemolytic–uremic syndrome: histopathologic changes in the colon over time. *Pediatr Dev Pathol*, 2000: 3: 232.

75 Isogai E, Isogai H, Kimura K *et al.* Role of tumor necrosis factor alpha in gnotobiotic mice infected with an *Escherichia coli* 0157:H7 strain. *Infect Immun*, 1998: 66: 197.

76 Guo X, Wang A, Chen S, Qiu Z. [The curative effects of anti-TNF monoclonal antibody in *E. coli* infected mice.] *Zhongguo Yi Xue Ke Xue Yuan Xue Bao*, 1997; 19: 312.

77 Candy DC, McNeish AS. Human *Escherichia coli* diarrhoea. *Arch Dis Child*, 1984; 59: 395.

78 Borriello SP. Clostridial disease of the gut. *Clin Infect Dis*, 1995; 20 (Suppl 2): S242.

79 Tsutaoka B, Hansen J, Johnson D, Holodniy M. Antibiotic-associated pseudomembranous enteritis due to *Clostridium difficile*. *Clin Infect Dis*, 1994; 18: 982.

80 Yee HF, Brown RS, Ostroff JW. Fatal *Clostridium difficile* enteritis after total abdominal colectomy. *J Clin Gastroenterol*, 1996; 22: 45.

81 Kralovich KA, Sacksner J, Karmy-Jones RA, Eggenberger JC. Pseudomembranous colitis with associated fulminant ileitis in the defunctionalized limb of a jejunal–ileal bypass. Report of a case. *Dis Colon Rectum*, 1997; 40: 622.

82 Vesoulis Z, Williams G, Matthews B. Pseudomembranous enteritis after proctocolectomy: report of a case. *Dis Colon Rectum*, 2000; 43: 551.

83 Torres J, Jennische E, Lange S, Lonnroth I. Enterotoxins from *Clostridium difficile*; diarrhoeogenic potency and morphological effects in the rat intestine. *Gut*, 1990; 31: 781.

84 Murrell TG, Walker PD. The pigbel story of Papua New Guinea. *Trans R Soc Trop Med Hyg*, 1991; 85: 119.

85 Butler T, Dahms B, Lindpaintner K, Islam M, Azad MA, Anton P. Segmental necrotising enterocolitis: pathological and clinical features of 22 cases in Bangladesh. *Gut*, 1987; 28: 1433.

86 Watson DA, Andrew JH, Banting S, Mackay JR, Stillwell RG, Merrett M. Pig-bel but no pig: enteritis necroticans acquired in Australia. *Med J Aust*, 1991; 155: 47.

87 Farrant JM, Traill Z, Conlon C *et al.* Pigbel-like syndrome in a vegetarian in Oxford. *Gut*, 1996; 39: 336.

88 Kreft B, Dalhoff K, Sack K. [Necrotizing enterocolitis: a historical and current review.] *Med Klin*, 2000; 95: 435.

89 Cooke R. The pathology of pig bel. *P N G Med J*, 1979; 22: 35.

90 Mintz AC, Applebaum H. Focal gastrointestinal perforations not associated with necrotizing enterocolitis in very low birth weight neonates. *J Pediatr Surg*, 1993; 28: 857.

91 Han SJ, Jung PM, Kim H *et al.* Multiple intestinal ulcerations and perforations secondary to methicillin-resistant *Staphylococcus aureus* enteritis in infants. *J Pediatr Surg*, 1999; 34: 381.

92 Altemeier WA, Hummel RP, Hill EO. Staphylococcal enterocolitis following antibiotic therapy. *Ann Surg* 1963; 157: 847–9.

93 Hummel RP, Altemeier WA, Hill EO. Iatrogenic staphylococcal enterocolitis. *Ann Surg*, 1964; 160: 551.

94 Bradford WD, Noce PS, Gutman LT. Pathologic features of enteric infection with *Yersinia enterocolitica*. *Arch Pathol*, 1974; 98: 17.

95 El Maraghi NR, Mair NS. The histopathology of enteric infection with *Yersinia pseudotuberculosis*. *Am J Clin Pathol*, 1979; 71: 631.

96 Anonymous. Yersiniosis today. *Lancet*, 1984; 1: 84.

97 Fenwick SG, McCarthy MD. *Yersinia enterocolitica* is a common cause of gastroenteritis in Auckland. *N Z Med J*, 1995; 108: 269.

98 Rabson AR, Hallett AF, Koornhof HJ. Generalized *Yersinia enterocolitica* infection. *J Infect Dis*, 1975; 131: 447.

99 Spira TJ, Kabins SA. *Yersinia enterocolitica* septicemia with septic arthritis. *Arch Intern Med*, 1976; 136: 1305.

100 Tauxe RV, Vandepitte J, Wauters G *et al.* *Yersinia enterocolitica* infections and pork: the missing link. *Lancet*, 1987; 1: 1129.

101 Satterthwaite P, Pritchard K, Floyd D, Law B. A case-control study of *Yersinia enterocolitica* infections in Auckland. *Aust N Z J Public Health*, 1999; 23: 482.

102 Arvastson B, Damgaard K, Winblad S. Clinical symptoms of infection with *Yersinia enterocolitica*. *Scand J Infect Dis*, 1971; 3: 37.

103 Gleason TH, Patterson SD. The pathology of *Yersinia enterocolitica* ileocolitis. *Am J Surg Pathol*, 1982; 6: 347.

104 Attwood SE, Mealy K, Cafferkey MT *et al.* *Yersinia* infection and acute abdominal pain. *Lancet*, 1987; 1: 529.

105 Karper CM, Boman I. The significance of *Klebsiella* enteritis. A study of seven cases. *Am J Clin Pathol*, 1966; 46: 632.

106 Janda JM, Abbott SL. Evolving concepts regarding the genus *Aeromonas*: an expanding panorama of species, disease presentations, and unanswered questions. *Clin Infect Dis*, 1998; 27: 332.

107 Merino S, Rubires X, Knochel S, Tomas JM. Emerging pathogens: *Aeromonas* spp. *Int J Food Microbiol*, 1995; 28: 157.

108 Alavandi S, Ananthan S, Kang G. Prevalence, in-vitro secretory activity, and cytotoxicity of *Aeromonas* species associated with childhood gastroenteritis in Chennai (Madras), India. *Jpn J Med Sci Biol*, 1998; 51: 1.

109 Jones BL, Wilcox MH. *Aeromonas* infections and their treatment. *J Antimicrob Chemother*, 1995; 35: 453.

110 Manley PN, Dhru R. Actinomycosis complicating Crohn's disease. *Gastroenterology*, 1980; 79: 934.

111 Piper JV, Stoner BA, Mitra SK, Talerman A. Ileo-vesical fistula associated with pelvic actinomycosis. *Br J Clin Pract*, 1969; 23: 341.

112 Uchiyama N, Ishikawa T, Miyakawa K *et al.* Abdominal actinomycosis: barium enema and computed tomography findings. *J Gastroenterol*, 1997; 32: 89.

113 Kirsch M. Bacterial overgrowth. *Am J Gastroenterol*, 1990; 85: 231.

114 Haboubi NY, Cowley PA, Lee GS. Small bowel bacterial overgrowth: a cause of malnutrition in the elderly? *Eur J Clin Nutr*, 1988; 42: 999.

115 Riordan SM, McIver CJ, Wakefield D, Duncombe VM, Bolin TD, Thomas MC. Luminal immunity in small-intestinal bacterial overgrowth and old age. *Scand J Gastroenterol*, 1996; 31: 1103.

116 Bragelmann R, Armbrecht U, Rosemeyer D, Schneider B, Zilly W, Stockbrugger RW. Small bowel bacterial overgrowth in patients after total gastrectomy. *Eur J Clin Invest*, 1997; 27: 409.

117 Kaye SA, Lim SG, Taylor M, Patel S, Gillespie S, Black CM. Small bowel bacterial overgrowth in systemic sclerosis: detection using direct and indirect methods and treatment outcome. *Br J Rheumatol*, 1995; 34: 265.

118 Mathias JR, Clench MH. Review: pathophysiology of diarrhea caused by bacterial overgrowth of the small intestine. *Am J Med Sci*, 1985; 289: 243.

119 Riordan SM, McIver CJ, Thomas DH, Duncombe VM, Bolin TD, Thomas MC. Luminal bacteria and small-intestinal permeability. *Scand J Gastroenterol*, 1997; 32: 556.

120 Haboubi NY, Lee GS, Montgomery RD. Duodenal mucosal morphometry of elderly patients with small intestinal bacterial overgrowth: response to antibiotic treatment. *Age Ageing*, 1991; 20: 29.

121 Kapoor VK. Abdominal tuberculosis. *Postgrad Med J*, 1998; 74: 459.

122 Klimach OE, Ormerod LP. Gastrointestinal tuberculosis: a retrospective review of 109 cases in a district general hospital. *Q J Med*, 1985; 56: 569.

123 Sherman S, Rohwedder JJ, Ravikrishnan KP, Weg JG. Tuberculous enteritis and peritonitis. Report of 36 general hospital cases. *Arch Intern Med*, 1980; 140: 506.

124 Koo J, Ho J, Ong GB. The value of colonoscopy in the diagnosis of ileo-caecal tuberculosis. *Endoscopy*, 1982; 14: 48.

125 Fukuya T, Yoshimitsu K, Kitagawa S, Masuda K, Ueyama T, Haraguchi Y. Single tuberculous stricture in the jejunum: report of 2 cases. *Gastrointest Radiol*, 1989; 14: 300.

126 Ha HK, Ko GY, Yu ES *et al*. Intestinal tuberculosis with abdominal complications: radiologic and pathologic features. *Abdom Imaging*, 1999; 24: 32.

127 Tandon HD, Prakash A. Pathology of intestinal tuberculosis and its distinction from Crohn's disease. *Gut*, 1972; 13: 260.

128 Gaffney EF, Condell D, Majmudar B *et al*. Modification of caecal lymphoid tissue and relationship to granuloma formation in sporadic ileocaecal tuberculosis. *Histopathology*, 1987; 11: 691.

129 Talwar S, Talwar R, Prasad P. Tuberculous perforations of the small intestine. *Int J Clin Pract*, 1999; 53: 514.

130 Riedel L, Segal I, Mohamed AE, Hale M, Mannell A. The prolonged course of gastrointestinal tuberculosis. *J Clin Gastroenterol*, 1989; 11: 671.

131 Kaushik SP, Bassett ML, McDonald C, Lin BP, Bokey EL. Case report: gastrointestinal tuberculosis simulating Crohn's disease. *J Gastroenterol Hepatol*, 1996; 11: 532.

132 Shepherd NA, Jass JR. Neuromuscular and vascular hamartoma of the small intestine: is it Crohn's disease? *Gut*, 1987; 28: 1663.

133 Lucas SB, De Cock KM, Hounnou A *et al*. Contribution of tuberculosis to slim disease in Africa. *Br Med J*, 1994; 308: 1531.

134 Rutstein RM, Cobb P, McGowan KL, Pinto-Martin J, Starr SE. *Mycobacterium avium intracellulare* complex infection in HIV-infected children. *AIDS*, 1993; 7: 507.

135 Hellyer TJ, Brown IN, Taylor MB, Allen BW, Easmon CS. Gastrointestinal involvement in *Mycobacterium avium-intracellulare* infection of patients with HIV. *J Infect*, 1993; 26: 55.

136 Horsburgh CR, Mason UG, Farhi DC, Iseman MD. Disseminated infection with *Mycobacterium avium-intracellulare*. A report of 13 cases and a review of the literature. *Medicine (Baltimore)*, 1985; 64: 36.

137 Maliha GM, Hepps KS, Maia DM, Gentry KR, Fraire AE, Goodgame RW. Whipple's disease can mimic chronic AIDS enteropathy. *Am J Gastroenterol*, 1991; 86: 79.

138 Boylston AW, Cook HT, Francis ND, Goldin RD. Biopsy pathology of acquired immune deficiency syndrome (AIDS). *J Clin Pathol*, 1987; 40: 1.

139 Whipple GH. A hitherto undescribed disease characterised anatomically by deposits of fat and fatty acids in the intestinal and mesenteric lymphatic tissues. *Johns Hopkins Hosp Bull* 1907; 18: 382.

140 Fleming JL, Wiesner RH, Shorter RG. Whipple's disease: clinical, biochemical, and histopathologic features and assessment of treatment in 29 patients. *Mayo Clin Proc*, 1988; 63: 539.

141 Carvati C, Litch M, Weisiger B, Regland S, Berliner H. Diagnosis of Whipple's disease by rectal biopsy with a report of three additional cases. *Ann Intern Med*, 1963; 58: 166.

142 Wilson KH, Blitchington R, Frothingham R, Wilson JA. Phylogeny of the Whipple's-disease-associated bacterium. *Lancet*, 1991; 338: 474.

143 Relman DA, Schmidt TM, MacDermott RP, Falkow S. Identification of the uncultured bacillus of Whipple's disease. *N Engl J Med*, 1992; 327: 293.

144 Chears W, Ashworth C. Electron microscopy study of the intestinal mucosa in Whipple's disease—demonstration of encapsulated bacilliform bodies in the lesion. *Gastroenterology*, 1961; 41: 129.

145 Yardley JH, Hendrix TR. Combined electron and light microscopy in Whipple's disease—demonstration of 'bacillary bodies' in the intestine. *Johns Hopkins Hosp Bull*, 1961; 109: 80.

146 Maiwald M, Schuhmacher F, Ditton HJ, von Herbay A. Environmental occurrence of the Whipple's disease bacterium (*Tropheryma whippelii*). *Appl Environ Microbiol*, 1998; 64: 760.

147 Dobbins WO. Current concepts of Whipple's disease. *J Clin Gastroenterol*, 1982; 4: 205.

148 Groll A, Valberg LS, Simon JB, Eidinger D, Wilson B, Forsdyke DR. Immunological defect in Whipple's disease. *Gastroenterology*, 1972; 63: 943.

149 Ectors N, Geboes K, De Vos R *et al*. Whipple's disease: a histological, immunocytochemical and electronmicroscopic study of the immune response in the small intestinal mucosa. *Histopathology*, 1992; 21: 1.

150 Martin FF, Vilseck J, Dobbins WO, Buckley CE, Tyor MP. Immunological alterations in patients with treated Whipple's disease. *Gastroenterology*, 1972; 63: 6.

151 Marth T, Roux M, von Herbay A, Meuer SC, Feurle GE. Persistent reduction of complement receptor 3 alpha-chain expressing mononuclear blood cells and transient inhibitory serum factors in Whipple's disease. *Clin Immunol Immunopathol*, 1994; 72: 217.

152 Bjerknes R, Odegaard S, Bjerkvig R, Borkje B, Laerum OD. Whipple's disease. Demonstration of a persisting monocyte and macrophage dysfunction. *Scand J Gastroenterol*, 1988; 23: 611.

153 Marth T, Neurath M, Cuccherini BA, Strober W. Defects of monocyte interleukin 12 production and humoral immunity in Whipple's disease. *Gastroenterology*, 1997; 113: 442.

154 Dobbins WO. Is there an immune deficit in Whipple's disease? *Dig Dis Sci*, 1981; 26: 247.

155 Geboes K, Ectors N, Heidbuchel H, Rutgeerts P, Desmet V, Vantrappen G. Whipple's disease: endoscopic aspects before and after therapy. *Gastrointest Endosc*, 1990; 36: 247.

156 Isenberg JI, Gilbert SB, Pitcher JL. Ascites with peritoneal involvement in Whipple's disease. Report of a case. *Gastroenterology*, 1971; 60: 305.

157 von Herbay A, Ditton HJ, Maiwald M. Diagnostic application of a polymerase chain reaction assay for the Whipple's disease bacterium to intestinal biopsies. *Gastroenterology*, 1996; 110: 1735.

158 Mansbach CM, Shelburne JD, Stevens RD, Dobbins WO. Lymph-node bacilliform bodies resembling those of Whipple's disease in a patient without intestinal involvement. *Ann Intern Med*, 1978; 89: 64.

159 Wilcox GM, Tronic BS, Schecter DJ, Arron MJ, Righi DF, Weiner NJ. Periodic acid–Schiff-negative granulomatous lymphadenopathy in patients with Whipple's disease. Localization of the Whipple bacillus to noncaseating granulomas by electron microscopy. *Am J Med*, 1987; 83: 165.

160 Moorthy S, Nolley G, Hermos JA. Whipple's disease with minimal intestinal involvement. *Gut*, 1977; 18: 152.

161 Dauga C, Miras I, Grimont PA. Strategy for detection and identification of bacteria based on 16S rRNA genes in suspected cases of Whipple's disease. *J Med Microbiol*, 1997; 46: 340.

162 Muller C, Petermann D, Stain C *et al.* Whipple's disease: comparison of histology with diagnosis based on polymerase chain reaction in four consecutive cases. *Gut*, 1997; 40: 425.

163 Gross M, Jung C, Zoller WG. Detection of *Tropheryma whippelii* DNA (Whipple's disease) in faeces. *Ital J Gastroenterol Hepatol*, 1999; 31: 70.

164 Gras E, Matias-Guiu X, Garcia A *et al.* PCR analysis in the pathological diagnosis of Whipple's disease: emphasis on extraintestinal involvement or atypical morphological features. *J Pathol*, 1999; 188: 318.

165 Morgenegg S, Dutly F, Altwegg M. Cloning and sequencing of a part of the heat shock protein 65 gene (hsp65) of '*Tropheryma whippelii*' and its use for detection of '*T. whippelii*' in clinical specimens by PCR. *J Clin Microbiol*, 2000; 38: 2248.

166 Keinath RD, Merrell DE, Vlietstra R, Dobbins WO. Antibiotic treatment and relapse in Whipple's disease. Long-term follow-up of 88 patients. *Gastroenterology*, 1985; 88: 1867.

167 Feurle GE, Marth T. An evaluation of antimicrobial treatment for Whipple's Disease. Tetracycline versus trimethoprim-sulfamethoxazole. *Dig Dis Sci*, 1994; 39: 1642.

168 Ramzan NN, Loftus E, Burgart LJ *et al.* Diagnosis and monitoring of Whipple disease by polymerase chain reaction. *Ann Intern Med*, 1997; 126: 520.

169 Geboes K, Ectors N, Heidbuchel H, Rutgeerts P, Desmet V, Vantrappen G. Whipple's disease: the value of upper gastrointestinal endoscopy for the diagnosis and follow-up. *Acta Gastroenterol Belg*, 1992; 55: 209.

170 Schneider T, Stallmach A, von Herbay A, Marth T, Strober W, Zeitz M. Treatment of refractory Whipple disease with interferon-gamma. *Ann Intern Med*, 1998; 129: 875.

171 Shepherd NA. What is the significance of muciphages in colorectal biopsies? Muciphages and other mucosal accumulations in the colorectal mucosa. *Histopathology*, 2000; 36: 559.

172 Rodarte JR, Garrison CO, Holley KE, Fontana RS. Whipple's disease simulating sarcoidosis. A case with unique clinical and histologic features. *Arch Intern Med*, 1972: 129, 479.

173 Prescott RJ, Harris M, Banerjee SS. Fungal infections of the small and large intestine. *J Clin Pathol*, 1992; 45: 806.

174 Radin DR, Fong TL, Halls JM, Pontrelli GN. Monilial enteritis in acquired immunodeficiency syndrome. *Am J Roentgenol*, 1983; 141: 1289.

175 Fischer D, Labayle D, Versapuech JM, Grange D, Kemeny F. [Candidiasis involvement of the small intestine complicated by perforation. A case of favorable course.] *Gastroenterol Clin Biol*, 1987; 11: 514.

176 Schulman A, Bornman P, Kaplan C, Morton P, Rose A. Gastrointestinal mucormycosis. *Gastrointest Radiol*, 1979; 4: 385.

177 Lyon DT, Schubert TT, Mantia AG, Kaplan MH. Phycomycosis of the gastrointestinal tract. *Am J Gastroenterol*, 1979; 72: 379.

178 Nagy-Agren SE, Chu P, Smith GJ, Waskin HA, Altice FL. Zygomycosis (mucormycosis) and HIV infection: report of three cases and review. *J Acquir Immune Defic Syndr Hum Retrovirol*, 1995; 10: 441.

179 Stringer JR. *Pneumocystis carinii*: what is it, exactly? *Clin Microbiol Rev*, 1996; 9: 489.

180 Carter TR, Cooper PH, Petri WA, Kim CK, Walzer PD, Guerrant RL. *Pneumocystis carinii* infection of the small intestine in a patient with acquired immune deficiency syndrome. *Am J Clin Pathol*, 1988; 89: 679.

181 Matsuda S, Urata Y, Shiota T *et al.* Disseminated infection of *Pneumocystis carinii* in a patient with the acquired immunodeficiency syndrome. *Virchows Arch A Pathol Anat Histopathol*, 1989; 414: 523.

182 Haws CC, Long RF, Caplan GE. *Histoplasma capsulatum* as a cause of ilecolitis. *Am J Roentgenol*, 1977; 128: 692.

183 Cappell MS, Mandell W, Grimes MM, Neu HC. Gastrointestinal histoplasmosis. *Dig Dis Sci*, 1988; 33: 353.

184 Orchard JL, Luparello F, Brunskill D. Malabsorption syndrome occurring in the course of disseminated histoplasmosis: case report and review of gastrointestinal histoplasmosis. *Am J Med*, 1979; 66: 331.

185 Ackers JP. Gut coccidia—*Isospora*, *Cryptosporidium*, *Cyclospora* and *Sarcocystis*. *Semin Gastrointest Dis*, 1997; 8: 33.

186 Farthing MJ. Diarrhoeal disease: current concepts and future challenges. Pathogenesis of giardiasis. *Trans R Soc Trop Med Hyg*, 1993; 87 (Suppl 3): 17.

187 Oberhuber G, Kastner N, Stolte M. Giardiasis: a histologic analysis of 567 cases. *Scand J Gastroenterol*, 1997; 32: 48.

188 Gillon J. Giardiasis: review of epidemiology, pathogenetic mechanisms and host responses. *Q J Med*, 1984; 53: 29.

189 Chester AC, MacMurray FG, Restifo MD, Mann O. Giardiasis as a chronic disease. *Dig Dis Sci*, 1985; 30: 215.

190 Ament ME, Rubin CE. Relation of giardiasis to abnormal intestinal structure and function in gastrointestinal immunodeficiency syndromes. *Gastroenterology*, 1972; 62: 216.

191 Oberhuber G, Vogelsang H, Stolte M, Muthenthaler S, Kummer AJ, Radaszkiewicz T. Evidence that intestinal intraepithelial lymphocytes are activated cytotoxic T cells in celiac disease but not in giardiasis. *Am J Pathol*, 1996; 148: 1351.

192 Katelaris PH, Farthing MJ. Diarrhoea and malabsorption in giardiasis: a multifactorial process? *Gut*, 1992; 33: 295.

193 Laurent F, McCole D, Eckmann L, Kagnoff MF. Pathogenesis of *Cryptosporidium parvum* infection. *Microbes Infect*, 1999; 1: 141.

194 Katsumata T, Hosea D, Ranuh IG, Uga S, Yanagi T, Kohno S. Short report: possible *Cryptosporidium muris* infection in humans. *Am J Trop Med Hyg*, 2000; 62: 70.

195 Blanshard C, Jackson AM, Shanson DC, Francis N, Gazzard BG. Cryptosporidiosis in HIV-seropositive patients. *Q J Med*, 1992; 85: 813.

196 Manabe YC, Clark DP, Moore RD *et al.* Cryptosporidiosis in patients with AIDS: correlates of disease and survival. *Clin Infect Dis*, 1998; 27: 536.

197 Goodgame RW, Kimball K, Ou CN *et al.* Intestinal function and injury in acquired immunodeficiency syndrome-related cryptosporidiosis. *Gastroenterology*, 1995; 108: 1075.

198 Genta RM, Chappell CL, White AC, Kimball KT, Goodgame RW. Duodenal morphology and intensity of infection in AIDS-

related intestinal cryptosporidiosis. *Gastroenterology*, 1993; 105: 1769.
199 Lumadue JA, Manabe YC, Moore RD, Belitsos PC, Sears CL, Clark DP. A clinicopathologic analysis of AIDS-related cryptosporidiosis. *AIDS*, 1998; 12: 2459.
200 Kelly P, Thillainayagam AV, Smithson J *et al*. Jejunal water and electrolyte transport in human cryptosporidiosis. *Dig Dis Sci*, 1996; 41: 2095.
201 Marcial MA, Madara JL. Cryptosporidium: cellular localization, structural analysis of absorptive cell–parasite membrane–membrane interactions in guinea pigs, and suggestion of protozoan transport by M cells. *Gastroenterology*, 1986; 90: 583.
202 Pape JW, Johnson WD. *Isospora belli* infections. *Prog Clin Parasitol*, 1991; 2: 119.
203 Bernard E, Delgiudice P, Carles M *et al*. Disseminated isosporiasis in an AIDS patient. *Eur J Clin Microbiol Infect Dis*, 1997; 16: 699.
204 Bendall RP, Lucas S, Moody A, Tovey G, Chiodini PL. Diarrhoea associated with cyanobacterium-like bodies: a new coccidian enteritis of man. *Lancet*, 1993; 341: 590.
205 Nhieu JT, Nin F, Fleury-Feith J, Chaumette MT, Schaeffer A, Bretagne S. Identification of intracellular stages of *Cyclospora* species by light microscopy of thick sections using hematoxylin. *Hum Pathol*, 1996; 27: 1107.
206 Green ST, McKendrick MW, Mohsen AH, Schmid ML, Prakasam SF. Two simultaneous cases of *Cyclospora cayatensis* enteritis returning from the Dominican Republic. *J Travel Med*, 2000; 7: 41.
207 Shlim DR, Hoge CW, Rajah R, Scott RM, Pandy P, Echeverria P. Persistent high risk of diarrhea among foreigners in Nepal during the first 2 years of residence. *Clin Infect Dis*, 1999; 29: 613.
208 Soave R, Herwaldt BL, Relman DA. *Cyclospora*. *Infect Dis Clin North Am*, 1998; 12: 1.
209 Looney WJ. *Cyclospora* species as a cause of diarrhoea in humans. *Br J Biomed Sci*, 1998; 55: 157.
210 Connor BA, Reidy J, Soave R. Cyclosporiasis: clinical and histopathologic correlates. *Clin Infect Dis*, 1999; 28: 1216.
211 Verdier RI, Fitzgerald DW, Johnson WD, Pape JW. Trimethoprim-sulfamethoxazole compared with ciprofloxacin for treatment and prophylaxis of *Isospora belli* and *Cyclospora cayetanensis* infection in HIV-infected patients. A randomized, controlled trial. *Ann Intern Med*, 2000; 132: 885.
212 Sturbaum GD, Ortega YR, Gilman RH, Sterling CR, Cabrera L, Klein DA. Detection of *Cyclospora cayetanensis* in wastewater. *Appl Environ Microbiol*, 1998; 64: 2284.
213 Fleming CA, Caron D, Gunn JE, Barry MA. A foodborne outbreak of *Cyclospora cayetanensis* at a wedding: clinical features and risk factors for illness. *Arch Intern Med*, 1998; 158: 1121.
214 Eberhard ML, Pieniazek NJ, Arrowood MJ. Laboratory diagnosis of *Cyclospora* infections. *Arch Pathol Lab Med*, 1997; 121: 792.
215 Lucas SB. Imported infectious diseases. In: Lowe DG, Underwood JCE, eds. *Recent Advances in Histopathology*. Edinburgh: Churchill Livingstone, 2000: 23.
216 Franzen C, Muller A. Molecular techniques for detection, species differentiation, and phylogenetic analysis of microsporidia. *Clin Microbiol Rev*, 1999; 12: 243.
217 Cali A, Kotler DP, Orenstein JM. *Septata intestinalis* N. G., N. Sp., an intestinal microsporidian associated with chronic diarrhea and dissemination in AIDS patients. *J Eukaryot Microbiol*, 1993; 40: 101.
218 Franzen C, Muller A, Schwenk A *et al*. Intestinal microsporidiosis with *Septata intestinalis* in a patient with AIDS—response to albendazole. *J Infect*, 1995; 31: 237.
219 Cotte L, Rabodonirina M, Chapuis F *et al*. Waterborne outbreak of intestinal microsporidiosis in persons with and without human immunodeficiency virus infection. *J Infect Dis*, 1999; 180: 2003.
220 Talal AH, Kotler DP, Orenstein JM, Weiss LM. Detection of *Enterocytozoon bieneusi* in fecal specimens by polymerase chain reaction analysis with primers to the small-subunit rRNA. *Clin Infect Dis*, 1998; 26: 673.
221 Schwartz DA, Abou-Elella A, Wilcox CM *et al*. The presence of *Enterocytozoon bieneusi* spores in the lamina propria of small bowel biopsies with no evidence of disseminated microsporidiosis. Enteric Opportunistic Infections Working Group. *Arch Pathol Lab Med*, 1995; 119: 424.
222 Albrecht H, Sobottka I, Emminger C *et al*. Visceral leishmaniasis emerging as an important opportunistic infection in HIV-infected persons living in areas nonendemic for *Leishmania donovani*. *Arch Pathol Lab Med*, 1996; 120: 189.
223 Alvar J, Canavate C, Gutierrez-Solar B *et al*. Leishmania and human immunodeficiency virus coinfection: the first 10 years. *Clin Microbiol Rev*, 1997; 10: 298.
224 Koberle F. Enteromegaly and cardiomegaly in Chagas' disease. *Gut*, 1963; 4: 42.
225 Binford CH, Connor DH. *Pathology of Tropical and Extraordinary Disease: an Atlas*. Washington DC: Armed Forces Institute of Pathology, 1976.
226 Sturchler D. Parasitic diseases of the small intestinal tract. *Baillieres Clin Gastroenterol*, 1987; 1: 397.
227 Grencis RK, Cooper ES. Enterobius, trichuris, capillaria, and hookworm including *Ancylostoma caninum*. *Gastroenterol Clin North Am*, 1996; 25: 579.
228 Albonico M, Savioli L. Hookworm infection and disease: advances for control. *Ann Ist Super Sanita*, 1997; 33: 567.
229 Stoltzfus RJ, Dreyfuss ML, Chwaya HM, Albonico M. Hookworm control as a strategy to prevent iron deficiency. *Nutr Rev*, 1997; 55: 223.
230 Banwell JG, Marsden PD, Blackman V, Leonard PJ, Hutt MS. Hookworm infection and intestinal absorption amongst Africans in Uganda. *Am J Trop Med Hyg*, 1967; 16: 304.
231 Salem SN, Truelove SC. Hookworm disease in immigrants. *Br Med J*, 1964; 1: 104.
232 Pawlowski ZS. Ascariasis. *Clin Gastroenterol*, 1978; 7: 157.
233 Embil JA, Pereira LH, White FM, Garner JB, Manuel FR. Prevalence of *Ascaris lumbricoides* infection in a small Nova Scotian community. *Am J Trop Med Hyg*, 1984; 33: 595.
234 Ihekwaba FN. Intestinal ascariasis and the acute abdomen in the tropics. *J R Coll Surg Edinb*, 1980; 25: 452.
235 Coskun A, Ozcan N, Durak AC, Tolu I, Gulec M, Turan C. Intestinal ascariasis as a cause of bowel obstruction in two patients: sonographic diagnosis. *J Clin Ultrasound*, 1996; 24: 326.
236 de Silva NR, Chan MS, Bundy DA. Morbidity and mortality due to ascariasis: re-estimation and sensitivity analysis of global numbers at risk. *Trop Med Int Health*, 1997; 2: 519.
237 Louw JH. Biliary ascariasis in childhood. *S Afr J Surg*, 1974; 12: 219.

238 Gomez B, Tabar AI, Tunon T *et al*. Eosinophilic gastroenteritis and *Anisakis*. *Allergy*, 1998; 53: 1148.

239 Garcia-Labairu C, Alonso-Martinez JL, Martinez-Echeverria A, Rubio-Vela T, Zozaya-Urmeneta JM. Asymptomatic gastroduodenal anisakiasis as the cause of anaphylaxis. *Eur J Gastroenterol Hepatol*, 1999; 11: 785.

240 Cespedes M, Saez A, Rodriguez I, Pinto JM, Rodriguez R. Chronic anisakiasis presenting as a mesenteric mass. *Abdom Imaging*, 2000; 25: 548.

241 Kakizoe S, Kakizoe H, Kakizoe K *et al*. Endoscopic findings and clinical manifestation of gastric anisakiasis. *Am J Gastroenterol*, 1995; 90: 761.

242 Cross JH. Intestinal capillariasis. *Clin Microbiol Rev*, 1992; 5: 120.

243 Dronda F, Chaves F, Sanz A, Lopez-Velez R. Human intestinal capillariasis in an area of nonendemicity: case report and review. *Clin Infect Dis*, 1993; 17: 909.

244 Halsted CH, Sheir S, Raasch FO. The small intestine in human schistosomiasis. *Gastroenterology*, 1969; 57: 622.

245 Elmasri SH, Boulos PB. Bilharzial granuloma of the gastrointestinal tract. *Br J Surg*, 1976; 63: 887.

246 Prata A. Schistosomiasis mansoni. *Clin Gastroenterol*, 1978; 7: 49.

247 Sherif SM. Malabsorption and schistosomal involvement of jejunum. *Br Med J*, 1970; 1: 671.

248 Iyer HV, Abaci IF, Rehnke EC, Enquist IF. Intestinal obstruction due to schistosomiasis. *Am J Surg*, 1985; 149: 409.

249 Mahmoud AA. Strongyloidiasis. *Clin Infect Dis*, 1996; 23: 949.

250 Berk SL, Verghese A, Alvarez S, Hall K, Smith B. Clinical and epidemiologic features of strongyloidiasis. A prospective study in rural Tennessee. *Arch Intern Med*, 1987; 147: 1257.

251 Sprott V, Selby CD, Ispahani P, Toghill PJ. Indigenous strongyloidiasis in Nottingham. *Br Med J (Clin Res Ed)*, 1987; 294: 741.

252 Gill GV, Bell DR. *Strongyloides stercoralis* infection in Burma Star veterans. *Br Med J (Clin Res Ed)*, 1987; 294: 1003.

253 Pelletier LL, Baker CB, Gam AA, Nutman TB, Neva FA. Diagnosis and evaluation of treatment of chronic strongyloidiasis in ex-prisoners of war. *J Infect Dis*, 1988; 157: 573.

254 Warren KS, Mahmoud AA. Algorithms in the diagnosis and management of exotic diseases. XXI. Liver, intestinal, and lung flukes. *J Infect Dis*, 1977; 135: 692.

255 Schantz PM. Tapeworms (cestodiasis). *Gastroenterol Clin North Am*, 1996; 25: 637.

256 Crohn BB, Ginzberg L, Oppenheimer GD. Regional ileitis: a pathological and clinical entity. *JAMA*, 1932; 99: 1323.

257 Dalziel TK. Chronic interstitial enteritis. *Br Med J*, 1913; ii: 1068.

258 Lockhart-Mummery HE, Morson BC. Crohn's disease (regional enteritis) of the large intestine and its distinction from ulcerative colitis. *Gut*, 1960; 1: 87.

259 Morson BC, Lockhart-Mummery HE. Anal lesions in Crohn's disease. *Lancet*, 1959; ii: 1122.

260 Fielding JF, Toye DK, Beton DC, Cooke WT. Crohn's disease of the stomach and duodenum. *Gut*, 1970; 11: 1001.

261 Basu MK, Asquith P, Thompson RA, Cooke WT. Proceedings: Oral lesions in patients with Crohn's disease. *Gut*, 1974; 15: 346.

262 Huchzermeyer H, Paul F, Seifert E, Frohlich H, Rasmussen CW. Endoscopic results in five patients with Crohn's disease of the esophagus. *Endoscopy*, 1977; 8: 75.

263 Rankin GB, Watts HD, Melnyk CS, Kelley ML Jr. National Cooperative Crohn's Disease Study: extraintestinal manifestations and perianal complications. *Gastroenterology*, 1979; 77: 914.

264 Greenstein AJ, Sachar DB, Smith H, Janowitz HD, Aufses AH Jr. Patterns of neoplasia in Crohn's disease and ulcerative colitis. *Cancer*, 1980; 46: 403.

265 Kirsner JB, Shorter RG. Recent developments in nonspecific inflammatory bowel disease (second of two parts). *N Engl J Med*, 1982; 306: 837.

266 Mayberry JF, Rhodes J. Epidemiological aspects of Crohn's disease: a review of the literature. *Gut*, 1984; 25: 886.

267 Lee FI, Costello FT. Crohn's disease in Blackpool—incidence and prevalence 1968. *Gut*, 1985; 26: 274.

268 Rose JD, Roberts GM, Williams G, Mayberry JF, Rhodes J. Cardiff Crohn's disease jubilee: the incidence over 50 years. *Gut*, 1988; 29: 346.

269 Shivananda S, Pena AS, Nap M *et al*. Epidemiology of Crohn's disease in Regio Leiden, The Netherlands. A population study from 1979 to 1983. *Gastroenterology*, 1987; 93: 966.

270 Satsangi J, Parkes M, Jewell DP. Molecular genetics of Crohn's disease: recent advances. *Eur J Surg*, 1998; 164: 887.

271 Farmer RG, Michener WM, Mortimer EA. Studies of family history among patients with inflammatory bowel disease. *Clin Gastroenterol*, 1980; 9: 271.

272 McConnell RB. The genetics of inflammatory bowel disease. In: Allan RN, Keighley MRB, Alexander-Williams J, Hawkins C, eds. *Inflammatory Bowel Disease*. Edinburgh: Churchill Livingstone, 1990: 11.

273 Satsangi J, Grootscholten C, Holt H, Jewell DP. Clinical patterns of familial inflammatory bowel disease. *Gut*, 1996; 38: 738.

274 Parkes M, Satsangi J. Do inflamatory bowel disease genes exist, and can we find them? In: Jewell DP, Mortensen NJ, Warren BF, eds. *Challenges in Inflammatory Bowel Disease*. Oxford: Blackwell Science, 2001: 20–34.

275 Probert CS, Jayanthi V, Hughes AO, Thompson JR, Wicks AC, Mayberry JF. Prevalence and family risk of ulcerative colitis and Crohn's disease: an epidemiological study among Europeans and south Asians in Leicestershire. *Gut*, 1993; 34: 1547.

276 Satsangi J, Parkes M, Louis E *et al*. Two stage genome-wide search in inflammatory bowel disease provides evidence for susceptibility loci on chromosomes 3, 7 and 12. *Nat Genet*, 1996; 14: 199.

277 Hugot JP, Laurent-Puig P, Gower-Rousseau C *et al*. Mapping of a susceptibility locus for Crohn's disease on chromosome 16. *Nature*, 1996; 379: 821.

278 Hugot J-P, Chamaillard M, Zouali H *et al*. Association of NOD2 leucine-rich repeat variants with susceptibility to Crohn's disease. *Nature*, 2001; 411: 599.

279 Ogura Y, Bonen DK, Inohara N *et al*. A frameshift mutation in *NOD2* associated with susceptibility to Crohn's disease. *Nature*, 2001; 411: 603.

280 Somerville KW, Logan RF, Edmond M, Langman MJ. Smoking and Crohn's disease. *Br Med J (Clin Res Ed)*, 1984; 289: 954.

281 Borley NR, Mortensen NJ, Jewell DP. Preventing postoperative recurrence of Crohn's disease. *Br J Surg*, 1997; 84: 1493.

282 Mayberry JF, Rhodes J, Newcombe RG. Increased sugar consumption in Crohn's disease. *Digestion*, 1980; 20: 323.

283 James AH. Breakfast and Crohn's disease. *Br Med J*, 1977; 1: 943.

284 Sullivan SN. Hypothesis revisited: toothpaste and the cause of Crohn's disease. *Lancet*, 1990; 336: 1096.
285 Levine J. Exogenous factors in Crohn's disease. A critical review. *J Clin Gastroenterol*, 1992; 14: 216.
286 O'Morain C, Segal AW, Levi AJ. Elemental diet as primary treatment of acute Crohn's disease: a controlled trial. *Br Med J (Clin Res Ed)*, 1984; 288: 1859.
287 Brown WR, Lee E. Radioimmunological measurements of bacterial antibodies. II. Human serum antibodies reactive with *Bacteroides fragilis* and *Enterococcus* in gastrointestinal and immunological disorders. *Gastroenterology*, 1974; 66: 1145.
288 Matthews N, Mayberry JF, Rhodes J *et al.* Agglutinins to bacteria in Crohn's disease. *Gut*, 1980; 21: 376.
289 Graham DY, Yoshimura HH, Estes MK. DNA hybridization studies of the association of *Pseudomonas maltophilia* with inflammatory bowel diseases. *J Lab Clin Med*, 1983; 101: 940.
290 Walmsley RS, Anthony A, Sim R, Pounder RE, Wakefield AJ. Absence of *Escherichia coli*, *Listeria monocytogenes*, and *Klebsiella pneumoniae* antigens within inflammatory bowel disease tissues. *J Clin Pathol*, 1998; 51: 657.
291 Prantera C, Scribano ML. Crohn's disease: the case for bacteria. *Ital J Gastroenterol Hepatol*, 1999; 31: 244.
292 Burnham WR, Lennard-Jones JE, Stanford JL, Bird RG. Mycobacteria as a possible cause of inflammatory bowel disease. *Lancet*, 1978; 2: 693.
293 Hermon-Taylor J, Bull TJ, Sheridan JM, Cheng J, Stellakis ML, Sumar N. Causation of Crohn's disease by *Mycobacterium avium* subspecies *paratuberculosis*. *Can J Gastroenterol*, 2000; 14: 521.
294 Moss MT, Sanderson JD, Tizard ML *et al.* Polymerase chain reaction detection of *Mycobacterium paratuberculosis* and *Mycobacterium avium* subsp *silvaticum* in long term cultures from Crohn's disease and control tissues. *Gut*, 1992; 33: 1209.
295 Fidler HM, Thurrell W, Johnson NM, Rook GA, McFadden JJ. Specific detection of *Mycobacterium paratuberculosis* DNA associated with granulomatous tissue in Crohn's disease. *Gut*, 1994; 35: 506.
296 Walmsley RS, Ibbotson JP, Chahal H, Allan RN. Antibodies against *Mycobacterium paratuberculosis* in Crohn's disease. *Q J Med*, 1996; 89: 217.
297 Frank TS, Cook SM. Analysis of paraffin sections of Crohn's disease for *Mycobacterium paratuberculosis* using polymerase chain reaction. *Mod Pathol*, 1996; 9: 32.
298 Chiba M, Fukushima T, Horie Y, Iizuka M, Masamune O. No *Mycobacterium paratuberculosis* detected in intestinal tissue, including Peyer's patches and lymph follicles, of Crohn's disease. *J Gastroenterol*, 1998; 33: 482.
299 Suenaga K, Yokoyama Y, Nishimori I *et al.* Serum antibodies to *Mycobacterium paratuberculosis* in patients with Crohn's disease. *Dig Dis Sci*, 1999; 44: 1202.
300 Kanazawa K, Haga Y, Funakoshi O, Nakajima H, Munakata A, Yoshida Y. Absence of *Mycobacterium paratuberculosis* DNA in intestinal tissues from Crohn's disease by nested polymerase chain reaction. *J Gastroenterol*, 1999; 34: 200.
301 Travis SP. Mycobacteria on trial: guilty or innocent in the pathogenesis of Crohn's disease? *Eur J Gastroenterol Hepatol*, 1995; 7: 1173.
302 Van Kruiningen HJ. Lack of support for a common etiology in Johne's disease of animals and Crohn's disease in humans. *Inflamm Bowel Dis*, 1999; 5: 183.
303 Wakefield AJ, Ekbom A, Dhillon AP, Pittilo RM, Pounder RE. Crohn's disease: pathogenesis and persistent measles virus infection. *Gastroenterology*, 1995; 108: 911.
304 Ekbom A, Daszak P, Kraaz W, Wakefield AJ. Crohn's disease after in-utero measles virus exposure. *Lancet*, 1996; 348: 515.
305 Montgomery SM, Morris DL, Pounder RE, Wakefield AJ. Paramyxovirus infections in childhood and subsequent inflammatory bowel disease. *Gastroenterology*, 1999; 116: 796.
306 Pardi DS, Tremaine WJ, Sandborn WJ *et al.* Early measles virus infection is associated with the development of inflammatory bowel disease. *Am J Gastroenterol*, 2000; 95: 1480.
307 Thompson NP, Montgomery SM, Pounder RE, Wakefield AJ. Is measles vaccination a risk factor for inflammatory bowel disease? *Lancet*, 1995; 345: 1071.
308 Wakefield AJ, Murch SH, Anthony A *et al.* Ileal-lymphoid-nodular hyperplasia, non-specific colitis, and pervasive developmental disorder in children. *Lancet*, 1998; 351: 637.
309 Anonymous. MMR vaccine coverage falls after adverse publicity. *Commun Dis Rep CDR Wkly*, 1998; 8 (41): 44.
310 Anonymous. WHO concludes that measles viruses are not associated with Crohn's disease. *Commun Dis Rep CDR Wkly*, 1998; 8 (75): 78.
311 Bookman MA, Bull DM. Characteristics of isolated intestinal mucosal lymphoid cells in inflammatory bowel disease. *Gastroenterology*, 1979; 77: 503.
312 MacDermott RP, Bragdon MJ, Thurmond RD. Peripheral blood mononuclear cells from patients with inflammatory bowel disease exhibit normal function in the allogeneic and autologous mixed leukocyte reaction and cell-mediated lympholysis. *Gastroenterology*, 1984; 86: 476.
313 Colombel JF, Reumaux D, Duthilleul P *et al.* Antineutrophil cytoplasmic autoantibodies in inflammatory bowel diseases. *Gastroenterol Clin Biol*, 1992; 16: 656.
314 Selby WS, Janossy G, Bofill M, Jewell DP. Intestinal lymphocyte subpopulations in inflammatory bowel disease: an analysis by immunohistological and cell isolation techniques. *Gut*, 1984; 25: 32.
315 Schreiber S, MacDermott RP, Raedler A, Pinnau R, Bertovich MJ, Nash GS. Increased activation of isolated intestinal lamina propria mononuclear cells in inflammatory bowel disease. *Gastroenterology*, 1991; 101: 1020.
316 Meuret G, Bitzi A, Hammer B. Macrophage turnover in Crohn's disease and ulcerative colitis. *Gastroenterology*, 1978; 74: 501.
317 Rugtveit J, Brandtzaeg P, Halstensen TS, Fausa O, Scott H. Increased macrophage subset in inflammatory bowel disease: apparent recruitment from peripheral blood monocytes. *Gut*, 1994; 35: 669.
318 Allison MC, Cornwall S, Poulter LW, Dhillon AP, Pounder RE. Macrophage heterogeneity in normal colonic mucosa and in inflammatory bowel disease. *Gut*, 1988; 29: 1531.
319 Sarsfield P, Jones DB, Wright DH. Accessory cells in Crohn's disease of the terminal ileum. *Histopathology*, 1996; 28: 213.
320 Rachmilewitz D, Stamler JS, Bachwich D, Karmeli F, Ackerman Z, Podolsky DK. Enhanced colonic nitric oxide generation and nitric oxide synthase activity in ulcerative colitis and Crohn's disease. *Gut*, 1995; 36: 718.
321 Buffinton GD, Doe WF. Depleted mucosal antioxidant defences in inflammatory bowel disease. *Free Radic Biol Med*, 1995; 19: 911.

322 Dubucquoi S, Janin A, Klein O *et al.* Activated eosinophils and interleukin 5 expression in early recurrence of Crohn's disease. *Gut*, 1995; 37: 242.

323 Dinarello CA. Interleukin-1 and its biologically related cytokines. *Adv Immunol*, 1989; 44: 153.

324 Nakamura M, Saito H, Kasanuki J, Tamura Y, Yoshida S. Cytokine production in patients with inflammatory bowel disease. *Gut*, 1992; 33: 933.

325 Mahida YR, Kurlac L, Gallagher A, Hawkey CJ. High circulating concentrations of interleukin-6 in active Crohn's disease but not ulcerative colitis. *Gut*, 1991; 32: 1531.

326 Stevens C, Walz G, Singaram C *et al.* Tumor necrosis factor-alpha, interleukin-1 beta, and interleukin-6 expression in inflammatory bowel disease. *Dig Dis Sci*, 1992; 37: 818.

327 Braegger CP, Nicholls S, Murch SH, Stephens S, MacDonald TT. Tumour necrosis factor alpha in stool as a marker of intestinal inflammation. *Lancet*, 1992; 339: 89.

328 Targan SR, Hanauer SB, van Deventer SJ *et al.* A short-term study of chimeric monoclonal antibody cA2 to tumor necrosis factor alpha for Crohn's disease. Crohn's Disease cA2 Study Group. *N Engl J Med*, 1997; 337: 1029.

329 Present DH, Rutgeerts P, Targan S *et al.* Infliximab for the treatment of fistulas in patients with Crohn's disease. *N Engl J Med*, 1999; 340: 1398.

330 Mullin GE, Lazenby AJ, Harris ML, Bayless TM, James SP. Increased interleukin-2 messenger RNA in the intestinal mucosal lesions of Crohn's disease but not ulcerative colitis. *Gastroenterology*, 1992; 102: 1620.

331 Sparano JA, Brandt LJ, Dutcher JP, DuBois JS, Atkins MB. Symptomatic exacerbation of Crohn disease after treatment with high-dose interleukin-2. *Ann Intern Med*, 1993; 118: 617.

332 Fais S, Capobianchi MR, Pallone F *et al.* Spontaneous release of interferon gamma by intestinal lamina propria lymphocytes in Crohn's disease. Kinetics of in vitro response to interferon gamma inducers. *Gut*, 1991; 32: 403.

333 Breese E, Braegger CP, Corrigan CJ, Walker-Smith JA, MacDonald TT. Interleukin-2- and interferon-gamma-secreting T cells in normal and diseased human intestinal mucosa. *Immunology*, 1993; 78: 127.

334 Kuhn R, Lohler J, Rennick D, Rajewsky K, Muller W. Interleukin-10-deficient mice develop chronic enterocolitis. *Cell*, 1993; 75: 263.

335 Sadlack B, Merz H, Schorle H, Schimpl A, Feller AC, Horak I. Ulcerative colitis-like disease in mice with a disrupted interleukin-2 gene. *Cell*, 1993; 75: 253.

336 Hermiston ML, Gordon JI. Inflammatory bowel disease and adenomas in mice expressing a dominant negative N-cadherin. *Science*, 1995; 270: 1203.

337 Rutgeerts P, Geboes K, Vantrappen G, Kerremans R, Coenegrachts JL, Coremans G. Natural history of recurrent Crohn's disease at the ileocolonic anastomosis after curative surgery. *Gut*, 1984; 25: 665.

338 Kelly JK, Sutherland LR. The chronological sequence in the pathology of Crohn's disease. *J Clin Gastroenterol*, 1988; 10: 28.

339 Zalev AH, Gardiner GW. Crohn's disease of the small intestine with polypoid configuration. *Gastrointest Radiol*, 1991; 16: 18.

340 Greenstein AJ, Lachman P, Sachar DB *et al.* Perforating and non-perforating indications for repeated operations in Crohn's disease: evidence for two clinical forms. *Gut*, 1988; 29: 588.

341 Pallone F, Boirivant M, Stazi MA, Cosintino R, Prantera C, Torsoli A. Analysis of clinical course of postoperative recurrence in Crohn's disease of distal ileum. *Dig Dis Sci*, 1992; 37: 215.

342 McDonald PJ, Fazio VW, Farmer RG *et al.* Perforating and non-perforating Crohn's disease. An unpredictable guide to recurrence after surgery. *Dis Colon Rectum*, 1989; 32: 117.

343 Borley NR, Mortensen NJ, Chaudry MA *et al.* Evidence for separate disease phenotypes in intestinal Crohn's disease. *Br J Surg* 2002; 89: 201.

344 Heaton KW, McCarthy CF, Horton RE, Cornes JS, Read AE. Miliary Crohn's disease. *Gut*, 1967; 8: 4.

345 Sheehan AL, Warren BF, Gear MW, Shepherd NA. Fat-wrapping in Crohn's disease: pathological basis and relevance to surgical practice. *Br J Surg*, 1992; 79: 955.

346 Borley NR, Mortensen NJ, Jewell DP, Warren BF. The relationship between inflammatory and serosal connective tissue changes in ileal Crohn's disease: evidence for a possible causative link. *J Pathol*, 2000; 190: 196.

347 Nugent FW, Roy MA. Duodenal Crohn's disease: an analysis of 89 cases. *Am J Gastroenterol*, 1989; 84: 249.

348 Oberhuber G, Hirsch M, Stolte M. High incidence of upper gastrointestinal tract involvement in Crohn's disease. *Virchows Arch*, 1998; 432: 49.

349 Wright CL, Riddell RH. Histology of the stomach and duodenum in Crohn's disease. *Am J Surg Pathol*, 1998; 22: 383.

350 Heimann TM, Miller F, Martinelli G, Szporn A, Greenstein AJ, Aufses AH Jr. Correlation of presence of granulomas with clinical and immunologic variables in Crohn's disease. *Arch Surg*, 1988; 123: 46.

351 Chambers TJ, Morson BC. The granuloma in Crohn's disease. *Gut*, 1979; 20: 269.

352 Schmitz-Moormann P, Pittner PM, Malchow H, Brandes JW. The granuloma in Crohn's disease. A bioptical study. *Pathol Res Pract*, 1984; 178: 467.

353 Wolfson DM, Sachar DB, Cohen A *et al.* Granulomas do not affect postoperative recurrence rates in Crohn's disease. *Gastroenterology*, 1982; 83: 405.

354 Hamilton SR. Pathologic features of Crohn's disease associated with recrudescence after resection. *Pathol Annu*, 1983; 18 Part 1: 191.

355 Chardavoyne R, Flint GW, Pollack S, Wise L. Factors affecting recurrence following resection for Crohn's disease. *Dis Colon Rectum*, 1986; 29: 495.

356 Kuramoto S, Oohara T, Ihara O, Shimazu R, Kondo Y. Granulomas of the gut in Crohn's disease. A step sectioning study. *Dis Colon Rectum*, 1987; 30: 6.

357 Mooney EE, Walker J, Hourihane DO. Relation of granulomas to lymphatic vessels in Crohn's disease. *J Clin Pathol*, 1995; 48: 335.

358 Wakefield AJ, Sankey EA, Dhillon AP *et al.* Granulomatous vasculitis in Crohn's disease. *Gastroenterology*, 1991; 100: 1279.

359 Matson AP, Van Kruiningen HJ, West AB, Cartun RW, Colombel JF, Cortot A. The relationship of granulomas to blood vessels in intestinal Crohn's disease. *Mod Pathol*, 1995; 8: 680.

360 Cook MG. The size and histological appearances of mesenteric lymph nodes in Crohn's disease. *Gut*, 1972; 13: 970.

361 Sankey EA, Dhillon AP, Anthony A *et al.* Early mucosal changes in Crohn's disease. *Gut*, 1993; 34: 375.

362 Wright NA, Pike C, Elia G. Induction of a novel epidermal growth factor-secreting cell lineage by mucosal ulceration in human gastrointestinal stem cells. *Nature*, 1990; 343: 82.

363 Hanby AM, Wright NA. The ulcer-associated cell lineage: the gastrointestinal repair kit? *J Pathol*, 1993; 171: 3.

364 Poulsom R, Chinery R, Sarraf C *et al*. Trefoil peptide gene expression in small intestinal Crohn's disease and dietary adaptation. *J Clin Gastroenterol*, 1993; 17 (Suppl 1): S78–S91.

365 Desreumaux P, Ernst O, Geboes K *et al*. Inflammatory alterations in mesenteric adipose tissue in Crohn's disease. *Gastroenterology*, 1999; 117: 73.

366 Geboes K, Collins S. Structural abnormalities of the nervous system in Crohn's disease and ulcerative colitis. *Neurogastroenterol Motil*, 1998; 10: 189.

367 Dvorak AM, Silen W. Differentiation between Crohn's disease and other inflammatory conditions by electron microscopy. *Ann Surg*, 1985; 201: 53.

368 Wakefield AJ, Sawyerr AM, Dhillon AP *et al*. Pathogenesis of Crohn's disease: multifocal gastrointestinal infarction. *Lancet*, 1989; 2: 1057.

369 Funayama Y, Sasaki I, Naito H, Fukushima K, Matsuno S, Masuda T. Remodeling of vascular wall in Crohn's disease. *Dig Dis Sci*, 1999; 44: 2319.

370 Desreumaux P, Huet G, Zerimech F *et al*. Acute inflammatory intestinal vascular lesions and in situ abnormalities of the plasminogen activation system in Crohn's disease. *Eur J Gastroenterol Hepatol*, 1999; 11: 1113.

371 Anthony A, Dhillon AP, Pounder RE, Wakefield AJ. Ulceration of the ileum in Crohn's disease: correlation with vascular anatomy. *J Clin Pathol*, 1997; 50: 1013.

372 Knutson H, Lunderquist A, Lunderquist A. Vascular changes in Crohn's disease. *Am J Roentgenol Radium Ther Nucl Med*, 1968; 103: 380.

373 Gad A. The diagnosis of gastroduodenal Crohn's disease by endoscopic biopsy. *Scand J Gastroenterol Suppl*, 1989; 167: 23.

374 Yao K, Yao T, Iwashita A, Matsui T, Kamachi S. Microaggregate of immunostained macrophages in noninflamed gastroduodenal mucosa: a new useful histological marker for differentiating Crohn's colitis from ulcerative colitis. *Am J Gastroenterol*, 2000; 95: 1967.

375 Schmidt-Sommerfeld E, Kirschner BS, Stephens JK. Endoscopic and histologic findings in the upper gastrointestinal tract of children with Crohn's disease. *J Pediatr Gastroenterol Nutr*, 1990; 11: 448.

376 Poggioli G, Stocchi L, Laureti S *et al*. Duodenal involvement of Crohn's disease: three different clinicopathologic patterns. *Dis Colon Rectum*, 1997; 40: 179.

377 Yamamoto T, Bain IM, Connolly AB, Keighley MR. Gastroduodenal fistulas in Crohn's disease: clinical features and management. *Dis Colon Rectum*, 1998; 41: 1287.

378 Spiess SE, Braun M, Vogelzang RL, Craig RM. Crohn's disease of the duodenum complicated by pancreatitis and common bile duct obstruction. *Am J Gastroenterol*, 1992; 87: 1033.

379 Rubio CA, Befritz R, Poppen B, Svenberg T, Slezak P. Crohn's disease and adenocarcinoma of the intestinal tract. Report of four cases. *Dis Colon Rectum*, 1991; 34: 174.

380 Geboes K, Ectors N, D'haens G, Rutgeerts P. Is ileoscopy with biopsy worthwhile in patients presenting with symptoms of inflammatory bowel disease? *Am J Gastroenterol*, 1998; 93: 201.

381 Pulimood AB, Ramakrishna BS, Kurian G *et al*. Endoscopic mucosal biopsies are useful in distinguishing granulomatous colitis due to Crohn's disease from tuberculosis. *Gut*, 1999; 45: 537.

382 Ament ME, Ochs HD. Gastrointestinal manifestations of chronic granulomatous disease. *N Engl J Med*, 1973; 288: 382.

383 Werlin SL, Chusid MJ, Caya J, Oechler HW. Colitis in chronic granulomatous disease. *Gastroenterology*, 1982; 82: 328.

384 Yogman MW, Touloukian RJ, Gallagher R. Letter: Intestinal granulomatosis in chronic granulomatous disease and in Crohn's disease. *N Engl J Med*, 1974; 290: 228.

385 Shepherd NA. The pelvic ileal reservoir: pathology and pouchitis. *Neth J Med*, 1990; 37 (Suppl 1): S57–S64.

386 Levison DA, Crocker PR, Smith A, Blackshaw AJ, Bartram CI. Varied light and scanning electron microscopic appearances of barium sulphate in smears and histological sections. *J Clin Pathol*, 1984; 37: 481.

387 Kewenter J, Hulten L, Kock NG. The relationship and epidemiology of acute terminal ileitis and Crohn's disease. *Gut*, 1974; 15: 801.

388 Warren BF, Shepherd NA. Surgical pathology of the intestines: the pelvic ileal reservoir and diversion proctocolitis. In: Lowe DG, Underwood JCE, eds. *Recent Advances in Histopathology. 18th ed.* Edinburgh: Churchill Livingstone, 2000: 63.

389 Wolff BG, Beart RW Jr, Frydenberg HB, Weiland LH, Agrez MV, Ilstrup DM. The importance of disease-free margins in resections for Crohn's disease. *Dis Colon Rectum*, 1983; 26: 239.

390 Fazio VW, Marchetti F. Recurrent Crohn's disease and resection margins: bigger is not better. *Adv Surg*, 1999; 32: 135.

391 Tytgat GN, Mulder CJ, Brummelkamp WH. Endoscopic lesions in Crohn's disease early after ileocecal resection. *Endoscopy*, 1988; 20: 260.

392 de Jong E, van Dullemen HM, Slors JF, Dekkers P, van Deventer SJ, Tytgat GN. Correlation between early recurrence and reoperation after ileocolonic resection in Crohn's disease: a prospective study. *J Am Coll Surg*, 1996; 182: 503.

393 Klein O, Colombel JF, Lescut D *et al*. Remaining small bowel endoscopic lesions at surgery have no influence on early anastomotic recurrences in Crohn's disease. *Am J Gastroenterol*, 1995; 90: 1949.

394 McLeod RS, Wolff BG, Steinhart AH *et al*. Risk and significance of endoscopic/radiological evidence of recurrent Crohn's disease. *Gastroenterology*, 1997; 113: 1823.

395 Rutgeerts P, Geboes K, Peeters M *et al*. Effect of faecal stream diversion on recurrence of Crohn's disease in the neoterminal ileum. *Lancet*, 1991; 338: 771.

396 D'Haens GR, Geboes K, Peeters M, Baert F, Penninckx F, Rutgeerts P. Early lesions of recurrent Crohn's disease caused by infusion of intestinal contents in excluded ileum. *Gastroenterology*, 1998; 114: 262.

397 Heuman R, Boeryd B, Bolin T, Sjodahl R. The influence of disease at the margin of resection on the outcome of Crohn's disease. *Br J Surg*, 1983; 70: 519.

398 Hamilton SR, Reese J, Pennington L, Boitnott JK, Bayless TM, Cameron JL. The role of resection margin frozen section in the surgical management of Crohn's disease. *Surg Gynecol Obstet*, 1985; 160: 57.

399 Cooper JC, Williams NS. The influence of microscopic disease at

the margin of resection on recurrence rates in Crohn's disease. *Ann R Coll Surg Engl*, 1986; 68: 23.
400 Adloff M, Arnaud JP, Ollier JC. Does the histologic appearance at the margin of resection affect the postoperative recurrence rate in Crohn's disease? *Am Surg*, 1987; 53: 543.
401 Kotanagi H, Kramer K, Fazio VW, Petras RE. Do microscopic abnormalities at resection margins correlate with increased anastomotic recurrence in Crohn's disease? Retrospective analysis of 100 cases. *Dis Colon Rectum*, 1991; 34: 909.
402 Fazio VW, Marchetti F, Church M *et al.* Effect of resection margins on the recurrence of Crohn's disease in the small bowel. A randomized controlled trial. *Ann Surg*, 1996; 224: 563.
403 Greenway SE, Buckmire MA, Marroquin C, Jadon L, Rolandelli RH. Clinical subtypes of Crohn's disease according to surgical outcome. *J Gastrointest Surg*, 1999; 3: 145.
404 Steinberg DM, Cooke WT, Alexander-Williams J. Free perforation in Crohn's disease. *Gut*, 1973; 14: 187.
405 Katz S, Schulman N, Levin L. Free perforation in Crohn's disease: a report of 33 cases and review of literature. *Am J Gastroenterol*, 1986; 81: 38.
406 Gyde SN, Prior P, Macartney JC, Thompson H, Waterhouse JA, Allan RN. Malignancy in Crohn's disease. *Gut*, 1980; 21: 1024.
407 Kvist N, Jacobsen O, Norgaard P *et al.* Malignancy in Crohn's disease. *Scand J Gastroenterol*, 1986; 21: 82.
408 Hoffman JP, Taft DA, Wheelis RF, Walker JH. Adenocarcinoma in regional enteritis of the small intestine. *Arch Surg*, 1977; 112: 606.
409 Hawker PC, Gyde SN, Thompson H, Allan RN. Adenocarcinoma of the small intestine complicating Crohn's disease. *Gut*, 1982; 23: 188.
410 Gillen CD, Wilson CA, Walmsley RS, Sanders DS, O'Dwyer ST, Allan RN. Occult small bowel adenocarcinoma complicating Crohn's disease: a report of three cases. *Postgrad Med J*, 1995; 71: 172.
411 Thompson EM, Clayden G, Price AB. Cancer in Crohn's disease—an 'occult' malignancy. *Histopathology*, 1983; 7: 365.
412 Simpson S, Traube J, Riddell RH. The histologic appearance of dysplasia (precarcinomatous change) in Crohn's disease of the small and large intestine. *Gastroenterology*, 1981; 81: 492.
413 Perzin KH, Peterson M, Castiglione CL, Fenoglio CM, Wolff M. Intramucosal carcinoma of the small intestine arising in regional enteritis (Crohn's disease). Report of a case studied for carcinoembryonic antigen and review of the literature. *Cancer*, 1984; 54: 151.
414 Sigel JE, Petras RE, Lashner BA, Fazio VW, Goldblum JR. Intestinal adenocarcinoma in Crohn's disease: a report of 30 cases with a focus on coexisting dysplasia. *Am J Surg Pathol*, 1999; 23: 651.
415 Sigel JE, Goldblum JR. Neuroendocrine neoplasms arising in inflammatory bowel disease: a report of 14 cases. *Mod Pathol*, 1998; 11: 537.
416 Perosio PM, Brooks JJ, Saul SH, Haller DG. Primary intestinal lymphoma in Crohn's disease: minute tumor with a fatal outcome. *Am J Gastroenterol*, 1992; 87: 894.
417 Brown I, Schofield JB, MacLennan KA, Tagart RE. Primary non-Hodgkin's lymphoma in ileal Crohn's disease. *Eur J Surg Oncol*, 1992; 18: 627.
418 Woodley HE, Spencer JA, MacLennan KA. Small-bowel lymphoma complicating long-standing Crohn's disease. *Am J Roentgenol*, 1997; 169: 1462.
419 Greenstein AJ, Janowitz HD, Sachar DB. The extra-intestinal complications of Crohn's disease and ulcerative colitis: a study of 700 patients. *Medicine (Baltimore)*, 1976; 55: 401.
420 Enlow RW, Bias WB, Arnett FC. The spondylitis of inflammatory bowel disease. Evidence for a non-HLA linked axial arthropathy. *Arthritis Rheum*, 1980; 23: 1359.
421 Ferguson RH. Arthritis associated with inflammatory bowel disease. *Minn Med*, 1981; 64: 165.
422 Lockhart-Mummery HE. Pathologic lesions of the anal region associated in Crohn's disease. *Dis Colon Rectum*, 1965; 8: 399.
423 McCallum DI, Kinmont PD. Dermatological manifestations of Crohn's disease. *Br J Dermatol*, 1968; 80: 1.
424 Burgdorf W. Cutaneous manifestations of Crohn's disease. *J Am Acad Dermatol*, 1981; 5: 689.
425 Tweedie JH, McCann BG. Metastatic Crohn's disease of thigh and forearm. *Gut*, 1984; 25: 213.
426 Eade MN, Cooke WT, Williams JA. Liver disease in Crohn's disease. A study of 100 consecutive patients. *Scand J Gastroenterol*, 1971; 6: 199.
427 Bjarnason I, Macpherson AJ. Intestinal toxicity of non-steroidal anti-inflammatory drugs. *Pharmacol Ther*, 1994; 62: 145.
428 Morris AJ. Nonsteroidal anti-inflammatory drug enteropathy. *Gastrointest Endosc Clin North Am*, 1999; 9: 125.
429 Allison MC, Howatson AG, Torrance CJ, Lee FD, Russell RI. Gastrointestinal damage associated with the use of nonsteroidal antiinflammatory drugs. *N Engl J Med*, 1992; 327: 749.
430 Davies NM, Saleh JY, Skjodt NM. Detection and prevention of NSAID-induced enteropathy. *J Pharm Pharm Sci*, 2000; 3: 137.
431 Taha AS. Histopathological aspects of mucosal injury related to non-steroidal anti-inflammatory drugs. *Ital J Gastroenterol*, 1996; 28 (Suppl 4): 12.
432 Schneider AR, Benz C, Riemann JF. Adverse effects of nonsteroidal anti-inflammatory drugs on the small and large bowel. *Endoscopy*, 1999; 31: 761.
433 Bjarnason I, Hayllar J, Macpherson AJ, Russell AS. Side effects of nonsteroidal anti-inflammatory drugs on the small and large intestine in humans. *Gastroenterology*, 1993; 104: 1832.
434 Levi S, Shaw-Smith C. Non-steroidal anti-inflammatory drugs: how do they damage the gut? *Br J Rheumatol*, 1994; 33: 605.
435 Anthony A, Dhillon AP, Thrasivoulou C, Pounder RE, Wakefield AJ. Pre-ulcerative villous contraction and microvascular occlusion induced by indomethacin in the rat jejunum: a detailed morphological study. *Aliment Pharmacol Ther*, 1995; 9: 605.
436 Anthony A, Pounder RE, Dhillon AP, Wakefield AJ. Vascular anatomy defines sites of indomethacin induced jejunal ulceration along the mesenteric margin. *Gut*, 1997; 41: 763.
437 Bjarnason I, Fehilly B, Smethurst P, Menzies IS, Levi AJ. Importance of local versus systemic effects of non-steroidal anti-inflammatory drugs in increasing small intestinal permeability in man. *Gut*, 1991; 32: 275.
438 Aabakken L. Small-bowel side-effects of non-steroidal anti-inflammatory drugs. *Eur J Gastroenterol Hepatol*, 1999; 11: 383.
439 Lee FD. Drug-related pathological lesions of the intestinal tract. *Histopathology*, 1994; 25: 303.
440 Lang J, Price AB, Levi AJ, Burke M, Gumpel JM, Bjarnason I. Diaphragm disease: pathology of disease of the small intestine induced by non-steroidal anti-inflammatory drugs. *J Clin Pathol*, 1988; 41: 516.

441 Levi S, de Lacey G, Price AB, Gumpel MJ, Levi AJ, Bjarnason I. "Diaphragm-like" strictures of the small bowel in patients treated with non-steroidal anti-inflammatory drugs. *Br J Radiol*, 1990; 63: 186.
442 Leijonmarck CE, Raf L. Ulceration of the small intestine due to slow-release potassium chloride tablets. *Acta Chir Scand*, 1985; 151: 273.
443 Rashid A, Hamilton SR. Necrosis of the gastrointestinal tract in uremic patients as a result of sodium polystyrene sulfonate (Kayexalate) in sorbitol: an underrecognized condition. *Am J Surg Pathol*, 1997; 21: 60.
444 Martin DM, Goldman JA, Gilliam J, Nasrallah SM. Gold-induced eosinophilic enterocolitis: response to oral cromolyn sodium. *Gastroenterology*, 1981; 80: 1567.
445 Jackson CW, Haboubi NY, Whorwell PJ, Schofield PF. Gold induced enterocolitis. *Gut*, 1986; 27: 452.
446 Cunningham D, Morgan RJ, Mills PR *et al*. Functional and structural changes of the human proximal small intestine after cytotoxic therapy. *J Clin Pathol*, 1985; 38: 265.
447 Smit JM, Mulder NH, Sleijfer DT *et al*. Gastrointestinal toxicity of chemotherapy and the influence of hyperalimentation. *Cancer*, 1986; 58: 1990.
448 Orazi AX, Yang Z, Kashai M, Williams DA. Interleukin-11 prevents apoptosis and accelerates recovery of small intestinal mucosa in mice treated with combined chemotherapy and radiation. *Lab Invest*, 1996; 75: 33.
449 Abratt RP, Pontin AR, Barnes RD. Chemotherapy, radical irradiation plus salvage cystectomy for bladder cancer—severe late small bowel morbidity. *Eur J Surg Oncol*, 1993; 19: 279.
450 Nagai Y, Horie T, Awazu S. Vitamin A, a useful biochemical modulator capable of preventing intestinal damage during methotrexate treatment. *Pharmacol Toxicol*, 1993; 73: 69.
451 Libicher M, Lamade W, Kasperk C, Grenacher L, Kauffmann GW. [Cicatricial small intestinal stenosis following chemotherapy for a gastrointestinal lymphoma.] *Deutsche Med Wochenschr*, 1996; 121: 1359.
452 Sakakura C, Hagiwara A, Nakanishi M *et al*. Bowel perforation during chemotherapy for non-Hodgkin's lymphoma. *Hepatogastroenterology*, 1999; 46: 3175.
453 Baba S, Maruta M, Ando K, Teramoto T, Endo I. Intestinal Behçet's disease: report of five cases. *Dis Colon Rectum*, 1976; 19: 428.
454 Sanderson IR, Risdon RA, Walker-Smith JA. Intractable ulcerating enterocolitis of infancy. *Arch Dis Child*, 1991; 66: 295.
455 Waxman I, Gardner JD, Jensen RT, Maton PN. Peptic ulcer perforation as the presentation of Zollinger–Ellison syndrome. *Dig Dis Sci*, 1991; 36: 19.
456 Meko JB, Norton JA. Management of patients with Zollinger–Ellison syndrome. *Annu Rev Med*, 1995; 46: 395.
457 Davies DR, Brightmore T. Idiopathic and drug-induced ulceration of the small intestine. *Br J Surg*, 1970; 57: 134.
458 Madhok R, MacKenzie JA, Lee FD, Bruckner FE, Terry TR, Sturrock RD. Small bowel ulceration in patients receiving non-steroidal anti-inflammatory drugs for rheumatoid arthritis. *Q J Med*, 1986; 58: 53.
459 Thomas WE, Williamson RC. Nonspecific small bowel ulceration. *Postgrad Med J*, 1985; 61: 587.
460 Harling H, Laustsen J. Primary non-specific ulcer of the small bowel. *Acta Chir Scand*, 1985; 151: 289.
461 Blackshaw AJ, Levison DA. Eosinophilic infiltrates of the gastrointestinal tract. *J Clin Pathol*, 1986; 39: 1.
462 Klein NC, Hargrove RL, Sleisenger MH, Jeffries GH. Eosinophilic gastroenteritis. *Medicine (Baltimore)*, 1970; 49: 299.
463 Kelly KJ. Eosinophilic gastroenteritis. *J Pediatr Gastroenterol Nutr*, 2000; 30 (Suppl): S28.
464 Johnstone JM, Morson BC. Eosinophilic gastroenteritis. *Histopathology*, 1978; 2: 335.
465 Karande T, Oak SN, Trivedi A, Karmarkar S, Kulkarni B, Kalgutkar A. Proximal jejunal obstruction due to eosinophilic gastroenteritis. *J Postgrad Med*, 1996; 42: 121.
466 Steele RJ, Mok SD, Crofts TJ, Li AK. Two cases of eosinophilic enteritis presenting as large bowel perforation and small bowel haemorrhage. *Aust N Z J Surg*, 1987; 57: 335.
467 Walia HS, Abraham TK, Walia HK. Eosinophilic enteritis with perforation. *Can J Surg*, 1988; 31: 268.
468 Beishuizen A, van Bodegraven AA, Bronsveld W, Sindram JW. Eosinophilic gastroenteritis—a disease with a wide clinical spectrum. *Neth J Med*, 1993; 42: 212.
469 Matsushita M, Hajiro K, Morita Y, Takakuwa H, Suzaki T. Eosinophilic gastroenteritis involving the entire digestive tract. *Am J Gastroenterol*, 1995; 90: 1868.
470 Buchman AL, Wolf D, Gramlich T. Eosinophilic gastrojejunitis associated with connective tissue disease. *South Med J*, 1996; 89: 327.
471 Suen KC, Burton JD. The spectrum of eosinophilic infiltration of the gastrointestinal tract and its relationship to other disorders of angiitis and granulomatosis. *Hum Pathol*, 1979; 10: 31.
472 Talley NJ, Shorter RG, Phillips SF, Zinsmeister AR. Eosinophilic gastroenteritis: a clinicopathological study of patients with disease of the mucosa, muscle layer, and subserosal tissues. *Gut*, 1990; 31: 54.
473 Lee CM, Changchien CS, Chen PC *et al*. Eosinophilic gastroenteritis: 10 years experience. *Am J Gastroenterol*, 1993; 88: 70.
474 Di Gioacchino M, Pizzicannella G, Fini N *et al*. Sodium cromoglycate in the treatment of eosinophilic gastroenteritis. *Allergy*, 1990; 45: 161.
475 Van Laethem JL, Jacobs F, Braude P, Van Gossum A, Deviere J. *Toxocara canis* infection presenting as eosinophilic ascites and gastroenteritis. *Dig Dis Sci*, 1994; 39: 1370.
476 Maluenda C, Phillips AD, Briddon A, Walker-Smith JA. Quantitative analysis of small intestinal mucosa in cow's milk-sensitive enteropathy. *J Pediatr Gastroenterol Nutr*, 1984; 3: 349.
477 Jenkins HR, Pincott JR, Soothill JF, Milla PJ, Harries JT. Food allergy: the major cause of infantile colitis. *Arch Dis Child*, 1984; 59: 326.
478 Berthrong M, Fajardo LF. Radiation injury in surgical pathology. Part II. Alimentary tract. *Am J Surg Pathol*, 1981; 5: 153.
479 MacNaughton WK. Review article: new insights into the pathogenesis of radiation-induced intestinal dysfunction. *Aliment Pharmacol Ther*, 2000; 14: 523.
480 Sher ME, Bauer J. Radiation-induced enteropathy. *Am J Gastroenterol*, 1990; 85: 121.
481 Oya M, Yao T, Tsuneyoshi M. Chronic irradiation enteritis: its correlation with the elapsed time interval and morphological changes. *Hum Pathol*, 1996; 27: 774.
482 Galland RB, Spencer J. Radiation-induced gastrointestinal fistulae. *Ann R Coll Surg Engl*, 1986; 68: 5.

483 Galland RB, Spencer J. The natural history of clinically established radiation enteritis. *Lancet*, 1985; 1: 1257.

484 Cohen SM. Radiation-induced jejunal mucosal vascular lesions as a cause of significant gastrointestinal hemorrhage. *Gastrointest Endosc*, 1997; 46: 183.

485 Hasleton PS, Carr N, Schofield PF. Vascular changes in radiation bowel disease. *Histopathology*, 1985; 9: 517.

486 Serdaroglu P. Behçet's disease and the nervous system. *J Neurol*, 1998; 245: 197.

487 Yurdakul S, Tuzuner N, Yurdakul I, Hamuryudan V, Yazici H. Gastrointestinal involvement in Behçet's syndrome: a controlled study. *Ann Rheum Dis*, 1996; 55: 208.

488 Pretorius ES, Hruban RH, Fishman EK. Inflammatory pseudotumor of the terminal ileum mimicking malignancy in a patient with Behçet's disease. CT and pathological findings. *Clin Imaging*, 1996; 20: 191.

489 Choi IJ, Kim JS, Cha SD *et al.* Long-term clinical course and prognostic factors in intestinal Behçet's disease. *Dis Colon Rectum*, 2000; 43: 692.

490 Kasahara Y, Tanaka S, Nishino M, Umemura H, Shiraha S, Kuyama T. Intestinal involvement in Behçet's disease: review of 136 surgical cases in the Japanese literature. *Dis Colon Rectum*, 1981; 24: 103.

491 Domizio P. Pathology of chronic inflammatory bowel disease in children. *Baillieres Clin Gastroenterol*, 1994; 8: 35.

492 Akpolat T, Koc Y, Yeniay I *et al.* Familial Behçet's disease. *Eur J Med*, 1992; 1: 391.

493 Sun A, Chang JG, Kao CL *et al.* Human cytomegalovirus as a potential etiologic agent in recurrent aphthous ulcers and Behçet's disease. *J Oral Pathol Med*, 1996; 25: 212.

494 Kahan A, Hamzaoui K, Ayed K. Abnormalities of T lymphocyte subsets in Behçet's disease demonstrated with anti-CD45RA and anti-CD29 monoclonal antibodies. *J Rheumatol*, 1992; 19: 742.

495 Hamzaoui K, Kahan A, Hamza M, Ayed K. Suppressive T cell function of Epstein–Barr virus induced B cell activation in active Behçet's disease. *Clin Exp Rheumatol*, 1991; 9: 131.

496 Yamashita S, Suzuki A, Yanagita T, Hirohata S, Kamada M, Toyoshima S. Analysis of neutrophil proteins of patients with Behçet's disease by two-dimensional gel electrophoresis. *Biol Pharm Bull*, 2000; 23: 519.

497 Yamashita S, Suzuki A, Yanagita T, Hirohata S, Toyoshima S. Characterization of a protease responsible for truncated actin increase in neutrophils of patients with Behçet's disease. *Biol Pharm Bull*, 2001; 24: 119.

498 Kobayashi M, Ito M, Nakagawa A *et al.* Neutrophil and endothelial cell activation in the vasa vasorum in vasculo-Behçet disease. *Histopathology*, 2000; 36: 362.

499 Sayek I, Aran O, Uzunalimoglu B, Hersek E. Intestinal Behçet's disease: surgical experience in seven cases. *Hepatogastroenterology*, 1991; 38: 81.

500 Takada Y, Fujita Y, Igarashi M *et al.* Intestinal Behçet's disease—pathognomonic changes in intramucosal lymphoid tissues and effect of a 'rest cure' on intestinal lesions. *J Gastroenterol*, 1997; 32: 598.

501 Hamza M, Eleuch M, Kchir N, Zitouna M. [Ileal perforation in three cases of Behçet disease.] *Ann Med Interne (Paris)*, 1994; 145: 99.

502 Roge J. [Behçet's syndrome and the digestive tract.] *J Mal Vasc*, 1988; 13: 235.

503 Kallinowski B, Noldge G, Stiehl A. Crohn's disease with Behçet's syndrome like appearance: a case report. *Z Gastroenterol*, 1994; 32: 642.

504 Parks AG, Nicholls RJ. Proctocolectomy without ileostomy for ulcerative colitis. *Br Med J*, 1978; 2: 85.

505 Shepherd NA, Jass JR, Duval I, Moskowitz RL, Nicholls RJ, Morson BC. Restorative proctocolectomy with ileal reservoir: pathological and histochemical study of mucosal biopsy specimens. *J Clin Pathol*, 1987; 40: 601.

506 de Silva HJ, Millard PR, Kettlewell M, Mortensen NJ, Prince C, Jewell DP. Mucosal characteristics of pelvic ileal pouches. *Gut*, 1991; 32: 61.

507 O'Connell PR, Rankin DR, Weiland LH, Kelly KA. Enteric bacteriology, absorption, morphology and emptying after ileal pouch–anal anastomosis. *Br J Surg*, 1986; 73: 909.

508 Warren BF, Shepherd NA. Pouch pathology. In: Nicholls RJ, Bartolo DCC, Mortensen NJ Mc C, eds. *Restorative Proctocolectomy*. Oxford: Blackwell Scientific Publications, 1993: 147.

509 Luukkonen P, Jarvinen H, Tanskanen M, Kahri A. Pouchitis—recurrence of the inflammatory bowel disease? *Gut*, 1994; 35: 243.

510 Nasmyth DG, Godwin PG, Dixon MF, Williams NS, Johnston D. Ileal ecology after pouch–anal anastomosis or ileostomy. A study of mucosal morphology, fecal bacteriology, fecal volatile fatty acids, and their interrelationship. *Gastroenterology*, 1989; 96: 817.

511 McLeod RS, Antonioli D, Cullen J *et al.* Histologic and microbiologic features of biopsy samples from patients with normal and inflamed pouches. *Dis Colon Rectum*, 1994; 37: 26.

512 Ruseler-van Embden JG, Schouten WR, van Lieshout LM. Pouchitis: result of microbial imbalance? *Gut*, 1994; 35: 658.

513 Moskowitz RL, Shepherd NA, Nicholls RJ. An assessment of inflammation in the reservoir after restorative proctocolectomy with ileoanal ileal reservoir. *Int J Colorectal Dis*, 1986; 1: 167.

514 Shepherd NA, Hulten L, Tytgat GN *et al.* Pouchitis. *Int J Colorectal Dis*, 1989; 4: 205.

515 Madden MV, Farthing MJ, Nicholls RJ. Inflammation in ileal reservoirs: 'pouchitis'. *Gut*, 1990; 31: 247.

516 Setti CP, Talbot IC, Nicholls RJ. Longterm appraisal of the histological appearances of the ileal reservoir mucosa after restorative proctocolectomy for ulcerative colitis. *Gut*, 1994; 35: 1721.

517 Veress B, Reinholt FP, Lindquist K, Lofberg R, Liljeqvist L. Long-term histomorphological surveillance of the pelvic ileal pouch: dysplasia develops in a subgroup of patients. *Gastroenterology*, 1995; 109: 1090.

518 Panis Y, Poupard B, Nemeth J, Lavergne A, Hautefeuille P, Valleur P. Ileal pouch/anal anastomosis for Crohn's disease. *Lancet*, 1996; 347: 854.

519 Warren BF, Shepherd NA. The role of pathology in pelvic ileal reservoir surgery. *Int J Colorectal Dis*, 1992; 7: 68.

520 Subramani K, Harpaz N, Bilotta J *et al.* Refractory pouchitis: does it reflect underlying Crohn's disease? *Gut*, 1993; 34: 1539.

521 Lohmuller JL, Pemberton JH, Dozois RR, Ilstrup D, van Heerden J. Pouchitis and extraintestinal manifestations of inflammatory bowel disease after ileal pouch–anal anastomosis. *Ann Surg*, 1990; 211: 622.

522 Penna C, Dozois R, Tremaine W *et al.* Pouchitis after ileal pouch–anal anastomosis for ulcerative colitis occurs with increased frequency in patients with associated primary sclerosing cholangitis. *Gut*, 1996; 38: 234.

523 Shepherd NA. The pelvic ileal reservoir: apocalypse later? *Br Med J*, 1990; 301: 886.

524 Gullberg K, Stahlberg D, Liljeqvist L *et al.* Neoplastic transformation of the pelvic pouch mucosa in patients with ulcerative colitis. *Gastroenterology*, 1997; 112: 1487.

525 Stern H, Walfisch S, Mullen B, McLeod R, Cohen Z. Cancer in an ileoanal reservoir: a new late complication? *Gut*, 1990; 31: 473.

526 Bassuini MM, Billings PJ. Carcinoma in an ileoanal pouch after restorative proctocolectomy for familial adenomatous polyposis. *Br J Surg*, 1996; 83: 506.

527 Vieth M, Grunewald M, Niemeyer C, Stolte M. Adenocarcinoma in an ileal pouch after prior proctocolectomy for carcinoma in a patient with ulcerative pancolitis. *Virchows Arch*, 1998; 433: 281.

528 Thompson-Fawcett MW, Mortensen NJ, Warren BF. 'Cuffitis' and inflammatory changes in the columnar cuff, anal transitional zone, and ileal reservoir after stapled pouch–anal anastomosis. *Dis Colon Rectum*, 1999; 42: 348.

529 Puthu D, Rajan N, Rao R, Rao L, Venugopal P. Carcinoma of the rectal pouch following restorative proctocolectomy. Report of a case. *Dis Colon Rectum*, 1992; 35: 257.

530 Ziv Y, Fazio VW, Sirimarco MT, Lavery IC, Goldblum JR, Petras RE. Incidence, risk factors, and treatment of dysplasia in the anal transitional zone after ileal pouch–anal anastomosis. *Dis Colon Rectum*, 1994; 37: 1281.

531 Sequens R. Cancer in the anal canal (transitional zone) after restorative proctocolectomy with stapled ileal pouch–anal anastomosis. *Int J Colorectal Dis*, 1997; 12: 254.

532 Helander KG, Ahren C, Philipson BM, Samuelsson BM, Ojerskog B. Structure of mucosa in continent ileal reservoirs 15–19 years after construction. *Hum Pathol*, 1990; 21: 1235.

533 Cox CL, Butts DR, Roberts MP, Wessels RA, Bailey HR. Development of invasive adenocarcinoma in a long-standing Kock continent ileostomy: report of a case. *Dis Colon Rectum*, 1997; 40: 500.

534 Price AB, Morson BC. Inflammatory bowel disease: the surgical pathology of Crohn's disease and ulcerative colitis. *Hum Pathol*, 1975; 6: 7.

535 Gardiner GA. 'Backwash ileitis' with pseudopolyposis. *Am J Roentgenol*, 1977; 129: 506.

536 Gustavsson S, Weiland LH, Kelly KA. Relationship of backwash ileitis to ileal pouchitis after ileal pouch–anal anastomosis. *Dis Colon Rectum*, 1987; 30: 25.

537 Schmidt CM, Lazenby AJ, Hendrickson RJ, Sitzmann JV. Preoperative terminal ileal and colonic resection histopathology predicts risk of pouchitis in patients after ileoanal pull-through procedure. *Ann Surg*, 1998; 227: 654.

538 Ferguson R, Allan RN, Cooke WT. A study of the cellular infiltrate of the proximal jejunal mucosa in ulcerative colitis and Crohn's disease. *Gut*, 1975; 16: 205.

539 Valdez R, Appelman HD, Bronner MP, Greenson JK. Diffuse duodenitis associated with ulcerative colitis. *Am J Surg Pathol*, 2000; 24: 1407.

540 Annese V, Caruso N, Bisceglia M *et al.* Fatal ulcerative panenteritis following colectomy in a patient with ulcerative colitis. *Dig Dis Sci*, 1999; 44: 1189.

541 Mitomi H, Atari E, Uesugi H *et al.* Distinctive diffuse duodenitis associated with ulcerative colitis. *Dig Dis Sci*, 1997; 42: 684.

542 Kaufman SS, Vanderhoof JA, Young R, Perry D, Raynor SC, Mack DR. Gastroenteric inflammation in children with ulcerative colitis. *Am J Gastroenterol*, 1997; 92: 1209.

543 Bechi P, Romagnoli P, Cortesini C. Ileal mucosal morphology after total colectomy in man. *Histopathology*, 1981; 5: 667.

544 Knill-Jones RP, Morson B, Williams R. Prestomal ileitis: clinical and pathological findings in five cases. *Q J Med*, 1970; 39: 287.

545 du Boulay CE, Fairbrother J, Isaacson PG. Mucosal prolapse syndrome—a unifying concept for solitary ulcer syndrome and related disorders. *J Clin Pathol*, 1983; 36: 1264.

546 Primrose JN, Quirke P, Johnston D. Carcinoma of the ileostomy in a patient with familial adenomatous polyposis. *Br J Surg*, 1988; 75: 384.

547 Attanoos R, Billings PJ, Hughes LE, Williams GT. Ileostomy polyps, adenomas, and adenocarcinomas. *Gut*, 1995; 37: 840.

548 Deane AM, Woodhouse CR, Parkinson MC. Histological changes in ileal conduits. *J Urol*, 1984; 132: 1108.

549 Mulholland C, McCallion WA, Biggart JD, Kennedy JA, Keane PF. Transitional cell carcinoma in an ileal conduit. *Br J Urol*, 1993; 71: 618.

550 Gratama S, Smedts F, Whitehead R. Obstructive colitis: an analysis of 50 cases and a review of the literature. *Pathology*, 1995; 27: 324.

551 Levine TS, Price AB. Obstructive enterocolitis: a clinico-pathological discussion. *Histopathology*, 1994; 25: 57.

552 Allibone RO, Hoffman J, Gosney JR, Helliwell TR. Granulation tissue polyposis associated with carcinoid tumours of the small intestine. *Histopathology*, 1993; 22: 475.

553 Ashton-Key M, Diss TC, Du Pan LMQ, Isaacson PG. Molecular analysis of T-cell clonality in ulcerative jejunitis and enteropathy-associated T-cell lymphoma. *Am J Pathol*, 1997; 151: 493.

554 Bagdi E, Diss TC, Munson P, Isaacson PG. Mucosal intra-epithelial lymphocytes in enteropathy-associated T-cell lymphoma, ulcerative jejunitis, and refractory celiac disease constitute a neoplastic population. *Blood*, 1999; 94: 260.

555 Chesler L, Hwang L, Patton W, Heyman MB. Henoch–Schönlein purpura with severe jejunitis and minimal skin lesions. *J Pediatr Gastroenterol Nutr*, 2000; 30: 92.

556 Radaelli F, Meucci G, Spinzi G *et al.* Acute self-limiting jejunitis as the first manifestation of microscopic polyangiitis associated with Sjögren's disease: report of one case and review of the literature. *Eur J Gastroenterol Hepatol*, 1999; 11: 931.

557 Sharma AK, Shekhawat NS, Behari S, Chandra S, Sogani KC. Nonspecific jejunitis—a challenging problem in children. *Am J Gastroenterol*, 1986; 81: 428.

558 Chen YM, King GT, Ott DJ, Marshall RB, Kerr RM. Infectious jejunitis with stricture after gastrojejunostomy. *Am J Gastroenterol*, 1985; 80: 334.

559 Adams JT, Skucas J. Corrosive jejunitis due to ingestion of nitric acid. *Am J Surg*, 1980; 139: 282.

560 Wyatt JI. Histopathology of gastroduodenal inflammation: the impact of *Helicobacter pylori*. *Histopathology*, 1995; 26: 1.

561 Caselli M, Gaudio M, Chiamenti CM *et al.* Histologic findings and *Helicobacter pylori* in duodenal biopsies. *J Clin Gastroenterol*, 1998; 26: 74.

562 Walker MM, Crabtree JE. *Helicobacter pylori* infection and the pathogenesis of duodenal ulceration. *Ann N Y Acad Sci*, 1998; 859: 96.

563 Sircus W. Duodenitis: a clinical, endoscopic and histopathologic study. *Q J Med*, 1985; 56: 593.

564 Day DW, Dixon MF. *Biopsy Pathology of the Oesophagus, Stomach and Duodenum*. London: Chapman & Hall Publishing Ltd, 1996.

565 Kreuning J, Bosman FT, Kuiper G, Wal AM, Lindeman J. Gastric and duodenal mucosa in 'healthy' individuals. An endoscopic and histopathological study of 50 volunteers. *J Clin Pathol*, 1978; 31: 69.

566 Jenkins D, Goodall A, Gillet FR, Scott BB. Defining duodenitis: quantitative histological study of mucosal responses and their correlations. *J Clin Pathol*, 1985; 38: 1119.

567 Jeffers MD, Hourihane DO. Coeliac disease with histological features of peptic duodenitis: value of assessment of intraepithelial lymphocytes. *J Clin Pathol*, 1993; 46: 420.

568 Walker MM, Dixon MF. Gastric metaplasia: its role in duodenal ulceration. *Aliment Pharmacol Ther*, 1996; 10 (Suppl 1): 119.

569 Phull PS, Price AB, Stephens J, Rathbone BJ, Jacyna MR. Histology of chronic gastritis with and without duodenitis in patients with *Helicobacter pylori* infection. *J Clin Pathol*, 1996; 49: 377.

570 Marshall BJ, McGechie DB, Rogers PA, Glancy RJ. Pyloric *Campylobacter* infection and gastroduodenal disease. *Med J Aust*, 1985; 142: 439.

571 Wyatt JI, Rathbone BJ, Dixon MF, Heatley RV. *Campylobacter pyloridis* and acid induced gastric metaplasia in the pathogenesis of duodenitis. *J Clin Pathol*, 1987; 40: 841.

572 Wyatt JI, Rathbone BJ, Sobala GM *et al*. Gastric epithelium in the duodenum: its association with *Helicobacter pylori* and inflammation. *J Clin Pathol*, 1990; 43: 981.

573 Hamlet A, Thoreson AC, Nilsson O, Svennerholm AM, Olbe L. Duodenal *Helicobacter pylori* infection differs in cagA genotype between asymptomatic subjects and patients with duodenal ulcers. *Gastroenterology*, 1999; 116: 259.

574 Crabtree JE, Shallcross TM, Wyatt JI *et al*. Mucosal humoral immune response to *Helicobacter pylori* in patients with duodenitis. *Dig Dis Sci*, 1991; 36: 1266.

575 Leonard N, Feighery CF, Hourihane DO. Peptic duodenitis—does it exist in the second part of the duodenum? *J Clin Pathol*, 1997; 50: 54.

22 Malnutrition, maldigestion and malabsorption

Adequate nutrition depends on the ingestion of a suitable diet and its proper digestion, absorption and metabolism. Malnutrition can result from inadequacy of one or more of these functions. In practice, it is helpful to consider differential diagnosis under the following four headings.

1 Malnutrition due to an unsatisfactory diet.

2 Malnutrition consequent on maldigestion. The primary disorder may involve the stomach, small bowel, pancreas, liver or biliary system.

3 Malnutrition due to malabsorption or to faulty intracellular metabolism: there are three principal categories to consider.

(a) Patients who have an inborn abnormality, often inherited, either of surface enterocytes with their associated enzyme systems which interferes with the final stages of digestion, absorption or intracellular metabolism, or of gut-associated lymphoid tissue which results in a hypersensitivity to particular ingested dietary components.

(b) Patients who sustain sufficient acquired damage either to surface enterocytes, producing interference with normal absorption or metabolism or to the crypt zone sufficient to disturb normal surface enterocyte replacement, or both.

(c) Patients with disorders usually associated with local organic disease or previous surgery, such as diverticula, strictures, fistulae, stagnant loops or short circuits of bowel, which reduce the surface area available for absorption. These patients often have concomitant disturbance of normal small bowel ecology (see p. 247).

4 Malnutrition due to miscellaneous disorders, some of which are of undetermined origin.

The separation of these groups depends on a careful clinical history and the proper use of radiological, laboratory and other techniques, including biopsy.

Malabsorption from whatever cause is usually accompanied by steatorrhoea and anaemia. Clinical investigation must always include naked-eye examination of stools which, if fat is present in excess, are characteristically frothy, bulky, offensive and silver-grey in colour and float in water. Haematological investigations to determine the pattern of any anaemia present are obligatory. Other selective techniques include radiology using barium meal and follow-through or small bowel barium enemas; ultrasound; measurement of small bowel transit times and carbohydrate absorption by means of hydrogen breath tests; the microscopic screening of stools for fat [1]; faecal fat estimations made over a number of days; and tests for calcium and bile absorption. The various techniques are reviewed in [2]. The choice of investigations rests with the clinician concerned, but many rely initially on a full clinical and haematological examination for all patients, followed by appropriate radiology for those in group 3(c) above, and intestinal biopsy for the remainder. They proceed to more complex investigations only if those used initially fail to suggest a diagnosis. In a textbook devoted primarily to histopathology only the macroscopic and histological findings in biopsies or resected specimens will be considered in detail in this chapter.

Histopathological diagnosis of malabsorptive states

Intestinal biopsy

Jejunal biopsy is a safe and straightforward procedure in adults and children; instruments are available for single and multiple biopsies [3,4] but sampling is 'blind' after positioning of the capsule. This can lead to sampling errors when lesions are patchily distributed [5,6] and a single negative biopsy does not necessarily exclude a particular disease. For this reason and because it allows direct visual assessment of the mucosa, many clinicians prefer endoscopic duodenal biopsy. This often presents problems in interpretation. The normal duodenum can include ridge and spade forms of villi closely resembling those seen in partial flattening caused by disease and a number of adult patients who are symptom free have some inflammatory cellular infiltration with or without a degree of flattening, usually referred to as 'duodenitis' [7,8] (see p. 308). These changes are unrelated to malabsorption but can be confusing to the pathologist since they cannot readily be distinguished histologically from the minor degrees of flattening with cellular infiltration sometimes seen in true malabsorption.

Dissecting microscopy

Considerable stress has been laid on the value of dissecting microscopy in the diagnosis of mucosal damage. Our own experience indicates that it has little value in differential diagnosis except as an aid to correct orientation of a biopsy for embedding prior to section. Minor degrees of pathological alteration in villus pattern cannot reliably be distinguished from normal variations, especially in those who live in tropical zones, and the presence of spade or leaf forms, and even ridges in children, is not a reliable indication of mucosal damage. There is no substitute for careful histological examination of correctly orientated serial or step-sections appropriately stained.

Microscopic pathology

Small bowel mucosa can only react to injury in a limited number of ways. In most cases there is excessive loss of enterocytes from the villi by a process of enhanced apoptosis [9]. If the damage is mild, increased activity of the crypt replication zone compensates for the increased cell loss and little detectable villous change results, though the crypt zone increases in length and in mitotic activity and enterocytes may appear crowded (Fig. 22.1). When cell loss is more severe and more rapid, crypt hyperplasia increases further, enterocytes migrating upwards to clothe villi do not have sufficient time to mature and tend to remain crowded together, and goblet cells are fewer. The villi become shorter and broader, probably because the enterocytes

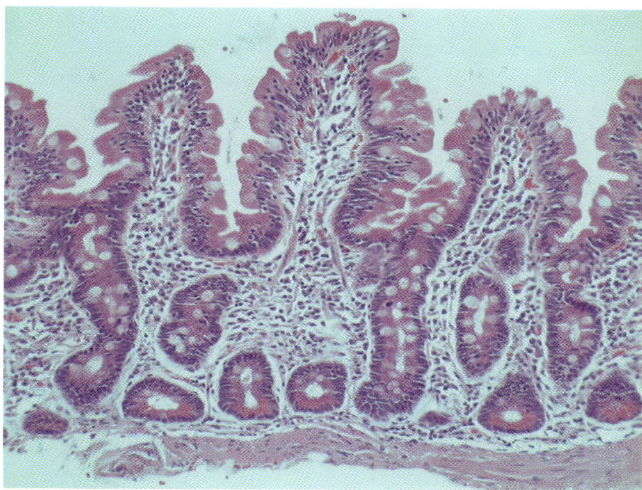

Fig. 22.1 A minor degree of villous change in gluten-induced enteropathy. Careful examination reveals slight shortening of surface enterocytes, increased crypt cell proliferation and slight thickening of the basal layer with crypt elongation.

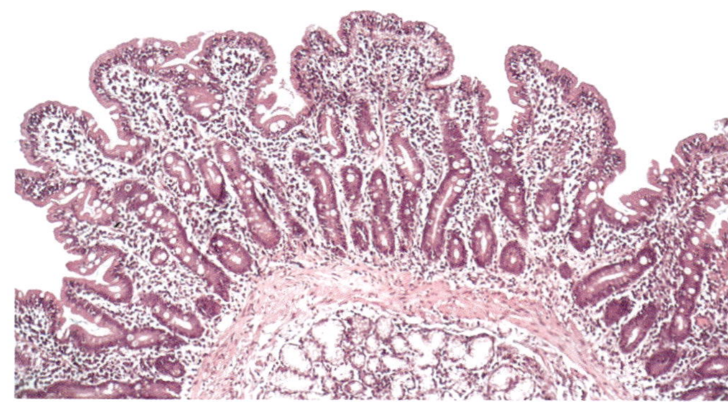

Fig. 22.2 There is shortening and blunting of villi with crypt hyperplasia in this duodenal biopsy from a patient with gluten-induced enteropathy. The enterocytes are crowded together and the basal layer is thickened. This picture is traditionally described as 'partial villous atrophy'.

can no longer cover them adequately (Fig. 22.2), and the basal layer begins to thicken, presumably as a direct result of the increased proliferation of the crypt zone. Continued inability of crypt cell proliferation to keep pace with enterocyte loss results in a flattened mucosa with a considerably thickened basal layer (Fig. 22.3); there may be complete loss of villi but because of the thickened basal layer the total width of the mucosa is little diminished; for this reason many workers, ourselves included, find the term 'mucosal atrophy' as opposed to 'flattening' inappropriate. At the same time there are alterations in the number both of intraepithelial lymphocytes and of lymphocytes and macrophages in the lamina propria;

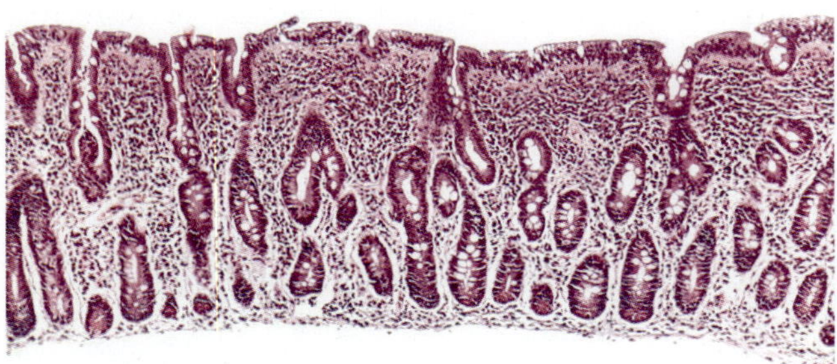

Fig. 22.3 Complete effacement of villi and thickening of the basal layer of the mucosa with crypt hyperplasia in a patient with gluten-induced enteropathy before dietary gluten exclusion. This picture is traditionally described as 'subtotal villous atrophy'.

plasma cell numbers also vary and there may be an increase or a decrease in the number of cells synthesizing particular immunoglobulins.

The picture here described is the basic common pattern of mucosal reaction to damage. Variations from it, which can be diagnostic, occur in different diseases. A number of disorders do not give rise to obvious morphological changes though specialized histochemical, ultrastructural, immunocytochemical and morphometric investigations can often detect them [10–12]. These are referred to in the text where appropriate (see also Chapter 2). At the risk of sounding banal there is now more truth than ever in the adage that 'all that flattens is not sprue' [13], and we now have available techniques which, properly used, can often distinguish many of the different patterns of mucosal damage.

Malnutrition due to unsatisfactory diet

Protein calorie malnutrition in children

Protein calorie malnutrition (Kwashiorkor) results from severe dietary protein deficiency and is found in Asia and in many African tribes, particularly in East and South Africa. It affects children and adults, but in humans and in experimental animals epithelial changes are more severe in the period of growth than in adult life or old age [14] All coats of the bowel are thinned and atrophic. Mucosal changes have to be interpreted with care since the 'normal' pattern for the region can be one of complex convolutions and some reduction in villous height, which is probably a manifestation of an almost universal degree of protein lack [15]; in severe protein calorie malnutrition jejunal and ileal villous height, surface area and the total volume of the lamina propria are all below normal. The mucosal flattening can be severe in children [16], sometimes mimicking gluten-induced enteropathy. Individual workers differ in the degree of crypt hyperplasia that they have described [17–21]: in the few cases which we have seen this has

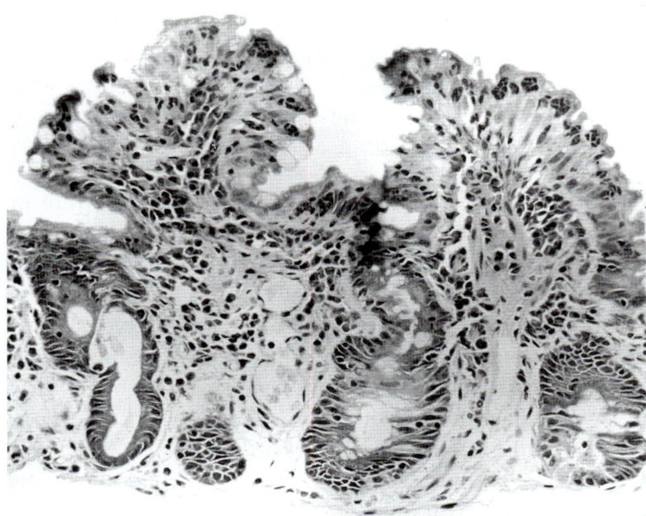

Fig. 22.4 Small intestine mucosa in protein calorie matnutrition. The villi show partial flettening but intra-epithelial lymphocytes are not numerous. The crypt zone shows no increase in activity and plasma cell numbers in the lamina propria are normal.

not been conspicuous and there has been no constant increase in intraepithelial lymphocytes or in the number of plasma cells in the lamina propria (Fig. 22.4); some workers have described a reduction in number of plasma cells, particularly those synthesizing immunoglobulin A (IgA), and a reduction of acid phosphatase activity within enterocytes [21]. The mucosa slowly reverts towards normal on an adequate diet [22]. Appearances suggest deficient replacement of the normal enterocyte loss due to failure in crypt cell proliferation, rather than an over-rapid loss of enterocytes [21].

Adult malnutrition

In the few examples of adult malnutrition which we have seen appearances have resembled those of protein calorie malnutrition in children and crypt cell hyperplasia has not been conspicuous. A single case of folate deficiency is reported [23] with villous flattening which improved and finally disappeared on dietary folate. This was presumably also the result of a failure of crypt zone regeneration.

Malnutrition consequent on maldigestion

Defects in gastric function

Deficiency of secretions

Acid and pepsinogen

Deficient secretion of acid and pepsinogen always occur after total and sometimes after partial gastrectomy, always in gastric atrophy, usually in chronic atrophic gastritis, and sometimes in advanced gastric carcinoma. Histological studies on small bowel mucosa after partial gastrectomy show either normal mucosa or mild patchy villous thickening and shortening. In some patients this may have preceded gastrectomy or be related to conditions such as alcohol ingestion which have also given rise to gastritis [24–26]. Linked absorption and histochemical studies suggest a correlation between impaired absorption and decrease in dehydrogenase activity in jejunal enterocytes.

Intrinsic factor

Deficient secretion of intrinsic factor occurs when there is atrophy of gastric body mucosa and loss of parietal cells as in pernicious anaemia, after total gastrectomy and in occasional patients after partial gastrectomy. In patients with untreated pernicious anaemia jejunal villi are often shorter and broader and cellular mitoses in crypts fewer than normal, suggesting, as in protein calorie malnutrition, that cell proliferation is insufficient to replace the normal enterocyte loss through wear and tear. There is increased lymphocyte and plasma cell infiltration in the lamina propria [27]. After appropriate treatment crypt mitotic rates return rapidly to normal, followed by normal villous regeneration over a period of 2–3 months.

Excess of secretions

Acid

Excessive acid secretion can lead to peptic ulceration in the upper small bowel, as in Zollinger–Ellison syndrome; enzyme systems in the brush border and in enterocytes may be temporarily or more permanently inactivated, but histological evidence of mucosal damage is unusual [28].

Defects in function in other organs

Defects in small intestinal digestion are discussed below. Those due to pancreatic or hepatobiliary malfunction are outside the scope of this book.

Malnutrition due to defects in absorption and metabolism

Mechanical defects

Local zones of disease in the small bowel can produce malabsorption in a limited number of ways.

1 They may give rise to sufficient local mucosal damage to impair absorption, particularly in sites where this is specialized, as in the terminal ileum.

2 They can lead to fistula formation with short circuiting, so that there is too little normal bowel available for absorption and/or the transit time is too short. They can also give rise to strictures with consequent stagnation of bowel content and disturbance of normal bowel ecology (see p. 246). The indigenous small intestinal flora are harmless but are supplanted by abnormal bacterial colonization of the small bowel in a large number of circumstances, including stagnant loops and fistulae. Although not necessarily invasive, or causing structural changes visible in haematoxylin and eosin (H&E)-stained sections, such infections damage the glycocalyx, producing a partial loss of disaccharide enzyme activity, resulting in maldigestion. In children this happens also in a large number of diarrhoeal illnesses, including food allergy [29]. It may also contribute to the clinical severity of the steatorrhoea in coeliac disease. The surgical resections and anastomoses which local disease may require can themselves produce similar effects.

Local disease is commonly associated with local mucosal ulceration, often with some distortion of the adjacent mucosa; there is rarely any generalized mucosal change and biopsies from uninvolved sites are usually normal. It will not be further discussed in this chapter.

Surgical resections

The average length of the small bowel in a live adult is about 280 cm. Because of marked individual variation it is difficult to say what length can be resected before malabsorption will regularly occur. Earlier studies suggested that about one-third of the upper small bowel could be resected with impunity and one-half with reasonable safety [30] and that survival is possible after a resection of 90% [31]. Ileal resections are less favourable than jejunal since, though the normal ileum can take over the absorptive functions of the jejunum, the reverse is not true; an intact ileocaecal valve is also important. There is some evidence that children tolerate massive resections better than adults, particularly as regards their long-term effects [32].

Biopsy studies on residual small intestinal mucosa following massive resection were originally claimed to show that villi were not hypertrophied though there was an increase in the number of absorptive enterocytes per unit length [33]. There is, however, increasing evidence, both from absorption and transit time studies on the one hand [34] and from experimental studies on rats who underwent surgical resections on the other [35], that adaptive changes certainly occur, with early crypt hyperplasia which may be regulated, at least in part, by endogenous enteroglucagon.

There has been a considerable interest in the last few years in the use of jejunoileal bypass operations for obesity, though the procedure is now less used than formerly because of the many complications that can ensue. Bypasses resemble resections to the extent that they reduce the length of bowel available for absorption, but since the operation is a bypass and not a resection a potentially functional loop of bowel is left intact and the two conditions are not strictly comparable. There is evidence that, if the bypass functions properly, there is crypt hyperplasia in the actively functional bowel, but we do not know of any detailed histological studies on the bypassed segments in humans.

Food intolerance

One of the major advances in gastrointestinal pathology in recent years has been a better understanding of, and a consequent improved interpretation of biopsy findings in patients who show an intolerance of ingested food. Such patients fall into two main categories.

First, there are those who lack certain necessary enzyme systems for digestion and metabolism of ingested food. Disaccharidase deficiency is an obvious example. The defects may be genetically inherited or may be acquired following exposure to infection, drugs or other toxic substances. They may be permanent or temporary and may or may not produce visible histological damage to enterocytes.

Second, there are those who appear to have a reaction which is immunologically based and manifests itself as an allergy to a particular ingested food or to its breakdown products; hypersensitivity to cow's milk protein in children and to shellfish in adults are well recognized examples.

Others seem to have a combined origin; an example is seen in coeliac disease in which a breakdown product of gluten acts as a toxic agent to enterocytes but only in a selected population which may be genetically determined (see p. 334).

Changes in histology can be severe but can also be minimal or non-existent, particularly in patients with enzyme defects. Confirmation of a suspected enzyme defect requires examination of unfixed tissue. This would usually be obtained by taking a second biopsy. Biochemical assay is the method of choice and falls outside the scope of this book. However, when specialized facilities are available, enzyme histochemistry can reveal subtle deficiencies of, for example, lactase.

Defects in enzyme systems

Enterocytes possess large numbers of enzyme systems, located in brush borders and in cell bodies; many are histochemically demonstrable and their distribution can also be recognized biochemically [36]. Their absence, however, is not usually accompanied by visible histological change. The principal patterns of abnormality are described below.

Disaccharidase deficiencies

Disaccharidase deficiency and disaccharide intolerance are not necessarily synonymous although they commonly coexist. The deficiency can occur in a primary inherited form due to an autosomally inherited recessive gene [37], in which case there is usually a specific deficiency in lactase while other disaccharidases are present in normal concentration. At all ages the condition can be secondary, usually to infection or to chemotherapy for cancer [38]. In adults primary deficiencies are more common amongst the black and Oriental populations than in Caucasians and usually affect more than one enzyme. There may also be a geographical incidence [39].

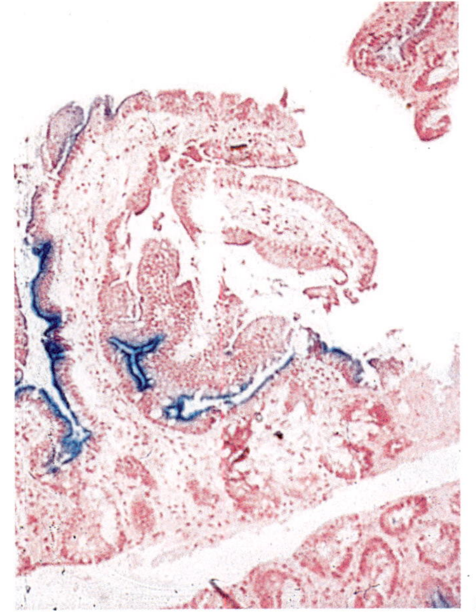

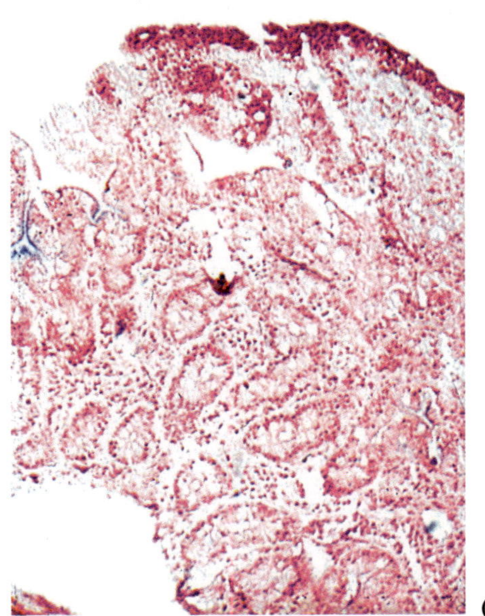

Fig. 22.5 Frozen sections of duodenal biopsies stained histochemically for N-lactase; (a) control, (b) biopsy from child with alactasia.

Biopsy interpretation is often difficult. In primary deficiencies the histology is usually normal and many children with genuine alactasia have been reported (by ourselves as well as others) simply as having no mucosal abnormality with the implication that there is therefore no disease process present. The enzymes are located in the brush border and there are histochemical techniques for their demonstration [40,41] (Fig. 22.5) though not all laboratories are equipped to perform them. Biochemical analysis of biopsy material is a practical alternative. Indeed, it has been suggested that the use of histochemistry for the diagnosis of inherited brush border enzyme deficiencies has no place in modern gastroenterological practice [42].

In secondary deficiencies histology may also appear normal, though biochemical analysis may confirm the deficiency [43]. Those that follow overt infection often show the inflammatory changes consequent on the infection (see Chapter 21).

Defects in lipid transport

Abetalipoproteinaemia

This rare disorder, also known as acanthocytosis, is probably transmitted by an autosomal recessive gene. There is inability to transfer preformed triglyceride from enterocytes to lymphatics in the lamina propria, probably due to failure to synthesize proteins known as apo-LP-ser, a group which includes chylomicron and β-lipoproteins and which forms the protein element of lipoprotein complexes [44]. The red cell envelope is abnormal, producing acanthocytes, and there may be retinopathy and central nervous system disease. Jejunal biopsy shows villi of relatively normal appearance but with marked foamy vacuolation of the cytoplasm of enterocytes covering the upper two-thirds of the villus (Fig. 22.6) [45]. In cryostat sections the vacuoles stain for neutral lipid [46] and must be distinguished in children from those sometimes seen in sensitivity to cow's milk [47,48]. Morphologically similar vacuolation of enterocytes has also been described in juvenile nutritional megaloblastic anaemia, coeliac disease and tropical sprue [49] and also after a fatty meal.

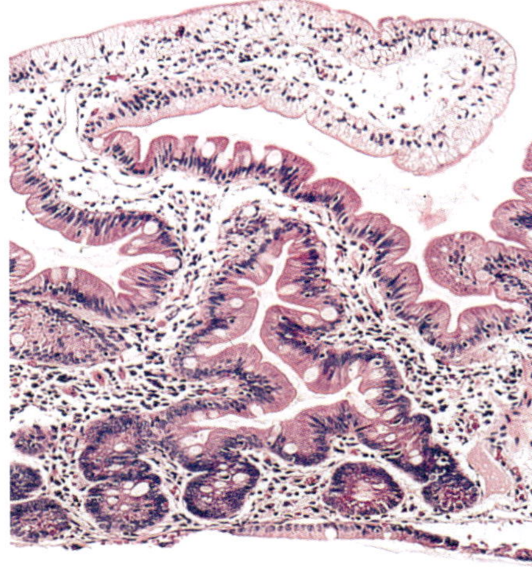

Fig. 22.6 Abetalipoproteinaemia. Biopsy of jejunal mucosa from a child. There is conspicuous fine vacuolation of the cytoplasm of the enterocytes of the upper two-thirds of the villi.

Other defects in lipid transport

These include homozygous hypobetalipoproteinaemia (a dominantly inherited condition) [50] and Andersen's disease (chylomicron retention disease) [51]. Both are associated with accumulation of esterified lipid in the enterocytes.

Immunological reactions to ingested food

Hypersensitivity reactions to ingested proteins and polypeptides are becoming increasingly recognized, especially in infants and children. The most common antigens are components of the proteins present in cow's milk [52] and in 'milk' derived from soy protein [52,53].

Cow's milk protein sensitivity in children

The jejunal lesions have been described as histologically and ultrastructurally similar to those seen in gluten-induced enteropathy [54]. In our experience they are usually less severe and a recent study using quantitative analysis has suggested that the total mucosal thickness is decreased (in contrast with the increase in thickness usually seen in childhood coeliac disease) because the capacity of the crypt zone to compensate for increased villous epithelial cell loss is limited [55], though other workers have described crypt cell hyperplasia [56]. There is partial villous flattening with an increase in intraepithelial lymphocyte number resembling that seen in gluten-induced enteropathy but quantitatively less numerous [57,58], combined with a marked increase in plasma cells containing IgE in the lamina propria. This is not a conspicuous feature of gluten-induced enteropathy and suggests a type I allergic response, a suggestion which is further borne out by the finding of increased numbers of eosinophils both intraepithelial [55] and, with increased numbers of mast cells, in the lamina propria [59]. Brush border alkaline phosphatase is also said to be reduced [60]. The clinical and histological criteria suggested for diagnosis [61] accord with our own experience.

Sensitivity to soy protein

Changes in small bowel mucosa after the ingestion of soy protein in sensitive individuals have been well described in calves [62] but reports on human infants are less reliable and sensitivity has been more often assessed by estimating serum antibody levels [63]. Significantly raised titres have predominated in patients with suspected gluten-induced enteropathy and especially in those who have not responded fully to a gluten-free diet; it may be that in this group some of the features attributed to gluten sensitivity were due, at least in part, to a separate or concomitant sensitivity to soy protein.

In both cow's milk and soy sensitivity a return to normal in the mucosa follows the withdrawal of the offending antigen.

Adults show sensitivity to other, more adult, dietary components, notably shellfish. Detailed studies have shown, as in childhood sensitivity to cow's milk, a marked increase in numbers of plasma cells synthesizing IgE in the lamina propria, but in adults, as opposed to children, intestinal morphology is usually, in our experience, normal. Nevertheless it is tempting to link these observations with those made on eosinophilic enteritis [64] and to suggest that this disorder represents a severe form of hypersensitivity to ingested antigenic food material.

Generalized damage to enterocytes

Coeliac syndromes

We use the term 'coeliac syndrome' to embrace the conditions alternatively termed 'coeliac sprue', 'non-tropical sprue', 'sprue syndrome' and 'gluten-sensitive' or 'gluten-induced enteropathy', and also 'refractory' or 'non-responsive coeliac disease'. *Coeliac disease* is an immunologically mediated inflammatory disease of the gastrointestinal mucosa due to intolerance to a component of gliadin, a storage protein of the cereals wheat, barley and rye, in genetically susceptible individuals. The precise pathogenesis is not completely understood but is considered in further detail on p. 334. Coeliac disease commonly presents in children, but in a significant minority of patients is first recognized in adolescence, in adult life, or even in old age. It is presumed that these patients probably had the disorder from early life, but with minimal symptoms. In 98% of patients there is a direct relationship which can be demonstrated by the beneficial effect of gluten withdrawal and conversely by the clinical test of gluten challenge [65]. The condition in these patients can be legitimately described as gluten-induced enteropathy. The 2% of patients who appear to have a disease in all other respects similar to gluten-induced enteropathy but in whom there is an incomplete or absent response to gluten withdrawal are classified as having refractory or non-responsive coeliac disease. In the past, the term 'idiopathic steatorrhoea' has been applied to this condition.

Gluten-induced enteropathy

There are three components necessary for complete certainty in diagnosis: an abnormal villous pattern on biopsy; clinical and some degree of mucosal improvement on removal of gluten from the diet; and clinical and mucosal relapse following its reintroduction [65], though either may be delayed for a time. Mucosal changes have in the past usually been assessed on jejunal biopsy; duodenal biopsy, although yielding less suitable samples, is now the method of choice, for reasons already discussed and, providing biopsies are only taken from the distal duodenum, is adequate for diagnosis in most cases [66]. In general, changes are most severe in the upper jejunum, decrease distally and may be minimal in the distal ileum [67]. The histological appearances are not uniform [4,6] and although a normal biopsy is unlikely, varying degrees of damage can be seen in multiple biopsies taken at the same time.

Appearances at dissecting microscopy are striking and can be seen also on magnifying endoscopy. We are not impressed by their diagnostic value but, since dissecting microscopy is practised by some endoscopists and may be useful for orientation, we include a short account of the principal findings.

Dissecting microscopic appearances

The following terms are commonly used.

1 *Normal villi* are finger-like and have slightly bulbous tips; if an appreciable number are present the biopsy is unlikely to show any major histological abnormality (see Fig. 18.4).

2 *Leaf or spade forms* are normal in height and width but increased in length. Some are present in most normal mucosae (Fig. 22.7).

3 *Ridges* are leaf forms in which the length and width are further increased. There is usually also a reduction in height and when this has occurred, they are always abnormal (Fig. 22.8).

4 *Convolutions* are long ridges reduced in height in which the straight luminal edge has become twisted and sometimes fused with itself to produce a surface rather resembling a cerebral hemisphere (Fig. 22.8). Occasionally a ridged or convoluted mucosa appears not to be reduced in height and then may appear normal on subsequent histological examination.

5 *A 'flat' mucosa* has lost its ridges and convolutions. It shows a mosaic pattern [67] in which clefts separate slightly raised mounds of epithelium, on the surface of which crypt openings may still be visible (Fig. 22.9). Submucosal vessels are often visible through it. These features are well seen with modern endoscopes (Fig. 22.10).

The disadvantages of relying on dissecting microscopic appearances for accurate diagnosis are:

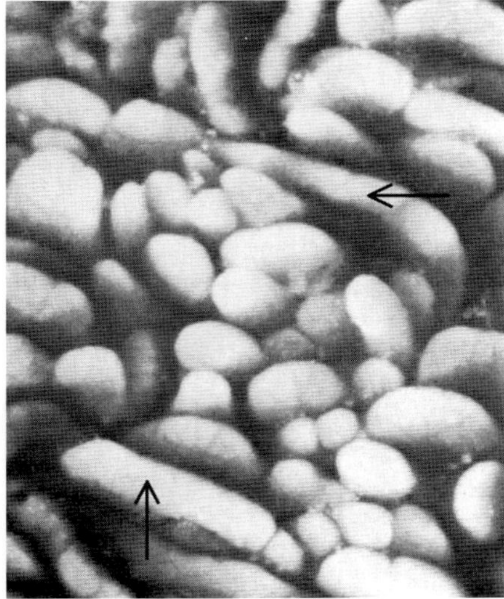

Fig. 22.7 Spade and ridge formation in a non-Caucasian. Occasional normal villi are present, there are numerous spade forms and long ridges, reduced in height compared with adjacent villi, arrowed.

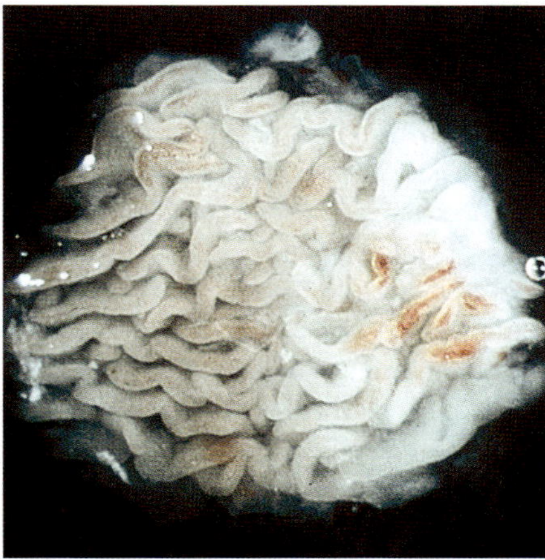

Fig. 22.8 A ridged and convoluted mucosa; the ridges are shortened in height and thickened and no spade or finger forms remain (dissecting microscope).

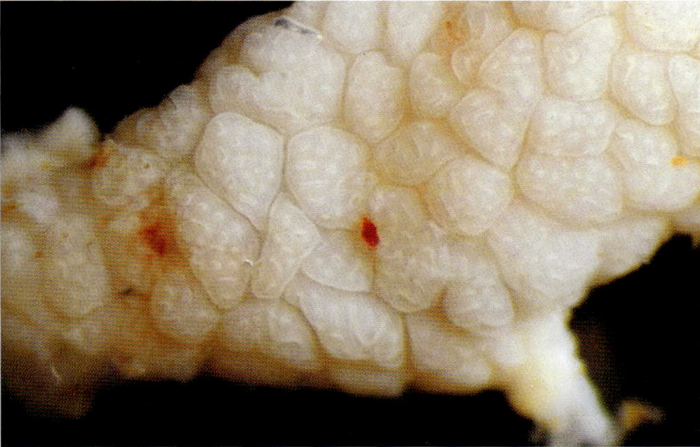

Fig. 22.9 A 'flat' mucosa showing a mosaic pattern. The raised mounds of epithelium with crypt openings in their centre are clearly visible (dissecting microscope).

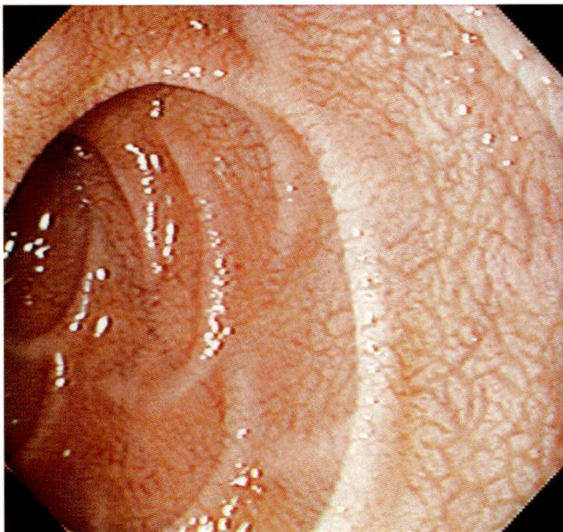

Fig. 22.10 Endoscopic appearance of a flat mucosa in gluten-induced enteropathy. There is a mosaic appearance (sometimes described as 'scalloping').

1 there is marked geographical and racial variation in the number of leaves and even ridges which can be seen in normal individuals. Asians and Africans have more than Caucasians, and those who live in tropical zones more than those who live in temperate regions;

2 it is difficult, when assessing leaf, spade and ridge forms, to be sure whether there is a diminution in villous height. This is all-important; many normal mucosae in which leaf and spade forms are present are diagnosed incorrectly as showing a degree of flattening because the fact that they are normal in height has not been appreciated; and

3 even if some degree of flattening is apparent, differential diagnosis between different patterns of mucosal damage is not possible except after careful histology with quantification; it cannot be made under the dissecting microscope.

Histological appearances

In assessing histological appearances it is vital to have correctly orientated specimens and to use step- or serial sections. Correct orientation is confirmed by seeing longitudinally sectioned crypts. Normal villi are slender, with a length of at least twice the depth of the basal part of the mucosa. It is conventionally stated that the presence of four normal consecutive villi indicates a normal biopsy [68]. However, in some patients there may be patchy disease and a single biopsy with apparently normal villi may reveal, on scrutiny, increased numbers of intraepithelial lymphocytes. The type and degree of abnormality require careful assessment.

The fundamental disorder in gluten-induced enteropathy is damage to enterocytes produced by breakdown products of gluten, and the failure of cell replication by the crypt zone to keep pace with this damage. The initial microscopic changes are those already described in detail on p. 325. The histological picture varies, depending on the stage of disease and its severity. The earliest changes seem to be an increase in number and immunoreactivity of intraepithelial lymphocytes (IELs) [69]. Past debate about the extent to which the increase in number is only apparent due to reduction in mucosal surface area has been superseded since it has been realized that lymphocyte density is also increased in the surface epithelium of gastric and colorectal mucosa in coeliac disease [70–72]. In the small intestinal mucosa there is an increase in IELs above the upper limit of normal of 40 lymphocytes per 100 enterocytes [73]. This makes assessment of duodenal and/or jejunal IEL density the earliest and most sensitive indicator of coeliac disease. IELs are also increased in asymptomatic relatives of patients with coeliac disease and in patients with dermatitis herpetiformis, even if there is no clinical evidence of enteropathy. To assist with counting, immunohistochemistry with CD3 may be useful. The IELs are a subpopulation of T lymphocytes that express a characteristic range of surface antigens, including HML-1 $\propto E\beta 7$ integrin [73a]. More than 95% of IELs are CD3 and CD2 positive. In gluten-induced enteropathy the proportion of IELs which express the $\gamma\delta$ T-cell receptor is increased above 10% (the upper limit of the normal range). The crypt zone is unable to keep pace with the increased rate of loss of damaged surface enterocytes. This leads to a shortening in height and apparent increase in width of individual villi, and an accompanying increase in the length of the crypts (Figs 22.2 & 22.3) resulting from increased mitotic activity [74,75]. This crypt hyperplasia is apparently driven by growth factors such as hepatocyte growth factor and keratinocyte growth factor, produced by mesenchymal cells and IELs [76,77]. The enterocytes forming the surface epithelium at the villous tips have not had time to mature and are consequently smaller, more squat and crowded together so that the epithelium appears more than one layer thick (Fig. 22.11) and the normal vertical orientation of cells is lost [78]. The increased depth of the crypts results in maintenance or even an increase of the total mucosal volume, despite the decrease in surface absorptive area.

In the lamina propria, lymphoid cell density also increases, mainly due to accumulation of plasma cells. The ratio of plasma cells containing IgA : IgG : IgM remains constant, the majority being responsible for production of the IgA antibodies to gliadin, to endomysium, and to tissue transglutaminase that are important serological markers of gluten-induced enteropathy [79–81] unless there is associated selective IgA deficiency [82–84]. Mast cells, basophils and eosinophils are all increased in number [85,86] though our experience has been that eosinophil numbers do not reach those seen in protein allergies; they revert to normal on a gluten-free diet.

Using conventional light microscopy Paneth cells may appear decreased in numbers but this is probably because they have a decreased lysozymal content and therefore stain less readily with conventional stains [87]. There are also reports that endocrine cell numbers are increased [84–91] with the possible exception of secretin-secreting cells [92]. Some of these reports must be treated with reservation since they depend on relative rather than absolute cell counts; in any event they are as likely to represent a secondary effect of crypt zone hyperplasia with increase in volume of the basal layer of cells from which endocrine cells develop as to be a specific primary response to gluten damage.

These are the basic histological features to be looked for in any gluten-induced enteropathy. Occasionally in a flat mucosa there may be a collagenous band of variable thickness between the surface enterocytes and the lamina propria (Fig. 22.12), a condition sometimes referred to as 'collagenous sprue'. Some workers have associated a broad band with a lack of response to a gluten-free diet and a consequent poor prognosis [2,93] while others, when it is present only in a minor degree, regard it as relatively common and probably reversible, conceding that marked deposition may indicate an unfavourable outlook [94]. Small intestinal mucosal biopsies in five out of a series of 10 patients with refractory sprue showed features of collagenous sprue [95]. Gastric metaplasia has been reported in 68% of upper small intestinal biopsies, of both endoscopic and Crosby capsule type, in gluten-induced enteropathy [96], though it is often mild and focal and it is generally much less striking than in peptic duodenitis (see pp. 150 and 308).

Intestinal biopsies allow only a study of the mucosa. At necropsy all coats of the bowel can be assessed, but such studies have generally been considered as of little value because of postmortem mucosal autolysis. While this is true for detailed mucosal microscopy, carefully performed autopsy studies allow estimation of the extent of the disease and the detection of associated neoplasms [97]. Lesions in the small bowel tend to diminish in severity distally, showing a flat mucosa in the proximal third, ridges and convolutions in the middle third, and digitate and leaf forms of villi in the distal third. Within each segment mucosal changes are patchy and variable. There is often associated thinning of the muscle coats [98] which may have a generalized brown colour due to the presence of lipochrome pigments (see p. 338). In one series [97] a malignant lymphoma was found in 10 out of 24 necropsies.

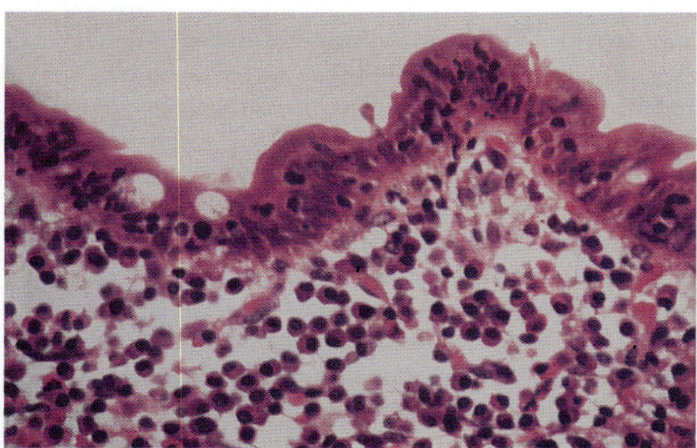

Fig. 22.11 Surface epithelium in gluten-induced enteropathy. The enterocytes are crowded and apparently multilayered.

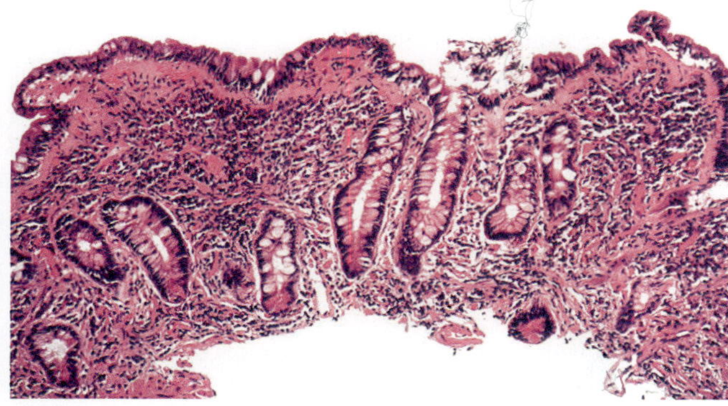

Fig. 22.12 Collagenous sprue. The subepithelial collagen plate is prominent. Crypt hyperplasia is less conspicuous than is usual for a flat mucosa.

Table 22.1 Grading of enteropathy (from [101]).

	0	1	2	3a	3b	3c
IEL	<40	>40	>40	>40	>40	>40
Crypts	Normal	Normal	Hypertrophic	Hypertrophic	Hypertrophic	Hypertrophic
Villi	Normal	Normal	Normal	Atrophy +	Atrophy ++	Absent

There have been a few patients reported, all female, who clinically have had gluten-induced enteropathy that has responded to a gluten-free diet but in whom the mucosa has been histologically normal apart from an increased cellularity of the lamina propria and an increase in number of intraepithelial lymphocytes; both of these changes reverted to normal on diet. They have been labelled as 'gluten-sensitive diarrhoea' [99]. When the affected patient shows the serological pattern of gluten-induced enteropathy, such as antigliadin, antiendomysial or antitissue transglutaminase antibodies, the term 'potential coeliac disease' has been suggested [100].

There may be advantages for clinicopathological liaison and communication between centres in using a grading system for the assessment of duodenal or jejunal biopsies from patients with gluten-induced enteropathy, as proposed by Marsh. The modified system of Oberhuber and colleagues has merit and is shown in Table 22.1 [101].

Such gradings, not based on actual measurements or cell counts, are naturally subjective but, if performed by the same pathologist, may allow some degree of comparison between repeat biopsies from a single patient.

Ultrastructural studies

There are good reports on scanning and transmission electron microscopic changes [102–105]. These show a reduction in number and size of microvilli that become short, irregular in shape and may fuse. Pinocytic vesicles decrease in number and the basement membrane is increased in width and in density and becomes disrupted. There is swelling of vascular endothelial cells, possibly secondary to a combination of gluten antigen with antibody [104].

Histochemical and chemical studies

Variations on the normal enzyme distribution described in Chapter 18 are well documented in coeliac syndromes [106]. Enterocyte content and surface expression of most enzymes is reduced [107–109].

The effects of gluten withdrawal and reintroduction

It is well known that adults and children who adhere strictly to a gluten-free diet usually improve clinically and the mucosa returns towards normal [110]. Scanning electron microscopic studies on children have shown that, in a previously flat mucosa, parallel ridges form by replication and migration of crypt cells; these twist, convolute and split to form spade-like villi, not all of which finally attain a finger shape [111]. Surface enterocytes mature, individual cells increase in height and the ratio of area of mucosal surface to area of crypt epithelium also increases [112]. The villous height: crypt length ratio, however, remains decreased and the raised number of IELs does not return to normal [113,114]. Variable results have been reported as regards immunoglobulin-containing plasma cells; in some series these have not often reverted entirely to normal [112–115], while in others the ratio and absolute number of these cells have been shown to revert to normal in children in remission [116]. This variability is no doubt due to the extreme difficulty in obtaining a completely gluten-free diet, as there are often tiny quantities of gluten in so-called 'gluten-free' foodstuffs. Future European Union regulations are expected to demand stricter definition of the term 'gluten-free', with a permissible level of gliadin likely to be set at 10 mg gliadin/100 g [116a].

The reintroduction of gluten after a period on a gluten-free diet can produce a variety of responses over a wide time scale [117–120] and clinical and mucosal improvement do not necessarily correlate. A very detailed study of 10 adults rechallenged by instillation of a single dose of gluten into the duodenum after being on a gluten-free diet showed immediate mucosal damage with falls in both brush border enzyme concentration and counts of villous cell population, thought to be due either to direct damage or to a type III immune response. There was some recovery of enzyme concentration after 24 hours, but not of the villous cell population [121]. Clinically most patients will relapse within 8 weeks and biopsy at that time will show mucosal flattening; others may have a flat mucosa without clinical relapse. Studies on children who appear to remain clinically well after reintroduction of gluten suggest that low lactate levels and increased intraepithelial lymphocyte counts indicate the probability of later relapse [114], and the presence of a raised number of IgG-containing plasma cells may have a similar significance. There is also a tendency in children for basement membranes to 'stain' for IgA complexes and for numbers of IgA-containing cells to be increased [118].

Dermatitis herpetiformis

It has long been recognized that there is a relationship between coeliac syndromes and dermatitis herpetiformis [122–125]. Some 60–80% of all patients with dermatitis herpetiformis also have true gluten-induced enteropathy which responds to gluten withdrawal [126,127], and enteropathy is also more common in their relatives than in the normal population [128].

About 80% also have antigen HLA-A8 [129], an incidence similar to that found in coeliac syndromes. Patients with dermatitis herpetiformis have raised serum antiendomysial antibodies [130] and increased numbers of intraepithelial lymphocytes in the small intestinal mucosa, particularly γδ T cells [131]. Approximately 90% of patients with gluten-induced enteropathy have some degree of epidermal ridge atrophy of the skin as is seen in dermatitis herpetiformis [132], and both groups have impaired glycine and L-alanine absorption [133]. A number of patients who have dermatitis herpetiformis but no mucosal abnormality on biopsy have developed mucosal flattening when fed a diet unusually high in gluten (latent coeliac disease [134]). This has reverted to normal on a normal diet [135]. Dermatitis herpetiformis appears to be a variant of coeliac disease in that the genetic profile of patients with the two conditions are very similar [136], although overt coeliac disease is expressed only in a percentage of patients with dermatitis herpetiformis [137]. It is of interest that the disease does not develop until after the first decade and is more common in males; an intestinal lymphoma has been recorded [138] and antral gastritis with hypochlorhydria is common [139].

Duodenal and jejunal biopsies have been used for diagnosis [140]; there is apparently no correlation between the severity of the skin lesions and the degree of mucosal flattening [141].

Aetiology [142]

The aetiology of gluten-induced enteropathy presents two major problems: what are the causative mechanisms [143–145]; and why does it involve only a small number of any population exposed to a gluten-containing diet?

Dealing with the second question first, there is clearly a genetic factor as relatives of patients show an increased prevalence of both mucosal abnormalities [146] and antigliadin and antiendomysial autoantibodies [147]. There is no doubt that the disease is closely linked with the possession of certain HLA antigens. The phenomenon of linkage disequilibrium has confounded investigation of association with specific HLA types but it has now emerged that there is genuine linkage with constitutional expression of the HLA class II molecules HLA-DQ2 and HLA-DQ8, both located on the short arm of chromosome 6, close to other HLA class II genes (in northern Europe HLA-A1, B8 and -DR3, and in Mediterranean races HLA-DR5 and -DR7). More specifically, the A1*0501,B1*0201 heterodimer of HLA-DQ2 is the genotype associated with gluten-induced enteropathy in 90% of patients [148]. It is likely that this gene functions in a recessive manner. However, it has become evident from genetic epidemiological studies that another gene, distinct from and unlinked to the HLA group, is likely to be a stronger determinant of disease susceptibility, probably by a factor of four [149]. This crucial gene has not been identified at the time of writing. It appears to be concerned with susceptibility or resistance of the small intestinal epithelium to the direct toxic effect of gliadin [150]. These authors suggest that presence of the susceptibility gene in the absence of HLA-DQ2 or -DQ8 or HLA-DR5 or -DR7 may result in gluten-induced diarrhoea without the immunological and full-blown clinical features of coeliac disease.

In an *in vitro* organ culture model it has been shown that within 1 hour of exposure to gliadin, duodenal enterocytes and adjacent macrophages showed marked expression of HLA-DR [151], suggesting that, in a susceptible subject, gliadin is directly toxic. Within a few hours of this, it has also been shown that HLA-DQ was up-regulated on mononuclear cells, activated CD4 helper T cells migrated to the subepithelial compartment and CD8 T cells began to invade the epithelium [152]. It is now known that there is a qualitative change in the IELs, which show up-regulation of CD5 [153] and synthesis of granzyme B [154]. Furthermore, there is an increase in the proportion of IELs that express γδ receptors from their normal value of less than 10% to up to 20% [155]. These activated lymphocytes may be responsible for cytolytic destruction of enterocytes.

As described above, most patients with gluten-induced enteropathy are constitutionally HLA-DQ2 positive. The remainder express HLA-DQ8. Both of these class II molecules are capable of presenting gluten peptides to the gluten-specific T cells that are uniquely found in the gut of gluten-induced enteropathy. It has been shown that tissue transglutaminase (tTG) deamidates gliadin [156] and two specific peptide fragments of gliadin then become the focus of DQ2-expressing T cells [157]. The apparently unique conformation of peptide–MHC complex that is produced seems to act as the trigger for an immune mechanism in which there a cytotoxic T-cell reaction against enterocytes.

Non-responsive coeliac syndrome/refractory sprue

Virtually all children with symptoms and biopsy findings suggestive of gluten-induced enteropathy respond to a gluten-free diet. A small number of adults with similar clinical and biopsy features do not respond, and non-committal terms such as 'idiopathic steatorrhoea' or 'refractory sprue' [158] have been applied. Great care must be taken to exclude concealed or inadvertent gluten ingestion, but when this is done an undoubted small group of non-responders exists. Although the numerous intraepithelial lymphocytes in refractory sprue are indistinguishable from those in coeliac disease on routine H&E staining, it has been shown that they have a phenotype distinct from gluten-induced enteropathy, with intracytoplasmic CD3ε receptors, absence of CD4, CD8 and surface T-cell receptors, and restricted rearrangements of the *TCRγ* gene [159]. It has also been claimed that, by taking biopsies from beyond the duodenum, using the technique of 'push' enteroscopy, features sufficiently characteristic to distinguish refractory sprue from gluten-induced enteropathy can be elicited [160]. Subcryptal chronic inflammation, neutrophilic infiltration and so-called collagenous sprue are claimed to be markers of refractory sprue in these circumstances.

The phenotype of the intraepithelial lymphocytes has been demonstrated to be identical with the cells of enteropathy-associated T-cell lymphoma (see p. 381), and intestinal lymphoma develops with increased frequency in these patients, suggesting that refractory sprue is a preinvasive, neoplastic condition [161].

Ulcerative jejunitis and malignant lymphoma

(see also p. 381)

Acute non-specific small intestinal ulceration has been described in patients with malabsorption [162–164] as well as in occasional patients with apparently normal mucosa. Of those with malabsorption, some have had proven gluten enteropathy, others unclassified sprue [163] or autoimmune enteropathy [165]. The mucosa surrounding the ulcers may be flat. Most of the ulcers have extended through the submucosa to involve the muscle coats, and perforation is common. Histological changes are usually non-specific, consisting of submucosal oedema and fibrosis with a marked non-specific inflammatory cell infiltrate in the base of the ulcer [166] (Fig. 22.13). Gastric metaplasia and drop-out of basal layer cells at the edge of the ulcer are common. Similar ulcers are described in dermatitis herpetiformis [167].

It is of great interest and practical importance that in the surface epithelium in refractory sprue, in the non-ulcerated mucosa in ulcerative jejunitis and in the non-tumorous mucosa adjacent to enteropathy-associated T-cell lymphoma, there is an identical aberrant monoclonal T-cell population, showing clonal identity with the cells of the lymphoma itself. Bagdi and colleagues [160] have shown that the monoclonal T-cell population is constituted by cytologically normal, non-invasive intraepithelial T lymphocytes that share an identical aberrant immunophenotype with enteropathy-associated T-cell lymphoma. Patients with refractory sprue and/or ulcerative jejunitis should therefore all be regarded as suffering from a neoplastic T-cell disorder at differing stages of development (see p. 381). The aberrant T cells lack expression of CD8 and show cytoplasmic rather than surface expression of CD3 [168]. This forms the basis of an immunohistochemical test that can be applied to paraffin sections of intestinal biopsies to confirm a suspected diagnosis of refractory sprue or enteropathy-associated T-cell lymphoma among patients with steatorrhoea [169].

As the constitutional HLA phenotype of patients with enteropathy-associated T-cell lymphoma is the same as that of most patients with gluten-induced enteropathy, it seems likely that enteropathy-associated T-cell lymphoma arises in patients with previous gluten-induced enteropathy by a process of evolution through intraepithelial lymphocytosis [170], at which stage there may be refractory sprue or ulcerative jejunitis. There do not seem to be any HLA markers specific for the development of malignancy [171], nor is hyposplenism associated with enteropathy-associated T-cell lymphoma [172,173].

Other tumours

An association with squamous carcinoma of the aerodigestive tract, including the upper oesophagus, is well established [174,175]. There is some doubt about an association with carci-

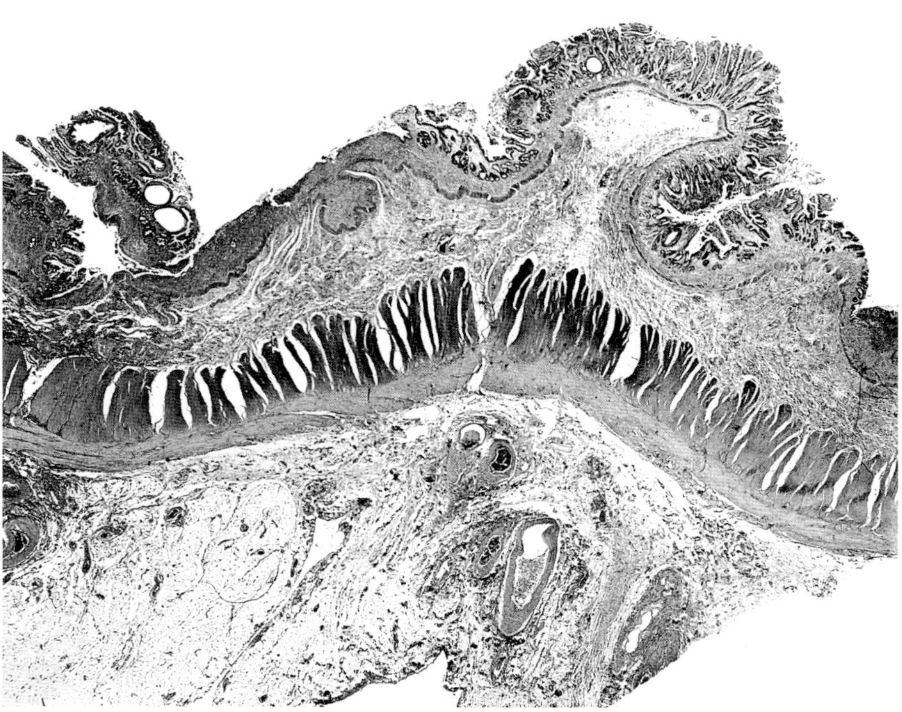

Fig. 22.13 Ulceration in coeliac disease. The ulcer has not yet affected the muscularis propria, but there is submucosal oedema, inflammation and early fibrosis. Drop-out of basal epithelium is conspicuous.

noma of small bowel, which could be fortuitous or due to genetic linkage rather than a direct consequence [176] (see p. 362).

Skin disorders

Gluten-induced enteropathy is associated with a range of skin disorders [177]. Besides dermatitis herpetiformis, which has a recognized relationship, patients with eczema [178], ichthyosis [179], psoriasis [180], rosacea [181] and urticaria pigmentosa [182] have been described as showing villous abnormalities, though these are not regularly associated with clinical evidence of malabsorption. While transient steatorrhoea can occur in direct relation to a rash, other dermatoses, with the possible exception of acrodermatitis enteropathica, are not specifically related to structural changes [183].

Other associated conditions

A number of less common complications or associations have also been described. These include granulomatous inflammation which has responded to gluten withdrawal [184,185], cavitation of mesenteric lymph nodes (especially in refractory sprue) [186], an association with cow's milk protein sensitivity [187], portal tract inflammation which can proceed to fibrosis [188], certain bronchopulmonary disorders [189] and a possible link with Down's syndrome [190].

Autoimmune enteropathy

There are occasional reports of patients, both adults and children, with a non-gluten-responsive enteropathy manifested by villous shortening, crypt hyperplasia and intraepithelial lymphocytosis in whom there are circulating antienterocyte antibodies of IgA and IgG class, sometimes in high titre, and no demonstrable antigliadin or antiendomysial antibodies [191,192]. Some of these patients have other organ-specific autoantibodies [192] and show a clinical and histological improvement with steroid therapy, suggesting an autoimmune enteropathy that is different from the coeliac syndromes. Immunophenotyping shows that the increased IELs differ from those seen in conventional gluten-induced enteropathy in that they do not express $\gamma\delta$ receptors.

Microvillous inclusion disease

This is a very rare autosomal recessive disorder that presents in neonates with refractory diarrhoea from birth, although occasional examples present a little later in infancy. It carries a very poor prognosis because a diffuse abnormality of the enterocytes in the small intestine results in severe intractable malabsorption that can only be controlled by lifelong total parenteral nutrition or small bowel transplantation. The disorder is primarily one of brush border assembly and differentiation, such that the normal microvilli of the cell surface become misplaced within the apical cytoplasm of the enterocytes to form the microvillous inclusions that give the condition its name [193]. These are best identified on electron microscopy as vesicles lined by microvilli that are often structurally unremarkable, and on light microscopy they are usually well demonstrated as PAS-positive inclusions in the supranuclear cytoplasm of the enterocytes that also stain strongly for carcinoembryonic antigen and alkaline phosphatase [194]. At lower-power magnification, the small bowel mucosa shows diffuse villous shortening with little or no crypt hyperplasia (so-called crypt hypoplastic villous atrophy) and there is no increase in mucosal inflammatory cells. Apart from the microvillous inclusions, PAS staining shows the enterocytes to have a poorly staining and discontinuous brush border, especially over the apices of any residual villi, but the other cellular components of the crypt, namely the goblet cells, Paneth cells and endocrine cells, are unremarkable [193]. However, cells in other areas of the gastrointestinal tract that normally harbour microvilli may also be affected, such that the microvillous inclusions may be found in gastric antral biopsies and in the large intestine, indicating that the defect in brush border assembly is more generalized.

Malabsorption related to infections

Temporary malabsorption is common in many patients with small intestinal infections and infestations, particularly giardiasis (see Chapter 21). It usually resolves when the infection is successfully treated.

Tropical sprue

Although tropical sprue is now recognized as infective [195], it remains in this chapter rather than in Chapter 21, because of its histological resemblance to gluten-sensitive enteropathy and its association with malabsorption. It is endemic in Puerto Rica, parts of the Caribbean, northern South America, Nigeria and other countries in West Africa, India, and much of south-east Asia and the Philippines (there is a valuable map in the article by Klipstein [196]) and is acquired by visitors to these regions. The cause is probably a persistent, as opposed to a transitory, contamination, initially of the proximal small bowel, by enteric pathogens, mostly coliforms, which the individual does not readily expel. These organisms produce enterotoxins that act directly on enterocytes and crypt cells. The intriguing suggestion has been made that the trigger for the continuing adverse response to such banal organisms may be a coccidial protozoon [197]. The condition, although often morphologically severe, may be symptomless, but gastrointestinal symptoms frequently result, with diarrhoea and steatorrhoea, and are followed by clinical evidence of malabsorption and nutritional deficiencies, including macrocytic anaemia; there is usually a good clinical and histopathological response to a combination of tetracycline or other suitable antibiotic and folic acid therapy.

The duodenum and jejunum are affected first, followed by involvement of the ileal mucosa. Dissecting microscopy shows partial rather than total villous flattening. Histologically the changes resemble those of gluten enteropathy, with crypt hyperplasia, broadening and shortening of villi, enterocyte distortion and crowding, an increase in number of intraepithelial lymphocytes which may also involve the crypt zone [198] and increased cellularity of the lamina propria with concomitant oedema and often eosinophilia. The histological features may closely resemble coeliac disease and, indeed, the two conditions are sometimes indistinguishable ([199]. Mucosal flattening is, however, rarely complete and at the less severe end of the spectrum appearances can merge with those seen in the indigenous population, so that biopsy is not always diagnostic [200,201].

Tropical sprue must be differentiated from giardiasis (see p. 283) and from genuine gluten enteropathy occurring in tropical zones [202,203]. Though the untreated condition is serious in itself, there are few important complications. We know of no reports of intestinal ulceration, associated skin conditions or increased risk of carcinoma or of lymphomas; this is probably because immunological disturbances are not a feature of tropical sprue.

Malabsorption related to drugs and chemicals

Antibiotics

Steatorrhoea has been reported following the administration of a number of broad-spectrum antibiotics [204], but there are few reliable reports on mucosal morphology. More important is the steatorrhoea, often accompanied by impaired absorption of xylose, sucrose and iron, which can follow the ingestion of neomycin and resembles that seen in idiopathic steatorrhoea [205]. There is clubbing of jejunal villi due to oedema, with round cell infiltration and vascular dilatation in the lamina propria [206] and the presence within it of macrophages containing intracytoplasmic particles thought to be of bacterial or lysosomal origin [205].

Other drugs

Steatorrhoea with mucosal lesions has been described in patients taking folic acid antagonists, probably due to inhibition of replication of crypt epithelium.

Alcohol

Many chronic alcohol abusers suffer from anorexia, abdominal discomfort, vomiting and diarrhoea, which may be related to gastritis or hepatic involvement. There are few reliable studies on human small bowel morphology, but alcohol dehydrogenase is demonstrable immunocytochemically in luminal enterocytes though not to any significant extent in crypt or goblet cells [207]. Concentrations are highest in the jejunum and decrease aborally. There is also evidence that alcohol disturbs the normal small bowel ecology, with significant increases in numbers of aerobic and anaerobic bacteria which may induce secondary functional and morphological changes [208] (see below). A study of enterocyte membranes has shown that alcohol acts as an acute dose-related toxin, causing increased static and dynamic membrane fluidity and decreased microvillous membrane cholesterol, leading to impaired absorption [209]. There is no adaptive mechanism to compensate for this effect and chronic alcoholics are just as susceptible as others.

Malabsorption related to disturbances in normal small bowel ecology

Normal small bowel ecology is discussed on p. 247. Although some of the normal indigenous organisms are capable of taking up and metabolizing vitamin B_{12} they are not present in sufficient numbers to give rise to vitamin deficiency or to steatorrhoea. When normal ecology is disturbed, non-indigenous organisms, mainly coliforms, colonize spaces normally occupied by indigenous anaerobes (see p. 279). They may then deconjugate sufficient bile acids to produce steatorrhoea and use up enough of the available oxygen to allow overgrowth of more strictly anaerobic *Bacteroides* species that readily bind B_{12} complex [210–213]. This accords with the clinical observation that antibiotics that are active against aerobes are not necessarily effective in improving vitamin B_{12} absorption.

Any mechanical condition that predisposes to overgrowth of coliforms is therefore likely to produce this type of malabsorption. Important examples include enterocolic fistula either due to organic disease such as Crohn's disease or to trauma, iatrogenic fistulas following surgery, as well as stagnant loops of bowel and short circuits. Bacterial overgrowth also occurs following stagnation of bowel contents, whether due to disturbances in intestinal motility, diverticula, strictures or areas of diseased mucosa due to organic diseases. Another cause is reduction in gastric acidity with consequent decreased power to destroy non-indigenous coliforms.

Histologically the mucosa may appear normal or can show a degree of flattening and inflammatory changes; these may simply be secondary to infection and resemble those seen in other infective disorders, but some may be primary [214] and there may be brush border damage with impaired sugar and amino acid uptake [215]. The steatorrhoea is likely to disappear temporarily on the exhibition of suitable antibiotics that inhibit intestinal bacterial growth.

Organic bowel disease

Secondary malabsorption syndromes can follow a number of organic diseases including Crohn's disease, tuberculosis, Whipple's disease, amyloid infiltration, progressive systemic sclerosis and primary or secondary lymphoid neoplasms. The malabsorption and steatorrhoea result from direct damage to the mucosal surface or from the complications described above; mucosa at a distance from the disease process is usually normal.

Miscellaneous causes of malnutrition

Diabetes mellitus

Occasionally patients with diabetes mellitus have steatorrhoea in the presence of normal pancreatic enzyme secretion. Few biopsy studies are available. In the majority the diabetes is poorly controlled and there is diarrhoea associated with diabetic neuropathy. Histologically dendritic swelling with the presence of giant sympathetic neurones is present in prevertebral and paravertebral sympathetic ganglia, but there is no specific lesion in the ganglion cells in submucosal and myenteric plexuses or in the mucosa [216]. Very rarely, patients have had a flat mucosa indistinguishable from gluten-induced enteropathy and have responded to a gluten-free diet [217–219]. These findings suggest that there may be two groups of patients with diabetes and steatorrhoea [216,220], one with loss of integration of postganglionic sympathetic function, the other with a coexistence of diabetes and gluten enteropathy. A greatly increased prevalence of gluten-induced enteropathy is reported among insulin-dependent diabetes [221], 2% compared with 0.05–0.5% in the European population at large [222,223], presumably due to genetic linkage, both diseases being linked with the major histocompatibility phenotype of HLA-DR3, B8 [224].

Other disorders associated with malabsorption

Abnormalities in absorption have also been described in haemochromatosis [225], α_1-antitrypsin deficiency [226] (which may be linked with IgA deficiency and respond to a gluten-free diet [227,228]) and chronic active hepatitis [229,230].

Villous abnormality without clinical malabsorption

Small intestinal mucosal abnormalities that include partial mucosal flattening have been described in postperinatal deaths, particularly in bottle-fed males [231], and have been attributed to overheating [232]. They are not obviously related to malabsorption.

Protein-losing enteropathies

The normal absorption of products of protein digestion is briefly discussed on p. 238. The total daily loss of protein from the small bowel in humans is about 84 g of which some comes

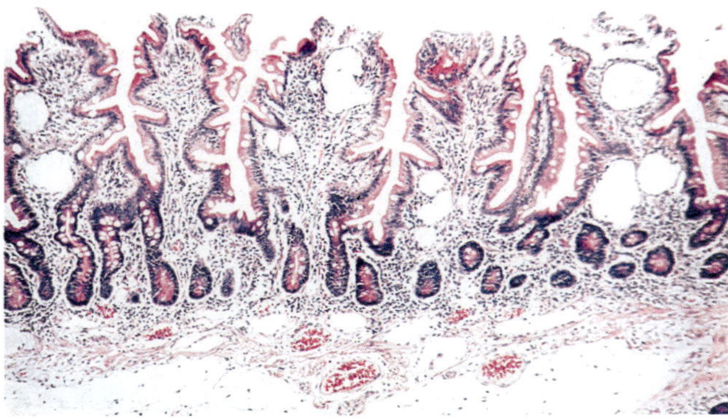

Fig. 22.14 Intestinal lymphangiectasia. Section of an ileal biopsy, showing numerous dilated lymphatic capillaries in the villi, which are abnormally broad as a consequence.

from exfoliated cells and the rest from extracellular sources [233]. The small bowel resorbs most of this. In a number of conditions there is excessive loss of protein from the gastrointestinal tract unmatched by an increase in protein synthesis, which leads to hypoproteinaemia in which various proteins are differently affected. One condition which causes this is intestinal lymphangiectasia. This may be the result of localized intra-abdominal lymphatic obstruction, for example by lymphatic permeation by carcinoma cells. Occasionally it develops as a congenital abnormality of intestinal lymphatics and presents in children and young adults as protein-losing enteropathy, although deficiencies of nutrients other than proteins are usual, particularly the lipid-soluble vitamins. Diagnosis is by small intestinal biopsy which, when informative, shows expansion of villi by multiple dilated lymphatic capillaries (Fig. 22.14). The ectatic lymphatics can be patchy and may be missed if only a single mucosal biopsy is taken. It is lymphorrhage from the distended lymphatics which leads to the protein loss. 'Protein-losing enteropathy', in fact, is not a single entity confined to the small intestine but a manifestation of many disorders, some of which (giant rugal hypertrophy of stomach, gastric carcinoma, ulcerative colitis, for example) are not primary in the small bowel; the term is now best reserved for a clinical syndrome which includes all those cases where no organic cause can be found for a protein loss.

The 'brown bowel' syndrome

Malabsorption from almost any cause is occasionally accompanied by a curious distinctive brown coloration of the small intestine and sometimes the stomach, clearly visible on the external surface at operation or autopsy [234,235]. The colour results from the deposition of small golden-yellow granules of pigment within the cytoplasm of muscle cells of muscularis propria and muscularis mucosae, and sometimes also in macrophages and in the smooth muscle of arterial walls. These granules are round or ovoid and 1–2 μm in diameter (Fig. 20.2); histochemically they fail to stain with techniques for melanin, iron or hydrophobic lipids but stain positively with PAS after diastase, and with Sudan black B in paraffin-embedded sections; they are autofluorescent [236,237]. These characteristics suggest a mixture of lipofuscins. There is no surrounding inflammation or necrosis and the bizarre appearance of the muscle fibres is solely due to the presence of pigment in the cytoplasm. The condition appears to be a mitochondrial myopathy related to vitamin E deficiency due to defective fat absorption, since the vitamin is known to be essential for stabilizing mitochondrial membranes [235].

Primary bile salt malabsorption [229]

Chronic diarrhoea may be due to excess bile acid loss, and with the advent of colonoscopy and ileoscopy it is possible to examine its effect on the terminal ileum. In such cases there is hyperplastic villous atrophy, colonization of the mucosa and increased numbers of plasma cells and lymphocytes in the lamina propria. The diagnosis should be suggested when there is a flat ileal biopsy in the presence of chronic unexplained diarrhoea. Cholestyramine may then produce a dramatic recovery.

References

1 Ghosh AK, Littlewood JM, Goddard D, Steel WF. Stool microscopy in screening for steatorrhoea. *J Clin Pathol*, 1977; 30: 749.

2 Russell RI. Small intestinal investigative tests and techniques. *Curr Opin Gastroenterol*, 1985; 1: 266.

3 Perrera D, Weinstein WM, Rubin CF. Small intestinal biopsy. *Hum Pathol*, 1975; 6: 157.

4 Scott BB, Losowsky MS. Peroral small intestinal biopsy: experience with the hydraulic multiple biopsy instrument in routine clinical practice. *Gut*, 1976; 17: 740.

5 Scott BB, Losowsky MS. Patchiness and duodenal jejunal variation of the mucosal abnormality in coeliac disease and dermatitis herpetiformis. *Gut*, 1977; 17: 984.

6 Manuel PD, Walker-Smith JA, France NE. Patchy enteropathy in childhood. *Gut*, 1979; 20: 211.

7 Hasan M, Ferguson A. Measurements of intestinal villi in non-specific and ulcer-associated duodenitis—correlation between area of microdissected villus and villous epithelial cell count. *J Clin Pathol*, 1981; 34: 1181.

8 Hasan M, Sircus W, Ferguson A. Duodenal mucosal architecture in non-specific and ulcer-associated duodenitis. *Gut*, 1981; 22: 637.

9 Moss SF, Attia L, Scholes JV, Walters JR, Holt PR. Increased small intestinal apoptosis in coeliac disease. *Gut*, 1996; 39: 811.

10 Doe WF, Hapel AJ. Intestinal immunity and malabsorption. *Clin Gastroenterol*, 1983; 12 (41): 5.

11 Guix M, Skinner JM, Whitehead R. Measuring intraepithelial lymphocytes, surface area and volume of lamina propria in the jejunal mucosa of coeliac patients. *Gut*, 1979; 20: 275.

12 Wright NA, Appleton DR, Marks J, Watson AJ. Cytokinetic studies of crypts in convoluted human small intestinal mucosa. *J Clin Pathol*, 1979; 32: 462.

13 Katz AJ, Grand RJ. All that flattens is not 'sprue'. *Gastroenterology*, 1979; 76: 375.

14 Rodrigues MAM, De Camargo JLV, Coelho KIR *et al*. Morphometric study of the small intestinal mucosa in young adult and old rats submitted to protein deficiency and rehabilitation. *Gut*, 1985; 26: 816.

15 Banwell JG, Hutt MS, Tunnicliffe R. Observations on jejunal biopsy in Ugandan Africans. *E Afr Med J*, 1964; 41: 46.

16 Barbezat GO, Bowie MD, Kaschula ROC. Studies on the small intestinal mucosa of children with protein calorie malnutrition. *S Afr Med J*, 1967; 41: 1031.

17 Stanfield JP, Hutt MSR, Tunnicliffe R. Intestinal biopsy in kwashiorkor. *Lancet*, 1965; ii: 519.

18 Burman D. The jejunal mucosa in Kwashiorkor. *Arch Dis Child*, 1965; 40: 526.

19 Brunser O, Reid A, Monckeberg F, Maccioni A, Contreras I. Jejunal mucosa in infant malnutrition. *Am J Clin Nutr*, 1968; 21: 976.

20 Kaschula ROC, Gajjar PD, Mann M *et al*. Infantile jejunal mucosa in infection and malnutrition. *Isr J Med Sci*, 1979; 15: 356.

21 Nassar AM, el Tantawy SA, Khalifa S, Abdel Fattab S, Abdel Hamid J. Ultrastructural changes in the mucosa of the small intestine due to protein calorie malnutrition. *J Trop Pediatr*, 1980; 26: 62.

22 Cook GC, Lee FD. The jejunum after kwashiorkor. *Lancet*, 1966; ii: 1263.

23 Dawson DW. Partial villous atrophy in nutritional megaloblastic anaemia corrected by folic acid therapy. *J Clin Pathol*, 1971; 24: 131.

24 Joske RA, Blackwell JB. Alimentary histology in the malabsorption syndrome following partial gastrectomy. *Lancet*, 1959; ii: 379.

25 Goldman H, Antonioli DA. Mucosal biopsy of the esophagus, stomach and duodenum. *Hum Pathol*, 1982; 13: 423.

26 Burhol PG, Myren J. Jejunal biopsy findings, mucosal dehydrogenase activity and intestinal absorption in patients with complications after partial gastrectomies. *Scand J Gastroenterol*, 1966; 1: 314.

27 Foroozan P, Trier JS. Mucosa of the small intestine in pernicious anaemia. *N Engl J Med*, 1967; 277: 553.

28 Mansbach CM II, Wilkins RM, Dobbins WO, Tyor MP. Intestinal mucosal function and structure in the steatorrhoea of Zollinger–Ellison syndrome. *Arch Intern Med*, 1968; 121: 487.

29 McClean P, Dodge JA, Nunn S, Carr KE, Sloane JM. Surface features of small-intestinal mucosa in childhood diarrheal disorders. *J Pediatr Gastroenterol Nutr*, 1996; 23: 538.

30 Haymond HE. Massive resections of the small intestine: an analysis of 257 collected cases. *Surg Gynecol Obstet*, 1935; 61: 693.

31 Pullan JM. Massive intestinal resection. *Proc R Soc Med*, 1959; 52: 31.

32 Rickham PP. Massive small intestinal resection in newborn infants. *Ann R Coll Surg*, 1967; 41: 480.

33 Porus RL. Epithelial hyperplasia following massive small bowel resection in man. *Gastroenterology*, 1965; 48: 753.

34 Curtis KJ, Sleisenger MH, Kim YS. Protein digestion and ab-

sorption after massive small bowel resection. *Dig Dis Sci*, 1984; 29: 834.

35 Gornacz GE, Al-Mukhtar MYT, Ghatai MA *et al*. Pattern of cell proliferation and enteroglucagon response following small bowel resection in the rat. *Digestion*, 1984; 29: 65.

36 Triadou N, Bataille J, Schmitz J. Longitudinal study of the human intestinal brush border membrane proteins: distribution of the main disaccharidases and peptidases. *Gastroenterology*, 1983; 85: 1326.

37 Sahi T. Progress report: dietary lactose and the aetiology of human small intestinal hypolactasia. *Gut*, 1978; 19: 1074.

38 Hyams JS, Batrus CL, Grand RJ, Sallan SE. Cancer chemotherapy-induced lactose malabsorption in children. *Cancer*, 1982; 49: 646.

39 Simoons FJ. The geographic hypothesis and lactose malabsorption. A weighing of the evidence. *Am J Dig Dis*, 1978; 23: 963.

40 Lojda Z. Suitability of the azocoupling reaction with 1-naphthyl-B-D-glucoside for the histochemical demonstration of lactase (lactase-β-glucosidase complex) in human enterobiopsies. *Histochemistry*, 1975; 43: 349.

41 Lojda Z. The application of enzyme histochemistry in diagnostic pathology. In: Stoward PJ, Polak JM, eds. *Histochemistry—the Widening Horizons*. Chichester: John Wiley, 1981: 205.

42 Lembcke B, Schneider H, Lankisch PG. Is the assay of disaccharidase activity in small bowel mucosal biopsy relevant for clinical gastroenterologists? *Klin Wochenschr*, 1989; 67: 568.

43 Ferguson A, MacDonald DM, Brydon WG. Prevalence of lactase deficiency in British adults. *Gut*, 1984; 25: 163.

44 Gotto A, Levy R, John K, Fredrickson L. On the protein defect in a-beta lipoproteinaemia. *N Engl J Med*, 1971; 284: 813.

45 Anonymous. Case records of the Massachusetts General Hospital. Weekly clinicopathological exercises. Case 35-1992. An eight-month-old boy with diarrhea and failure to thrive. *N Engl J Med*, 1992; 327: 628.

46 Greenwood N. The jejunal mucosa in two cases of a-beta-lipoproteinemia. *Am J Gastroenterol*, 1976; 65: 160.

47 Variend S, Placzec M, Raafat F, Walker-Smith JA. Small intestinal mucosal fat in childhood enteropathies. *J Clin Pathol*, 1984; 37: 373.

48 Scott BB, Miller JP, Losowsky MS. Hypo-β-lipoproteinaemia—a variant of the Bassen–Kornzweig syndrome. *Gut*, 1979; 20: 163.

49 Joshi M, Hyams J, Treem W, Ricci A Jr. Cytoplasmic vacuolization of enterocytes: an unusual histopathologic finding in juvenile nutritional megaloblastic anemia. *Mod Pathol*, 1991; 4: 62.

50 Scott BB, Miller JP, Losowsky MS. Hypobetalipoproteinaemia—a variant of the Bassen–Kornzweig syndrome. *Gut*, 1979; 20: 163.

51 Bouma ME, Beucler I, Aggerbeck LP, Infante R, Schmitz J. Hypobetalipoproteinemia with accumulation of an apoprotein B-like protein in intestinal cells. Immunoenzymatic and biochemical characterization of seven cases of Anderson's disease. *J Clin Invest*, 1986; 78: 398.

52 Kuitunen P, Visakorpi JK, Savilahti E, Pelkenen P. Malabsorption syndrome with cow's milk intolerance. *Arch Dis Child*, 1975; 50: 351.

53 Ament ME, Rubin CE. Soy protein—another cause of the flat intestinal lesion. *Gastroenterology*, 1972; 62: 227.

54 Walker-Smith JA. Gastrointestinal food allergy in childhood. *Ann Allergy*, 1987; 59: 166.

55 Maluenda C, Phillips AD, Briddon A, Walker-Smith JA. Quantitative analysis of small intestinal mucosa in cows' milk sensitive enteropathy. *J Pediatr Gastroenterol Nutr*, 1984; 3: 349.

56 Kosnai I, Kuitunen P, Savilahti E, Rapola J, Koheygi J. Cell kinetics in the jejunal crypt epithelium in malabsorption syndrome with cow's milk protein intolerance and in coeliac disease in childhood. *Gut*, 1980; 21: 1041.

57 Phillips AD, Rice SJ, France NE, Walker-Smith JA. Small intestinal intraepithelial lymphocyte levels in cows' milk protein intolerance. *Gut*, 1979; 20: 509.

58 Rosencranz PCM, Meijer CJLM, Connelisse CJ, van de Wal AM. Use of morphometry and immunohistochemistry of small intestinal biopsy specimens in the diagnosis of food allergy. *J Clin Pathol*, 1980; 33: 125.

59 Kesuaai I, Kuitonen P, Savilahti E, Sippenen P. Mast cells and eosinophils in the jejunal mucosa of patients with intestinal cows' milk allergy and coeliac disease of childhood. *J Pediatr Gastroenterol Nutr*, 1984; 3: 368.

60 Jyngkaran N, Yadav M, Balabaskaran S, Sumithran F. In vitro diagnosis of cow's milk protein sensitive enteropathy by organ culture method. *Gut*, 1980; 22: 199.

61 Jyngkaran N, Robinson MJ, Prathap K, Sumithran E, Yadav M. Cow's milk protein sensitive enteropathy; combined clinical and histological criteria for diagnosis. *Arch Dis Child*, 1978; 53: 20.

62 Barratt MEJ, Porter P. Immunoglobulin classes implicated in intestinal disturbances of calves associated with soya protein antigens. *J Immunol*, 1979; 123: 676.

63 Haeney MR, Goodwin BJF, Barratt MEJ, Mike N, Asquith P. Soya protein antibodies in man; their occurrence and possible relevance in coeliac disease. *J Clin Pathol*, 1982; 3: 319.

64 Blackshaw AJ, Levison DA. Eosinophilic infiltrates of the gastrointestinal tract. *J Clin Pathol*, 1986; 39: 1.

65 Rubin CF, Eidelman S, Weinstein WM. Sprue by any other name. *Gastroenterology*, 1970; 58: 409.

66 Rubin CE, Brandborg LL, Phelps PC, Taylor HC Jr. Studies of celiac disease. I. The apparent identical and specific nature of the duodenal and proximal jejunal lesion in celiac disease and idiopathic sprue. *Gastroenterology*, 1968; 54 (4) (Suppl): 800.

67 Stewart JS, Pollock DJ, Hoffbrand AV, Mollin DL, Booth CC. A study of proximal and distal intestinal structure and absorptive function in idiopathic steatorrhoea. *Q J Med*, 1967; 36: 425.

68 Rubin CE, Dobbins WO III. Peroral biopsy of the small intestine. A review of its diagnostic usefulness. *Gastroenterology*, 1965; 49: 676.

69 Marsh MN. Gluten, major histocompatibility complex, and the small intestine. A molecular and immunobiologic approach to the spectrum of gluten sensitivity ('celiac sprue'). *Gastroenterology*, 1992; 102: 330.

70 Oberhuber G, Bodingbauer M, Mosberger I, Stolte M, Vogelsang H. High proportion of granzyme B-positive (activated) intraepithelial and lamina propria lymphocytes in lymphocytic gastritis. *Am J Surg Pathol*, 1998; 22: 450.

71 Cellier C, Patey N, Mauvieux L *et al*. Abnormal intestinal intraepithelial lymphocytes in refractory sprue. *Gastroenterology*, 1998; 114: 471.

72 Vogelsang H, Oberhuber G, Wyatt J. Lymphocytic gastritis and gastric permeability in patients with celiac disease. *Gastroenterology*, 1996; 111: 73.

73 Ferguson A, Murray D. Quantitation of intraepithelial lymphocytes in human jejunum. *Gut*, 1971; 12: 988.

73a Kohme G, Schneider T, Zeitz M. Special features of the intestinal lymphocytic system. *Ballieres Clinical Gastroenterology* 1996; 10: 427.

74 Wright N, Watson A, Morley A, Appleton D, Marks J, Douglas A. The cell cycle time in the flat (avillous) mucosa of the human small intestine. *Gut*, 1973; 14: 603.

75 Wright N, Watson A, Morley A, Appleton D, Marks J. Cell kinetics in flat (avillous) mucosa of the human small intestine. *Gut*, 1973; 14: 701.

76 Chedid M, Rubin JS, Csaky KG, Aaronson SA. Regulation of keratinocyte growth factor gene expression by interleukin 1. *J Biol Chem*, 1994; 269: 10753.

77 MacDonald TT. Oxpentifylline, tumour necrosis factor-alpha and Crohn's disease. *Gut*, 1997; 40: 559.

78 Watson AJ, Wright NA. Morphology and cell kinetics of the jejunal mucosa in untreated patients. *Clin Gastroenterol*, 1974; 3: 11.

79 Picarelli A, Maiuri L, Frate A, Greco M, Auricchio S, Londei M. Production of antiendomysial antibodies after in-vitro gliadin challenge of small intestine biopsy samples from patients with coeliac disease. *Lancet*, 1996; 348: 1065.

80 Dieterich W, Ehnis T, Bauer M *et al.* Identification of tissue transglutaminase as the autoantigen of celiac disease. *Nat Med*, 1997; 3: 797.

81 Falchuk ZM, Strober W. Gluten-sensitive enteropathy: synthesis of antigliadin antibody in vitro. *Gut*, 1974; 15: 947.

82 Holmes GKT, Asquith P, Stokes PL, Cooke WT. Cellular infiltrate of jejunal biopsies in adult coeliac disease in relation to gluten withdrawal. *Gut*, 1974; 15: 278.

83 Lancaster-Smith M, Kumar P, Marks R, Clark ML, Dawson AM. Jejunal mucosal immunoglobulin-containing cell, and jejunal fluid immunoglobulins in adult coeliac disease and dermatitis herpetiformis. *Gut*, 1974; 15: 371.

84 Scott BB, Goodall A, Stephenson P, Jenkins D. Small intestinal plasma cells in coeliac disease. *Gut*, 1984; 25: 41.

85 Strobel S, Busuttil A, Ferguson A. Human intestinal mucosal mast cells: expanded population in untreated coeliac disease. *Gut*, 1983; 24: 222.

86 Marsh MN, Hinde J. Inflammatory component of celiac sprue mucosa. I. Mast cells, basophils and eosinophils. *Gastroenterology*, 1985; 89: 92.

87 Scott H, Brandtzaeg P. Enumeration of Paneth cells in coeliac disease: comparison of conventional light microscopy and immunofluorescence staining for lysozyme. *Gut*, 1981; 22: 812.

88 Challacombe DN, Robertson K. Enterochromaffin cells in the duodenal mucosa of children with coeliac disease. *Gut*, 1977; 18: 373.

89 Sjolund K, Alumets J, Berg N-O, Hakanson R, Sundler F. Enteropathy of coeliac disease in adults; increased number of enterochromaffin cells in the duodenal mucosa. 1982; 23: 42.

90 Enerback LP, Hallert C, Norrby K. Raised 5-hydroxytryptamine concentrations in enterochromaffin cells in adult coeliac disease. *J Clin Pathol*, 1983; 36: 499.

91 Sjolund K, Hakanson R, Lundqvist G, Sundlar F. Duodenal somatostatin in coeliac disease. *Scand J Gastroenterol*, 1982; 17: 969.

92 Polak JM, Pearce AGE, Van Noorden S, Bloom SR, Rossiter MA. Secretin cells in coeliac disease. *Gut*, 1973; 14: 870.

93 Weinstein WM, Saunders DR, Tytgat GN, Rubin CE. Collagenous sprue—an unrecognised type of malabsorption. *N Engl J Med*, 1970; 283: 1297.

94 Bossart R, Henry K, Booth CC, Doe WF. Subepithelial collagen in intestinal malabsorption. *Gut*, 1975; 16: 18.

95 Robert ME, Ament ME, Weinstein WM. The histologic spectrum and clinical outcome of refractory and unclassified sprue. *Am J Surg Pathol*, 2000; 24: 676.

96 Shaoul R, Marcon MA, Okada Y, Cutz E, Forstner G. Gastric metaplasia: a frequently overlooked feature of duodenal biopsy specimens in untreated celiac disease. *J Pediatr Gastroenterol Nutr*, 2000; 30: 397.

97 Thompson H. Necropsy studies on adult coeliac disease. *J Clin Pathol*, 1974; 27: 710.

98 Himes HW, Adlersberg D. Pathologic changes in the small bowel in idiopathic sprue; biopsy and autopsy findings. *Gastroenterology*, 1958; 35: 142.

99 Cooper BT, Holmes GKT, Ferguson R *et al.* Gluten-sensitive diarrhoea without evidence of coeliac disease. *Gastroenterology*, 1980; 79: 801.

100 Ferguson A. Coeliac disease research and clinical practice: maintaining momentum into the twenty-first century. *Baillieres Clin Gastroenterol*, 1995; 9: 395.

101 Oberhuber G, Granditsch G, Vogelsang H. The histopathology of coeliac disease: time for a standardized report scheme for pathologists. *Eur J Gastroenterol Hepatol*, 1999; 11: 1185.

102 Asquith P, Johnson AG, Cooke WT. Scanning electron microscopy of normal and coeliac jejunal mucosa. *Am J Dig Dis*, 1970; 15: 511.

103 Shiner M. Electron microscopy of jejunal mucosa in coeliac disease. *Clin Gastroenterol*, 1974; 3: 33.

104 Shiner M. Ultrastructural changes suggestive of immune reactions in the jejunal mucosa of coeliac children following gluten challenge. *Gut*, 1973; 14: 1.

105 Mantzaris G, Jewell DP. In vivo toxicity of a synthetic dodecapeptide from A gliadin in patients with coeliac disease. *Scand J Gastroenterol*, 1991; 26: 392.

106 O'Grady JG, Stevens EM, Keane R *et al.* Intestinal lactase, sucrase, and alkaline phosphatase in 373 patients with coeliac disease. *J Clin Pathol*, 1984; 37: 298.

107 Berg NO, Dahlqvist A, Lindberg T, Norden A. Intestinal dipeptidases and disaccharidases in coeliac disease in adults. *Gastroenterology*, 1970; 59: 575.

108 Woodley JG, Keane F. Enterokinase on normal intestinal biopsies and those from patients with untreated coeliac disease. *Gut*, 1972; 13: 900.

109 Riecken EO, Stewart JS, Booth CC, Pearse AGE. A histochemical study on the role of lysosomal enzymes in idiopathic steatorrhoea before and during a gluten-free diet. *Gut*, 1966; 7: 317.

110 Dissanyake AS, Truelove SC, Whitehead F. Jejunal mucosal recovery in coeliac edisease in relation to the degree of adherence to a gluten free diet. *Q J Med N S*, 1974; 161: 185.

111 Halter SA, Greene IHLI, Helinek G. Gluten-sensitive enteropathy; sequence of villous regrowth as viewed by scanning electron microscopy. *Hum Pathol*, 1982; 13: 811.

112 Chapman BLH, Henry K, Paice F, Coghill NF, Stewart JS.

Measuring the response of the jejunal mucosa in adult coeliac disease to treatment with a gluten free diet. *Gut*, 1974; 15: 870.
113 Lancaster-Smith M, Kumar PJ, Dawson AM. The cellular infiltrate of the jejunum in adult coeliac disease and dermatitis herpetiformis following the re-introduction of dietary gluten. *Gut*, 1975; 16: 683.
114 Lancaster-Smith M, Packer S, Kumar PJ, Harries JT. Cellular infiltrate of the jejunum after reintroduction of dietary gluten in children with treated coeliac disease. *J Clin Pathol*, 1976; 29: 587.
115 Holmes GKT, Asquith P, Stokes PL, Cooke WT. Cellular infiltrate of jejunal biopsies in adult coeliac disease in relation to gluten withdrawal. *Gut*, 1974; 15: 278.
116 Scott H, Ek J, Baklein K, Brandtzaeg P. Immunoglobulin-producing cells in jejunal mucosa of children with coeliac disease on a gluten-free diet and after gluten challenge. *Scand J Gastroenterol*, 1980; 15: 81.
116a Caspary WF, Stein J. Diseases of the small intestine. *Eur J Gastroenterol Hepatol*, 1999; 11: 21.
117 Pollock DJ, Nagle RE, Jeejeebhoy KN, Coghill NE. The effect on jejunal mucosa of withdrawing and adding dietary gluten in cases of idiopathic steatorrhoea. *Gut*, 1971; 11: 567.
118 Lancaster-Smith M, Packer S, Kumar P, Harries JT. Immunological phenomena in the jejunum and serum after reintroduction of dietary gluten in children with treated coeliac disease. *J Clin Pathol*, 1976; 29: 592.
119 McNicholl B, Egan-Mitchell B, Fottrell PF. Variability of gluten intolerance in treated childhood coeliac disease. *Gut*, 1979; 20: 126.
120 Kumar PJ, O'Donoghue DP, Stenson K, Dawson AM. Reintroduction of gluten in adults and children with treated coeliac disease. *Gut*, 1979; 20: 743.
121 Bramble MG, Zucoloto S, Wright NA, Record CO. Acute gluten challenge in treated adult coeliac disease; a morphometric and enzymatic study. *Gut*, 1985; 26: 169.
122 Shuster S, Watson A, Marks J. Coeliac syndrome in dermatitis herpetiformis. *Lancet*, 1968; i: 1101.
123 Meyerson LB, Stagnone JJ. Small bowel changes in dermatitis herpetiformis. *South Med J*, 1969; 62: 971.
124 Fry L, Keir P, McMinn RMH, Cowan J, Hoffbrand AV. Small intestinal structure and function and haematological changes in dermatitis herpetiformis. *Lancet*, 1967; ii: 729.
125 Weinstein WM, Brow JR, Parker F, Rubin CF. The small intestinal mucosa in dermatitis herpetiformis. II. Relationship of the small intestinal lesion to gluten. *Gastroenterology*, 1971; 60: 362.
126 Brow JR, Parker F, Weinstein WM, Rubin CE. The small intestinal mucosa in dermatitis herpetiformis. I. Severity and distribution of the small intestinal lesion and associated malabsorption. *Gastroenterology*, 1971; 60: 335.
127 Fry L, Seals PP, Harper PG, Hoffbrand AV, McMinn RMH. The small intestine in dermatitis herpetiformis. *J Clin Pathol*, 1974; 27: 817.
128 Marks J, Birkell D, Shuster S, Roberts DF. Small intestinal mucosal abnormalities in relatives of patients with dermatitis herpetiformis. *Gut*, 1970; 11: 493.
129 Scott BB, Young S, Rajals SM, Marks J, Losowsky MS. Coeliac disease and dermatitis herpetiformis; further studies on their relationship. *Gut*, 1976; 17: 759.
130 Chorzelski TP, Sulej J, Tchorzewska H, Jablonska S, Beutner EH, Kumar V. IgA class endomysium antibodies in dermatitis herpetiformis and coeliac disease. *Ann N Y Acad Sci*, 1983; 420: 325.
131 Vecchi M, Crosti L, Berti E, Agape D, Cerri A, De Franchis R. Increased jejunal intraepithelial lymphocytes bearing gamma / delta T-cell receptor in dermatitis herpetiformis. *Gastroenterology*, 1992; 102: 1499.
132 David TJ, Ajdukiewicz AB, Read AE. Dermal and epidermal ridge atrophy in celiac sprue. *Gastroenterology*, 1973; 64: 539.
133 Silk DBA, Kumar PJ, Perrett D, Clark ML, Dawson AM. Amino acid and peptide absorption in patients with coeliac disease and dermatitis herpetiformis. *Gut*, 1974; 15: 1.
134 Ferguson A. Coeliac disease research and clinical practice: maintaining momentum into the twenty-first century. *Baillieres Clin Gastroenterol*, 1995; 9: 395.
135 Weinstein WM. Latent coeliac sprue. *Gastroenterology*, 1974; 66: 489.
136 Loft DE, Nwokolo CU, Ciclitira PJ. The diagnosis of gluten sensitivity and coeliac disease—the two are not mutually inclusive. *Eur J Gastroenterol Hepatol*, 1998; 10: 911.
137 Fry L. Dermatitis herpetiformis. *Baillieres Clin Gastroenterol*, 1995; 9: 371.
138 Gawkrodger DJ, Blackwell JN, Gilmour HM *et al*. Dermatitis herpetiformis; diagnosis, diet and demography. *Gut*, 1984; 25: 151.
139 Gillberg R, Kastnup W, Mobacken H, Stockbrugger R, Ahren C. Gastric morphology and function in dermatitis herpetiformis and in coeliac disease. *Scand J Gastroenterol*, 1985; 20: 133.
140 Gillberg R, Kastnup W, Mobacken H, Stockbrugger R, Ahren C. Endoscopic duodenal biopsy compared with biopsy with the Watson capsule from the upper jejunum in patients with dermatitis herpetiformis. *Scand J Gastroenterol*, 1982; 17: 305.
141 Cooney T, Doyle CT, Buckley D, Whelton MJ. Dermatitis herpetiformis; a comparative assessment of skin and bowel abnormality. *J Clin Pathol*, 1977; 30: 749.
142 Parnell ND, Ciclitira PJ. Review article: coeliac disease and its management. *Aliment Pharmacol Ther*, 1999; 13: 1.
143 Kumar PJ. The enigma of coeliac disease. *Gastroenterology*, 1985; 89 (214): 136.
144 Cole SG, Kagnoff ME. Celiac disease. *Ann Rev Nutr*, 1985; 5: 241.
145 Davidson AGF, Bridges MA. Coeliac disease: a critical review of aetiology and pathogenesis. *Clin Chim Acta*, 1987; 163: 1.
146 Robinson DC, Watson AJ, Wyatt FH, Marks JM, Roberts DF. Incidence of small intestinal mucosal abnormalities and of clinical coeliac disease in the relatives of children with coeliac disease. *Gut*, 1971; 12: 789.
147 Ferreira M, Davies SL, Butler M, Scott D, Clark M, Kumar P. Endomysial antibody: is it the best screening test for coeliac disease? *Gut*, 1992; 33: 1633.
148 Sollid LM, Thorsby E. HLA susceptibility genes in celiac disease: genetic mapping and role in pathogenesis. *Gastroenterology*, 1996; 105: 910.
149 Houlston RS, Ford D. Genetics of coeliac disease. *Q J Med*, 1996; 89: 737.
150 Godkin A, Jewell D. The pathogenesis of celiac disease. *Gastroenterology*, 1998; 115: 206.
151 Maiuri L, Picarelli A, Boirivant M *et al*. Definition of the initial immunologic modifications upon in vitro gliadin challenge in

the small intestine of celiac patients. *Gastroenterology*, 1996; 110: 1368.

152 Picarelli A, Maiuri L, Frate A, Greco M, Auricchio S, Londei M. Production of antiendomysial antibodies after in-vitro gliadin challenge of small intestine biopsy samples from patients with coeliac disease. *Lancet*, 1996; 348: 1065.

153 Selby WS, Janossy G, Goldstein G, Jewell DP. T lymphocyte subsets in human intestinal mucosa: the distribution and relationship to MHC-derived antigens. *Clin Exp Immunol*, 1981; 44: 453.

154 Oberhuber G, Vogelsang H, Stolte M, Muthenthaler S, Kummer AJ, Radaszkiewicz T. Evidence that intestinal intraepithelial lymphocytes are activated cytotoxic T cells in celiac disease but not in giardiasis. *Am J Pathol*, 1996; 148: 1351.

155 Halstensen TS, Scott H, Brandtzaeg P. Intraepithelial T cells of the TcR gamma/delta+ CD8– and V delta 1/J delta 1+ phenotypes are increased in coeliac disease. *Scand J Immunol*, 1989; 30: 665.

156 Anderson RP, Degano P, Godkin AJ, Jewell DP, Hill AV. In vivo antigen challenge in celiac disease identifies a single transglutaminase-modified peptide as the dominant A-gliadin T-cell epitope. *Nat Med*, 2000; 6: 337.

157 Arentz-Hansen H, Korner R, Molberg O *et al*. The intestinal T-cell response to alpha-gliadin in adult celiac disease is focused on a single deamidated glutamine targeted by tissue transglutaminase. *J Exp Med*, 2000; 191: 603.

158 Trier JS, Falchuk ZM, Carey MC, Schreiber DS. Coeliac sprue and refractory sprue. *Gastroenterology*, 1978; 75: 307.

159 Cellier C, Patey N, Mauvieux L *et al*. Abnormal intestinal intraepithelial lymphocytes in refractory sprue. *Gastroenterology*, 1998; 114: 471.

160 Robert ME, Ament ME, Weinstein WM. The histologic spectrum and clinical outcome of refractory and unclassified sprue. *Am J Surg Pathol*, 2000; 24: 676.

161 Bagdi E, Diss TC, Munson P, Isaacson PG. Mucosal intra-epithelial lymphocytes in enteropathy-associated T-cell lymphoma, ulcerative jejunitis, and refractory celiac disease constitute a neoplastic population. *Blood*, 1999; 94: 260.

162 Modigliani R, Poitras P, Galiama A *et al*. Chronic, non-specific ulcerative duodeno-jejuno-ileitis: report of four cases. *Gut*, 1979; 20: 318.

163 Baer AN, Bayless TM, Yardley JH. Intestinal ulceration and malabsorption syndromes. *Gastroenterology*, 1980; 79: 754.

164 Robertson DAF, Dixon MF, Scott BB, Simpson FG, Losowsky MS. Small intestinal ulceration; diagnostic difficulties in relation to coeliac disease. *Gut*, 1983; 24: 565.

165 Ryan BM, Kelleher D. Refractory celiac disease. [Review] *Gastroenterology*, 2000; 119: 243.

166 Isaacson P, Wright DH. Malignant histiocytosis of the intestine. Its relationship to malabsorption and ulcerative jejunitis. *Hum Pathol*, 1978; 9: 661.

167 Tönder M, Sørlie D, Kearney MS. Adult coeliac disease. A case with ulceration, dermatitis herpetiformis and reticulosarcoma. *Scand J Gastroenterol*, 1976; 2: 107.

168 Brousse N, Verkarre V, Patey-Mariaud de Serre N *et al*. Is complicated celiac disease or refractory sprue an intestinal intraepithelial cryptic T-cell lymphoma? *Blood*, 1999; 93: 3154.

169 Patey-Mariaud de Serre N, Cellier C, Jabri B *et al*. Distinction between coeliac disease and refractory sprue: a simple immunohistochemical method. *Histopathology*, 2000; 37: 70.

170 Wright DH. Enteropathy associated T cell lymphoma. [Review] *Cancer Surv*, 1997; 30: 249.

171 Isaacson PG. Intestinal lymphoma and enteropathy. *J Pathol*, 1995; 177: 111.

172 Robertson DAF, Swinson CM, Hall R, Losowsky MS. Coeliac disease, splenic function and malignancy. *Gut*, 1982; 23: 666.

173 O'Gardy JG, Stevens FM, Harding B *et al*. Hyposplenism and gluten sensitive enteropathy. Natural history, incidence and relationship to diet and small bowel morphology. *Gastroenterology*, 1984; 87: 1326.

174 Holmes GK, Prior P, Lane MR, Pope D, Allan RN. Malignancy in coeliac disease—effect of a gluten free diet. *Gut*, 1989; 30: 333.

175 Ribeiro U Jr, Posner MC, Safatle-Ribeiro AV, Reynolds JC. Risk factors for squamous cell carcinoma of the oesophagus. [Review] *Br J Surg*, 1996; 83: 1174.

176 Kingham JG, Ramanaden D, Dawson A. Metachronous small-bowel adenocarcinoma in coeliac disease: gluten-free diet is not protective. *Scand J Gastroenterol*, 1998; 33: 218.

177 Fry L. The skin and the small intestine. *Curr Opin Gastroenterol*, 1986; 2: 223.

178 Third Leader. Eczema and gastrointestinal malabsorption. *Br Med J*, 1965; i: 941.

179 Fry L, McMinn RMH, Shuster S. The small intestine in skin diseases. *Arch Dermatol*, 1966; 93: 647.

180 Barry RE, Salmon PR, Read AE, Warin RP. Mucosal architecture of the small bowel in cases of psoriasis. *Gut*, 1971; 12: 873.

181 Watson WC, Paton E, Murray D. Small bowel disease in rosacea. *Lancet*, 1965; ii: 47.

182 Bank S, Marks IN. Malabsorption in systemic mast cell disease. *Gastroenterology*, 1963; 45: 535.

183 Marks J, Shuster S. Small intestinal mucosal abnormalities in various skin diseases—fact or fancy? *Gut*, 1970; 11: 281.

184 Bjorneklett A, Facosa O, Refsum EB, Torsvik H, Sigstad H. Jejunal villous atrophy and granulomatous inflammation responding to a gluten-free diet. *Gut*, 1977; 18: 814.

185 Rubin LA, Little LH, Kolin A, Keystone EC. Lymphomatoid granulomatosis involving the gastrointestinal tract. Two case reports and a review of the literature. *Gastroenterology*, 1983; 84: 829.

186 Matuchansky C, Colin R, Hemet J *et al*. Cavitation of mesenteric lymph nodes, splenic atrophy and a flat small intestinal mucosa. Report of six cases. *Gastroenterology*, 1984; 87: 606.

187 Watt J, Pincott JR, Harries JT. Combined cows' milk protein and gluten-induced enteropathy; common or rare? *Gut*, 1983; 24: 165.

188 Pollock DJ. The liver in coeliac disease. *Histopathology*, 1977; 1: 421.

189 Edwards C, Williams A, Asquith P. Bronchopulmonary disease in coeliac patients. *J Clin Pathol*, 1985; 38: 361.

190 Nowak TV, Ghisham FK, Schulze-Delrieu K. Celiac syndrome in Down's syndrome; considerations of a pathogenetic link. *Am J Gastroenterol*, 1983; 78: 280.

191 Unsworth DJ, Walker-Smith JA. Autoimmunity in diarrhoeal disease. *J Pediatr Gastroenterol Nutr*, 1985; 4: 375.

192 Corazza GR, Biagi F, Volta U *et al*. Autoimmune enteropathy and villous atrophy in adults. *Lancet*, 1997; 350: 106.

193 Cutz E, Rhoads JM, Drumm B *et al*. Microvillous inclusion dis-

ease: an inherited defect of brush border assembly and differentiation. *N Engl J Med*, 1989; 320: 646.
194 Groisman G, Ben-Izhak O, Schwersenz A, Berant M, Fyfe M. The value of polyclonal carcinoembryonic antigen immunostaining in the diagnosis of microvillous inclusion disease. *Hum Pathol*, 1993; 24: 1232.
195 Haghighi P, Wolf PL. Tropical sprue and subclinical enteropathy: a vision for the nineties. *Crit Rev Clin Lab Sci*, 1997; 34: 313.
196 Klipstein FA. Tropical sprue in travellers and ex-patriates living abroad. *Gastroenterology*, 1981; 80: 590.
197 Cook GC. 'Tropical sprue': some early investigators favoured an infective cause, but was a coccidian protozoan involved? *Gut*, 1997; 40: 428.
198 Ross IM, Mathan VI. Immunological changes in tropical sprue. *Q J Med*, 1981; 50: 435.
199 Schenk EA, Samloff IM, Klipstein FA. Morphologic characteristics of jejunal biopsies in celiac disease and in tropical sprue. *Am J Pathol*, 1965; 47: 765.
200 Brunser O, Eidelman S, Klipstein FA. Intestinal morphology of rural Haitians: a comparison between overt tropical sprue and asymptomatic subjects. *Gastroenterology*, 1970; 58: 655.
201 Mongomery RD, Shearer ACI. The cell population of the upper jejunal mucosa in tropical sprue and post infective malabsorption. *Gut*, 1974; 15: 387.
202 Walia BNS, Sidhu JK, Tandon BN, Ghai OI, Bhargava S. Coeliac disease in North Indian children. *Br Med J*, 1966; ii: 1233.
203 Misra RC, Kasthuri P, Chuttanni HK. Adult coeliac disease in tropics. *Br Med J*, 1966; ii: I230.
204 Merliss RRI, Hoffman A. Steatorrhea following the use of antibiotics. *N Engl J Med*, 1951; 245: 328.
205 Keusch GT, Troncale FJ, Plaut AG. Neomycin-induced malabsorption in a tropical population. *Gastroenterology*, 1970; 58: 197.
206 Jacobson ID, Prior JT, Faloon WW. Malabsorptive syndrome induced by neomycin: morphologic alterations in the jejunal mucosa. *J Lab Clin Med*, 1960; 56: 245.
207 Pestalozzi DM, Buhler R, von Wartburg JP, Hess M. Immunohistochemical localization of alcohol dehydrogenase in the human gastrointestinal tract. *Gastroenterology*, 1983; 85: 1011.
208 Bode JC, Bode C, Heidelbach R, Deurr H-K, Martin GA. Jejunal microflora in patients with chronic alcohol abuse. *Hepatogastroenterology*, 1984; 31: 30.
209 Bjorkman DJ, Jessop LD. Effects of acute and chronic ethanol exposure on intestinal microvillus membrane lipid composition and fluidity. *Alcohol Clin Exp Res*, 1994; 18: 560.
210 King CF, Tooskes PP. Small intestinal bacterial overgrowth. *Gastroenterology*, 1978; 76: 1035.
211 Banwell JG, Kistler LA, Gianella RA *et al*. Small intestinal bacterial overgrowth syndrome. *Gastroenterology*, 1981; 80: 834.
212 Isaacs PFT, Kim YS. Blind loop syndrome and small bowel bacterial contamination. *Clin Gastroenterol*, 1983; 12: 395.
213 Barry RE. Small bowel bacteriology/overgrowth. *Cur Opin Gastroenterol*, 1985; 2: 241.
214 Ament ME, Shimoda SS, Saunders DR, Rubin CE. Pathogenesis of steatorrhoea in 3 cases of small intestinal stasis syndrome. *Gastroenterology*, 1972; 63: 728.
215 Giannella RA, Rout WR, Toskes PP. Jejunal brush border injury and impaired sugar and amino acid uptake in the blind loop syndrome. *Gastroenterology*, 1974; 67: 965.
216 Hensley GT, Soergel KH. Neuropathologic findings in diabetic diarrhoea. *Arch Pathol*, 1968; 85: 587.
217 Malins JM, Maynne N. Diabetic diarrhoea: a study of 13 patients with jejunal biopsy. *Diabetes*, 1969; 18: 858.
218 Berge KG, Sprague RC, Bennett WA. The intestinal tract in diabetic diarrhoea. A pathologic study. *Diabetes*, 1956; 5: 289.
219 Ellenberg M, Bookman JJ. Diabetic diarrhoea with malabsorption syndrome. *Diabetes*, 1961; 9: 14.
220 Vinnik IF, Kern J Jr, Struthers JE Jr. Malabsorption and the diarrhea of diabetes mellitus. *Gastroenterology*, 1962; 43: 507.
221 Page SR, Lloyd CA, Hill PG, Peacock I, Holmes GK. The prevalence of coeliac disease in adult diabetes mellitus. *Q J Med*, 1994; 87: 631.
222 Logan RFA. *Descriptive epidemiology of coeliac disease*. In: Branski D, Rozen P, Kagnoff MF, eds. *Gluten-sensitive Enteropathy*. Basel: Karger, 1992: 1.
223 Catassi C, Ratsch IM, Fabiani E *et al*. High prevalence of undiagnosed coeliac disease in 5280 Italian students screened by antigliadin antibodies. *Acta Paediatr*, 1995; 84: 672.
224 Collin P, Reunala T, Pukkala E, Laippala P, Keyrilainen O, Pasternack A. Coeliac disease—associated disorders and survival. *Gut*, 1994; 35: 1215.
225 Powell EW, Campbell CB, Wilson E. Intestinal mucosal uptake of iron and iron retention in idiopathic haemochromatosis as evidence for a mucosal abnormality. *Gut*, 1970; 11: 727.
226 Greenwald AJ, Johnson DS, Oskvig RM, Aschenbrener CA, Randa DC. Antitrypsin deficiency, emphysema, cirrhosis and intestinal mucosal atrophy. *JAMA*, 1975; 231: 273.
227 Dura WT, Bernatowska E. Secretory compound α-1-antitrypsin and lysozyme in IgA-deficient children. An immunohistochemical evaluation of intestinal mucosa. *Histopathology*, 1984; 8: 747.
228 Nielson K. Coeliac disease: alpha-1-antitrypsin contents in jejunal mucosa before and after gluten-free diet. *Histopathology*, 1984; 8: 759.
229 Popovic OS, Milumalavic VB, Milutinovic-Djuric S *et al*. Primary bile acid malabsorption. *Gastroenterology*, 1987; 92: 1851.
230 Lindberg J, Ahren C, Iwarson S. Intestinal villous atrophy in chronic active hepatitis. *Scand J Gastroenterol*, 1979; 15: 1015.
231 Variend S, Sunderland R. Small intestinal mucosal abnormalities in post-perinatal deaths. *J Clin Pathol*, 1984; 37: 283.
232 Stanton AN, Scott DJ, Downham MAPS. Is over-heating a factor in unexpected infant deaths? *Lancet*, 1980; i: 1054.
233 Da Costa LR, Croft DN, Creamer B. Protein loss and cell loss from the small intestinal mucosa. *Gut*, 1971; 12: 179.
234 Toffler AH, Hukill PB, Spiro HM. Brown-bowel syndrome. *Ann Intern Med*, 1963; 58: 872.
235 Foster CS. The brown bowel syndrome: a possible smooth muscle mitochondrial myopathy. *Histopathology*, 1979; 3: 1.
236 Fox B. Lipofuscinosis of the gastrointestinal tract in man. *J Clin Pathol*, 1967; 20: 806.
237 Bauman MB, DiMase JD, Oski F, Senior JR. Brown bowel and skeletal myopathy associated with Vitamin E depletion in pancreatic insufficiency. *Gastroenterology*, 1968; 54: 93.

23 Vascular disorders of the small intestine

Anatomy

Except for the first part of the duodenum, which is supplied through the coeliac axis, the whole small intestine receives its blood supply from the superior mesenteric artery. This vessel runs in a curved course through the mesentery, and branches, the intestinal arteries, arise from its convex aspect and join together to form arcades; from these arcades, short straight branches, which do not anastomose to a significant extent, supply the jejunum and most of the ileum. Each branch ramifies in the serosa and passes through the muscle coat to the submucosa; arterioles arise from them to supply the villi. The presence of arteriovenous anastomoses is controversial and if present they are few and probably not of great functional importance [1]. There are free anastomoses between branches from the coeliac and inferior mesenteric arteries around the duodenum, head of the pancreas and the splenic flexure, respectively [2]. Arising from the concave aspect of the superior mesenteric artery high up is the inferior pancreaticoduodenal artery and then the middle colic, right colic and ileocolic arteries distally. The ileocolic artery supplies the caecum, ascending colon and terminal ileum. It follows from this that occlusion of the superior mesenteric at its origin is likely to cause widespread infarction, that occlusion of a major branch may be silent or produce infarction according to the state of the collateral circulation in the arcades, and that occlusion of a short straight branch is likely to produce local infarction of the whole or part of a segment of bowel.

The venous drainage is through the portal system via the superior mesenteric vein; some portal–systemic anastomoses are available around the lower end of the oesophagus, the umbilicus and the anorectal region. Venous obstruction is just as capable as arterial of producing infarction, but the infarcts develop more slowly and are always haemorrhagic.

In a vascular perfusion study of normal ileum in hospital postmortem cases using India ink, it has been shown that the antimesenteric half of the ileum (but not the jejunum) has a paradoxically more robust arterial supply, with numerous 'vasa recta', passing straight from the superior mesenteric artery arcades, in comparison with the shorter arteries which serve the mesenteric border, which are smaller and more tortuous [3]. Investigation of surgically resected specimens in this way, before fixation, permits areas of vascular constriction or even luminal obliteration to be readily recognized so that sections can be taken from the appropriate segments. An alternative technique is to use silicone rubber for the perfusion [4].

Physiology

The measurement of intestinal blood flow is important

because up to 50% of all cases of intestinal ischaemia might be the result of a reduced flow [5,6]. The splanchnic blood flow at the origin of the main mesenteric vessel does not vary much with alterations of blood pressure within the normal physiological range, but at extremely low pressures there is a rapid fall-off in the amount of blood supplied to the gut. About one-fifth of the total cardiac output normally goes to the splanchnic areas; if this has to be redistributed (as, for example, in shock) the splanchnic area contributes significantly because the flow through it can be decreased markedly by vasoconstriction of peripheral vessels which are very sensitive to pressor amines. If hypotension from any cause produces a marked drop in arterial pressure, particularly across a partial occlusion of a main stem of a mesenteric artery, it is possible for the perfusion pressure to drop below the critical closing pressure of the mesenteric vessels even if there are no measurable changes in blood flow. This can result in functional closure of arterioles with deprivation of blood supply to the gut, particularly the mucous membrane. Approximately 10–15% of cardiac output goes to the small intestine and 5–10% to the large intestine [7].

Of greater importance than the total amount of blood reaching the alimentary tract is the distribution of blood throughout the different layers of the bowel wall, and experimental clearance studies in the cat have shown that 75–85% of the blood goes to the mucosa and submucosa with about 20% of total flow passing through the villi. An increasing proportion of the total flow passes to the villi during arterial hypotension and under these circumstances the mean transit time is considerably prolonged [8]. The close association of afferent and efferent vessels running in different directions in the small intestinal villus has led to the proposition that a countercurrent exchange mechanism operates [7,9]. If so, it would play a crucial role in digestive metabolism. In ischaemia increased shunting of oxygen across the base of the villus in situations where the transit time was prolonged would result in necrosis, particularly at the tips of the villi.

The mesenteric circulation is under the control of the autonomic nervous system as well as being profoundly influenced by the general state of the circulation and the presence of vasoactive agents, such as histamine, 5-hydroxytryptamine and noradrenaline [7]. Disturbances in the normal control of the splanchnic circulation can be used to explain the pathogenesis of some cases of intestinal ischaemia in which no organic vascular block is demonstrated. A finely balanced system of mediators of smooth muscle tone is involved, the final common pathway being nitric oxide, which has a profoundly relaxing effect on both the bowel wall and the vasculature. Injurious stimuli such as endotoxic shock, result in production of tumour necrosis factor alpha (TNF-α) which down-regulates nitric oxide synthase (NOS) in vascular endothelial cells, effectively increasing arterial tone and producing inappropriate tissue hypoxia in the small bowel and its mucosa [10]. Direct damage to endothelial cells due, for example, to ischaemia itself, has a similar effect and no doubt explains many of the circumstances in which disproportionate ischaemic damage may occur in the small bowel, with or without overt vascular occlusion.

Pathogenesis

The essential factor in all forms of intestinal ischaemia is that the affected segment of gut receives less blood than it requires to maintain its proper structure and function. The two main causative factors are vascular occlusion and hypotension, which together can result in disturbances in the control of the mesenteric circulation. It is appropriate to mention in this context that tissues have needs other than oxygen such as proteins, carbohydrates, lipids, water, electrolytes, vitamins, etc. The capacity of cells to obtain these nutrients and to extract oxygen from the blood is intimately associated with their membrane structure and internal metabolism. Ischaemia and inflammation profoundly affect these structures and their function. The mucosal defences weakened by any ischaemic insult will be more susceptible to bacterial invasion, a particular problem in the colon.

The causes (Table 23.1) can be divided into those that are extrinsic to the bowel and those that are intrinsic. Within this division is the important distinction between an occlusive and a non-occlusive aetiology [11]. Non-occlusive or 'low flow' states operate at both extrinsic and intrinsic levels. It is the balance between the two mechanisms, vessel wall disease versus flow, that determines the clinical presentation and the pathology [11–14]. For example, there are patients with two of the three major mesenteric vessels narrowed by over 50% at their origins, yet who are without symptoms and signs of ischaemia [15].

Whatever the mechanism that ultimately reduces the mucosal blood flow the net result is tissue hypoxia and damage. A large number of variables influence the severity of the insult and the length of time it acts. Thus, canine gut can revert to normal after up to 6 hours of severe ischaemia [16]. However, reversal of the ischaemia is unsafe after a more prolonged period, with ensuing haemorrhage and perhaps absorption of toxic metabolites [12]. The vascular endothelium becomes damaged, probably more through the local activation of complement than through the effect of oxygen free radicals [17]. This is the condition of 'reperfusion injury' and it explains the high mortality of mesenteric embolectomy in clinical practice. There is therefore a complex interaction of events already in motion at the time the patient clinically presents with ischaemia.

Occlusive ischaemia

Arterial occlusion

About half of all cases of intestinal ischaemia have an asso-

Table 23.1 Causes of ischaemic bowel disease.

Arterial occlusion
Atherosclerosis
Thrombosis
Embolism
Mesenteric vascular compression tumours, aneurysm, haematoma, etc.
Takayasu's disease
Iatrogenic causes, e.g. ligation at reconstructive vascular surgery, angiography
Venous occlusion
Mesenteric thrombosis
Portal thrombosis, e.g. cirrhosis
Pyelothrombosis, e.g. appendicitis
Mesenteric vascular compression (as for arterial occlusion)
Hypercoagulable states, e.g. polycythaemia rubra vera
Oral contraceptives
Increased luminal pressure due to intestinal obstruction
Carcinoma
Faecal impaction
Hirschsprung's disease
Diverticular disease
Low flow states
Cardiogenic
Haemorrhage
Dehydration
Septic shock
Drugs—functional: vasospasm with hypotension, e.g. ergotamine, digitalis
Small vessel disease
Vasculitis
Rheumatoid arthritis
Systemic lupus erythematosus
Polyarteritis nodosa
Progressive systemic sclerosis
Henoch–Schönlein purpura
Thromboangiitis obliterans
Post irradiation
Ehlers–Danlos syndrome
Kohlmeier–Degos syndrome
Disseminated intravascular coagulation

ciated vascular block, usually due to atheroma [18], thrombus or embolus but occasionally the result of an arteritis or other condition [19]. As just mentioned, arterial narrowing by itself must be extremely severe before symptoms or pathological changes develop [15,20] and reduction of the blood flow also plays a part in most cases. Careful necropsy studies show that atheromatous lesions are most common and severe in the proximal 2 cm of the superior and inferior mesenteric arteries, leaving the most distal vessels relatively uninvolved [15]. Such narrowing is more common in men than women and is usually associated with severe aortic atheroma, coronary atheroma and often diabetes [21]. Attempts to measure the cross-sectional area of the superior mesenteric artery in unselected cases show a remarkable variation in the degree of narrowing from patient to patient [15,22]. Aortography in life and the injection of radio-opaque material into the main arteries at necropsy [23] confirm that narrowing is most common at the ostia and first centimetre of the superior mesenteric artery [24]. These studies suggest that ischaemic symptoms do not occur while two-thirds of the cross-sectional area remain patent and are unlikely until patency is reduced by 50–80% [20,25,26]; below this symptoms are to be expected, but cross-sectional area has always to be balanced against blood pressure and other extraneous factors. Infarction as opposed to anginal symptoms need not necessarily occur, even when the main stem of the superior mesenteric artery is occluded [23].

Complete occlusion of an artery is usually the result of intravascular thrombosis, embolism or haemorrhage beneath an atheromatous plaque. In the main trunk of the superior mesenteric or its major branches thrombosis on a basis of pre-existing atheroma is the most common lesion, particularly in men [18], though in some patients thrombosis follows operation or trauma without significant preceding arterial disease. In smaller branches, in which atheroma is less common, thrombosis is rarer but may be found in elderly patients. Thrombosis accounts for about 25% of cases of acute ischaemia [27].

An embolus can effectively block the superior mesenteric artery or its branches, whether there is pre-existing arterial disease or not. Emboli account for between 20 and 33% of acute intestinal ischaemia [18,27]. Common preceding conditions are atrial fibrillation with thrombus formation in the left atrium or myocardial infarction with thrombus adherent to the infarcted area [28].

Although atheroma is much the commonest cause of arterial narrowing of the superior mesenteric artery there are other causes. In the controversial 'coeliac axis syndrome' there is said to be stenosis, due to an anomalous origin of the coeliac axis, at or above the level of the lower border of the 12th thoracic vertebra. This is above the diaphragm instead of opposite the first lumbar vertebra below the diaphragm. When this happens, the artery passes beneath the median arcuate ligament and may be constricted by it [29,30].

Following aortic resection and grafting, ischaemic small bowel lesions can arise either directly or because, in generalized severe constrictive atheroma, the viability of the small bowel depends on anastomoses between coeliac, superior mesenteric and inferior mesenteric arteries [31]. More commonly, ischaemia of the colon and rectum follows such operations [32], and ischaemic colitis has also occurred at varying intervals after abdominoperineal excision of the rectum [33]. Ischaemia has also resulted from an aortography [34], successful operative treatment of aortic coarctation and infusion of vasopressin into the superior mesenteric artery to control bleeding oesophageal varices [35]. In severe occlusive disease of the lower aorta the legs may be supplied by the mesenteric system, usually via the marginal artery. Intestinal ischaemic pain may then occur on exercise. This is the mesenteric steal syndrome [36].

Venous occlusion

Bowel ischaemia secondary to venous occlusion accounts for approximately 5–15% of cases of mesenteric ischaemia [37] and, unless diagnosed promptly, carries a mortality of 20–50% [38]. Among the most common causes are external lesions producing pressure, either the margins of hernial sacs or large abdominal lymph nodes [39], intra-abdominal trauma, inflammatory conditions including appendicitis, pelvic inflammation and peritonitis, and prothrombotic states due to inherited or acquired disorders of coagulation. The latter include side-effects of oral contraceptives [40,41] and inherited defects of prothrombin and protein C [38], and mesenteric thrombosis in these disorders begins in small veins and progresses into larger vessels. Cirrhosis or a hepatic tumour may initially cause a portal vein thrombosis that can then propagate back to the mesenteric veins.

Non-occlusive ischaemia

The arterial pressure at the origin of the superior mesenteric artery is the same as in the aorta, while the portal venous pressure is about 10% of this. There is considerable peripheral resistance in the splanchnic bed [7], the vessels of which are sensitive to pressor amines. In any situation causing hypotension or 'low flow' states the splanchnic vessels are likely to constrict in an attempt to maintain normal blood pressure. Thus both the initial hypotension and the subsequent vascular constriction reduce markedly the effective flow to the bowel.

The most common hypotensive disorders that lead to bowel ischaemia are left ventricular failure, aortic insufficiency and shock. In 25–50% [5,27,42] of all patients with clinical and pathological evidence of bowel ischaemia no significant organic vascular block is demonstrated though minor vascular narrowing is often present. The role of shock has been hotly disputed. Experience from young war casualties who lost blood because of wounds produced no convincing evidence that bowel infarction is an important cause of death [43]. There are, however, reports that show that intestinal necrosis can develop after multiple injuries that did not involve the abdomen and in patients with circulatory depletion [5,44]. The majority of patients in whom shock is associated with bowel infarction are elderly. They are likely to have accompanying mesenteric vessel atherosclerosis. In such circumstances, any major hypotensive episode is more likely to precipitate mucosal damage and allow invasion by intestinal bacterial flora, in particular *Clostridium* species [45]. Paracrine mediators of damage to endothelial cells, alluded to earlier, contribute to a vicious circle. It has been shown that reperfusion injury can be alleviated by transforming growth factor beta (TGF-β), through its effect in stimulating nitric oxide synthase [46]. Pure shock, in the absence of any background of mesenteric vascular insufficiency, is probably only rarely a cause of non-occlusive ischaemia.

There is some evidence that haemoconcentration [47] and polycythemia [48] may predispose to ischaemic lesions, presumably by increasing blood viscosity. Acute small intestinal ischaemia is also a recognized complication of open cardiac surgery in the elderly [49]. In these patients perioperative dehydration appears to be an important pathogenetic factor. However, the mesenteric ischaemia appears to be restricted to patients with atheromatous constriction of the origin of the superior mesenteric artery. Ischaemia can also be associated with widespread microthrombi in other organs as part of disseminated intravascular coagulation [50]. The role of digitalis in the production of non-occlusive mesenteric ischaemia is debatable since any local vasoconstrictive effect that the drug might have is probably counterbalanced by the increased cardiac output resulting from treatment of left ventricular failure [51]. Other factors that may play a crucial or contributory role in the development of intestinal ischaemia include small vessel occlusion due to increased intraluminal pressure (see p. 545) and the bacterial content of the gut.

Nomenclature

When the intestine is deprived of blood histological changes follow which vary, as mentioned, with the acuteness and severity of the ischaemia. The considerable variation in the clinical presentation as well as the pathology are the main explanations for a confusing nomenclature covering a spectrum ranging from acute infarction, through transient subclinical episodes to the chronic evolution of a fibrotic stricture. The expressions gangrene, haemorrhagic necrosis [52–54], necrotizing enterocolitis [55–59], pseudomembranous enterocolitis [55,60,61] and ischaemic enterocolitis [62] have all been used to describe different clinicopathological manifestations of acute severe ischaemia. Moreover, some cases reported in the past as segmental enteritis or colitis were probably also due to ischaemic disease. Uraemic enterocolitis is an expression that was used to describe a clinical picture that nowadays might be regarded as having an ischaemic basis. The majority of these acute forms of intestinal ischaemia have been grouped together as 'acute intestinal failure' [1] but pseudomembranous colitis is placed in a separate group now that the aetiological role of *Clostridium difficile* is understood (see p. 516).

The chronic variety of ischaemia is best known as ischaemic stricture. However, the histopathology of acute ischaemia and ischaemic stricture merge into one another and the appearances seen in surgical specimens depend on the stage at which the operation is performed, as well as on the severity and duration of the ischaemic episode. Between the clinical emergency of acute infarction and a chronic ischaemic stricture exists an ill-defined stage manifest by transient ischaemic episodes. These may be single subclinical reversible thrombotic events perhaps, for example, due to the contraceptive pill, or be attacks of recurrent 'intestinal angina' in patients with chronic arterial obstruction [15].

The clinical patterns of mesenteric vascular disease have been classified by Marston [63] in the following way.

1 Acute intestinal ischaemia:
  (a) with arterial occlusion;
  (b) non-occlusive.
2 Chronic arterial obstruction.
3 Focal ischaemia:
  (a) of the small bowel;
  (b) of the colon.

Acute intestinal ischaemia refers to infarction of major lengths of bowel, chronic obstruction refers to the controversial subclinical preinfarctive state of 'intestinal angina', and focal ischaemia covers the main local causes of ischaemic bowel disease (see Table 23.1).

Histopathology of intestinal ischaemia

Macroscopic appearances

Infarction requires little explanation. The bowel becomes oedematous and plum coloured (Fig. 23.1). The mucosa is necrotic and has a nodular surface appearance due to extensive submucosal haemorrhage but the deep muscle layers may initially appear well preserved. As necrosis becomes more complete or gangrene develops, all layers of the intestinal wall are affected. The external surface has a mottled purple or greenish hue and the tissues of the bowel are thin and friable. The mucosal surface becomes covered by patches of white slough. Bubbles of gas may be present within mesenteric veins [64].

In some cases of acute ischaemic enterocolitis only the mucosa is affected with quite good preservation of the deeper layers of the bowel wall. This is particularly characteristic of the non-occlusive type of intestinal ischaemia and is due to the muscularis propria being relatively more resistant to acute deprivation of blood than the mucosa and submucosa. The bowel may be a normal colour from the outside, although usually dilated, or it may be reddened and show focal areas of violet discoloration where full-thickness necrosis has occurred. The mucosal surface is haemorrhagic with superficial pinpoint ulcers or deeper longitudinal and serpiginous ulceration. In other cases, necrosis of the mucosa gives rise to diffuse ill-defined yellow (Fig. 23.2), greenish or tan-coloured plaques which have sloughed into the bowel lumen or can be easily scraped off the underlying viable tissue. Membranous or pseudomembranous enterocolitis has been used to describe this appearance of ischaemic mucosal necrosis in the past, but the term is now applied to the focal raised creamy yellow plaques that predominantly affect the large bowel and are due to *C. difficile* toxin, although ischaemia may be a contributory factor (see Chapter 36).

The distribution and type of lesion in the small intestine and proximal colon will depend on the cause of the ischaemia. If the latter is due to a vascular block then the pathological changes will have a uniform appearance and a segmental distribution that reflects a shutdown in the blood supply to a particular part of the gut. In non-occlusive intestinal ischaemia, however, the lesions are often patchy and very widespread and vary in their severity [5].

Microscopic appearances

Early mucosal lesions are usually patchy, with almost normal mucosa separating diseased areas in which crypts show necrosis and there is a surface membrane composed of mucus, fibrin, blood cells and necrotic tissue. Sometimes, only the tips of the intestinal villi are affected (Fig. 23.3). There is vascular

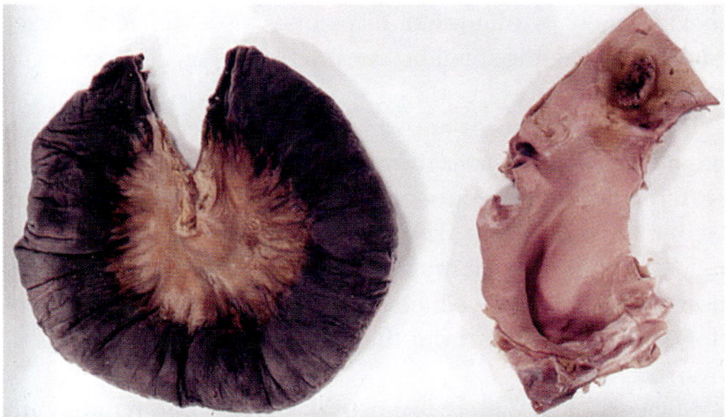

Fig. 23.1 Infarction of small bowel following embolism to superior mesenteric artery from thrombus in aortic arch (right). The bowel is swollen and haemorrhagic.

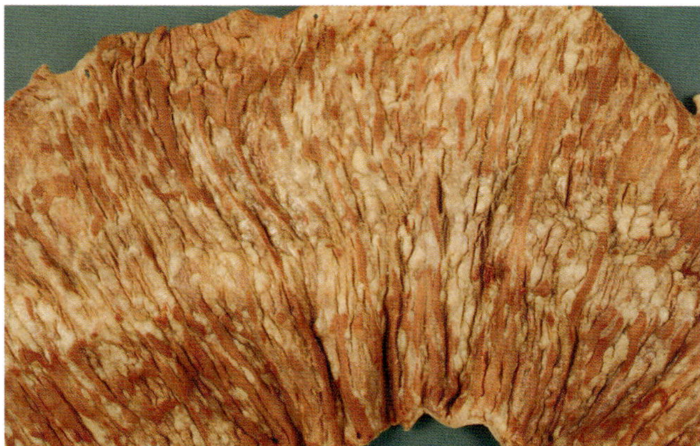

Fig. 23.2 Acute ischaemia of small intestine showing extensive yellow plaques of mucosal necrosis.

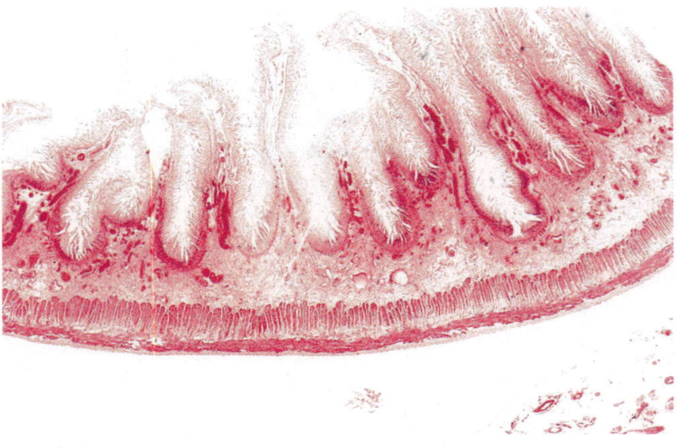

Fig. 23.3 Acute ischaemia of small intestine, showing necrosis of the upper half of the villi but sparing the basal half of the mucosa.

congestion with oedema and occasional haemorrhages in the submucosal layer. It is common to see fibrin thrombi within the blood vessels of both the mucosa and submucosa, and in non-occlusive ischaemia a significant number will have thrombi in other organs. This pattern might be a manifestation of disseminated intravascular coagulation centred on the gut [50]. A search for minute ischaemic lesions in the mucosa should be made in which the only features are capillary congestion, necrosis of a few crypts and erosions of the surface epithelium.

With increasing severity of ischaemia the deeper layers of the bowel wall become affected. There should always be a careful inspection of the muscularis even when the most obvious changes are mucosal and submucosal because in the early stages of acute deprivation of blood the muscle layers show only poor staining with loss of nuclei and little other abnormality. Later, lysis of muscle cells is more obvious with separation and thinning of fibres by oedema and the beginning of an inflammatory infiltrate.

Infarction is manifested by haemorrhage into the bowel wall, particularly the submucosa, with intravascular thrombosis and mucosal ulceration. In cases of intestinal gangrene widespread necrosis is apparent and this is accompanied by secondary infection which often extends through the bowel wall to involve mesenteric tissues and engulf the mesenteric vessels. The latter then show intravascular thrombosis and varying degrees of arteritis. This is more usually secondary than a primary cause of the ischaemic bowel disease. In any one case the histology of the affected gut only exceptionally reveals the primary cause or causes of the intestinal ischaemia. More often this is explained by consideration of the clinical history. However, it is important to exclude the various types of primary vasculitis which can lead to ischaemic bowel disease, such as the collagen disorders including polyarteritis nodosa, systemic sclerosis and systemic lupus erythematosus (see below). An opinion on whether the vascular changes are the result of venous or arterial occlusion can be useful, but this is only possible if the mesenteric vasculature has been carefully examined.

All the features of ischaemic necrosis, however severe, can go through a process of resolution and repair. Granulation tissue replaces the layers of the bowel, often patchily. The whole process is essentially the same for the small intestine and colon (see Chapter 37) and a stricture is often the end-result [65]. We have observed, in several cases, considerable degrees of mesenteric fat necrosis accompanying major vessel occlusion.

Ischaemic strictures and ulcers

Ischaemic strictures occur in the small bowel or colon (see also p. 543). Within the small intestine they have been classified into primary and secondary [65]. The primary causes are small mesenteric vessel emboli, trauma and the sequelae of herniae or bands. Secondary ischaemic strictures are due to drugs, in particular potassium chloride tablets [66] (see p. 299), the contraceptive pill [67] and non-steroidal anti-inflammatory drugs [68] (p. 298), or irradiation [69]; there are a small number whose origin is unknown [70,71].

The strictures can be short or long, single or multiple. Occasionally they present with a malabsorption syndrome but more often they produce signs and symptoms of intestinal obstruction, usually subacute. It is probable that the episodes of acute ischaemia that eventually give rise to a stricture are subclinical. Several evanescent or transient patterns of enterocolitis, which may be ischaemic, are described (see pp. 351 and 544). Alternatively, ischaemic strictures may be the result of a slowly developing chronic ischaemic process corresponding to the clinical state of 'intestinal angina' [15]. Partial vascular occlusion and emboli can sometimes be found [65,72]. They can be produced by specific causes of peripheral arteritis such as polyarteritis nodosa. These are usually obvious on histological examination though there may be difficulty recognizing burnt-out cases of arteritis. Volvulus of the small intestine and obstruction of the blood supply due to internal herniae are also possible causes. Cholesterol emboli due to dislodgement of atheromatous plaques are a well recognized cause of ischaemic small bowel strictures (Fig. 23.4), particularly in the elderly [73,74].

Ischaemic strictures are concentric. The serosal surface is often whiter than normal due to serosal fibrosis. The mucosal surface may be atrophic or may show one or more small, clearly demarcated ulcers. The cut surface of the stricture will reveal a prominent submucosa that is filled with white fibrous tissue (Fig. 23.5). If possible, sections for microscopic examination should be taken from the mesenteric vessels as well as from the stricture.

Microscopically, there is mucosal necrosis, commonly with ulceration. The submucosal layer is filled with granulation tissue of a very uniform character containing many new blood vessels and a sprinkling of inflammatory cells some-

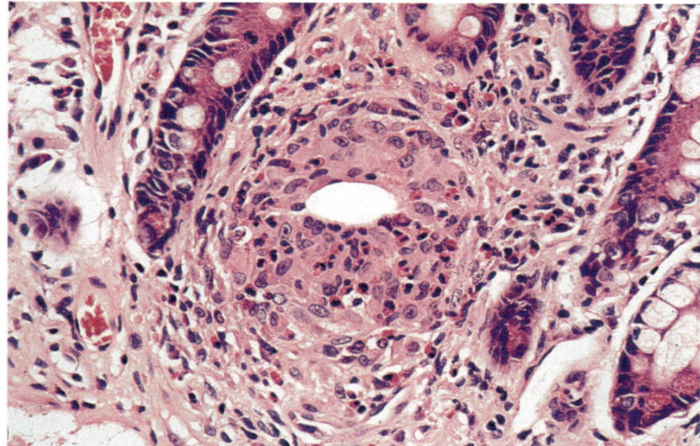

Fig. 23.4 Histological section of a duodenal mucosal biopsy from an arteriopathic patient. A cholesterol cleft surrounded by foamy macrophages and inflammatory cells marks the site of embolized material from an atheromatous plaque in a major afferent artery.

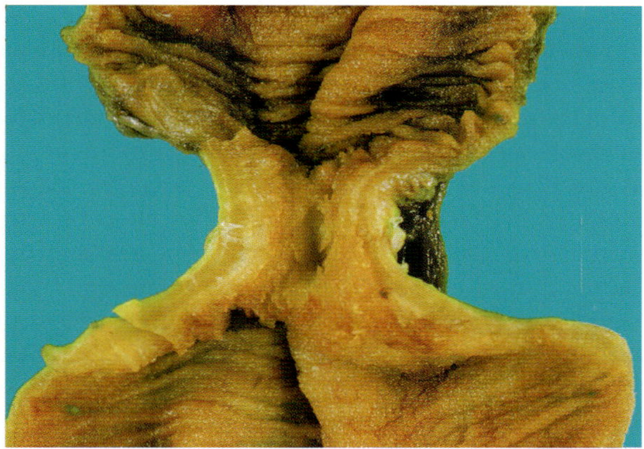

Fig. 23.5 Ileum opened through an ischaemic stricture. Note the mural thickening, particularly the white fibrous tissue in submucosa, at the site of the stricture.

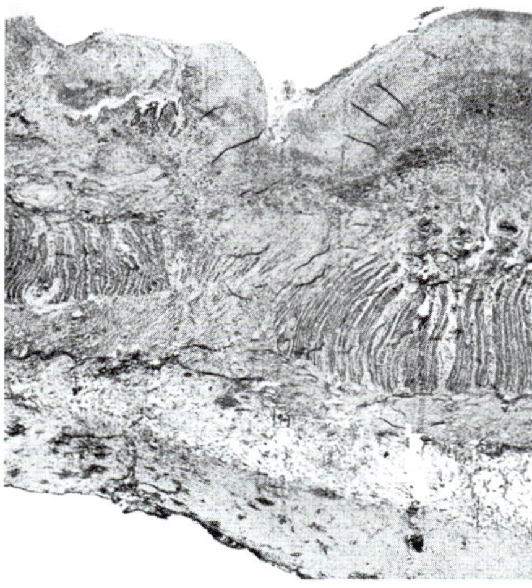

Fig. 23.6 Histological section of an ischaemic stricture, showing disorganization of the muscularis propria, with fibrous tissue extending from the submucosa between the bundles of the inner part of the circular muscle layer. There is necrosis and ulceration of the more delicate mucosa.

times including haemosiderin-laden macrophages, an indication of former submucosal haemorrhage during the acute phase of the illness. This granulation tissue spreads beneath intact mucosa beyond the macroscopic limits of the stricture. The deep muscle layers can be normal or show varying degrees of disorganization by granulation tissue. A useful sign is to see the inner bundles of the circular muscle layer being nipped off by fibrous tissue (Fig. 23.6). The serosa will often contain granulation tissue similar to that seen in the submucosal layer. It is unusual to find vascular changes unless the stricture has been caused by a specific type of arteritis.

Ischaemic stricture of the small bowel has to be distinguished from other causes of intestinal stenosis. These include Crohn's disease, tuberculosis, carcinoma and malignant lymphoma. The correct diagnosis is usually apparent from microscopic examination with particular emphasis on the study of the deep muscle layer. It is only as a result of ischaemia that much fibrosis of the muscularis propria occurs.

Chronic intestinal ischaemia (intestinal angina)

This term covers what is coming to be accepted as the preinfarction stage of intestinal ischaemia; the stage when symptoms might occur due to reduction in blood flow but the stage of infarction has not been reached. An attempt to study this problem in an unselected autopsy series found there was no correlation between degree of stenosis of the main mesenteric vessels and antemortem gastrointestinal symptoms. A 50% reduction in intraluminal diameter, corresponding to an 80% reduction in cross-sectional area, was taken as a critical stenosis but even then no clinical correlations could be made [15]. In a clinical study [63], it was possible to identify a small group of patients with symptoms prior to infarction who had varying degrees of mesenteric vessel stenosis and/or occlusion in whom surgical reconstruction of the visceral arteries relieved symptoms. Such patients are rare and the relation between symptoms and pathology in chronic ischaemia still remains uncertain [15,25,26].

The relation of symptoms and radiological signs to lesions

It cannot be too strongly emphasized that anoxia must be severe before any symptoms, signs or visible lesions become apparent. In severe anoxia without complete cessation of blood flow, vague abdominal symptoms appear, of which the most significant is abdominal (visceral) angina. This consists of severe, cramp-like, colicky upper abdominal pain, often with diarrhoea and sometimes with vomiting and melaena. It occurs shortly after food and persists for 1–3 hours, being much more severe after a large meal [75,76]. Early barium studies may show either no abnormality or transverse ridging and 'thumbprinting'. When present, this corresponds with the fluid transudation and mucosal and submucosal haemorrhage of the early ischaemic lesion. In later lesions radiology may show one or more solitary ulcers or strictures with proximal bowel dilatation.

When the anoxia is severe enough to produce full-thickness infarction, peristalsis is interrupted with consequent clinical evidence of obstruction and peritonitis. There is usually severe continuous abdominal pain with distension and vomiting. There may also be evidence of shock or hypertension that on careful enquiry has usually preceded rather than followed abdominal symptoms. The history may suggest a likely source of an embolus. Plain X-rays of the abdomen are negative and the only useful laboratory findings are a leucocytosis and a raised haematocrit. Prior to irreversible bowel necrosis the serum phosphate can be raised and may be of great diagnostic value [77]. A number of cases of severe ischaemic enterocolitis mimic acute ulcerative colitis except that there is hypotension and the small intestine is also involved [62].

Mesenteric venous thrombosis, like arterial occlusion, produces colicky abdominal pain, nausea, vomiting and bloody diarrhoea, but the clinical course is usually more gradual [78].

Thus there are two broad clinical patterns of ischaemic enteritis, though neither is clear cut. When the onset is gradual or the anoxia short-lasting, as in vascular narrowing and in some patients with hypotensive episodes, symptoms tend to be absent or of an anginal type. Radiology may be negative or demonstrate thumbprinting. The lesion is superficial within the mucosa and submucosa and healing can lead to stricture formation. Occasionally such patients eventually present with painless watery diarrhoea [49]. When anoxia is acute in onset, severe or long-lasting, as in patients with complete occlusions or severe hypotension, symptoms are of more continuous abdominal pain, severe bloody diarrhoea, intestinal obstruction and collapse with corresponding full-thickness infarction. Many patients in the first group recover spontaneously, but may later show evidence of a solitary ulcer or stricture; in the second group, death is common and embolectomy, thrombectomy or resection offer the only rational treatment.

Ischaemic enterocolitis and Hirschsprung's disease

The macroscopic and microscopic pathology of the enterocolitis of Hirschsprung's disease seems to be almost identical with that seen in the acute ischaemic enterocolitis of adults [79,80]. It has been suggested that a vascular event associated with a period of circulatory collapse might explain the onset of mucosal necrosis. Experimental studies lend support to the idea that a Schwarzman reaction might be involved. This complication of Hirschsprung's disease is further considered in the discussion of obstructive colitis (see p. 545).

Neonatal necrotizing enterocolitis

Although this entity may well have an ischaemic element, it has been shown that infants with this condition have a deficiency in Paneth cells [81] and it appears to be an infective condition. It is therefore considered on p. 522.

'Necrotizing' enteritis

Conditions which come under the umbrella of this term are considered on pp. 277 and 521. They are necrotizing lesions of the small or large bowel most commonly associated with clostridial organisms, but not necessarily so [82]. Because many of the cases occur in children they would seem unlikely to have solely a primary vascular aetiology. An initial infectious insult to the mucosa followed by ischaemic damage precipitated by the known vasoconstrictive effect of certain clostridial toxins seems a likely pathogenetic mechanism. In the adult it is of course possible to postulate the reverse: ischaemic damage to the mucosa could be an initial event, due to atherosclerosis of the mesenteric circulation, that allows invasion by organisms of the necrotic tissue. Whether the initial insult is ischaemic or infective cannot be resolved by pathological examination at present, for such cases are only studied after surgical excision or death when the bowel is at the 'end-stage'.

Possible drug-induced ischaemic lesions

The small bowel circulation is sensitive to many pharmacological agents and it is not surprising therefore that drugs have been implicated in ischaemic damage. Cocaine, potassium chloride, non-steroidal anti-inflammatory drugs and oral contraceptives are the best documented. The pathology is difficult if not impossible to distinguish from that of either infarction or a chronic ischaemic stricture and ulceration. It is partly on this basis that the pathogenesis is believed to be ischaemic.

Cocaine-induced intestinal ischaemia

Cocaine addicts frequently develop systemic arterial thrombotic occlusions and occasionally the mesenteric arteries can be affected [83]. The small bowel may show sharply demarcated patches of 'pseudomembranous' enteritis or even extensive regional infarction [84].

So-called 'thiazide' or 'potassium' ulcers

A small group of patients can be recognized with solitary or multiple ulcers of the small bowel associated with the taking of enteric-coated tablets of potassium chloride with hydrochlorothiazide for systemic hypertension [66,85,86]. Macroscopically and histologically these are very similar to the ischaemic ulcers that accompany strictures. We believe with others [87] that these are essentially ischaemic in origin, either due to relative hypotension as the blood pressure is lowered or to arterial or venous spasm [88] set up as tablets stick in the small bowel and release a high local concentration of the potassium. The majority of such patients have advanced cardiovascular disease [89,90] so that the pathogenesis is likely to be multifactorial.

Non-steroidal anti-inflammatory drugs

Among the reports of solitary ulcers of the small intestine are cases incriminating non-steroidal anti-inflammatory drugs (NSAIDs) [66,68,91]. There are no experimental data to suggest the lesions are ischaemic, the evidence being based on the morphological similarity with known ischaemic ulceration. A more likely mechanism is via the effects these drugs have on prostaglandin metabolism which in turn affects mucosal integrity although ischaemia may have a secondary role. The pathology of NSAID damage to the small bowel is discussed in detail on p. 295.

The contraceptive pill

It is well known that oral contraceptive use increases the risk of vascular disease in many systems [67], although the risk seems to be considerably less with modern low-dose regimens. Ischaemia, both acute and chronic, has been documented in the small intestine and colon [92]. Massive infarction of the small bowel may be due to mesenteric arterial or venous thrombosis [92,93]. The patients have often had symptoms prior to presentation, and if the diagnosis is considered and the oral contraceptive stopped the ischaemia is reversed [41].

Other primary vascular lesions in the small intestine

The gastrointestinal tract is involved in many conditions in which there is a vasculitis as part of the disease. The classification of vasculitic disorders has become rationalized following the realization that the necrotizing vasculitides (Wegener's granulomatosis, microscopic polyangiitis and Churg–Strauss syndrome) share the feature of raised serum antineutrophil cytoplasmic antibodies (ANCA) [94,95]. Behçet's disease is a distinct microscopic vasculitic disease but the ulceration resulting from the vasculitis is more conspicuous than the vasculitis itself (p. 302) [96]. Systemic lupus erythematosus, rheumatoid arthritis, systemic sclerosis and Henoch–Schönlein purpura are separate entities, each associated with a microangiopathy that can affect the small bowel. Classical polyarteritis nodosa and Takayasu's disease are very rare in the small intestine [97]. The diagnoses are difficult to make from biopsy material [98], though deep rectal biopsies are said to be helpful in rheumatoid arthritis [99,100]. Surgery is for the complications of haemorrhage, perforation, infarction and occasionally a stricture. The distinction between these conditions is usually made on clinical grounds and the vasculitis in these diseases seldom has distinguishing features. Finally, when it is difficult to establish the underlying disease in a patient with mesenteric vasculitis causing small intestinal ischaemia, it should be remembered that occult malignancy can sometimes be responsible [101].

Progressive systemic sclerosis (scleroderma)

As well as muscle atrophy and replacement by fibrous tissue a vasculitis can accompany progressive systemic sclerosis and cause a range of ischaemic pathology in the gut [102]. In the CREST syndrome (calcinosis, Raynaud's phenomenon, oesophageal dysmotility, sclerodactyly and telangiectasia) ectatic vascular lesions can be seen at many sites in the gastrointestinal tract [103,104] They are similar to the vascular ectasias in the Rendu–Osler–Weber syndrome. Pneumatosis intestinalis has also been documented, perhaps as a result of obstruction and bacterial overgrowth [105].

Rheumatoid arthritis

Approximately 1% of patients with rheumatoid arthritis show a clinical vasculitis and one-fifth of these will demonstrate gastrointestinal involvement [106]. Although infarction and an acute abdomen are recorded [107,108], in general the symptoms are less dramatic than in polyarteritis nodosa [99], though a pancolitis with multiple discrete ulcers can occur [106]. Involvement is more likely in patients with long-standing arthritis, a high rheumatoid factor and subcutaneous nodules. Where there is clinical evidence of vasculitis, a deep rectal biopsy may show a vasculitis in submucosal vessels in up to 40% of cases [100].

Systemic lupus erythematosus

Gastrointestinal symptoms in systemic lupus erythematosus are common, occurring in from 10 to 34% of patients [109]. The predominant pathology identified is a vasculitis [110], either an arteritis [111] or a venulitis [112,113]. The vasculitis can lead to infarction [114] of the small or large bowel [115] but haemorrhage from ischaemic ulcers may be the presenting feature [112,114]. Immune complexes can be demonstrated within the inflamed vessels and also in the basement membrane beneath the mucosal epithelial cells [112,113].

Henoch–Schönlein purpura

Henoch–Schönlein purpura is a hypersensitivity disease of childhood characterized by immune complex deposition beneath vascular basement membrane, with diverse haemorrhagic leucocytoclastic vasculitic lesions in the skin, kidneys, joints and alimentary tract. Clinically, gut involvement occurs in from 35 to 85% [116]. However, surgery is only required in 2–6% [117]. The vasculitis can cause haemorrhage, initiating intussusception, as well as perforation and infarction [117]. If the acute phase passes then a chronic intestinal ischaemic stricture can follow [118]. It may be possible to demonstrate immunoglobulin A (IgA) and complement (C3) in involved vessels.

Polyarteritis nodosa

Abdominal pain, often of anginal type, diarrhoea and the passage of blood are common symptoms in polyarteritis nodosa [119]. Between 40 and 70% of patients show gastrointestinal involvement. The complete spectrum of ischaemic changes due to an arteriolar or venous vasculitis can be seen. This includes steatorrhoea [120], perforation [121], strictures, ulcerative enteritis, intussusception and ischaemic necrosis [122]. It may affect large or small bowel.

At laparotomy or necropsy a careful search will usually disclose lesions but a number of patients have abdominal symptoms without visible disease or vice versa. Macroscopically the principal findings are nodules along the course of the mesenteric vessels [122], and localized mucosal ulcers that lie along the antimesenteric border and can penetrate deeply and perforate; the bowel is often friable. There can be localized haemorrhagic infarcts that are seen in various stages of activity and may show healing with fibrosis. Microscopically there is an acute arteritis (Fig. 23.7) with fibrinoid necrosis of the vessel wall and often superimposed thrombus formation. Disease may involve any size of vessel, though it usually affects the small, straight arteries; veins can be affected. Infarction is described, with uniform intimal hyperplasia of small arteries that may represent a healing phase [123]. There can be diagnostic difficulty after steroid therapy in which the inflammatory infiltrate has subsided. Here an elastic stain may be helpful to demonstrate destruction of the internal elastic lamina.

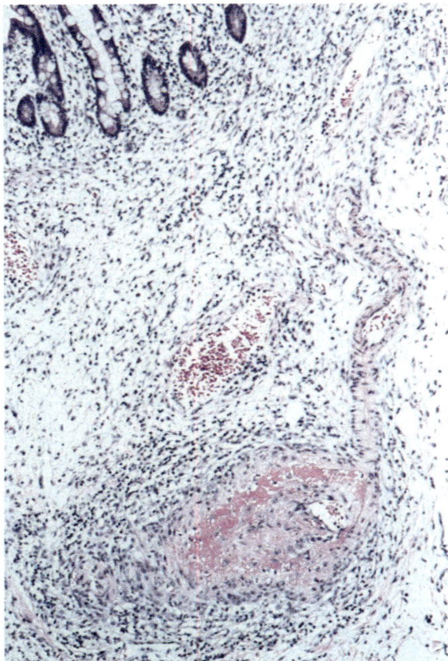

Fig. 23.7 Polyarteritis nodosa with involvement of small ileal submucosal arteries. There is fibrinoid necrosis of the vessel wall and periarterial inflammation.

Allergic granulomatous vasculitis (Churg–Strauss syndrome)

A polyarteritis nodosa-like picture accompanied by asthma and eosinophilia, the Churg–Strauss syndrome can include gastrointestinal involvement [124]. Discrete nodules are seen along the course of the vessels and the vasculitis is characterized by a heavy eosinophil infiltrate and granuloma formation in relation to vessels and in extravascular positions [125].

Thromboangiitis obliterans (Buerger's disease)

This disease rarely involves the distal branches of the superior mesenteric artery producing local ischaemia. It may present after the diagnosis of limb disease has been made but cases are described with intestinal ischaemia occurring prior to any signs of limb claudication [126,127]. Characteristic vascular lesions are present in smaller submucosal and serosal vessels, producing local occlusion of lumina by organizing thrombi. There is endothelial proliferation and medial fibrosis but in all vessels the internal elastic lamina is intact. This is characteristic of the disease and distinguishes it from other forms of vasculitis. There can also be perivascular inflammation. Both small and large bowel can be involved.

Kohlmier–Degos syndrome (progressive arterial occlusive disease)

In this condition, which affects particularly the skin and gastrointestinal tract, the intima of small and medium-sized arteries undergoes progressive occlusive sclerosis leading to localized zones of infarction [128]. The condition is probably a form of vasculitis and leads to multiple zones of fibrosis throughout the tract, presumably the end-result of ischaemia with or without infarction.

Ehlers–Danlos syndrome

Patients with Ehlers–Danlos syndrome have hypermobile joints and hyperextensibility of the skin which are the visible results of a generalized tissue 'fragility', probably itself the result of a defect in collagen metabolism. Vessels are characteristically affected in the type IV variety of the Ehlers–Danlos syndrome in which they are abnormally fragile, the defect being in type III collagen. Instances have been described of severe intramural haemorrhage and of spontaneous perforations of the bowel [129]. There are occasional recorded cases of perforation being the presenting illness [130–132]. The correct diagnosis, in one case [130], was made 5 years later when the patient re-presented with an aortic aneurysm. In the cases where pathology of the gut is documented, the muscle coat is thinned with loss of the submucosa, fibrosis of the circular muscle is apparent and defects in the media of mural arterioles [130–132] can be found.

Intramural haematomas of the small intestine

Bleeding into the wall of the small intestine from any cause is likely to result in swelling and obstruction and to produce a characteristic 'coiled spring' pattern on X-ray. In adults such haemorrhage, though occasionally traumatic, more commonly follows the use of anticoagulants [133,134] and may involve many parts of the small intestine. It can follow endoscopic biopsy [135]. The bleeding associated with the use of NSAIDs is more usually mucosal. In children the haemorrhage is more often duodenal and is the result of 'blunt trauma' without penetrating injury [135,136]; the duodenum is fixed both at the pylorus and at the end of the fourth part. It is therefore particularly liable to damage in childhood where it crosses an unyielding vertebral column [137,138].

Macroscopically the affected bowel is swollen and dark red and may appear gangrenous; on incision, blood and blood clot exude, but the mucosa usually remains intact and peritonitis is not a common feature. Acute pancreatitis is a recognized complication. Some cases may be examples of Ehlers–Danlos syndrome.

Mycotic aneurysm

Mycotic aneurysms are rare in the superior mesenteric artery or its branches and are related to bacterial endocarditis [139,140]. The aneurysm may rupture but secondary lesions in the gastrointestinal tract are rare.

Mesenteric inflammatory veno-occlusive disease

Mesenteric inflammatory veno-occlusive disease (MIVOD) is a recently described condition characterized by subacute intestinal ischaemia that is reported to be associated with, and possibly caused by, marked phlebitis and venulitis affecting the veins of the bowel and mesentery [141,142]. Arteries are unaffected and while there was no involvement of extraintestinal veins in one series of seven cases [142], one out of three patients in a second publication had recurrent peripheral thrombophlebitis and pulmonary embolism [141]. The phlebitis is described as lymphocytic, or occasionally necrotizing or even granulomatous, and affected veins may show myointimal hyperplasia. Presenting symptoms are most commonly those of abdominal pain and nausea for a period of a few weeks; men and women appear to be equally affected, with a wide age-span from the third to the eighth decade, and most make an uneventful recovery following surgical resection of the affected segment. Apart from the phlebitis and venulitis, and the superimposed occlusive venous thrombosis, histological examination of the affected bowel has shown a spectrum of lesions from acute congestion and transmural haemorrhagic infarction to more chronic strictures with intramural fibrosis.

The authors have also seen similar cases, but have found it difficult in many to be certain that the inflammatory venous changes are not secondary to the bowel ischaemia, and not *vice versa*. It is not uncommon to find inflammatory infiltration of the walls of mesenteric veins within a segment of infarcted bowel when another primary cause is established (such as entrapment within a hernia). Great care must therefore be taken to exclude other causes before attributing a case to inflammatory veno-occlusive disease.

References

1 Marston A. Applied anatomy of the intestinal circulation. In: Marston A, ed. *Vascular Disease of the Gut: Pathophysiology, Recognition and Management*. London: Edward Arnold, 1986: 1.

2 Reiner L, Platt L, Rodriguez FL, Jimenez FA. Injection studies on the mesenteric arterial circulation, II. Intestinal infarction. *Gastroenterology*, 1960; 39: 747.

3 Anthony A, Dhillon AP, Pounder RE, Wakefield AJ. Ulceration of the ileum in Crohn's disease: correlation with vascular anatomy. *J Clin Pathol*, 1997; 50: 1013.

4 Reynolds DG. Injection techniques in the study of intestinal vascular tree under normal conditions and in ulcerative colitis. In: Boley SJ, Schwartz SS, Williams LF, eds. *Vascular Disorders of the Intestine*. London: Butterworths, 1971: 383.

5 Renton CJC. Non-occlusive intestinal infarction. *Clin Gastroenterol*, 1972; 1 (3): 655.

6 Williams LF, Anastasia LF, Hasiotis C, Bosniak MA, Byrne JJ. Non-occlusive mesenteric infection. *Am J Surg*, 1967; 114: 376.

7 Lundgren O. The regulation and distribution of intestinal blood flow. In: Marston A, ed. *Vascular Disease of the Gut: Pathophysiology, Recognition and Management*. London: Edward Arnold, 1986: 16.

8 Lundgren O, Svanvik J. Mucosal hemodynamics in the small intestine of the cat during reduced perfusion pressure. *Acta Physiol Scand*, 1973; 88: 551.

9 Jodal M, Haglund V, Lundgren O. Counter-current exchange mechanisms in the small intestine. In: Shepherd AR, Granger DN, eds. *Physiology of the Intestinal Circulation*. New York: Raven Press, 1984: 83.

10 Fong YM, Marano MA, Moldawer LL *et al*. The acute splanchnic and peripheral tissue metabolic response to endotoxin in humans. *J Clin Invest*, 1990; 85: 1896.

11 Reeders JWAJ, Tytgat GNJ, Rosenbusch G, Gratama S. *Ischaemic Colitis*. The Hague: Martinus-Nijhoff, 1984.

12 Marston A. Ischaemia. *Clin Gastroenterol*, 1985; 14 (4): 847.

13 Thompson H. Vascular pathology of the splanchnic circulation. *Clin Gastroenterol*, 1972; 1 (3): 597.

14 Marston A. Basic structure and function of the intestinal circulation. *Clin Gastroenterol*, 1972; 1 (3): 539.

15 Croft RJ, Menon GP, Marston A. Does 'intestinal angina' exist? A critical study of obstructed visceral arteries. *Br J Surg*, 1981; 68: 316.

16 Chiu CJ, McArdle AH, Brown R, Scott HJ, Gurd FN. Intestinal mucosal lesion in low-flow states. *Arch Surg*, 1970; 101: 478.

17 Spain DA, Fruchterman TM, Matheson PJ, Wilson MA, Martin AW, Garrison RN. Complement activation mediates intestinal injury after resuscitation from hemorrhagic shock. *J Trauma Inj Infect Crit Care*, 1999; 46: 224.

18 Kairaluoma MI, Karkola P, Heikkinen E, Huttunen R, Mokka REM, Larmi TKI. Mesenteric infarction. *Am J Surg*, 1977; 133: 188.

19 Kumar PJ, Dawson AM. Vasculitis of the alimentary tract. *Clin Gastroenterol*, 1972; 1 (3): 719.

20 May GM, De Weese JA, Rob CG. Haemodynamic effects of arterial stenosis. *Surgery*, 1963; 53: 513.

21 Reiner L, Jimenez FA, Rodriguez FL. Atherosclerosis in the mesenteric circulation. Observations and correlations with aortic and coronary atherosclerosis. *Am Heart J*, 1963; 66: 200.

22 Derrick JR, Pollard HS, Moore RM. The pattern of arteriosclerotic narrowing of the coeliac and superior mesenteric arteries. *Ann Surg*, 1959; 149: 684.

23 Reiner L, Rodriguez FL, Jimenez FA, Platt R. Injection studies on mesenteric arterial circulation. III. Occlusions without intestinal infarction. *Arch Pathol*, 1962; 73: 461.

24 Price WG, Rohrer GV, Jacobsen ED. Mesenteric vascular disease. *Gastroenterology*, 1969; 57: 599.

25 Dick AP, Gregg D. Chronic occlusions of the visceral arteries. *Clin Gastroenterol*, 1972; 1 (3): 689.

26 Dick AP, Graff R, Gregg D, Peters N, Sarner M. An arteriographic study of mesenteric arterial disease. 1. Large vessel changes. *Gut*, 1967; 8: 206.

27 Wilson C, Gupta R, Gilmour DG, Imrie CW. Acute superior mesenteric ischaemia. *Br J Surg*, 1987; 74: 279.

28 Bergan JJ, Yao JS. Acute intestinal ischaemia. In: Rutherford P, ed. *Vascular Surgery*, 2nd edn. Philadelphia: W.B. Saunders, 1981: 948.

29 Szilagyi DE, Rian RL, Elliot JP, Smith RF. The coeliac artery compression syndrome: Does it exist? *Surgery*, 1972; 72: 849.

30 Evans W. Long-term evaluation of the coeliac band syndrome. *Surgery*, 1974; 76: 867.

31 Orr NWN, Ware CC. Some gastrointestinal complications of abdominal surgery (summary). *Proc R Soc Med*, 1968; 61: 342.

32 Ernst CB, Hagihara PF, Daugherty ME, Sachatello CR, Griffin WOJR. Ischaemic colitis incidence following abdominal aortic reconstruction: a prospective study. *Surgery*, 1976; 80: 417.

33 Wittenberg J, O'Sullivan P, Williams L Jr. Ischaemic colitis after abdominal perineal resection. *Gastroenterology*, 1975; 69: 1321.

34 Wilder RJ, Steichen FM. Necrosis of the entire gastrointestinal tract following translumbar aortography. *Arch Surg*, 1960; 80: 198.

35 Roberts C, Maddison FE. Partial mesenteric arterial occlusion with subsequent ischaemic bowel damage due to pitressin infusion. *Am J Roentgenol Radium Ther Nucl Med*, 1976; 126: 829.

36 Harris PL, Charlesworth D. Chronic intestinal ischaemia due to aorta—deal steal. *J Cardiovasc Surg*, 1974; 15: 122.

37 Grendell JH, Ockner RK. Mesenteric venous thrombosis. *Gastroenterology*, 1982; 82: 358.

38 Kumar S, Sarr MG, Kamath PS. Mesenteric venous thrombosis. *N Engl J Med*, 2001; 345: 1683.

39 Schwartzchild W, Myerson RM. Venous insufficiency of the small intestine secondary to sarcoidosis of mesenteric lymph nodes. *Am J Gastroenterol*, 1968; 50: 69.

40 Civetta JM, Kolodny M. Mesenteric venous thrombosis association with oral contraceptives. *Gastroenterology*, 1970; 58: 713.

41 Cotton PB, Thomas ML. Ischaemic colitis and the contraceptive pill. *Br Med J*, 1971; 3: 27.

42 Ottinger LW. Nonocclusive mesenteric infarction. *Surg Clin North Am*, 1974; 54: 689.

43 Moossa AR, Shackford S, Sise MJ. Acute intestinal ischaemia. In: Marston A, ed. *Vascular Disease of the Gut: Pathophysiology, Recognition and Management*. London: Edward Arnold, 1986: 64.

44 Haglund V, Hulten L, Asken C, Lundgren O. Mucosal lesions in the human small intestine in shock. *Gut*, 1976; 16: 979.

45 Marston A. The bowel in shock. *Lancet*, 1962; ii: 365.

46 Thomas GR, Thibodaux H. Transforming growth factor-beta 1 inhibits postischemic increases in splanchnic vascular resistance. *Biotechnol Ther*, 1992; 3: 91.

47 Fogarty TJ, Fletcher WS. Non-occlusive mesenteric ischaemia. *Am J Surg*, 1965; 111: 130.

48 Schwartz CJ, Acheson ED, Webster CV. Chronic mid gut ischaemia with steatorrhoea in polycythemia rubra vera. *Am J Med*, 1961; 32: 950.

49 Schutz A, Eichinger W, Breuer M, Gansera B, Kemkes BM. Acute mesenteric ischemia after open heart surgery. *Angiology*, 1998; 49: 267.

50 Whitehead R. Ischaemic enterocolitis an expression of the intravascular coagulation syndrome. *Gut*, 1971; 12: 912.

51 Polansky BJ, Berger RL, Byrne JJ. Massive nonocclusive intestinal infarction associated with digitalis toxicity. *Circulation (Suppl)*, 1964; 30: 141.

52 Ming SC. Haemorrhagic necrosis of the gastrointestinal tract and its relation to cardiovascular status. *Circulation*, 1965; 32: 332.

53 Drucker WR, Davies JH, Holden WD, Reagan JR. Haemorrhagic necrosis of the intestine. *Arch Surg*, 1964; 89: 42.

54 Freiman DG. Haemorrhagic necrosis of the gastrointestinal tract. *Circulation*, 1965; 32: 329.

55 Kay AW, Richards RL, Watson AJ. Acute necrotizing (pseudomembranous) enterocolitis. *Br J Surg*, 1958; 46: 45.

56 Wiklander O. Phlegmonous or necrotizing enterocolitis. *Acta Chir Scand Suppl*, 1964: 328.

57 Mizrahi A, Barlow O, Berdon W, Bland WA, Silverman WA. Necrotising enterocolitis in premature infants. *J Paediatr*, 1965; 66: 697.

58 Tanner NC, Hardy KJ. Acute necrotizing enterocolitis. *Br J Surg*, 1968; 55: 381.

59 Killingback MJ, Williams KL. Necrotising colitis. *Br J Surg*, 1961; 49: 175.

60 Carroll PT, Van Der Hoeven LM. Pseudomembranous enterocolitis. *Dis Colon Rectum*, 1959; 2: 264.

61 Goulston SJM, McGovern VJ. Pseudomembranous enterocolitis. *Dis Colon Rectum*, 1965; 2: 264.

62 McGovern VJ, Goulston SJM. Ischaemic enterocolitis. *Gut*, 1965; 6: 213.

63 Marston A, Clarke JMF, Garcia S, Miller AL. Intestinal function and intestinal blood supply: a 20 year surgical study. *Gut*, 1985; 26: 656.

64 Stewart JOR. Portal gas embolism: a prognostic sign in mesenteric vascular occlusion. *Br Med J*, 1963; i: 1328.

65 Windsor CWO. Ischaemic strictures of the small bowel. *Clin Gastroenterol*, 1972; 1 (3): 707.

66 Davies DR, Brightmore T. Idiopathic and drug induced ulceration of the small intestine. *Br J Surg*, 1970; 57: 134.

67 Kay CR. The Royal College of General Practitioners Oral Contraception Study: some recent observations. *Clin Obstet Gynaecol*, 1984; II (30): 759.

68 Lang J, Price AB, Levi AJ, Burke M, Gumpel JM, Bjarnason I. Diaphragm disease: pathology of the small intestine induced by non-steroidal anti-inflammatory drugs. *J Clin Pathol*, 1988; 41: 516.

69 Berthrong M, Fajardo LF. Radiation injury in surgical pathology. Part II, Alimentary Tract. *Am J Surg Pathol*, 1981; 5: 163.

70 Brookes VS, Windsor CWO, Howell JS. Ischaemic ulceration with stricture formation in the small bowel. *Br J Surg*, 1966; 53: 583.

71 Boydstun JS, Gaffey TA, Bartholomew LG. Clinicopathologic study of non-specific ulcers of the small intestine. *JAMA*, 1981; 192: 763.

72 Darjee JR. Cholesterol embolism: the great masquerader. *South Med J*, 1979; 12: 174.

73 Blundell JW. Small bowel stricture secondary to multiple cholesterol emboli. *Histopathology*, 1988; 13: 459.

74 Mulliken JB, Marshall K, Bartlett MD. Small bowel obstruction secondary to atheromatous embolism. *Ann Surg*, 1971; 174: 145.

75 Rob C. Diseases of the coeliac and mesenteric arteries. *Surg Gynecol Obstet*, 1967; 124: 118.

76 Rob C. Stenosis and thrombosis of the coeliac and mesenteric arteries. *Am J Surg*, 1967; 114: 363.

77 Jamieson WG, Marchuk S, Rowsom J, Durand D. The early diagnosis of massive intestinal ischaemia. *Br J Surg*, 1982; 69: 952.

78 Cokkinis A. Intestinal ischaemia. *Proc R Soc Med*, 1961; 54: 354.

79 Berry CL, Fraser GC. The experimental production of colitis in the rabbit with particular reference to Hirschsprung's disease. *J Pediatr Surg*, 1968; 3: 36.

80 Teich S, Schisgall RM, Anderson KD. Ischemic enterocolitis as a complication of Hirschsprung's disease. *J Pediatr Surg*, 1986; 21: 143.

81 Coutinho HB, da Mota HC, Coutinho VB *et al*. Absence of lysozyme (muramidase) in the intestinal Paneth cells of newborn infants with necrotising enterocolitis. *J Clin Pathol*, 1998; 51: 512.

82 Butler T, Dahms B, Lindpainter K, Islam M, Azad MAK, Anton P. Segmental necrotizing enterocolitis: pathological and clinical features of 22 cases in Bangladesh. *Gut*, 1987; 28: 1433.

83 Hoang MP, Lee EL, Anand A. Histologic spectrum of arterial and arteriolar lesions in acute and chronic cocaine-induced mesenteric ischemia: report of three cases and literature review. *Am J Surg Pathol*, 1998; 22: 1404.

84 Freudenberger RS, Cappell MS, Hutt DA. Intestinal infarction after intravenous cocaine administration. *Ann Intern Med*, 1990; 113: 715.

85 Baker DR, Schradar WH, Hitchcock CR. Small bowel ulceration apparently associated with thiazide and potassium therapy. *JAMA*, 1964; 190: 586.

86 Sharefkin JB, Silen W. Diuretic agents. Inciting factors in non-occlusive mesenteric infarction. *JAMA*, 1974; 229: 1451.

87 Kradjian RM. Ischaemic stenosis of small intestine. *Arch Surg*, 1965; 91: 829.

88 Boley SJ, Schultz S, Krieger H, Schwartz S, Elguezabal A, Allen AC. Evaluation of thiazides and potassium as a cause of small bowel ulcer. *JAMA*, 1965; 192: 763.

89 Lawrason FD, Alpert E, Mohr FL, McMahon FG. Ulcerative obstructive lesions of the small intestine. *JAMA*, 1965; 191: 641.

90 Wayte DM, Helwig EB. Small bowel ulceration—iatrogenic or multifactorial origin. *Am J Clin Pathol*, 1968; 49: 26.

91 Madhok R, Mackenzie JA, Lee FD, Bruckner FE, Terry TR, Sturrock RD. Small bowel ulceration in patients receiving non-steroidal anti-inflammatory drugs for rheumatoid arthritis. *Q J Med*, 1986; 255: 53.

92 Hoyle M, Kennedy A, Prior AL, Thomas GE. Small bowel ischaemia and infarction in young women taking oral contraceptives and progestational agents. *Br J Surg*, 1977; 64: 533.

93 Rose MB. Superior mesenteric vein thrombosis and oral contraceptive. *Postgrad Med J*, 1972; 48: 430.

94 Jennette JC, Falk RJ. Small-vessel vasculitis. *N Engl J Med*, 1997; 337: 1512.

95 Gross WL. Systemic necrotizing vasculitis. *Baillieres Clin Rheumatol*, 1997; 11: 259.

96 Ehrlich GE. Vasculitis in Behçet's disease. *Int Rev Immunol*, 1997; 14: 81.

97 Watts RA, Scott DG. Classification and epidemiology of the vasculitides. *Baillieres Clin Rheumatol*, 1997; 11: 191.

98 Camilleri M, Pusey CD, Chadwick VS, Rees AJ. Gastrointestinal manifestations of systemic vasculitis. *Q J Med*, 1983; 52: 141.

99 Scott DGI, Bacon PA, Elliott PJ, Tribe CR, Wallington TB. Systemic vasculitis in a District General Hospital 1972–1980: clinical and laboratory features, classification and prognosis of 80 cases. *Q J Med*, 1982; 51: 299.

100 Tribe CR, Scott DGI, Bacon PI. Rectal biopsy in the diagnosis of systemic vasculitis. *J Clin Pathol*, 1981; 34: 843.

101 Sanchez-Guerrero J, Gutierrez-Urena S, Vidaller A, Reyes E, Iglesias A, Alarcon-Segovia D. Vasculitis as a paraneoplastic syndrome. Report of 11 cases and review of the literature. *J Rheumatol*, 1990; 17: 1458.

102 Fisher RS, Myers AR. Progressive systemic sclerosis (scleroderma). In: Bouchier IAD, Allan RN, Hodgson HJF, Keighley MRB, eds. *Textbook of Gastroenterology*. London: Baillière Tindall, 1984: 642.

103 Baron M, Srolovitz H. Colonic telangiectasias in a patient with progressive systemic sclerosis. *Arthritis Rheum*, 1986; 29: 282.

104 Rosekrans PC, de Rooy DJ, Bosman FT, Eulderink F, Cats A. Gastrointestinal telangiectasia as a cause of severe blood loss in systemic sclerosis. *Endoscopy*, 1980; 12: 200.
105 Meihoff WE, Hirschfield JS, Kern F. Small intestinal scleroderma with malabsorption and pneumatosis cystoides intestinalis. *JAMA*, 1968; 204: 854.
106 Burt RW, Berenson MM, Samuelson CO, Cathey WJ. Rheumatoid vasculitis of the colon presenting as pancolitis. *Dig Dis Sci*, 1983; 28: 183.
107 Lindsay MK, Tavadia HB, Whyte AS, Lee P, Webb J. Acute abdomen in rheumatoid arthritis due to necrotizing arteritis. *Br Med J*, 1973; ii: 592.
108 Bienenstock H, Minick R, Rogoff B. Mesenteric arteritis and intestinal infarction in rheumatoid disease. *Arch Intern Med*, 1967; 119: 359.
109 Joviasis A, Kraag G. Acute gastrointestinal manifestations of systemic lupus erythematosus. *Can J Surg*, 1987; 30: 185.
110 Hoffman BI, Katz WA. The gastrointestinal manifestations of systemic lupus erythematosus: a review of the literature. *Semin Arthritis Rheum*, 1980; 9: 237.
111 Prouse PJ, Thompson EM, Gumpel JM. Systemic lupus erythematosus and abdominal pain. *Br J Rheumatol*, 1983; 22: 172.
112 Helliwell TR, Flook D, Whitworth J, Day DW. Arteritis and venulitis in systemic lupus erythematosus resulting in massive lower intestinal haemorrhage. *Histopathology*, 1985; 9: 1103.
113 Weiser MM, Andres GA, Brentjens JR, Evans JT, Rachlin M. Systemic lupus erythematosus and intestinal venulitis. *Gastroenterology*, 1981; 81: 570.
114 Stoddard CJ, Kay PH, Simms JM, Kennedy A, Hugher P. Acute abdominal complications of systemic lupus erythematosus. *Br J Surg*, 1978; 65: 625.
115 Papa MZ, Shiloni E, McDonald HD. Total colonic necrosis: a catastrophic complication of systemic lupus erythematosus. *Dis Colon Rectum*, 1986; 29: 576.
116 Feldt RH, Sholder GB. The gastrointestinal manifestations of anaphylactoid purpura in children. *Staff Meet Mayo Clin*, 1962; 37: 465.
117 Martinez-Frontanilla LA, Haase GM, Ernster JA, Bailey WC. Surgical complications of Henoch–Schonlein purpura. *J Pediatr Surg*, 1984; 19: 434.
118 Lombard KA, Shah PC, Thrasher TV, Grill BB. Ileal stricture as a late complication of Henoch–Schonlein purpura. *Paediatrics*, 1986; 77: 396.
119 Savage COS, Lockwood CM, Hodgson HJF. Vasculitic and connective tissue disorders. In: Bouchier IAD, Allan RN, Hodgson HJF, Keighley MRB, eds. *Textbook of Gastroenterology*. London: Baillière-Tindall, 1984: 652.
120 Carron DB, Douglas AP. Steatorrhoea in vascular insufficiency of the small intestine. *Q J Med*, 1965; 34: 331.
121 Roikjaer O. Perforation and necrosis of the colon complicating polyarteritis nodosa. *Acta Chir Scand*, 1987; 153: 385.
122 Wood MK, Read DR, Kraft AR, Barreta TM. A rare cause of ischaemic colitis. Polyarteritis nodosa. *Dis Colon Rectum*, 1979; 22: 428.
123 Aboumrad MH, Fine G, Horn RC Jr. Intimal hyperplasia of small mesenteric arteries. *Arch Pathol*, 1963; 75: 196.
124 Chumley LC, Harrison EG, de Rernee RA. Allergic granulomatosis and angiitis (Churg–Strauss syndrome). Report and analysis of 30 cases. *Mayo Clin Proc*, 1977; 52: 477.
125 Modigliani R, Muschart J, Galian A, Clauval JP, Piel-Desriusseaux JL. Allergic granulomatous vasculitis (Churg–Strauss syndrome). Report of a case with widespread digestive involvement. *Dig Dis Sci*, 1981; 26: 264.
126 Deitch EA, Sikkema WW. Intestinal manifestations of Buerger's disease: case report and literature review. *Am Surg*, 1981; 47: 326.
127 Rosen N, Sommer I, Knobel B. Intestinal Buerger's disease. *Arch Pathol Lab Med*, 1985; 109: 962.
128 Strole WG Jr, Clark WH Jr, Isselbacher KJ. Progressive arterial occlusive disease (Kohlmeier–Degos). *N Engl J Med*, 1967; 276: 195.
129 Beighton PH, Murdoch JL, Votteler T. Gastrointestinal complications of the Ehlers–Danlos syndrome. *Gut*, 1969; 10: 1004.
130 Gertsch P, Loup PW, Lochman A, Anani P. Changing patterns in the vascular form of Ehlers–Danlos syndrome. *Arch Surg*, 1986; 121: 1061.
131 Sykes EM Jr. Colon perforation in Ehlers–Danlos syndrome. *Am J Surg*, 1984; 147: 410.
132 Silva R, Coghill TH, Hansbrough JF, Zapata-Sirvent RL, Harrington DS. Intestinal perforation and vascular rupture in Ehlers–Danlos syndrome. *Int Surg*, 1986; 71: 48.
133 Beamish RE, McCreath ND. Intestinal obstruction complicating anticoagulant therapy. *Lancet*, 1961; ii: 390.
134 Levine S, Whelan TJ Jr. Small bowel infarction due to intramural haematoma during anticoagulant therapy. *Arch Surg*, 1967; 95: 245.
135 Ben-Baruch D, Powsner E, Cohen M, Dintsman M. Intramural haematoma of duodenum following endoscopic intestinal biopsy. *J Pediatr Surg*, 1987; 22: 1009.
136 Bailey WC, Akers DR. Traumatic intramural hematoma of the duodenum in children: a report of 5 cases. *Am J Surg*, 1965; 110: 695.
137 Moore SW, Erlandson ME. Intramural hematoma of the duodenum. *Ann Surg*, 1963; 157: 573.
138 Golding MR, de Jong Parker JW. Intramural hematoma of the duodenum. *Ann Surg*, 1963; 157: 573.
139 DeBakey ME, Cooley DA. Successful resection of mycotic aneurysm of superior mesenteric artery. *Ann Surg*, 1953; 19: 202.
140 Buchman RJ, Martin GW. Management of mycotic aneurysm of the superior mesenteric artery. *Ann Surg*, 1962; 155: 620.
141 Saraga EP, Costa J. Idiopathic entero-colic lymphocytic phlebitis: a cause of ischemic intestinal necrosis. *Am J Surg Pathol*, 1989; 13: 303.
142 Flaherty MJ, Lie JT, Haggitt RC. Mesenteric inflammatory veno-occlusive disease: a seldom recognized cause of intestinal ischemia. *Am J Surg Pathol*, 1994; 18: 779.

24 Epithelial tumours of the small intestine

Introduction

Epithelial tumours are rare in the small intestine in comparison with the large bowel. In an analysis of data from multiple tumour registries in the USA [1], small bowel tumours occurred with an average annual incidence rate of 9.9 per million people. Carcinoid tumours and adenocarcinomas were the most common histological subtypes, with average annual incidence rates of 3.8 and 3.7 per million people, respectively, followed by sarcomas (1.3 per million people) and lymphomas (1.1 per million people). One study [2] found that adenocarcinoma and carcinoid tumour is four times as common in cigarette smokers as in non-smokers. There was also occasionally a history of previous cholecystectomy in patients with both of these tumours but not with lymphoma or sarcoma. There is good evidence for an adenoma–carcinoma sequence in the small bowel, just as in the large intestine [3]. Although carcinoid tumours, lymphomas and sarcomas occur most frequently in the distal small bowel and least frequently in the duodenum, the opposite is true for adenomas and adenocarcinomas [4]. Adenomas are present in the duodenum in over 90% of patients with familial adenomatous polyposis [5] and there is a high incidence of duodenal adenocarcinomas in these individuals. It is remarkable that the relatively small area of the duodenum is the site for more epithelial neoplasms than the whole of the rest of the small bowel. There is a phenomenon of clustering around the influx of undiluted bile from the ampulla of Vater [6] and it appears that bile salts act as tumour-promoting agents, especially in conjunction with acid from the stomach. It has been shown that bile is capable of inducing the formation of DNA adducts in the duodenal epithelium [7]. Despite the influence of bile, DNA adducts are reported to be found far less frequently in the epithelium of the small bowel than in the large bowel, suggesting that the small intestinal epithelium is less susceptible to the effects of environmental carcinogens [8]. A possible explanation for this is that, in contrast to the large bowel, the apoptosis-suppressing protein bcl-2 is not expressed in the epithelium of the normal small intestinal mucosa [9] so that cells affected by genotoxic damage can be eliminated from the small intestinal epithelium by unrestrained apoptosis.

Adenomas

Adenomas are found more frequently in the duodenum, especially the periampullary area, than in the more distal small bowel [10]. Although sporadic lesions are rare in the duodenum, in familial adenomatous polyposis they are found in most adult patients [5]. As in the large bowel, they take the form of tubular, tubulovillous or villous lesions [11]. Villous adenomas have been more frequently reported in the literature [12–16], but experience with familial adenomatous polyposis [5] suggests that, as in the colon and rectum, a tubular growth pattern is more common. It is likely that the vast majority of small intestinal adenomas are never clinically discovered and that those that have been documented are the ones large enough to cause symptoms by obstructing the lumen [10]. Thus there has probably been a reporting bias towards large and villous adenomas, which are relatively more frequently moderately or severely dysplastic. The true picture awaits systematic study of the small bowel at autopsy.

Most small bowel adenomas are single, though occasional multiple examples have been described. They can be pedunculated (Fig. 24.1) or sessile (when they may surround the bowel lumen) and can bleed and cause obstruction [12]. Macroscopically small bowel adenomas have a coarse lobulated appearance rather like their large bowel counterparts, though some of the duodenal ones may have a more villous appearance [13–15].

Microscopically they are separable into tubular, tubulovillous and villous adenomas. In one thoroughly investigated duodenal example, cells showing absorptive, goblet, endocrine and Paneth cell differentiation were all present [16]. There is no doubt that many of these adenomas have malig-

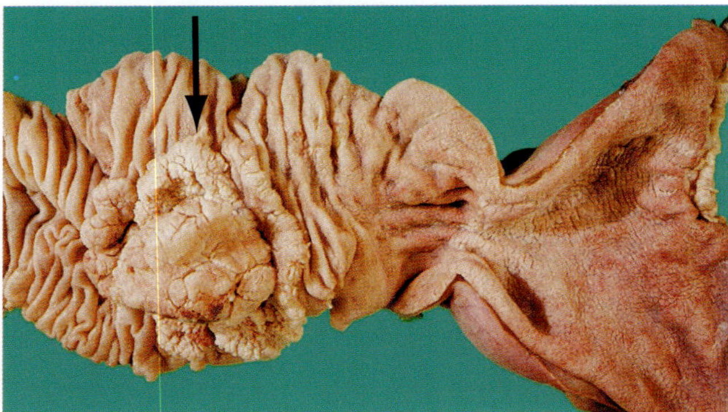

Fig. 24.1 Adenomatous polyp arising at the duodenal papilla. The lobulated surface is typical. The stomach and pylorus are indicated by the arrowhead and arrow, respectively.

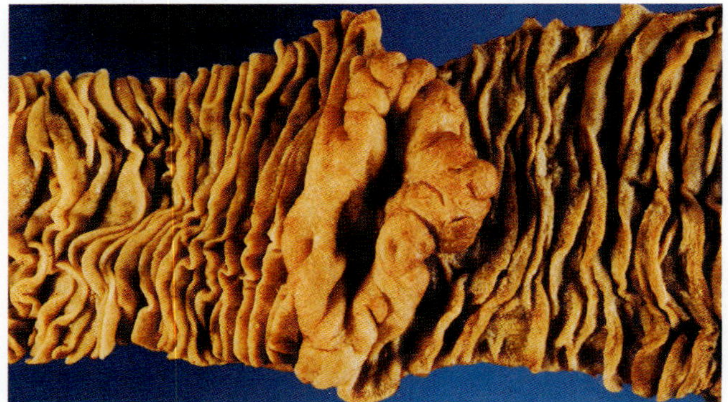

(a)

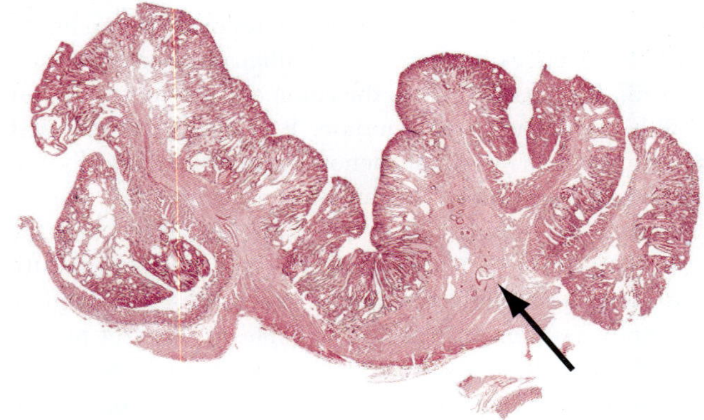

(b)

Fig. 24.2 (a) A tubular adenoma of ileum, with adenocarcinoma arising in its centre, which is depressed. (b) Section of the tubular adenoma in (a), with the focus of adenocarcinoma arrowed.

nant potential [11,15,17], and in many one can find small zones of undoubted carcinoma (Fig. 24.2a,b).

Adenomas in familial adenomatous polyposis

The majority of adult patients with familial adenomatous

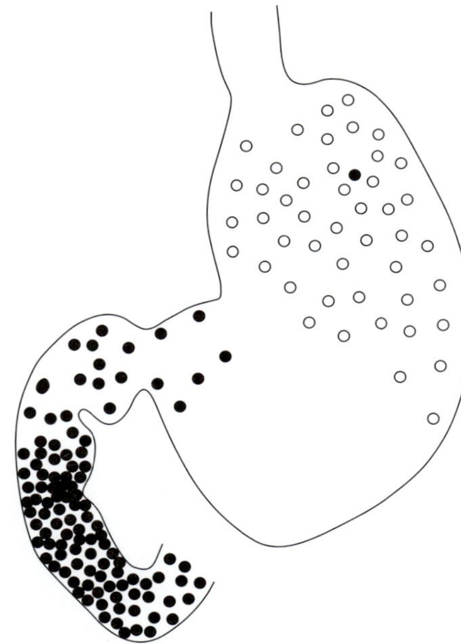

Fig. 24.3 Diagram illustrating the frequency of occurrence of duodenal and gastric adenomas (solid circles) in a series of 102 patients with FAP. the open circles represent fundic gland polyps.

polyposis (FAP) have multiple adenomas in the duodenal mucosa [5]. The lesions tend to be clustered around the duodenal papilla and frequently involve the ampulla of Vater (Fig. 24.3). The mucosa can be carpeted with adenomas but they are rarely pedunculated and may only be discovered as a result of random biopsy of endoscopically normal mucosa in this region. They are usually only a few millimetres in diameter and are composed of dysplastic epithelium, most frequently with a tubular pattern (Fig. 24.4). The underlying villous architecture of the duodenal mucosa may confound the tubular nature of small lesions but 10% of these lesions are genuinely villous in structure and 20% are tubulovillous [18]. The dysplasia in most of these lesions is only of mild grade but occasionally there is moderate or even severe dysplasia, as in adenomas of the large bowel (see p. 559). Given the evidence that periampullary adenocarcinoma arises as the result of an adenoma–carcinoma sequence [3], duodenal adenomas pose a difficult management problem in patients with FAP [19]. Their complete removal by anything less than major surgery is impracticable [20] and the risk of duodenal cancer relative to the risk of surgery is small (3.1% of all individuals with FAP developed duodenal cancer in one series) [21]. Spigelman has devised a staging scheme for classification of duodenal adenomas in accordance with their malignant potential [22], shown in Table 24.1. This scheme provides useful guidelines to assist in the clinical management of these lesions. Stage IV disease is only found in about 10% of patients with FAP [18] but should be regarded as a marker of high risk for development of duodenal carcinoma.

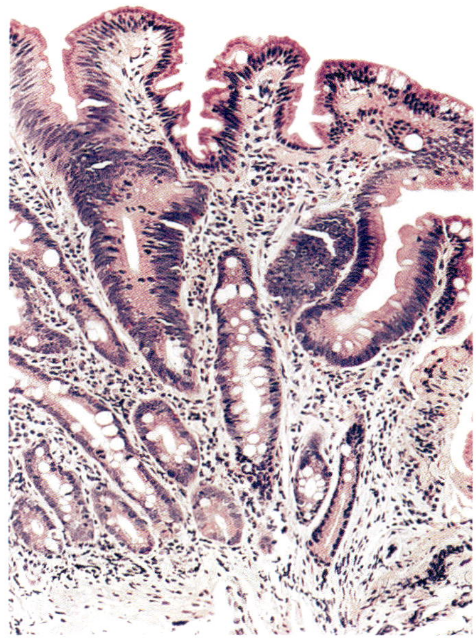

Fig. 24.4 A small adenoma of duodenal mucosa from a patient with FAP. Although probably tubular, there is ambivalence of structure due to the villous nature of the normal mucosa.

Table 24.1 Staging system for severity of duodenal polyposis in FAP. From [22].

Duodenal disease grading: points			
	1	2	3
Polyp number	1–4	5–20	> 20
Polyp size (mm)	1–4	5–10	> 10
Histology	Tubular	Tubulovillous	Villous
Dysplasia	Mild	Moderate	Severe
Stages			
O	0 points		
I	1–4 points		
II	5–6 points		
III	7–8 points		
IV	9–12 points		

Patients with FAP also have an increased risk of developing adenomas in the ileum, the incidence being between 10 and 21% [23].

Adenocarcinoma

Incidence

It has been pointed out that although the small intestine contributes 75% of the mucosal surface area of the gastrointestinal tract, malignancies of the large bowel are 50 times more numerous [2] and the small bowel is the site of only 1% of all gastrointestinal carcinomas [24,25]. Probably for similar reasons to those responsible for the large size, frequent villous architecture and severe dysplasia displayed by small intestinal adenomas described above, adenocarcinoma is clinically more frequent in the small bowel than symptomatic sporadic adenoma. Baillie and Williams [26] found that only 14% of small intestinal tumours are benign. Adenocarcinomas of small bowel are most frequent in the duodenum and are increasingly less common at more distal sites [4]. They are usually single, and reports of multiple small intestinal carcinomas are a rarity [27,28]. On the other hand, small intestinal carcinoma is often associated with a second (synchronous or metachronous) primary malignancy at another site, occurring in 20% of cases in one series [24]. The age incidence is similar to or slightly later than for large bowel adenocarcinoma, the average age at presentation in one series being 72 years (range 62–78). Men are eight times more likely to be affected than women [26].

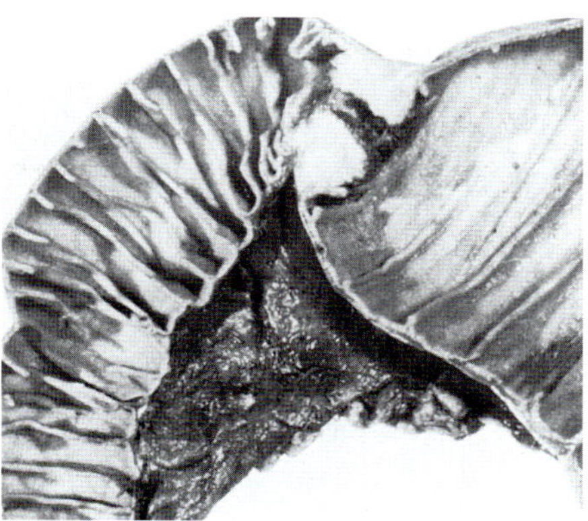

Fig. 24.5 A stenosing carcinoma of the jejunum which presented with obstructive symptoms.

Gross appearances

Most small intestinal carcinomas are annular and constricting (Fig. 24.5), although a minority are polypoid or fungating.

Histology

Microscopically, small intestinal adenocarcinomas closely resemble adenocarcinomas of the large bowel (Fig. 24.6), the majority being moderately differentiated and some showing mucinous characteristics. Despite their differentiation, most of these tumours are at an advanced stage of development when clinically diagnosed and prognosis is poor. This is probably related to the liquid content of the small bowel, so that signs of obstruction, a common presenting feature in large bowel carcinomas, are late or absent with small bowel tumours. Spread is to local lymph nodes, and transperitoneal spread with seedling growth on the peritoneal surface of the bowel is not uncommon.

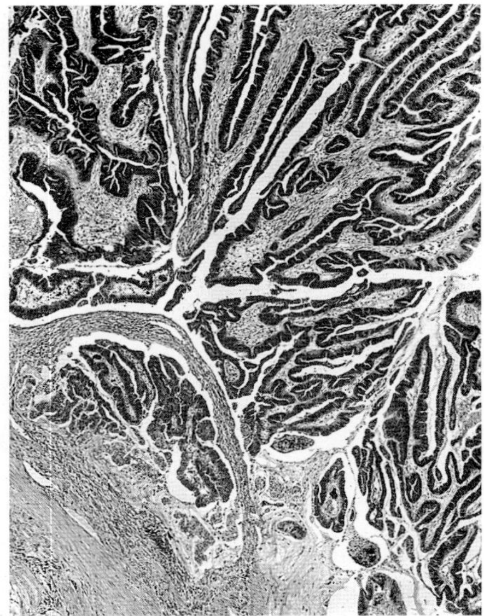

Fig. 24.6 Adenocarcinoma of jejunum arising in a pre-existing adenoma. The upper and right-hand aspects of the section show an adenoma with a villous pattern; in the lower aspect there is carcinomatous change with some mucus secretion, part of which lies deep to the muscularis mucosae.

Staging

In several series, 5-year survival rates of only 20–25% are recorded [4,29]. A Dutch study showed that, although prognosis could not be predicted by extent of local spread as classified by the TNM system, when tumour was present in mesenteric lymph nodes the prognosis was particularly poor, not one out of 64 patients surviving 5 years [29]. In the special case of adenocarcinoma of the ampulla of Vater, for early tumours, when the growth is confined to the wall of the ampulla or common bile duct or immediately surrounding tissues and does not involve the pancreatic parenchyma or lymph nodes, unless poorly differentiated, the prognosis is excellent [30]. A staging system has been devised to take the above factors into account (Fig. 24.7).

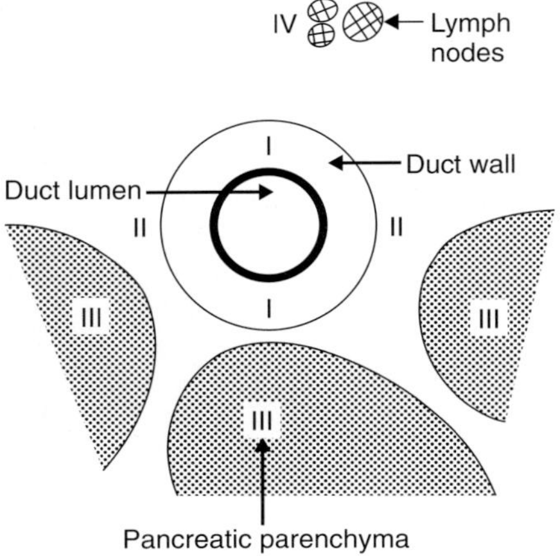

Fig. 24.7 Diagram of staging of carcinoma of the ampulla of Vater. Addition of the staging values to the grading score provides a precise prognostic index (from [30]).

Precancerous conditions

The incidence of periampullary cancer in FAP is estimated to be 100 times that of the rest of the population [21]. The risk in Crohn's disease has already been mentioned. Carcinoma should be suspected in a patient with long-standing Crohn's disease who has a sudden worsening of obstructive symptoms [31]. Tumours occur in diseased zones such as strictures and care on the part of the surgeon is needed to avoid missing a diffuse stricturing tumour at stricturoplasty. Because these tumours arise in a background of abnormal mucosa and can be well differentiated their diagnosis may also pose a problem for the pathologist. The ileum is most frequently involved and coexisting epithelial dysplasia may be present [32,33]. Carcinoma can also arise in bypassed segments [34] and even uninvolved regions of small bowel are not immune.

Small intestinal adenocarcinoma is also well recognized in association with long-standing gluten enteropathy and with idiopathic steatorrhoea, particularly in patients in whom the mucosa remains flat even after appropriate dietary treatment [35].

Complications

Few complications are recorded [36]; an interesting one is the unexplained coexistence of digital ischaemia [37]. Adherence to another part of the small or large bowel with the formation of an internal fistula can occur.

Endocrine cell tumours

The endocrine cells dispersed within the epithelium of the small intestinal mucosa constitute a major part of the diffuse endocrine system that is distributed throughout the endodermally derived mucosa and together forms the largest endocrine organ in the body. The cells contributing to this system are functionally diverse, synthesizing a variety of peptide hormone products. Their salient features are described in Chapter 18. Tumours of the diffuse endocrine system have been variously termed 'carcinoid tumours' or 'endocrine tumours', and reflect this diversity. The generic term, neuroendocrine tumours, embraces the heterogeneous collection of tumours defined by their predominantly diffuse endocrine cell differentiation. The most common differentiated tumour within this group is the enterochromaffin cell (EC-cell) tumour, traditionally known as the classical carcinoid tumour. Less common are G-cell tumours (gastrinomas), D-cell tumours (somatostatinomas) and L-cell tumours (non-argentaffin tumours that synthesize enteroglucagon and peptide YY and are mainly found in the mid- and hindgut). Occasionally one of the above tumours will be less well differentiated, but the archetypal poorly differentiated neuroendocrine tumour is the small cell ('oat cell') carcinoma. Subdivision according to ontogeny (foregut, midgut and hindgut) [38] provides a theoretical basis for classification. Foregut carcinoids include those of the bronchus, stomach, pancreas and duodenum.

Duodenal endocrine tumours

Only 2% of neuroendocrine tumours arise in the duodenum, but those that do are unusual and present fascinating diagnostic challenges to the histopathologist. Unusual morphological features and unusual histochemical reactions and specific clinical syndromes, while fascinating, can cause diagnostic confusion unless properly understood. There are five groups: gastrin-containing G-cell tumours, somatostatin-containing D-cell tumours, other well differentiated endocrine cell tumours, the gangliocytic paraganglioma and poorly differentiated endocrine carcinomas/small cell carcinomas. Gangliocytic paragangliomas are always benign but the behaviour of all the other tumours depends on their size, extent of spread in the duodenal wall, vascular invasion and hormonal function, which may result in a clinical peptide hormone hypersecretion syndrome.

Based on proposals by Burke and colleagues [39], Capella and colleagues [40] and Kloppel and colleagues [41], Table 24.2 gives guidelines on the behaviour of these tumours.

G-cell tumours

Approximately 60% of duodenal endocrine tumours are G-cell tumours (gastrinomas), more frequent in men. They are slow growing, low-grade neoplasms that usually measure less than 1 cm and can be confused endoscopically with Brunner's gland hamartomas or gastric heterotopia. A 2-cm peri-ampullary tumour reported to obstruct the bile duct [42] is exceptional.

Approximately one-third of duodenal G-cell tumours, and particularly those occurring distal to the duodenal bulb, are functioning neoplasms, giving rise to the Zollinger–Ellison syndrome (ZES). Moreover, in about 40% of patients with sporadic (non-inherited) ZES the causative tumour is located in the duodenum (the remainder are pancreatic). Systemic manifestations do not correlate well with tumour size and some patients with ZES have minute duodenal gastrinomas as small as 2 mm in diameter that can be easily overlooked at endoscopy or surgical exploration [43,44]. Moreover, many of these small functioning tumours have already metastasized to the regional lymph nodes at diagnosis. The volume of such metastatic tumours is often much larger than that of the duodenal primary. Despite this, duodenal tumours causing ZES usually follow an indolent course with generally good outcome after surgery [45]. Even distant spread to the liver or elsewhere, which is uncommon and occurs late in the course of the disease, may be associated with long survival, provided that the effects of hypergastrinaemia are controlled by gastric acid suppression and therapeutic somatostatin analogues. Histological features are generally not useful in predicting which tumours are likely to be metastatic, but one study has suggested that flow cytometric identification of tumour cell aneuploidy might be valuable [46]. Non-functioning sporadic G-cell tumours, by contrast, are usually small, benign-behaving lesions in the bulbar (first) part of the duodenum; they are said to occur in much older individuals (median age 66 years compared with 36 years for functioning tumours in one study) [47]. The rare cases that measure more than 2 cm in diameter and invade the muscularis propria have metastatic potential [39] (Table 24.2).

Multiple small gastrin-producing carcinoids may be found in the proximal duodenum of up to 90% of patients with multiple endocrine neoplasia type I (MEN-I) [48,49]. More than 60% of individuals affected by this autosomal dominant condition have hypergastrinaemia or a full-blown ZES. This was previously thought to be the result of gastrin secretion from one or more of the pancreatic endocrine cell tumours that occur in MEN-I. However, it is now apparent that one or more minute duodenal gastrin-secreting tumours are responsible. These often measure less than 5 mm in diameter (Fig. 24.8) [48], and are too small to be identified endoscopically unless random biopsies of the duodenal bulb are taken. At least some appear to arise in a background of duodenal mucosal endocrine cell hyperplasia, allowing a spectrum to be recognized from hyperplasia through multiple intramucosal microcarcinoids to macroscopic infiltrative tumours [49]. Recognition of these tiny lesions, and their endoscopic or surgical extirpation, is important in the clinical management of ZES in MEN-I patients.

Table 24.2 Prognostic classification of duodenal endocrine cell tumours (from [40] and [41]).

Benign
Non-functioning well differentiated endocrine cell tumour measuring up to 1 cm within the mucosa/submucosa and without angioinvasion
Gangliocytic paraganglioma, any size
Benign or low-grade malignant
Non-functioning well differentiated tumour within the mucosa/submucosa measuring > 1–2 cm without angioinvasion OR up to 2 cm with angioinvasion
Low-grade malignant
Non-functioning well differentiated tumour measuring > 2 cm or extending beyond submucosa
Functioning well differentiated tumour of any size and extent
High-grade malignant
Functioning or non-functioning poorly differentiated intermediate or small cell carcinoma

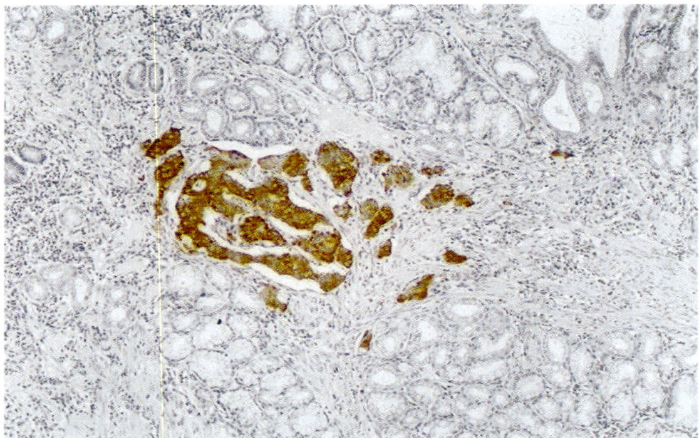

Fig. 24.8 Microscopic duodenal G-cell tumour in a patient with Zollinger–Ellison syndrome and type I multiple endocrine neoplasia. No macroscopic abnormality was visible. Gastrin immunostaining.

Microscopically, duodenal G-cell tumours are infiltrative neoplasms that are usually composed of trabeculae or acini of uniform cells separated by a delicate and vascular stroma that allows them to be easily recognized as endocrine cell tumours (Fig. 24.9). Necrosis is virtually never seen. The tumour cells have round nuclei containing stippled chromatin and inconspicuous nucleoli, few or no mitoses, and lightly eosinophilic or amphophilic cytoplasm in which argyrophil peptide hormone granules can usually be demonstrated by the Grimelius or Churukian–Schenk silver impregnation techniques and by immunocytochemistry for chromogranin and gastrin [50,49]. Tumour cells containing other peptide hormones, including somatostatin, calcitonin, insulin, pancreatic polypeptide, cholecystokinin, vasoactive intestinal polypeptide (VIP), serotonin, substance P and peptide YY, are frequently present as minority components [48,49,51]. Sometimes stromal deposits of amyloid may be present.

D-cell tumours

These somatostatin-containing tumours make up approximately 15–20% of duodenal endocrine cell neoplasms. They occur almost exclusively at or around the ampulla of Vater and local effects, notably obstructive jaundice, pancreatitis or haemorrhage, are responsible for the clinical presentation. Systemic manifestations attributable to somatostatin hypersecretion have not been described [39], suggesting that the tumours are usually non-functioning, although a number of reported patients have had either gallstones or diabetes. Nevertheless, in one published case, a diabetic with gallstones, removal of the tumour was followed by correction of the abnormal glucose tolerance [52] and in another, also presenting with gallstones and glucose intolerance, elevated blood somatostatin levels returned to normal after surgical excision [53].

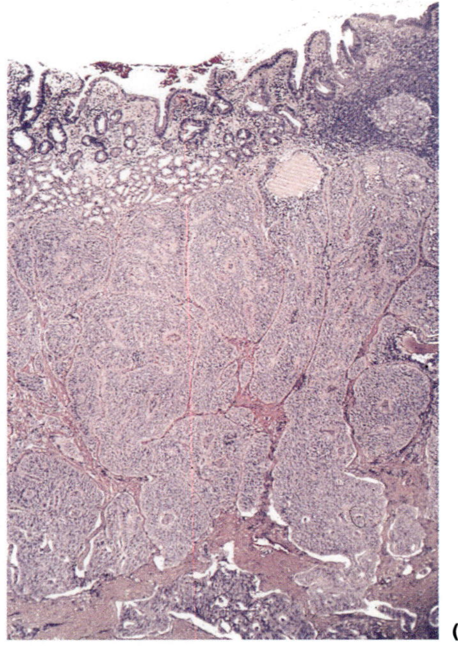

(a)

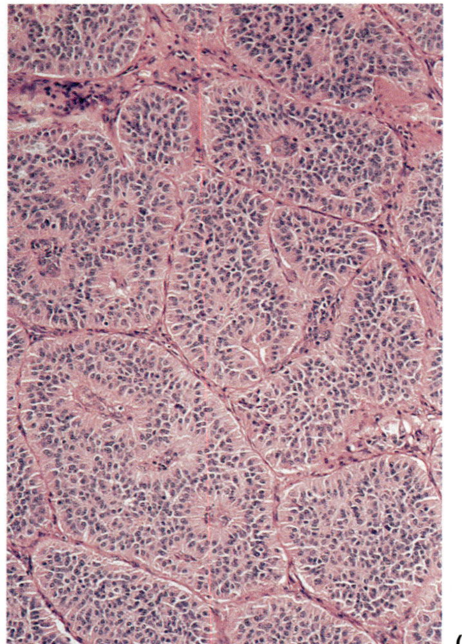

(b)

Fig. 24.9 Duodenal G-cell tumour. (a) Low-power view showing a well differentiated endocrine cell neoplasm with a mixed trabecular and acinar architecture. (b) Higher power shows regular tumour cells with granular eosinophilic cytoplasm that is most abundant at the periphery of the cellular aggregates, a typical feature of gastrointestinal endocrine neoplasms.

An association with type 1 neurofibromatosis (NF-1, von Recklinghausen's disease) is well established [54], and in one published series 50% of patients with duodenal D-cell tumours suffered from this condition [55]. Phaeochromocytoma has also been described in such patients, occurring in six of 27 cases in one literature review, raising the possibility that NF-1 patients with duodenal D-cell tumours have a special propensity for developing this neoplasm [56]. However, there is as yet no information on the molecular genetic basis for these associations. While tumours in NF-1 patients do not arise in a background of overt duodenal or periampullary D-cell hyperplasia, one of the authors has seen one resection specimen from an NF-1 patient in which there were two independent D-cell tumours, one situated at the ampulla of Vater and the second at the duodenal opening of a separate accessory pancreatic duct. Another interesting facet is the coexistence of a duodenal D-cell tumour with an ampullary gangliocytic paraganglioma in an NF-1 patient [57].

Macroscopically, duodenal D-cell tumours are 1–2-cm homogeneous tan-coloured intramural ampullary or periampullary nodules [58,59], though larger polypoid or ulcerated lesions have been described [60]. Histologically, neoplastic glandular structures intermingle with the ducts and smooth muscle of the ampulla of Vater and extend into the mucosa and the wall of the duodenum (Fig. 24.10). The neoplastic glands are made up of uniform cuboidal or low columnar cells with abundant finely granular eosinophilic cytoplasm and small, basally located vesicular nuclei with small nucleoli. Mitotic figures are scanty. The glandular lumina frequently contain amorphous eosinophilic PAS-positive, diastase-resistant, material. Densely calcified, concentrically laminated psammoma bodies measuring 5–30 μm in diameter are sometimes present (Fig. 24.10) [49,58–61]. Confusion with adenocarcinoma is possible unless focal solid, acinar or even trabecular growth patterns, typical of conventional endocrine cell tumours, are seen. In purely glandular tumours, however, the diagnostic difficulty may be compounded by the fact that the tumour cells are usually neither argentaffin nor argyrophil with the routinely used silver impregnation techniques, including the Grimelius reaction. It is only the Hellerstrom–Hellman argyrophil technique that consistently gives positive results [55], in keeping with the presence of somatostatin within the cells. Immunocytochemistry resolves the difficulty, with positive staining for neurone-specific enolase or N-Cam (CD56), chromogranin A and synaptophysin, and specific staining for somatostatin (Fig. 24.10b). Unusually for endocrine cell tumours, there is binding for WGA and PNA lectins [62]. Occasional cells may also be reactive for calcitonin, insulin or gastrin, particularly in tumours not associated with NF-1 [55], but the majority of tumours contain somatostatin alone. Electron microscopy confirms the presence of dense core granules and may also demonstrate a microvillous border and glycocalyceal bodies at the luminal aspect of the cells [62].

It is important that glandular D-cell endocrine tumours are distinguished from adenocarcinoma of the periampullary region as the prognosis is completely different. Although metastasis to regional lymph nodes is recorded in approximately a quarter of D-cell tumours [56], usually from lesions larger than 2 cm [55], and liver metastasis has been described rarely [52], fatalities are rare and local resection is usually curative. Accordingly, most examples are classified (Table 24.2) as non-functioning well differentiated tumours of low-grade malignancy.

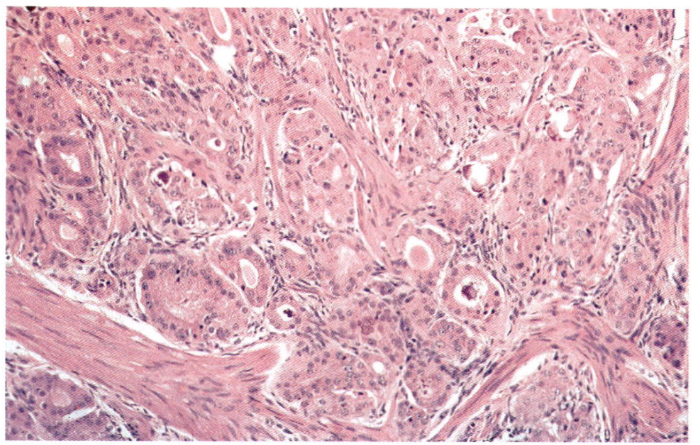

(a)

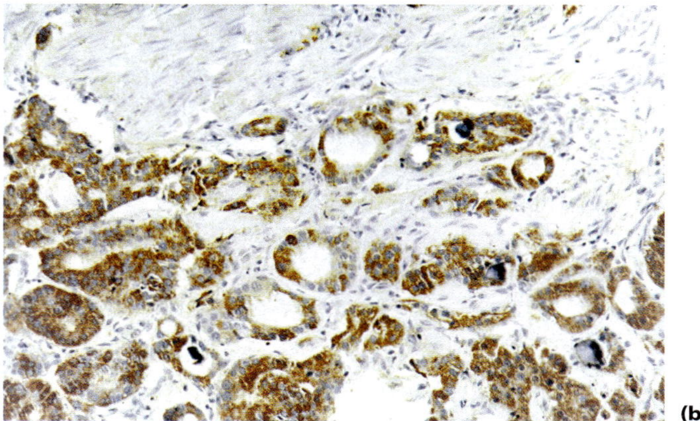

(b)

Fig. 24.10 Duodenal ampullary D-cell tumour with a prominent glandular architecture (a) and showing strong immunopositivity for somatostatin (b). Intraluminal calcified psammoma bodies are seen in both images.

Other differential diagnoses are Brunner's gland hamartoma and metastatic carcinoma. The ampullary or periampullary location, the infiltrative growth pattern, the psammoma bodies and the immunocytochemical characteristics allow Brunner's gland hamartoma to be excluded. Metastatic carcinomas should be distinguishable by their cytological atypia and mitotic activity. Those containing psammoma bodies usually show a papillary architecture, not seen in glandular carcinoids, their psammoma bodies are usually stromal rather than intraluminal and histochemical and ultrastructural features of endocrine cell tumour are lacking.

In contrast to the rarity of clinically apparent ampullary endocrine cell tumours, a meticulous histological study from Japan [63] has suggested that small asymptomatic aggregates or micronests of somatostatin and / or pancreatic polypeptide-containing endocrine cells may not be uncommon at the duodenal papilla. Their relationship to overt D-cell tumours is uncertain.

Other well differentiated endocrine (carcinoid) tumours

Rare duodenal endocrine cell tumours containing immunodetectable serotonin, calcitonin, cholecystokinin, VIP, bombesin or pancreatic polypeptide, but without a significant content of gastrin or somatostatin, may involve the ampulla or elsewhere [50,64]. Many are multihormonal. Those outside the ampulla are usually small and lack infiltrative growth [41] while those at the ampulla have produced clinical obstructive effects [64,65]. An example is the duodenal argentaffin EC-cell tumour containing serotonin, indistinguishable, both pathologically and in its behaviour, from the much commoner EC-cell tumour of the jejunum and ileum, described below. One such reported case gave rise to the carcinoid syndrome after metastasizing to the liver [66].

Also recorded are case reports of duodenal insulin- and glucagon-producing tumours. The former was a functioning, encapsulated 2-cm insulinoma in the wall of the third part of the duodenum that contained immunoreactive insulin and beta islet cell granules on electron microscopy [67]. Occasional somatostatin and glucagon-containing cells were also present. The lack of any mucosal component and the morphology of the lesion suggested that it might represent an 'ectopic' pancreatic islet cell tumour. The glucagon-producing tumour was a 1.4-cm intramural nodule that had a trabecular architecture and was associated with a 'glucagonoma syndrome' [68].

Gangliocytic paraganglioma

This rare benign tumour has been the subject of much interest because of its uncertain histogenesis, its peculiar histological appearance and its almost exclusive location in the periampullary portion of the duodenum [69–74]. There is no particular age or sex predilection; the tumour has been reported in patients ranging from 17 to 84 years of age, with only slightly more in men than in women. Gangliocytic paragangliomas are generally solitary, sporadic lesions, though multiple tumours have been recorded in one report [75]. Associations with neurofibromatosis, with [57] or without [76] a somatostatin-rich glandular duodenal carcinoid, and with duodenal adenocarcinoma [77,78], have been described.

Gangliocytic paragangliomas are sessile, or more usually polypoid, exophytic lesions that protrude into the lumen of the intestine. They can measure up to 7 cm in diameter and usually present with overt haemorrhage or anaemia. Less frequently they may give rise to clinical features of duodenal or biliary obstruction. Grossly, the tumour mass appears to be centred on the submucosa of the intestinal wall and is covered by mucosa that may be focally eroded or ulcerated. Although the tumours typically produce peptide hormones, these do not lead to a clinically overt endocrine hypersecretion syndrome.

Microscopically, gangliocytic paragangliomas appear as infiltrative lesions composed of an admixture of three cell types: spindle cells, ganglion cells and epithelioid cells with morphological and histochemical features of endocrine differentiation (Fig. 24.11) [69–74,77,78]. These three components may vary greatly in their relative proportions from case to case and in different areas of the same lesion.

The spindle cells, which usually form the major component of the tumour, have a neural phenotype. They have thin, elongated wavy nuclei resembling Schwann cells, show strong immunoreactivity for S-100 and neurofilament, and are arranged in broad intertwining fascicles that contain numerous argyrophil nerve fibres. Sometimes they envelop individual or aggregated clusters of the epithelioid cells and ganglion cells, in a manner resembling sustentacular cells.

The epithelioid cells are larger cells with finely granular eosinophilic or amphophilic cytoplasm and uniform ovoid

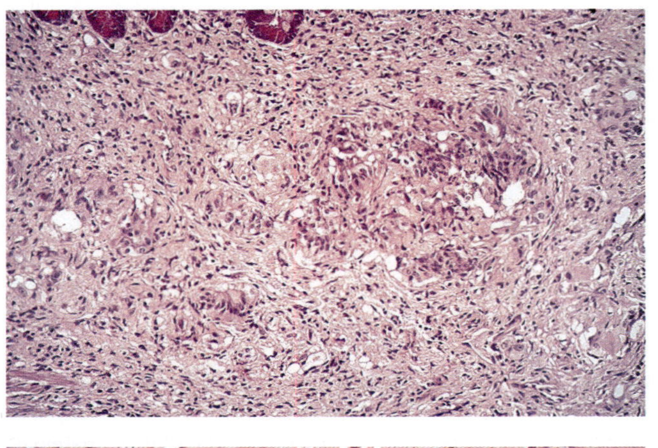
(a)

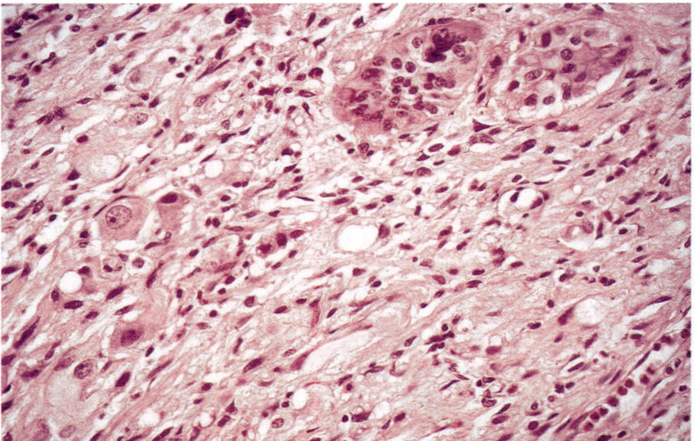
(b)

Fig. 24.11 Gangliocytic paraganglioma of the duodenum. (a) Low-power view showing a spindle cell lesion with loose collections of epithelioid endocrine cells. (b) Higher power shows more compact groups of endocrine cells (top right) and scattered ganglion-like cells (left) in a background of spindle cells of neural type.

nuclei with finely stippled chromatin that are arranged in solid nests or ribbons, or pseudoglandular or papillary structures (Fig. 24.11). Although undoubtedly endocrine in nature, being neurone-specific enolase positive and typically containing immunoreactive pancreatic polypeptide and somatostatin (and occasionally serotonin, glucagon, VIP, insulin, gastrin or calcitonin), they are non-argentaffin and frequently non-argyrophil, and only sometimes give a positive reaction on immunostaining for chromogranin. They usually stain for low and intermediate molecular weight cytokeratins [78] but they are S-100 protein negative. Amyloid may be found in relation to the epithelioid cells [73], and also concentrically laminated psammoma bodies, especially if the endocrine cells contain somatostatin [78].

The ganglion cells of gangliocytic paragangliomas are of two types [69]. Some appear as typical ganglion cells surrounded by satellite cells that are scattered singly in neural tissue and are synaptophysin or glial fibrillary acidic protein positive. Others are not so typical, appearing to form part of a morphological continuum with the epithelioid cells (though having more vesicular nuclei and rather more prominent nucleoli) and they may contain immunoreactive pancreatic polypeptide or somatostatin. They are often arranged in well demarcated nests, when the appearances can be highly reminiscent of the *Zellballen* of classical paragangliomas.

Mitotic figures and tumour necrosis are virtually never seen in gangliocytic paragangliomas, though a moderate degree of cytonuclear pleomorphism may be present. The three cellular components also intermingle with the normal smooth muscle and small pancreatic ducts at the ampulla to produce a very complex lesion. Despite their characteristic histological appearance, gangliocytic paragangliomas may be mistaken for carcinoids, smooth muscle tumours or gastrointestinal stromal tumours, nerve sheath tumours, adenocarcinomas and extra-adrenal paragangliomas. The triphasic pattern of gangliocytic paraganglioma is the main diagnostic aid to differentiation but this should be complemented by immunocytochemistry when there is any doubt about the diagnosis.

The histogenesis of these neoplasms requires further elucidation but two broad theories exist. The first proposes that they are derived from pancreatic maldevelopment [72] and this is corroborated by the frequent presence within the tumour of misplaced pancreatic tissue and the high incidence of immunoreactivity for pancreatic polypeptide and somatostatin. The alternative theory suggests a neoplastic lesion [73,74], with a complex triphasic growth pattern. Rare reports of local lymph node deposits composed of the endocrine cell component, either alone [79,80], or with sparse spindle cell or ganglion cell elements [69], support this. It is also remarkable to note that an identical tumour occurs in the cauda equina region [81] whose origin is difficult to explain on the basis of pancreatic maldevelopment.

Whatever their nature, duodenal gangliocytic paragangliomas have an excellent prognosis following complete surgical excision, even if there is lymph node metastasis. While local recurrence has been recorded 11 years after an initial excision [82], we are not aware of a recorded case that led to distant metastasis and the death of the patient.

Poorly differentiated endocrine carcinoma/small cell carcinoma

Four cases of this exceptionally rare and highly aggressive periampullary tumour have been recorded in the literature, all in men who presented with obstructive jaundice, abdominal pain and weight loss and who followed a rapidly fatal course surviving only 6 weeks to 17 months [83,84]. Grossly the tumours were relatively small (2–3-cm), focally ulcerated or protuberant lesions which on histological examination revealed sheets or nests of small, mitotically active cells with round or oval hyperchromatic nuclei and scanty cytoplasm, foci of necrosis and conspicuous vascular invasion. Malignant lymphoma was excluded by immunocytochemistry and metastatic tumours by clinical examination, radiology and, in one case, autopsy. The endocrine nature of the tumour cells was confirmed by immunoreactivity for neurone-specific enolase and Leu-7 and by the finding of cytoplasmic membrane-bound dense core endocrine granules on electron microscopy [84]. Low molecular weight cytokeratins were also present. A minority of cells in one case showed cytoplasmic argyrophilia and positive immunostaining for chromogranin and neurofilament [84]; VIP was demonstrated in liver metastases of a second [83].

Goblet cell carcinoid (mucinous carcinoid, adenocarcinoid, microglandular goblet cell carcinoma)

Two cases of this rare tumour have been reported within the duodenum, one at the ampulla of Vater [85] and one within the duodenal bulb [86]. Morphologically, these were small tumours that appeared identical histologically to their commoner counterparts in the appendix (see Chapter 31), being composed of small infiltrative nests of cytologically bland sialomucin-containing goblet cells, signet ring cells and argyrophil endocrine cells. By analogy with appendiceal goblet cell carcinoids their prognosis should be intermediate between those of well differentiated endocrine cell tumours and adenocarcinomas of the duodenum.

Composite carcinoid–adenocarcinoma

In this neoplasm islands of endocrine cell tumour are intermingled with neoplastic glandular structures typical of adenocarcinoma. We are aware of a single case report of such a tumour in the periampullary region of the duodenum [87]. It was an aggressive neoplasm that resulted in death from widespread metastases.

Endocrine cell tumours of the jejunum and ileum

Endocrine cell tumours of the jejunum and ileum account for about 30% of all gastrointestinal endocrine cell tumours [88] and for a large proportion of all neoplasms arising in the jejunum and ileum [89]. The great majority are serotonin- and substance P-containing EC-cell tumours, with the morphology and argentaffinity of classical carcinoids, and may give rise to the carcinoid syndrome following liver metastasis. The remainder comprise uncommon non-argentaffin, well differentiated tumours such as gastrin-containing G-cell tumours, L-cell tumours that contain enteroglucagon/PP/PYY, and the very rare, poorly differentiated/small cell endocrine carcinoma.

The main factors governing the behaviour of this group of tumours are their size, extent of infiltration into the intestinal wall, angioinvasion, and whether or not they are producing a clinical hypersecretion syndrome (i.e. functioning). Table 24.3 derived from Capella *et al.* [40] and Kloppel *et al.* [41] provides a useful classification.

EC-cell tumours (so-called classical carcinoids)

Serotonin-containing endocrine cell tumours that show EC cell differentiation are the tumours traditionally termed classical carcinoid tumours.

These tumours arise most commonly in the mid or distal ileum [90], but they also occur more proximally in the ileum, in the jejunum, in Meckel's diverticula [91] and even in small intestinal duplication cysts [92]. A number of cases have been reported arising in ileum affected by Crohn's disease [93,94], including one case with multiple tumours [95] but any pathogenetic relationship between these two conditions is uncertain. While mucosal endocrine cell hyperplasia has been described in some cases of Crohn's disease [96], there is no mention of this in reports of coexisting endocrine cell neoplasia. A reported case of synchronous EC-cell carcinoid of the ileum and L-cell carcinoid of the rectum [97] is most likely a chance association.

It has been suggested in a number of series that carcinoid tumours of the small intestine may be associated with an increased frequency of malignant neoplasms elsewhere in the body, especially in the gastrointestinal tract [90,98,99]. However, it is unclear whether this represents a genuine association or a reflection of increased clinical investigation of the gut in carcinoid cases.

Jejunoileal EC-cell tumours occur with similar frequency in males and females; the age incidence ranges widely from the third to tenth decade, with a peak in the sixth and seventh decades. Small tumours are often discovered incidentally at autopsy or laparotomy while larger neoplasms present with either abdominal pain, intestinal obstruction or ischaemia from the local effects of the tumour. Multiple tumours are found in approximately 30% of ileal EC-cell neoplasia [90,98,99], and sometimes dozens of tumours are present, including tiny intramucosal microtumours. One study has suggested that this multifocal neoplasia results from an underlying background endocrine cell hyperplasia [100].

Table 24.3 Prognostic classification of jejunoileal endocrine cell tumours (from [40] and [41]).

Benign
Non-functioning well differentiated endocrine cell tumour measuring up to 1 cm within the mucosa/submucosa and without angioinvasion
Benign or low-grade malignant
Non-functioning well-differentiated tumour within the mucosa/submucosa measuring > 1–2 cm without angioinvasion
Low-grade malignant
Non-functioning well differentiated tumour measuring > 2 cm or extending beyond submucosa
Functioning or angioinvasive well differentiated tumour of any size and extent
High-grade malignant
Functioning or non-functioning poorly differentiated intermediate or small cell carcinoma

Macroscopic appearances

EC-cell tumours usually appear as firm nodules that are embedded in the bowel wall and bulge slightly into the bowel lumen. The overlying mucosa is usually intact, but is occasionally ulcerated. Some form polypoid masses (Fig. 24.12) that may lead to intussusception. The primary lesions in the bowel wall range from barely palpable foci of thickening to nodules measuring up to 3.5 cm; rarely do the primary tumours exceed this size. Typically, the cut surface is tan, yellow or grey-brown in colour.

Microscopic appearances

Histologically, the typical appearances are of classical carcinoids with multiple, solid, somewhat rounded, acinar or 'insular' nests of closely packed cells that may show peripheral nuclear palisading, set in a rather fibrotic stroma (Fig. 24.13).

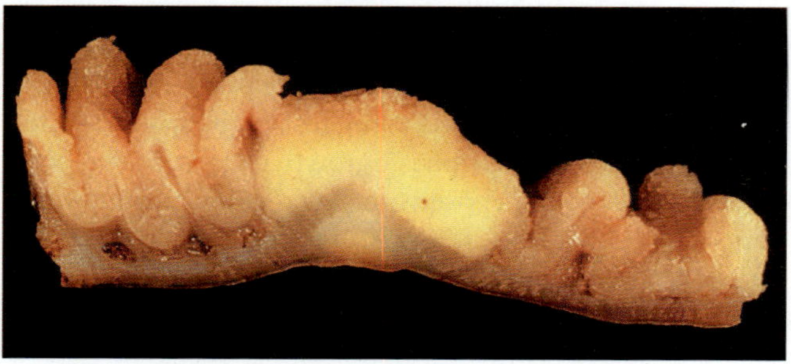

Fig. 24.12 Gross appearance of EC-cell tumour (carcinoid) of jejunum. The cut surface typically has a yellow or tan colour.

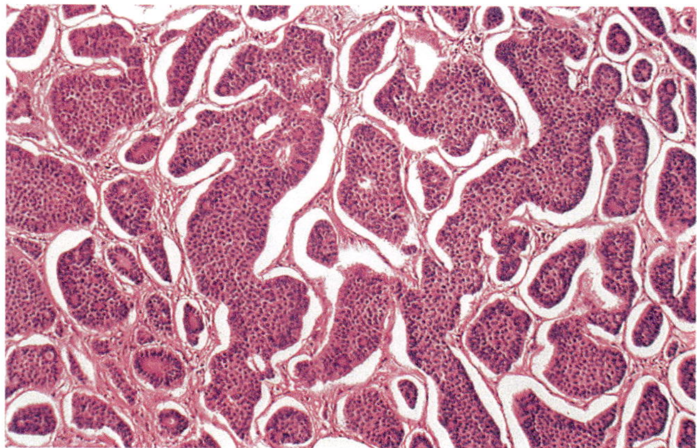

Fig. 24.13 Histology of an EC-cell tumour of the ileum. Note the insular pattern with solid packets of cells showing deep eosinophilic peripheral staining of the cytoplasm.

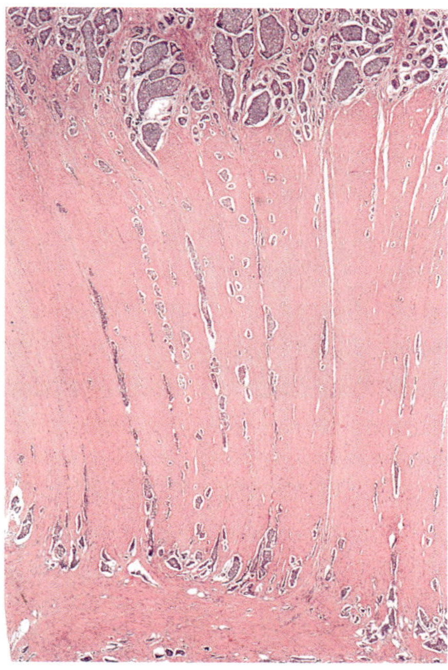

Fig. 24.14 Small intestinal EC-cell (carcinoid) tumour showing how the neoplastic cells insinuate themselves between undamaged smooth muscle fibres.

The tumour cells are uniform, with little or no pleomorphism, nuclear hyperchromasia or mitotic activity. Their nuclei are rounded or ovoid with finely stippled chromatin. They have moderate amounts of cytoplasm containing granules that vary from fine and lightly eosinophilic to coarse and bright red (Fig. 24.13). These are both argentaffin and argyrophil by all conventional silver impregnation techniques and on immunostaining they show strong positivity for chromogranin A, synaptophysin PGP 9.5 and neurone-specific enolase or N-Cam (CD56). Their content of serotonin, substance P and tachykinins can be readily confirmed immunohistochemically; a minority population of other peptide hormones is found only infrequently, including somatostatin, gastrin, bombesin, pancreatic polypeptide, calcitonin, cholecystokinin (CCK), ACTH, enteroglucagon, motilin and neurotensin [98,101–103]. Dopamine and noradrenaline were present in one reported case [104]. Approximately two-thirds also stain for carcinoembryonic antigen and about 20% for prostatic acid phosphatase (but not prostatic-specific antigen) [98]. Another interesting feature is the expression of acidic fibroblast growth factor by EC-cell tumours, which correlates with the amount of fibrous stroma [105]. On ultrastructural examination, most of these tumours have large, pleomorphic intensely osmiophilic secretory granules, typical of those found in normal EC cells. However, some cells contain secretory granules that more resemble the granules found in other types of endocrine cells, probably corresponding to the minority populations found on immunostaining.

Infiltration of the bowel wall by EC-cell tumours is frequently in the form of distinct masses or cords that insinuate themselves between undamaged muscle bundles (Fig. 24.14). By contrast, in the submucosa and extramural tissues they are often accompanied by dense fibrosis, perineural infiltration and invasion of lymphatics and blood vessels.

As EC-cell tumours increase in size, they infiltrate locally into the submucosa, into the muscularis propria, eventually reaching the adjacent serosa and mesentery and sometimes projecting into the peritoneal cavity. Sometimes they produce a circumferential mass that constricts the bowel lumen. Erosion of the serosal surface may lead to solitary peritoneal deposits [106], or to a diffuse peritoneal carcinomatosis [107] and, rarely, serotonin release from these, presumably directly into the systemic circulation, may lead to the carcinoid syndrome in the absence of liver metastases [108]. Extension into the mesentery is often associated with a florid desmoplastic and/or elastotic reaction that causes the adjacent bowel wall to become angulated, kinked or retracted (Fig. 24.15), compromises the blood supply to the intestine, and promotes the formation of serosal adhesions. Clinically, then, patients may present with intestinal obstruction, volvulus or ischaemia. Sometimes there is more widespread ischaemic necrosis of the bowel due to a peculiar occlusive elastic sclerosis affecting the adventitia and intima of medium-sized mesenteric arteries and veins located away from the tumour (Fig. 24.16) [109–112], presumably a paracrine effect of a substance produced by the tumour.

Spread of jejunoileal carcinoid tumours

Surgically resected EC-cell tumours of the jejunum and ileum have frequently metastasized to regional lymph nodes [90]. This seems to be related to the size of the primary tumour [90,99], and does not appear to have a significant influence on survival [98]. Involved lymph nodes may become large, mea-

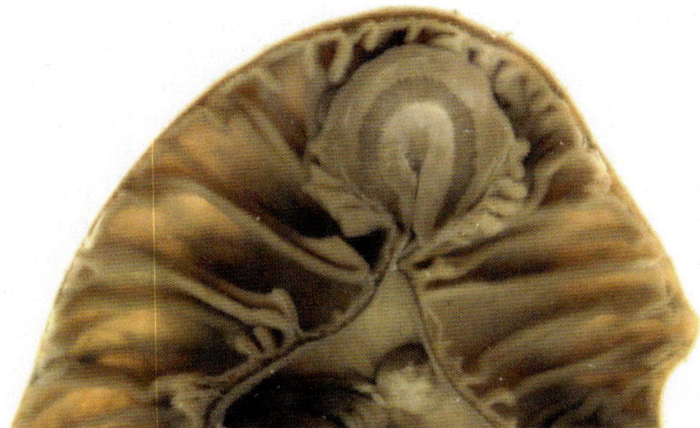

Fig. 24.15 Ileal EC-cell (carcinoid) tumour showing how such tumours often cause retraction and kinking of the bowel wall. There is often thickening of the muscularis propria within these tumours.

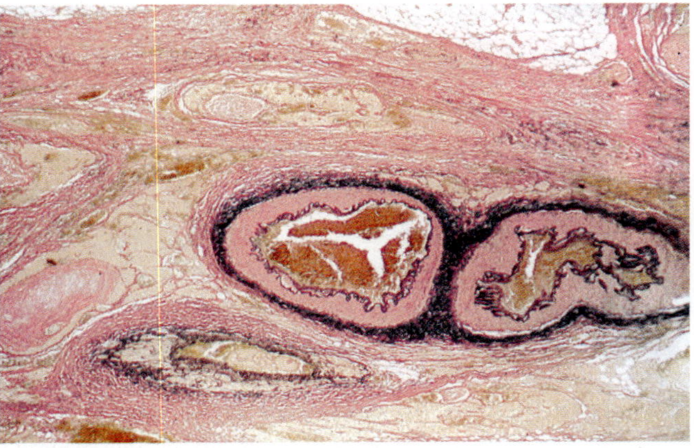

Fig. 24.16 Elastic vascular sclerosis associated with an ileal EC-cell tumour. Elastic–van Gieson staining reveals adventitial elastic sclerosis of both mesenteric arteries and veins, with luminal venous thrombosis. The patient presented with acute small bowel infarction. Ghosts of necrotic tumour cell islands (yellow) are seen among the perivascular fibrous tissue.

suring up to 6 cm in diameter, and are frequently considerably larger than the primary tumour in the bowel wall. They often become matted together by the fibrosis that is associated with the tumour.

By far the commonest site for distant metastases is the liver, the right lobe more often than the left. The incidence varies greatly between different published series, partly depending on the proportion of symptomatic cases studied [98,90], but is again related to the size of the primary tumour. In one series of 78 cases 53% of tumours measuring more than 2 cm had liver metastases compared with 20% of smaller tumours [99]. On the other hand, very small (0.5-cm) primaries can be accompanied by liver metastases.

Metastasis from jejunoileal EC-cell carcinoids at locations other than the regional lymph nodes and the liver are uncommon, but reported sites include the ovaries [113], the spleen [114], the pleura [90], the heart [115], the breast [116], the skin and subcutaneous tissues [117], the uveal tract [118], the cervical lymph nodes [119] and the bone marrow [90].

Carcinoid syndrome

Most tumours are functional and secrete 5-hydroxytryptamine (5-HT) which, with its breakdown product 5-hydroxyindoleacetic acid (5-HIAA), can be detected biochemically; some also secrete kallikreins, but the secretion of other peptides is uncommon. A minority of carcinoids show no demonstrable functional activity. The carcinoid syndrome results from release of serotonin and other tumour-derived vasoactive substances from liver metastases directly into the systemic circulation via the hepatic vein. The syndrome does not occur if the tumour is confined to the bowel wall or mesentery because its secretory products drain into the portal venous system and are inactivated in the liver. Consequently, only 5–7% of patients with small intestinal carcinoid tumours actually present with the carcinoid syndrome. The syndrome consists of episodic cutaneous flushing of the face and neck, sweating, diarrhoea, wheezing, hypotension and, in about half of the cases, right-sided heart disease, due to fibrosis of the ventricular surface of the tricuspid valve, the pulmonary arterial surface of the pulmonary valve and the subendocardium of the right side of the heart [108]. Such cardiac disease is a major cause of death in affected patients [120]. The diagnosis of carcinoid syndrome can usually be established by demonstrating elevated levels of the serotonin metabolite 5-HIAA in a 24-hour urine sample.

Behavour of jejunoileal carcinoid tumours

Despite frequent metastasis, small intestinal carcinoid tumours generally behave in an indolent fashion and their prognosis is much better than conventional adenocarcinomas. For example, data from the US SEER programme show a 5-year survival with distant metastasis of 40%, compared with 5% for adenocarcinoma [89]. For carcinoids localized to the primary site it is 92% and for those with regional spread 86%. Overall, the outcome is also better for ileal tumours (71%) than for jejunal neoplasms (49%). Small intestinal carcinoid tumours that infiltrate only the submucosa or extend partly into the muscularis propria are unlikely to metastasize, whereas those that have infiltrated through the bowel wall into the extramural fat are frequently associated with metastases in regional lymph nodes and at distant sites [121,122]. Features reported to be of prognostic significance include tumour size, depth of invasion into the bowel wall [122], metastatic disease at the time of surgery, a mitotic rate of more than 4 mitoses per 50 high-power fields and the presence of a carcinoid syndrome. The last three of these were found to have independent significance in multivariate analysis of 167 cases [98]. In that study no patient with an initial tumour less than 1 cm in diameter, or without nodal or liver metastases at the time of diagnosis, died of disease. Outcome has also been reported to correlate with DNA content assessed by flow cytometry [123]. Other adverse prognostic factors include extra-abdominal spread, substantial (>9-kg) weight loss, intestinal ischaemia and carcinoid valvular heart disease [120].

Other well differentiated jejunoileal endocrine cell tumours

Well differentiated jejunoileal endocrine cell tumours that are non-argentaffin but argyrophil are uncommon. Gastrin-producing G-cell tumours of the jejunum are particularly likely to be functional, giving rise to a clinical Zollinger–Ellison syndrome [61]. Compared with their counterparts in the proximal duodenum, with which they are morphologically similar, they tend to occur in younger individuals, to be larger neoplasms, and to be more aggressive, frequently giving rise to metastases [61]. Small L-cell tumours that contain enteroglucagon and related peptides, morphologically identical to L-cell carcinoids of the large bowel, may arise rarely in the ileum [102].

Other rarities include a jejunal endocrine tumour that produced VIP and gave rise to severe watery diarrhoea (pancreatic cholera syndrome) [124], another jejunal tumour in which somatostatin was the major peptide product [125] and an ileal tumour that produced both serotonin and insulin and gave rise to clinical features of both the carcinoid syndrome and hypoglycaemia [126].

Endocrine cell tumours in Meckel's diverticula must not be confused histologically with intramural or extramural nests of heterotopic pancreatic islets of Langerhans. The latter may or may not be accompanied by foci of exocrine pancreas, but it is when they are absent that diagnostic difficulty may arise. The endocrine cell nests are usually small, rounded and unassociated with a desmoplastic stromal reaction. Immunostaining for normal pancreatic islet cell hormones demonstrates the typical islet configuration, with insulin-containing B cells predominating in the central portion of the nests and somatostatin-containing D cells more peripherally.

Gangliocytic paraganglioma

Two cases of gangliocytic paraganglioma of the jejunum have been reported, one arising in association with pancreatic heterotopia [73,127]. In all other respects they are identical to their periampullary counterparts (see above).

Poorly differentiated endocrine carcinoma/small cell carcinoma

Jejunoileal tumours of this sort are exceedingly rare. Toker [128] reported an 'oat cell tumour' of the small bowel that had the histological appearance of a small cell carcinoma and contained endocrine granules on ultrastructural examination. Another biologically aggressive poorly differentiated endocrine carcinoma of the jejunum contained scattered, multinucleated, osteoclast-like giant cells [129]. This was described as an ileal 'atypical carcinoid tumour', complicating coeliac disease. It was non-argyrophil but neurone-specific enolase positive and also contained neuroendocrine granules on electron microscopy. The authors suggested that the tumour had arisen in a background of intracryptal endocrine cell hyperplasia, which is reported to occur in some patients with coeliac disease [130]. A further type of malignant endocrine cell tumour that has been described is a mixed endocrine carcinoma and adenocarcinoma, arising at a long-standing ileostomy site [131].

Fenoglio-Preiser *et al.* [132] have described and illustrated another rare ileal neoplasm that they termed pleomorphic giant cell neuroendocrine carcinoma. This highly aggressive tumour is composed of large pleomorphic cells with abundant eosinophilic cytoplasm that may be focally PAS positive. The nuclei are also large or multiple with chromatin clumping and prominent nucleoli, and mitoses are plentiful. Scanty neuroendocrine granules were demonstrated by electron microscopy and the tumour cells were said to be immunoreactive for unspecified 'various hormones' and 'neuroendocrine markers'. The differential diagnosis includes other highly pleomorphic malignant neoplasms and metastatic amelanotic malignant melanoma.

Goblet cell carcinoid (mucinous carcinoid, adenocarcinoid, microglandular goblet cell carcinoma)

We are aware of only one publication describing goblet cell carcinoids arising in the ileum [133]. This report details one patient with a 6-cm 'multicentric' goblet cell carcinoid of the ileum, and another patient with a 4-cm ileal tumour accompanied by a similar tumour of the appendix. The morphology of the ileal tumours was identical to those described in the appendix (see Chapter 31).

Composite carcinoid–adenoma

Varghese *et al.* [134] reported a polypoid terminal ileal tumour in which a metastasizing argyrophil (but non-argentaffin) endocrine cell neoplasm was associated with a surface tubular adenoma. Interestingly, endocrine cells were not prominent within the adenomatous component. The relationship between the two elements is uncertain, but given the rarity of adenomas in the terminal ileum a chance collision of two neoplasms would seem unlikely. Similar composite neoplasms can occur in the large bowel [135,136].

Metastatic epithelial tumours

In the small intestine, metastatic tumours are slightly more common than primary malignancies, with a ratio of 61 : 51 in one series [26]. We have seen them from primary tumours in bronchus, adrenal, ovary, stomach and large bowel, and they are also reported from uterus, cervix, kidney and testis [137]. Secondary mucosal ulceration occurs but is not invariable and careful examination will usually suggest whether a tumour is primary or secondary. Multiple small or seedling deposits must be distinguished from fat necrosis, and larger haemorrhagic ones from endometriosis.

References

1 Chow JS, Chen CC, Ahsan H, Neugut AI. A population-based study of the incidence of malignant small bowel tumours: SEER, 1973–1990. *Int J Epidemiol*, 1996; 25 (4): 722.

2 Chen CC, Neugut AI, Rotterdam H. Risk factors for adenocarcinomas and malignant carcinoids of the small intestine: preliminary findings. *Cancer Epidemiol Biomarkers Prev*, 1994; 3 (3): 205.

3 Spigelman AD, Talbot IC, Penna C *et al.* Evidence for adenoma–carcinoma sequence in the duodenum of patients with familial adenomatous polyposis. The Leeds Castle Polyposis Group (Upper Gastrointestinal Committee). *J Clin Pathol*, 1994; 47 (8): 709.

4 DiSario JA, Burt RW, Vargas H, McWhorter WP. Small bowel cancer: epidemiological and clinical characteristics from a population-based registry. *Am J Gastroenterol*, 1994; 89 (5): 699.

5 Domizio P, Talbot IC, Spigelman AD, Williams CB, Phillips RK. Upper gastrointestinal pathology in familial adenomatous polyposis: results from a prospective study of 102 patients. *J Clin Pathol*, 1990; 43: 738.

6 Spigelman AD. Familial adenomatous polyposis: recent genetic advances [editorial]. *Br J Surg*, 1994; 81 (3): 321.

7 Scates DK, Spigelman AD, Phillips RK, Venitt S. DNA adducts detected by 32P-postlabelling, in the intestine of rats given bile from patients with familial adenomatous polyposis and from unaffected controls. *Carcinogenesis*, 1992; 13 (4): 731.

8 Hamada K, Umemoto A, Kajikawa A *et al.* Mucosa-specific DNA adducts in human small intestine: a comparison with the colon. *Carcinogenesis*, 1994; 15 (11): 2677.

9 Potten CS. Stem cells in the gastrointestinal epithelium: numbers, characteristics and death. *Philos Trans R Soc Biol Sci*, 1998; 353: 821.

10 Matsuo S, Eto T, Tsunoda T, Kanematsu T, Shinozaki T. Small bowel tumors: an analysis of tumor-like lesions, benign and malignant neoplasms. *Eur J Surg Oncol*, 1994; 20 (1): 47.

11 Perzin KH, Bridge MF. Adenomas of the small intestine: a clinicopathological review of 51 cases and a study of their relationship to carcinoma. *Cancer*, 1981; 48: 799.

12 Delevett AF, Cuello R. True villous adenoma of the jejunum. *Gastroenterology*, 1975; 69 (1): 217.

13 Komorowski RA, Cohen EB. Villous tumors of the duodenum: a clinicopathologic study. *Cancer*, 1981; 47 (6): 1377.

14 Geier GE, Gashti EN, Houin HP, Johnloz D, Madura JA. Villous adenoma of the duodenum. A clinicopathologic study of five cases. *Am Surg*, 1984; 50 (11): 617.

15 Haglund U, Fork FT, Genell S, Rehnberg O. Villous adenomas in the duodenum. *Br J Surg*, 1985; 72 (1): 26.

16 Mingazzini PL, Malchiodi Albedi F, Blandamura V. Villous adenoma of the duodenum: cellular composition and histochemical findings. *Histopathology*, 1982; 6 (2): 235.

17 Johansen A, Larsen E. Adenomas of the small intestine. A report of four cases with special reference to their relation to carcinomas. *Acta Pathol Microbiol Scand*, 1969; 75 (2): 247.

18 Spigelman AD, Phillips RKS. The upper gastrointestinal tract. In: Phillips RKSP, Spigelman AD, Thomson JPS, eds. *Familial Adenomatous Polyposis*. London, Boston, Melbourne, Auckland: Edward Arnold, 1994: 111.

19 Spigelman AD. Screening modalities in familial adenomatous polyposis and hereditary nonpolyposis colorectal cancer. [Review] [27 references] *Gastrointest Endosc Clin North Am*, 1997; 7 (1): 81.

20 Spigelman AD, Phillips RKS. The upper gastrointestinal tract. In: Phillips RKSP, Spigelman AD, Thomson JPS, eds. *Familial Adenomatous Polyposis*. London, Boston, Melbourne, Auckland: Edward Arnold, 1994: 117.

21 Jagelman DG, DeCosse JJ, Bussey HJ. Upper gastrointestinal cancer in familial adenomatous polyposis. *Lancet*, 1988; 1 (8595): 1149.

22 Spigelman AD, Williams CB, Talbot IC, Domizio P, Phillips RK. Upper gastrointestinal cancer in patients with familial adenomatous polyposis. *Lancet*, 1989; 2 (8666): 783.

23 Spigelman AD, Phillips RKSP. The upper gastrointestinal tract. In: Phillips RKSP, Spigelman AD, Thomson JPS, eds. *Familial Adenomatous Polyposis*. London, Boston, Melbourne, Auckland: Edward Arnold, 1994: 114.

24 Barclay TH, Schapira DV. Malignant tumors of the small intestine. *Cancer*, 1983; 51 (5): 878.

25 Weiss NS, Yang CP. Incidence of histologic types of cancer of the small intestine. *J Natl Cancer Inst*, 1987; 78 (4): 653.

26 Baillie CT, Williams A. Small bowel tumours: a diagnostic challenge. *J R Coll Surg Edinb*, 1994; 39 (1): 8.

27 Warner TF, Peralta J. Multifocal adenocarcinoma of the jejunum. *Cancer*, 1979; 44 (3): 1142.

28 Wagner KM, Thompson J, Herlinger H, Caroline D. Thirteen primary adenocarcinomas of the ileum and appendix: a case report. *Cancer*, 1982; 49 (4): 797.

29 Contant CM, Damhuis RA, van Geel AN, van Eijck CH, Wiggers T. Prognostic value of the TNM-classification for small bowel cancer. *Hepatogastroenterology*, 1997; 44 (14): 430.

30 Talbot IC, Neoptolemos JP, Shaw DE, Carr-Locke D. The histopathology and staging of carcinoma of the ampulla of Vater. *Histopathology*, 1988; 12: 155.

31 Ribeiro MB, Greenstein AJ, Heimann TM, Yamazaki Y, Aufses A Jr. Adenocarcinoma of the small intestine in Crohn's disease. *Surg Gynecol Obstet*, 1991; 173 (5): 343.

32 Leader M, Jass JR. Increased alpha-fetoprotein concentration in association with ileal adenocarcinoma complicating Crohn's disease. *J Clin Pathol*, 1984; 37 (3): 293.

33 Fell J, Snooks S. Small bowel adenocarcinoma complicating Crohn's disease. *J R Soc Med*, 1987; 80 (1): 51.

34 Bearzi I, Ranaldi R. Small bowel adenocarcinoma and Crohn's disease: report of a case with differing histogenetic patterns. *Histopathology*, 1985; 9 (3): 345.

35 Wright DH. The major complications of coeliac disease. *Baillieres Clin Gastroenterol*, 1995; 9 (2): 351.

36 O'Riordan BG, Vilor M, Herrera L. Small bowel tumors: an overview. [Review] [41 references] *Dig Dis*, 1996; 14 (4): 245.

37 Wytock DH, Bartholomew LG, Sheps SG. Digital ischemia associated with small bowel malignancy. *Gastroenterology*, 1983; 84 (5 Part 1): 1025.

38 Williams ED, Sandler M. The classification of carcinoid tumours. *Lancet*, 1963; 1: 238.

39 Burke AP, Sobin LH, Federspiel BH, Shekitka KM, Helwig EB. Carcinoid tumors of the duodenum. A clinicopathologic study of 99 cases. *Arch Pathol Lab Med*, 1990; 114 (7): 700.

40 Capella C, Heitz PU, Hofler H, Solcia E, Kloppel G. Revised classification of neuroendocrine tumours of the lung, pancreas and gut. *Virchows Arch*, 1995; 425 (6): 547.

41 Kloppel G, Heitz PU, Capella C, Solcia E. Pathology and nomenclature of human gastrointestinal neuroendocrine (carcinoid) tumors and related lesions. *World J Surg*, 1996; 20 (2): 132.

42 Lee WM, Silva F, Price JB Jr. Gastrin-secreting tumor of the duodenum (G-cell apudoma) associated with secondary biliary cirrhosis. *Cancer*, 1982; 49 (12): 2596.

43 Vesoulis Z, Petras RE. Duodenal microgastrinoma producing the Zollinger–Ellison syndrome. *Arch Pathol Lab Med*, 1985; 109 (1): 40.

44 Thompson NW, Vinik AI, Eckhauser FE. Microgastrinomas of the duodenum. A cause of failed operations for the Zollinger–Ellison syndrome. *Ann Surg*, 1989; 209 (4): 396.

45 Bonfils S, Landor JH, Mignon M, Hervoir P. Results of surgical management in 92 consecutive patients with Zollinger–Ellison syndrome. *Ann Surg*, 1981; 194 (6): 692.

46 Metz DC, Kuchnio M, Fraker DL *et al.* Flow cytometry and Zollinger–Ellison syndrome: relationship to clinical course. *Gastroenterology*, 1993; 105 (3): 799.

47 Solcia E, Fiocca R, Rindi G, Villani L, Cornaggia M, Capella C. The pathology of the gastrointestinal endocrine system. *Endocrinol Metab Clin North Am*, 1993; 22 (4): 795.

48 Pipeleers-Marichal M, Somers G, Willems G *et al.* Gastrinomas in the duodenums of patients with multiple endocrine neoplasia type 1 and the Zollinger–Ellison syndrome [see comments]. *N Engl J Med*, 1990; 322 (11): 723.

49 Stamm B, Hedinger CE, Saremaslani P. Duodenal and ampullary carcinoid tumors. A report of 12 cases with pathological characteristics, polypeptide content and relation to the MEN I syndrome and von Recklinghausen's disease (neurofibromatosis). *Virchows Arch A Pathol Anat Histopathol*, 1986; 408 (5): 475.

50 Burke AP, Federspiel BH, Sobin LH, Shekitka KM, Helwig EB. Carcinoids of the duodenum. A histologic and immunohistochemical study of 65 tumors. *Am J Surg Pathol*, 1989; 13 (10): 828.

51 Wilander E, Grimelius L, Lundqvist G, Skoog V. Polypeptide hormones in argentaffin and argyrophil gastroduodenal endocrine tumors. *Am J Pathol*, 1979; 96 (2): 519.

52 Swinburn BA, Yeong ML, Lane MR, Nicholson GI, Holdaway IM. Neurofibromatosis associated with somatostatinoma: a report of two patients. *Clin Endocrinol (Oxf)*, 1988; 28 (4): 353.

53 Yoshida T, Matsumoto T, Morii Y *et al.* Carcinoid somatostatinoma of the papilla of Vater: a case report. *Hepatogastroenterology*, 1998; 45 (20): 451.

54 Griffiths DF, Williams GT, Williams ED. Multiple endocrine neoplasia associated with von Recklinghausen's disease. *Br Med J (Clin Res Ed)*, 1983; 287 (6402): 1341.

55 Dayal Y, Tallberg KA, Nunnemacher G, DeLellis RA, Wolfe HJ. Duodenal carcinoids in patients with and without neurofibromatosis. A comparative study. *Am J Surg Pathol*, 1986; 10 (5): 348.

56 Griffiths DF, Williams GT, Williams ED. Duodenal carcinoid tumours, phaeochromocytoma and neurofibromatosis: islet cell tumour, phaeochromocytoma and the von Hippel–Lindau complex: two distinctive neuroendocrine syndromes. [Review] [62 references] *Q J Med*, 1987; 64 (245): 769.

57 Stephens M, Williams GT, Jasani B, Williams ED. Synchronous duodenal neuroendocrine tumours in von Recklinghausen's disease—a case report of co-existing gangliocytic paraganglioma and somatostatin-rich glandular carcinoid. *Histopathology*, 1987; 11 (12): 1331.

58 Dayal Y, Doos WG, O'Brien MJ, Nunnemacher G, DeLellis RA, Wolfe HJ. Psammomatous somatostatinomas of the duodenum. *Am J Surg Pathol*, 1983; 7 (7): 653.

59 Griffiths DF, Jasani B, Newman GR, Williams ED, Williams GT. Glandular duodenal carcinoid—a somatostatin rich tumour with neuroendocrine associations. *J Clin Pathol*, 1984; 37 (2): 163.

60 Makhlouf HR, Burke AP, Sobin LH. Carcinoid tumors of the ampulla of Vater: a comparison with duodenal carcinoid tumors. *Cancer*, 1999; 85 (6): 1241.

61 Capella C, Riva C, Rindi G *et al.* Histopathology, hormone products and clinicopathologic profile of endocrine tumors of the upper small intestine. *Endocrine Pathol*, 1991; 2: 92.

62 Ranaldi R, Bearzi I, Cinti S, Suraci V. Ampullary somatostatinoma. An immunohistochemical and ultrastructural study. *Pathol Res Pract*, 1988; 183 (1): 8.

63 Noda Y, Watanabe H, Iwafuchi M *et al.* Carcinoids and endocrine cell micronests of the minor and major duodenal papillae. Their incidence and characteristics. *Cancer*, 1992; 70 (7): 1825.

64 Sanchez-Sosa S, Angeles Angeles A, Orozco H, Larriva-Sahd J. Neuroendocrine carcinoma of the ampulla of Vater. A case of absence of somatostatin in a vasoactive intestinal polypeptide-, bombesin-, and cholecystokinin-producing tumor. *Am J Clin Pathol*, 1991; 95 (1): 51.

65 Ricci JL. Carcinoid of the ampulla of Vater. Local resection or pancreaticoduodenectomy. *Cancer*, 1993; 71 (3): 686.

66 Warren KW, McDonald WM, Logan CJH. Periampullary and duodenal carcinoid tumours. *Gut*, 1964; 5: 448.

67 Miyazaki K, Funakoshi A, Nishihara S, Wasada T, Koga A, Ibayashi H. Aberrant insulinoma in the duodenum. *Gastroenterology*, 1986; 90 (5 Part 1): 1280.

68 Roggli VL, Judge DM, McGavran MH. Duodenal glucagonoma: a case report. *Hum Pathol*, 1979; 10 (3): 350.

69 Burke AP, Helwig EB. Gangliocytic paraganglioma. *Am J Clin Pathol*, 1989; 92 (1): 1.

70 Hamid QA, Bishop AE, Rode J *et al.* Duodenal gangliocytic paragangliomas: a study of 10 cases with immunocytochemical neuroendocrine markers. *Hum Pathol*, 1986; 17 (11): 1151.

71 Kepes JJ, Zacharias DL. Gangliocytic paragangliomas of the duodenum. A report of two cases with light and electron microscopic examination. *Cancer*, 1971; 27 (1): 61.

72 Perrone T, Sibley RK, Rosai J. Duodenal gangliocytic paraganglioma. An immunohistochemical and ultrastructural study and a hypothesis concerning its origin. *Am J Surg Pathol*, 1985; 9 (1): 31.

73 Reed RJ, Caroca PJ Jr, Harkin JC. Gangliocytic paraganglioma. *Am J Surg Pathol*, 1977; 1 (3): 207.

74 Scheithauer BW, Nora FE, LeChago J *et al*. Duodenal gangliocytic paraganglioma. Clinicopathologic and immunocytochemical study of 11 cases. *Am J Clin Pathol*, 1986; 86 (5): 559.

75 Kawaguchi K, Takizawa T, Koike M, Tabata I, Goseki N. Multiple paraganglioneuromas. *Virchows Arch A Pathol Anat Histopathol*, 1985; 406 (3): 373.

76 Kheir SM, Halpern NB. Paraganglioma of the duodenum in association with congenital neurofibromatosis. Possible relationship. *Cancer*, 1984; 53 (11): 2491.

77 Anders KH, Glasgow BJ, Lewin KJ. Gangliocytic paraganglioma associated with duodenal adenocarcinoma. Case report with immunohistochemical evaluation. *Arch Pathol Lab Med*, 1987; 111 (1): 49.

78 Collina G, Maiorana A, Trentini GP. Duodenal gangliocytic paraganglioma. Case report with immunohistochemical study on the expression of keratin polypeptides. *Histopathology*, 1991; 19 (5): 476.

79 Buchler M, Malfertheiner P, Baczako K, Krautzberger W, Beger HG. A metastatic endocrine-neurogenic tumor of the ampulla of Vater with multiple endocrine immunoreaction—malignant paraganglioma? *Digestion*, 1985; 31 (1): 54.

80 Inai K, Kobuke T, Yonehara S, Tokuoka S. Duodenal gangliocytic paraganglioma with lymph node metastasis in a 17-year-old boy. [Review] [29 references] *Cancer*, 1989; 63 (12): 2540.

81 Sonneland PR, Scheithauer BW, LeChago J, Crawford BG, Onofrio BM. Paraganglioma of the cauda equina region. Clinicopathologic study of 31 cases with special reference to immunocytology and ultrastructure. *Cancer*, 1986; 58 (8): 1720.

82 Dookhan DB, Miettinen M, Finkel G, Gibas Z. Recurrent duodenal gangliocytic paraganglioma with lymph node metastases. *Histopathology*, 1993; 22 (4): 399.

83 Swanson PE, Dykoski D, Wick MR, Snover DC. Primary duodenal small-cell neuroendocrine carcinoma with production of vasoactive intestinal polypeptide. *Arch Pathol Lab Med*, 1986; 110 (4): 317.

84 Zamboni G, Franzin G, Bonetti F *et al*. Small-cell neuroendocrine carcinoma of the ampullary region. A clinicopathologic, immunohistochemical, and ultrastructural study of three cases. *Am J Surg Pathol*, 1990; 14 (8): 703.

85 Jones MA, Griffith LM, West AB. Adenocarcinoid tumor of the periampullary region: a novel duodenal neoplasm presenting as biliary tract obstruction. *Hum Pathol*, 1989; 20 (2): 198.

86 Burke A, Lee YK. Adenocarcinoid (goblet cell carcinoid) of the duodenum presenting as gastric outlet obstruction. *Hum Pathol*, 1990; 21 (2): 238.

87 Shah IA, Schlageter MO, Boehm N. Composite carcinoid-adenocarcinoma of ampulla of Vater. *Hum Pathol*, 1990; 21 (11): 1188.

88 Modlin IM, Sandor A. An analysis of 8305 cases of carcinoid tumors. *Cancer*, 1997; 79 (4): 813.

89 Thomas RM, Sobin LH. Gastrointestinal cancer. *Cancer*, 1995; 75 (1 Suppl): 154.

90 Moertel CG, Dockerty MB, Judd ES, Baggenstoss AH. Life history of the carcinoid tumor of the small intestine. *Cancer*, 1961; 14: 901.

91 Moyana TN. Carcinoid tumors arising from Meckel's diverticulum. A clinical, morphologic, and immunohistochemical study. *Am J Clin Pathol*, 1989; 91 (1): 52.

92 Smith JH, Hope PG. Carcinoid tumor arising in a cystic duplication of the small bowel. *Arch Pathol Lab Med*, 1985; 109 (1): 95.

93 Greenstein AJ, Balasubramanian S, Harpaz N, Rizwan M, Sachar DB. Carcinoid tumor and inflammatory bowel disease: a study of eleven cases and review of the literature. *Am J Gastroenterol*, 1997; 92 (4): 682.

94 Van Landingham SB, Kluppel S, Symmonds R Jr, Snyder SK. Coexisting carcinoid tumor and Crohn's disease. *J Surg Oncol*, 1983; 24 (4): 310.

95 Tehrani MA, Carfrae DC. Carcinoid tumour and Crohn's disease. *Br J Clin Pract*, 1975; 29 (5): 123.

96 Bishop AE, Pietroletti R, Taat CW, Brummelkamp WH, Polak JM. Increased populations of endocrine cells in Crohn's ileitis. *Virchows Arch A Pathol Anat Histopathol*, 1987; 410 (5): 391.

97 Colbert PM. Primary carcinoids of the ileum and rectum. A simultaneous occurrence. *JAMA*, 1976; 236 (19): 2201.

98 Burke AP, Thomas RM, Elsayed AM, Sobin LH. Carcinoids of the jejunum and ileum: an immunohistochemical and clinicopathologic study of 167 cases. *Cancer*, 1997; 79 (6): 1086.

99 Strodel WE, Talpos G, Eckhauser F, Thompson N. Surgical therapy for small-bowel carcinoid tumors. *Arch Surg*, 1983; 118 (4): 391.

100 Moyana TN, Satkunam N. A comparative immunohistochemical study of jejunoileal and appendiceal carcinoids. Implications for histogenesis and pathogenesis. *Cancer*, 1992; 70 (5): 1081.

101 Bostwick DG, Roth KA, Barchas JD, Bensch KG. Gastrin-releasing peptide immunoreactivity in intestinal carcinoids. *Am J Clin Pathol*, 1984; 82 (4): 428.

102 Wilander E, Grimelius L, Portela-Gomes G, Lundqvist G, Skoog V, Westermark P. Substance P and enteroglucagon-like immunoreactivity in argentaffin and argyrophil midgut carcinoid tumours. *Scand J Gastroenterol Suppl*, 1979; 53: 19.

103 Yang K, Ulich T, Cheng L, Lewin KJ. The neuroendocrine products of intestinal carcinoids. An immunoperoxidase study of 35 carcinoid tumors stained for serotonin and eight polypeptide hormones. *Cancer*, 1983; 51 (10): 1918.

104 Goedert M, Otten U, Suda K *et al*. Dopamine, norepinephrine and serotonin production by an intestinal carcinoid tumor. *Cancer*, 1980; 45 (1): 104.

105 La Rosa S, Chiaravalli AM, Capella C, Uccella S, Sessa F. Immunohistochemical localization of acidic fibroblast growth factor in normal human enterochromaffin cells and related gastrointestinal tumours. *Virchows Arch*, 1997; 430 (2): 117.

106 Robb JA, Kuster GG, Bordin GM, Unni KK. Polypoid peritoneal metastases from carcinoid neoplasms. *Hum Pathol*, 1984; 15 (10): 1002.

107 Vasseur B, Cadiot G, Zins M *et al*. Peritoneal carcinomatosis in patients with digestive endocrine tumors. *Cancer*, 1996; 78 (8): 1686.

108 Davis Z, Moertel CG, McIlrath DC. The malignant carcinoid syndrome. *Surg Gynecol Obstet*, 1973; 137 (4): 637.

109 Anthony PP, Drury RA. Elastic vascular sclerosis of mesenteric blood vessels in argentaffin carcinoma. *J Clin Pathol*, 1970; 23 (2): 110.

110 Eckhauser FE, Argenta LC, Strodel WE *et al.* Mesenteric angiopathy, intestinal gangrene, and midgut carcinoids. *Surgery*, 1981; 90 (4): 720.

111 Qizilbash AH. Carcinoid tumors, vascular elastosis, and ischemic disease of the small intestine. *Dis Colon Rectum*, 1977; 20 (7): 554.

112 Warner TF, O'Reilly G, Lee GA. Mesenteric occlusive lesion and ileal carcinoids. [Review] [28 references] *Cancer*, 1979; 44 (2): 758.

113 Robboy SJ, Scully RE, Norris HJ. Carcinoid metastatic to the ovary. A clinicopathologic analysis of 35 cases. *Cancer*, 1974; 33 (3): 798.

114 Falk S, Stutte HJ. Splenic metastasis in an ileal carcinoid tumor. *Pathol Res Pract*, 1989; 185 (2): 238; discussion 242.

115 Fine SN, Gaynor ML, Isom OW, Dannenberg AJ. Carcinoid tumor metastatic to the heart. *Am J Med*, 1990; 89 (5): 690.

116 Schurch W, Lamoureux E, Lefebvre R, Fauteux JP. Solitary breast metastasis: first manifestation of an occult carcinoid of the ileum. *Virchows Arch A Pathol Anat Histol*, 1980; 386 (1): 117.

117 Norman JL, Cunningham PJ, Cleveland BR. Skin and subcutaneous metastases from gastrointestinal carcinoid tumors. *Arch Surg*, 1971; 103 (6): 767.

118 Harbour JW, De Potter P, Shields CL, Shields JA. Uveal metastasis from carcinoid tumor. Clinical observations in nine cases. *Ophthalmology*, 1994; 101 (6): 1084.

119 Marks WH, Strodel WE, Lloyd RV, Eckhauser FE, Thompson NW, Vinik AI. Cervical metastases from small bowel carcinoid tumors. *J Surg Oncol*, 1983; 24 (2): 135.

120 Makridis C, Ekbom A, Bring J *et al.* Survival and daily physical activity in patients treated for advanced midgut carcinoid tumors. *Surgery*, 1997; 122 (6): 1075.

121 Zakariai YM, Quan SH, Hajdu S. Carcinoid tumors of the gastrointestinal tract. *Cancer*, 1975; 35: 588.

122 Hajdu SI, Winawer SJ, Myers WP. Carcinoid tumors. A study of 204 cases. *Am J Clin Pathol*, 1974; 61 (4): 521.

123 Cohn G, Erhardt K, Cedermark B, Hamberger B, Auer G. DNA distribution pattern in intestinal carcinoid tumors. *World J Surg*, 1986; 10 (4): 548.

124 Capella C, Polak JM, Buffa R *et al.* Morphologic patterns and diagnostic criteria of VIP-producing endocrine tumors. A histologic, histochemical, ultrastructural, and biochemical study of 32 cases. *Cancer*, 1983; 52 (10): 1860.

125 Alumets J, Ekelund G, Hakanson R *et al.* Jejunal endocrine tumor composed of somatostatin and gastrin cells and associated with duodenal ulcer disease. *Virchows Arch A Pathol Anat Histol*, 1978; 378 (1): 17.

126 Pelletier G, Cortot A, Launay JM *et al.* Serotonin-secreting and insulin-secreting ileal carcinoid tumor and the use of in vitro culture of tumoral cells. *Cancer*, 1984; 54 (2): 319.

127 Aung W, Gallagher HJ, Joyce WP, Hayes DB, Leader M. Gastrointestinal haemorrhage from a jejunal gangliocytic paraganglioma. *J Clin Pathol*, 1995; 48 (1): 84.

128 Toker C. Oat cell tumor of the small bowel. *Am J Gastroenterol*, 1974; 61 (6): 481.

129 Gardiner GW, Van Patter T, Murray D. Atypical carcinoid tumor of the small bowel complicating celiac disease. *Cancer*, 1985; 56 (11): 2716.

130 Challacombe DN, Robertson K. Enterochromaffin cells in the duodenal mucosa of children with coeliac disease. *Gut*, 1977; 18 (5): 373.

131 Listinsky CM, Halpern NB, Workman RB, Herrera GA. Ultrastructural and immunocytochemical features of a case of neuroendocrine carcinoma developing in a prior ileostomy site. *Ultrastruct Pathol*, 1994; 18 (5): 503.

132 Fenoglio-Preiser CM, Pascal RR, Perzin KH. 1990 *Tumors of the Intestines*, 2nd edn. Washington: Armed Forces Institute of Pathology, 1990 Atlas of Tumor Pathology: Volume Fascicle 27.

133 Hofler H, Kloppel G, Heitz PU. Combined production of mucus, amines and peptides by goblet-cell carcinoids of the appendix and ileum. *Pathol Res Pract*, 1984; 178 (6): 555.

134 Varghese NM, Zaitoun AM, Thomas SM, Senapati A, Theodossi A. Composite glandular-carcinoid tumour of the terminal ileum. *J Clin Pathol*, 1994; 47 (5): 427.

135 Lyda MH, Fenoglio-Preiser CM. Adenoma-carcinoid tumors of the colon. *Arch Pathol Lab Med*, 1998; 122 (3): 262.

136 Moyana TN, Qizilbash AH, Murphy F. Composite glandular-carcinoid tumors of the colon and rectum. Report of two cases. *Am J Surg Pathol*, 1988; 12 (8): 607.

137 Chait MM, Kurtz RC, Hajdu SI. Gastrointestinal tract metastasis in patients with germ-cell tumor of the testis. *Am J Dig Dis*, 1978; 23 (10): 925.

25 Non-epithelial tumours of the small intestine

Benign lymphoid proliferations

Whilst a comprehensive account of the lymphoid tissue of the small intestine and its organization is presented in Chapter 18, it is appropriate to emphasize certain aspects here to further understanding of the pathology of the small intestinal lymphoid tissue. The small intestine contains a large amount of lymphoid tissue. Within the mucosa, lymphoid tissue is diffusely dispersed but is also organized into follicles. The mucosa of the terminal ileum contains larger aggregations of lymphoid tissue, known as Peyer's patches, which measure up to 20 × 12 mm in diameter. These are often clearly visible macroscopically as elevations on the mucosal surface. The dome epithelium overlying the lymphoid follicles of Peyer's patches and other lymphoid aggregates possess a population of specialized phagocytic columnar cells, known as M (standing for microfold) cells, which act as gateways for luminal antigens. These antigens are processed and presented by specialized dendritic histiocytes to lymphoid cells, which are capable of eliciting an immune response [1]. One attribute of these histiocytes is their ability to sample particulate matter, as well as smaller antigen material, in a process known as persorption [2]. One characteristic, and apparently unique, feature of Peyer's patches is their ability to take up and concentrate such particulate matter, within histiocytes toward the base of the lymphoid tissue. Thus in our experience all adults possess black granular material, which on X-ray analysis contains silicon, aluminium and titanium (presumably deriving from soil contamination of food), at this site in Peyer's patches [3]. This black pigment allows the positive identification of Peyer's patches in biopsy material.

There is now a substantial body of evidence to support the concept of mucosa-associated lymphoid tissue (MALT) and that the lymphoid tissue throughout the small bowel conforms to such a concept [4]. Thus the lymphoid aggregates within the small bowel contain large lymphoid follicles with germinal centres and adjacent marginal zone, and a mantle containing cells with their characteristic morphology and immunohistochemistry [5,6]. Of the primary lymphomas arising in the small intestine, MALT lymphomas are the largest single group and these are characterized by neoplastic marginal zone cells, with a centrocyte-like morphology, often around reactive germinal centres [5]. The neoplastic marginal zone cells are able to infiltrate epithelium, producing the characteristic lymphoepithelial lesions, in a similar way to the physiological involvement of dome epithelium seen in Peyer's patches, once again recapitulating physiological MALT [7]. Unlike other parts of the gut, in which T-cell lymphomas are distinctly rare, these are relatively common in the small intestine, both associated with coeliac disease and without such a relationship. The reasons for this are not entirely clear, as the small intestine possesses similar amounts of T lymphocytes and in a similar proportion to other parts of the alimentary tract.

Lymphoid hyperplasia in the terminal ileum

This condition has two presentation forms. The first is a rare lesion of infants and children, presenting as a tumour-like mass of the terminal ileum, which may cause obstruction due to intussusception or lead to haemorrhage [8,9]. It is more common in male children. Peyer's patches become polypoid and project as papillary folds into the lumen, exacerbating the potential for obstruction [9]. Histologically the lymphoid tissue demonstrates pronounced hyperplasia with prominent germinal centre formation. There is no disorganization of the lymphoid tissue, there is no extension of the lymphoid tissue deep to the submucosa and ulceration is absent unless the secondary effects of obstruction and/or intussusception have supervened. These features help to differentiate the condition from lymphoma. The condition almost always represents an exaggerated response of the lymphoid tissue to viral infection; echovirus or adenovirus are usually implicated in its cause [9].

The second form of lymphoid hyperplasia in the terminal ileum occurs in adults, especially the elderly, but is again rare [10]. It usually presents with abdominal pain associated with a right iliac fossa mass. It is sometimes known as 'florid lymphoid hyperplasia' and is characterized by deep extension of the hyperplastic lymphoid tissue into the muscularis propria and may be accompanied by ulceration [10]. A pronounced eosinophil polymorph and an interfollicular lymphoplasmacytic infiltrate between follicles are often present. The disease may closely mimic both MALT-type lymphoma and follicle centre cell-derived lymphoma (follicular lymphoma). Indeed it may be difficult to distinguish these conditions on morphological grounds. This is one area where molecular biological investigation may be required to differentiate between these conditions.

Diffuse nodular lymphoid hyperplasia of the small intestine

There are two major forms of this disease, which affects long segments of the small intestine [11,12]. Although still rare, the disease is most commonly seen as a complication of congenital or acquired immunodeficiency [11,13,14]. Patients with these immune deficiencies suffer recurrent infections: in the UK bacterial enteritis is most common, particularly *Campylobacter*, but other infections, notably giardiasis, may also occur. About 20% of adults with primary hypogammaglobulinaemia will show nodular lymphoid hyperplasia [11,13]. The nodules, measuring up to about 5 mm in diameter, are most prominent in the small bowel but can occur in the large intestine and more rarely in the stomach. They consist of hyperplastic lymphoid follicles with prominent germinal centres (Fig. 25.1). The adjacent mantle zone appears normal and ulceration is not a feature: these findings aid in the distinction from lymphoma [6]. The nodules lack the features of Peyer's patches, being devoid of overlying specialized epithelium (Fig. 25.1).

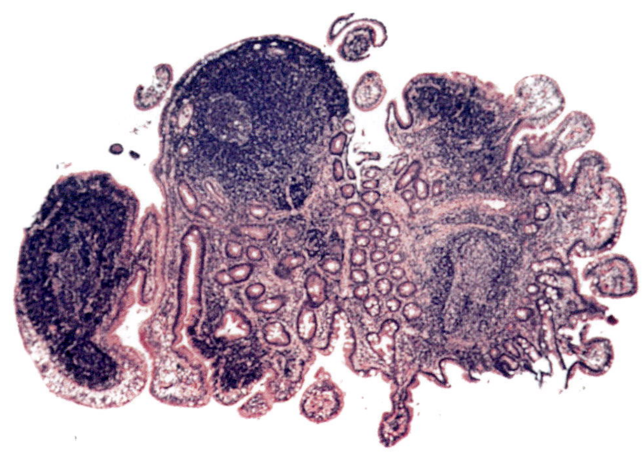

Fig. 25.1 Nodular lymphoid hyperplasia on biopsy. There is lymphoid follicular hyperplasia with prominent germinal centre formation.

Nodular lymphoid hyperplasia may also occur outwith the hypogammaglobulinaemia syndromes [15,16]. Whilst the macroscopic and microscopic features are similar in the two clinical settings, acquired nodular lymphoid hyperplasia without dysgammaglobulinaemia is much more closely associated with development of malignant lymphoma [12,16–18]. In this situation, the lymphoma is of MALT type and, like other MALT-type lymphomas in the gut and elsewhere, the tumour arises on a basis of long-term lymphoid hyperplasia [6]. Indeed it has been shown that the hyperplastic follicles and the associated lymphoma demonstrate the same monoclonal expansion of B cells [17]. Whilst most of these lymphomas show the expected B-cell phenotype, T-cell lymphoma arising on a basis of nodular lymphoid hyperplasia has been described [16].

Immunodeficiency-related lymphoproliferative disease

Lymphoma complicating congenital immunodeficiency and nodular lymphoid hyperplasia has been dealt with in the preceding sections. There remain two other entities in which lymphoma complicates immunological pathology. As in the stomach and large intestine, lymphoid hyperplasia and malignant lymphoma are well recognized complications of the acquired immune deficiency syndrome (AIDS) [19]. Intestinal lymphomas in AIDS are usually of high-grade B-cell type. In the REAL classification, most fall into the diffuse large B-cell category. These are highly aggressive tumours with a poor prognosis [20].

Post-transplant lymphoproliferative disease (PTLD) is an Epstein–Barr virus (EBV)-driven lymphoid proliferation that occurs in all forms of transplantation where immunosuppression is required to prevent rejection [21,22]. Whilst all parts of the gut may be affected, the disease is commonest in the small intestine, presumably because of the wealth of lymphoid tissue here [23]. The morphological features of the disease would suggest high-grade malignant lymphoma with a predominant B-cell phenotype (although some cases show a T-cell phenotype) as there are numerous activated blast-type cells amongst the infiltrate [22]. Restoration of immune function or adequate treatment of the disease by chemotherapy often occasions a remarkably good prognosis, in the early stages of disease, compared with *de novo* high-grade malignant lymphomas at this site, although in some cases, true high-grade lymphoma supervenes [22,23]. There is some evidence that the behaviour of this tumour relates to the clonal nature of the lesion. Early good prognosis disease is polyclonal despite the number of activated lymphoid cells, whereas monoclonality presages the development of high-grade lymphoma with a rapidly progressive behaviour and poor prognosis [22].

Primary malignant lymphoma of the small intestine

Primary small intestinal lymphoma accounts for less than 2% of all gastrointestinal malignancies but it does account for between 20% and 30% of all primary lymphomas of the gut [24,25]. Thus its incidence is intermediate, in Western populations, between that of the stomach (at around 60%) and large intestine (less than 10%). However, in the eastern Mediterranean, Middle East and South Africa, the small intestine is the commonest site for primary lymphoma because of the predominance of immunoproliferative small intestinal disease (IPSID), a low-grade MALT-type lymphoma. The preferred sites of involvement, within the small intestine, are often type dependent. For instance, IPSID usually presents with duodenal or jejunal disease whilst T-cell lymphomas, such as those complicating enteropathy, are most common in the jejunum (Fig. 25.2) [5]. Low-grade B-cell lymphomas are most commonly found in the distal, or terminal, ileum [26,27]. As it is the type of lymphoma that primarily determines the site of origin and therefore presentation, the morphological features, the treatment and the prognosis, each major type of primary lymphoma arising in the small intestine will be considered separately. Initially, however, the interested reader is invited to study the 'Lymphoma' section in the 'Stomach' section of this book (p. 196) for a fuller account of the concepts and classification of primary gastrointestinal lymphoma.

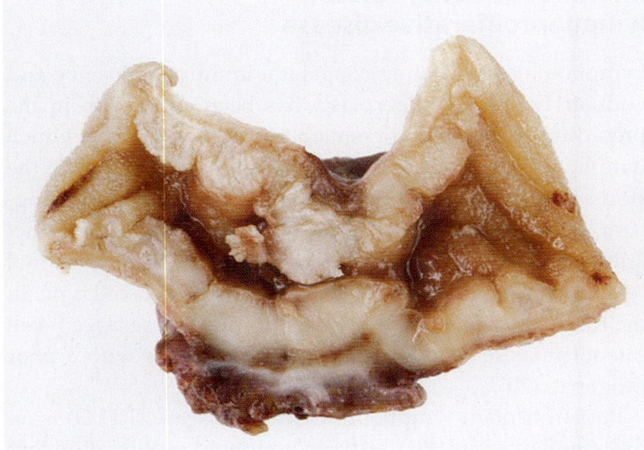

Fig. 25.2 A stricturing ulcerating malignant lymphoma of the jejunum. The patient had a long history of coeliac disease and presented with small bowel obstruction. The tumour was confirmed histologically as EATL (enteropathy-associated T-cell lymphoma).

Primary MALT lymphoma of the small intestine

B-cell MALT-type lymphomas constitute the largest single group of primary lymphomas in the small intestine. In one major and well characterized series, 45% of small bowel lymphomas fulfilled criteria for this type [27]. These data derive from a Western series and it should be emphasized that, in certain populations, immunoproliferative small intestinal disease (IPSID), a low-grade MALT-type lymphoma, is overwhelmingly the commonest type of primary lymphoma in the entire gut. This discussion will concentrate on MALT-type lymphoma of Western type, whereas IPSID will be considered separately because of its very specific clinical and pathological characteristics.

Whilst the terminal ileum is undoubtedly the commonest site for Western MALT-type lymphoma (Fig. 25.3), these lymphomas may also occur in the duodenum and jejunum [7,27]. Unlike in the stomach, low-grade MALT lymphomas are not predominant in the small intestine: tumours which fulfil criteria for high-grade diffuse large B-cell lymphoma are commoner [27–29], in one series accounting for two-thirds of all the small intestinal MALT tumours [27]. There are also intermediate cases where there are low-grade areas with foci

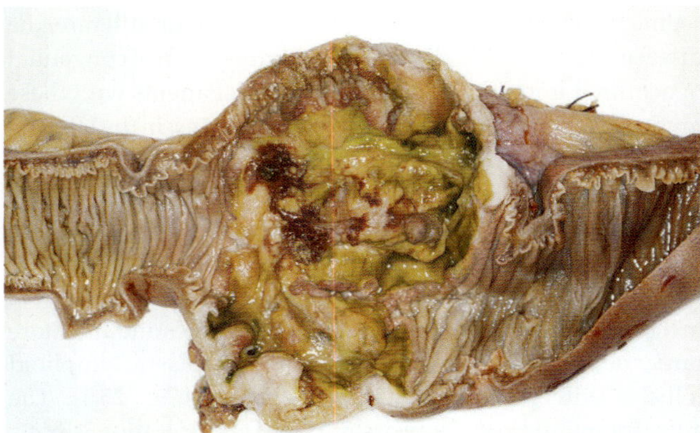

Fig. 25.3 A large ulcerating high-grade B-cell lymphoma of the terminal ileum, the commonest site for B-cell tumours of the small intestine in Western countries.

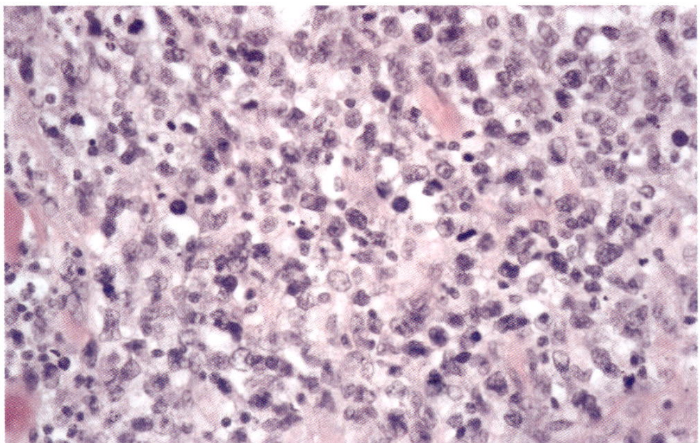

Fig. 25.4 Histology of the high-grade lymphoma shown in Fig. 25.3. There are sheets of transformed cells, some with centroblast-like morphology. Even at this power, the substantial mitotic and apoptotic activity is obvious.

of blast cell infiltrate [27]. Although grading of these tumours remains a subject of some controversy, grade provides useful prognostic information with resected low-grade tumours having a much better prognosis than their high-grade counterparts [27–29].

MALT-type lymphoma is primarily a disease of adults, especially the elderly, although high-grade tumours may also occur in young adults [27]. Males are more likely to be affected, with a ratio of about 2 : 1. The disease usually presents with abdominal pain, often with the symptoms and signs of obstruction. Perforation does not usually occur with low-grade tumours but is a significant adverse prognostic factor in high-grade lymphomas [27]. Low-grade MALT lymphoma shows identical features to those seen elsewhere, especially the stomach. A diffuse infiltrate of neoplastic marginal zone cells, the centrocyte-like cells, is a prerequisite for the diagnosis [6]. In addition there is the typical cellular polymorphism with neoplastic plasma cells and activated blast cells also present. Furthermore lymphoepithelial lesions, in which the neoplastic marginal zone cells infiltrate and destroy the small intestinal epithelium, are a typical feature. Although less common than in primary gastric lymphoma, lymphoepithelial lesions are seen in up to 80% of low-grade MALT-type lymphomas of the small intestine [27]. The presence of large reactive lymphoid follicles, with infiltration and destruction by the neoplastic marginal zone cells, is also a very common feature of low-grade lymphoma in the small intestine [6].

The differentiation of low-grade lymphoma from high-grade disease is usually straightforward. The diagnosis of high-grade lymphoma requires the presence of sheets of transformed, blast-type cells (Fig. 25.4) [5]. These have a morphology similar to centroblasts although nucleoli are often less conspicuous (Fig. 25.4) [30]. Lymphoepithelial lesions, due to such transformed cells, may be present but they are much less numerous than in low-grade MALT lymphoma. Reactive lymphoid follicles may be present; however, these characteristic components of MALT-type lymphoma and the associated low-grade component of the disease may be destroyed by the high-grade tumour.

No specific initiating factor has yet been discovered for Western-type MALT lymphoma of the small intestine. Unlike in the stomach, there is no clear relationship between *Helicobacter* infection and the disease. As far as is known at the current time, the lymphoma shares the immunohistochemical, cytogenetic and molecular pathological features of primary gastric lymphoma (see p. 196). The behaviour of small intestinal MALT-type lymphoma is not as favourable as its gastric counterpart. Firstly the predominance of high-grade tumours is a major factor. These tumours have a 5-year survival rate of around 30% whereas low-grade disease has a range from around 50 to 75% [27–29]. Other important prognostic factors indicating a good prognosis are resectability, early stage, the lack of tumour perforation, terminal ileal site and lack of multiplicity [27,28]. There is also some developing evidence that radical resection followed by chemotherapy may enhance survival rates, especially in high-grade disease [29,31].

Immunoproliferative small intestinal disease

Immunoproliferative small intestinal disease (IPSID) is a low-grade MALT-type lymphoma, characterized by a presentation with malabsorption and a specific geographical location. Although the disease has now been described from several continents, it is most common in the eastern Mediterranean, the Middle East and in the Cape region of South Africa. The disease was first described in the Middle East in 1962 [32] and further characterized from Israel in 1965 [33]. It usually occurs in young adults and presents with malabsorption or alternatively with the symptoms and signs of malignant lymphoma but with a long history of diarrhoea, steatorrhoea and weight loss [34–36].

The lymphoma is a MALT-type lymphoma but with prominent plasma cell differentiation: a highly characteristic feature of the tumour is that the lymphoma cells secrete heavy chains, α-immunoglobulin, but without light chain production [37]. In about 60% of cases, the heavy chains are detectable in either the small intestinal secretion or in the blood [36,38]. In the remaining cases the immunoglobulin is detectable in the neoplastic plasma cells but not secreted [39,40]. This production of α-immunoglobulin has led to the alternative name of the disease: α-chain disease [38]. IPSID has also been previously termed Mediterranean lymphoma [36].

The lymphoma primarily affects the jejunum, although the duodenum and ileum may also be involved. Indeed duodenal biopsy is usually the mode of diagnosis. The small intestine shows a characteristic diffuse thickening and there is usually mesenteric lymphadenopathy. The thickening of the jejunum may be circumferential and cause obstruction due to stricturing [41]. Tumorous masses, some of which may be expansile and polypoid, are usually the portent of high-grade transfor-

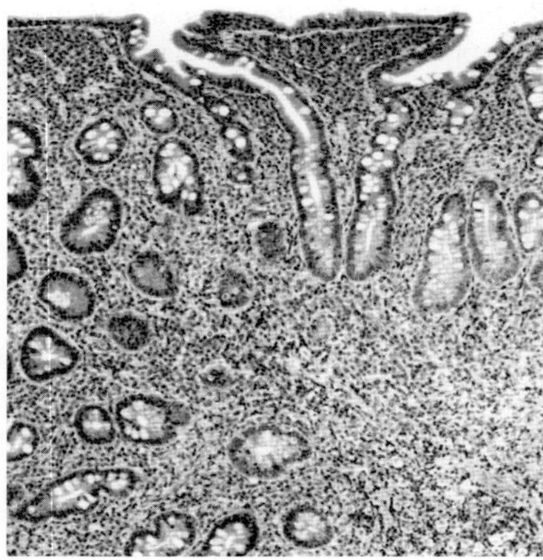

Fig. 25.5 Alpha-chain disease in which the lamina propria is expanded by heavy infiltrate of plasma cells. Villi can still be discerned and the surface enterocytes are relatively normal (H&E × 150).

mation. Histologically the lymphoma is a low-grade MALT-type lymphoma but with extreme plasmacytic differentiation (Fig. 25.5). Thus the mucosa of the small intestine is expanded by a predominant lymphoplasmacytic infiltrate, which results in villous architectural abnormalities (Fig. 25.5) [5,41]. Nevertheless other features of MALT lymphoma are usually present, including sheets of centrocyte-like cells, lymphoepithelial lesions and destruction of reactive lymphoid follicles [5].

Immunohistochemical analysis shows the lymphocytes and plasma cells stain strongly for CD20 whilst cytokeratin markers will serve to highlight lymphoepithelial lesions. Neoplastic lymphocytes and plasma cells both produce α-chain, which can be demonstrated immunohistochemically [42,43]. Although some have questioned the neoplastic nature of the disease in its early stages, molecular analysis has demonstrated that the plasmacytic infiltrate is monoclonal, confirming its neoplastic nature even in the early stages and confirming the similarities with *Helicobacter*-driven primary gastric lymphoma [44]. Various cytogenetic abnormalities have also been described including chromosomal translocations [45].

Three stages of the disease are recognized and these correlate well with clinical features and macroscopic appearances [5,40,46]. Initially the disease is solely mucosal and presents with malabsorptive features. Eventually there is expansion of disease into the submucosa and nodules form. These nodules comprise follicular colonization of reactive lymphoid aggregates by the neoplastic cells. Finally high-grade transformation results in the large tumour masses with deep involvement of the bowel wall [46]. Notwithstanding these local stages of disease, mesenteric lymph nodes are involved early in the disease, with an initial plasmacytic infiltrate detectable in sinuses. Eventually high-grade disease overruns the lymph nodes and then systemic spread is likely.

IPSID, in its early stages, shows a capacity for clinical remission and, some have suggested, cure when treated with broad-spectrum antibiotics, such as tetracyclines [46,47]. This has allowed comparisons with *Helicobacter* and primary gastric lymphoma. It suggests that in certain geographical locations, a bacterial agent or agents is responsible for chronic immunological stimulation, which eventually results in a monoclonal expansion of immunoglobulin heavy chain-secreting plasma cells. Even then, these plasma cells may respond to removal of the antigen stimulus, the (presumed) bacterium, with clinical remission of the disease. As yet, no single bacterial agent has been found responsible for IPSID. A major confounding factor is the small intestine's colonization with numerous different bacteria and this makes detection of a single responsible microorganism so much more difficult than in the stomach.

IPSID has a long, relapsing and remitting course especially when appropriately treated [40,46,47]. Although the malabsorption itself is associated with morbidity and some mortality, it is the onset of high-grade transformation that is a grave prognostic occurrence: systemic spread with bone marrow involvement may then rapidly supervene [6]. The morphology of such high-grade tumours is often bizarre, although some may show typical immunoblastic and/or plasmablastic morphology.

Burkitt's lymphoma

Two major subtypes of this tumour are recognized. Whilst there are many similarities, the two subtypes show subtle differences in clinical, molecular and immunophenotypical features but they are most usefully considered together [5]. Endemic Burkitt's lymphoma is most common in central Africa and is strongly associated with pandemic malaria infection; Epstein–Barr virus (EBV) is implicated in its aetiology [48]. Although the jaw is the classical site of involvement, the terminal ileum is a recognized site for the tumour. On the other hand, the terminal ileum is the commonest site for sporadic Burkitt's lymphoma. Burkitt's lymphoma is a disease of childhood, usually between the ages of 2 and 12 years. Macroscopically there is usually a large ulcerating mass of the ileocaecal region although long segment involvement of the small intestine is well described. The histological features are characteristic: there is a monotonous infiltrate of intermediate-sized blast cells, which appear tightly packed [49]. The nuclei are rounded with small nucleoli (numbering between two and five) which are diffusely dispersed within the nucleus and do not touch the membrane. The tumour cells show prodigious mitotic activity and the numerous tingible body macrophages, containing numerous apoptotic bodies, impart the highly typical 'starry-sky' appearance to the tumour. Smears or imprints of the tumour cells demonstrate intracytoplasmic lipid droplets, a useful diagnostic feature in these preparations [5]. Although the tumour is usually deeply invasive in the intestinal wall, there is often a curious preservation of muscularis propria cells with the tumour dissecting between muscle cells but not destroying them (singly unlike other high-grade lymphomas in the gut) [50].

The immunophenotype of Burkitt's lymphoma is remarkably consistent, with the tumour cells expressing pan B-cell markers, including CD20, and demonstrating detectable intracytoplasmic immunoglobulin [5,51]. The two subtypes differ in their expression of certain B-cell markers, especially CD23 and CD30 [5]. Endemic Burkitt's lymphoma usually expresses CD30 (especially with the monoclonal antibody Ber-H2) whereas the sporadic disease shows this much less commonly [5]. More than 90% of endemic cases will show the presence of EBV whereas less than 20% of sporadic cases will demonstrate the virus [48,52]. The most important molecular abnormalities of both types of lymphoma are translocations between immunoglobulin gene loci (either the heavy chain on chromosome 14 or the light chain loci on chromosomes 2 and 22) and the *c-myc* oncogene locus on chromosome 8 [53,54]. Thus t(8;14), t(8;22) and t(2;8) translocations result in activation of the *c-myc* gene with overexpression of its protein [53,55,56]. There are some differences in the gene breakpoints between the two forms of the disease although the actual translocations (and their molecular effects) are the same [54,56,57].

Unlike many high-grade lymphomas of the gut, Burkitt's lymphoma shows a pronounced sensitivity to chemotherapy [58]. Whilst of benefit for prognosis, the extensive tumour lysis that can occur during treatment means that small bowel perforation is a considerable risk, if the disease is not fully removed at the time of operative surgery [59]. Although endemic Burkitt's lymphoma continues to have a relatively poor prognosis in Africa, the Western-type sporadic disease is associated with a much better prognosis with cure rates of up to 70% regularly recorded [5,58].

Enteropathy-associated T-cell lymphoma

Enteropathy-associated T-cell lymphoma (EATL) accounts for only a small proportion of primary gastrointestinal lymphomas but it is a disease of considerable pathological importance because of its relationships with coeliac disease, the controversies concerning this relationship, the difficulties of its clinical and pathological diagnosis, controversy concerning its true histogenesis and its adverse prognosis. Primary T-cell lymphoma is most unusual in the stomach and large intestine, whereas in the small intestine, T-cell neoplasms account for up to 30% of the total [27]. Not all of these tumours are associated with coeliac disease although more than half are probably complications of this enteropathy [6,27].

Few tumours have undergone such a rapid re-evaluation of their histogenesis as EATL. It was termed 'malignant histiocytosis of the intestines' by Isaacson and Wright because of the tumour cells' morphological appearances and immunohistochemical expression of histiocytic markers such as lysozyme [60]; subsequent molecular analyses by Isaacson and colleagues [61] convincingly demonstrated its T-cell origin. More recently molecular evidence has suggested that two conditions with previously uncertain relationships with EATL, refractory coeliac disease, in which there is an unexplained failure to sustain a clinical response to a gluten-free diet without demonstration of a specific additional pathology of the small bowel, and ulcerative jejunitis, in which there is also failure of response to gluten-free diet but with ulceration of the jejunum, also represent neoplastic T-cell conditions with identical aberrant immunophenotype and molecular pathology to EATL [62–64].

There remains some controversy concerning the relationship between coeliac disease and EATL [65]. There is little doubt that cases do exist that represent *de novo* lymphoma with a low-grade T-cell lymphoma component mimicking coeliac disease both clinically and pathologically [66]. This particularly occurs in the elderly. In contrast, there is now compelling evidence that coeliac disease precedes most cases conforming to the pathological, immunohistochemical and molecular features of EATL and that adequate control of coeliac disease, by gluten-free diet, substantially reduces the incidence of the lymphoma [67]. For instance, there is evidence that many patients with coeliac disease and EATL have a common HLA phenotype [68] and EATL patients share other pathological manifestations of the enteropathy, such as dermatitis herpetiformis and splenic atrophy [69]. Most would now accept that a large proportion of T-cell lymphomas of the small intestine are associated with pre-existing coeliac disease, whether the enteropathy has been previously diagnosed or not. A small proportion of T-cell lymphomas do represent *de novo* disease with clinical and/or pathological mimicry of coeliac disease [66]. Furthermore it is clear that not all T-cell lymphomas are associated with enteropathy, although the true proportion of such tumours is difficult to determine because of difficulties in defining the diseases and because of incomplete documentation of what is a rare condition.

EATL presents clinically in diverse ways. It can present as a complication of long-term coeliac disease with failure of response to a gluten-free diet and worsening malabsorption. Subsequent investigation may reveal a tumour mass or alternatively non-specific, often multiple ulceration (ulcerative jejunitis) or no specific pathology (refractory coeliac disease). Alternatively there may be presentation with the direct effects of the tumour with abdominal pain, small intestinal obstruction, perforation and/or haemorrhage [70]. The commonest site for EATL is the jejunum (Fig. 25.2). Whilst a single tumour mass may occur, EATL is often multifocal and the duodenum and/or the ileum can be involved. Ulceration and the destructive infiltration of the intestinal wall may cause perforation and strictures are common (Fig. 25.2). Wide dissemination at the time of initial diagnosis is the rule, with involvement of liver, spleen and bone marrow common [60,70]. Close attention should be paid to the assessment of the adjacent mucosa, whether in biopsies or at dissection of resection specimens, for evidence of coeliac disease, notably villous atrophy and intraepithelial lymphocytic infiltration [60]. It should be emphasized, however, that non-specific changes, especially in villous architecture, may be observed proximal to any obstructing lesion of the small bowel, as a result of stasis and/or bacterial overgrowth. Biopsies of the proximal small bowel, especially the duodenum, are recommended to confirm or refute an association of the tumour with coeliac disease [60].

Most EATLs are high-grade T-cell lymphomas composed of large cells with highly pleomorphic nuclei. Some show T immunoblastic features whilst a minority show a predominance of intermediate and small T lymphocytes. In the latter there is often a florid intraepithelial component [65]. EATL discloses a characteristic destructive morphology with deep fissuring ulcers, necrosis and destruction of the muscularis propria. It cannot be overemphasized that EATL should be strongly considered with any destructive ulcerative condition of the small intestine, especially if associated with coeliac disease. This is because the neoplastic T cells may be scanty and camouflaged by an associated inflammatory cell component, especially eosinophils, which may be numerous [71].

Immunohistochemistry shows that the tumour cells of EATL usually express CD3 with variable expression of CD8; they are negative for CD4 [72]. They usually show the immunophenotype of intraepithelial T cells of the gut and there is some evidence that EATL arises from these cells [64,65,73,74]. Molecular analysis has demonstrated that EATL shows clonal rearrangement of T-cell receptor (TCR)-β or TCR-γ genes [61,62,72,75]. These same abnormalities have also been demonstrated in refractory coeliac disease (refractory sprue) and ulcerative jejunitis, lending further evidence that these conditions do indeed represent neoplastic complications of coeliac disease [64].

Adverse prognostic features in small bowel lymphoma (as a whole) are a T-cell phenotype, multifocality, perforation and advanced stage [27]. EATL is strongly associated with all of these features. Thus EATL has a particularly gloomy prognosis with 5-year survival rates of 20% or less [5,27]. There is little evidence of a good response of the disease to any form of adjuvant therapy [27].

Other primary lymphomas of the small intestine

Mantle cell lymphoma, also known as malignant (multiple) lymphomatous polyposis, is a lymphoma characterized by multiple polypoid tumours composed of monotonous neoplastic mantle cells, which have a centrocyte-like morphology [3,76–78]. Massive terminal ileal involvement is a distinguishing feature of the disease, and multiple polyps of the ileum and jejunum, and less commonly the duodenum and stomach, are prevalent. Sometimes the tumour produces a more generalized thickening of the mucosa and submucosa (Fig. 25.6). Nevertheless the disease usually presents with large bowel

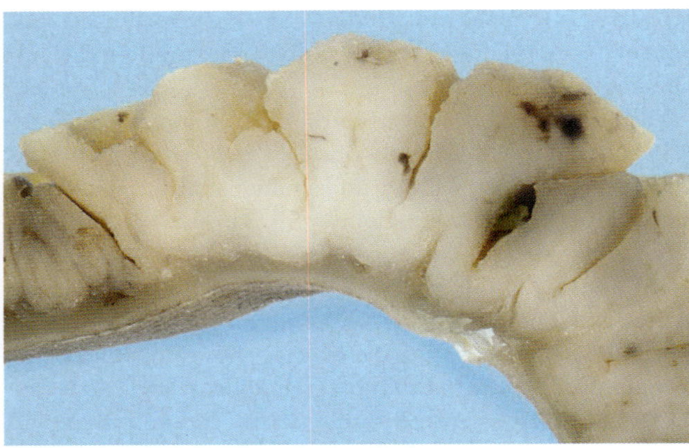

Fig. 25.6 Mantle zone lymphoma of the jejunum producing band-like thickening of the mucosa and submucosa. The relative sparing of the deeper layers of the bowel wall is a common feature of this tumour.

involvement and is therefore much more comprehensively covered elsewhere (see p. 613).

Although follicle centre cell lymphoma is the most common non-Hodgkin's lymphoma in nodal disease, it is curiously rare as a primary lymphoma of the gut [26]. In one series these tumours accounted for just 2% of primary lymphomas of the small bowel [27]. Follicular lymphomas are extremely unusual at all sites of the gut except the terminal ileum where they arise from the follicles of Peyer's patches [26,79]. Their follicle cell centre origin is supported by the expression of *bcl-2* in the majority of cases in the largest fully substantiated series in the literature [26]. Whilst such tumours are usually single, of early stage and have a relatively good prognosis, multifocality with 'lymphomatous polyposis' has been ascribed to follicle centre cell lymphomas in the small intestine [26,80]. There is a report of malignant lymphoma occurring in an ileal reservoir but the surgery is unlikely to be causal in this case [81].

About 20% of small intestinal lymphomas will show a T-cell phenotype and many of these represent EATL. Sporadic T-cell lymphomas are predominantly high-grade tumours with few specific pathological features: they have a poor prognosis and are likely to be multifocal [27,82]. There is some evidence that many of these sporadic T-cell tumours may arise from intraepithelial T-lymphocytes [82]. Whilst EATLs occasionally show tumour cell epitheliotropism, there are occasional reports of T-cell neoplasms, in which this epitheliotropism is the most pronounced feature [83]. These tumours demonstrate a T-cell cytotoxic/suppressor immunophenotype, being CD8 positive [83]. There are reports of a novel chromosomal translocation in a primary low-grade T-cell lymphoma of the small bowel [84] and of a primary T-lymphoblastic lymphoma without evidence of thymic involvement [85].

There is an unusual group of T-cell lymphomas, primarily of small intestinal origin but occasionally arising in the stomach, that is characterized by a marked, often intense, eosinophil infiltrate [71]. This may be so marked as to conceal the

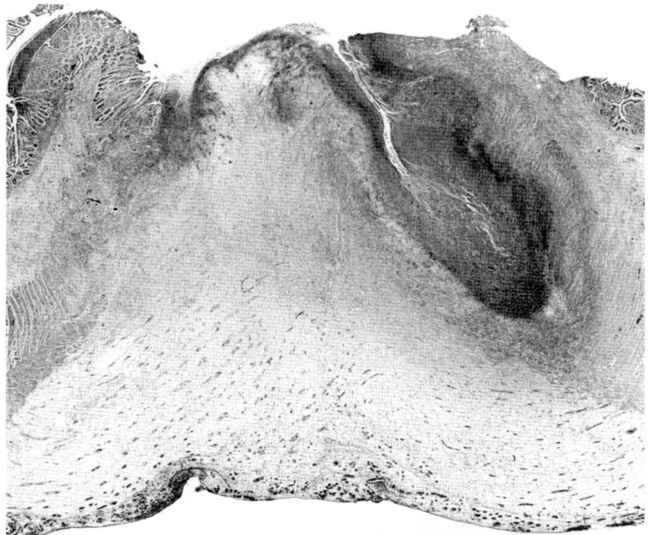

Fig. 25.7 High-grade lymphoma in the small intestine. The deep fissuring ulceration is a characteristic feature. The zoning phenomenon so prominent here is a typical feature of 'malignant lymphoma with eosinophilia' of the small intestine.

neoplastic cells. Occasionally this 'malignant lymphoma with eosinophilia' occurs in patients with known coeliac disease and thus represents one variant of EATL [71]. However, many of these cases show no evidence of an associated enteropathy. The lymphoma is distinguished by a zoning phenomenon with fissuring ulceration, transmural bowel wall involvement with a propensity to perforation, multifocality and a very poor prognosis with 5-year survival rates of less than 10% (Fig. 25.7). Malignant lymphoma should always be considered in small bowel disease with a pronounced eosinophil infiltrate along with the other well recognized causes of small intestinal tissue eosinophilia such as eosinophilic enteritis, infections and infestations, inflammatory bowel disease, vasculitis and arteritis and inflammatory fibroid polyp [86].

Secondary lymphomatous and leukaemic involvement of the small intestine

Secondary involvement of the small intestine by lymphoma is common in clinical and autopsy practice. Indeed such secondary involvement, in strict numerical terms, is commoner than primary tumours. Secondary involvement of the small intestine is especially common in high-grade lymphomas and it may be difficult on morphological and immunohistochemical grounds to differentiate these from primary tumours. The distinctive features of primary MALT lymphoma, including lymphoepithelial lesions, a low-grade component and the immunohistochemical and molecular phenotype, may help to differentiate the conditions. Acute myeloblastic leukaemia can present as a myeloblastic sarcoma in the small intestine, often before the presentation of leukaemia [87,88]. The neoplasm can mimic primary lymphoma, for the cells show a diffuse infiltrate of blast cells, often with some plasmacytoid appearances. Evidence of eosinophil precursors, within the tumour, should be sought whilst histochemical analysis for chloroacetate esterase and lysozyme is usually confirmatory. Chronic lymphocytic leukaemia (CLL) is an important pathological differential diagnosis of primary low-grade MALT lymphoma [6]. Often immunophenotypic analysis is required to confirm the diagnosis: expression of CD5 and CD23 by CLL is perhaps the most useful means of differentiating CLL from MALT lymphoma.

Gastrointestinal stromal tumours

Our understanding of the histogenesis of spindle cell tumours of the gut has changed considerably in the last decade or so. Whilst the previous edition of this textbook, published just over a decade ago, regards smooth muscle tumours of the small bowel as the commonest spindle cell tumours, immunohistochemical and molecular evidence have necessitated a profound rethink. We, and others, believe that most, if not all, tumours with a spindle cell morphology and without identifying features indicating an origin from specific connective tissue cells should be regarded as gastrointestinal stromal tumours (GISTs) [89,90]. For a comprehensive account of current theories of the histogenesis of GISTs, and a general overview of the histological and immunohistochemical features, the interested reader is referred to the equivalent chapter in the 'Stomach' section (p. 204), as this is the commonest site for GISTs. Nevertheless the small intestine is a relatively common site for such tumours and there are several important site-specific aspects of GISTs for the small intestine.

Perhaps not surprisingly, given its length and therefore its content of connective tissue, the small intestine is a relatively common site for GISTs. About 25–30% of all GISTs arise here, with ileum being overall the commonest site within the small intestine [89]. Specific mention should be made of the duodenum, however, for a disproportionately large number of GISTs arise here [91]. In general the histological spectrum of stromal tumours of the small intestine is similar to that of the stomach. However, the proportion of subtypes is notably different: epithelioid GISTs are unusual in the small bowel compared with the stomach, apart from the epithelioid tumour known as gastrointestinal autonomic nerve tumour (GANT) which, although rare in terms of total numbers of GISTs, is commonest in the small bowel (see below). Thus most small bowel GISTs are spindle cell stromal tumours [92].

Stromal tumours in the duodenum

GISTs arising in the duodenum are usually spindle cell tumours; epithelioid tumours are very unusual [92]. Approximately half the tumours are of uniform spindle cell morphology, with low cellularity, organoid morphology and less than 2 mitoses per 50 high-power fields (hpf) [91]. They tend to show plentiful eosinophilic extracellular material, which almost certainly represents skeinoid fibres on ultrastructural examination [93,94]. These tumours are generally benign in behaviour and are characteristically small in size (less than 5 cm in diameter) [91]. One the other hand, those duodenal GISTs with more aggressive natural history are large, and histological examination shows high cellularity with mitotic activity in excess of 2 per 50 hpf. Such malignant duodenal GISTs may focally demonstrate the more 'benign' morphological appearances already described. Only when these areas are present do these more aggressive GISTs contain skeinoid fibres: these benign foci within otherwise aggressive tumours, are most commonly seen, seemingly, in the submucosa [91]. GISTs in the duodenum share the immunohistochemical and molecular pathology of GISTs at other sites (see p. 203). Their principal differential diagnosis is from gangliocytic paraganglioma and other tumours of neural origin (see below).

GISTs in the jejunum and ileum

Like the duodenum, most GISTs in the jejunum and ileum are of spindle cell type (Fig. 25.8) [95]. In general, epithelioid morphology is unusual in the jejunal and ileal GISTs, although it should be remembered that one epithelioid tumour, GANT, makes up a modest proportion of GISTs at this site [96]. As in the duodenum, small GISTs are relatively common in the jejunum and ileum [92]. They show an organoid, paucicellular morphology with low mitotic indices [95,97]. On the other hand, large tumours are characterized by high cellularity, less organoid morphology, necrosis and high mitotic rates [97,98]. In one study, dense cellularity, mitotic activity, epithelioid cell shape, mucosal infiltration and size were univariate prognostic determinants [97]. Multivariate analysis revealed that only dense cellularity and mitotic counts were independent predictors for metastatic disease [97]. Thus it would appear that size, cellularity and mitotic index are the most important factors for prognosis in jejunal and ileal GISTs. These tumours tend to share the immunohistochemical and molecular pathology of GISTs at other sites (see p. 204).

Gastrointestinal autonomic nerve tumours (GANTs)

GANTs were first identified as malignant stromal tumours of the small bowel and were initially termed plexosarcomas by Herrera and colleagues [99]. Walker and Dvorak introduced the term 'gastrointestinal autonomic nerve tumour' because of evidence of axonal differentiation and the presence of dense core granules on electron microscopic analysis [100]. It has subsequently been demonstrated that such tumours arise in the stomach and in the proximal colon but the small bowel re-

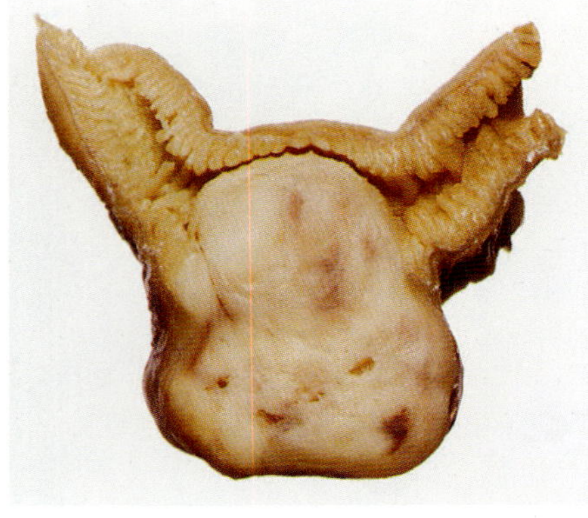

(a)

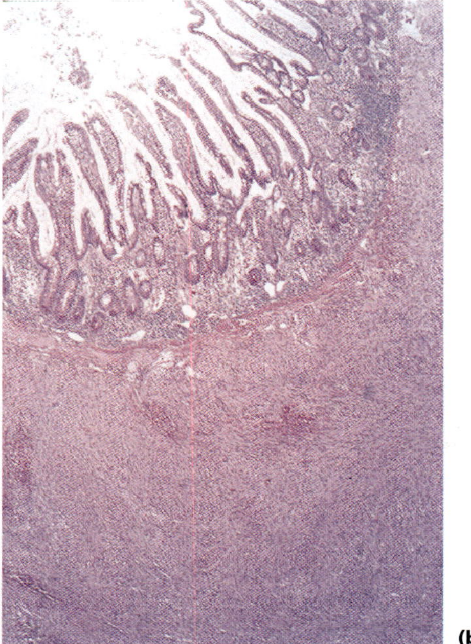

(b)

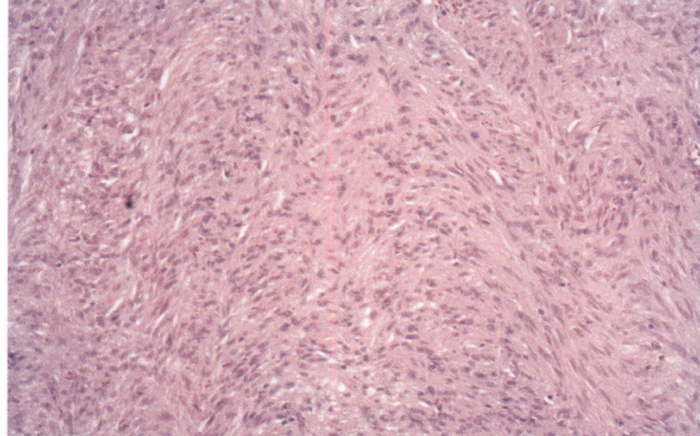

(c)

Fig. 25.8 A gastrointestinal stromal tumour (GIST) of the jejunum. (a) Macroscopic assessment shows the dumb-bell shape with expansion of the submucosa and subserosa by the tumour, which shows a pale fibroid-like cut surface with some central haemorrhage. (b) As might be expected, the tumour shows early involvement of the overlying mucosa. (c) The GIST shows a spindle cell morphology.

mains the most common site for this aggressive form of GIST [90,94,96,101–104].

GANTs are relatively large tumours of the small intestine, which may be intramural or predominantly subserosal or may arise in the mesenteric tissues of the bowel (Fig. 25.9) [96,102]. They may have a uniform cut surface, often tan or pink in colour, but there are often cystic and/or haemorrhagic areas (Fig. 25.9) [96,102]. Their histological appearances are characteristic: they are composed of sheets and nests of epithelioid or spindle cells often in an interfasciculating pattern [96,102]. GANTs have a pronounced vascularity (Fig. 25.10) and also have dispersed lymphocytes, sometimes in small aggregates, throughout the tumour. Electron microscopic analysis shows the presence of dendritic structures, synapse-like structures containing dense core granules and endocytoplasmic vesicles [96,101,105].

Immunohistochemical evidence shows that, while fundamentally similar to other GISTs, GANTs show evidence of neural differentiation. Thus they are usually positive for vimentin and CD117 (c-kit) (as are most GISTs) but may also show staining for chromogranin, S-100, neurone-specific enolase, synaptophysin and PGP 9.5 [104]. CD 34 shows variable staining: whilst many GISTs are positive for this marker, negativity for CD34, in GANTs, is a feature that appears to be more prevalent in the more aggressive tumours (Fig. 25.11) [106]. GANTs are negative for smooth muscle actin, desmin and cytokeratins [96]. There is little doubt that, as a whole, these tumours are very much disposed toward the malignant end of the spectrum of GISTs in general. Many of the papers in the literature testify to their high mitotic activity, which in itself may be an important prognostic indicator, their large size, their propensity toward intraperitoneal spread and their metastatic liability [90,94,96,101–104]. It is now clear that there is a close interrelationship between GISTs, as a whole, and GANTs, particularly now further immunohistochemical evidence is available [89,90]. For instance, most tumours in both groups express CD117 (c-kit) whilst some GANTs also demonstrate skeinoid fibres, a feature characteristic of GISTs, especially in the small intestine [94,104].

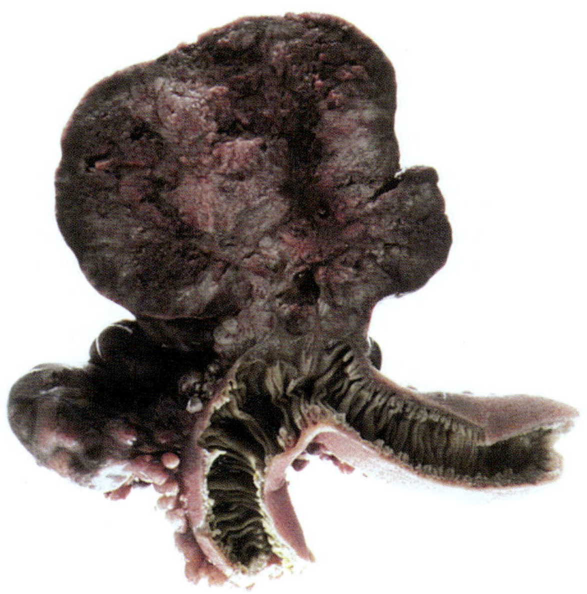

Fig. 25.9 A gastrointestinal autonomic nerve tumour (GANT) of the jejunum. The tumour is typically large, transmural and has a relatively uniform cut surface, tan in colour, with focal haemorrhagic areas.

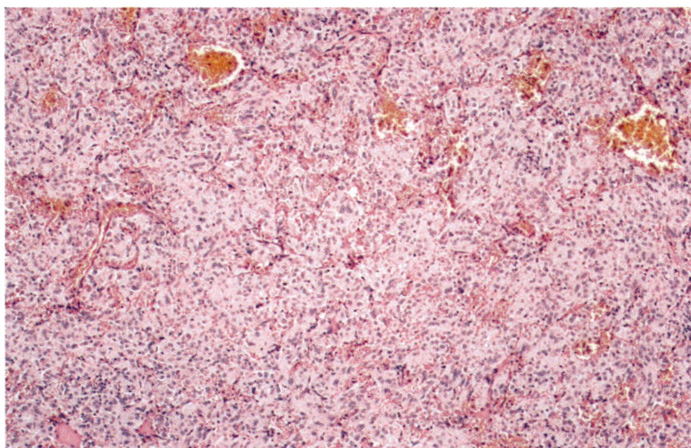

Fig. 25.10 Gastrointestinal autonomic nerve tumour (GANT) composed of eosinophilic epithelioid tumour cells with marked vascularity.

Gastrointestinal stromal tumours with skeinoid fibres

Gastrointestinal stromal tumours with skeinoid fibres

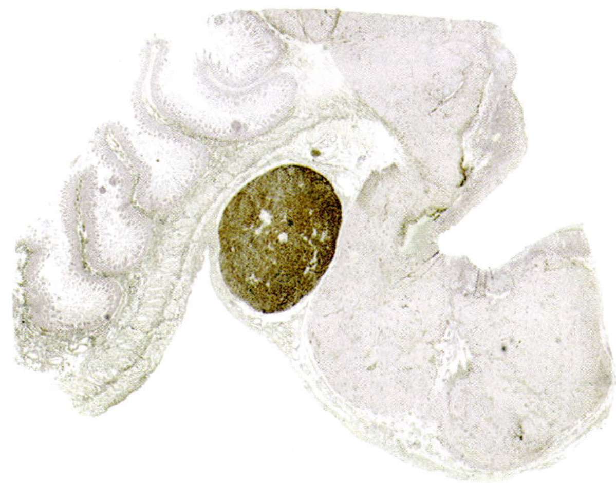

Fig. 25.11 A wholemount section, stained immunohistochemically for CD34, in a gastrointestinal autonomic nerve tumour (GANT) of the ileum. Much of the tumour appears negative but there is one clone that is strikingly positive. Intriguingly, it was this clone of the tumour that had metastasized across the peritoneum, a typical feature of GANTs, and to a local lymph node.

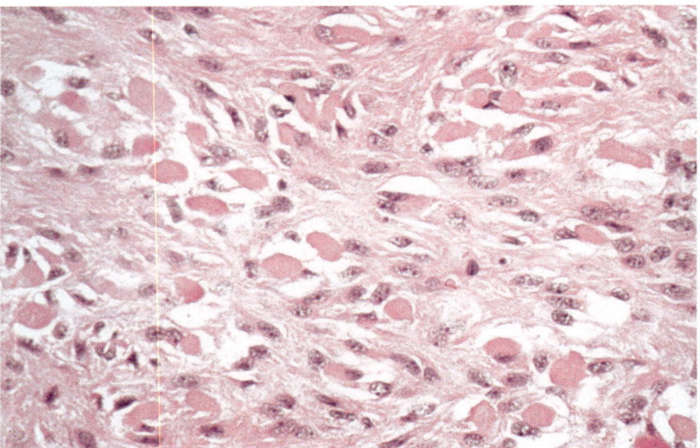

Fig. 25.12 Large numbers of eosinophilic skeinoid fibres are seen in this gastrointestinal stromal tumour of the ileum.

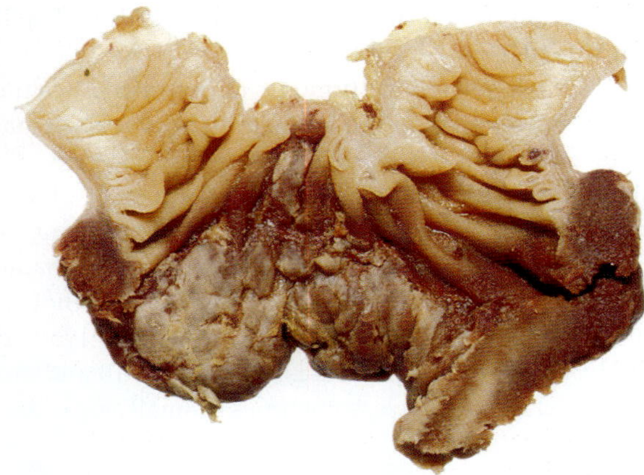

Fig. 25.13 An angiosarcoma of the jejunum. A large haemorrhagic tumour replaces much of the wall of the intestine in this resection specimen. These are rare but aggressive tumours. The patient died of metastatic angiosarcoma within 1 year of this resection.

(GISTSFs) are a GIST subtype apparently more specific to the small bowel [93]. Whilst they have many of the morphological features of standard GISTs, they have whorled extracellular collagen-like material, which stains eosinophilic in histological sections (Fig. 25.12). The term skeinoid derives from their resemblance to skeins, or yarns of wool, on ultrastructural examination [93]. It is now questioned whether skeinoid fibres are of any specific significance (apart from enabling a diagnosis of GIST) because such formations have been demonstrated in GANTs and are also demonstrable ultrastructurally in most small intestinal GISTs [89,94].

Tumours of adipose tissue

Lipomas are relatively common in the colon but are less often seen in the small bowel. Most are discovered incidentally and are symptomless: occasionally they present with obstruction and/or intussusception [107,108]. There is an extraordinary report of an ileal lipoma being expulsed per rectum [109]. Macroscopically they are yellowish in colour and histologically they show mature adipose tissue. They are usually submucosal but are on occasion subserosal. There is the occasional report of primary liposarcoma of the small intestine but such tumours are exceptionally rare [110].

Vascular tumours

Haemangiomas are still rare lesions in the small intestine, even though they do account for about 10% of all benign tumours of the small bowel [111]. They are usually classified into three major types: cavernous, capillary or mixed; the type tends to determine the size of the lesions. Most are small and of capillary type whilst cavernous tumours may involve long segments of the ileum, in particular, and may involve all layers of the bowel wall [112]. Most haemangiomas are benign and may be incidental findings at necropsy. However, a significant number present with haemorrhage, which may be cryptic, and thus presentation is with severe recalcitrant iron deficiency anaemia or with obstruction or intussusception [112–114]. Protein-losing enteropathy is also a recognized presenting feature of larger haemangiomas [115,116].

Multiple haemangiomas can be seen in the intestines in several conditions, some well defined and others less so. The blue rubber bleb naevus syndrome [117] is associated with cutaneous vascular naevi and, often life-threatening, gastrointestinal haemorrhage. The lesions are small capillary angiomas and have a blue wrinkled surface. The Klippel–Trenaunay–Weber syndrome associates soft tissue and bone hypertrophy, varicose veins and port wine haemangiomas with vascular malformations of the gut. An apparent *forme fruste* of Peutz–Jeghers syndrome, due to incomplete penetrance of the gene, may result in multiple intestinal haemangiomas [117]. Most of these lesions simply show the features of cavernous haemangiomas [118].

Haemangiopericytomas are described as primary tumours of the small intestine [119], although it could be that now some of the tumours would be regarded as GISTs with a prominent vascular component. The small bowel is a common site for gastrointestinal involvement by Kaposi's sarcoma (KS) in the context of AIDS [120,121]. This disease is almost always in homosexuals with AIDS: about 20% of these patients with advanced immune paresis will show intestinal involvement by KS [122,123]. The lesions of KS are usually submucosal but extensively involve the bowel wall. Perforation may occur, although this may be an effect of other, coincident, opportunistic infections rather than directly related to KS. Histologically, KS demonstrates pleomorphic spindle cells with clefts in which erythrocytes are entrapped. The tumour cells often demonstrate intracytoplasmic hyaline droplets. Whilst the presence of intestinal KS indicates advanced immunosuppression, the prognosis is not usually further adversely influenced by the presence of gastrointestinal KS [122]. Primary angiosarcomas of the small bowel are described (Fig. 25.13), including some after previous radiotherapy [124–126], but such lesions are exceptionally rare.

Lymphangiomas

These very rare anomalies, which are probably hamartomatous, are usually solitary and mostly occur in the duodenum [127–129]. They are often incidental findings but they can present with small bowel obstruction [130] or rarely with chronic bleeding [131]. The diagnosis of duodenal lymphangioma is usually achieved at the time of endoscopy, when the characteristic elevated yellow-tan lesions are seen, often with satellite lesions, which can be impressed by an endoscopic biopsy forceps [128]. Biopsy results in the exudation of yellow chylous liquid [128]. Histologically lymphangiomas consist of dilated lymphatic channels interspersed with more solid 'angiomatous'-type tissue and some smooth muscle: the presence of lymphocytes helps to differentiate these lesions from true haemangiomas.

Lymphangiectasia

Although the presentation of this small bowel pathology is not necessarily with a tumour-like mass, it is best considered here. These lesions can be solitary and then tumour-like, or the disease can be more diffuse. Solitary lymphangiectasia has considerable overlap with lymphangioma and with lymphatic cysts (see above and below). Furthermore it must be emphasized that localized lymphangiectasia is relatively commonplace in duodenal biopsies and may be considered functional and part of the normal range of appearances in such biopsies [132]. Only if the disease is diffuse throughout the mucosa and pronounced, should the condition of diffuse lymphangiectasia be strongly considered.

Diffuse lymphangiectasia was first described by Waldmann [133]. It is a disease of infants, children and young adults; common presentations are malabsorption, protein-losing enteropathy, hypoalbuminaemia, chylous ascites, intermittent diarrhoea and/or steatorrhoea and failure to thrive [134,135]. Occasionally it can present with obscure bleeding which may be fatal [136]. Macroscopically, usually at the time of laparotomy, the small bowel shows a curious brown thickening of the serosal surface with dilated lymphatics; tumorous masses are not a feature [135,137]. Histological examination reveals distortion of villi with often grossly dilated lacteals and lymphatics in the lamina propria (Fig. 25.14) [138]. There is associated oedema, presumably due to the hypoproteinaemia. The dilatation may be restricted to the mucosa and submucosa but usually there is lymphangiectasia in transmural lymphatics with extension to mesenteric vessels and lymph nodes [137]. Although lymphangiectasia can be seen as a consequence of acquired obstruction of the lymphatic system (Fig. 25.14), most cases are congenital in origin and are probably due to failure in the proper formation of lymphatic vessels [137]. Treatment is generally supportive with restriction of triglyceride intake: this may result in normalization of weight and loss of symptoms [135].

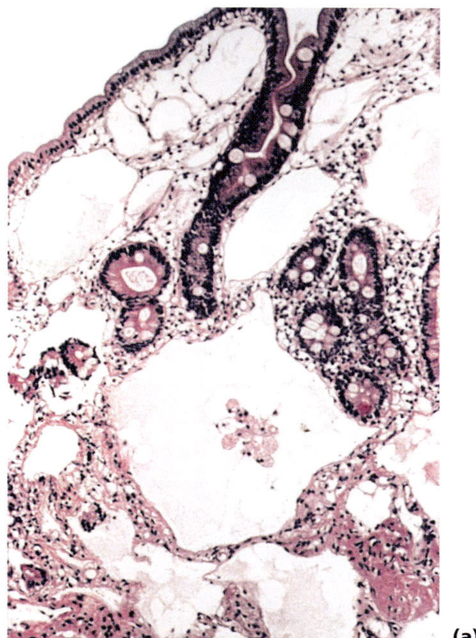

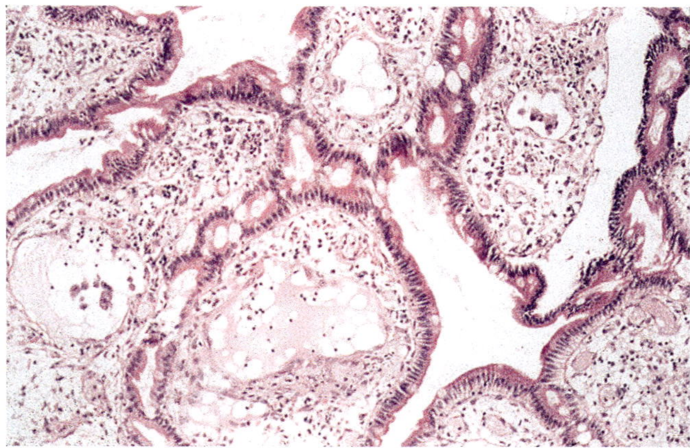

Fig. 25.14 Primary and secondary lymphangiectasia of the duodenum. (a) In primary lymphangiectasia, there are grossly dilated lacteals and lymphatics in the lamina propria. (b) Similar changes are seen in secondary lymphangiectasia but, in this case, the cause is discernible. There are papillary groupings of metastatic pancreatic adenocarcinoma within some of the lymphatics.

Lymphatic cysts

Lymphatic cysts can occur in the wall of the small intestine or

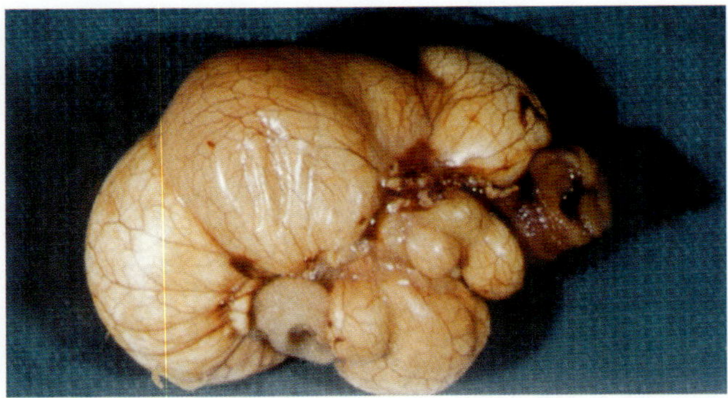

Fig. 25.15 A small intestinal mesenteric lymphatic cyst. It is large and multiloculated. Presentation was with small intestinal obstruction.

in the mesentery [139,140]. They have been described as lymphangiectatic cysts and thus there is some confusion with intestinal lymphangiectasia; we believe the latter term is best reserved for the diffuse paediatric pathology and that other solitary lesions are best termed lymphatic (or mesenteric) cysts. In the wall of the bowel, the cysts present as small, usually symptomless, nodules up to 1.0 cm in diameter; they are usually in the submucosa and contain thick, creamy fluid [140]. They are usually single, but multiple lesions do occur in a small proportion of cases [140]. They are most often unilocular and are lined by flattened endothelial cells. There may be some ectasia of afferent lymphatics in the mucosa but this is always localized to the lesion. The condition is not associated with protein-losing enteropathy or malabsorption. Mesenteric lymphatic cysts are usually multiple and may reach a considerable size, with consequent risk of rupture, small intestinal volvulus or obstruction (Fig. 25.15) [141]. Most mesenteric cysts are probably lymphatic in type although it is possible that some derive from mesothelial inclusion. The pathogenesis is obscure: the growth and dilatation of embryologically deformed lymphatics, cystic degeneration of mesenteric lymph nodes and dysfunctional fusion of mesenteric leaves have all been proposed as possible causes [141,142]. They may be associated with intramural lymphangiectasia. Microscopically the cyst is lined by flattened cells, which are usually demonstrably endothelial in nature by immunohistochemistry, seemingly confirming the lymphatic nature of the cyst.

Neural tumours of the small intestine

It is difficult to ascertain the true incidence of sporadic nerve sheath tumours of the small intestine because many will have been classified as gastrointestinal stromal tumours (GISTs) as the morphological and immunohistochemical features can be similar. Occasional examples of neurilemmoma are described, often presenting with haemorrhage [143], and there are also examples of malignant nerve sheath tumours primary in the small intestine [144,145]. Granular cell tumours, now undeniably of nerve sheath origin, are very occasionally described in the small intestine but are much more common in the oesophagus [146].

Solitary neurofibromas of the small intestine do occur but are excessively rare, presenting either incidentally or with obstruction/intussusception [147]. However, small intestinal neurofibromas are more likely to be seen in the context of von Recklinghausen's disease (neurofibromatosis): the small intestine is the commonest site in the gut for neurofibromas in the syndrome [148]. The neurofibromas of von Recklinghausen's disease present with bleeding or obstruction [149–151]. Patients with von Recklinghausen's disease may also suffer other tumours of the small bowel; these include gastrointestinal stromal tumours, with or without skeinoid fibres, ganglioneuromas, gangliocytic paragangliomas of the duodenum and carcinoid tumours [148,152–156]. Solitary ganglioneuromas and ganglioneuromatosis do occur in the small intestine but these confusing conditions are more fully dealt with in the section on the large intestine (see p. 619).

Neuromuscular and vascular hamartoma is a title given to a condition of the small bowel characterized by a haphazard arrangement of neural, muscular and vascular elements, in the submucosa, muscularis and subserosa [157–160]. Although it is possible that some of these cases are truly hamartomatous, we believe it more likely that most cases represent connective tissue disorganization as a result of previous inflammatory insults, especially Crohn's disease, in a burnt-out phase of the disease [159]. This is supported by recent evidence of an overlap between the features described as neuromuscular and vascular hamartoma and changes seen as a consequence of non-steroidal anti-inflammatory drug-induced diaphragm disease [161].

Gangliocytic paraganglioma

This histologically distinctive tumour [162–165], which occurs most commonly in the periampullary region of the duodenum, is described fully in the section on neuroendocrine tumours on p. 365. It is characteristically composed of a combination of three cell types in varying proportions: S-100-positive neural elements in intertwining fascicles, ganglion cells and chromogranin-staining endocrine cells. When the latter are inconspicuous, confusion with other neural tumours is understandable, and the diagnosis should be seriously considered in every periampullary tumour with neural features.

Metastatic disease to the small bowel

Although theoretically any malignant tumour can metastasize to the small bowel, specific mention should be made of two malignancies which show a particular propensity so to do. Firstly, one epithelial malignancy, lobular carcinoma of the

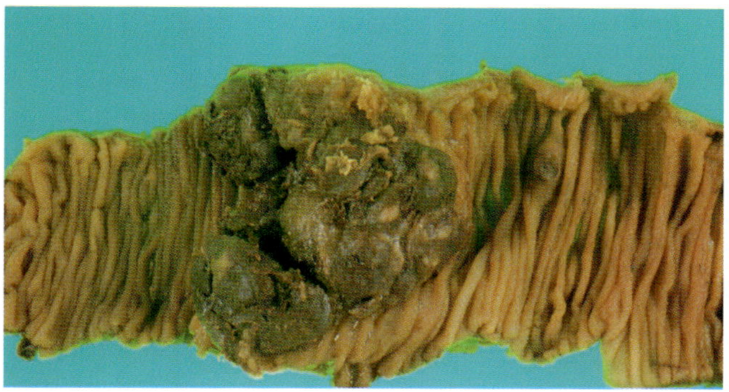

Fig. 25.16 Metastatic malignant melanoma in the ileum, easily mistaken for a primary tumour, particularly malignant lymphoma.

breast, may present obscurely with multiple strictures of the small bowel. Secondly, metastatic malignant melanoma shows an especial predilection for metastasis to the small intestine (Fig. 25.16). It should also be noted that apparently primary malignant melanomas are described in the small intestine without history of an antecedent primary [166]. We believe it most likely that most of the latter represent metastatic disease with an undetectable, or perhaps regressed, cutaneous primary melanoma. Nevertheless there are exceptional cases which do, apparently, represent true primary malignant melanomas of the small intestine [166]. There are two important properties of metastatic malignant melanoma: firstly, their propensity to multiplicity and their predominant location in the submucosa produces a polyposis-like syndrome in the small intestine; secondly, they are an important histological mimic of high-grade malignant lymphoma and the possible diagnosis of metastatic melanoma should always be considered and investigated in this situation [167].

References

1 Owen RL, Jones AL. Epithelial cell specialization within human Peyer's patches: an ultrastructural study of intestinal lymphoid follicles. *Gastroenterology*, 1974; 66: 189.

2 Volkheimer G. Persorption of particles: physiology and pharmacology. *Adv Pharmacol Chemother*, 1977; 14: 163.

3 Shepherd NA, Crocker PR, Smith AP, Levison DA. Exogenous pigment in Peyer's patches. *Hum Pathol*, 1987; 18: 50.

4 Isaacson P, Wright DH. Extranodal malignant lymphoma arising from mucosa-associated lymphoid tissue. *Cancer*, 1984; 53: 2515.

5 Isaacson PG, Norton AJ. *Extranodal Lymphomas*. Edinburgh: Churchill Livingstone, 1994: 15.

6 Isaacson PG. Lymphoproliferative disorders of the gastrointestinal tract. In: Ming S, Goldman H, eds. *Pathology of the Gastrointestinal Tract*. Baltimore: Williams & Wilkins, 1998: 339.

7 Isaacson PG. Gastrointestinal lymphomas of T- and B-cell types. *Mod Pathol*, 1999; 12: 151.

8 Fieber SS, Schaefer HJ. Lymphoid hyperplasia of the terminal ileum—a clinical entity? *Gastroenterology*, 1966; 50: 83.

9 Atwell JD, Burge D, Wright D. Nodular lymphoid hyperplasia of the intestinal tract in infancy and childhood. *J Pediatr Surg*, 1985; 20: 25.

10 Rubin A, Isaacson PG. Florid reactive lymphoid hyperplasia of the terminal ileum in adults: a condition bearing a close resemblance to low-grade malignant lymphoma. *Histopathology*, 1990; 17: 19.

11 Hermans PE, Huizenga KA, Hoffman HN, Brown AL Jr, Markowitz H. Dysgammaglobulinemia associated with nodular lymphoid hyperplasia of the small intestine. *Am J Med*, 1966; 40: 78.

12 Rambaud JC, Saint-Louvent P, Marti R *et al*. Diffuse follicular lymphoid hyperplasia of the small intestine without primary immunoglobulin deficiency. *Am J Med*, 1982; 73: 125.

13 Webster AD, Kenwright S, Ballard J *et al*. Nodular lymphoid hyperplasia of the bowel in primary hypogammaglobulinaemia: study of in vivo and in vitro lymphocyte function. *Gut*, 1977; 18: 364.

14 Lamers CB, Wagener T, Assmann KJ, van Tongeren JH. Jejunal lymphoma in a patient with primary adult-onset hypogammaglobulinemia and nodular lymphoid hyperplasia of the small intestine. *Dig Dis Sci*, 1980; 25: 553.

15 Kahn LB, Novis BH. Nodular lymphoid hyperplasia of the small bowel associated with primary small bowel reticulum cell lymphoma. *Cancer*, 1974; 33: 837.

16 Matuchansky C, Touchard G, Lemaire M *et al*. Malignant lymphoma of the small bowel associated with diffuse nodular lymphoid hyperplasia. *N Engl J Med*, 1985; 313: 166.

17 Matuchansky C, Morichau-Beauchant M, Touchard G *et al*. Nodular lymphoid hyperplasia of the small bowel associated with primary jejunal malignant lymphoma. Evidence favoring a cytogenetic relationship. *Gastroenterology*, 1980; 78: 1587.

18 Harris M, Blewitt RW, Davies VJ, Steward WP. High-grade non-Hodgkin's lymphoma complicating polypoid nodular lymphoid hyperplasia and multiple lymphomatous polyposis of the intestine. *Histopathology*, 1989; 15: 339.

19 Steinberg JJ, Bridges N, Feiner HD, Valensi Q. Small intestinal lymphoma in three patients with acquired immune deficiency syndrome. *Am J Gastroenterol*, 1985; 80: 21.

20 Levine AM. AIDS-associated malignant lymphoma. *Med Clin North Am*, 1992; 76: 253.

21 Craig FE, Gulley ML, Banks PM. Posttransplantation lymphoproliferative disorders. *Am J Clin Pathol*, 1993; 99: 265.

22 Nalesnik MA. Clinical and pathological features of post-transplant lymphoproliferative disorders (PTLD). *Semin Immunopathol*, 1998; 20: 325.

23 Nalesnik MA. Involvement of the gastrointestinal tract by Epstein–Barr virus—associated posttransplant lymphoproliferative disorders. *Am J Surg Pathol*, 1990; 14 (Suppl 1): 92.

24 Freeman C, Berg JW, Cutler SJ. Occurrence and prognosis of extranodal lymphomas. *Cancer*, 1972; 29: 252.

25 Otter R, Bieger R, Kluin PM, Hermans J, Willemze R. Primary gastrointestinal non-Hodgkin's lymphoma in a population-based registry. *Br J Cancer*, 1989; 60: 745.

26 LeBrun DP, Kamel OW, Cleary ML, Dorfman RF, Warnke RA. Follicular lymphomas of the gastrointestinal tract. Pathologic features in 31 cases and bcl-2 oncogenic protein expression. *Am J Pathol*, 1992; 140: 1327.

27 Domizio P, Owen RA, Shepherd NA, Talbot IC, Norton AJ.

Primary lymphoma of the small intestine. A clinicopathological study of 119 cases. *Am J Surg Pathol*, 1993; 17: 429.

28 Radaszkiewicz T, Dragosics B, Bauer P. Gastrointestinal malignant lymphomas of the mucosa-associated lymphoid tissue: factors relevant to prognosis. *Gastroenterology*, 1992; 102: 1628.

29 Zinzani PL, Magagnoli M, Pagliani G *et al*. Primary intestinal lymphoma: clinical and therapeutic features of 32 patients. *Haematologica*, 1997; 82: 305.

30 Isaacson PG. Gastrointestinal lymphoma. *Hum Pathol*, 1994; 25: 1020.

31 Pandey M, Wadhwa MK, Patel HP, Kothari KC, Shah M, Patel DD. Malignant lymphoma of the gastrointestinal tract. *Eur J Surg Oncol*, 1999; 25: 164.

32 Azar HA. Cancer in Lebanon and the Near East. *Cancer*, 1962; 15: 16.

33 Ramot B, Shahin N, Bubis JJ. Malabsorption syndrome in lymphoma of the small intestine. A study of 13 cases. *Isr J Med Sci*, 1965; 1: 221.

34 Doe WF, Henry K, Hobbs JR, Jones FA, Dent CE, Booth CC. Five cases of alpha chain disease. *Gut*, 1972; 13: 947.

35 Lewin KJ, Kahn LB, Novis BH. Primary intestinal lymphoma of 'Western' and 'Mediterranean' type, alpha chain disease and massive plasma cell infiltration: a comparative study of 37 cases. *Cancer*, 1976; 38: 2511.

36 Salem PA, Nassar VH, Shahid MJ *et al*. 'Mediterranean abdominal lymphoma', or immunoproliferative small intestinal disease. Part I: clinical aspects. *Cancer*, 1977; 40: 2941.

37 Seligmann M. Alpha chain disease: immunoglobulin abnormalities, pathogenesis and current concepts. *Br J Cancer*, 1975; 31 (Suppl 2): 356.

38 Seligmann M, Danon F, Hurez D, Mihaesco E, Preud'homme, JL. Alpha-chain disease: a new immunoglobulin abnormality. *Science*, 1968; 162: 1396.

39 Rambaud JC, Modigliani R, Phuoc BK *et al*. Non-secretory alpha-chain disease in intestinal lymphoma [letter]. *N Engl J Med*, 1980; 303: 53.

40 Rambaud JC. Small intestinal lymphomas and alpha-chain disease. *Clin Gastroenterol*, 1983; 12: 743.

41 Nassar VH, Salem PA, Shahid MJ *et al*. 'Mediterranean abdominal lymphoma' or immunoproliferative small intestinal disease. Part II: pathological aspects. *Cancer*, 1978; 41: 1340.

42 Isaacson PG, Price SK. Light chains in Mediterranean lymphoma. *J Clin Pathol*, 1985; 38: 601.

43 Isaacson PG, Dogan A, Price SK, Spencer J. Immunoproliferative small-intestinal disease. An immunohistochemical study. *Am J Surg Pathol*, 1989; 13: 1023.

44 Smith WJ, Price SK, Isaacson PG. Immunoglobulin gene rearrangement in immunoproliferative small intestinal disease (IPSID). *J Clin Pathol*, 1987; 40: 1291.

45 Berger R, Bernheim A, Tsapis A, Brouet JC, Seligmann M. Cytogenetic studies in four cases of alpha chain disease. *Cancer Genet Cytogenet*, 1986; 22: 219.

46 Gilinsky NH, Novis BH, Wright JP, Dent DM, King H, Marks IN. Immunoproliferative small-intestinal disease: clinical features and outcome in 30 cases. *Medicine*, 1987; 66: 438.

47 Ben Ayed F, Halphen M, Najjar T *et al*. Treatment of alpha chain disease. Results of a prospective study in 21 Tunisian patients by the Tunisian-French Intestinal Lymphoma Study Group. *Cancer*, 1989; 63: 1251.

48 zur Hausen H. The role of Epstein Barr virus (EBV) in Burkitt's lymphomas. *Jpn J Cancer Res*, 1998; 89: inside.

49 Banks PM, Arseneau JC, Gralnick HR, Canellos GP, DeVita VT Jr, Berard CW. American Burkitt's lymphoma: a clinicopathologic study of 30 cases. II. Pathologic correlations. *Am J Med*, 1975; 58: 322.

50 Levison DA, Hall PA, Blackshaw AJ. The gut-associated lymphoid tissue and its tumours. In: Williams GT, ed. *Current Topics in Gastrointestinal Pathology*. Berlin: Springer-Verlag, 1989: 134.

51 Payne CM, Grogan TM, Cromey DW, Bjore CG, Kerrigan DP. An ultrastructural morphometric and immunophenotypic evaluation of Burkitt's and Burkitt's-like lymphomas. *Lab Invest*, 1987; 57: 200.

52 Philip T, Lenoir GM, Bryon PA *et al*. Burkitt-type lymphoma in France among non-Hodgkin malignant lymphomas in Caucasian children. *Br J Cancer*, 1982; 45: 670.

53 Lenoir GM, Land H, Parada LF, Cunningham JM, Weinberg RA. Activated oncogenes in Burkitt's lymphoma. *Curr Top Microbiol Immunol*, 1984; 113: 6.

54 Pelicci PG, Knowles DM, Magrath I, Dalla-Favera R. Chromosomal breakpoints and structural alterations of the c-myc locus differ in endemic and sporadic forms of Burkitt lymphoma. *Proc Natl Acad Sci USA*, 1986; 83: 2984.

55 Zimber-Strobl U, Strobl L, Hofelmayr H *et al*. EBNA2 and c-myc in B cell immortalization by Epstein–Barr virus and in the pathogenesis of Burkitt's lymphoma. *Curr Top Microbiol Immunol*, 1999; 246: 315.

56 Glassman AB, Hopwood V, Hayes KJ. Cytogenetics as an aid in the diagnosis of lymphomas. *Ann Clin Lab Sci*, 2000; 30: 72.

57 Neri A, Barriga F, Knowles DM, Magrath IT, Dalla FR. Different regions of the immunoglobulin heavy-chain locus are involved in chromosomal translocations in distinct pathogenetic forms of Burkitt lymphoma. *Proc Natl Acad Sci USA*, 1988; 85: 2748.

58 Patte C, Michon J, Frappaz D *et al*. Therapy of Burkitt and other B-cell acute lymphoblastic leukaemia and lymphoma: experience with the LMB protocols of the SFOP (French Paediatric Oncology Society) in children and adults. *Baillieres Clin Haematol*, 1994; 7: 339.

59 Veenstra J, Krediet RT, Somers R, Arisz L. Tumour lysis syndrome and acute renal failure in Burkitt's lymphoma. Description of 2 cases and a review of the literature on prevention and management. *Neth J Med*, 1994; 45: 211.

60 Isaacson P, Wright DH. Malignant histiocytosis of the intestine. Its relationship to malabsorption and ulcerative jejunitis. *Hum Pathol*, 1978; 9: 661.

61 Isaacson PG, O'Connor NT, Spencer J *et al*. Malignant histiocytosis of the intestine: a T-cell lymphoma. *Lancet*, 1985; 2: 688.

62 Ashton-Key M, Diss TC, Du Pan LMQ, Isaacson PG. Molecular analysis of T-cell clonality in ulcerative jejunitis and enteropathy-associated T-cell lymphoma. *Am J Pathol*, 1997; 151: 493.

63 Carbonnel F, Grollet-Bioul L, Brouet JC *et al*. Are complicated forms of celiac disease cryptic T-cell lymphomas? *Blood*, 1998; 92: 3879.

64 Bagdi E, Diss TC, Munson P, Isaacson PG. Mucosal intra-

epithelial lymphocytes in enteropathy-associated T-cell lymphoma, ulcerative jejunitis, and refractory celiac disease constitute a neoplastic population. *Blood*, 1999; 94: 260.

65 Wright DH. Enteropathy associated T cell lymphoma. *Cancer Surv*, 1997; 30: 249.

66 Wright DH, Jones DB, Clark H, Mead GM, Hodges E, Howell WM. Is adult-onset coeliac disease due to a low-grade lymphoma of intraepithelial T lymphocytes? *Lancet*, 1991; 337: 1373.

67 Holmes GK, Prior P, Lane MR, Pope D, Allan RN. Malignancy in coeliac disease—effect of a gluten free diet. *Gut*, 1989; 30: 333.

68 Howell WM, Leung ST, Jones DB *et al*. HLA-DRB, -DQA, and -DQB polymorphism in celiac disease and enteropathy-associated T-cell lymphoma. Common features and additional risk factors for malignancy. *Hum Immunol*, 1995; 43: 29.

69 Freeman HJ, Weinstein WM, Shnitka TK, Piercey JR, Wensel RH. Primary abdominal lymphoma. Presenting manifestation of celiac sprue or complicating dermatitis herpetiformis. *Am J Med*, 1977; 63: 585.

70 Isaacson P, Wright DH. Intestinal lymphoma associated with malabsorption. *Lancet*, 1978; 1: 67.

71 Shepherd NA, Blackshaw AJ, Hall PA *et al*. Malignant lymphoma with eosinophilia of the gastrointestinal tract. *Histopathology*, 1987; 11: 115.

72 Murray A, Cuevas EC, Jones DB, Wright DH. Study of the immunohistochemistry and T cell clonality of enteropathy-associated T cell lymphoma. *Am J Pathol*, 1995; 146: 509.

73 Russell GJ, Nagler-Anderson C, Anderson P, Bhan AK. Cytotoxic potential of intraepithelial lymphocytes (IELs). Presence of TIA-1, the cytolytic granule-associated protein, in human IELs in normal and diseased intestine. *Am J Pathol*, 1993; 143: 350.

74 de Bruin PC, Connolly CE, Oudejans JJ *et al*. Enteropathy-associated T-cell lymphomas have a cytotoxic T-cell phenotype. *Histopathology*, 1997; 31: 313.

75 Diss TC, Watts M, Pan LX *et al*. The polymerase chain reaction in the demonstration of monoclonality in T cell lymphomas. *J Clin Pathol*, 1995; 48: 1045.

76 Isaacson PG, MacLennan KA, Subbuswamy SG. Multiple lymphomatous polyposis of the gastrointestinal tract. *Histopathology*, 1984; 8: 641.

77 Lavergne A, Brouland JP, Launay E, Nemeth J, Ruskone-Fourmestraux A, Galian A. Multiple lymphomatous polyposis of the gastrointestinal tract. An extensive histopathologic and immunohistochemical study of 12 cases. *Cancer*, 1994; 74: 3042.

78 Ruskone-Fourmestraux A, Delmer A, Lavergne A *et al*. Multiple lymphomatous polyposis of the gastrointestinal tract: prospective clinicopathologic study of 31 cases. Groupe d'Etude des Lymphomes Digestifs. *Gastroenterology*, 1997; 112: 7.

79 Freeman HJ, Anderson ME, Gascoyne RD. Clinical, pathological and molecular genetic findings in small intestinal follicle centre cell lymphoma. *Can J Gastroenterol*, 1997; 11: 31.

80 Moynihan MJ, Bast MA, Chan WC *et al*. Lymphomatous polyposis. A neoplasm of either follicular mantle or germinal center cell origin. *Am J Surg Pathol*, 1996; 20: 442.

81 Nyam DC, Pemberton JH, Sandborn WJ, Savcenko M. Lymphoma of the pouch after ileal pouch–anal anastomosis: report of a case. *Dis Colon Rectum*, 1997; 40: 971.

82 Schmitt GA, Hummel M, Zemlin M *et al*. Intestinal T-cell lymphoma: a reassessment of cytomorphological and phenotypic features in relation to patterns of small bowel remodelling. *Virchows Arch*, 1996; 429: 27.

83 Foucar K, Foucar E, Mitros F, Clamon G, Goeken J, Crossett J. Epitheliotropic lymphoma of the small bowel. Report of a fatal case with cytotoxic/suppressor T-cell immunotype. *Cancer*, 1984; 54: 54.

84 Carbonnel F, Lavergne A, Messing B *et al*. Extensive small intestinal T-cell lymphoma of low-grade malignancy associated with a new chromosomal translocation. *Cancer*, 1994; 73: 1286.

85 Chiu EK, Loke SL, Chan AC, Liang RH. T-lymphoblastic lymphoma arising in the small intestine. *Pathology*, 1991; 23: 356.

86 Blackshaw AJ, Levison DA. Eosinophilic infiltrates of the gastrointestinal tract. *J Clin Pathol*, 1986; 39: 1.

87 Brugo EA, Larkin E, Molina-Escobar J, Contanzi J. Primary granulocytic sarcoma of the small bowel. *Cancer*, 1975; 35: 1333.

88 Brugo EA, Marshall RB, Riberi AM, Pautasso OE. Preleukemic granulocytic sarcomas of the gastrointestinal tract. Report of two cases. *Am J Clin Pathol*, 1977; 68: 616.

89 Miettinen M, Sarlomo-Rikala M, Lasota J. Gastrointestinal stromal tumors: recent advances in understanding of their biology. *Hum Pathol*, 1999; 30: 1213.

90 Chan JK. Mesenchymal tumors of the gastrointestinal tract: a paradise for acronyms (STUMP, GIST, GANT, and now GIPACT), implication of c-kit in genesis, and yet another of the many emerging roles of the interstitial cell of Cajal in the pathogenesis of gastrointestinal diseases? *Adv Anat Pathol*, 1999; 6: 19.

91 Goldblum JR, Appelman HD. Stromal tumors of the duodenum. A histologic and immunohistochemical study of 20 cases. *Am J Surg Pathol*, 1995; 19: 71.

92 Appelman HD. Mesenchymal tumors of the gastrointestinal tract. In: Ming S, Goldman H, eds. *Pathology of the Gastrointestinal Tract*. Baltimore: Williams & Wilkins, 1998: 361.

93 Min KW. Small intestinal stromal tumors with skeinoid fibers. Clinicopathological, immunohistochemical, and ultrastructural investigations. *Am J Surg Pathol*, 1992; 16: 145.

94 Ojanguren I, Ariza A, Navas-Palacios JJ. Gastrointestinal autonomic nerve tumor: further observations regarding an ultrastructural and immunohistochemical analysis of six cases. *Hum Pathol*, 1996; 27: 1311.

95 Appelman HD. Smooth muscle tumors of the gastrointestinal tract. What we know now that Stout didn't know. *Am J Surg Pathol*, 1986; 10 (Suppl 1): 83.

96 Lauwers GY, Erlandson RA, Casper ES, Brennan MF, Woodruff JM. Gastrointestinal autonomic nerve tumors. A clinicopathological, immunohistochemical, and ultrastructural study of 12 cases. *Am J Surg Pathol*, 1993; 17: 887.

97 Tworek JA, Appelman HD, Singleton TP, Greenson JK. Stromal tumors of the jejunum and ileum. *Mod Pathol*, 1997; 10: 200.

98 Akwari OE, Dozois RR, Weiland LH, Beahrs OH. Leiomyosarcoma of the small and large bowel. *Cancer*, 1978; 42: 1375.

99 Herrera GA, Pinto DM, Grizzle WE, Han SG. Malignant small bowel neoplasm of enteric plexus derivation (plexosarcoma). Light and electron microscopic study confirming the origin of the neoplasm. *Dig Dis Sci*, 1984; 29: 275.

100 Walker P, Dvorak AM. Gastrointestinal autonomic nerve (GAN) tumor. Ultrastructural evidence for a newly recognized entity. *Arch Pathol Lab Med*, 1986; 110: 309.

101 Dhimes P, Lopez CM, Ortega-Serrano MP, Garcia MH, Martinez-Gonzalez MA, Ballestin C. Gastrointestinal autonomic nerve tumours and their separation from other gastrointestinal stromal tumours: an ultrastructural and immunohistochemical study of seven cases. *Virchows Arch*, 1995; 426: 27.

102 Shanks JH, Harris M, Banerjee SS, Eyden BP. Gastrointestinal autonomic nerve tumours: a report of nine cases. *Histopathology*, 1996; 29: 111.

103 Kerr JZ, Hicks MJ, Nuchtern JG *et al*. Gastrointestinal autonomic nerve tumors in the pediatric population: a report of four cases and a review of the literature. *Cancer*, 1999; 85: 220.

104 Tornoczky T, Kalman E, Hegedus G *et al*. High mitotic index associated with poor prognosis in gastrointestinal autonomic nerve tumour. *Histopathology*, 1999; 35: 121.

105 Matsumoto K, Min W, Yamada N, Asano G. Gastrointestinal autonomic nerve tumors: immunohistochemical and ultrastructural studies in cases of gastrointestinal stromal tumor. *Pathol Int*, 1997; 47: 308.

106 Sircar K, Hewlett BR, Huizinga JD, Chorneyko K, Berezin I, Riddell RH. Interstitial cells of Cajal as precursors of gastrointestinal stromal tumors. *Am J Surg Pathol*, 1999; 23: 377.

107 Brzezinski W, Bailey RJ, Besney M, Turner G. Small-bowel lipoma: an uncommon cause of obstruction. *Can J Surg*, 1990; 33: 423.

108 Urbano J, Serantes A, Hernandez L, Turegano F. Lipoma-induced jejunojejunal intussusception. US and CT diagnosis. *Abdom Imaging*, 1996; 21: 522.

109 Misra SP, Singh SK, Thorat VK, Gulati P, Malhotra V, Anand BS. Spontaneous expulsion per rectum of an ileal lipoma. *Postgrad Med J*, 1988; 64: 718.

110 Mohandas D, Chandra RS, Srinivasan V, Bhaskar AG. Liposarcoma of the ileum with secondaries in the liver. *Am J Gastroenterol*, 1972; 58: 172.

111 Baird DB, Norris HT. Vascular disorders. In: Ming S, Goldman H, eds. *Pathology of the Gastrointestinal Tract*. Baltimore: Williams & Wilkins, 1998: 267.

112 Boyle L, Lack EE. Solitary cavernous hemangioma of small intestine. Case report and literature review. *Arch Pathol Lab Med*, 1993; 117: 939.

113 Pradhan DJ, Juanteguy M, Musikabhumma S, Ulfohn A. Gastrointestinal hemangiomas. *Arch Surg*, 1972; 104: 704.

114 Taylor TV, Torrance HB. Haemangiomas of the gastro-intestinal tract. *Br J Surg*, 1974; 61: 236.

115 Jackson AE, Peterson C. Hemangioma of the small intestine causing protein-losing enteropathy. *Ann Intern Med*, 1967; 66: 1190.

116 Sasaki M, Nakamura F, Koyama S, Fujiyama Y, Bamba T, Okabe H. Case report. Haemangioma of the small intestine complicated by protein-losing gastroenteropathy. *J Gastroenterol Hepatol*, 1998; 13: 387.

117 Camilleri M, Chadwick VS, Hodgson HJ. Vascular anomalies of the gastrointestinal tract. *Hepatogastroenterology*, 1984; 31: 149.

118 Boley SJ, Brandt LJ, Mitsudo SM. Vascular lesions of the colon. *Adv Intern Med*, 1984; 29: 301.

119 Olsen EG, Wellwood JM. Haemangiopericytoma of the small intestine. A report of three cases. *Br J Surg*, 1970; 57: 66.

120 Rotterdam H, Sommers SC. Alimentary tract biopsy lesions in the acquired immune deficiency syndrome. *Pathology*, 1985; 17: 181.

121 Ell C, Matek W, Gramatzki M, Kaduk B, Demling L. Endoscopic findings in a case of Kaposi's sarcoma with involvement of the large and small bowel. *Endoscopy*, 1985; 17: 161.

122 Parente F, Cernuschi M, Orlando G, Rizzardini G, Lazzarin A, Bianchi PG. Kaposi's sarcoma and AIDS: frequency of gastrointestinal involvement and its effect on survival. A prospective study in a heterogeneous population. *Scand J Gastroenterol*, 1991; 26: 1007.

123 Friedman SL. Kaposi's sarcoma and lymphoma of the gut in AIDS. *Baillieres Clin Gastroenterol*, 1990; 4: 455.

124 Murray-Lyon IM, Doyle D, Philpott RM, Porter NH. Haemangiomatosis of the small and large bowel with histological malignant change. *J Pathol*, 1971; 105: 295.

125 Chen KT, Hoffman KD, Hendricks EJ. Angiosarcoma following therapeutic irradiation. *Cancer*, 1979; 44: 2044.

126 Nanus DM, Kelsen D, Clark DG. Radiation-induced angiosarcoma. *Cancer*, 1987; 60: 777.

127 Elliott RL, Williams RD, Bayles D, Griffin J. Lymphangioma of the duodenum: case report with light and electron microscopic observation. *Ann Surg*, 1966; 163: 86.

128 Shigematsu A, Iida M, Hatanaka M *et al*. Endoscopic diagnosis of lymphangioma of the small intestine. *Am J Gastroenterol*, 1988; 83: 1289.

129 Singh S, Maghrabi M. Small bowel obstruction caused by recurrent cystic lymphangioma. *Br J Surg*, 1993; 80: 1012.

130 Kok KY, Mathew VV, Yapp SK. Lymphangioma of the small-bowel mesentery: unusual cause of intestinal obstruction. *J Clin Gastroenterol*, 1997; 24: 186.

131 Barquist ES, Apple SK, Jensen DM, Ashley SW. Jejunal lymphangioma. An unusual cause of chronic gastrointestinal bleeding. *Dig Dis Sci*, 1997; 42: 1179.

132 Patel AS, de Ridder PH. Endoscopic appearance and significance of functional lymphangiectasia of the duodenal mucosa. *Gastrointest Endosc*, 1990; 36: 376.

133 Waldmann TA, Steinfeld JL, Dutcher TF, Davidson JD, Gordon RS Jr. The role of the gastrointestinal system in 'idiopathic hypoproteinemia'. *Gastroenterology*, 1968; 54: Suppl 6.

134 Fadell EJ, Dame RW, Wolford JL. Chronic hypoalbuminemia and edema associated with intestinal lymphangiectasia. *JAMA*, 1965; 194: 917.

135 Bujanover Y, Liebman WM, Goodman JR, Thaler MM. Primary intestinal lymphangiectasia. Case report with radiological and ultrastructural study. *Digestion*, 1981; 21: 107.

136 Poirier VC, Alfidi RJ. Intestinal lymphangiectasia associated with fatal gastrointestinal bleeding. *Am J Dig Dis*, 1973; 18: 54.

137 Olmsted WW, Madewell JE. Lymphangiectasia of the small intestine: description and pathophysiology of the roentgenographic signs. *Gastrointest Radiol*, 1976; 1: 241.

138 Asakura H, Miura S, Morishita T *et al*. Endoscopic and histopathological study on primary and secondary intestinal lymphangiectasia. *Dig Dis Sci*, 1981; 26: 312.

139 Shilkin KB, Zerman BJ, Blackwell JB. Lymphangiectatic cysts of the small bowel. *J Pathol Bacteriol*, 1968; 96: 353.

140 Aase S, Gundersen R. Submucous lymphatic cysts of the small intestine. An autopsy study. *Acta Pathol Microbiol Immunol Scand A Pathol*, 1983; 91: 191.

141 Bliss DP, Coffin CM, Bower RJ, Stockmann PT, Ternberg JL. Mesenteric cysts in children. *Surgery*, 1994; 115: 571.

142 Liew SC, Glenn DC, Storey DW. Mesenteric cyst. *Aust N Z J Surg*, 1994; 64: 741.

143 Hesselfeldt-Nielsen J, Geerdsen JP, Pedersen VM. Bleeding schwannoma of the small intestine: a diagnostic problem. Case report. *Acta Chir Scand*, 1987; 153: 623.
144 Hansen D, Pedersen A, Pedersen KM. Malignant intestinal schwannoma. Case report. *Acta Chir Scand*, 1990; 156: 729.
145 Eskelinen M, Pasanen P, Kosma VM, Alhava E. Primary malignant schwannoma of the small bowel. *Ann Chir Gynaecol*, 1992; 81: 326.
146 Johnston J, Helwig EB. Granular cell tumors of the gastrointestinal tract and perianal region: a study of 74 cases. *Dig Dis Sci*, 1981; 26: 807.
147 Watanuki F, Ohwada S, Hosomura Y *et al*. Small ileal neurofibroma causing intussusception in a non-neurofibromatosis patient. *J Gastroenterol*, 1995; 30: 113.
148 Fuller CE, Williams GT. Gastrointestinal manifestations of type 1 neurofibromatosis (von Recklinghausen's disease). *Histopathology*, 1991; 19: 1.
149 Petersen JM, Ferguson DR. Gastrointestinal neurofibromatosis. *J Clin Gastroenterol*, 1984; 6: 529.
150 Waxman BP, Buzzard AJ, Cox J, Stephens MJ. Gastric and intestinal bleeding in multiple neurofibromatosis with cardiomyopathy. *Aust N Z J Surg*, 1986; 56: 171.
151 Melin MM, Grotz RL, Nivatvongs S. Gastrointestinal hemorrhage complicating systemic neurofibromatosis. *Am J Gastroenterol*, 1994; 89: 1888.
152 Hough DR, Chan A, Davidson H. Von Recklinghausen's disease associated with gastrointestinal carcinoid tumors. *Cancer*, 1983; 51: 2206.
153 Stephens M, Williams GT, Jasani B, Williams ED. Synchronous duodenal neuroendocrine tumours in von Recklinghausen's disease—a case report of co-existing gangliocytic paraganglioma and somatostatin-rich glandular carcinoid. *Histopathology*, 1987; 11: 1331.
154 Min KW, Balaton AJ. Small intestinal stromal tumors with skeinoid fibers in neurofibromatosis: report of four cases with ultrastructural study of skeinoid fibers from paraffin blocks. *Ultrastruct Pathol*, 1993; 17: 307.
155 Shekitka KM, Sobin LH. Ganglioneuromas of the gastrointestinal tract. Relation to Von Recklinghausen disease and other multiple tumor syndromes. *Am J Surg Pathol*, 1994; 18: 250.
156 Ishida T, Wada I, Horiuchi H, Oka T, Machinami R. Multiple small intestinal stromal tumors with skeinoid fibers in association with neurofibromatosis 1 (von Recklinghausen's disease). *Pathol Int*, 1996; 46: 689.
157 Fernando SS, McGovern VJ. Neuromuscular and vascular hamartoma of small bowel. *Gut*, 1982; 23: 1008.
158 Smith CE, Filipe MI, Owen WJ. Neuromuscular and vascular hamartoma of small bowel presenting as inflammatory bowel disease. *Gut*, 1986; 27: 964.
159 Shepherd NA, Jass JR. Neuromuscular and vascular hamartoma of the small intestine: is it Crohn's disease? *Gut*, 1987; 28: 1663.
160 Kwasnik EM, Tahan SR, Lowell JA, Weinstein B. Neuromuscular and vascular hamartoma of the small bowel. *Dig Dis Sci*, 1989; 34: 108.
161 Cortina G, Wren S, Armstrong B, Lewin K, Fajardo L. Clinical and pathologic overlap in nonsteroidal anti-inflammatory drug-related small bowel diaphragm disease and the neuromuscular and vascular hamartoma of the small bowel. *Am J Surg Pathol*, 1999; 23: 1414.
162 Perrone T, Sibley RK, Rosai J. Duodenal gangliocytic paraganglioma. An immunohistochemical and ultrastructural study and a hypothesis concerning its origin. *Am J Surg Pathol*, 1985; 9: 31.
163 Scheithauer BW, Nora FE, LeChago J *et al*. Duodenal gangliocytic paraganglioma. Clinicopathologic and immunocytochemical study of 11 cases. *Am J Clin Pathol*, 1986; 86: 559.
164 Burke AP, Helwig EB. Gangliocytic paraganglioma. *Am J Clin Pathol*, 1989; 92: 1.
165 Attanoos R, Williams GT. Epithelial and neuroendocrine tumors of the duodenum. *Semin Diagn Pathol*, 1991; 8: 149.
166 Elsayed AM, Albahra M, Nzeako UC, Sobin LH. Malignant melanomas in the small intestine: a study of 103 patients. *Am J Gastroenterol*, 1996; 91: 1001.
167 Shepherd NA. Polyps and polyposis syndromes of the intestines. *Curr Diag Pathol*, 1997; 5: 222.

26 Tumour-like lesions of the small intestine

Brunner's gland hyperplasia/hamartoma/adenoma

These uncommon lesions are really hamartomas and can present at any age, but are most frequently found during the fifth and sixth decades. Both sexes are equally affected. There is no known genetic basis and they are not associated with oral pigmentation. In one series of 27 cases, the lesion was symptomless and found incidentally in seven cases but 10 cases presented with haemorrhage and there were 10 patients with obstruction [1]. Macroscopically, Brunner's gland hamartomas protrude into the lumen of the first or second part of the duodenum as single (rarely multiple) polyps that are frequently pedunculated. They may measure up to 6 cm in diameter (Fig. 26.1), although most examples are much smaller. Histologically (Fig. 26.2) they are purely epithelial lesions consisting of groups or clumps of Brunner's glands separated by septa of proliferated smooth muscle derived from and lying deep to the muscularis mucosae [1]. Focal cystic change may be seen. The epithelium of the lesions is of normal Brunner's gland type, with basal nuclei, without atypia. Mitoses are very scanty and there is no tendency to neoplastic change. Paneth cells are often present.

Periampullary myoepithelial hamartoma

Small myoepithelial hamartomas composed of dilated gland elements and surrounded by muscle occur in the duodenum, usually in relation to the ampulla of Vater. Most cases are asymptomatic and discovered incidentally; larger pedunculated lesions may cause intermittent biliary or pancreatic obstruction. The sexes appear equally affected. The macroscopic appearances are usually of an umbilicated sessile polyp. Histological examination reveals a submucosal admixture of hypertrophic smooth muscle bundles together with cystic glands lined by cytologically benign low columnar epithelium (Fig. 26.3), Brunner's glands and variable numbers of pancreatic acini and ducts. Islets of Langerhans are present in approximately one-third of cases and their presence greatly facilitates the diagnosis. Neoplastic change has not been reported. The complex admixture of epithelial and smooth muscle elements in a periampullary mass may persuade the unwary into a diagnosis of malignancy, especially in frozen sections. Important differentiating features of this lesion are a lack of cytological atypia and the absence of a desmoplastic reaction in relation to the glandular elements.

Peutz–Jeghers polyp

Peutz–Jeghers syndrome

The classical Peutz–Jeghers syndrome has three components—gastrointestinal polyposis, oral pigmentation and an autosomal dominant pattern of inheritance. It results from germline mutation affecting the serine/threonine kinase 11 (*LKB1/STK11*) gene on the short arm of chromosome 19 [2] All three components are present in some 55% of patients, while *formes frustes*, in which the pigmentation or the polyps appear to be absent, are well described [3]; some of these represent a non-coterminous development in which the pigment is usually visible before the polyps present clinically. The sex incidence is equal. Polyps can develop anywhere in the gut, but small bowel is the most common site, with the jejunum predominating, followed by ileum and duodenum. They tend to appear sequentially in crops in different regions. Presenting features are haemorrhage with consequent anaemia, and recurrent attacks of severe colic, sometimes with recurring intussusception, especially after a meal. Before this was recognized, multiple resections were often performed resulting eventually in malabsorption syndromes; once the condition is

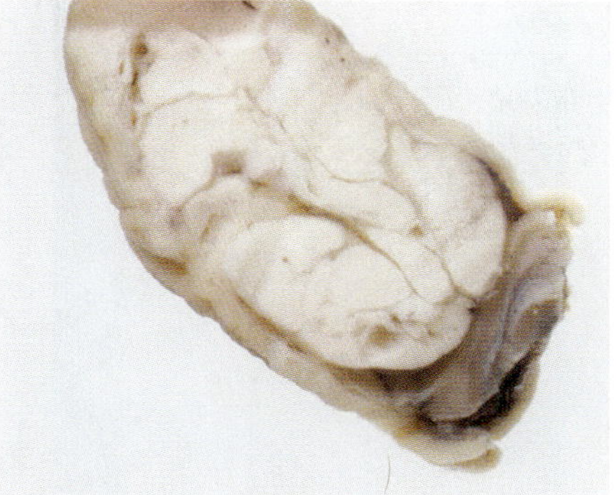

Fig. 26.1 Brunner's gland hamartoma. This particular lesion is unusually large and polypoid, sufficient to cause duodenal obstruction. The lobulated structure is well seen on the cut surface.

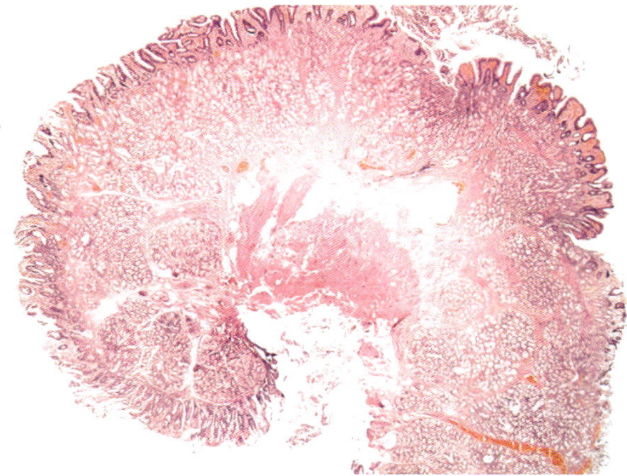

Fig. 26.2 Histological section of a biopsy of a hamartoma of Brunner's glands. The lobules of proliferated glands are divided by thin smooth muscle septa. A few of the glands are cystically dilated.

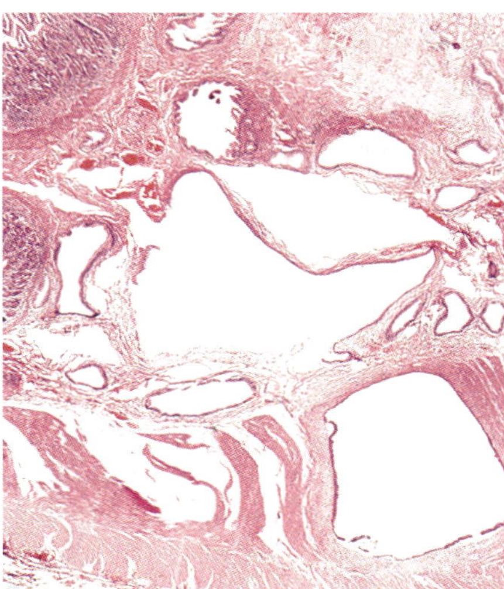

Fig. 26.3 Duodenal 'myoepithelial hamartoma'. The lesion consists of dilated gland elements lined by flattened epithelium and surrounded by smooth muscle.

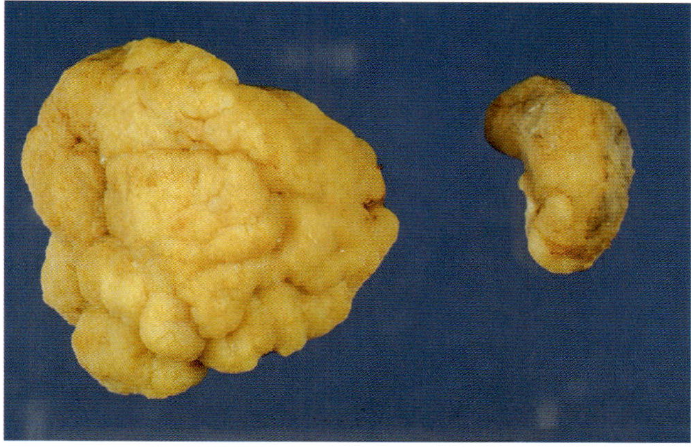

Fig. 26.4 Peutz–Jeghers polyps from the small bowel. The surface shows characteristic coarse lobulation.

recognized a conservative attitude is often justified as many intussusceptions will reduce themselves and local mucosal stripping may provide an alternative treatment.

Macroscopically, the surface of a Peutz–Jeghers polyp has a coarse lobulation, resembling that of an adenoma but with larger lobules and in marked contrast with the smooth surface of a juvenile polyp (Fig. 26.4). The polyps may or may not be pedunculated; when they are the stalk is often short, broad and poorly formed. The polyps vary in size from a few millimetres to several centimetres. When they are over 0.5 cm the typical histological features are easily identified, but when small, the polyps can be little more than tags of mucosa that do not show diagnostic features.

Microscopically the essential feature is a branching core of muscle derived from the muscularis mucosae (Figs 26.5 & 26.6); the branches become thinner and eventually disappear as they reach the periphery of the polyp. Each branch is covered by histologically normal epithelium with a normal lamina propria; Paneth and endocrine cells are present in their normal sites at the base of the crypts. Small areas of normal superficial gastric-type epithelium are often found in duodenal and jejunal polyps and there is no excess of lamina propria and no nuclear hyperchromatism or glandular irregularity such as is seen in adenomas. The whole appearance irresistibly suggests a tree-like overgrowth of the muscularis mucosae, which has carried with it a covering of normal gland elements set in a normal lamina propria (Figs 26.5 & 26.6). The hamartomatous condition seems to involve the whole bowel wall and there is often apparent misplacement of glands and lamina propria within or even through the muscularis propria, a feature that can mimic adenocarcinoma (Fig. 26.7), especially as epithelial dysplasia may occasionally develop in these polyps (see below).

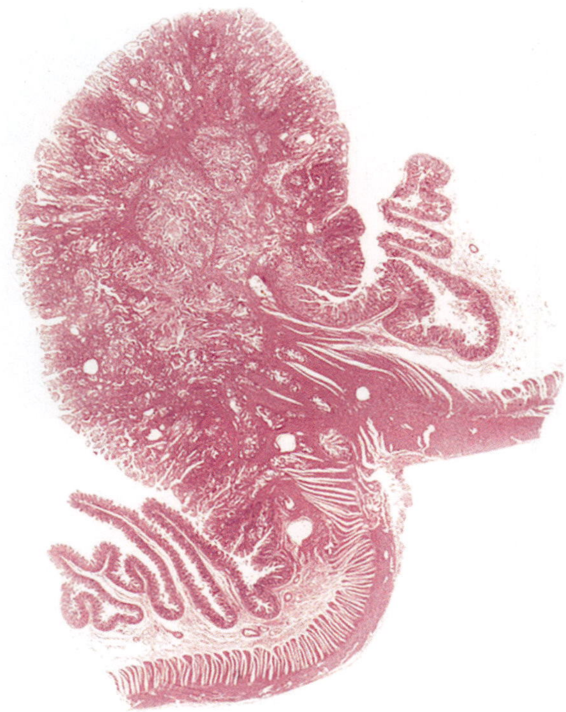

Fig. 26.5 Peutz–Jeghers polyp of jejunum, showing tree-like arborization, with much-folded normal small intestinal epithelium lying on a core of muscle.

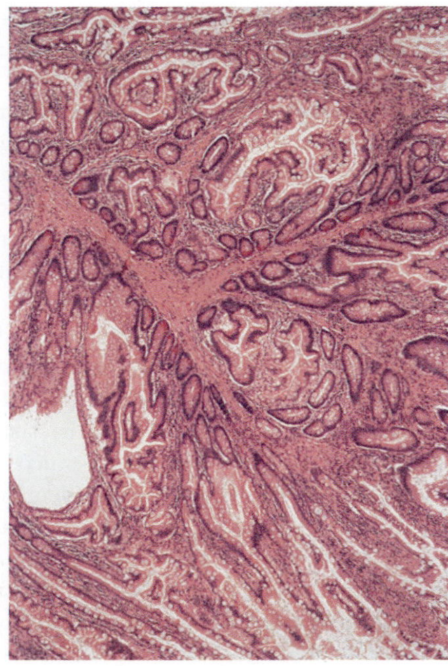

Fig. 26.6 Part of a Peutz–Jeghers polyp at higher magnification. The epithelium is not dysplastic. The branching smooth muscle core is displayed.

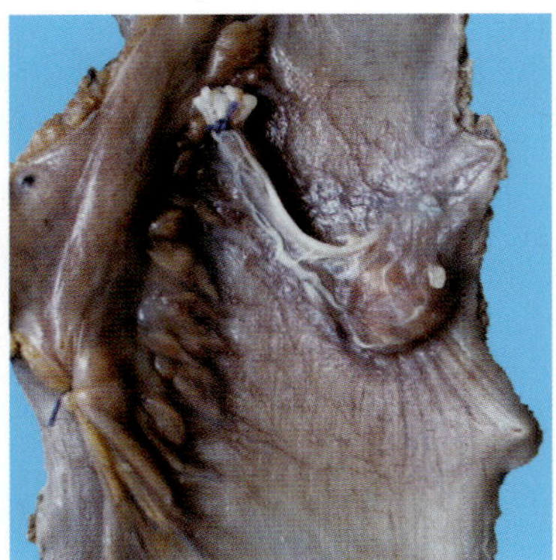

Fig. 26.7 Extension of the hamartomatous glands of a Peutz–Jeghers polyp through the small intestinal wall has resulted in a serosal nodule, easily confused with a malignant tumour.

Complications

Intussusception has already been mentioned. Malignant change in the epithelium is uncommon but well recognized, particularly in gastric and duodenal polyps [4–6]. Foci of dysplasia can be found in a minority of both small bowel and large bowel polyps [7,8]. Care in diagnosis of malignancy is necessary since hypersecretion of mucin is common and this can become trapped between mucosal folds, causing misplacement of epithelium with histological appearances that the unwary can interpret as carcinoma [9–11].

It has become clear that it is not only the hamartomatous lesions themselves that are at risk of neoplasia. Although Peutz–Jeghers syndrome is associated with a risk of death from gastrointestinal cancer 13 times that of the general population, there is also an increased incidence of neoplasms at other sites. The chance of dying of cancer by the age of 57 is 48% [12] and the relative risk of death from cancer at any site is nine, suggesting that the gene locus is relevant to the development of malignancy in general. Interesting associations have been demonstrated between Peutz–Jeghers syndrome and breast cancer, which is usually bilateral [13,14], and also with sex cord tumours of the ovary [15] and feminizing Sertoli cell tumours of the testis [16,17].

Juvenile polyp

We are not aware of the occurrence of juvenile polyps in the small bowel, other than in the context of juvenile polyposis, which occurs in two forms. One is a generalized form that occurs in infancy in which polyps are present in the stomach, small bowel and colon [18]. The polyps vary in size from 1 to 30 mm and may be sessile or pedunculated (Fig. 26.8). Clinically the infants have diarrhoea, haemorrhage, malnutrition and intussusception, and death is usual at an early age. The second form usually presents later in childhood or in adult life and

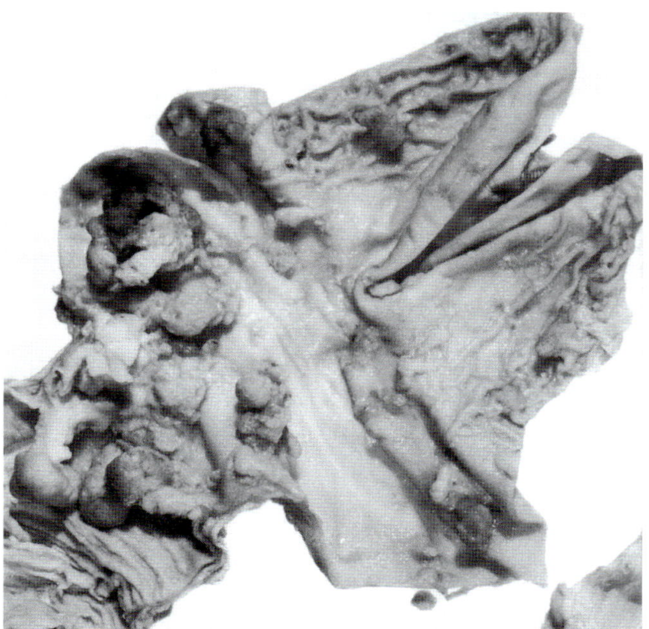

Fig. 26.8 Postmortem specimen from a child aged 1 year with juvenile polyposis of infancy. There are occasional polyps in the body and antrum of the stomach and a large number of polyps in the first part of the duodenum (bottom left).

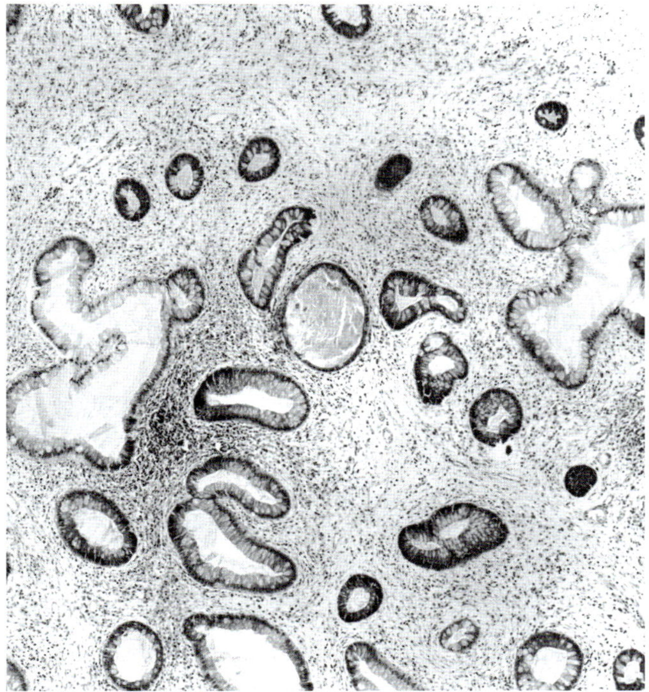

Fig. 26.9 Histology of duodenal polyp shown in Fig. 26.8. Appearances are similar to juvenile polyps of large bowel except that appropriate endocrine cells and Paneth cells may be present.

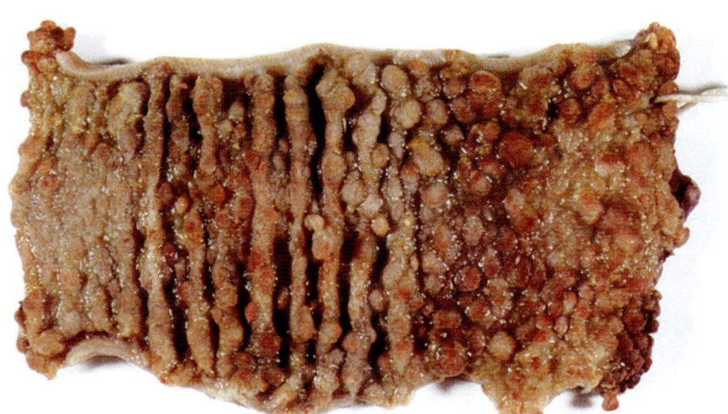

Fig. 26.10 Ileum from a patient with Cronkhite–Canada syndrome. The mucosa is diffusely inflamed and carpeted with small polyps.

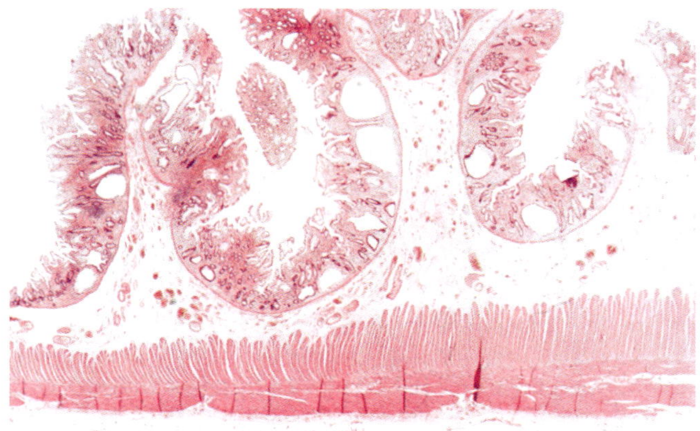

Fig. 26.11 Histology of the ileum shown in Fig. 26.10. There is conspicuous and random cystic dilatation of glands. The lamina propria is oedematous.

may be sporadic or inherited. In this form the colon is predominantly affected (see p. 628), but occasional patients have small bowel polyps [19,20] and other congenital anomalies are common [21]. Histological studies on juvenile polyps of the small intestine are few [22]. In cases of infantile type we have seen jejunal polyps closely resembling those seen in the large intestine (Fig. 26.9). Small intestinal carcinoma has not been reported in juvenile polyposis.

Cronkhite–Canada syndrome

This excessively rare syndrome combines diffuse polypoid thickening of the small bowel mucosa with ectodermal changes that include alopecia, hyperpigmentation and atrophy of the nails. There is loss of protein from the gut [23,24]. The mucosa appears grossly to be diffusely inflamed and is carpeted with small rounded polyps (Fig. 26.10) that are composed of dilated glands surrounded by an oedematous stroma (Fig. 26.11). There is a histological similarity to juvenile polyps

[25] and also to the stomach in Ménétrier's disease [26]. Endocrine and Paneth cells are reduced or absent [27]. Whether the ectodermal changes are the result of the loss of essential amino acids in excessive secretion of glycoprotein [28] or whether all the manifestations of the syndrome, including the small intestinal changes, are the result of impaired growth, possibly due to a deficiency state [27], is unknown.

Inflammatory fibroid polyp

Inflammatory fibroid polyp is the name given to a group of tumour-like masses that occur in the stomach, ileum and (rarely) the right side of the colon [29,30]. They mostly present in adults with a median age of 60 and show a slight male preponderance. In the small bowel they occur as rounded, circumscribed, greyish-white rubbery masses that appear to originate within the submucosa of the intestine but expand to form a polypoid intraluminal mass and often extend into, and even through, the muscularis propria. Smaller lesions are sessile but larger lesions are polypoid (Fig. 26.12). They vary in size from about 2 cm to 5 cm in diameter. Occasional examples show a dumb-bell shape with an intraluminal, mucosal and submucosal portion, a narrow neck and an intramural portion. They are usually single, but occasionally can be multiple, and most commonly present with obstruction and/or intussusception (Fig. 26.12a). Ulceration is a relatively common accompaniment. Excisional surgery is curative.

While inflammatory fibroid polyps at different sites show similar pathological features, it is debatable whether all such lesions represent a single entity [31]. What is clear is the lesion is not really a neoplasm, in the true sense of the word, but is a reactive overgrowth of fibrovascular connective tissue. It has been intimated that inflammatory fibroid polyp represents an exaggerated response of fibroblasts and myofibroblasts to unidentified stimuli, possibly mechanical in nature [32]. The fact that inflammatory fibroid polyps have been described after previous surgery, notably in the pelvic ileal reservoir, gives some credence to this notion [33,34]. Although ileal inflammatory fibroid polyps are usually single, there is a remarkable Devon, UK, family in whom multiple inflammatory fibroid polyps occur, usually in females, suggesting that the factors that produce inflammatory fibroid polyps may be genetically determined: sadly this family have not been willing to undergo genetic analysis [35,36].

Microscopically, inflammatory fibroid polyps of the small bowel are composed of loose connective tissue containing thin-walled blood vessels (Fig. 26.12b), surrounded by an onion-skin arrangement of palisaded spindle and stellate fibroblasts and myofibroblasts [37]. There is a background of collagen bundles with wavy fibres and myxoid areas infiltrated by inflammatory cells including plentiful mast cells and eosinophils (Fig. 26.12c). However, unlike eosinophilic gastroenteritis, which sometimes enters the differential diagnosis [38], there is no blood eosinophilia or other specific clinical abnormality. Ileal inflammatory fibroid polyps tend to be more oedematous than their gastric counterparts and their appearance has been likened to that of excessive granulation tissue [31]. Sometimes the palisading elongated cells are reminiscent of nerve sheath tumours but they are consistently S-100 protein negative. Similarly, they differ from gastrointestinal stromal tumours by being c-kit and CD34 negative.

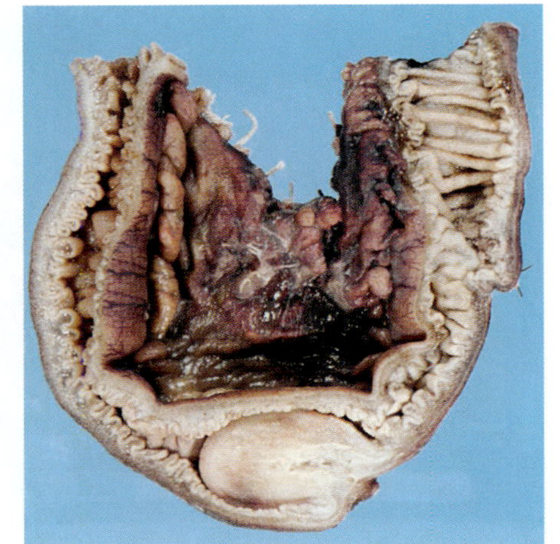

(a)

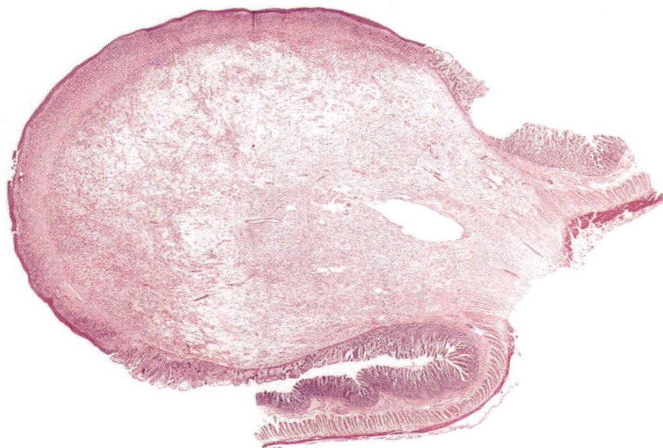

(b)

Fig. 26.12 (a) An inflammatory fibroid polyp which had intussuscepted and caused small intestinal obstruction. (b) Histological appearance of the inflammatory fibroid polyp shown in (a). The lesion is a mass of loosely arranged connective tissue containing thin-walled blood vessels (H&E × 23). (c) Higher magnification shows a mixture of spindle cells and inflammatory cells including eosinophils, with a myxoid background containing wavy collagen fibres (H&E × 100).

Pyogenic granuloma

Pyogenic granuloma has been described in the small bowel [39]. It resembles pyogenic granuloma at other sites, being a polypoid mass of granulation tissue with a narrow stalk

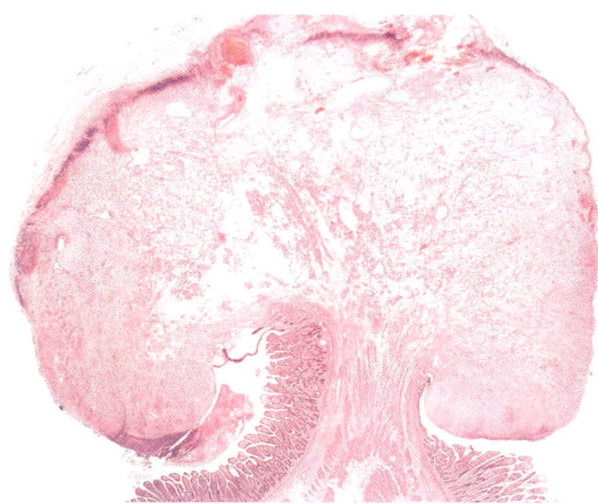

Fig. 26.13 Pyogenic granuloma of small intestine. The lesion is a narrow-necked polyp composed of granulation tissue (H&E × 4.5).

(Fig. 26.13). Whether it represents an early stage in the formation of an inflammatory fibroid polyp is uncertain.

References

1 Levine JA, Burgart LJ, Batts KP, Wang KK. Brunner's gland hamartomas: clinical presentation and pathological features of 27 cases. *Am J Gastroenterol*, 1995; 90: 290.

2 Jenne DE, Reimann H, Nezu J *et al*. Peutz–Jeghers syndrome is caused by mutations in a novel serine threonine kinase. *Nat Genet*, 1998; 18: 38.

3 Bartholomew LG, Dahlin DC, Waugh JM. Intestinal polyposis associated with mucocutaneous melanin pigmentation (Peutz–Jeghers syndrome). *Gastroenterology*, 1957; 32: 434.

4 Bussey HJR. Gastrointestinal polyposis syndromes. In: Anthony PP, MacSween RNM, eds. *Recent Advances in Histopathology 12*. Edinburgh: Churchill Livingstone, 1984: 169.

5 Hsu S-D, Zaharopoulos P, May JT, Costanzi JJ. Peutz–Jeghers syndrome with intestinal carcinoma. Report of the association in one family. *Cancer*, 1979; 44: 1527.

6 Burdick D, Prior JT. Peutz–Jeghers syndrome. A clinicopathologic study of a large family with a 27 year follow-up. *Cancer*, 1982; 50: 2139.

7 Hizawa K, Iida M, Matsumoto T, Kohrogi N, Yao T, Fujishima M. Neoplastic transformation arising in Peutz–Jeghers polyposis. *Dis Colon Rectum*, 1993; 36: 953.

8 Flageole H, Raptis S, Trudel JL, Lough JO. Progression toward malignancy of hamartomas in a patient with Peutz–Jeghers syndrome: case report and literature review. *Can J Surg*, 1994; 37: 231.

9 Rintala A. The histological appearances of gastrointestinal polyps in the Peutz–Jeghers syndrome. *Acta Chir Scand*, 1959; 117: 366.

10 Morson BC. Precancerous lesions of upper gastrointestinal tract. *JAMA*, 1962; 179: 311.

11 Shepherd NA, Bussey HVR, Jass JR. Epithelial misplacement in Peutz–Jeghers polyps. *Am J Surg Pathol*, 1987; 11: 743.

12 Spigelman AD, Murday V, Phillips RK. Cancer and the Peutz–Jeghers syndrome. *Gut*, 1989; 30: 1588.

13 Riley E, Swift EC. A family with Peutz–Jeghers syndrome and bilateral breast cancer. *Cancer*, 1980; 46: 815.

14 Trau H, Schewach-Millet M, Fisher BK, Tour H. Peutz–Jeghers syndrome and bilateral breast carcinoma. *Cancer*, 1982; 50: 788.

15 Young RH, Welch WR, Dickersin GR, Scully RE. Ovarian sex-cord tumour with annular tubules. Review of 74 cases including 27 with Peutz–Jeghers syndrome and 4 with adenoma malignum of the cervix. *Cancer*, 1982; 50: 1384.

16 Cantu JM, Rivera H, Ocampo-Campos R *et al*. Peutz–Jeghers syndrome with femininising sertoli cell tumour. *Cancer*, 1980; 46: 223.

17 Young S, Gooneratne S, Straus FHII, Zeller WP, Bulun SE, Rosenthal IM. Feminizing sertoli cell tumors in boys with Peutz–Jeghers syndrome. *Am J Surg Pathol*, 1995; 19: 50.

18 Sachetello CR, Pickren JW, Grance JT Jr. Generalised juvenile gastrointestinal polyposis. *Gastroenterology*, 1970; 58: 699.

19 Stemper TJ, Kent TH, Summers NW. Juvenile polyposis and gastrointestinal carcinoma; a study of a kindred. *Ann Intern Med*, 1975; 83: 639.

20 Grotsky HW, Richert RR, Smith WD, Newsome JF. Familial juvenile polyposis coli. A clinical and pathological study of a large kindred. *Gastroenterology*, 1982; 82: 494.

21 Grigioni WF, Alampi G, Martinelli G, Piccaluga A. Atypical juvenile polyposis. *Histopathology*, 1981; 5: 361.

22 Sachetello CR, Hahn IS, Carrington CB. Juvenile gastrointestinal polyposis in a female infant. Report of a case and review of the literature of a recently recognised syndrome. *Surgery*, 1974; 75: 107.

23 Johnston MM, Vosburgh JW, Weins AT, Walsh GC. Gastrointestinal polyposis associated with alopecia, pigmentation and atrophy of the fingernails and toenails. *Ann Intern Med*, 1962; 56: 935.

24 Jamum S, Jensen H. Diffuse gastrointestinal polyposis with ectodermal changes. *Gastroenterology*, 1966; 50: 107.

25 Ruymann FB. Juvenile polyps with cachexia. Report of an infant and comparison with Cronkhite–Canada syndrome in adults. *Gastroenterology*, 1969; 57: 431.

26 Gill WJ, Wilken BJ. Diffuse gastrointestinal polyposis associated with hypoproteinaemia. *J R Coll Surg Edinb*, 1967; 12: 149.

27 Freeman K, Anthony PP, Miller DS, Warin AP. Cronkhite Canada syndrome: a new hypothesis. *Gut*, 1985; 26: 531.

28 Manousos O, Webster CU. Diffuse gastrointestinal polyposis with ectodermal changes. *Gut*, 1966; 7: 375.

29 Johnstone JM, Morson BC. Inflammatory fibroid polyp of the gastrointestinal tract. *Histopathology*, 1978; 2: 349.

30 Navas-Palacios JJ, Colina-Ruizdelgado F, Sanchez-Larrea MD, Cortes CJ. Inflammatory fibroid polyps of the gastrointestinal tract. An immunohistochemical and electron microscopic study. *Cancer*, 1983; 51: 1682.

31 Appelman HD. Mesenchymal tumors of the gastrointestinal tract. In: Ming S, Goldman H, eds. *Pathology of the Gastrointestinal Tract*. Baltimore: Williams & Wilkins, 1998: 361.

32 Widgren S, Pizzolato GP. Inflammatory fibroid polyp of the gastrointestinal tract: possible origin in myofibroblasts? A study of twelve cases. *Ann Pathol*, 1987; 7: 184.

33 Tysk C, Schnurer LB, Wickbom G. Obstructing inflammatory fibroid polyp in pelvic ileal reservoir after restorative proctocolectomy in ulcerative colitis. Report of a case. *Dis Colon Rectum*, 1994; 37: 1034.
34 Widgren S, Cox JN. Inflammatory fibroid polyp in a continent ileo-anal pouch after colectomy for ulcerative colitis—case report. *Pathol Res Pract*, 1997; 193: 643.
35 Anthony PP, Morris DS, Vowles KD. Multiple and recurrent inflammatory fibroid polyps in three generations of a Devon family: a new syndrome. *Gut*, 1984; 25: 854.
36 Allibone RO, Nanson JK, Anthony PP. Multiple and recurrent inflammatory fibroid polyps in a Devon family ('Devon polyposis syndrome'): an update. *Gut*, 1992; 33: 1004.
37 Kolodziejczyk P, Yao T, Tsuneyoshi M. Inflammatory fibroid polyp of the stomach. A special reference to an immunohistochemical profile of 42 cases. *Am J Surg Pathol*, 1993; 17: 1159.
38 Blackshaw AJ, Levison DA. Eosinophilic infiltrates of the gastrointestinal tract. *J Clin Pathol*, 1986; 39: 1.
39 Yao T, Nagai E, Utsunomiya T, Tsuneyoshi M. An intestinal counterpart of pyogenic granuloma of the skin. A newly proposed entity. *Am J Surg Pathol*, 1995; 19: 1054.

27 Miscellaneous conditions of the small intestine

Amyloid

Amyloid in the small bowel may be predominantly mucosal and subepithelial in distribution, confined to the vasculature, or deposited in the muscularis mucosae and the muscularis propria (Fig. 27.1). The distribution is partly related to the nature of the underlying systemic amyloidosis. Clinical effects depend on the pattern of involvement, and include malabsorption, ischaemia and motility disorders. Gastrointestinal amyloidosis is discussed more fully in Chapter 41 (see p. 634).

Bypass operations

Obesity surgery with bypass of small bowel segments is performed rarely now, but many individuals exist who have had this surgery performed in the past. The non-bypassed functioning segments of ileum show a gradual increase in length and diameter. In both the functioning and excluded or diverted segments there is an increase in mucosal height due to lengthening and broadening of the villi and an increase in the number of mucosal folds [1,2]. These changes are considered to be adaptive and may explain the failure of many patients to continue to lose weight after a satisfactory initial weight loss. We have seen one case in which the excluded segment developed not only hyperplastic villous changes but also increased numbers of lymphoid follicles and mild diffuse chronic mucosal inflammation reminiscent of the changes seen in diverted colonic segments (see p. 520) (Fig. 27.2), although there was also an intraepithelial lymphocytosis (but no evidence of gluten sensitivity).

Complications of intestinal bypass surgery may occur both within the excluded segment and outside the gastrointestinal tract. Enteric hyperoxaluria may produce acute renal failure [3]. Other complications include electrolyte imbalance, malnutrition, diarrhoea, liver disease including cirrhosis, nephrolithiasis, arthritis and pathological fractures. Of these complications, the electrolyte imbalance, malnutrition and diarrhoea usually improve after reversal [4]. A dermal leucocytoclastic vasculitis that is responsive to tetracycline may also occur as part of the so-called 'bowel bypass arthritis dermatitis syndrome' [5]. Within the bypassed segment itself pneumatosis cystoides intestinalis, severe blood loss, localized ulceration, intussusception, adhesions and bacterial overgrowth have all been observed [6,7].

Cholesterol ester storage disease

This is a very rare inherited disorder of lipid metabolism in which the liver and spleen are enlarged, serum cholesterol is raised and cholesterol esters are stored in various body tissues. Macroscopically the small bowel mucosa has a yellow tinge. Microscopically the epithelium is normal but foamy macrophages may be seen in considerable numbers in the lamina propria at the tips of villi [8].

Endometriosis

The small bowel is very much less commonly affected by endometriosis than the large bowel (see p. 635). Lesions are recognized on finding endometrial glands and stroma, most frequently in the serosa but occasionally intramurally,

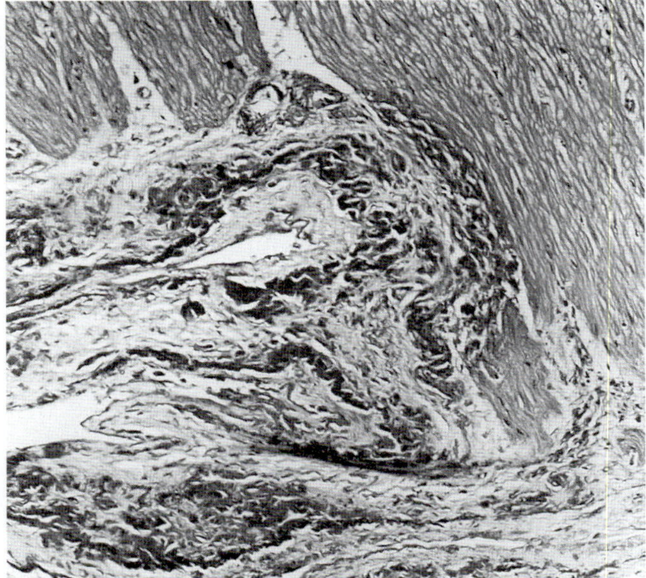

(a)

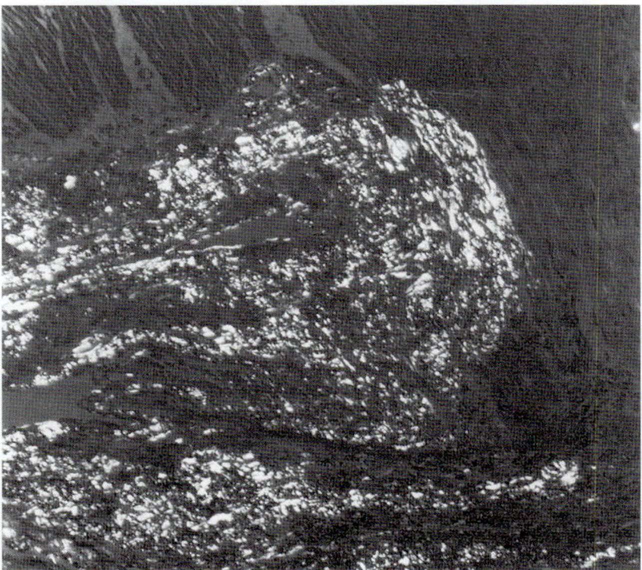

(b)

Fig. 27.1 (a) Amyloid deposits stained by Congo red are present between muscle fibres. The pattern is commonest in primary amyloidosis. No amyloid was found in other organs at autopsy, but the patient had chronic fibrocaseous tuberculosis and it remains uncertain whether his amyloid was primary or secondary. (b) The same field under polarized light to show birefringence.

and sometimes in association with haemosiderin-laden macrophages. Dense stromal fibrosis may lead to multiple complex adhesions, especially after laparoscopic surgery for endometriosis. In postmenopausal women inactive endometriotic foci composed of glands but little stroma should not be confused with deposits of adenocarcinoma.

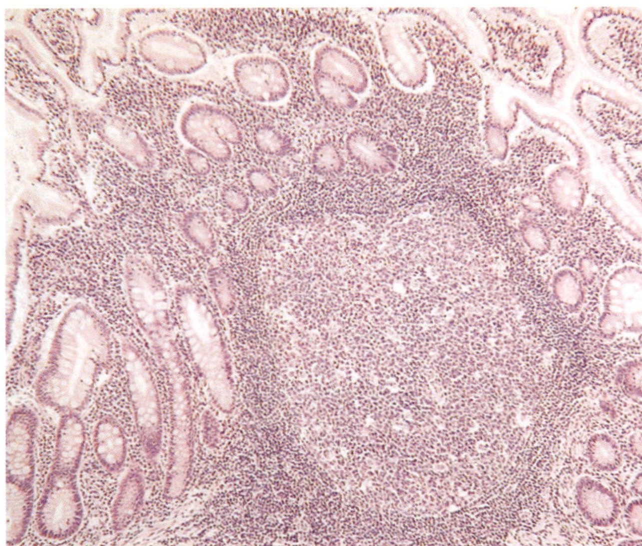

Fig. 27.2 Bypassed jejunum with lymphoid follicular hyperplasia and diffuse mucosal chronic inflammation.

Gas cysts—pneumatosis cystoides intestinalis

Pneumatosis cystoides intestinalis of the small bowel occurs in two forms [9–11]. The first, in patients with chronic obstructive pulmonary disease, is the result of gaseous dissection through the perivascular space of intra-abdominal blood vessels. The second occurs in infants with necrotizing enterocolitis and in adults with ischaemic bowel and is the result of intramural gas-forming organisms (*Clostridium perfringens, Enterobacter aerogenes* and *Escherichia coli*). The cysts are found in the mucosa, submucosa and subserosa, they may be single or multiple, and they may give rise to sessile or even pedunculated mucosal polyps. They are usually lined by mixed inflammatory cells, macrophages or foreign body giant cells (Fig. 27.3) but occasionally those associated with lung disease have an apparent lining of endothelial cells. In mucosal biopsies they are recognized as incomplete cysts surrounded by macrophages in the submucosa.

Malakoplakia

Malakoplakia is rarer in the small intestine than in the large bowel. It may be seen complicating pre-existing chronic inflammatory bowel disease or arising in isolation in adults, often in association with *E. coli* infection [12].

Systemic mastocytosis

Steatorrhoea may occasionally complicate urticaria pigmen-

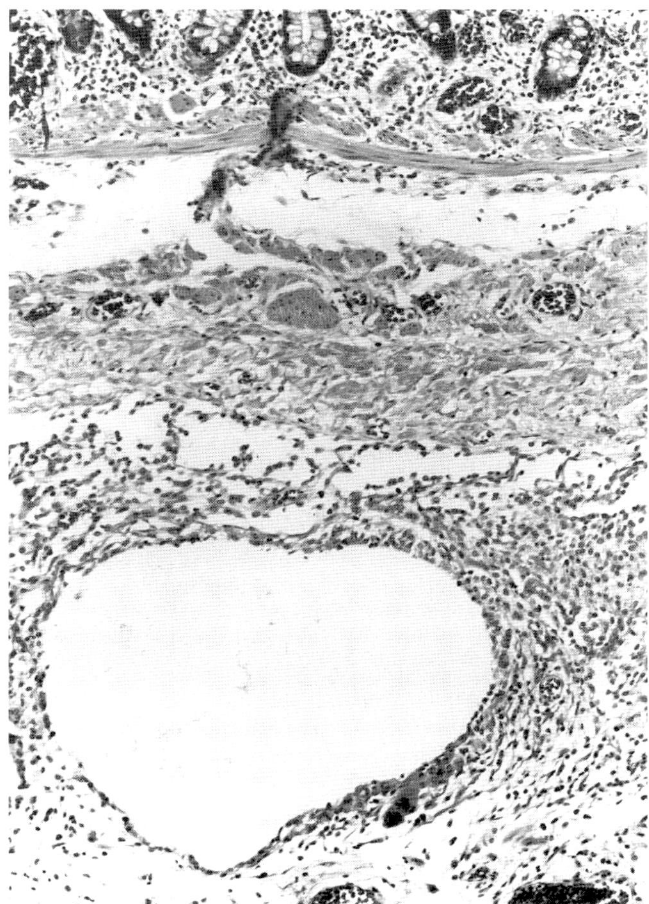

Fig. 27.3 A gas cyst in the serosa of a 50-year-old man with chronic obstructive airway disease who developed abdominal symptoms. Numerous cysts were present in the illeum. Note the lack of lining epithelium and the inflammatory and giant cell reaction around the cyst.

tosa and systemic mastocytosis, and some such cases show small intestinal mucosal flattening with infiltration by mast cells, accompanied by eosinophils and neutrophils [13]. Mast cells may be identified by metachromatic staining with toluidine blue or with immunohistochemistry using antibodies to mast cell tryptase and CD68 [14].

Melanosis and pseudomelanosis

Melanosis (or more accurately pseudomelanosis) due to lipofuscin deposition in mucosal macrophages, which is commonly seen in the large bowel (see p. 635) of patients taking anthraquinone laxatives, virtually never occurs in the small bowel. However, a melanin-like pigmentation of the duodenal mucosa has been described rarely in association with peptic ulcer and folate deficiency [15] and in patients with AIDS or those receiving haemodialysis [16]. This appears to begin with iron deposition and the pigment later stains with the Masson Fontana reaction. These rare cases of mucosal pigmentation should be distinguished from the brown bowel syndrome that is seen in association with severe malabsorption, in which the lipofuscin pigmentation occurs within the intramural musculature (see Chapter 22, p. 338).

Zinc deficiency

A rare autosomal recessive disorder—acrodermatitis enteropathica—results in zinc malabsorption [17] and morphological effects on the small bowel mucosa including focal villous atrophy with crypt hyperplasia, reduced brush border enzymes, and mild focal chronic inflammation in the lamina propria. Electron microscopy shows Paneth cells to contain characteristic pleomorphic cytoplasmic inclusions [18].

Pseudolipomatosis

This is another condition that is common in the colorectum but rarely reported in the duodenum [19]. There are numerous tiny gas bubbles, usually measuring less than 50 μm in diameter, in the lamina propria of the mucosa. On superficial examination they resemble adipocytes; hence the term pseudolipomatosis. They may cause expansion of the villous cores and separation of the crypts and must be distinguished from lymphangiectasia and Whipple's disease, if necessary by immunostaining. Pseudolipomatosis is now considered to be an artefact of mucosal biopsies that results from penetration of gas into the mucosa during endoscopy (see Chapter 41, p. 636).

Graft-versus-host disease

The small intestine, like other parts of the gastrointestinal tract, may be involved in graft-versus-host disease following bone marrow transplantation, when it gives rise to malabsorption and/or diarrhoea. Changes in the duodenum are best reported, being most amenable to biopsy, and these closely reflect those seen more regularly in the large intestine [20] (see p. 637). They include villous atrophy, epithelial degeneration and crypt loss consequent upon damage to crypt stem cells, along with an increase in chronic inflammatory cells. Sometimes there are erosions or frank ulcers and the changes may be diffuse or patchy. Typically apoptotic bodies are conspicuous within the crypt proliferative zones. Endocrine cells, having a longer lifespan than other crypt cell constituents, may form isolated aggregates in the lamina propria that represent the graveyards of pre-existing crypts that have been wiped out by the immunological attack [21].

References

1 Solhaug JH, Tvelte S. Adaptive changes in the small intestine following bypass operation for obesity: a radiological and histological study. *Scand J Gastroenterol*, 1978; 13: 401.

2 Asp N-G, Gudmand-Hoyer E, Andersen B, Berg NO. Enzyme activities and morphological appearance in functioning and excluded segments of the small intestine after shunt operation for obesity. *Gut*, 1979; 20: 553.

3 Wharton R, D'Agati V, Magun AM, Whitlock R, Kunis CL, Appel GB. Acute deterioration of renal function associated with enteric hyperoxaluria. *Clin Nephrol*, 1990; 34: 116.

4 Dean P, Joshi S, Kaminski DL. Long term outcome of reversal of small intestinal bypass operations. *Am J Surg*, 1990; 159: 118.

5 Sandbank M, Weltfriend S, Wolf R. Bowel bypass arthritis dermatitis syndrome: a histological and electron microscopical study. *Acta Derm Venereol*, 1984; 64: 79.

6 Leung FW, Drenick EJ, Stanley TM. Intestinal bypass complications involving the excluded small bowel segment. *Am J Gastroenterol*, 1982; 77: 67.

7 Ikard RW. Pneumatosis cystoides intestinalis following intestinal bypass. *Am J Surg*, 1977; 43: 467.

8 Partin JC, Schubert WK. Small intestinal mucosa in cholesterol ester storage disease: a light and electron microscopic study. *Gastroenterology*, 1969; 57: 542.

9 Galandiuk S, Fazio VW. Pneumatosis cystoides intestinalis. *Dis Colon Rectum*, 1986; 29: 358.

10 Koss LK. Abdominal gas cysts (pneumatosis cystoides intestinorum hominis): an analysis with a report of a case and a critical review of the literature. *Arch Pathol*, 1952; 53: 523.

11 Hughes DTD, Gordon KCD, Swann JC, Bolt GL. Pneumatosis cystoides intestinalis. *Gut*, 1966; 7: 553.

12 McClure J. Malakoplakia of the gastrointestinal tract. *Postgrad Med J*, 1981; 57: 95.

13 Braverman DZ, Dollbergh L, Shiner M. Clinical, histological and electron microscopic study of mast cell disease of the small bowel. *Am J Gastroenterol*, 1985; 80: 30.

14 Li W, Kapadia S, Sonmez-Alpan E *et al*. Immunohistochemical characterisation of mast cell disease in paraffin sections using tryptase, CD68, myeloperoxidase, lysosyme, and CD20 antibodies. *Mod Pathol*, 1996; 9: 982.

15 Sharp JR, Insalaco DJ, Johnson LJ. Melanosis of the duodenum associated with a gastric ulcer and folic acid deficiency. *Gastroenterology*, 1980; 78: 366.

16 Kang JY, Wu AYT, Chia JLS *et al*. Clinical and ultrastructural studies in duodenal pseudomelanosis. *Gut*, 1987; 28: 1673.

17 Danbolt N, Closs K. Acrodermatitis enteropathica. *Acta Derm Venereol*, 1942; 23: 127.

18 Bohane TD, Cutz E, Hamilton JR *et al*. Acrodermatitis enteropathica, zinc and the Paneth cell. *Gastroenterology*, 1977; 73: 587.

19 Cook DS, Williams GT. Duodenal 'pseudolipomatosis'. *Histopathology*, 1998; 33: 394.

20 Ponec RJ, Hackman RC, McDonald GB. Endoscopic and histologic diagnosis of intestinal graft-versus-host disease after marrow transplantation. *Gastrointest Endosc*, 1999; 49: 612.

21 Bryan RL, Antonakopoulos GN, Newman J, Milligan DW. Intestinal graft versus host disease. *J Clin Pathol*, 1991; 44: 866.

PART
5 Appendix

28 Normal appendix

Anatomy

The appendix in an adult has an average length of 7 cm, though variations between 5 cm and 12 cm are common, and lengths of up to 20 cm have been recorded. It is correspondingly shorter in children. The external diameter varies from 3 to 8 mm, reaching a maximum transverse diameter by the age of 4 years [1]. It arises from the posteromedial wall of the caecum, usually at a point about 2.5 cm below the ileocaecal valve, but detailed anatomical studies [2,3] have shown that four types of caecoappendiceal junction are possible, though only two are common. In type 1, seen in fetuses and in many young children, the caecum is funnel-shaped and the appendix arises from its apical end, as one might expect from its embryological derivation (see p. 410). In type 3, the common type in adults, the lateral aspect of the caecum has undergone sacculation, because it grows more rapidly than the medial, forcing the appendicular opening away from the apex and towards the ileocaecal valve. The actual orifice may be round, oval, irregular or slit-like, and in over 80% of patients in one large series [3] there were one or more valvular folds of mucosa, which did not contain any muscle, arising from the superior caecal wall and overhanging the orifice. The appendiceal lumen normally varies from 1 to 2 mm and the tip is often obliterated. The lumen tends to be triangular or stellate in shape in childhood, adolescence and early adulthood, but with diminution in the amount of lymphoid tissue with age it assumes a circular or ovoid appearance. A short mesoappendix, which is a prolongation of the mesentery of the terminal ileum, attaches the base of the appendix to the superior abdominal wall; the tip is free.

The relation of the appendix to other organs in the abdominal cavity is variable [4,5]. It normally lies behind the caecum and ascending colon, but may lie on the psoas muscle near to or overhanging the pelvic brim, behind or in front of the terminal ileum, or beside the ascending colon. It receives its blood supply from a branch of the posterior caecal artery that runs in the mesentery and its venous drainage is to the portal system. Lymphatics drain first into nodes in the mesoappendix and from there to right paracolic nodes and those in the ileocaecal angle.

Physiology

In herbivorous animals the appendix is commonly a large structure which is concerned in the digestion of cellulose and perhaps plays some part in the maintenance of a normal bacterial flora in the small intestine. In humans it is not known to serve any definite purpose. It may be merely vestigial, but the presence of large amounts of lymphoid tissue in its wall suggests an immunological role that may be related to the recognition of foreign protein and bacteria in the bowel and the formation of IgA immunoglobulins. It secretes 1–2 mm^3 of mucoid fluid daily, and the studies on exteriorized appendices indicate that, if this is not free to escape, considerable intraluminal pressures may be built up [6] which may seriously compress mucosal vessels. The appendix can be shown radiologically to fill and empty at regular intervals, and irregular peristaltic movements running from tip to luminal orifice appear in it.

Histology

The appendiceal mucosal lining is large intestinal in pattern, but less thick than that lining the colon or rectum. Nonbranching crypts lined predominantly by mucus-secreting columnar cells extend from the surface down to the muscularis mucosae, which is poorly developed and can be absent in places. Absorptive cells cover the luminal surface and the upper part of the crypts. Epithelial endocrine cells, most of which are argentaffin and almost all of the remainder argyrophil, are present at the base of the crypts, and in about 50% of all appendices similar cells lie free, deep in the lamina propria [7] (*see* below). Paneth cells are sometimes present in small numbers; they are more common in chronic inflammation and in ulcerative colitis and it is uncertain whether they are normally present in an appendix that is not diseased. The mucosa contains numerous lymphoid follicles that are conspicuous in children and disappear gradually in old age. In structure they resemble the lymphoid tissue of the small intestine. The surface epithelial cells that overlie them are modified to form M cells [8] which transmit potentially antigenic protein. Between the M cells and the small lymphocytes which form the mantle of the follicle is a mixed cell zone which contains follicle-centre-like B cells, numerous T helper cells and HLA-DR containing macrophages, suggesting that antigen from the gut is transferred across the mucosa by M cells to a milieu capable of mounting an immune response [9]. Numerous intraepithelial lymphocytes of B-cell type are present throughout the surface mucosa, especially in the suprafollicular epithelium.

The lamina propria resembles that of the large bowel; in places where the muscularis mucosae is deficient it cannot readily be distinguished from the underlying submucosa. Its contained nerve plexus is discussed below. A circular and a longitudinal muscle coat, which is not split into taeniae, are present and there is a well defined serosa. Cells with periodic acid–Schiff (PAS)-positive granules are found singly or in small clusters in the circular muscle coat close to, or extending into, the submucosa in up to 5% of appendices [10,11]. Ultrastructural studies suggest they represent a degenerative change in smooth muscle cells.

The appendix and the adjacent region of the caecum from which it arises have an intrinsic autonomic nervous system different from the remainder of the large bowel. The submucosal plexus consists only of a few scattered ganglion cells, and the cells of the myenteric plexus are also scattered diffusely instead of having a plexiform arrangement [12]. Much debate has arisen about the derivation and function of the endocrine cells in the appendiceal lamina propria. There is general agreement that these cells are present in a number, though apparently not all, of histologically normal appendices and, in others, in the connective tissue where the lumen has been obliterated. The granules present in the majority show the histochemical and ultrastructural characteristics of serotonin (5-hydroxytryptamine), and can be demonstrated by immunohistochemical techniques for neurone-specific enolase (NSE) and chromogranin [7,13–16], and some contain somatostatin and perhaps substance P [17]. They appear always to be associated with Schwann cells (immunoreactive with S-100) and with a meshwork of fine non-myelinated nerve fibrils that often show varicose axonal swellings. The whole has been called an *enterochromaffin cell–nerve fibre complex* [13]. Mast cells are a frequent accompaniment [18]. These appearances were first described many years ago [19] in appendices with obliterated lumina and were then considered to be the end-result of a mild inflammation with partial mucosal damage, followed by connective tissue and neurogenous reparative proliferation and scarring; the endocrine cells were considered to be of epithelial origin and the condition was named *appendicite neurogène*, or neurogenous appendicitis. This view is still held by many pathologists [7]. The fact that endocrine cells, always associated with non-myelinated fibres and Schwann cells, are present in the lamina propria of many histologically normal appendices [15], however, suggests that a peptidergic neuroendocrine complex of neuroectodermal rather than epithelial origin is normally present and may proliferate under certain as yet undetermined circumstances. This suggestion seems inherently more probable, but is not yet proven; nor do we know whether any of the 'carcinoid' tumours arise from extraepithelial endocrine cells. The possibility that appendiceal pain in the absence of histological evidence of active inflammation could result from neural proliferations in the appendix has been reviewed recently [20].

References

1 Dhillon AP, Williams RA, Rode J. Age, site and distribution of subepithelial neurosecretory cells in the appendix. *Pathology*, 1992; 24: 56.

2 Treves F. Lectures on the anatomy of the intestinal canal and peritoneum in man. *Br Med J*, 1885; i: 415, 470, 527 & 580.

3 Wangensteen OH, Buirge RE, Dennis C, Ritchie WP. Studies in the aetiology of acute appendicitis. The significance of the structure and function of the vermiform appendix in the genesis of appendicitis. A preliminary report. *Ann Surg*, 1937; 106: 910.

4 Wakeley CPG, Gladstone RJ. The relative frequency of the various positions of the vermiform appendix, as ascertained by an analysis of 5000 cases. *Lancet*, 1928; i: 178.

5 Wakeley C, Childs P. Appendicitis. *Br Med J*, 1960; ii: 1347.

6 Wangensteen OH, Dennis C. Experimental proof of the obstructive origin of appendicitis in man. *Ann Surg*, 1939; 110: 629.

7 Millikin PD. Extra-epithelial enterochromaffin cells and Schwann cells in the human appendix. *Arch Pathol Lab Med*, 1983; 107: 189.

8 Bockman DE, Cooper MD. Early lymphoepithelial relationships in human appendix. A combined light and electron microscope study. *Gastroenterology*, 1975; 68: 1160.

9 Spencer J, Finn T, Isaacson PG. Gut-associated lymphoid tissue: a morphological and immunocytochemical study of the human appendix. *Gut*, 1985; 26: 672.

10 Husman R. Granular cells in musculature of the appendix. *Arch Pathol*, 1963; 75: 360.

11 Sobel HJ, Marquet E, Schwarz R. Granular degeneration of appendiceal smooth muscle. *Arch Pathol*, 1971; 92: 427.

12 Emery JL, Underwood J. The neurological junction between the appendix and ascending colon. *Gut*, 1970; 11: 118.

13 Aubock L, Ratzenhofer M. 'Extra-epithelial enterochromaffin cell–nerve fibre complexes' in the normal human appendix and in neurogenous appendicopathy. *J Pathol*, 1982; 136: 217.

14 Rode J, Dhillon AP, Papadaki L, Griffiths D. Neurosecretory cells of the lamina propria of the appendix and their possible relationship to carcinoid. *Histopathology*, 1982; 6: 69.

15 Papadaki L, Rode J, Dhillon AP, Dische FE. Fine structure of a neuro-endocrine complex in the mucosa of the appendix. *Gastroenterology*, 1983; 84: 490.

16 Rode J, Dhillon AP, Papadaki L. Serotonin-immunoreactive cells in the lamina propria plexus of the appendix. *Hum Pathol*, 1983; 14: 464.

17 Hofler H, Kasper M, Heitz PU. The neuroendocrine system of the normal human appendix, ileum and colon and in neurogenic appendicopathy. *Virchows Arch Pathol Anat*, 1983; 399: 127.

18 Stead RH, Dixon MF, Bramwell NH, Riddell RH, Bienenstock J. Mast cells are closely apposed to nerves in the human gastrointestinal mucosa. *Gastroenterology*, 1989; 97: 575.

19 Masson P. Appendicite neurogène et carcinoides. *Ann Anat Pathol*, 1924; 1: 3.

20 Williams RA. Neuroma of the appendix. In: Williams RA, Myers P, eds. *Pathology of the Appendix*. London: Chapman & Hall Medical, 1994: 126.

29 Normal embryology and fetal development; developmental abnormalities of the appendix

Normal development

The appendix is a derivative of the caecum; the two organs have a common pattern of autonomic innervation in which ganglion cells are scattered rather than grouped into plexuses [1] and there is something to be said for considering them as a single organ. The caecum appears as an outgrowth from the wall of the primitive midgut at the end of the 5th week, before the latter differentiates into small and large intestines [2]. The distal three-quarters of this outgrowth elongate rapidly to form a conical caecum, the tip of which extends further to form a narrow, tubular primitive appendix. This arrangement persists throughout fetal life and is often present at birth. At term and subsequently, the lateral wall of the caecum grows faster than the medial, so that the appendix is 'pushed' round to approach the ileocaecal valve, in relation to which it can adopt a number of positions. At the same time it narrows and becomes a more definitely separate, thin tube-like structure.

There is little available information about the development of the mucosa [3,4]; a little lymphoid tissue is present in the lamina propria in the fetus at the 108-mm crown–rump stage [5], but there are no germinal centres present at birth [6]. These develop rapidly between the 3rd and 6th weeks of postnatal life, presumably following the introduction of foreign proteins into the gut in ingested food and milk.

Maldevelopments

Duplications, diverticula and cysts

Caecal duplication is extremely rare, but in view of the derivation of the appendix from its conical tip it is not surprising that appendiceal duplication is commonly associated with it [7–9]. Three patterns of appendiceal duplication can occur in the presence of a normal caecum [10]. In the first, or 'double-barrelled' appendix, two separate tubes, each lined by mucosa and separated by submucosa, are enclosed in a single common muscle coat. In the second, described only in infants with multiple abnormalities, there are two symmetrically placed appendices, one on either side of the ileocaecal valve. In the third, a normal appendix is present in the usual position while a rudimentary second appendix arises separately from the caecum, usually in relation to one of the taeniae. Triplication of the appendix [11] and a horseshoe anomaly with two separate openings of the appendix into the lumen [12] have also been described.

The great majority of diverticula are acquired (*see* Chapter 32). In one series of 71 000 appendices studied there were said to be 14 congenital diverticula [13,14], and occasional individual reports are recorded [15], some of which have been linked to trisomy 13 [16]. The criteria for separating them from the acquired type are the absence of inflammation and the presence of all the coats of the appendix in the wall of the diverticulum. We know of no reliable reports of congenital cysts in the appendix.

Absence of the appendix

Agenesis and congenital absence of the appendix, though rare, are well documented [17–19]; some at least appeared to represent a thalidomide-induced anomaly [20]. Agenesis must be separated from hypoplasia in which, though the caecum is fully developed, only rudimentary appendiceal tissue is present. It can be associated with a normal caecum or with caecal dysgenesis, and other congenital anomalies may be present [21]. Agenesis has also to be distinguished from autoamputation secondary to inflammation, intussusception or volvulus. We know of no proven examples of atresia or stenoses, but diaphragms, which may represent a form of atresia, are described [22].

Malpositions

Occasional examples of acute appendicitis have been described in which the appendix is subhepatic. These are associated with maldescent of the caecum and subsequent malfixation, which of necessity leads to maldescent of the appendix [23,24].

Appendix helicus

There is a description of a single example of a helically twisted appendix in a 13-month-old male with an associated meningomyelocoele [25].

Heterotopias in the appendix

Heterotopic epithelium is rare in the appendix but gastric, oesophageal and pancreatic tissue have been reported [14,26,27].

Hamartomas

Peutz–Jeghers and juvenile-type polyps are both well recognized in the appendix [28,29]. They are sometimes wrongly referred to as adenomatous polyps, and here, as elsewhere, must be clearly distinguished from neoplasms. Their structure is similar to Peutz–Jeghers and juvenile polyps elsewhere in the gut. We have not seen haemangiomas or lymphangiomas, although they are said to occur [14]. The so-called lymphoid polyps are reactive and not hamartomatous.

References

1 Emery JL, Underwood J. The neurological junction between the appendix and ascending colon. *Gut*, 1970; 11: 118.
2 Wakeley C, Childs P. Appendicitis. *Br Med J*, 1960; ii: 1347.
3 Johnson FK. The development of the mucous membrane of the large intestine and vermiform process in the human embryo. *Am J Anat*, 1913; 14: 187.
4 Jit I. Histogenesis of the human vermiform appendix. *Indian J Med Res*, 1954; 42: 17.
5 Jit I. The development of lymph nodes in the human vermiform appendix. *Indian J Surg*, 1953; 15: 217.
6 Erdohazi M, Read CR. A histological study of the appendix vermiformis. *Dev Med Child Neurol*, 1967; 9: 98.
7 Aitken AB. Case of doubling of the great intestine. *Glas Med J*, 1912; 78: 431.
8 Cave AJE. Appendix vermiformis duplex. *J Anat*, 1936; 70: 283.
9 Wallbridge PH. Double appendix. *Br J Surg*, 1963; 50: 346.
10 Waugh TR. Appendix vermiformis duplex. *Arch Surg*, 1941; 42: 311.
11 Tinckler LF. Triple appendix vermiformis—a unique case. *Br J Surg*, 1968; 55: 79.
12 Mesko TW, Lugo R, Breitholtz T. Horseshoe anomaly of the appendix: a previously undescribed entity. *Surgery*, 1989; 106: 563.
13 Collins DC. Diverticula of the vermiform appendix. A study based on 30 cases. *Ann Surg*, 1936; 104: 1001.
14 Collins DC. 71,000 human appendix specimens: a final report, summarizing forty years' study. *Am J Proctocol*, 1963; 14: 365.
15 Hedinger E. Kongenitale Divertikehbildung im Processus vermiformis. *Virch Arch Pathol Anat Physiol*, 1904; 178: 25.
16 Favara BE. Multiple congenital diverticula of the vermiform appendix. *Am J Clin Pathol*, 1968; 49: 60.
17 Collins DC. Agenesis of vermiform appendix. *Am J Surg*, 1951; 82: 689.
18 Halim M, Clough DM. Congenital absence of the vermiform appendix with a twisted ovarian teratoma. *Guthrie Clin Bull*, 1960; 30: 15.
19 Yokose Y, Maruyama H, Tsutsumi M *et al*. Ileal atresia and absence of appendix. *Acta Pathol Jpn*, 1986; 36: 1403.
20 Bremner DM, Mooney G. Agenesis of appendix; a further thalidomide anomaly (letter). *Lancet*, 1978; i: 826.
21 Elias RG, Hults R. Congenital absence of vermiform appendix. *Arch Surg*, 1967; 95: 257.
22 Chou ST, Hall J. An appendicular diaphragm: a unique case. *Pathology*, 1978; 10: 83.
23 King A. Subhepatic appendicitis. *Arch Surg*, 1955; 71: 265.
24 Scott KJ, Sacks AJ, Goldschmidt RP. Subhepatic appendicitis. *Am J Gastroenterol*, 1993; 88: 1773.
25 Mikat DM, Mikat KW. Appendix helicus; a unique anomaly of the vermiform appendix. *Gastroenterology*, 1967; 71: 303.
26 Droga BW, Levine S, Baber JJ. Heterotopic gastric and esophageal tissue in the vermiform appendix. *Am J Clin Pathol*, 1963; 40: 190.
27 Aubrey DA. Gastric mucosa in the vermiform appendix. *Arch Surg*, 1970; 101: 628.
28 Kitchin AP. Polyposis of small intestine with pigmentation of oral mucosa. Report of 2 cases. *Br Med J*, 1953; i: 658.
29 Shnitka TK, Sherbaniuk RW. Adenomatous polyps of the appendix in children. *Gastroenterology*, 1957; 32: 462.

30 Inflammatory disorders of the appendix

Acute non-specific appendicitis

Acute appendicitis is the most common abdominal emergency in childhood, adolescence and young adult life; it is interesting and humiliating that a small organ, which in humans performs no known useful function, can so frequently give rise to problems which, if not promptly and correctly treated, may even have fatal complications, and of which we still do not fully know the cause.

Incidence

Acute appendicitis is common in Western Europe, North America and Australia, but is rare in tropical Africa [1] and India. Its precise incidence is not known; approximately 46000 appendicectomies were carried out in England in 1985 for presumptive appendicitis but no statistics are available as to how many of the patients had the disease [2]. Based on the numbers of operations carried out, however, there appears to be a recent fall in the incidence of the disease. Thus, in one district general hospital with a stable population, the number of cases of acute appendicitis (based on pathological records) fell from 100 to 52 per 100000 between the years 1975–91 [3]. Acute appendicitis is rare before the age of 5 years and has its peak incidence in the second and third decades [4]; it is slightly more common in males and this sex difference is accentuated in early childhood. Deaths from appendicitis are very rare, and usually occur in the elderly, in whom the symptoms are less striking in relation to the severity of the disease, and in whom 'silent' perforation of the appendix with peritonitis is more common. Thus in England and Wales in 1983, 83 out of the 136 deaths from acute appendicitis occurred in patients over the age of 70 years [5]. The mortality from acute appendicitis has fallen by about 20 times over the last 50 years, largely because of earlier diagnosis and surgical intervention and the use of antibiotics.

Aetiology and pathogenesis

Acute appendicitis is not thought to be regularly associated with any specific bacterial, viral or protozoal invader, though a number of claims for particular organisms have been made. Outbreaks of dysentery are not normally associated with an increased incidence of appendicitis, though there is good evidence that a few cases may be so precipitated [6,7]. Immunological studies have shown a raised antibody titre to mumps V antigen [8] and the presence of serum agglutinins to *Yersinia enterocolitica* (formerly *Pasteurella pseudotuberculosis X*) [9]. Bacteriological studies usually show a wide variety of organisms drawn from those normally present in the caecum, which suggests that these are secondary invaders into tissues already damaged.

The most likely precipitating factor is obstruction of the appendiceal lumen. There are a number of possible causes for this [10]. The mucosa can undergo inflammatory changes with oedema; lymphoid tissues in the lamina propria and submucosa may hypertrophy; foreign material, particularly food residues, can lodge in the lumen and become surrounded by faecal material to form a slowly growing laminated faecolith, which can subsequently calcify to form a stone; kinks and adhesions may angulate the organ upon itself; a low-residue diet may predispose to exaggerated muscle activity and muscle spasm in the wall of the appendix or at its base; tumours in the caecum or appendix may block the lumen of the appendix. Appendicitis has also followed barium enema examinations [11] and colonoscopy [12]. All these factors have in common the single feature that they obstruct the lumen, and so interfere with normal peristaltic drainage. The role of some of them is fairly readily assessable; for example, faecoliths are commonly present in appendices removed for proven acute appendicitis, although estimates of their frequency have varied considerably [13,14]. It is also of interest that the presence of faecoliths is geographically distributed and appears to correlate with the incidence of appendicitis in a population [15].

However, in one study their prevalence was greater in an autopsy population when compared with a younger surgically resected group, implying that they were not a major cause of appendicitis [16]. It is well known that the age of greatest liability to acute appendicitis coincides with the age of maximal development of appendiceal lymphoid tissue, which tends to bulge into and narrow the lumen [17]. One hypothesis to explain the time trends of acute appendicitis in Britain proposes that the rise in incidence of the disease in the late 19th century was primarily a consequence of improved living standards and sanitation, resulting in reduced exposure of infants and young children to enteric organisms. This altered the pattern of immunity so that later systemic infection with viruses or bacteria triggered appendicitis [18,19]. It is more difficult to assess the degree of mucosal oedema present in a resected specimen, and oedema at the caecoappendiceal junction cannot be assessed at all, since this part of the appendix is invaginated into the caecum at operation and is not available for examination.

Bacterial infection is probably important as a concomitant factor. There is good experimental evidence that in dogs, rabbits, apes and humans bacterial infection will not by itself cause acute appendicitis. Artificially produced obstruction also rarely does so when the appendix has previously been washed free of faecal material. Combined obstruction and bacterial infection, however, nearly always result in lesions [20,21]. The likely course of events is obstruction, damming up of normal mucus secretions, distension of the lumen with ischaemic damage of the mucosa, access into the tissues of bacteria normally confined to the lumen, and secondary bacterial infection leading first to non-suppurative, then to suppurative appendicitis. The common causes of the initial obstruction are likely to be enlargement of lymphoid tissue, mucosal oedema and faecolith formation. Oxyuris infestation is probably not a causative factor [22] and there is little positive evidence to support a primary blood-borne infection [23].

Once an infection has become established, microangiographic studies suggest that the occlusion of arterioles either by intravascular thrombus or by pressure from inflammatory oedema or a faecolith may increase the liability to rapid perforation and gangrene [24].

Macroscopic appearances

The earliest visible external macroscopic change is dilatation and congestion of the small vessels on the serosal surface, which gives rise to a localized or generalized hyperaemia. The distal part may be swollen and if the appendix is opened longitudinally, particularly after fixation, the distal lumen is often dilated and contains purulent material. A patchy purulent exudate commonly forms on the serosal surface, dulling it. Later the tip, and sometimes the whole organ, becomes soft, purplish and haemorrhagic as necrosis supervenes. The lumen becomes more markedly distended with pus, often blood stained, and suppurative foci are often visible in the wall; there is visible thrombosis in the veins of the mesoappendix [25]. It is difficult to give an accurate time scale for these events. It is well known that gangrenous changes can be present within a few hours of the onset of symptoms, but these may be related to concomitant ischaemia.

Microscopic appearances

Acute appendicitis is characterized by oedema and congestion of the wall, a transmural infiltration of polymorphs, often forming small intramural abscesses, ulceration of the mucosa and a local fibrinopurulent peritonitis. Vascular thrombosis is often present and, in the most florid examples, the combination of suppurative inflammation and ischaemia leads to gangrenous appendicitis with necrosis of the wall and perforation [26]. Occasional cases of xanthogranulomatous inflammation of the appendix have also been reported [27].

While the histological diagnosis of established appendicitis is easy, difficulties may arise when an appendix removed from a patient with the clinical features of acute appendicitis shows only mild inflammation confined to the mucosa. Although it is tempting to regard this as early appendicitis, a number of studies have shown that up to 35% of appendices removed electively show small collections of neutrophil polymorphs in the lumen, focal ulceration of the surface epithelium with pus cells in the adjacent lamina propria, and even a few crypt abscesses [28]. On the other hand, studies of experimental appendicitis have shown that identical mucosal lesions can progress rapidly to established acute appendicitis with gangrene and perforation [21]. It is obviously not possible to dismiss acute inflammation, even if confined to the mucosa, in patients with clinical features of appendicitis, but in such cases it is prudent to exclude other causes for acute abdominal pain. To confound the issue further a recent study has shown that a significant proportion of histologically normal appendices from patients with a clinical diagnosis of acute appendicitis have expressed abnormal amounts of cytokines (tumour necrosis factor alpha (TNF-α) and interleukin-2), sensitive markers of inflammation, when examined using *in situ* hybridization [29].

On occasion, examination of appendicectomy specimens shows the features of an infective colitis with diffuse active inflammation confined to the mucosa (*see* Chapter 36). Causative agents which have resulted in this presentation of acute appendicitis include salmonella, shigella and campylobacter organisms [7,30,31].

Complications and sequelae

Perforation, peritonitis and abscess formation

It is probable that resolution occurs in some cases of early acute appendicitis, but once any significant amount of pus has formed there are likely to be complications if the appendix is not removed quickly. Perforation is the most common and serious. It occurs most frequently in children under the age of 5 years in whom appendicitis itself is uncommon [32]. When associated with fulminating inflammation and gangrene it commonly leads to peritonitis; if the patient survives, pus tends to localize in the pelvis or beneath the diaphragm. When the inflammation is less acute or when the appendix is retrocaecal or retrocolic, or subhepatic in maldescent of the caecum [33], localized adhesions form and wall off the perforation, leading to a localized appendix abscess. Once formed, such an abscess may persist after appendicectomy; it can localize in the pelvis and secondarily involve the bladder [34] or the caecum, where it gives rise to so-called appendicular granuloma (see p. 416). Pelvic abscesses can 'point' and perforate into the rectum or vagina with subsequent resolution, but periappendicular abscesses and subdiaphragmatic collections of pus tend to remain localized and become walled off by fibrous tissue. Fistula formation can occur between the appendix and gastrointestinal tract or bladder [35]. Appendicitis with perforation in women is associated with an increased risk of tubal infertility [36] or ectopic pregnancy due to peritubal adhesions [37]. Appendicitis and its complications may also occur in appendices sited in hernial sacs [38,39].

Suppurative pylephlebitis

Infected thrombi in the small vessels of the serosa and mesoappendix are common in acute appendicitis. Rarely the thrombus extends into larger vessels, and pieces of infected clot occasionally break off and are carried to the liver, where they set up metastatic abscesses [40]. This complication is rare since the advent of efficient antibiotics.

Ileocolic intussusception

Rare examples of ileocolic intussusception have been reported following inversion of the appendiceal stump into the caecum at appendicectomy [41].

The development of 'chronic appendicitis'

There has been considerable doubt and controversy whether acute appendicitis can progress to a chronic form and whether some of the vague abdominal symptoms which go to make the diagnosis of a 'grumbling appendix' have any pathological basis. There is no doubt that many appendices seen at necropsy [16] or removed electively are small, shrunken and without lumina, and that histologically the mucosa and lymphoid tissue are atrophic and the submucosa often virtually replaced by fibrous tissue and fat. The difficulty is to decide whether these changes are the result of physiological atrophy or previous acute inflammation. Studies comparing the appendices from patients with symptoms suggesting appendicitis with electively removed appendices from patients without symptoms, have shown little difference in pathology [42]. We believe that there must be evidence of active chronic inflammation with infiltration of the muscle coats and serosa by lymphocytes and plasma cells before one can diagnose chronic appendicitis, though there is one report which suggests that the presence of stainable iron is a reliable indication of inflammation within the previous 6 months [43].

The presence of other sequelae of previous acute appendicitis, such as old adhesions, is evidence of previous inflammation, whether the appendix is histologically normal or not [44]. These adhesions can predispose to volvulus and obstruction but such a condition should not be called chronic appendicitis.

Obstructive appendicopathy

It is common for pathologists to report an appendicectomy specimen as histologically normal when there have undoubtedly been symptoms and signs of 'appendicitis' or 'appendicular colic'. In such cases a careful search should be made for evidence of obstruction or narrowing of the lumen by fibrosis, a faecolith or a foreign body. In some specimens the lumen is slightly dilated and packed with soft faeces and it may be that this is the cause of the obstructive symptoms, among other possibilities.

Simple mucocoele

Mucocoele is defined as distension of part or all of the appendix by accumulation of mucus within the lumen. It is not a specific diagnosis but merely a description of a gross appearance that is common to simple mucocoele, mucinous cystadenoma and mucinous cystadenocarcinoma of the appendix.

About 0.2% of all appendices examined at operation or necropsy have a dilated distal lumen which is distended with mucus [45,46]. This dilatation or simple mucocoele, which is most common in the middle-aged and has an equal sex incidence, is thought by many to follow attacks of acute appendicitis with obstruction of the lumen. Postinflammatory fibrosis and faecolith are mentioned in the literature as the commonest causes, and in our experience both can be seen in association with excess mucus in the lumen. Most mucocoeles are small and symptomless but occasionally they are larger (Fig. 30.1), containing thick, gelatinous mucin which occasionally forms numerous, small discrete globules, like fish eggs, so-called myxoglobulosis [47].

The microscopic appearances of simple mucocoele have to be distinguished from mucinous cystadenoma and this is not always straightforward. In our opinion it is best to restrict the diagnosis of simple mucocoele to those cases in which there is no evidence of any epithelial abnormality in the mucosal

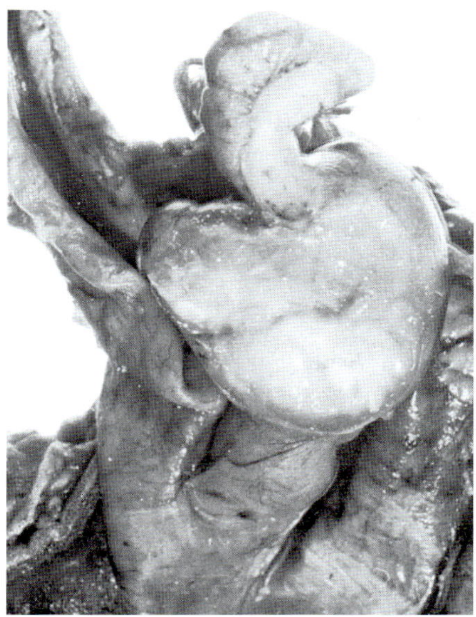

Fig. 30.1 Mucocoele of the tip of the appendix.

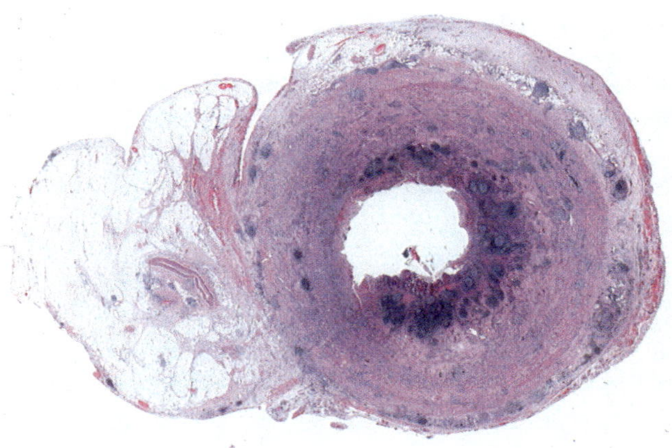

Fig. 30.2 Crohn's disease. There is complete mucosal ulceration and transmural inflammation with many prominent lymphoid aggregates in the submucosa.

lining of the appendix other than flattening. If there is any evidence of epithelial dysplasia, papillary infoldings or a multiloculated appearance, then the diagnosis of mucinous cystadenoma at an early stage of development should be made.

Mucocoeles can become secondarily infected, producing an empyema. Uncommonly, they rupture, discharging mucin and possibly epithelial cells, to form either a local collection of mucus around the appendix or more widespread deposits of gelatinous mucin throughout the peritoneal cavity, a condition sometimes known as pseudomyxoma peritonei. It should be emphasized here that removal of the appendix leads to regression of pseudomyxoma peritonei if the underlying condition is benign.

Prognosis

The mortality for uncomplicated acute appendicitis at all ages is extremely low, being 0.24% in two recent analyses [48,49]. Once complications ensue it rises rapidly, especially in those under 5 years and in the elderly [50]. Rupture alone can be associated with a 6% mortality and generalized peritonitis can have a mortality as high as 12% [51]. There is no doubt that early operation to minimize these risks is the most important single factor in prognosis.

Other forms of appendicitis

Tuberculous appendicitis

Tuberculosis of the appendix is described in association with local tuberculous disease in the ileocaecal region and as secondary to pulmonary tuberculosis [52,53]; examples of apparent primary lesions have also been described. Macroscopically the appendix can form part of a mass of granulomatous tissue which also involves the caecum and mesoappendix [54], or can be indistinguishable from acute purulent appendicitis. Histology reveals characteristic tuberculoid follicles that may also be present in mesenteric lymph nodes.

The appendix in Crohn's disease

Involvement of the appendix is found in about one-quarter of all cases of Crohn's disease of the terminal ileum, but is also found synchronously with disease at a considerable distance from the ileocaecal region, for example in the rectum or upper small intestine. The histology of Crohn's disease of the appendix (Fig. 30.2) in no way differs from the appearances in other parts of the intestinal tract, with acute inflammatory changes of the mucosa, including cryptitis, erosion, and ulceration which may be fissuring, and transmural inflammation with scattered aggregates of lymphoid tissue. Granulomas are seen in a minority of cases. Secondary adhesion formation is common.

Identical histological features, often associated with prominent numbers of granulomas, are occasionally seen in appendicectomy specimens from patients without a history of Crohn's disease. Most have presented with the typical symptoms of acute appendicitis and the postoperative course has usually been uneventful. Although Crohn's disease may appear at a later date elsewhere in the gastrointestinal tract in a minority [55–57], follow-up studies have shown that this sequence is distinctly unusual [58,59]. The term idiopathic granulomatous appendicitis has been used in this context when other causes of granulomatous inflammation and coexistent Crohn's disease have been excluded.

Acute suppurative (non-granulomatous) appendicitis can occur in patients with Crohn's disease but appears to be rare [60].

Sarcoid lesions in the appendix

There are occasional case reports of sarcoid granulomas in the appendix in patients with other stigmata of sarcoidosis [61,62].

The appendix in ulcerative colitis

Involvement of the appendix has been variably reported in 28–86% of patients with pancolitis, although this is seldom obvious macroscopically [63–65]. The microscopic features are no different from those seen in the colon and, since they are confined to the mucosa, do not result in any of the complications associated with ordinary appendicitis. There has been a more recent appreciation that appendiceal inflammation may be present as a discontinuous 'skip' lesion in colitics in the absence of either active or quiescent changes of ulcerative colitis in the caecum [64–68]. It may even be present in patients with colitis restricted to the distal colon and rectum and be apparent at endoscopic examination as small erosions or ulcers identified at the mouth of the appendix [69]. Another recent observation, derived from case-control studies, suggests that previous appendicectomy is rare in patients with ulcerative colitis [70–72], raising the possibility that the appendix may play an initiating role in the subsequent development of colorectal inflammation in this disease.

Actinomycosis

True acute actinomycotic inflammation of the appendix must be distinguished from ileocaecal actinomycosis and from the presence of actinomyces in the appendiceal lumen. *Actinomyces israelii*, which is the only species pathogenic to humans, is present in the mouth of 5% of normal people. It can survive passage through the acid gastric juice and reach the appendiceal lumen, where it may lodge without causing disease. It is sometimes seen in stained sections of normal appendices, and even when present in acute appendicitis it cannot be identified as the causative organism unless it is actually present in the inflamed tissues. True acute actinomycotic appendicitis is extremely rare, but it is important to diagnose it, since failure to treat it adequately may result in protracted illness with extensive local spread and the risk of metastatic abscesses.

Chronic suppurative appendicitis can follow the acute condition and, though rare, is the form most often seen. Chronic abscesses, in which colonies of organisms can readily be identified, develop in the coats of the appendix and become surrounded by dense fibrous tissue in which the organisms and consequent inflammation spread to produce sinus tracks and fistulae between the appendix, adjacent bowel and other organs and skin surfaces. The possibility of actinomycosis should be considered in all patients who develop faecal fistulae after appendicectomy. The infection may spread into veins and give rise to metastatic abscesses in the liver.

Yersiniasis

The appendix is not infrequently involved in ileal and mesenteric lymph nodal yersiniasis. Lesions are similar to those described in the ileum (see p. 277) and are usually located in the submucosa.

Schistosomiasis

In endemic areas schistosomes have been found in 1–2% of appendicectomy specimens [73,74], although not necessarily from symptomatic individuals. Results of a study from Saudi Arabia [74] suggested that the clinical picture of acute appendicitis could result from schistosomal infection via one of two possible pathogenetic pathways. Granulomatous appendicitis occurs in younger patients during the early phase of egg-laying in the appendix and is associated with acute granulomatous inflammation around viable ova, with tissue necrosis and a tissue eosinophilia, although neutrophil exudation is not a feature. So-called obstructive appendicitis, which tended to occur in an older age group, was a secondary suppurative bacterial inflammation consequent upon fibrosis of a portion of the wall of the appendix as a result of long-standing inflammation to schistosomal ova, which appear calcified in tissue sections.

Spirochaetosis

Spirochaetosis of the appendix has not been associated with histological evidence of acute appendicitis, although its prevalence is greater in non-inflamed appendices from individuals clinically suspected of appendicitis compared with incidentally removed organs [75].

'Appendicular granuloma' (ligneous caecitis, pseudoneoplastic appendicitis)

In this unusual form of inflammatory disease, which presents clinically as carcinoma of the caecum, usually in patients over the age of 70 years [76–78], the appendix is either incorporated into, or replaced by, a large mass of granulation or fibrous tissue which also grows around the adjacent caecum or ileum, binding the appendix to them so that separation by dissection is impossible. There is no specific causative factor and it is probable that the condition results from incomplete resolution of an abscess in a retrocaecal appendix.

Miscellaneous forms of appendicitis

Polyarteritis nodosa can occasionally present as acute appendicitis without specific histological lesions in the appendix [79]. However, a similar focal necrotizing arteritis of the appendix also occurs as an incidental finding, usually in young women, unrelated to appendicitis or any systemic disease [80]. Isolated cases of appendicitis secondary to metastatic carcinoma [81,82], and to lymphoma [83,84] have been reported. Kaposi's sarcoma presenting as acute appendicitis in HIV-1-positive patients has also been described [85,86]. Other causes of appendicitis include amoebic dysentery [87,88], balantidial infection [89], strongyloidiasis [90] and pinworm infestation [91,92], although the appendix is histologically normal in most patients with pinworms in the lumen. The appendix may be involved in cases of pseudomembranous colitis [93].

References

1 Walker AR, Segal I. Appendicitis: an African perspective. *J R Soc Med*, 1995; 88: 616.

2 Hospital in-patient enquiry (England): trends 1979–85. *OCPS Monitor*, May 1987.

3 McCahy P. Continuing fall in the incidence of acute appendicitis. *Ann R Coll Surg Engl*, 1994; 76: 282.

4 Lee JAH. The influence of sex and age on appendicitis in children and young adults. *Gut*, 1962; 3: 80.

5 Mortality statistics—cause: review of the Registrar General on deaths by cause, sex and age in England and Wales, 1983. London: Series DH2, no. 11, 1984.

6 White MEE, Lord MD, Rogers KB. Bowel infection and acute appendicitis. *Arch Dis Child*, 1961; 36: 394.

7 Thompson RG, Harper IA. Acute appendicitis and salmonella infections. *Br Med J*, 1973; ii: 300.

8 Jackson RH, Gardner PS, Kennedy J, McQuillin J. Viruses in the aetiology of acute appendicitis. *Lancet*, 1966; ii: 711.

9 Winblad S, Nilehn B, Sternby NH. *Yersinia enterocolitica (Pasteurella X)* in human enteric infections. *Br Med J*, 1966; ii: 1363.

10 Burkitt DP. The aetiology of appendicitis. *Br J Surg*, 1971; 58: 695.

11 Sisley JF, Wagner CW. Barium appendicitis. *South Med J*, 1982; 75: 498.

12 Hirata K, Noguchi J, Yoshikawa I *et al*. Acute appendicitis immediately after colonoscopy. *Am J Gastroenterol*, 1996; 91: 2239.

13 Bowers WF. Appendicitis: with special reference to pathogenesis, bacteriology and healing. *Arch Surg*, 1939; 39: 362.

14 Horton LWL. Pathogenesis of acute appendicitis. *Br Med J*, 1977; iii: 1672.

15 Jones BA, Demetriades D, Segal I, Burkitt DP. The prevalence of appendiceal faecoliths in patients with and without appendicitis. *Ann Surg*, 1985; 202: 80.

16 Andreou P, Blain S, du Boulay CEH. A histopathological study of the appendix at autopsy and after surgical resection. *Histopathology*, 1990; 17: 427.

17 Bohrod MG. The pathogenesis of acute appendicitis. *Am J Clin Pathol*, 1946; 16: 752.

18 Barker DJP. Acute appendicitis and dietary fibre: an alternative hypothesis. *Br Med J*, 1985; 290: 1125.

19 Heaton KW. Aetiology of acute appendicitis. *Br Med J*, 1987; 294: 1632.

20 Wangensteen OH, Bowers WF. Significance of the obstructive factor in the genesis of acute appendicitis. An experimental study. *Arch Surg*, 1937; 34: 496.

21 Buirge RE, Dennis C, Varco RL, Wangensteen OH. Histology of experimental appendiceal obstruction (rabbit, ape and man). *Arch Pathol*, 1940; 30: 481.

22 Symmers WStC. Pathology of oxyuriasis. *Arch Pathol*, 1950; 50: 475.

23 Wakeley C, Childs P. Appendicitis. *Br Med J*, 1950; ii: 1347.

24 Lindgren I, Aho AJ. Microangiographic investigations on acute appendicitis. *Acta Chir Scand*, 1969; 135: 77.

25 Remington JH, MacDonald JR. Vascular thrombosis in acute appendicitis. *Surgery*, 1948; 24: 787.

26 Butler C. Surgical pathology of acute appendicitis. *Hum Pathol*, 1981; 12: 870.

27 Birch PJ, Richmond I, Bennett MK. Xanthogranulomatous appendicitis. *Histopathology*, 1993; 22: 597.

28 Pieper R, Kager L, Nasman P. Clinical significance of mucosal inflammation of the vermiform appendix. *Ann Surg*, 1983; 197: 368.

29 Wang Y, Reen DJ, Puri P. Is a histologically normal appendix following emergency appendicectomy always normal? *Lancet*, 1996; 347: 1076.

30 Sanders DY, Cort CR, Stubbs AJ. Shigellosis associated with appendicitis. *J Pediatr Surg*, 1972; 7: 315.

31 van Spreeuwel JP, Lindeman J, Bax R, Elbers HJR, Sybrandy R, Meijer CJLM. *Campylobacter*-associated appendicitis: prevalence and clinicopathologic features. *Pathol Annu*, 1987; 22: 55.

32 Gilbert SR, Emmens RW, Putman TC. Appendicitis in children. *Surg Gynecol Obstet*, 1985; 161: 261.

33 Scott KJ, Sacks AJ, Goldschmidt RP. Subhepatic appendicitis. *Am J Gastroenterol*, 1993; 88: 1773.

34 Fox M. Appendix abscess with stone formation and traction diverticulum of bladder. *Br Med J*, 1962; ii: 1731.

35 Walker LG Jr, Rhame DW, Smith RB III. Enteric and cutaneous appendiceal fistulae. *Arch Surg*, 1969; 99: 585.

36 Mueller BA, Daling JR, Moore DE *et al*. Appendectomy and the risk of tubal infertility. *N Engl J Med*, 1986; 315: 1506.

37 Lehmann WE, Mecke H, Riedel HH. Sequelae of appendectomy, with special reference to intra-abdominal adhesions, chronic abdominal pain, and infertility. *Gynecol Obstet Invest*, 1990; 29: 241.

38 Thomas WEG, Vowles KDJ, Williamson RCN. Appendicitis in external herniae. *Ann R Coll Surg Engl*, 1982; 64: 121.

39 Lyass S, Kim A, Bauer J. Perforated appendicitis within an inguinal hernia: case report and review of the literature. *Am J Gastroenterol*, 1997; 92: 700.

40 Milliken NT, Stryker HB Jr. Suppurative pylethrombophlebitis and multiple liver abscesses following acute appendicitis. Report of case with recovery. *N Engl J Med*, 1951; 244: 52.

41 Harson EL, Goodkin L, Pfeffer RB. Ileocolic intussusception in an adult caused by a granuloma of the appendiceal stump. *Ann Surg*, 1967; 166: 150.

42 Thackray AC. 'Chronic appendicitis'—some pathological observations. *Br J Radiol*, 1959; 32: 180.
43 Howie JGR. The Prussian-Blue reaction in the diagnosis of previous appendicitis. *J Pathol Bacteriol*, 1966; 91: 85.
44 Muller S. Macroscopic changes in so-called 'chronic appendicitis'. *Acta Chir Scand*, 1959; 118: 146.
45 Carleton CC. Mucoceles of appendix and peritoneal pseudomyxoma. *Arch Pathol*, 1955; 60: 39.
46 Wesser DR, Edelman S. Experiences with mucoceles of the appendix. *Ann Surg*, 1961; 153: 272.
47 Gonzalez JEG, Hann SE, Trujillo YP. Myxoglobulosis of the appendix. *Am J Surg Pathol*, 1988; 12: 962.
48 Velanovich V, Satava R. Balancing the normal appendectomy rate with the perforated appendicitis rate: implications for quality assurance. *Am Surg*, 1992; 58: 264.
49 Baigrie RJ, Dehn TCB, Fowler SM, Dunn DC. Analysis of 8651 appendicectomies in England and Wales during 1992. *Br J Surg*, 1995; 82: 933.
50 Sherlock DJ. Acute appendicitis in the over-sixty age group. *Br J Surg*, 1985; 72: 245.
51 Egdahl RH. Current mortality in appendicitis. *Am J Surg*, 1964; 107: 757.
52 Carson WJ. Tuberculosis of appendix. *Am J Surg*, 1936; 34: 379.
53 Bobrow ML, Friedman S. Tuberculosis appendicitis. *Am J Surg*, 1956; 91: 389.
54 Patkin M, Robinson BL. Tuberculosis of the appendix. *Br J Clin Pract*, 1964; 18: 741.
55 Ewen SWB, Anderson J, Galloway JMD, Miller JDB, Kyle J. Crohn's disease confined to the appendix. *Gastroenterology*, 1971; 60: 853.
56 Yang SS, Gibson P, McCaughey RS, Arcari FA, Bernstein J. Primary Crohn's disease of the appendix: report of 14 cases and review of the literature. *Ann Surg*, 1979; 189: 384.
57 Allen DC, Biggart JD. Granulomatous disease in the vermiform appendix. *J Clin Pathol*, 1983; 36: 632.
58 Ariel I, Vinograd I, Hershlag A *et al*. Crohn's disease isolated to the appendix: truths and fallacies. *Hum Pathol*, 1986; 17: 1116.
59 Dudley TH Jr, Dean PJ. Idiopathic granulomatous appendicitis, or Crohn's disease of the appendix revisited. *Hum Pathol*, 1993; 24: 595.
60 Rawlinson J, Hughes RG. Acute suppurative appendicitis—a rare associate of Crohn's disease. *Dis Colon Rectum*, 1985; 28: 608.
61 Macleod IB, Jenkins AM, Gill W. Sarcoidosis involving the vermiform appendix. *J R Coll Surg Edinb*, 1965; 10: 319.
62 Tinker MA, Viswanathan B, Laufer H, Margolis IB. Acute appendicitis and pernicious anaemia as complications of gastrointestinal sarcoidosis. *Am J Gastroenterol*, 1984; 79: 868.
63 Saltzstein SL, Rosenberg BP. Ulcerative colitis of the ileum, and regional enteritis of the colon: a comparative histopathologic study. *Am J Clin Pathol*, 1963; 40: 60.
64 Davison AM, Dixon MF. The appendix as a 'skip lesion' in ulcerative colitis. *Histopathology*, 1990; 16: 93.
65 Groisman GM, George J, Harpaz N. Ulcerative appendicitis in universal and nonuniversal ulcerative colitis. *Mod Pathol*, 1994; 7: 322.
66 Cohen T, Pfeffer RB, Valensi O. 'Ulcerative appendicitis' occurring as a skip lesion in ulcerative colitis: report of a case. *Am J Gastroenterol*, 1974; 62: 151.
67 Kroff SH, Stryker SJ, Rao MS. Appendiceal involvement as a skip lesion in ulcerative colitis. *Mod Pathol*, 1994; 7: 912.
68 Scott IS, Sheaff M, Coumbe A, Feakins RM, Rampton DS. Appendiceal inflammation in ulcerative colitis. *Histopathology*, 1998; 33: 168.
69 Okawa K, Aoki T, Sano K, Harihara S, Kitano A, Kuroki T. Ulcerative colitis with skip lesions at the mouth of the appendix: a clinical study. *Am J Gastroenterol*, 1998; 93: 2405.
70 Gilat T, Hacohen D, Lilos P, Langman MJ. Childhood factors in ulcerative colitis and Crohn's disease. An international cooperative study. *Scand J Gastroenterol*, 1987; 22: 1009.
71 Rutgeerts P, D'Haens G, Hiele M, Geboes K, Vantrappen G. Appendectomy protects against ulcerative colitis. *Gastroenterology*, 1994; 106: 1251.
72 Russel MG, Dorant E, Brummer R-JM. Appendectomy and the risk of developing ulcerative colitis or Crohn's disease: results of a large case-control study. *Gastroenterology*, 1997; 113: 377.
73 Onuigbo WIB. Appendiceal schistosomiasis—method of classifying oviposition and inflammation. *Dis Colon Rectum*, 1985; 28: 397.
74 Satti MB, Tamimi DB, Al Sohaibani MO, Al Quorain A. Appendicular schistosomiasis: a cause of clinical acute appendicitis? *J Clin Pathol*, 1987; 40: 424.
75 Henrik-Nielsen R, Lundbeck FA, Teglbjaerg PS, Ginnerup P, Hovind-Hougen K. Intestinal spirochetosis of the vermiform appendix. *Gastroenterology*, 1985; 88: 971.
76 Le Brun HI. Appendicular granuloma. *Br J Surg*, 1958; 46: 32.
77 Gruhn J, Tetlow F. Granulomatous pseudoneoplastic appendicitis. *Am J Surg*, 1960; 99: 358.
78 Rex JC, Harrison EG, Priestley JT. Appendicitis and ligneous perityphlitis. *Arch Surg*, 1961; 82: 735.
79 Gallagher EW, Hanna WA. Polyarteritis presenting as acute appendicitis. *J R Coll Surg Edinb*, 1964; 9: 294.
80 Plaut A. Asymptomatic focal arteritis of the appendix (88 cases). *Am J Pathol*, 1951; 27: 247.
81 Latchis KS, Canter JW. Acute appendicitis secondary to metastatic carcinoma. *Am J Surg*, 1966; 111: 220.
82 Ramia JM, Alcalde J, Dhimes P, Cubedo R. Metastasis from choriocarcinoma of the mediastinum producing acute appendicitis. *Dig Dis Sci*, 1998; 43: 332.
83 Pasquale MD, Shabahang M, Bitterman P, Lack EE, Evans SR. Primary lymphoma of the appendix. Case report and review of the literature. *Surg Oncol*, 1994; 3: 243.
84 Huh J, Hong S-M, Kim SS *et al*. Angiocentric lymphoma masquerading as acute appendicitis. *Histopathology*, 1999; 34: 373.
85 Ravalli S, Vincent RA, Beaton H. Primary Kaposi's sarcoma of the gastrointestinal tract presenting as acute appendicitis. *Am J Gastroenterol*, 1990; 85: 772.
86 Chetty R, Slavin JL, Miller RA. Kaposi's sarcoma presenting as acute appendicitis in an HIV-1 positive patient. *Histopathology*, 1993; 23: 590.
87 Peison B. Acute localised amebic appendicitis. *Dis Colon Rectum*, 1973; 16: 532.
88 Malik AK, Hanum N, Yip CH. Acute isolated amoebic appendicitis. *Histopathology*, 1994; 24: 87.

89 Dorfman S, Rangelo O, Bravo LG. Balantidiasis: report of a fatal case with appendicular and pulmonary involvement. *Trans R Soc Trop Med Hyg*, 1984; 78: 833.
90 Noodleman JS. Eosinophilic appendicitis—demonstration of *Strongyloides stercoralis* as a causative agent. *Arch Pathol*, 1981; 105: 148.
91 Boulos PB, Cowie AGA. Pinworm infestation of the appendix. *Br J Surg*, 1973; 60: 975.
92 Sterba J, Vlcek M. Appendiceal enterobiasis—its incidence and relationships to appendicitis. *Folia Parasitol*, 1984; 31: 311.
93 Coyne JD, Dervan PA, Haboubi NY. Involvement of the appendix in pseudomembranous colitis. *J Clin Pathol*, 1997; 50: 70.

31 Tumours and tumour-like lesions of the appendix

The infrequency with which tumours are found in the vermiform appendix is probably only a reflection of the small size of the organ. Four main types of primary neoplasia are found: carcinoids, adenomas, adenocarcinomas and a miscellaneous group of tumours.

Epithelial neoplasms of the appendix

Carcinoid tumours

Carcinoid (endocrine cell) tumours are the most common neoplasms arising in the appendix, accounting for about 85% of all tumours seen in surgical pathology practice [1] and occurring in 0.02–1.5% of all appendicectomy specimens [1–6]. They occur in all age groups, including childhood [7,8], but are most common in the third, fourth and fifth decades of life [2,4,6,9]. Many series show a preponderance of carcinoids in women [2–6,10,11], probably representing a true increased incidence in females [6,11], although this is exaggerated by the fact that incidental appendicectomy during laparotomy for unrelated gallbladder or gynaecological conditions is more common in women [1].

Most carcinoids are found either in appendices removed incidentally at laparotomy for some unrelated condition or in appendicectomy specimens for acute appendicitis. In the latter situation the coexistence of the tumour with appendicitis is usually coincidental, although when the neoplasm is close to the base of the appendix (which occurs in some 10% of cases), it may at least contribute to the onset of inflammation by causing obstruction of the lumen [2]. In other rare cases asymptomatic luminal obstruction may account for the occasional finding of simple mucocoele distal to an appendiceal carcinoid. Carcinoid syndrome, resulting from the systemic effects of serotonin secretion by the tumour, is an extremely rare complication [12], due to the small size of the majority of appendiceal tumours and the rarity of liver metastases. However, Cushing's syndrome, resulting from the ectopic secretion of corticotrophin by an appendiceal carcinoid, has been reported [13].

The majority of carcinoids (70% or more) are found near the tip of the appendix [1,2]. In the fresh state they are firm and grey-white but characteristically assume a yellow colour after formaldehyde fixation. They usually measure less than 1 cm in diameter and rarely more than 2 cm [1–6], and not infrequently are discovered only as a result of microscopic examination. They are usually round and quite well demarcated, but can be diffuse within the wall and along the lumen of the appendix (Fig. 31.1).

The precise origin of carcinoids in the appendiceal mucosa is controversial [14]. Endocrine cells occur normally both within the crypts and scattered singly or in small clusters in the lamina propria, where they form complexes with intramucosal nerve fibres and sustentacular cells [15–17]. The relationship of the cells in the two sites is unknown. Some microscopic tumours show an intimate relationship with the basal parts of the crypts [3], suggesting that they are derived from the cryptal endocrine cell population. Despite evidence of hyperplasia of these cryptal endocrine cells in the background mucosa in appendices containing carcinoids, suggesting a possible preneoplastic endocrine cell proliferation [18], most carcinoids are now thought to originate from the subepithelial neuroendocrine complexes. This is based on the fact that the carcinoid tumour cells are usually associated with small nerves and S-100 protein-positive sustentacular cells, recapitulating the structure of the normal lamina propria neuroendocrine complex [14,15,17,19,20]. The anatomical and age-related distribution of lamina propria endocrine cells also supports this view [21].

Histology

Appendiceal carcinoids are usually divided into three distinct

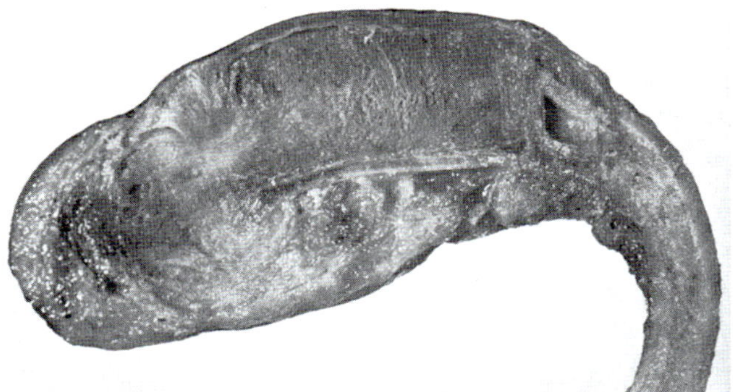

Fig. 31.1 Carcinoid tumour of appendix, filling the lumen at the tip.

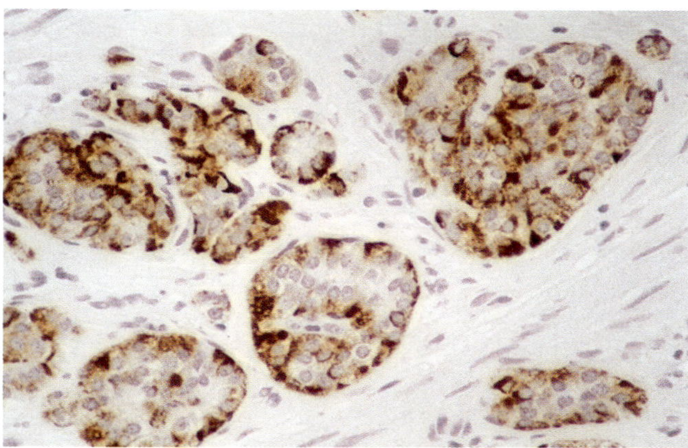

Fig. 31.3 Carcinoid of the appendix composed predominantly of solid islands in which the peripheral cells are chromogranin A positive.

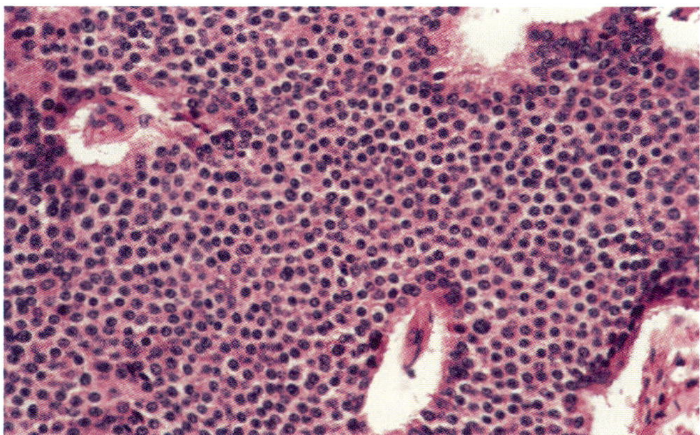

Fig. 31.2 Classical argentaffin carcinoid tumour of appendix. The palisading of the outermost layer is clearly shown.

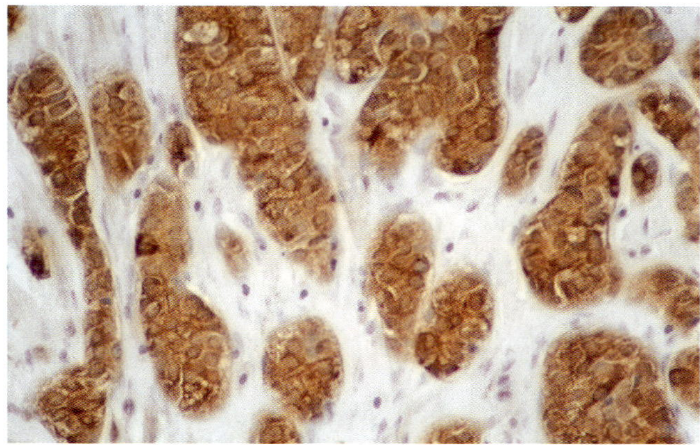

Fig. 31.4 Carcinoid formed of solid islands that are diffusely positive for neurone-specific enolase.

histological patterns, the typical argentaffin enterochromaffin (EC)-cell carcinoid, the non-argentaffin L-cell carcinoid [3], and the more recently described mucinous, goblet cell or adenocarcinoid [22–28]. Apart from differences in histological structure the former two varieties are similar in behaviour, but the third variety is a somewhat different, rather controversial, and biologically more aggressive lesion.

The classical argentaffin carcinoid (Fig. 31.2) in no way differs from its counterpart in the ileum and exhibits the histochemical features and electron microscopic appearances of a so-called EC-cell carcinoid (see p. 367). It is composed of solid clumps of uniform polygonal cells with granular eosinophilic cytoplasm, the outermost layers of which often show a tendency to palisading. The cells show little nuclear pleomorphism or mitotic activity, and have many similarities with enterochromaffin (EC) cells of the normal gut, the cytoplasmic granules giving positive argentaffin and diazo reactions and containing 5-hydroxytryptamine. Other peptides, such as somatostatin, neurotensin, motilin, pancreatic polypeptide and substance P, may also be demonstrated in some tumours by immunohistochemistry [17,29]. The granules may be scattered evenly throughout the cytoplasm of the neoplastic cells or, more frequently, they are concentrated at the periphery of the tumour clumps. They are chromogranin A positive (Fig. 31.3). The cytoplasm is uniformly positive for neurone-specific enolase (NSE) (Fig. 31.4). Occasionally the cytoplasm may show vacuolation, possibly a degenerative phenomenon (Fig. 31.5) [3]. Although arising in the mucosa, the bulk of most appendiceal carcinoids lies in the deeper layers of the wall, often accompanied by hypertrophy of the smooth muscle of the muscularis propria, and frequently extending into the mesoappendix to reach the serosal surface. A retraction artefact of fixation around the tumour clumps in paraffin sections commonly gives a false impression of lymphatic invasion, although true lymphatic permeation, where the spaces around tumour clumps are lined by lymphatic endothelium, is not rare. Perineural invasion may also be found.

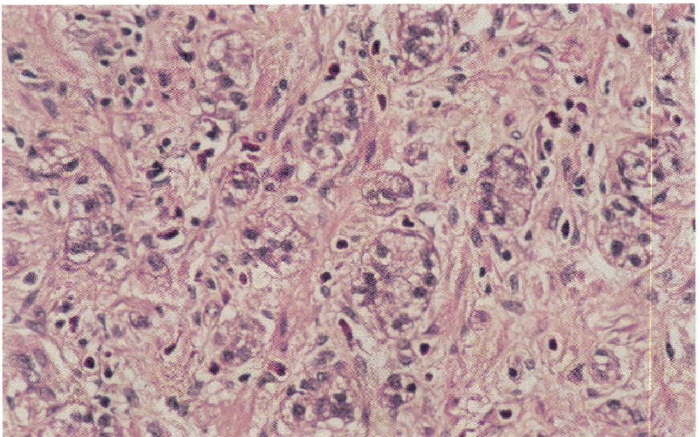

Fig. 31.5 Carcinoid formed of small acini and showing cytoplasmic vacuolation.

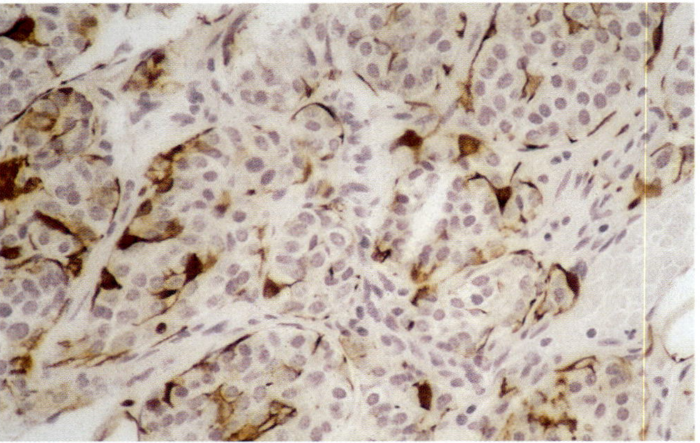

Fig. 31.6 Carcinoid showing S-100 sustentacular cells surrounding small islands.

Most argentaffin carcinoids show a solid, packeted structure in a pure form although where tumour infiltrates muscle the cells may be arranged in narrow cords or ribbons. The packets are surrounded by S-100-positive sustentacular cells (Fig. 31.6). A minority have an acinar element that exceptionally may dominate the histological picture (Fig. 31.5). In this variant the cells differentiate either into solid rosettes with no lumen, or into small blind acini containing a little inspissated periodic acid–Schiff (PAS)-positive material. In some examples it is possible to find a spectrum of differentiation from solid packets to rosettes and finally to acini [3]. Argentaffinity and argyrophilia is present in the acinar areas as well as among the solid clumps of cells; they are positive for chromogranin A and serotonin but negative for S-100 [20]. In some instances the acinar differentiation may be so marked that the tumour superficially resembles and may be mistaken for goblet cell carcinoid (see below) or adenocarcinoma [30], but the lack of intracytoplasmic mucin in acinar carcinoids allows the distinction to be made.

Non-argentaffin L-cell carcinoids are usually small and consequently often missed on gross examination of the appendix. They have a histological structure similar to rectal or so-called hindgut carcinoids, being composed of columns, ribbons, acini or small tubular or glandular structures of small neoplastic endocrine cells that are regular and show little mitotic activity. Round solid clumps typical of argentaffin carcinoids are not a feature. Although non-argentaffin their cytoplasmic granules are frequently, but not always, strongly argyrophil, and may be shown by immunohistochemistry to contain a variety of peptides including glucagon-like peptides, pancreatic polypeptide, motilin, somatostatin, gastrin, neurotensin, and even 5-hydroxytryptamine [29,31–33]. They are neurone-specific enolase (NSE) and synaptophysin positive, and are often chromogranin A negative but chromogranin B positive. Intracytoplasmic mucin secretion is not seen.

Goblet cell carcinoids, mucinous carcinoids or adenocarcinoids of the appendix [22–28] show striking differences in histology from the other two varieties, despite the fact that they have a similar macroscopic appearance and pattern of infiltration. They occur in any portion of the appendix. The term carcinoid is often a misnomer, since these tumours are frequently composed predominantly of small clumps, strands or microglandular collections of mucus-secreting epithelial cells which are distended with mucin, giving a striking resemblance to goblet cells or signet ring cells (Fig. 31.7a). Indeed it is the presence of these cells with intracytoplasmic mucin vacuoles that allows goblet cell carcinoids to be distinguished from conventional carcinoids with an acinar or tubular growth pattern (see above). Mucin production by the neoplastic cells may sometimes be so abundant that pools of extracellular mucus form within the deeper layers of the appendiceal wall. Endocrine cells, argyrophil more than argentaffin, are usually but not invariably present (Fig. 31.7b); they rarely form the majority population and scattered Paneth cells may also be found. In one series all tumours stained positively for NSE, chromogranin A or PGP 9.5 [28]. Nuclear pleomorphism and mitotic activity are usually inconspicuous and the muscular hypertrophy typical of conventional carcinoids is often lacking.

Goblet cell carcinoids are therefore neoplasms composed of cells which show the various types of divergent differentiation of normal crypt epithelial cells [34]. Following the functional demonstration of four lineages: columnar, Paneth, endocrine and goblet cell, the name 'crypt cell carcinoma' was suggested as being more appropriate than a term including the word 'carcinoid' [35]. Although 'goblet cell carcinoid' has emerged as the preferred term, the concept of 'crypt cell carcinoma' emphasizes the crypt base origin in contrast with the likely origin of classical carcinoid tumours from the subepithelial neuroendocrine complex. The microglandular structures, clumps and strands may sometimes include a relatively high proportion of eosinophilic columnar cells (Fig. 31.8). This pattern may be associated with a more aggressive behaviour. One study using

(a)

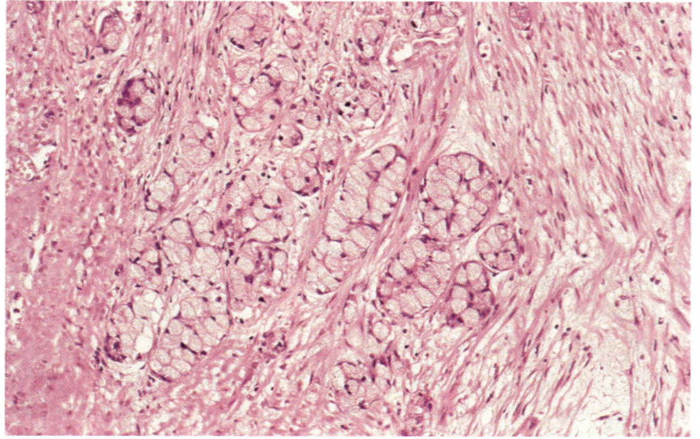

(b)

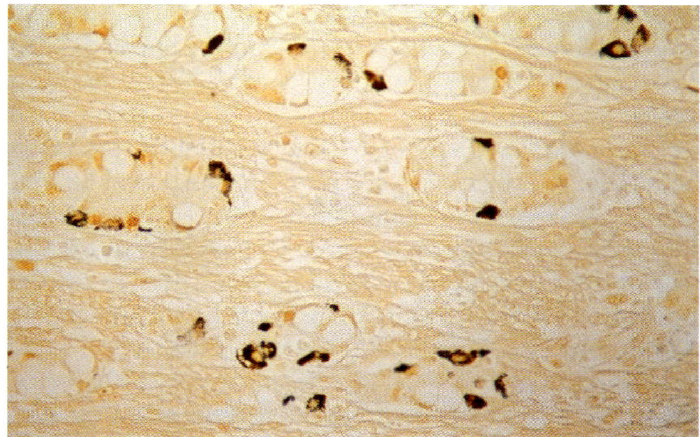

Fig. 31.7 Goblet cell carcinoid of appendix. Although distended mucous cells are most conspicuous on routine staining (a), Grimelius argyrophil silver impregnation (b) reveals considerable numbers of endocrine cells.

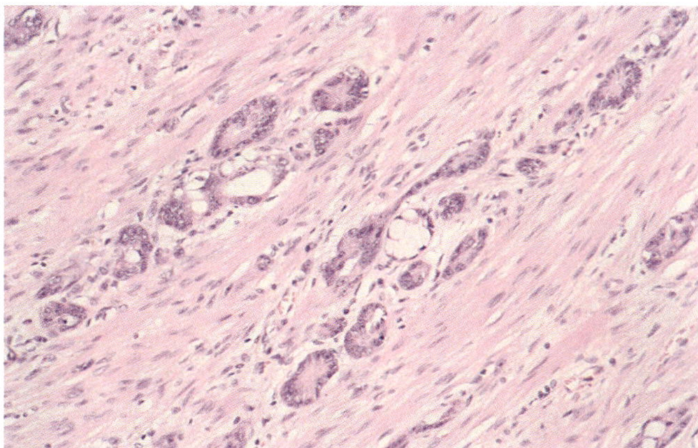

Fig. 31.8 Microacinar variant of goblet cell carcinoid.

immunohistochemistry at ultrastructural level demonstrated both mucin granules and endocrine granules within the cytoplasm of a single tumour cell [36]. In fact the degree of endocrine cell differentiation varies greatly both between and within tumours. In a minority it is predominant and those parts of the lesion are indistinguishable from a conventional carcinoid [37], while in most cases it is inconspicuous, often being appreciated only after histochemical reactions for argentaffin and argyrophil granules have been examined. In some examples, endocrine cells cannot be found at all [24] and in these cases the histological picture is one of a pure signet ring cell carcinoma that can mimic metastatic carcinoma. The term mixed carcinoid–adenocarcinoma has been employed with respect to signet ring cell carcinoma arising in a pre-existing goblet cell carcinoid [30].

Spread and prognosis

The behaviour of argentaffin and non-argentaffin carcinoid tumours is similar. Despite the fact that they are invasive neoplasms, often showing perineural or lymphatic invasion and extending through the wall of the appendix to the serosa or mesoappendix, the vast majority are cured by simple appendicectomy; metastases to the peritoneum, regional lymph nodes and the liver are very rare [6,38]. Moreover, the histological appearances of the primary tumours, including the demonstration of lymphatic invasion, have been found to be of no value in predicting the small number of cases that do metastasize [1,2,5,8]. The only firm indications for further surgery are incomplete excision of the primary tumour or strong clinical evidence of metastases to regional lymph nodes, preferably supported by histological proof. Nevertheless there is considerable evidence to show that the likelihood of metastasis to the regional lymph nodes is governed by the size of the primary tumour, in that such spread virtually never occurs in lesions of less than 1.0 cm in diameter, is rare in tumours of 1.0–2.0 cm [4,6], but is not infrequent in those rare tumours which measure 2.0 cm or more in maximum diameter [1,2,5]. In one large series 31% of tumours measuring 2 cm or more metastasized [1]. Consequently, it is often stated that tumours larger than 2.0 cm should also be treated by radical surgery [1,2,5,10]. However, in the majority of cases with metastatic appendiceal carcinoids the extra-appendiceal spread has been apparent at the time of the primary surgery [2,6], and there is little evidence that radical operations alter the course of the disease in patients with large tumours which are apparently confined to the appendix at diagnosis. In 12 such patients followed for a median period of 28 years local recurrence with regional lymph node metastases occurred in just one, and only then after a period of 29 years from the original operation [2]. Furthermore, patients can survive for many years even in the presence of quite extensive secondary deposits [2]. It would seem reasonable, therefore, that if further surgery for large appendiceal carcinoid tumours is to be recommended at all, it should only be contemplated in the young or middle-aged patient who has an otherwise long life expectancy.

The situation is rather different for goblet cell carcinoids. Although the early reports of these neoplasms suggested an indolent behaviour similar to conventional carcinoids [22,23], more recent publications have indicated that they are more aggressive, with extra-appendiceal spread occurring in up to 20% of cases [24,26–28]. In some the regional lymph nodes and the liver may be involved as a result of lymphatic or vascular dissemination [28,39], but there appears to be a special propensity to transcoelomic spread, especially to the ovaries and, less frequently, to the peritoneal surfaces [39–42]. Histologically the metastases may have the appearances of pure carcinoid, goblet cell carcinoid containing variable proportions of endocrine cells, or of pure carcinoma, usually of signet ring cell type [24,39]. The presence or prominence of the endocrine cell component in the primary tumour does not correlate with the malignant behaviour and, as in conventional carcinoids, perineural or lymphatic invasion is a poor marker of unfavourable prognosis. The more aggressive tumours often show nuclear pleomorphism, a higher mitotic rate (2 or more per 10 high-power fields) [24,26] and a 'carcinomatous' growth pattern, defined as fused or cribriform glands, single-file structures, diffusely infiltrating signet ring cells, or sheets of solid cells [30]. These histological features, if present in more than 50% of the tumour, along with incomplete removal of the primary tumour and the presence of lymph node metastases, have been suggested as indications for radical treatment by right hemicolectomy. However the potential for transcoelomic spread exists in any tumour which has reached and ulcerated the serosal surface, irrespective of other histological features, and it is doubtful whether further surgery is likely to affect this complication. Nevertheless, some advocate right hemicolectomy for all goblet cell carcinoids [27]. It is important for the pathologist to distinguish goblet cell carcinoids, and even those tumours with the pattern of mucinous carcinoid but without demonstrable endocrine cells (i.e. signet ring cell carcinomas), from conventional colonic-type mucinous adenocarcinomas of the appendix, since the latter are much more aggressive tumours that warrant correspondingly more radical surgery. The frequent presence of a pre-existing mucosal adenoma is a useful marker for mucinous adenocarcinoma. However, an association between usual carcinoids and epithelial neoplasia within the appendix has been recorded [43]. Goblet cell carcinoids, like conventional carcinoids, are not associated with any recognizable preinvasive lesion [37].

Adenoma

The appendix, as part of the large intestine, is susceptible to the same influences that cause neoplasia of the colon or rectum. It is not surprising therefore that colonic-type adenomas and carcinomas occur in the appendix though, because of the small size of the organ, they are infrequent.

Appendiceal adenomas are of two main types [44,45]. A few are tiny, localized, pedunculated or sessile lesions that are nearly always asymptomatic and discovered incidentally on routine microscopy. However, the majority involve the appendiceal mucosa in a widespread, diffuse fashion. In these, exuberant secretion of mucus by the neoplastic epithelium within the confined space of the appendiceal lumen frequently gives rise to cystic dilatation and the formation of so-called mucocoele of the appendix [46,47]. Such tumours, which are often termed mucinous cystadenomas, may convert the whole appendix into a large, sausage-shaped or roughly spherical mass laden with viscid mucus. In occasional cases calcification of this mucus can result in the formation of a calculus and this may be detected radiologically [45]. Mucinous cystadenomas occur a little more commonly in women, with a wide age range. They are often discovered incidentally during laparotomy for some other abdominal condition, but occasionally secondary infection may lead to a preoperative diagnosis of appendicitis.

Like colorectal tumours, adenomas of the appendix may have a tubular, tubulovillous or villous configuration, and a similar spectrum of mild, moderate and severe epithelial dysplasia or cytological atypia may be found [44–47]. Small pedunculated lesions usually have a tubular pattern and low-grade dysplasia while the more diffuse mucinous cystadenomas show a tubulovillous or villous architecture with a more variable degree of dysplasia (Figs 31.9–31.12). The superficial villous fronds covered by prominent mucus-secreting cells often appear deceptively bland, but examination of the basal part of the mucosa allows the true neoplastic nature of the lesion to be recognized (Fig. 31.12). Lymphoid tissue is absent in the area of adenomatous change [48].

Two other special histological features may occur in appendiceal adenomas, both of which may lead to misdiagnosis. The first is the development of a serrated architecture, with formation of elongated, serrated crypts similar to colorectal hyperplastic polyps [46,48]. Similar lesions in the colorectum have been described as mixed hyperplastic polyps/adenomas or

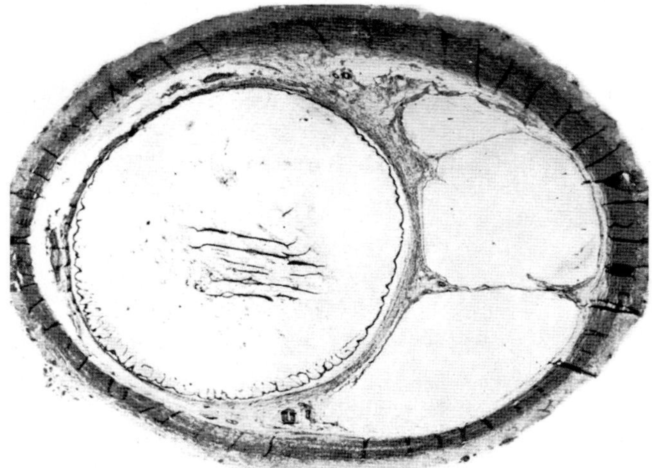

Fig. 31.9 Mucinous cystadenoma of appendix with mucocoele. The lumen of the appendix is replaced by a multiloculated cyst lined by flattened epithelium with small papillary infoldings.

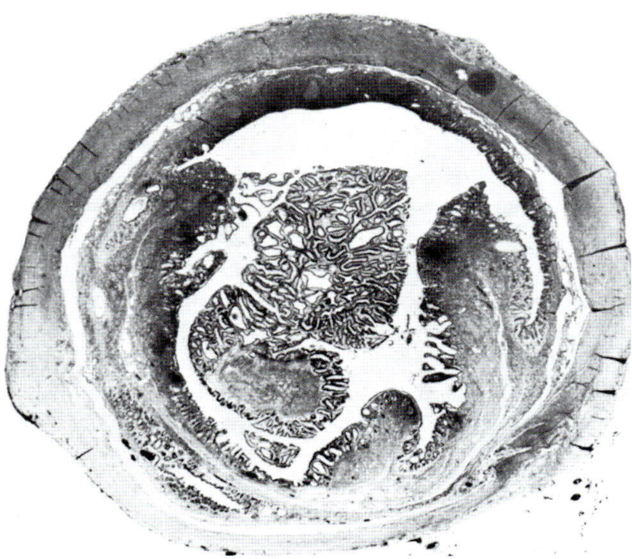

Fig. 31.10 Tubulovillous cystadenoma of appendix. The lumen was distended with mucin but this is not apparent in the section.

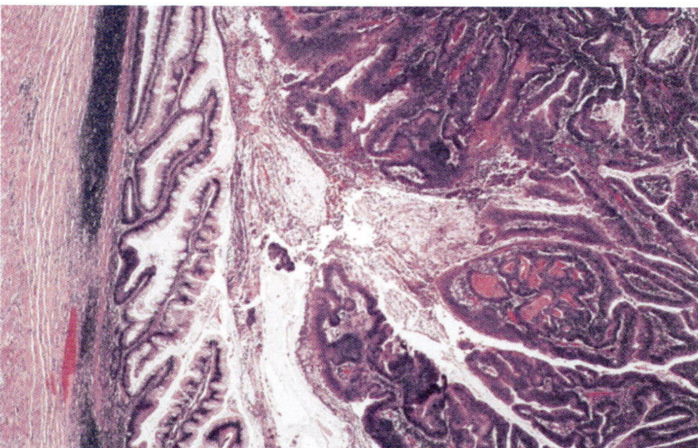

Fig. 31.11 Mucinous cystadenoma of appendix. The lumen is filled with a severely dysplastic tubulovillous adenoma.

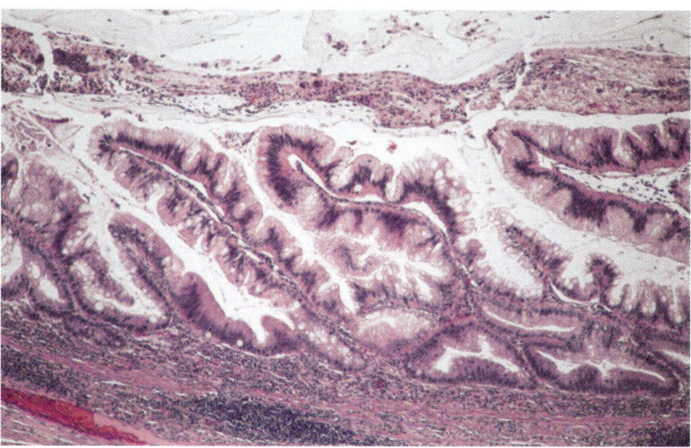

Fig. 31.12 Detail from Fig. 31.11 showing villous processes covered by mildly dysplastic epithelium. Appearances are identical with those that may be seen in villous adenoma of the colorectum. The epithelium covering the villi shows serration and this lesion could be classed as a serrated adenoma.

serrated adenomas (Fig. 31.12) [49,50]. The other change occurs when a mucinous cystadenoma gives rise to a so-called mucocoele. Distension of the appendiceal lumen by mucus then compresses the neoplastic epithelium, flattening it to a single cell layer and thereby obscuring the features of dysplasia [47,48]. This change is often focal, and examination of multiple sections of an appendiceal mucocoele, which may at first appear to have a bland and atrophic epithelial lining, will prevent misdiagnosis. Non-neoplastic (i.e. obstructive) mucocoeles of the appendix rarely cause dilatation of the lumen to more than 1 cm in diameter. It is therefore highly likely that a mucocoele of any substantial size is a mucinous cystadenoma and multiple sections should be taken to establish the correct diagnosis [48].

As with other colorectal epithelial tumours, appendiceal adenomas are preinvasive neoplasms that have the potential to progress to invasive adenocarcinomas or cystadenocarcinomas. They are also associated with synchronous or metachronous adenomas or carcinomas elsewhere in the large intestine—in one series about 20% of patients were found to have an associated and quite separate primary adenocarcinoma of the colon [45]. When a benign adenoma of the appendix is found it is important that the whole lesion is carefully examined for focal malignant invasion of the wall and the remainder of the colon and rectum should be carefully screened for other neoplasms. The appendix is consistently involved by adenomas in familial adenomatous polyposis coli, but in these patients small, localized adenomas are most prevalent [51]. Appendiceal neoplasia has also been documented in subjects with long-standing ulcerative colitis [52].

The distinction between epithelial misplacement and genuine invasion in appendiceal neoplasms is not always straightforward, especially in mucinous cystadenomas. To establish malignancy it is essential to demonstrate invasion of neoplastic epithelium through the muscularis mucosae into the submucosa, but occasionally this may be mimicked by displacement of mucin-secreting adenomatous epithelium into the wall of the appendix as a consequence of raised intraluminal pressure from mucus hypersecretion or from episodes of inflammation [47]. Acellular mucin may also dissect through the appendiceal wall. Displacement of cellular or acellular mucin is often accompanied by inflammation, abscess formation or diverticulosis, and the presence of these features may help to exclude malignant change. Invasive carcinoma is often surrounded by a dense, desmoplastic reaction while the epithelial components of displaced adenomatous mucosa retain their surrounding lamina propria made up of loose connective tissue. However, well differentiated mucinous adenocarcinomas may lack desmoplasia and invade on a broad front. Conclusive evidence of tissue invasion must be found before a diagnosis of cystadenocarcinoma is made because adenomas and cystadenomas are treated by simple appendicectomy whereas right hemicolectomy and regional lymphadenectomy are required for adenocarcinoma. In cases where it is not possible to achieve a definitive diagnosis, the term 'mucinous tumour of uncertain malignant potential' may be employed.

Molecular genetic changes in appendiceal adenomas are similar to those described in their colorectal counterparts: K-*ras* mutation and allelic imbalance (loss of heterozygosity) on chromosomes 5q22, 6q, 17p13 and 18q21 [53].

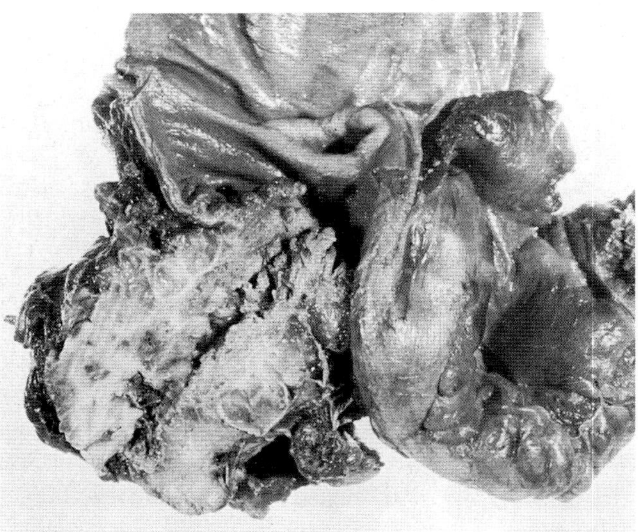

Fig. 31.13 Primary mucinous cystadenocarcinoma of appendix.

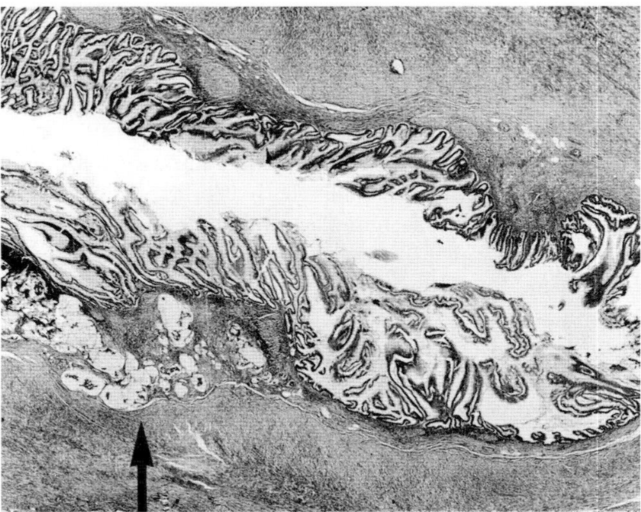

Fig. 31.14 Mucinous cystadenoma of appendix with early carcinomatous change (arrowed).

Adenocarcinoma

Invasive adenocarcinoma of the appendix is a rare tumour that presents either as acute appendicitis or as an abdominal mass in a middle-aged or elderly patient [54]. The most common type is a well differentiated mucinous adenocarcinoma (Fig. 31.13), in which exuberant mucus secretion often gives rise to the gross appearance of a mucocoele [44,46,55,56]. The tumour shows no fundamental difference histologically from mucinous adenocarcinoma of the remainder of the large intestine and there is often clear evidence of an origin from a mucinous cystadenoma (Fig. 31.14) [56]. Tubular or papillary types of adenocarcinoma without excessive production of extracellular mucin [55] are less frequent in the appendix. They cause thickening of the appendiceal wall, which may lead to obstructive appendicitis. A case of adenocarcinoma with squamous differentiation, termed adenoacanthoma by the authors, has also been described [57].

The behaviour of appendiceal adenocarcinoma closely resembles that of colorectal cancer with prognosis varying with the grade of malignancy, non-mucinous histology and extent of spread [56,58,59]. Lymph node metastases are present in about a quarter of resection specimens and the overall 5-year survival rate in one series was 60% [60]. Other authors have reported a much poorer outlook, especially for tumours that present with perforation of the appendix [54].

Reports of signet ring carcinoma [56], microglandular carcinoma [55] and linitis plastica of the appendix [55] usually describe variants of goblet cell carcinoid of the appendix in which the mucinous component is dominant (see above), or metastases from primary tumours of the stomach, breast or ovary.

The boundary between adenocarcinoma of the appendix and mucinous carcinoids has become less clear cut in recent years with the recognition that on the one hand well differentiated colonic-type adenocarcinomas may contain variable numbers of endocrine cells [55,56], while on the other hand tumours with the infiltrative pattern of carcinoids may have very few, or even no, endocrine cells and consist largely of mucous cells [24]. The realization that such goblet cell carcinoids do not have the excellent prognosis of classical carcinoids (see above) suggests that they might be better regarded as special variants of appendiceal carcinoma, especially if they demonstrate the 'carcinomatous' growth pattern described above [30]. However, we believe that the relatively good prognosis of completely excised goblet cell carcinoids that have no such features, along with the special propensity for transcoelomic spread with frequent ovarian involvement in those that do, warrants their continued separation from typical colonic-type adenocarcinomas.

Pseudomyxoma peritonei

Mucinous tumours of the appendix are not infrequently associated with escape of mucus through the appendiceal wall into the peritoneal cavity, a condition described as pseudomyxoma peritonei [44]. This may be either localized to the right iliac fossa or more generalized. When the cause is simple displacement of mucus through the wall of a benign cystadenoma due to raised intraluminal pressure the condition is often localized [46] and usually regresses after resection of the primary lesion. Other cases follow a less indolent course that may require additional surgery, and fatal outcomes have been recorded [61,62]. These slowly progressing cases are probably the result of an underlying well differentiated mucinous adenocarcinoma. In more aggressive cases, the peritoneal involvement is diffuse and ultimately proves fatal, obliterating the abdominal cavity and leading to recurrent attacks of intestinal obstruction. Poor prognostic features include abdominal distension, weight loss, high histological grade and invasion of underlying structures. The ovary was once considered to be a common primary site of mucinous neoplasia associated with pseudomyxoma peritonei. There is now good evidence that the appendix is the usual primary site of pseudomyxoma peritonei, with any ovarian involvement being secondary [53,61,62].

Miscellaneous tumours

Neuromas

Well demarcated, macroscopically distinct neurofibromas of the appendix are uncommon [63]; many of those reported have occurred in a background of von Recklinghausen's neurofibromatosis. We are aware of one report of an appendiceal ganglioneuroma [64]. However, a more ill-defined, diffuse neuronal proliferation, frequently accompanied by endocrine cells, may be found in a high proportion of appendicectomy specimens, especially those with fibrous obliteration of the lumen at the appendiceal tip [65]. Their frequency increases with age. Such lesions have been termed axial neuromas, but there is considerable controversy over whether they represent true neoplasms or a non-neoplastic neuronal proliferation, possibly induced by previous episodes of inflammation [65,66]. The lesions are often multiple, and the terms neuromatosis of the appendix, neurogenic appendicitis or neurogenic appendicopathy [17] have been applied by those who consider that they may provide some explanation for the symptoms and signs of so-called chronic appendicitis. A small proportion have been associated with carcinoid tumours, especially microcarcinoids of the appendiceal mucosa [17], and it is conceivable that some carcinoid tumours arise from endocrine cell proliferation within such lesions.

Other non-epithelial tumours

There are infrequent reports of primary smooth muscle tumours of the appendix [67], primary appendiceal malignant lymphomas, especially Burkitt's lymphoma [68], granular cell tumours [69] and so-called dermoid cysts of the appendix [70], and inflammatory pseudotumours [71].

Non-neoplastic epithelial polyps

Hamartomatous polyps of both Peutz–Jeghers [72] and juvenile [73] types may occur rarely in the appendix, nearly always in association with more widespread gastrointestinal involvement. They may give rise to appendiceal intussusception.

Hyperplastic (metaplastic) polyps with their characteristic histological appearances of serrated crypts, although common in the colon and rectum, are found only infrequently as discrete, well demarcated localized mucosal lesions in the appendix (Fig. 31.15). However, it is not uncommon to find a more diffuse hyperplastic-like change extending over a wide area of the appendiceal mucosa, either in an otherwise normal appendix or in association with luminal distension with mucin (mucocoele) [74,75]. The true nature of this hyperplastic-like change is uncertain. Careful examination shows that although the affected crypts have a serrated appearance, their epithelial lining is not typical of colonic hyperplastic polyps in that there is often a predominance of mucus-secreting cells and sometimes nuclear stratification [48]. Occasionally the change is accompanied by or may merge with an obvious appendiceal villous adenoma [46], raising the possibility that it may represent not conventional large intestinal-type hyperplasia, but a very well differentiated adenoma with a serrated villous growth pattern (serrated adenoma of the appendix). In view of this, it is advisable to search carefully for true adenomatous change in any appendix lined by such diffuse hyperplastic-type mucosa. Diffuse hyperplastic change in the appendix may be associated with colonic adenocarcinoma [76].

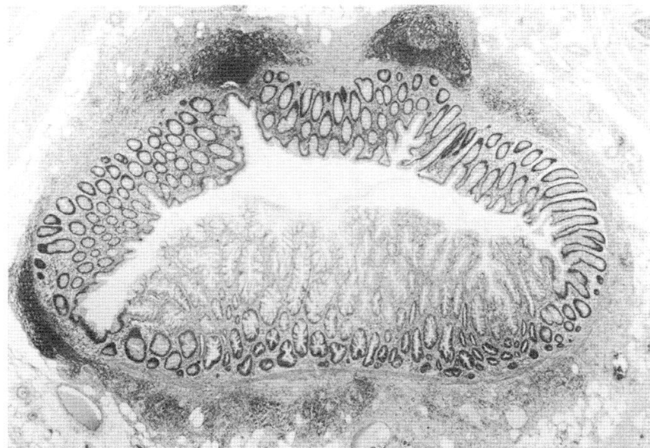

Fig. 31.15 Discrete metaplastic polyp of the appendix, occupying the lower half of the luminal circumference.

Metastatic tumours

The appendix is a well recognized site of spread from carcinoma of the ovary [77]. Secondary carcinoma in the appendix has also been described from tumours of the breast, stomach or bronchus [78,79]; superimposed acute appendicitis is usually responsible for bringing to light the appendiceal involvement and the outlook is poor.

References

1 Moertel CG, Dockerty MB, Judd ES. Carcinoid tumours of the vermiform appendix. *Cancer*, 1968; 21: 270.

2 Moertel CG, Weiland LH, Nagorney DM, Dockerty MB. Carcinoid tumor of the appendix: treatment and prognosis. *N Engl J Med*, 1987; 317: 1699.

3 Dische FE. Argentaffin and non-argentaffin carcinoid tumours of the appendix. *J Clin Pathol*, 1968; 21: 60.

4 Syracuse DC, Perzin KH, Price JB, Wiedel PD, Mesa-Tejada R. Carcinoid tumours of the appendix. *Ann Surg*, 1979; 190: 58.

5 Glasser CM, Bhagavan BS. Carcinoid tumours of the appendix. *Arch Pathol Lab Med*, 1980; 104: 272.

6 Anderson JR, Wilson BG. Carcinoid tumours of the appendix. *Br J Surg*, 1985; 72: 545.

7 Willcox SW. Carcinoid tumours of the appendix in childhood. *Br J Surg*, 1964; 51: 110.

8 Ryden SE, Drake RM, Franciosi RA. Carcinoid tumours of the appendix in children. *Cancer*, 1975; 36: 1538.

9 Ponka JL. Carcinoid tumours of the appendix: report of 35 cases. *Am J Surg*, 1973; 126: 77.

10 Bowman GA, Rosenthal D. Carcinoid tumours of the appendix. *Am J Surg*, 1983; 146: 700.

11 Modin IM, Sandor A. An analysis of 8305 cases of carcinoid tumors. *Cancer*, 1997; 79: 813.

12 Markgraf WH, Dunn TM. Appendiceal carcinoid with carcinoid syndrome. *Am J Surg*, 1964; 107: 730.

13 Johnston WH, Waisman J. Carcinoid tumour of the vermiform appendix with Cushing's syndrome. *Cancer*, 1971; 27: 681.

14 Moyana TN, Satkunam N. A comparative immunohistochemical study of jejunoileal and appendiceal carcinoids. *Cancer*, 1992; 70: 1081.

15 Rode J, Dhillon AP, Papadaki L, Griffiths D. Neurosecretory cells of the lamina propria of the appendix and their possible relationship to carcinoids. *Histopathology*, 1982; 6: 69.

16 Papadaki L, Rode J, Dhillon AP, Dische FE. Fine structure of a neuroendocrine complex in the mucosa of the appendix. *Gastroenterology*, 1983; 84: 490.

17 Hofler H, Kasper M, Heitz PU. The neuroendocrine system of normal human appendix, ileum and colon, and in neurogenic appendicopathy. *Virchows Arch A*, 1983; 399: 127.

18 Cross SS, Hughes AD, Williams GT, Williams ED. Endocrine cell hyperplasia and appendiceal carcinoids. *J Pathol*, 1988; 156: 325.

19 Lundqvist M, Wilander E. Subepithelial neuroendocrine cells and carcinoid tumours of the human small intestine and appendix. A comparative immunohistochemical study with regard to serotonin, neuron-specific enolase and S-100 protein reactivity. *J Pathol*, 1986; 148: 141.

20 Goddard MJ, Lonsdale RN. The histogenesis of appendiceal carcinoid tumours. *Histopathology*, 1992; 20: 345.

21 Shaw PAV. The topographical and age distributions of neuroendocrine cells in the normal human appendix. *J Pathol*, 1991; 164: 235.

22 Klein HZ. Mucinous carcinoid tumour of the vermiform appendix. *Cancer*, 1970; 33: 770.

23 Subbuswamy SG, Gibbs NM, Ross CF, Morson BC. Goblet carcinoid of the appendix. *Cancer*, 1978; 34: 338.

24 Warkel RL, Cooper RH, Helwig EB. Adenocarcinoid, a mucin-producing carcinoid tumor of the appendix. *Cancer*, 1978; 42: 2781.

25 Olsson B, Ljungberg O. Adenocarcinoid of the vermiform appendix. *Virchows Arch*, 1980; 386: 201.

26 Edmonds P, Merrino MJ, LiVolsi VA, Duray DH. Adenocarcinoid (mucinous carcinoid) of the appendix. *Gastroenterology*, 1984; 86: 302.

27 Park K, Blessing K, Kerr K, Chetty U, Gilmour H. Goblet cell carcinoid of the appendix. *Gut*, 1990; 31: 322.

28 Anderson NH, Somerville JE, Johnston CF *et al*. Appendiceal goblet cell carcinoids: a clinicopathological and immunohistochemical study. *Histopathology*, 1991; 18: 61.

29 Yang K, Ulich T, Cheng L, Lewin KJ. The neuroendocrine products of intestinal carcinoids. An immunoperoxidase study of 35 carcinoid tumors stained for serotonin and eight polypeptide hormones. *Cancer*, 1983; 51: 1918.

30 Burke AP, Sobin LH, Federspiel BH, Shekitka KM, Helwig EB. Goblet cell carcinoids and related tumors of the vermiform appendix. *Am J Clin Pathol*, 1990; 94: 27.

31 Iwafuchi M, Watanabe H, Ajioka Y *et al*. Immunohistochemical and ultrastructural studies of twelve argentaffin and six argyrophil carcinoids of the appendix vermiformis. *Hum Pathol*, 1990; 21: 773.

32 Shaw PA, Pringle JH. The demonstration of a subset of carcinoid tumours of the appendix by in situ hybridization using synthetic probes to proglucagon mRNA. *J Pathol*, 1992; 167: 375.

33 Solcia E, Fiocca R, Rindi G *et al*. The pathology of the gastrointestinal endocrine system. *Endocrinol Metab Clin North Am*, 1993; 22: 795.

34 Warner TFCS, Seo IS. Goblet cell carcinoid of the appendix. Ultrastructural features and histogenetic aspects. *Cancer*, 1979; 44: 1700.

35 Isaacson P. Crypt cell carcinoma of the appendix (so-called adenocarcinoid tumor). *Am J Surg Pathol*, 1981; 5: 213.

36 Hofler H, Kloppel G, Heitz PU. Combined production of mucus, amines and peptides by goblet-cell carcinoid of the appendix and ileum. *Pathol Res Pract*, 1984; 178: 555.

37 Chen V, Qizilbash AH. Goblet cell carcinoid tumor of the appendix. *Arch Pathol Lab Med*, 1979; 103: 180.

38 Knowles CHR, McCrea AN, Davis A. Metastasis from argentaffinoma of the appendix. *J Pathol Bacteriol*, 1956; 29: 326.

39 Bak M, Jorgensen LJ. Adenocarcinoid of the appendix presenting with metastases to the liver. *Dis Colon Rectum*, 1987; 30: 112.

40 Heisterberg L, Wahlin A, Nielsen KS. Two cases of goblet cell carcinoid tumor of the appendix with bilateral ovarian metastasis. *Acta Obstet Gynecol Scand*, 1982; 61: 153.

41 Hirschfield LS, Kahn LB, Winkler B, Bochner RZ, Gibstein AA. Adenocarcinoid of the appendix presenting as bilateral Krukenberg's tumor of the ovaries. *Arch Pathol Lab Med*, 1985; 109: 930.

42 Hood IC, Jones BA, Watts JC. Mucinous carcinoid tumor of the appendix presenting as bilateral ovarian tumors. *Arch Pathol Lab Med*, 1986; 109: 336.

43 Carr NJ, Remotti H, Sobin LH. Dual carcinoid/epithelial neoplasia of the appendix. *Histopathology*, 1995; 27: 557.

44 Higa E, Rosai J, Pizzimbono CA, Wise L. Mucosal hyperplasia mucinous cystadenoma, and mucinous cystadenocarcinoma of the appendix. *Cancer*, 1973; 32: 1525.

45 Wolff M, Ahmed N. Epithelial neoplasms of the vermiform appendix (exclusive of carcinoid). II. Cystadenomas, papillary adenomas and adenomatous polyps of the appendix. *Cancer*, 1976; 37: 2511.

46 Qizilbash AH. Mucoceles of the appendix. Their relationship to hyperplastic polyps, mucinous cystadenomas, and cystadenocarcinomas. *Arch Pathol*, 1975; 99: 548.

47 Gibbs NM. Mucinous cystadenoma and cystadenocarcinoma of the vermiform appendix with particular reference to mucocoele and pseudomyxoma peritonei. *J Clin Pathol*, 1973; 26: 413.

48 Appelman HD. Epithelial neoplasia of the appendix. In: Norris HT, ed. *Pathology of the Small Intestine, Colon and Anus*, 2nd edn. New York: Churchill Livingstone, 1991: 263.

49 Carr NJ, Sobin LH. Epithelial noncarcinoid tumors and tumor-like lesions of the appendix. *Cancer*, 1995; 76: 757.

50 Williams GR, Du Boulay CEH, Roche WR. Benign epithelial neoplasms of the appendix: classification and clinical associations. *Histopathology*, 1992; 21: 447.

51 Bussey HJR. *Familial Polyposis Coli*. Baltimore: Johns Hopkins University Press, 1975.

52 Odze RD, Medline P, Cohen Z. Adenocarcinoma arising in an appendix involved with chronic ulcerative colitis. *Am J Gastroenterol*, 1994; 89: 1905.

53 Szych C, Staebler A, Connolly DC *et al*. Molecular genetic evidence supporting the clonality and appendiceal origin of pseudomyxoma peritonei in women. *Am J Pathol*, 1999; 154: 1849.

54 Gilhome RW, Johnston DH, Clark J, Kyle J. Primary adenocarcinoma of the vermiform appendix: report of a series of ten cases, and review of the literature. *Br J Surg*, 1984; 71: 553.

55 Qizilbash AH. Primary adenocarcinoma of the appendix. *Arch Pathol*, 1975; 99: 556.

56 Wolff M, Ahmed N. Epithelial neoplasms of the vermiform appendix (exclusive of carcinoid). I. Adenocarcinoma of the appendix. *Cancer*, 1976; 37: 2493.

57 Schulte WJ, Pintar K, Schmahl T. Adenoacanthoma of the appendix. *J Surg Oncol*, 1974; 6: 93.

58 Cortina R, McCormick J, Kolm P, Perry RR. Management and prognosis of adenocarcinoma of the appendix. *Dis Colon Rectum*, 1995; 38: 848.

59 Nitecki SS, Wolff BG, Schlinkert R, Sarr MG. The natural history of surgically treated primary adenocarcinoma of the appendix. *Ann Surg*, 1994; 219: 51.

60 Hesketh KT. The management of primary adenocarcinoma of the vermiform appendix. *Gut*, 1963; 4: 158.

61 Prayson RA, Hart WR, Petras RE. Pseudomyxoma peritonei. A clinicopathologic study of 19 cases with emphasis on site of origin and nature of associated ovarian tumors. *Am J Surg Pathol*, 1994; 18: 591.

62 Ronnett BM, Kurman RJ, Zahn CM *et al*. Pseudomyxoma peritonei in women: a clinicopathologic analysis of 30 cases with emphasis on site of origin, prognosis, and relationship to ovarian mucinous tumors of low malignant potential. *Hum Pathol*, 1995; 26: 509.

63 Olsen BS. Giant appendicular neurofibroma. A light and immunohistochemical study. *Histopathology*, 1987; 11: 851.

64 Zarabi M, LaBach JP. Ganglioneuroma causing acute appendicitis. *Hum Pathol*, 1982; 13: 1143.

65 Olsen BS, Holck S. Neurogenous hyperplasia leading to appendiceal obliteration. an immunohistochemical study of 237 cases. *Histopathology*, 1987; 11: 843.

66 Stanley MW, Cherwitz D, Hagen K, Snover DC. Neuromas of the appendix. *Am J Surg Pathol*, 1986; 10: 801.

67 Jones PA. Leiomyosarcoma of the appendix: report of two cases. *Dis Colon Rectum*, 1979; 22: 175.

68 Sin IC, Ling E-T, Prentice RSA. Burkitt's lymphoma of the appendix: report of two cases. *Hum Pathol*, 1980; 11: 465.

69 Johnston J, Helwig EB. Granular cell tumors of the gastrointestinal tract and perianal region. *Dig Dis Sci*, 1981; 26: 807.

70 Cotton MH, Blake JR. Dermoid cyst: a rare tumour of the appendix. *Gut*, 1986; 27: 334.

71 Yamagiwa Y, Terada N, Hashimoto O, Itano S. An inflammatory pseudotumor of the appendix. *Gan-No-Rinsho*, 1990; 36: 1059.

72 Kitchin AP. Polyposis of small intestine with pigmentation of oral mucosa. *Br Med J*, 1953; i: 658.

73 Shnitka TK, Sherbaniuk RW. Adenomatous polyps of the appendix in children. *Gastroenterology*, 1957; 32: 462.

74 MacGillivray JB. Mucosal metaplasia in the appendix. *J Clin Pathol*, 1922; 25: 809.

75 Qizilbash AH. Hyperplastic (metaplastic) polyps of the appendix. *Arch Pathol*, 1974; 97: 385.

76 Younes M, Katikaneni PR, Lechago J. Association between mucosal hyperplasia of the appendix and adenocarcinoma of the colon. *Histopathology*, 1995; 26: 33.

77 Malfetano JH. The appendix and its metastatic potential in epithelial ovarian cancer. *Obstet Gynecol*, 1987; 69: 396.

78 Latchis KS, Canter JW. Acute appendicitis secondary to metastatic carcinoma. *Am J Surg*, 1966; 111: 220.

79 Dieter RA. Carcinoma metastatic to the vermiform appendix: report of three cases. *Dis Colon Rectum*, 1970; 13: 336.

32 Miscellaneous conditions of the appendix

Diverticular disease

Diverticula are found within surgically removed appendices in up to 2% of specimens [1]. Appendiceal diverticula may be congenital or acquired.

Congenital diverticula

In congenital diverticula of the appendix the muscularis propria is continuous around the diverticulum. Only some 3% of the reported cases of appendiceal diverticula are of this variety; they are apparently commoner in males and the diverticula are usually solitary [2,3]. Favara (1968) has reported congenital appendiceal diverticula in association with the trisomy 13 syndrome [4].

Acquired diverticula

These are outpouchings of mucosa through the appendiceal wall, which are typically not invested by muscularis propria although occasionally a few strands of the longitudinal muscle coat may be present (Fig. 32.1). They may occur on the mesenteric or on the antimesenteric border of the appendix, usually in the distal third, and are more often multiple than single giving the appendix a curious beaded appearance externally [1]. They often contain faecoliths. Microscopically they are lined by appendiceal mucosa.

Acquired diverticula probably result from increased intraluminal pressure due to distension combined with muscular contraction. They are not uncommon in young adults and an association with cystic fibrosis has been recorded in children [5]. Weakening of the appendiceal wall from previous inflammation or an abnormally large perivascular space may also contribute to the mucosal herniation through the muscular propria, as may traction from adhesions.

Appendiceal diverticulitis

Histological examination of some appendicectomy specimens for clinical acute appendicitis reveals diverticulitis and peridiverticulitis at the appendiceal tip, and the thin wall of an acquired diverticulum means that there is little barrier to perforation and consequent peritonitis or peridiverticular abscess formation. Diverticulitis of the appendix generally occurs in older patients than those with typical acute appendicitis and occasionally it is found in appendices removed incidentally [1,6,7].

Appendiceal septa

Single or multiple, complete or incomplete septa consisting of mucosa and submucosa have been described in appendices showing acute inflammation [8]. When complete septa were present the inflammatory process was frequently confined to one compartment. Most cases occurred in the 15–19 age group and there was a clear male predominance.

Intussusception

Appendiceal intussusception is extremely uncommon. It was first reported in 1859 in a male child who died 1 month after presentation with abdominal pain [9]. It may involve either a normal [10] or an abnormal appendix [11], and its recognition in right hemicolectomy specimens can be difficult unless it is suspected. Clinical presentation is usually with blood-stained faeces [12,13] or with features of acute appendicitis [13], and sometimes a preoperative diagnosis can be made radiologically [14].

McSwain classified appendiceal intussusception into four

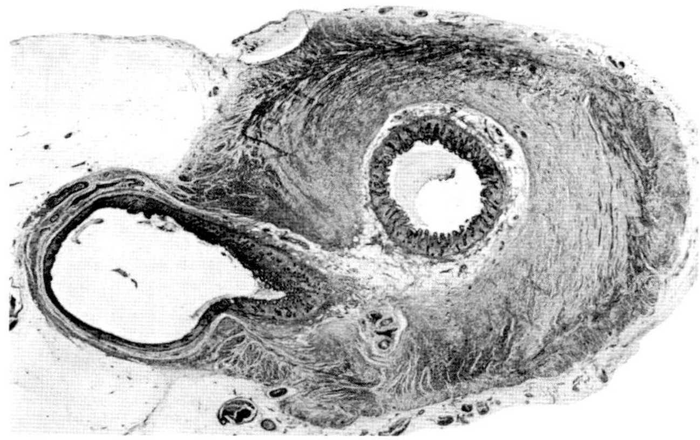

Fig. 32.1 Muscular thickening of wall of appendix, with formation of a diverticulum.

types [15]. In Type 1 there is intussusception of the distal appendix into the proximal appendix; in Type 2 there is intussusception of the distal appendix into the caecoappendiceal valvular opening; in Type 3 there is intussusception of the proximal appendix into the distal appendix; and in Type 4 there is complete inversion of the appendix, usually as part of ileocaecal intussusception.

Most cases of appendiceal intussusception occur in childhood and it is likely that persistence of a fetal cone-shaped pattern to the caecum, or an unusually thin mesoappendix, are predisposing factors. Some cases have been linked to adenovirus-related lymphoid hyperplasia [16] or to *Yersinia enterocolitica* infection [17]. Mass lesions including endometriosis [18], adenomas [19] or Peutz–Jeghers polyps [20] are sometimes responsible, and in all resections for appendiceal intussusception it is important for the pathologist to exclude these.

Torsion

Torsion of the appendix is rare. It leads to ischaemic necrosis and presents clinically as acute appendicitis. It is more common in long subhepatic appendices and intracaecal appendices [21].

Endometriosis

The appendix is involved in approximately 1% of cases of pelvic endometriosis and usually represents an incidental finding at laparotomy [22]. Occasionally symptoms of appendicitis may be present, especially if there is intramural haemorrhage that has occluded the appendiceal lumen [23], and in one case report this was associated with an obstructing decidual polyp in a pregnant woman [24]. Severe haemorrhage leading to massive lower gastrointestinal haemorrhage has also been reported [25]. Most endometriotic deposits are subserosal or intramuscular and, as elsewhere in the large bowel, they are associated with gross thickening of the muscularis propria. A case of dysplastic change in mucinous epithelium in appendiceal endometriosis has been reported [26].

Malakoplakia

The appendix is an exceptionally rare site for malakoplakia. One case with malakoplakia apparently confined to the appendix was reported in a woman who died from pulmonary nocardia infection [27].

References

1 Lipton S, Estrin J, Glasser I. Diverticular disease of the appendix. *Surg Gynecol Obstet*, 1989; 168: 13.
2 Beswick JS, Desai S. Diverticular disease of the vermiform appendix and its clinical relevance. *Australas Radiol*, 1994; 38: 260.
3 Trollope ML, Lindenauer SM. Diverticulosis of the appendix; a collective review. *Dis Colon Rectum*, 1974; 17: 200.
4 Favara BE. Multiple congenital diverticula of the vermiform appendix. *Am J Clin Pathol*, 1968; 49: 60.
5 George DH. Diverticulosis of the vermiform appendix in patients with cystic fibrosis. *Hum Pathol*, 1987; 18: 75.
6 Delikaris P, Tegbjaerg PS, Fisker-Sorensen P, Balsley I. Diverticula of the vermiform appendix. Alternatives of clinical presentations and significance. *Dis Colon Rectum*, 1983; 26: 374.
7 Place RJ, Simmang CI, Huber PJ Jr. Appendiceal diverticulitis. *South Med J*, 2000; 93: 76.
8 De la Fuente AA. Septa in the appendix: a previously undescribed condition. *Histopathology*, 1985; 9: 1329.
9 McKidd J. Case of invagination of caecum and appendix. *Edinb Med J*, 1859; 4: 793.
10 Patton KR, Ferrera PC. Intussusception of a normal appendix. *Am J Emerg Med*, 2000; 18: 115.
11 Desai N, Wayne MG, Taub PJ, Levitt MA, Spiegel R, Kim U. Intussusception in adults. *Mt Sinai J Med*, 1999; 66: 336.
12 Langsam LB, Raj PK, Galang CF. Intussusception of the appendix. *Dis Colon Rectum*, 1984; 27: 387.
13 Yates LN. Intussusception of the appendix. *Int Surg*, 1983; 68: 231.
14 Levine MS, Trenkner SW, Herlinger H *et al.* Coiled spring sign of intussusception. *Radiology*, 1985; 155: 41.
15 McSwain B. Intussusception of the appendix. Review of the literature and report of a case. *South Med J*, 1941; 34: 263.
16 Porter HJ, Padfield CJH, Peres LC *et al.* Adenovirus and intranuclear inclusions in appendices in intussusception. *J Clin Pathol*, 1993; 46: 154.
17 Winesett MP, Pietsch JB, Barnard JA. *Yersinia enterocolitica* in a child with intussusception. *J Pediatr Gastroenterol Nutr*, 1996; 23: 77.
18 Nycum LR, Moss H, Adams JQ, Macri CI. Asymptomatic intussusception of the appendix due to endometriosis. *South Med J*, 1999; 92: 524.
19 Ohno M, Nakamura T, Hori H, Tabuchi Y, Kuroda Y. Appendiceal

intussusception induced by a villous adenoma with carcinoma; report of a case. *Surg Today*, 2000; 30: 441.

20 Yoshikawa A, Kuramoto S, Mimura T *et al*. Peutz–Jeghers syndrome manifesting complete intussusception of the appendix associated with a focal cancer of the duodenum and a cystadenocarcinoma of the pancreas: report of a case. *Dis Colon Rectum*, 1998; 41: 517.

21 De Bruin AJ. Torsion of the appendix. *Med J Aust*, 1969; 1: 581.

22 Ortiz-Hidalgo C, Cortes-Aguilar D, Ortiz de la Pena J. Endometriosis of the vermiform appendix (EVA) is an uncommon lesion with a frequency <1% of all cases of pelvic endometriosis. Recent case. *World J Surg*, 1999; 23: 427.

23 Mittal VK, Choudhury SP, Cortez JA. Endometriosis of the appendix presenting as acute appendicitis. *Am J Surg*, 1981; 142: 519.

24 Silvestrini IE, Marcial MA. Endometriosis of the appendix with decidual polyp formation: a rare cause of acute appendicitis during pregnancy. *P R Health Sci J*, 1995; 14: 223.

25 Shome GP, Nagaraju M, Munis A, Wiese D. Appendiceal endometriosis presenting as massive lower intestinal haemorrhage. *Am J Gastroenterol*, 1995; 90: 1881.

26 Mai KT, Burns BF. Development of dysplastic mucinous epithelium from endometriosis of the appendix. *Histopathology*, 1999; 35: 368.

27 Blackshear WM Jr. Malakoplakia of the appendix: a case report. *Am J Clin Pathol*, 1970; 53: 284.

PART

6 Large intestine

33 Normal large intestine

Knowledge of the anatomy of the colon and rectum is of importance to the diagnostic pathologist, providing the baseline from which the abnormal can be observed to deviate. This statement is especially pertinent today in view of the ever-increasing availability of techniques to probe cell structure and function. When investigating disease processes one must always be mindful of the normal organization of tissues, distribution of cells and expression of cell products. These may be influenced by anatomical region, genetic and racial heterogeneity, age, sex and iatrogenic factors.

Anatomical relationships and gross appearance

The large intestine is approximately 150 cm in length from the lower pole of the caecum to the anus. Its transverse diameter is much greater than that of the small bowel, but like the latter it diminishes continuously towards its distal end, except for the dilation known as the rectal ampulla. The colon is divided into the caecum, which is that part below a horizontal line across the bowel at the level of the ileocaecal valve; the ascending colon that extends from this line to the hepatic flexure; the transverse colon from the hepatic to the splenic flexure; and the descending colon from the splenic flexure to that point where the colon crosses the brim of the pelvis. The sigmoid colon extends from the latter point to the rectosigmoid junction, which is arbitrarily but usefully defined as being opposite the promontory of the sacrum.

The large bowel is invested by peritoneum to a variable degree. The caecum is completely invested but the ascending colon, hepatic flexure and descending colon are covered on their anterior sides only. The transverse and sigmoid colon are completely invested apart from their mesenteric attachments. The rectum is covered by peritoneum on the anterior and lateral sides of the upper third and anteriorly only for its middle third; the lower third is entirely subperitoneal. The colon from the caecum to the rectosigmoid is covered by pouches of fat, the epiploic appendages. The wall of the colon and rectum consists of a mucous membrane, of which the muscularis mucosae is a part, separated from the deep muscle layers or muscularis propria by the submucosal layer of loose connective tissue. The muscularis propria is separated from the peritoneum by the serosa, which contains a variable amount of fat and connective tissue.

The mucous membrane has a smooth surface but careful inspection shows the presence of innumerable furrows known as innominate grooves about 0.5 mm apart and resembling fingerprint dermatoglyphs. These can be appreciated microscopically as clefts between mucosal hillocks.

The muscularis propria consists of two muscle layers each forming a continuous sheath around the bowel, the inner circular muscle and the much thinner outer or longitudinal muscle that is mainly concentrated into three narrow bands or taeniae coli. Their position relative to the circumference of the bowel varies in different segments and they fuse in the region of the rectosigmoid junction and about 15 cm above the peritoneal reflection. Both circular muscle and taeniae coli are thin in the proximal colon and become gradually thicker towards the rectosigmoid junction.

The taeniae coli are generally credited with the function of shortening the colon because they are about one-sixth shorter than the intestine to which they belong and consequently the circular muscle is puckered into sacculations and haustral clefts. Some haustra are permanent, especially those in the proximal colon where the circular muscle is thinnest. Others, mostly in the left colon, are produced by active muscle contraction. The mucosa is thrown into transverse folds, the plicae semilunares, as a result of this longitudinal shortening. The plicae are gathered along three longitudinal parallel lines, representing the midpoints of the taeniae. These lines are typically the sites of ulceration in ulcerative colitis. The taeniae seem to act not only as shortening bands but also as strong longitudinal cables upon which the circular muscle is fixed. The muscle fibres of the circular layer and the taeniae coli are intimately mixed and this linkage is sufficiently strong to allow the circular muscle points of purchase on the taeniae for contraction [1]. There is a very considerable amount of elastic tissue in the muscularis propria and this increases with age [2]. These observations on the anatomy of the colon muscle and haustra are relevant to the pathogenesis of diverticular disease of the colon (see p. 457).

The rectum has complete layers of circular and longitudinal muscle but the latter has anterior and posterior thickenings which cause some shortening and give rise to the three lateral flexures with their corresponding crescentic shelves composed of circular muscle and mucous membrane known as the valves of Houston.

Blood supply

The ileocolic, right colic and middle colic branches of the superior mesenteric artery supply the colon from the caecum to the splenic flexure. The remainder of the colon is supplied by the inferior mesenteric artery through its left colic and sigmoid branches. The rectum is supplied by the superior rectal branch of the inferior mesenteric artery, the middle rectal arteries from the internal iliac vessels and the inferior rectal arteries from the internal pudendal vessels [3]. There is a continuous marginal artery along the mesenteric border of the colon that is of great surgical importance. This vessel is often small in the region of the splenic flexure [4], which accounts for the precariousness of the blood supply to this part of the colon. The blood supply to the colon pierces the muscularis propria through well defined defects in the muscle and enters the submucosal layer from which a network of capillaries ramifies in the mucous membrane. It is through the same defects that mucosal sacs herniate in diverticular disease.

The arteries are accompanied, as components of neurovascular bundles, by veins, lymphatics and nerves. These bear the same names as the arteries. The veins form a well developed submucosal plexus and another, less well developed plexus outside the muscularis propria. They are tributaries of the portal system. Portal–systemic anastomoses occur by communication of the superior rectal with the middle and inferior rectal veins.

Lymphatic drainage

The lymph nodes of the large intestine can be divided into those that lie close to the bowel wall (the paracolic and pararectal nodes) and those that follow the course of the blood supply. The lymph vessels of the caecum and ascending colon pass through nodes along the course of the ileocolic and right colic vessels; those in the transverse colon through nodes along the middle colic artery; and those from the descending and sigmoid colon through nodes along the left colic and sigmoid arteries which join the main stream of lymph vessels from the upper rectum along the course of the superior rectal artery. The lymphatic drainage of the lower rectum is through the nodes along the superior rectal artery, and through nodes along the middle rectal vessels to the internal iliac nodes and, to a much lesser extent, to the inguinal nodes probably via presacral lymphatics.

Nerve supply

Important insights into the organization of the enteric nervous system have been made recently. It used to be thought that the gut was regulated by opposing excitatory (sympathetic) and inhibitory (sympathetic) systems, with the central nervous system being the seat of control and integration. It is now understood that the intrinsic enteric nervous system provides the major controlling network. This may be readily appreciated by observing the co-ordinated peristaltic movements of denervated colon.

As in the rest of the gut, the nerve supply to the large intestine may be divided into extrinsic and intrinsic components [5]. The extrinsic supply comprises the two arms of the autonomic nervous system, sympathetic and parasympathetic. The parasympathetic supply is via the vagus for the proximal colon and via sacral spinal nerves for the distal colon and rectum. The preganglionic fibres terminate in the myenteric plexus between the longitudinal and circular muscle coats. The nerves contain afferent as well as efferent fibres, the former being essential for the completion of reflex loops. The sympathetic supply is through lower thoracic spinal nerves that mainly end in the superior mesenteric ganglion and lumbar spinal nerves that end in the inferior mesenteric ganglion. These prevertebral ganglia lie closer to the spinal cord than the colon. From them the postganglionic fibres terminate in either the myenteric (Auerbach's) or submucosal (Meissner's) plexus. Like the parasympathetic nerves, sympathetic nerves also contain afferent fibres whose cell bodies may reside either within the wall of the bowel (e.g. acting as mechanoreceptors) or within the dorsal root ganglia of the spinal cord. These will complete short and long reflex loops, respectively. The smooth muscle of the internal anal sphincter is supplied by both sympathetic and parasympathetic fibres.

The myenteric and submucosal plexuses together comprise a network of intercommunicating ganglia. Within each ganglion are nerve (ganglion) cell bodies, nerve processes and glia (Fig. 33.1). Most of the direct innervation of the smooth muscle of the bowel wall is through the intrinsic neurones of the two plexuses. Excitatory neurones are mainly cholinergic whereas the inhibitory neurones are non-adrenergic non-cholinergic (NANC) [6]. Neurones innervating smooth muscle directly

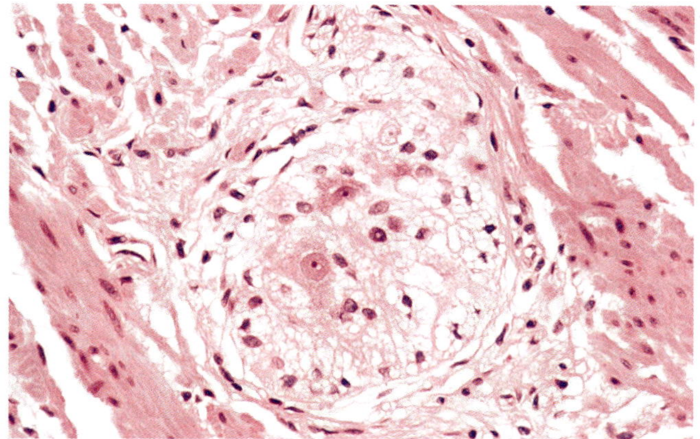

Fig. 33.1 Ganglion of myenteric plexus comprising glia and nerve (ganglion) cell bodies. The latter have abundant cytoplasm and a vesicular nucleus with a prominent nucleolus.

are in turn driven, inhibited or modulated by intrinsic interneurones or extrinsic parasympathetic fibres. The neurotransmitter associated with inhibitory NANC neurones may be vasoactive intestinal polypeptide, whereas substance P has been proposed as an alternative excitatory neurotransmitter to acetylcholine [7]. The list of putative neurotransmitters or coneurotransmitters also includes adenosine triphosphate [6], 5-hydroxytryptamine [8], enkephalin [9], somatostatin and nitric oxide [10]. The neurones of the myenteric plexus were formerly classified according to whether or not they were argyrophil and cholinesterase positive [11]. These classical studies show no clear correlation with modern functional classifications in which neurotransmitters are identified immunohistochemically and ultrastructurally [12]. More details on the enteric nervous system may be found in a monograph [13].

Individual smooth muscle cells are not supplied by nerve terminals. Nerve processes with bead-like varicosities surround groups of muscle fibres, and neurotransmitters are released into tissue spaces to reach target cells by diffusion. Electrical coupling from cell to cell is achieved through the junctional complexes which are of three types—interdigitations, gap junctions (nexuses) and intermediate junctions [14].

Physiology

The functions of the colon are complex and not completely understood [15]. The essential function is to receive the fluid chyme from the small intestine and by extracting water prepare the faeces for defecation at a socially acceptable time and at the discretion of the individual. Although the colon is an important site for absorption of electrolytes and water, it can also secrete fluid, particularly under pathological conditions [16]. Diarrhoea should not be viewed simply as a failure to absorb [17].

The different regions of the large bowel subserve different functions. Fluid chyme entering the right colon is altered both by absorption of fluid and electrolytes and by the fermentative breakdown of carbohydrate into short-chain fatty acids. Most of the carbohydrate will be derived from plant cell walls ('fibre') and undigested starch. These substrates are converted by anaerobic bacteria into butyric, propionic and acetic acid [18]. Short-chain fatty acids function as anions in fluid and electrolyte balance [19] and as an important energy source for colorectal epithelium [20]. The transverse and descending colon serve mainly as organs of storage and propulsion. Little or no absorption takes place in the sigmoid colon and rectum, the latter region being important in the control of continence.

The normal person has an evacuation about once a day, but the limits of normal seem to vary between three per day and three per week. In healthy individuals the rectum is normally empty and the desire to defecate occurs only as a result of movements of the colon causing faeces to enter the rectum. The faeces leave the rectum as the result of contraction of the distal large bowel aided by straining which causes an increase in abdominal pressure and by relaxation of the anal sphincters. Movements of the colon can be divided into intermittent muscular activity of a segmental type, which results in to-and-fro contractions over a short distance, and mass peristalsis, which probably accounts for the passage of faeces along the colon.

The study of transit times has shown that food residue may remain in the colon from meals taken as much as a week previously, but most is evacuated within 4 days. It is likely that segmental activity is responsible for impeding transit and mixing of the faeces. However, radiological studies have shown that the progression of radio-opaque markers is surprisingly smooth. In diarrhoea there is, paradoxically, a great decrease in muscular activity of the colon whereas in constipation it is often increased. The movements of the colon are influenced by many factors of which the most important are eating, posture, colonic distension, hormones, drugs and emotion. The so-called gastrocolic reflex is the mass movement occurring after meals, which provokes a desire to defecate. Interestingly this will occur without the presence of a stomach. Much remains to be learned about colonic motility and the physiology of the smooth muscle of the large intestine in health and disease. There are conditions (such as diverticular disease, the irritable bowel syndrome, ulcerative colitis and various forms of megacolon) which may be due, at least partly, to abnormal muscle or neuromuscular function. Until more is known of normal physiological processes in the colon it will be difficult to unravel the pathogenesis of these conditions.

Histology

The mucosa

Although there has been little study of the dissecting microscope appearances of the mucosal surface of the colon and rectum over the years [21], this is becoming increasingly important in both research and practice. The high resolution and magnification achieved through modern videoendoscopy allows the surface microanatomy to be studied *in situ* [22]. The orifices of the crypts can be seen as regularly spaced round depressions of uniform size. These are surrounded by interconnecting furrows, delimiting the areae colonicae of the mucosal surface (Fig. 33.2). Within the areae colonicae, a honeycomb pattern is formed by the vascular network surrounding the crypt orifices [23]. Characteristic alterations in the normal surface topography have been described in hyperplastic polyps, tubular adenomas and villous adenomas [22,24]. More recently, attention has focused on aberrant crypt foci and microadenomas, in both experimental models [25] and humans [26].

The large intestinal mucosa as seen by the light microscope is composed of epithelial tubules embedded in a connective tissue framework (the lamina propria) and resting on the muscularis mucosae (Fig. 33.3). The latter is composed of longitudinal, transverse and oblique muscle fibres that are pierced by the small vessels supplying the mucous membrane. Lymphatics have been described within the muscularis mucosae, but very few appear to pass into the lamina propria [27]. This may explain why neoplastic lesions confined to the mucosa are never associated with lymph node metastasis. The only other structures which interfere with the continuity of the muscularis mucosae are foci of lymphoid tissue which lie astride it and cause its fibres to become splayed out. These dome-like aggregates of gut-associated lymphoid tissue (GALT) have been described as lymphoglandular or lymphoepithelial complexes as they are associated with a specialized form of surface and crypt epithelium (dome epithelium) which participates in the translocation of antigenic material from the bowel lumen [28,29]. Dome epithelium comprises colonocytes and specialized columnar cells called M cells [29,30]. Antigenic material is modified by cathepsin E and passed in pinocytotic vesicles to the invaginating lymphoid cells [31]. M stands for 'microfold' which refers to folds of the apical membrane resembling short microvilli. M also stands for 'membranous' which describes the thin rim of M-cell cytoplasm overlying evaginating lymphocytes (T and B) and dendritic cell process (Fig. 33.4) [32,33].

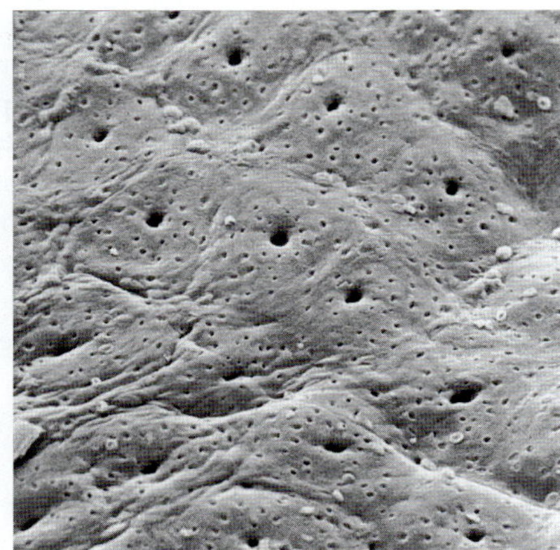

Fig. 33.2 Scanning electron micrograph of surface of large bowel mucosa. The large depressions are the openings of crypts. Furrows delineate the areae colonicae. The small openings are the mouths of goblet cells.

The lymphoglandular complexes extend into the submucosa and it is important that the presence of epithelium within such structures is not misinterpreted as malignant invasion. This can easily occur when the lymphoglandular complex epithelium becomes dysplastic (e.g. in ulcerative colitis) and sections are cut tangentially. Lymphoglandular complexes are normally located within the clefts (innominate grooves) between mucosal hillocks. B lymphocytes are found in the

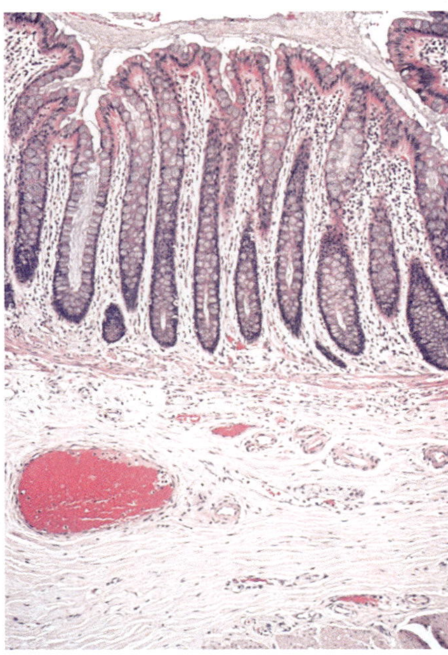

Fig. 33.3 Normal large bowel mucosa.

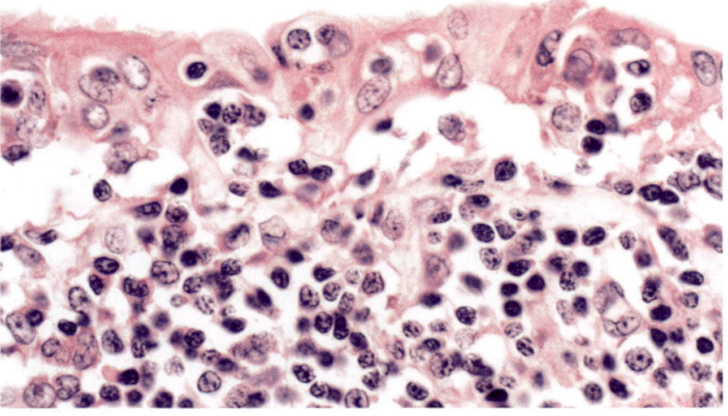

Fig. 33.4 Dome epithelium of lymphoglandular complex showing intraepithelial lymphocytes within M cells.

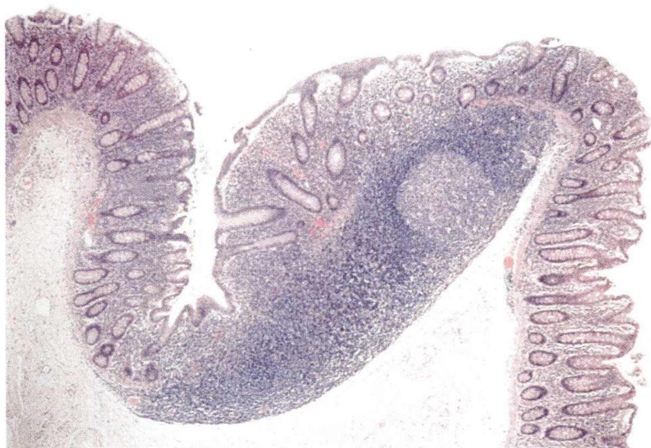

Fig. 33.5 Lymphoglandular complex with germinal centre formation.

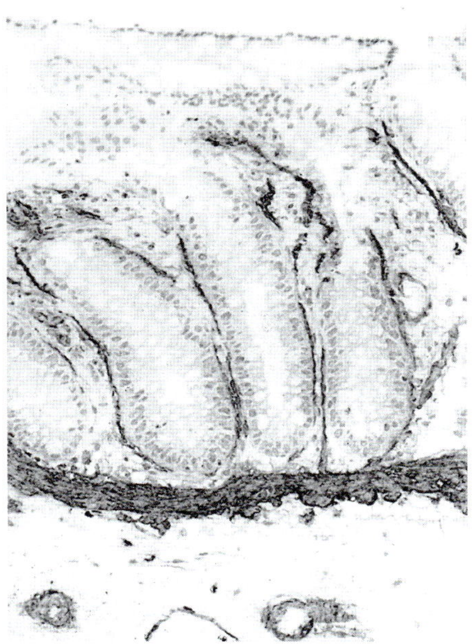

Fig. 33.6 Immunoperoxidase demonstration (monoclonal antibody PR2D3) of smooth muscle cells of the pericryptal sheath, muscularis mucosae and blood vessel walls.

central and subepithelial zones and T lymphocytes are found in the peripheral rim. In the normal adult colon germinal centre formation is evident in approximately 1% of lymphoglandular complexes (Fig. 33.5), but this figure rises to about 10% in inflammatory bowel disease and carcinoma of the large bowel [29]. Lymphoglandular complexes attain their largest size in young children and adolescents. In some young patients they may be so prominent that a state of 'lymphoid polyposis' is present (see p. 611). It is important to recognize this as a benign condition, probably of a viral aetiology, and unrelated to malignant lymphoma. The number of lymphoglandular complexes steadily increases from the caecum to the rectum [34,35] and they are particularly noticeable just above the dentate line of the anal canal ('anal tonsils').

The connective tissue or lamina propria of the colonic mucosa is composed of a stroma of argyrophilic (reticulin) fibres containing fibroblasts, lymphocytes, plasma cells, mast cells, eosinophils, and macrophages. Very few neutrophils are seen except within capillaries. Lymphocytes are predominantly T cells and plasma cells mainly produce immunoglobulin A (IgA), though IgM and IgG isotypes are represented [36]. It is generally believed that plasma cells are not seeded directly into the lamina propria from the lymphoepithelial complexes, but that transformed B cells mature whilst migrating via lymphatics and the circulatory system, before finally homing back to the lamina propria. This mechanism, based on studies of Peyer's patches in laboratory animals, would serve to increase the sphere of influence of a clone of transformed B cells [37]. In humans such a process may apply only to IgA-producing cells, with other idiotypes being seeded directly into the lamina propria [36]. Doubts have been raised as to whether even IgA immunocytes enter such a cycle in humans [38]. These issues are of importance and warrant further research. Such studies, for example, have provided insight into the pathogenesis and anatomical distribution of intestinal lymphoma. It is clear that the colon, like the rest of the gastrointestinal tract, is an important lymphoid organ whose functional organization is comparable to that of other organs in which mucosa and lymphoid tissue come into intimate contact. The number of leucocytes in the lamina propria varies greatly under normal conditions. The experience of looking at normal mucosa is essential if subjective assessments of the state of the lamina propria are to be reasonably accurate. Morphological studies may be useful in this context.

The epithelial component of the colonic and rectal mucosa consists of straight, perpendicular tubules or crypts, which lie strictly parallel and close to one another and do not exhibit any branching (Fig. 33.3). There are no villi and the crypt and surface epithelium are one cell thick. It has been shown recently that the crypts are ensheathed by smooth muscle cells or myofibroblasts (Fig. 33.6) [39] rather than by fibroblasts. This pericryptal sheath is unlikely to be an inert scaffold, but may serve to propel the secreted contents of distended crypts into the bowel lumen. Contraction of the smooth muscle sheath may possibly be mediated by 5-hydroxytryptamine released by immediately subjacent crypt enterochromaffin cells [39]. The suggestion that the pericryptal cells migrate from the crypt base to the luminal surface in company with the migration of epithelial cells [40] has not been confirmed.

Four main cell types are represented within the crypt and surface epithelium. First, and most numerous, are the columnar cells, outnumbering mucin-distended goblet cells by at least 3 : 1 [41]. The crypt columnar cells are compressed inconspicuously between goblet cells and therefore appear less numerous than they in fact are. The structure and function of the columnar cell is altered as it leaves the crypt to occupy the surface epithelium (Fig. 33.7). Crypt columnar cells have a pri-

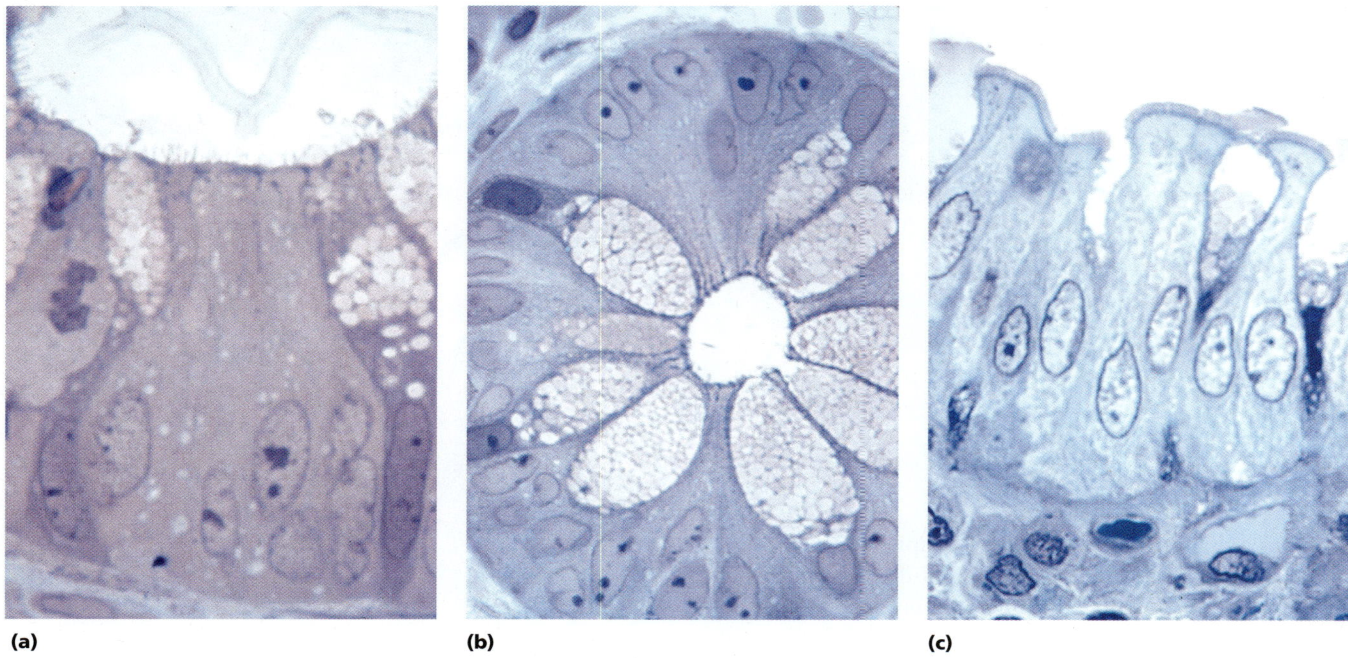

Fig. 33.7 Semithin sections (toluidine blue stain) to show (a) crypt base, (b) midcrypt and (c) surface epithelium. Within the crypt base (a) are differentiating, vacuolated columnar cells with scalloped, vesicular nuclei and immature goblet cells with condensed chromatin. A mitotic figure is shown. Within the midcrypt (b) several immature columnar cells are compressed between mature goblet cells containing pale mucin droplets. The surface epithelium (c) includes senescent goblet cells and columnar cells with a well developed microvillous brush border.

marily secretory role elaborating secretory component which participates in the epithelial translocation of IgA [42], and glycoproteins that are destined to form the glycocalyx or fuzzy coat [43,44], as well as being involved in the cellular movement of water and electrolytes. Surface columnar cells function as absorptive units and are characterized by a well developed microvillous brush border and a relatively filled-out cytoplasm as compared to their crypt counterparts. The surface columnar cells are homologues of the columnar cells lining small intestinal villi, but are less well endowed with brush border enzymes [45]. Paneth cells with large, supranuclear eosinophilic granules are the third cell type; they are normally limited to the right colon. Endocrine cells with small, subnuclear eosinophilic granules are the fourth type of epithelial cell. They are more common in the rectum than the colon and secrete enteroglucagon, neurotensin, somatostatin, vasoactive intestinal polypeptide-like peptide and 5-hydroxytryptamine [46,47]. It is now accepted that the four end-cells (columnar, goblet, Paneth and endocrine) are derived from a common stem cell and that the latter reside at or near the crypt base [48,49]. Furthermore, the entire cellular population of a crypt is clonal and maintained by a single stem cell [50–52]. However, mathematical models of crypt cell kinetics provide evidence of small numbers of stem cells per crypt [53], possibly organized into a stem cell 'niche' [80], or at least a population of cells with an extended half-life [54].

Semithin sections (Fig. 33.7) and ultrastructural studies have provided useful insights into the organization of the crypt cell populations [55,56]. Undifferentiated cells and cells in the earliest stages of differentiation are found in the lower third of the crypt. Undifferentiated cells have a relatively pale or electron lucent cytoplasm containing mitochondria, free ribosomes and polysomes and glycoprotein-containing vacuoles in the apical and supranuclear cytoplasm. Stubby microvilli bearing glycocalyceal material arise from the apical cell membrane. The nucleus is large and scalloped and contains finely dispersed heterochromatin and a large nucleolus. The foregoing features and the presence of a Golgi apparatus indicate that these cells are not truly undifferentiated. As differentiation continues the cytoplasmic vesicles become larger and more numerous. These cells have been termed differentiating cells [55], intermediate cells [56] and, in species other than humans, vacuolated-columnar cells [57]. In spite of this sign of cytoplasmic maturation these cells retain the ability to replicate. Most are probably destined to become columnar cells [57]. Certainly the nuclear and cytoplasmic features of the vacuolated intermediate cells are more akin to columnar cells than goblet cells [56]. In the middle and upper third of the crypt the structural dichotomy of columnar cells and goblet cells is complete. However, whereas goblet cells are fully mature and distended with mucus at this stage, the final form of the columnar cell is not attained until it migrates from the crypt to the surface. Its functions then switch from secretory to absorptive and this is accompanied by the development of a well formed microvillous brush border. The suggestion that surface columnar cells represent goblet cells that have discharged their mucus [58] cannot be sustained. The glycoprotein secretions within the crypt columnar cells of the left and right colon differ in their electron density. In the right colon the material is electron dense and in the left colon it is electron lucent [58]. This may be related to the differing blood group antigen expression of secreted glycoproteins in the left and right colon (see below).

The mucin histochemistry of large bowel epithelium has been studied intensively, particularly in the last few years with the increasing availability of new probes including lectins and monoclonal antibodies of defined specificities [59]. Mucins are glycoprotein macromolecules formed by the sequential addition of monosaccharides into chains that are attached to a polypeptide backbone [60]. Genes coding for the polypeptide component (apomucin) have been cloned and monoclonal antibodies to the repetitive amino acid sequences specific to various apomucins are available. Goblet cells secrete MUC1, MUC2, MUC3 and MUC4 mucin, with MUC2 predominating (Fig. 33.8) [61–63]. Columnar cells secrete MUC1, MUC3 and MUC4, MUC1 being restricted to the crypt base [61,63,64]. The histochemical reactivity of the carbohydrate component of epithelial mucus is determined by the more peripheral sugars since these will be accessible to specific reagents. Neutral sugars include fucose, N-acetyl galactosamine, N-acetyl glucosamine and galactose. Sialic acid is an acid sugar and acidity may also be conferred by the addition of sulphate ester, either to sialic acid or to a neutral sugar. It is an oversimplification to refer to mucins as either neutral or acidic. Reactive neutral sugars are

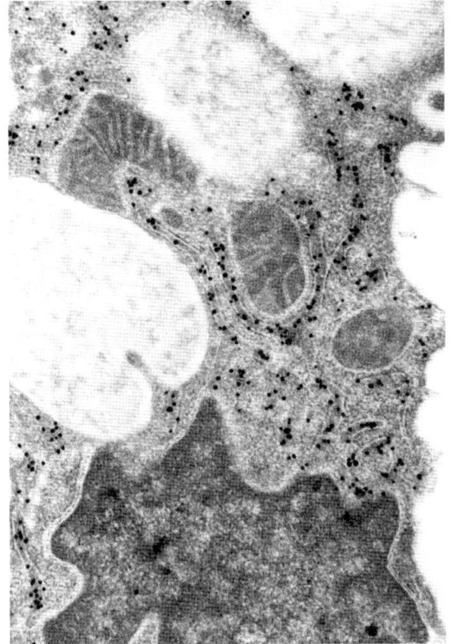

Fig. 33.8 Demonstration of MUC2 (MoAb 3A2) within rough endoplasmic reticulum of goblet cells (immunogold electron microscopy).

present in all mucins, but in colorectal goblet cell mucus sialic acid is well represented as a peripheral sugar within the saccharide chain. Nevertheless, the presence of neutral sugars is appreciated by the diastase/PAS (periodic acid–Schiff) reaction associated with colorectal goblet cells. This relatively weak PAS reaction may be confirmed as due to neutral sugars by blocking the Schiff effect with phenylhydrazine. More specifically, fucose can be detected, at least in the proximal colon, by means of the lectin derived from *Ulex europaeus* (UEA-1) [65]. Similarly, fucose-rich blood group substances are expressed by the mucous secretions of the proximal colon [66]. Lectins with an affinity for N-acetyl galactosamine, such as *Dolichos biflorus* agglutinin (DBA), will also bind to goblet cell mucus [67,68]. DBA shows a pancolorectal pattern of binding, but limited to goblet cells within the upper crypt and surface epithelium [59]. Galactose can be demonstrated by means of the lectin peanut agglutinin (PNA), but only following the removal of terminal sialic acid with neuraminidase.

Sialic acid within mucus of the large bowel shows O-acetyl substitution of the sidearm (C7, 8 and 9) and/or at position C4. These modifications render colonic sialic acid resistant to the bacterial enzyme neuraminidase (sialidase). However, in 9% of Caucasians and 40% of Sino-Japanese individuals sialic acid does not show O-acetyl substitution, being instead structurally similar to sialic acid within the proximal small intestine [69,81]. This heterogeneity is genetic in origin, but there is no evidence that subjects with the non-O-acetylated form of sialic acid are at increased risk of colorectal disease [69]. It is important to heed this constitutional variation when studying the acquired loss of O-acetyl substituents that occurs in such diseases as colorectal cancer [69] or ulcerative colitis [70]. Furthermore, O-acetylation influences the antigenicity of sialic acid [71,72].

It is possible to demonstrate focal (usually unicryptal) alterations in sialic structure by both conventional mucin histochemistry and immunohistochemistry [69,73,74] (Fig. 33.9). As the change affects all the goblet cells within a crypt, it is probably caused by a stem cell mutation implicating the gene that codes for O-acetyl transferase (OAT). However, as this would be a mutation at the somatic level, only heterozygous individuals (OAT+/OAT–) would be implicated, i.e. it is far less likely that the same mutation would occur twice within a single stem cell of a homozygous subject (OAT+/OAT+). The demonstration of unicryptal alterations is of considerable interest as it corroborates animal studies that have shown that all cells within a crypt are maintained by a single stem cell [51,73].

The goblet cell has at least one function over and above the secretion of mucus, namely the secretion of the proteolytic enzyme kallikrein [75]. This enzyme may have a cytoprotective function and has also been implicated in the transport of electrolytes.

The submucosa

This is composed of collagen and reticulin fibres, blood

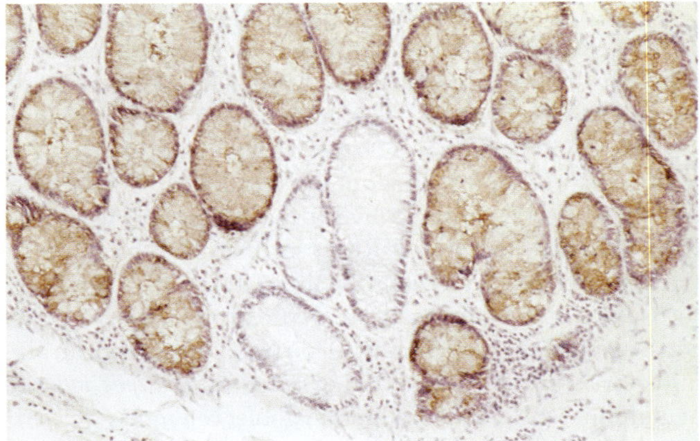

(a)

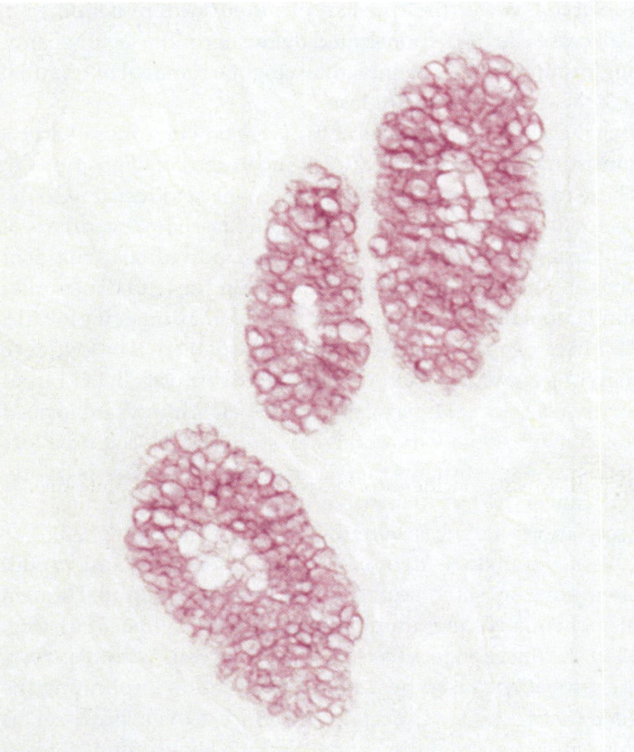

(b)

Fig. 33.9 (a) With monoclonal antibody PR3A5, which recognizes a colon-specific form of O-acetyl sialic acid, single crypts may contain unreactive goblet cell mucus (immunoperoxidase). (b) The same goblet cells give a positive result with mild PAS, which stains N-acetyl but not O-acetyl sialic acid.

vessels, lymphatics and nerves as well as small groups of ganglion cells, most of which lie just beneath the muscularis mucosae in the superficial submucosa. It is normal to find a little adipose tissue in the submucosa but this can be greatly increased in pathological conditions such as the defunctioned bowel. There is a well developed plexus of thin-walled veins in the submucosa, which can be seen through the mucous membrane at sigmoidoscopy.

The value of scanning electron microscopy is illustrated by a study of the histology of the large intestinal submucosa using this technique [76]. This showed that the submucosal collagen is a pliable network of fibres that is arranged differently at different levels. There is a fine reticular pattern of collagen close to the mucosa, a coarse arrangement of fibres beneath this, and a loose reticular pattern of thick fibres adjacent to the circular muscle layer. It is interesting that this arrangement of collagen is similar to that in the skin. The strength, natural tension and extensibility of the submucosa is a reflection of the physical properties of collagen and its arrangement in the form of a pliable honeycomb through which the vascular channels pass. This has surgical importance in the provision of a layer able to hold sutures during the construction of an intestinal anastomosis.

The muscularis propria

The circular muscle layer is divided into bands of smooth muscle cells separated by connective tissue, including collagen and elastic fibres. These bands are divisible into smaller units, the fasciculi, of which there are about four to six in each band. There are no connective tissue septa between the fasciculi. Dissection studies have shown that the circular muscle is an expanding meshwork of interlinked bundles [1]. The muscle of the longitudinal layer, particularly the taeniae coli, is extremely tough and contains more collagen and elastic tissue than the circular muscle. Smooth muscle cells are spindle-shaped and covered by a thin basement membrane. At the cell surface are caveolae or pinocytotic invaginations that may be associated with the smooth endoplasmic reticulum. These are probably involved with Ca^{2+} transport. Within the cytoplasm are thin (actin) and thick (myosin) contractile filaments. Dense bands are present, but without the regular organization of striated muscle. Cytoskeletal intermediate filaments (desmin) anchor the condensations of dense material on the cytoplasmic side of the intermediate junctions. Cell to cell electrical coupling is achieved through the intermediate junctions and other types of junctional complexes known as interdigitations and gap junctions (nexuses) [14].

The muscularis propria is pierced at regular intervals by the main arterial supply and venous drainage of the mucous membrane. Between the two layers is the myenteric plexus, whose structure and organization has been described above. Situated between the smooth muscle fasciculi and the nerves of the myenteric plexus are the interstitial cells of Cajal, spindle-shaped cells with several long, anastomosing processes. They are thought to be the pacemaker cells of the gut musculature [77,78] and stain for CD34 and CD117 (c-kit) [79].

The serosa

The serosa is a thin sheet of connective tissue containing blood vessels and lymphatics and covered by the peritoneum, a layer of flattened mesothelium resting upon a well developed elastic lamina.

References

1 Pace JL, Williams I. Organisation of the muscular wall of the human colon. *Gut*, 1969; 10: 352.

2 Pace JL. The anatomy of the haustra of the human colon. *Proc R Soc Med*, 1968; 61: 934.

3 Griffiths JD. Extramural and intramural blood supply of the colon. *Br Med J*, 1961; i: 323.

4 Griffiths JD. Surgical anatomy of the blood supply of the distal colon. *Ann R Coll Surg*, 1956; 19: 241.

5 Baumgarten HG. Morphological basis of gastrointestinal motility: structure and innervation of gastrointestinal tract. In: Bertaccini G, ed. *Mediators and Drugs in Gastrointestinal Motility I. Morphological Basis and Neurophysiological Control*. New York: Springer-Verlag, 1982.

6 Burnstock G. Autonomic innervation and transmission. *Br Med J*, 1979; 35: 255.

7 Furness JB, Costa M. Identification of gastrointestinal neurotransmitters. In: Bertaccini G, ed. *Mediators and Drugs in Gastrointestinal Motility I. Morphological Basis and Neurophysiological Control*. New York: Springer-Verlag, 1982.

8 Gershon MD, Erde SM. The nervous system of the gut. *Gastroenterology*, 1981; 80: 1571.

9 Hoyle CHV, Burnstock G, Jass JR, Leonard-Jones JE. Enkephalins inhibit non-adrenergic, non-cholinergic neuromuscular transmission in the human colon. *Eur J Pharmacol*, 1986; 131: 159.

10 Boeckxstaens GE, Pelckmans PA, Herman AG, Van Maercke YM. Involvement of nitric oxide in the inhibitory innervation of the human isolated colon. *Gastroenterology*, 1993; 104: 690.

11 Smith B. Disorders of the myenteric plexus. *Gut*, 1970; 11: 271.

12 Burnstock G. Ultrastructural identification and neurotransmitters. *Scand J Gastroenterol*, 1981; 16: 1.

13 Furness JB, Costa M. *The Enteric Nervous System*. Edinburgh: Churchill Livingstone, 1987.

14 Gabella G. Smooth muscle cell junctions and structural aspects of contraction. *Br Med Bull*, 1979; 35: 213.

15 Moran BJ, Jackson AA. Function of the human colon. *Br J Surg*, 1992; 79: 1132.

16 Asakura H, Yoshioka M. Cholera toxin and diarrhoea. *J Gastroenterol Hepatol*, 1994; 9: 186.

17 Phillips SF. Functions of the large bowel: an overview. In: Polak JM, Bloom SR, Wright NA, Butler AG, eds. *Basic Science in Gastroenterology. Physiology of the Gut*. Glaxo Group Research Ltd, Royal Postgraduate Medical School, 1984: 283.

18 Cummings JH. Colonic absorption; the importance of short chain fatty acids in man. In: Polak JM, Bloom SR, Wright NA, Butler AG, eds. *Basic Science in Gastroenterology. Physiology of the Gut*. Glaxo Group Research Ltd, Royal Postgraduate Medical School, 1984: 371.

19 Roediger WEW, Moore A. Effect of short chain fatty acid on sodium absorption in isolated human colon perfused through the vascular bed. *Dig Dis Sci*, 1981; 26: 100.

20 Roediger WEW. Anaerobic bacteria support the metabolic welfare of the colonic mucosa in man. *Gut*, 1980; 21: 793.

21 Fabrini A, Torsoli A, Allessandrini A *et al*. Surface microscopy of the large bowel. *Separatum Experientia*, 1966; 22: 408.

22 Jaramillo E, Watanabe M, Slezak P, Rubio C. Flat neoplastic lesions of the colon and rectum detected by high-resolution video endoscopy and chromoscopy. *Gastrointest Endosc*, 1995; 42: 114.

23 Bank S, Cobb JS, Burns DG, Marks IN. Dissecting microscopy of rectal mucosa. *Lancet*, 1970; i: 64.

24 Thompson JJ, Enterline HT. The macroscopic appearance of colorectal polyps. *Cancer*, 1981; 48: 151.

25 McLellan EA, Bird RP. Aberrant crypts: potential preneoplastic lesions in the murine colon. *Cancer Res*, 1988; 48: 6187.

26 Roncucci L, Stamp D, Medline A, Cullen JB, Bruce WR. Identification and quantification of aberrant crypt foci and microadenomas in the human colon. *Hum Pathol*, 1991; 22: 287.

27 Fenoglio CM, Kaye GI, Lane N. Distribution of human colonic lymphatics in normal, hyperplastic and adenomatous tissue. *Gastroenterology*, 1973; 64: 51.

28 Kealy WF. Lymphoid tissue and lymphoid glandular complexes of the colon: relation to diverticulosis. *J Clin Pathol*, 1976; 29: 245.

29 O'Leary AD, Sweeney EC. Lymphoglandular complexes of the colon: structure and distribution. *Histopathology*, 1986; 10: 267.

30 Jacob E, Baker SJ, Swaminathan SP. 'M' cells in the follicle associated epithelium of the human colon. *Histopathology*, 1987; 11: 941.

31 Finzi G, Cornaggia M, Capella C *et al*. Cathepsin E in follicle associated epithelium of intestine and tonsils: localization to M cells and possible role in antigen processing. *Histochemistry*, 1993; 99: 201.

32 Gebert A, Rothkötter H-J, Pabst R. M cells in Peyer's patches of the intestine. *Int Rev Cytol*, 1996; 167: 91.

33 Neutra MR. Current concepts in mucosal immunity v. role of M cells in transepithelial transport of antigens and pathogens to the mucosal immune system. *Gastrointest Liver Physiol*, 1998; 37: G785.

34 Dukes C, Bussey HJR. The number of lymphoid follicles of the human large intestine. *J Pathol Bacteriol*, 1926; 29: 111.

35 Traill MA. The incidence of lymphoid foci in the large intestine. *Med J Aust*, 1976; ii: 809.

36 Bjerke K, Brandtzaeg P, Rognum TO. Distribution of immunoglobulin producing cells is different in normal human appendix and colon mucosa. *Gut*, 1986; 27: 667.

37 Parrott DMV. The gut-associated lymphoid tissues and gastrointestinal immunity. In: Ferguson A, MacSween RNM, eds. *Immunological Aspects of the Liver and Gastrointestinal Tract*. Lancaster: MTP, 1976.

38 Spencer J, Finn T, Issacson PG. Human Peyer's patches: an immunohistochemical study. *Gut*, 1986; 27: 405.

39 Richman PI, Tilly R, Jass JR, Bodmer WF. The colonic pericrypt sheath: characterisation of cell type with a novel monoclonal antibody. *J Clin Pathol*, 1987; 40: 593.

40 Pascal RR, Kaye GI, Lane N. Colonic pericryptal fibroblast sheath: replication, migration and cytodifferentiation and mesenchymal cell system in adult tissue I and II. *Gastroenterology*, 1968; 54: 852.

41 Cheng H, Bjerknes M, Amar J. Methods for the determination of epithelial cell kinetic parameters of human colonic epithelium isolated from surgical and biopsy specimens. *Gastroenterology*, 1984; 86: 78.

42 Brandtzaeg P. Human secretory component VI immunoglobulin-binding properties. *Immunochemistry*, 1977; 14: 179.

43 Michaels JE. Glycoprotein containing vesicles in the surface epithelial cells of the ascending colon of the rat. *Anat Rec*, 1977; 188: 525.

44 Thomopoulous GN, Schulte BA, Spicer SS. The influence of embedding media and fixation on the postembedment ultrastructural demonstration of complex carbohydrates, I. Morphology and periodic acid–thiocarbohydraxide–silver proteinate staining of vicinal diols. *Histochem J*, 1983; 15: 763.

45 Abe M, Ohuchi N, Sakano H. Enzyme histo- and biochemistry of intestinalized gastric mucosa. *Acta Histochem Cytochem*, 1974; 7: 282.

46 Bloom SR, Polak JM. *Gut Hormones*. Edinburgh: Churchill Livingstone, 1981.

47 Sjöjund K, Sandén GH, Håkanson R, Sundler F. Endocrine cells in human intestine: an immunocytochemical study. *Gastroenterology*, 1983; 85: 1120.

48 Cheng H, Leblond CF. Origin, differentiation and renewal of the four main epithelial cell types in the mouse small intestine V. Unitarian theory of the origin of the four epithelial cell types. *Am J Anat*, 1974; 141: 537.

49 Garcia SB, Park HS, Novelli M, Wright NA. Field cancerization, clonality, and epithelial stem cells: the spread of mutated clones in epithelial sheets. *J Pathol*, 1999; 187: 61.

50 Griffiths DFR, Davies SJ, Williams D, Williams GT, Williams ED. Demonstration of somatic mutation and colonic crypt clonality by X-linked enzyme histochemistry. *Nature*, 1988; 333: 461.

51 Campbell F, Fuller CE, Williams GT, Williams ED. Human colonic stem cell mutation frequency with and without irradiation. *J Pathol*, 1994; 174: 175.

52 Endo Y, Sugimura H, Kino I. Monoclonality of normal human colonic crypts. *Pathol Int*, 1995; 45: 602.

53 Loeffler M, Birke A, Winton D, Potten C. Somatic mutation, monoclonality and stochastic models of stem cell organisation in the intestinal crypt. *J Theor Biol*, 1993; 160: 471.

54 Bjerknes M, Cheng H. Clonal analysis of mouse intestinal epithelial progenitors. *Gastroenterology*, 1999; 116: 7.

55 Lorenzsonn V, Trier JS. The fine structure of human rectal mucosa. The epithelial lining of the base of the crypt. *Gastroenterology*, 1968; 55: 88.

56 Kaye GI, Fenoglio CM, Pascal RR, Lane N. Comparative electron microscopic features of normal, hyperplastic and adenomatous human colonic epithelium. *Gastroenterology*, 1973; 64: 926.

57 Chang WWL, Leblond CP. Renewal of the epithelium in the descending colon of the mouse. I. Presence of three cell populations: vacuolated-columnar, mucous and argentaffin. *Am J Anat*, 1971; 131: 73.

58 Shamsuddin AM, Phelps PC, Trump BF. Human large intestinal epithelium: light microscopy, histochemistry and ultrastructure. *Hum Pathol*, 1982; 13: 790.

59 Jass JR, Roberton AM. Colorectal mucin histochemistry in health and disease: a critical review. *Pathol Int*, 1994; 44: 487.

60 Hounsell EF, Feizi T. Gastrointestinal mucus. Structures and antigenicities of their carbohydrate chains in health and disease. *Med Biol*, 1982; 60: 227.

61 Chang S-K, Dohrman AF, Basbaum CB *et al*. Localization of mucin (MUC2 and MUC3) messenger RNA and peptide expression in human normal intestine and colon cancer. *Gastroenterology*, 1994; 107: 28.

62 Ogata S, Uehara H, Chen A, Itzkowitz SH. Mucin gene expression in colonic tissues and cell lines. *Cancer Res*, 1992; 52: 5971.

63 Winterford CM, Walsh MD, Leggett BA, Jass JR. Ultrastructural localization of epithelial mucin core proteins in colorectal tissues. *J Histochem Cytochem*, 1999; 47: 1063.

64 Ajioka Y, Allison LJ, Jass JR. Significance of MUC1 and MUC2 mucin expression in colorectal cancer. *J Clin Pathol*, 1996; 49: 560.

65 Yonezawa S, Nakamura T, Tanaka S, Sato E. Glycoconjugate with *Ulex europaeus* agglutinin-I-binding site in normal mucosa, adenoma and carcinoma of the human large bowel. *J Natl Cancer Inst*, 1977; 69: 777.

66 Denk H, Tappeiner S, Holzner JH. Blood group substances (BGS) as carcinofetal antigens in carcinomas of the distal colon. *Eur J Cancer*, 1974; 10: 487.

67 Boland CR, Montgomery CK, Kim YS. Alterations in human colonic mucin occurring with cellular differentiation and malignant transformation. *Proc Natl Acad Sci USA*, 1982; 79: 2051.

68 Jass JR, Allison LJ, Stewart SM, Lane MR. *Dolichos biflorus* agglutinin binding in hereditary bowel cancer. *Pathology*, 1994; 26: 110.

69 Sugihara K, Jass JR. Heterogeneity of colorectal goblet cell mucus and its relation to neoplastic disease. *J Pathol*, 1986; 148: 83.

70 Jass JR, England J, Miller K. Value of mucin histochemistry in follow up surveillance of patients with long standing ulcerative colitis. *J Clin Pathol*, 1986; 39: 393.

71 Jass JR, Allison LJ, Edgar SG. Distribution of sialosyl Tn and Tn antigens within normal and malignant colorectal epithelium. *J Pathol*, 1995; 176: 143.

72 Ogata S, Ho I, Chen A *et al*. Tumor-associated sialylated antigens are constitutively expressed in normal human colonic mucosa. *Cancer Res*, 1995; 55: 1869.

73 Fuller CE, Davies RP, Williams GT, Williams ED. Crypt restricted heterogeneity of goblet cell mucus glycoprotein in histologically normal human colonic mucosa: a potential marker of somatic mutation. *Br J Cancer*, 1990; 61: 382.

74 Hughes NR, Walls RS, Newland RC, Payne JE. Gland to gland heterogeneity in histologically normal mucosa of colon cancer patients demonstrated by monoclonal antibodies to tissue-specific antigens. *Cancer Res*, 1986; 46: 5993.

75 Schachter M, Peret MW, Billing AG, Wheeler GD. Immunolocalization of the protease kallikrein in the colon. *J Histochem Cytochem*, 1983; 31: 1255.

76 Lord MG, Valies P, Broughton AC. A morphologic study of the submucosa of the large intestine. *Surg Gynecol Obstet*, 1977; 145: 55.

77 Thomsen TL, Robinson TL, Lee JCF *et al*. Interstitial cells of Cajal generate a rhythmic pacemaker current. *Nat Med*, 1998; 4: 848.

78 Rumessen JJ. Identification of interstitial cells of Cajal. Significance for studies of human small intestine and colon. *Dan Med Bull*, 1994; 41: 275.

79 Sanders KM. A case for interstitial cells of Cajal as pacemakers and mediators of neurotransmission in the gastrointestinal tract. *Gastroenterology*, 1996; 111: 492.

80 Williams ED, Lowes AP, Williams D, Williams GT. A stem cell niche theory of intestinal crypt maintenance based on a study of somatic mutation in colonic mucosa. *Am J Pathol*, 1992; 141: 773.

81 Campbell F, Appleton MAC, Fuller CE *et al*. Racial variation in the O-acetylation phenotype of human colonic mucosa. *J Pathol*, 1994; 174: 169.

34 Normal embryology and fetal development; developmental abnormalities of the large intestine and the anal region

Normal development

Details of normal embryological development are available in standard texts, some of which also describe the more common aberrations which can occur [1,2]. Many of the papers describing individual anomalies cited below also give a detailed account of the relevant normal development.

Proximal large intestine

The caecum, appendix, ascending colon and a variable length of the transverse colon are of midgut origin. Originally they share a mesentery with the small intestine, derive their blood supply from the superior mesenteric artery and are included in the physiological herniation and return of the midgut between the 6th and 10th weeks (see Chapter 19). The further development of the caecum and appendix is described in Chapter 29. The mesentery attached to the caecum and ascending colon is normally absorbed after they return to the abdomen, anchoring them to the posterior abdominal wall, while the transverse colon retains its mesentery.

Distal large intestine

The descending and sigmoid colons, the rectum and the upper two-thirds of the anal canal are derived from the hindgut and are supplied by the inferior mesenteric artery. Anastomoses between superior and inferior mesenteric arteries are not well developed and the splenic flexure can be a relatively poorly vascularized zone.

Anorectal region

During the 4th to 5th week the hindgut, allantois and urogenital tract end in a common *cloaca* lined by endoderm. The ventral cloacal wall is formed by the cloacal membrane, which is bounded on its external (ectodermal) aspect by the genital swellings and folds. A vertical partition, the *urorectal septum*, develops in the angle between the allantois and the hindgut and grows transversely and caudally, separating a *urogenital sinus* ventrally from the developing rectum dorsally; it fuses caudally with the cloacal membrane, thus dividing it into dorsal and ventral parts (Fig. 34.1). Two *anal tubercles* develop beneath the ectoderm posterior to the ventral cloaca and fuse with the urorectal septum to form the *proctodeum;* here the ectoderm and the endoderm are in direct contact. The proctodeum is later invaded by mesoderm that will form the external anal sphincter. The whole mass then moves backwards and grows inwards to fuse with the rectum as a solid plug, the future anus; it canalizes during the 3rd month.

Microscopic appearances

At the 20-mm stage, villous structures resembling those in the developing small bowel are found throughout the large bowel; as growth proceeds they thicken, shorten and gradually disappear with the development of the mucosal crypts. Brush border enzyme systems begin to develop at about 8 weeks in oral–anal direction [3]. Tubular glands grow outwards from the cloacogenic zone of the anal canal and penetrate through the submucosa into the internal sphincter.

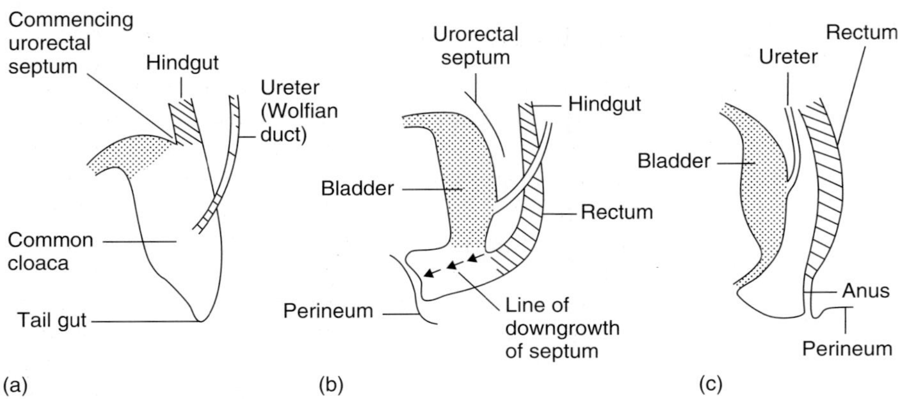

Fig. 34.1 Development of normal rectum and bladder from cloaca.

Malpositions

Most malpositions of large intestine are consequent on malrotation of the small bowel occurring at the time when the contents of the physiological hernia return to the alimentary cavity in the 10th–11th week (see p. 253). The small bowel may come to lie superficial to the transverse colon, which then usually passes through an aperture in the mesentery; the caecum and ascending colon often retain their mesentery and are not anchored to the posterior abdominal wall. If the small bowel fails to rotate, the caecum may lie in the left iliac fossa or in the midline, in which case both it and the ascending colon retain a mesentery and the ascending colon is connected to a normal descending colon by a shortened transverse length; the whole bowel from duodenum to splenic flexure is then supported by a single mesentery with a narrow base, prone to volvulus [1,4]. Among the more common minor anomalies is failure of absorption of the caecal and ascending colonic mesentery with development of fibrous bands between colon and abdominal wall; these can cross and compress the duodenum or upper jejunum, leading to high intestinal obstruction, the cause of which may not be obvious at laparotomy. A useful general review is available [5].

Vestigial remnants

At the 4–6-mm stage, the embryo possesses a definite tail that has totally regressed by the 30–35-mm stage. During the formation of the cloacal septum, a small part of the distal hindgut becomes separated and lies isolated as the *tailgut*; it has normally disappeared by the 8-mm stage. Microscopically a number of types of epithelium can be recognized, including mucin-containing cells, but muscle coats are not present although there may be clumps of smooth muscle cells [6]. A number of postanal cysts without muscle coats and lined by a variety of epithelial cells, including squamous and columnar cells, sometimes ciliated, have been described [6], and carcinomatous epithelial changes have been reported in them [6]. They are probably of tailgut origin.

Maldevelopments

Atresias and stenoses

Atresia (absence of bowel lumen) and stenosis (narrowing of bowel lumen) are extremely rare in the caecum, colon and upper rectum; we know of one example in the colon [7] and of a congenital diaphragm in the upper rectum [8].

Atresia and stenosis of the lower rectum and anal canal occur about once in every 5000 births. A number of different classifications exist [9,10]; an international one has been suggested and is reproduced in Table 34.1; the important differentiation appears to be between 'high' and 'low' anomalies, that is, those above and below the pelvic floor [9,10]. In the high anomalies there is often a considerable gap between the lower end of the rectum and the anal canal, which is usually normally formed, and fistulae between the rectum and some part of the urogenital apparatus are relatively common. In males these are usually rectourethral or rectourethral and rectovesical, and the anus is usually normal; in females they are rectovaginal, rectovestibular or rectoperineal and anal stenosis is not uncommon [11]. Occasional cases of persistent cloaca occur in association with multiple anomalies which are usually inoperable [12,13].

Duplications, diverticula and cysts

Duplications

These are extremely uncommon in the large bowel. There is compete or partial formation of a second tube with its own mucosa and submucosa but often with incomplete separation of muscle coats; the duplicated segment is always on the mesenteric aspect of the normal bowel. Examples are described in caecum, transverse colon, rectum and anus [14], and there are more complex examples associated with duplications in the

Table 34.1 Anorectal anomalies: a suggested international classification.

Male	Female
1 Low (translevator)	
(a) *At normal anal site*	(a) *Same*
(i) Anal stenosis	(i) Same
(ii) Covered anus: complete	(ii) Same
(b) *At perineal site*	(b) *Same*
(i) Anocutaneous fistula (covered anus: incomplete)	(i) Same
(ii) Anterior perineal anus	(ii) Same
	(c) *At vulvar site*
	(i) Anovulvar fistula
	(ii) Anovestibular fistula
	(iii) Vestibular anus
2 Intermediate	
(a) *Anal agenesis*	(a) *Same*
(i) Without fistula	(i) Without fistula
(ii) With fistula (rectobulbar)	(ii) With fistula (rectovestibular; rectovaginal: low)
(b) *Anorectal stenosis*	(b) *Same*
3 High (supralevator)	
(a) *Anorectal agenesis*	(a) *Same*
(i) Without fistula	(i) Without fistula
(ii) With fistula (rectourethral; rectovesical)	(ii) With fistula (rectovaginal high; rectocloacal; rectovesical)
(b) *Rectal atresia*	(b) *Same*
4 Miscellaneous	*Same*
Imperforate anal membrane	
Cloacal extrophy	
Others	

From [10].

urinary and genital tracts [15]. Triplications have been described [16]. Squamous cell [17] and adenocarcinoma [18] have been recorded as complications and it is possible that some of the anorectal 'fistulae' in which adenocarcinomas have occurred may in fact represent duplications [19].

Diverticula

Congenital diverticula are very rare in the large bowel [20] and when present in the rectum can be associated with vertebral anomalies. They commonly have a more or less complete covering of all bowel coats.

Cysts

Developmental cysts localized within the bowel wall are extremely rare [21]; many of them almost certainly represent remnants of the tailgut [22] (see above).

Heterotopia and metaplasia

Heterotopic tissue is rare in the large bowel and is usually associated with malformations such as duplications, diverticula or cysts. Every example that we have seen has been in the rectum, which agrees with the findings of others [23–25], though occasional examples are reported in the colon [26,27]. Virtually all the epithelia described are gastric in type and the difficulty is in knowing whether this is heterotopic or metaplastic. Points in favour of a heterotopia are the presence of more than one type of epithelium or of full-thickness and perfectly structured fundic mucosa; the presence of appreciable pyloric-type mucosa suggests an acquired lesion [23]. Pancreatic elements are occasionally seen [28]. Gastric mucosa in the rectum presents endoscopically as a well demarcated area of granularity or as a polypoid lesion.

Disturbances of innervation

New insight into the innervation of the gut has broadened our understanding of Hirschsprung's disease and of many related disorders.

In the complete absence of a nerve supply, bowel muscle will still contract, but not in a co-ordinated fashion; an intact nervous system is needed for co-ordinated peristalsis. This system has three components: a sympathetic and a parasympathetic inflow and a widespread intrinsic peptidergic system that allows much more local control of bowel movement than earlier workers appreciated [29]. Within the bowel wall there are two plexuses of ganglion cells and neurones, a submucosal and a myenteric, which are more independent of each other than has been sometimes realized. The myenteric plexus contains ganglia in which are two types of neurone: argyrophil cells which have well stained nerve processes, many of which are multiaxonal and branch frequently, terminate on other argyrophil and on argyrophobe cells, but do not supply muscle fibres directly; and argyrophobe cells which are acetylcholinesterase (AChE) positive and have axons, some of which appear to end directly on muscle fibres. The myenteric nerve trunks are made up of axons from the argyrophil cells and extrinsic nerve fibres. These are of two kinds: sympathetic (which show catecholamine fluorescence and end around neurones) and parasympathetic (which end on intrinsic neurones which are probably all argyrophilic) [30]. All the intrinsic neurones and nerve fibres are probably peptidergic, non-adrenergic and non-cholinergic, and this system can function autonomously; substance P and enkephalin probably act as excitatory factors in the myenteric plexus while vasoactive intestinal polypeptide (VIP), which is mainly located in the submucosal plexus, is probably inhibitory. It appears that nerve cells and fibres which are cholinergic are actually responsible for muscle contraction, and that cells and fibres which are adrenergic and sympathetic or peptidergic and intrinsic exert a controlling influence [31].

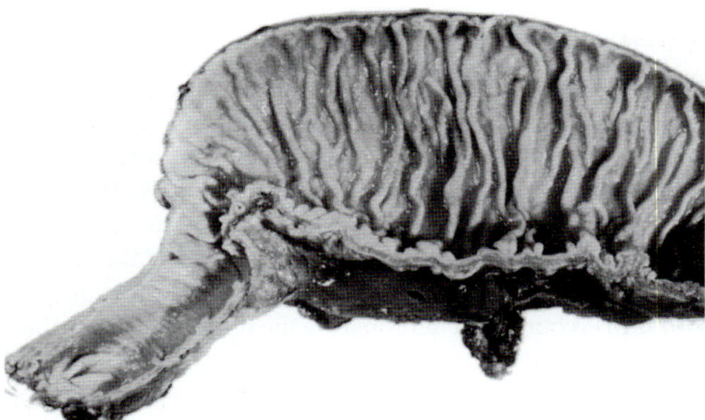

Fig. 34.2 Resected rectum and sigmoid colon in Hirschsprung's disease, showing the narrowed aganglionic distal segment on the left, and the dilated normally innervated proximal bowel on the right.

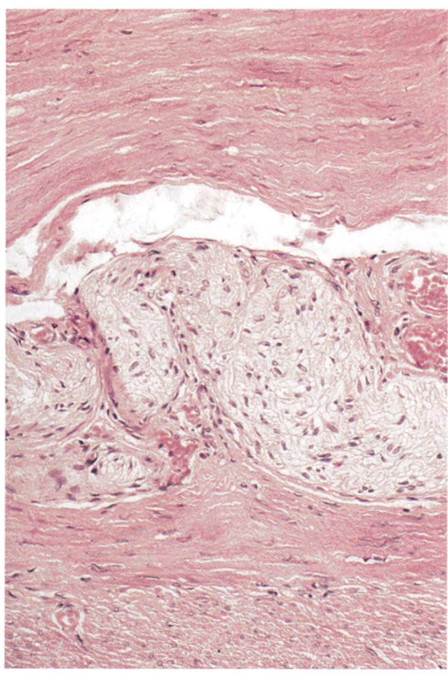

Fig. 34.3 Myenteric plexus in Hirschsprung's disease. The enlarged wavy nerve trunks without ganglion cells are well shown.

It is clear that if the account given above is correct, any factors that damage these nerve cells or fibres or interfere with their development can disturb gut motility and lead to chronic constipation or diarrhoea. A number of syndromes are being recognized in which different components of the systems are damaged; they are discussed below.

Hirschsprung's disease

Over one hundred years ago Hirschsprung first described a condition in children in which a widely dilated and hypertrophied colon ended in a narrowed segment of rectum that extended to the anus [32]. It occurs once in every 20 000–30 000 live births [33] and is six to nine times more common in boys than in girls. There is evidence for a familial incidence but most cases are sporadic [34]. At least three genes have been implicated, including the tyrosine kinase receptor Ret [35], endothelin receptor B and its ligand endothelin 3 (EDN3) [36]. Ten per cent of all cases occur in children with Down's syndrome and 5% of cases are associated with other congenital abnormalities [37]. Most patients present in infancy with constipation and gaseous abdominal distension, and repeated episodes of intestinal obstruction are common. There may be an accompanying colitis which can be severe, leading to perforation. Others present with persistent constipation in later childhood or even adulthood [38]. On clinical examination the anus is normal while the anal canal and a variable length of affected rectum are small and empty. At the junction of the diseased and unaffected bowel, the enormously dilated proximal part empties into the contracted lower segment in a funnel-shaped manner (Fig. 34.2). In virtually all cases the narrowed segment extends proximally from the anus. Its length varies. In one large series of 1560 cases [39], 53.8% involved rectum and sigmoid, 25.6% had ultrashort segments and 20.6% were so-called 'long segment' in that they extended proximal to the sigmoid and some involved the whole large and sometimes the small bowel.

Microscopically, in the classical disease and using conventionally stained sections, there are two principal abnormalities in the affected bowel. The first is a total absence of ganglion cells in both the submucosal and myenteric plexuses. The second is the presence of increased numbers of enlarged wavy nerve trunks, most conspicuous in the myenteric plexus but present also in the submucosa (Figs 34.3 & 34.4). Muscle coats are essentially normal, and inflammatory changes, if present, are secondary. Some children show a form of arteritis that may present as intimal or adventitial fibroplasia or medial fibromuscular dysplasia [39]. At the junction of the narrowed affected bowel with the normal is a transitional zone of variable length in which occasional ganglion cells are present and in which the nerve fibres have a more normal appearance, although some thickening and waviness persists [40]. Until histochemical techniques became available diagnosis was either by a full-thickness biopsy which included the myenteric plexus or by submucosal biopsy which allowed assessment of the submucosal plexus only.

Techniques using methods to demonstrate cholinesterase render submucosal biopsies much simpler to interpret. They also reveal the presence of fine cholinergic nerve fibres extending through the muscularis mucosae into the lamina propria [40–43]; these fibres are greatly increased in number, thicker and more tortuous in Hirschsprung's disease (see Figs 2.7 & 2.10) and in many workers' opinion are sufficiently

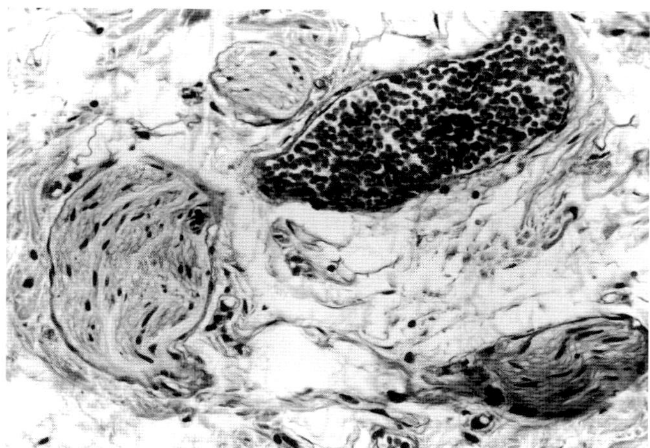

Fig. 34.4 Submucosal plexus in Hirschsprung's disease. The nerves are less enlarged than in the myenteric plexus but are still larger than normal and a wavy pattern is evident.

characteristic to allow diagnosis on mucosal punch biopsy (see below). If these fibres are present the diagnosis is reasonably certain, but if they are absent and the clinical picture is suggestive, a submucosal biopsy should be taken. The advent of immunocytochemical techniques for demonstrating peptidergic nerves and nerve cells [44] has shown that in Hirschsprung's disease substance P and VIP are both diminished. The number of enteroglucagon- and somatostatin-containing cells in the mucosa is also reduced [44]; this may be a secondary effect.

The pathogenesis of Hirschsprung's disease is not fully understood. There is a failure of migration of neurones from the neural crest that would normally form the intrinsic nervous system [39,40]. Possible explanations could be a primary shortage of neuroblasts, failure of neuroblast survival during the process of migration or a defect in microenvironment sensing following successful migration. A number of nerve growth factors are critical for this process, including glial cell line-derived neurotrophic factor (GDNF), which is the ligand for Ret, and EDN3. Disruption of these genes or genes implicated in the associated cell signalling pathways could result in apoptotic deletion of the neuroblasts [36]. Whatever the mechanism, the loss of neuroblasts results in secondary hyperplasia and ingrowth of preganglionic fibres which can be visualized through the AChE technique [40].

Allied Hirschsprung's disorders

This term covers a number of conditions in which patients have had all or some of the clinical features of Hirschsprung's disease but in whom at least some ganglion cells have been found on biopsy and abnormal nerve trunks are not always present. The nature of some of them is becoming clearer and their classification is now possible [45].

Hypoganglionosis

A number of neonates with symptoms suggestive of Hirschsprung's disease have a reduction in the number of ganglion cells immediately above the dentate line; there are no abnormal AChE-positive fibres in the lamina propria in early biopsies, though these appear in some patients by the age of 9 months [45,46]. Appearances closely resemble those seen in the transitional zone of Hirschsprung's disease and hypoganglionosis may represent a form of Hirschsprung's disease. A deficiency of c-kit-positive pacemaker cells of Cajal has been described in hypoganglionosis, neuronal intestinal dysplasia and subjects with immature ganglia [47].

Zonal aganglionosis

Patients have been described in whom there are zones of aganglionosis, usually narrow, with normal ganglion cells above and below the zones [39,48–50]; in these zones abnormal nerve trunks can also be present [50,51].

Other forms

Hirschsprung-like syndromes have also been described in patients who on investigation have hyperplasia of ganglion cells in submucosal and muscle coats [50] along with the formation of giant ganglia and the presence of occasional ganglion cells in the lamina propria [52]. Occasional patients with apparently immature ganglion cells are also described [45]. This rare condition is described as neuronal intestinal dysplasia or hyperganglionosis [53].

Diagnostic techniques for Hirschsprung's disease and allied disorders

Ideally, the maximum information would be gained from a full-thickness biopsy and the application of the AChE technique. It is usually necessary to examine multiple levels to confirm the presence or absence of ganglion cells. In practice, diagnosis of Hirschsprung's disease, but not of the related conditions, can be made on mucosal biopsies using the AChE technique to demonstrate abnormal nerve fibres ramifying within the lamina propria [40]. This technique has to be performed on frozen sections, but is superior to immunoperoxidase methods (e.g. PGP 9.5 or S-100) [54]. Detailed studies of normal and abnormal biopsies have shown AChE to be reliable, except when biopsies are taken within 1 cm of the dentate line (due to the normal paucity of ganglion cells in this region). A positive finding is diagnostic, but a negative one does not exclude a neuronal abnormality and full-thickness biopsy is then necessary [41,55,56]. This technique may fail in the case of ultrashort segment Hirschsprung's disease when one may need to rely on manometry and clinical history. Intraoperative frozen section biopsies may be taken to confirm the presence of ganglion cells. Again, it will usually be necessary to examine multiple levels.

References

1 Synder WH. The embryology of the alimentary tract with special emphasis on the colon and rectum. *Surg Gynecol Obstet*, 1958; 106: 311.

2 Willis RA. *The Borderland of Embryology and Pathology*, 2nd edn. London: Butterworths, 1962.

3 Lacroix B, Kedinger M, Simon-Assman P *et al*. Developmental patterns of brush border enzymes in the human fetal colon. Correlation with some morphological events. *Early Hum Dev*, 1984; 9: 95.

4 Thorlakson PHT, Monie IW, Thorlakson TK. Anomalous peritoneal encapsulation of small intestine; report of 3 cases. *Br J Surg*, 1953; 40: 490.

5 Filston HC, Kirk DR. Malrotation: the ubiquitous anomaly. *J Pediatr Surg*, 1981; 16: 614.

6 Marco V, Autonell J, Farre J, Fernandez-Layos M, Doncel F. Retrorectal cyst hamartomas. Report of two cases with adenocarcinoma developing in one. *Am J Surg Pathol*, 1982; 6: 707.

7 Peck DA, Lynn HB, Harris LE. Congenital atresia and stenosis of the colon. *Arch Surg*, 1963; 87: 428.

8 Cole GJ. Congenital diaphragm in the upper rectum. *Br J Surg*, 1963; 50: 523.

9 Partridge JP, Gough MH. Congenital abnormalities of the anus and rectum. *Br J Surg*, 1961; 49: 37.

10 Santulli TV, Keisewetter WB, Bill AH Jr. Anorectal anomalies: a suggested international classification. *J Pediatr Surg*, 1970; 5: 281.

11 Chatterjee SK. Double termination of the alimentary tract—a second look. *J Pediatr Surg*, 1980; 15: 623.

12 Koffler H, Aase JM, Papile LuA, Coen RW. Persistent cloaca with absent penis and anal atresia in one of idential twins. *J Pediatr*, 1978; 93: 821.

13 Williams DA, Weiss T, Wade E, Dignan P. Prune perineum syndrome: report of a second case. *Teratology*, 1983; 28: 145.

14 Teja K, Geissinger WT, Shaw A. Duplication of the transverse colon. Report of a case. *Dis Colon Rectum*, 1975; 18: 430.

15 Beach PD, Brascho DJ, Hein WR, Nichol WW, Geppert LJ. Duplications of the primitive hindgut of the human being. *Surgery*, 1961; 49: 779.

16 Ravitch MM. Hindgut duplication—doubling of colon and of genital and lower urinary tracts. *Ann Surg*, 1953; 137: 588.

17 Hickey WF, Corson JM. Squamous cell carcinoma arising in a duplication of the colon; case report and literature review of malignancy complicating colonic duplication. *Cancer*, 1981; 47: 602.

18 Weitzel RA, Breed JR. Carcinoma arising in a rectal duplication (enterocystoma). *Ann Surg*, 1963; 157: 476.

19 Jones EA, Morson BC. Mucinous adenocarcinoma in anorectal fistulae. *Histopathology*, 1984; 8: 279.

20 Morison JE. Giant congenital diverticula and neonatal rupture of colon: a case associated with true congenital partial hypertrophy of the crossed type. *Arch Dis Child*, 1944; 19: 135.

21 Singh S, Minor CL. Cystic duplication of the rectum. A case report. *J Pediatr Surg*, 1980; 15: 205.

22 Caropreso PR, Wengert PA Jr, Milford HE. Tailgut cyst—a rare retrorectal tumour. Report of a case and review. *Dis Colon Rectum*, 1975; 18: 597.

23 Wolf M. Heterotopic gastric epithelium in the rectum. *Am J Clin Pathol*, 1971; 55: 604.

24 Picard EJ, Picard JJ, Jorissen J, Jardon M. Heterotopic gastric mucosa in the epiglottis and rectum. *Am J Dig Dis*, 1978; 23: 217.

25 Debas HT, Chaun H, Thomson FB, Soon-Shiong P. Functioning heterotopic oxyntic mucosa in the rectum. *Gastroenterology*, 1980; 79: 1300.

26 Dubilier LD, Caffrey PR, Hyde GL. Multifocal gastric heterotopia in a malformation of the colon presenting as a megacolon. *Am J Clin Pathol*, 1969; 51: 646.

27 Taylor FM, Swank RI. Epithelial heterotopia in the colon of a child; a case presentation and review of the literature. *J Fla Med Assoc*, 1982; 69: 788.

28 Willis RA. Some unusual developmental heterotopias. *Br Med J*, 1968; iii: 627.

29 Bishop AE, Ferri G-L, Probert L, Bloom SR, Polak JM. Peptidergic nerves. *Scand J Gastroenterol*, 1982; 17: 43.

30 Smith B. The neuropathology of pseudo-obstruction of the intestine. *Scand J Gastroenterol*, 1982; 17: 103.

31 Goyal RK, Hirano I. The enteric nervous system. *N Engl J Med*, 1996; 334: 1106.

32 Hirschsprung H. Stuhltragheit Neugeborener in Folge von Dilatation und Hypertrophic des Colons. *J Kinderheilk*, 1888; 27: 1.

33 Bodian M, Carter CO, Ward BCH. Hirschsprung's disease. *Lancet*, 1951; i: 302.

34 Bodian M, Carter CO. A family study of Hirschsprung's disease. *Ann Hum Genet*, 1963; 26: 261.

35 Edery P, Lyonnet S, Mulligan LM *et al*. Mutations of the RET proto-oncogene in Hirschsprung's disease. *Nature*, 1994; 367: 378.

36 Wartiovaara K, Salo M, Sariola H. Hirschsprung's disease genes and the development of the enteric nervous system. *Ann Med*, 1998; 30: 66.

37 Blisard KS, Kleinman R. Hirschsprung's disease: a clinical and pathological overview. *Hum Pathol*, 1986; 17: 1189.

38 Wu JS, Schoetz DJ Jr, Coller JA, Veidenheimer MC. Treatment of Hirschsprung's disease in the adult. Report of five cases. *Dis Colon Rectum*, 1995; 38: 655.

39 Taguchi T, Tanaka K, Ikeda K. Fibromuscular dysplasia of arteries in Hirschsprung's disease. *Gastroenterology*, 1985; 88: 1099.

40 Meier-Ruge W. Hirschsprung's disease: its aetiology, pathogenesis and differential diagnosis. *Curr Top Pathol*, 1974; 59: 131.

41 Trigg PH, Belin R, Haberkorn S *et al*. Experience with a cholinesterase histochemical technique for rectal suction biopsies in the diagnosis of Hirschsprung's disease. *J Clin Pathol*, 1974; 27: 207.

42 Lake BD, Puri P, Nixon HH, Claireaux AE. Hirschsprung's disease. An appraisal of histochemically demonstrated acetyl cholinesterase activity in suction rectal biopsy specimens as an aid to diagnosis. *Arch Pathol Lab Med*, 1978; 102: 244.

43 Patrick WJA, Besley GTN, Smith II. Histochemical diagnosis of Hirschsprung's disease and a comparison of the histochemical and biochemical activity of acetylcholine. *J Clin Pathol*, 1980; 33: 336.

44 Bishop AE, Polak JM, Lake BD, Bryant MG, Bloom SR. Abnormalities of the colonic regulatory peptides in Hirschsprung's disease. *Histopathology*, 1981; 5: 679.

45 Munakata K, Okabe I, Morita K. Histologic studies of rectocolic aganglionosis and allied diseases. *J Pediatr Surg*, 1978; 13: 67.

46 Scharli AF, Sossai R. Hypoganglionosis. *Semin Pediatr Surg*, 1998; 7: 187.

47 Yamataka A, Ohshiro K, Kobayashi H *et al*. Intestinal pacemaker C-KIT+ cells and synapses in allied Hirschsprung's disorders. *J Pediatr Surg*, 1997; 32: 1069.

48 MacIver AG, Whitehead R. Zonal colonic aganglionosis, a variant of Hirschsprung's disease. *Arch Dis Child*, 1972; 47: 233.

49 Kadair RG, Sims JE, Critchfield CF. Zonal colonic hypoganglionosis. *JAMA*, 1977; 238: 1838.

50 MacMahon RA, Moore CCM, Cussen LJ. Hirschsprung-like syndromes in patients with normal ganglion cells on suction rectal biopsy. *J Pediatr Surg*, 1981; 16: 835.

51 Fu CG, Muto T, Masaki T, Nagawa H. Zonal adult Hirschsprung's disease. *Gut*, 1996; 39: 765.

52 Scharli AF, Meier-Ruge W. Localized and disseminated forms of neuronal intestinal dysplasia mimicking Hirschsprung's disease. *J Pediatr Surg*, 1981; 16: 164.

53 Meier-Ruge WA, Bronnimann PB, Gambazzi F *et al*. Histopathological criteria for intestinal neuronal dysplasia of the submucosal plexus (type B). *Virchows Arch*, 1995; 426: 549.

54 Robey SS, Kuhajda FP, Yardley JH. Immunoperoxidase stains of ganglion cells and abnormal mucosal nerve proliferations in Hirschsprung's disease. *Hum Pathol*, 1988; 19: 432.

55 Chow CW, Chan WC, Yue PCK. Histochemical criteria for the diagnosis of Hirschsprung's disease in rectal suction biopsies by acetylcholinesterase activity. *J Pediatr Surg*, 1977; 12: 675.

56 Venugopal S, Mancer K, Shandling B. The validity of rectal biopsy in relation to morphology and distribution of ganglion cells. *J Pediatr Surg*, 1981; 16: 433.

35 Neuromuscular and mechanical disorders of the large intestine

Diverticular disease of the colon

This is a common and important condition in most Western countries which is responsible for considerable morbidity and has a low, but significant, mortality in the older members of the population.

Terminology

Terminology has been a cause of much confusion. The name diverticulosis is used merely to indicate the presence of multiple diverticula in the large intestine, with or without the accompanying muscle abnormality found in classical diverticular disease, and irrespective of aetiology or symptomatology. Consequently it has no clinical connotation. Diverticular disease, on the other hand, is used to describe a specific clinical disorder with defined radiological and pathological appearances, in which there is a characteristic muscle abnormality, usually, but not invariably, accompanied by the presence of diverticula which may or may not be inflamed. When this muscular abnormality occurs in the absence of established diverticula the term prediverticular disease is sometimes used. Diverticulitis is applied when one or more diverticula are the source of visible macroscopic inflammation. It is often accompanied by pericolic abscess formation.

Incidence

The assessment of incidence of diverticular disease is made difficult because it is not always clear whether individual workers are referring to the incidence of diverticula, inflamed diverticula, muscle abnormality or combinations of these. The frequency of diverticula in Western countries has been calculated from radiological studies [1–6] and at necropsy [7–9]. Probably at least one in three of all persons over 60 years of age have diverticula and the incidence steadily rises with increasing age. In the fifth and sixth decades the condition is present in about one in 10 and below the age of 40 diverticula are rarely seen. Population studies suggest that only 1–2% of individuals with diverticular disease develop symptoms and that only about 0.5% ever require surgery [10], but one study of the natural history of diverticular disease suggests that the disease is complicated by diverticulitis in 10–25% of patients [11]. The disease or its complications was said to account for 4% of all hospital discharges among those aged over 65 in the New England States of the USA in 1980 [12]. Consequently it is responsible for a significant proportion of health care spending in the Western world. There are no major differences in the incidence in males and females.

While diverticula are common in northern Europe, North America and Australia [13,14], they are less numerous in southern Europe and South America, where the population is mainly of Latin origin, and rare in the Middle East, Africa, India and the Orient [12,15]. Indeed, only eight cases were identified in a retrospective review of 6896 autopsies performed over 60 years at one Chinese hospital [16]. There are also variations, both racial and socioeconomic, within national boundaries. Diverticulosis is eight times more common in white persons than among the black population of Johannesburg, where the condition is much more common in urban communities than in rural areas [17]. In Israel it is much more common among the Ashkenazim than in Sephardic and Oriental Jews and Arabs; the incidence is increasing in the latter groups but stable in the Ashkenazic population [18].

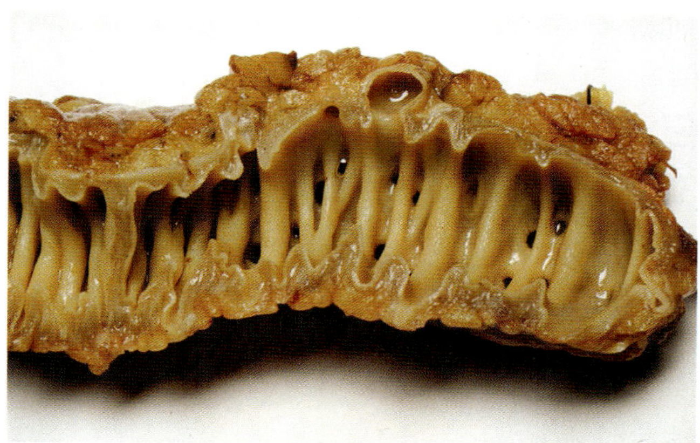

Fig. 35.1 Diverticular disease of colon. Note the concertina-like appearance produced by hypertrophy of the circular muscle coat. The mouths of diverticula lie between the corrugations, reaching the pericolic fat.

Macroscopic and microscopic appearances

The diverticula

From an anatomical point of view diverticula of the colon are of typical pulsion type consisting of a pouch of mucous membrane (including muscularis mucosae) projecting through and beyond the circular muscle layers of the bowel wall so that they come to lie in the pericolic fat and appendices epiploicae. They remain covered by the investing layer of longitudinal muscle, but this is extremely thin. It has been confirmed that the majority of diverticula pass through the bowel wall at weak points in the circular muscle layer through which the main blood vessels pass to supply the colonic mucosa [19]. This is an important anatomical fact, and it is also relevant to the complication of haemorrhage from diverticula of the colon, discussed later. It is usual to find two rows of diverticula, one on each side of the bowel wall between the mesenteric and antimesenteric taeniae [19] (Fig. 35.1). In about 50% of cases a third row of very small diverticula can be found between the two antimesenteric taeniae [20].

Diverticula are most common in the sigmoid part of the colon; indeed they are confined to this segment in the majority of cases. More proximal involvement occurs only when the sigmoid is also affected and always seems to involve the various parts of the proximal colon in continuity; total diverticulosis of the colon is not so very uncommon. The rectum is never involved. Regardless of the length of colon affected the number of diverticula found is variable. They can be very few or present in large numbers. We have seen a few examples of diverticulosis confined to the right colon, but this seems to be a separate condition (see below). So-called diverticula of the rectum are congenital duplications and are unrelated to the condition of diverticular disease of the colon.

The muscle

The muscle abnormality is the most striking and consistent abnormality in diverticular disease of the sigmoid colon [21,22]. The taeniae coli appear thick, assuming an almost cartilaginous consistency in some cases. The circular muscle is also much thicker than normal and has a corrugated or concertina-like appearance (the so-called sawtooth sign on barium enema radiographs). In between these muscular corrugations the mouths of the diverticula are found penetrating the bowel wall to reach the pericolic fat. Sometimes, the bowel wall between the corrugations shows no diverticulum formation but rather a tendency to sacculation. These sacs are outbulgings that retain the circular muscle coat in their walls. In some specimens the mucosal surface between the corrugations appears trabeculated and looks very similar to the trabeculation of the bladder seen in chronic prostatic obstruction. The corrugations are interdigitating processes of circular muscle. If the structure of the bowel is studied in transverse section or by opening longitudinally without bisection it can be seen that these interdigitating processes are not continuous around the circumference of the bowel wall. They are, in fact, semilunar arcs of muscle confined to the zone between the mesenteric and antimesenteric taeniae. Each consists of two layers of circular muscle in apposition. In some specimens of long-standing disease the number of arcs of circular muscle is so great that they appear fused. The circular muscle between the antimesenteric taeniae of the sigmoid shows only small muscle ridges projecting into the lumen of the bowel. The degree of muscular thickening is variable, being particularly obvious in specimens from the sigmoid. It has been suggested that a ridge width of 1.8 mm might be regarded as the dividing line between normal and abnormal [22]. Corrugation is never present to the same degree in other parts of the colon containing diverticula, although slight muscle thickening with an increase in the number of haustral clefts can be seen in the ascending and transverse colon of some specimens.

A considerable excess of fat around the sigmoid colon has been described in many cases of diverticular disease. This has been explained away as a local response to chronic inflammation and to the alleged susceptibility of fat, middle-aged persons to the disease. It is probably more apparent than real and is due to bunching of the pericolic and mesenteric tissues consequent upon shortening of the bowel by muscle contraction.

The muscle abnormality of diverticular disease is recognizable in surgical specimens and at autopsy [9,23]. However, it cannot be well demonstrated unless the colon is distended with formalin under pressure for purposes of fixation and then cut longitudinally when the abnormality is seen to correlate very well with the appearance in barium enema radiographs [24,25]. Occasionally, the muscle abnormality is seen in the absence of diverticula [26,27], a fact which is important in the pathogenesis of diverticular disease. Histologically, the

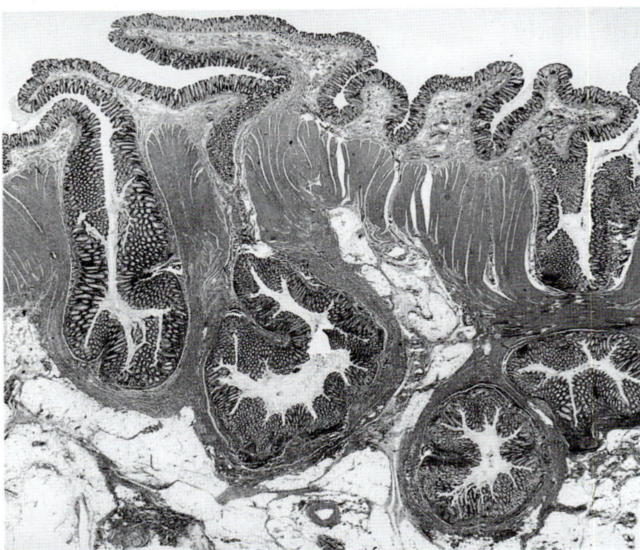

Fig. 35.2 Diverticular disease of sigmoid colon showing mucosal redundancy, thickened circular muscle coat and extramural diverticula still bounded by the longitudinal muscle coat.

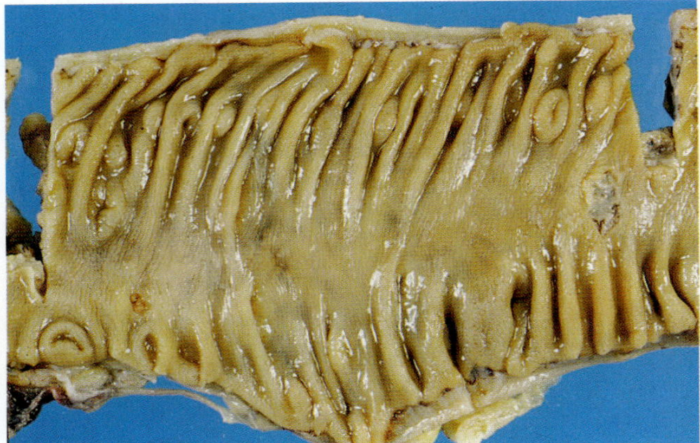

(a)

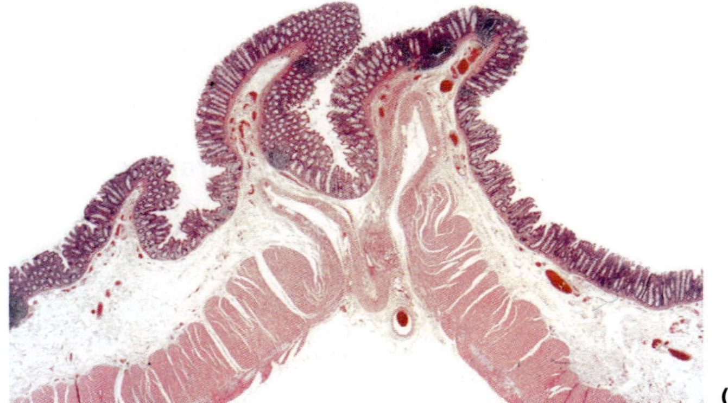

(b)

Fig. 35.3 (a) Nipple-like tags of mucosa formed by everted colonic mucosal diverticula. (b) Histological appearances of everted diverticulum (a 'pseudopolyp').

muscle in diverticular disease shows thickening but no evidence of hyperplasia or hypertrophy of muscle cells [28,29]. The circular muscle is broken up into well demarcated fasciculi separated from one another by loose connective tissue that is probably only an exaggeration of the normal structure (Fig. 35.2). In the longitudinal taeniae, however, there is a significant increase in both coarse and fine elastic fibres which distorts the normal fascicular pattern [29]. This elastosis of the taeniae appears to be an early manifestation of diverticular disease, being consistently found in uncomplicated cases, and may even be the primary lesion. It has been suggested that contraction of the elastic fibres produces shortening of the taeniae and consequently is responsible for the concertina-like corrugation of the circular muscle [29]. There does not seem to be any abnormality of the submucosal and myenteric nerve plexuses in diverticular disease. Although there may appear to be some excess of nervous tissue this is likely to be due to shortening of the bowel rather than to any true thickening of nerve trunks or an increase in neuronal numbers.

The mucosa

In the absence of complications, particularly inflammation, the diverticula themselves have a lining of colonic mucous membrane which is entirely normal apart from an increase in size and number of lymphoid follicles which are especially prominent if a faecolith is present. This excess of lymphoid tissue is probably a response to faecal stasis within the diverticulum, analogous with the appendix. Sometimes diverticula can become everted, the result being nipple-like tags of redundant mucosa on the mucosal lining of the colon, which can be mistaken for polyps and could, indeed, truly be described as 'pseudopolyps' (Fig. 35.3a.b). These tags are also often composed of entirely normal mucosa. A further distinctive feature of some specimens of diverticular disease of the sigmoid and, to a lesser extent of prediverticular disease, is the way the lumen of the bowel is filled with redundant folds of mucous membrane, gathered as a result of shortening of the bowel by muscle contraction. The lumen may be so obliterated by these folds of mucosa that it is difficult to pass even a narrow probe from one end of the specimen to the other. The luminal narrowing cannot be described as a stricture but the folds add to the stenosis caused by the muscle thickening. Hence, diverticular disease is a common cause of intestinal obstruction and features of obstructive colitis are frequently found in the proximal mucosa (see pp. 525 and 545).

The mucosa of the gathered folds may be subjected to mechanical stress from peristalsis, particularly when the stool is firm, and localized mucosal ischaemia may develop. The folds may then become congested or haemorrhagic and even ulcerated, a condition for which the term 'crescentic fold colitis' has been coined [30]. More diffuse inflammation, involving the whole segment of bowel affected by diverticular disease, is the condition of 'segmental' or diverticular colitis (see p. 511) [31,32] (Fig. 35.4a.b). This must be distinguished from ulcerative colitis by its relatively mild distortion of mucosal architecture and mild activity but particularly by its segmental distribution.

Chronic mechanical stress to the redundant folds leads to the state of mucosal prolapse and polypoid tags of prolapsed mucosa are frequently found in bowel affected by diverticular disease [33,34]. These show histological features indistinguishable from so-called inflammatory 'myoglandular' polyps [35] or so-called 'cap' polyps (see p. 630) (Fig. 35.5).

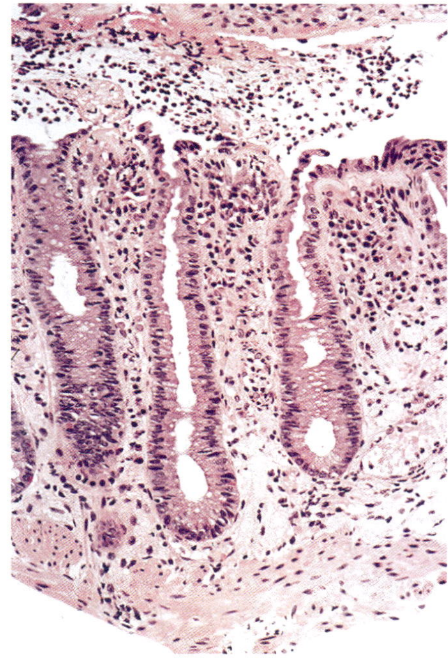

Fig. 35.4 (a) Inflammation of sigmoid colonic mucosa thrown into redundant folds by foreshortening of the colon by diverticular disease ('segmental colitis' or 'crescentic colitis'). (b) Histology of a biopsy of sigmoid colon from a patient with segmental colitis associated with diverticular disease. There is mild diffuse chronic inflammation with a surface exudate of pus but the architecture is not disturbed.

Complications

Inflammation (diverticulitis)

Diverticula are mainly extramural structures and since inflammation commonly begins at the apex and rarely involves the mucosa proximal to the neck of the sac the inflammatory process commonly involves only the pericolic and mesenteric fat (Fig. 35.6). Diverticula become inflamed because faecal matter is not discharged through the narrow neck, becomes inspissated to produce a faecolith and abrades the mucosal lining of the sac to produce low-grade, chronic inflammation. The mucosal lymphoid tissue undergoes hyperplasia and the earliest signs of inflammation are often found in lymphoid tissue at the apices of diverticula [21]. Commonly only one diverticulum becomes inflamed and it is unusual for more than three or four to be affected. Because the coats of the sac are thin there is early involvement of pericolic fat and local peritonitis is common [36]; free perforation into the peritoneal cavity is a recognized complication and there may be adherence of the colon to other intra-abdominal structures such as small intestine or bladder with subsequent fistula formation.

The inflammation often spreads longitudinally from the apex of the diverticulum parallel to the outer aspect of the deep muscle layers to form a dissecting abscess. With

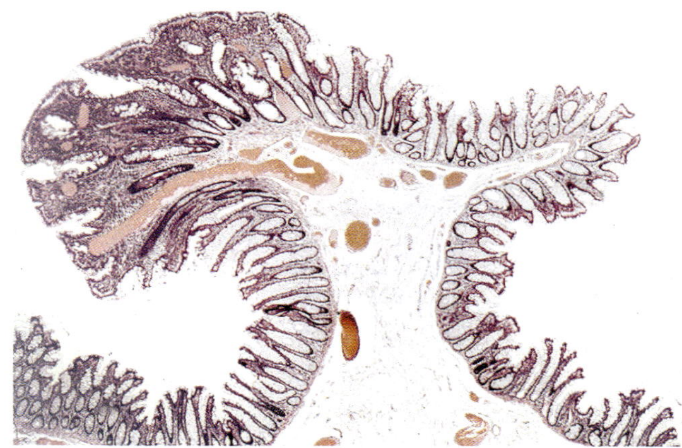

Fig. 35.5 A redundant tag of mucosa in sigmoid diverticular disease showing features of mucosal prolapse and forming an inflammatory myoglandular polyp.

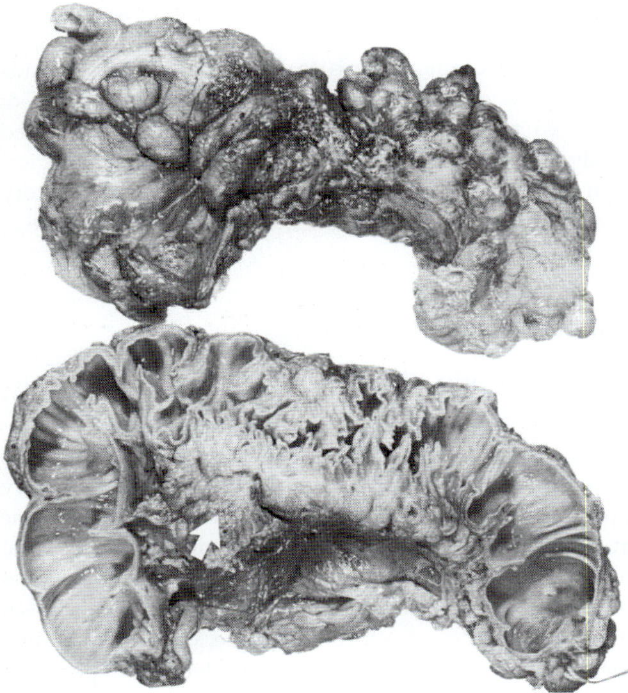

Fig. 35.6 Diverticular disease of sigmoid colon with pericolic abscess formation and fibrosis, with stricturing. Obstruction of the lumen is the result of both the stricturing and plugging by folds of redundant mucosa.

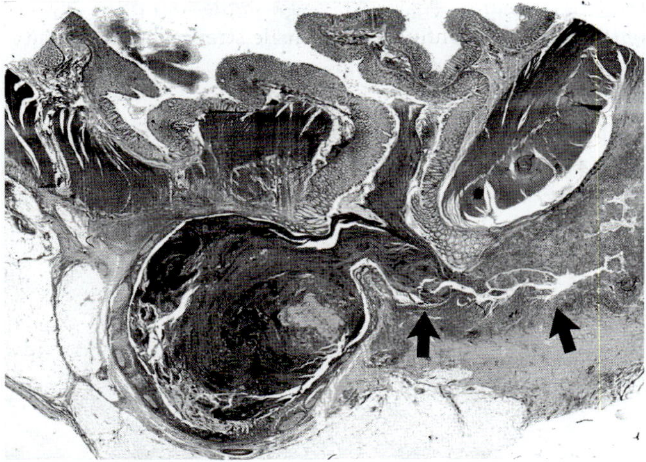

Fig. 35.7 Diverticular disease with diverticulitis. A diverticulum containing a faecolith communicates with a pericolic abscess (arrowed) in the extramural tissues. Note the marked circular muscle hypertrophy.

its source in only one diverticulum inflammation may thus spread widely up and down immediately outside the bowel wall, ensheathing it with inflammatory and later fibrous tissue and forming a large mass around the colon (Fig. 35.7).

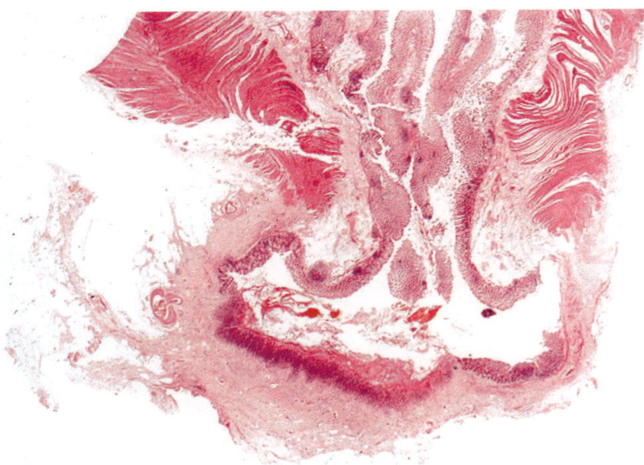

Fig. 35.8 Erosion of mucosa within a diverticulum. Bleeding from the granulation tissue lining the ulcer is a common source of blood loss in diverticular disease.

The clinical, surgical or radiological diagnosis of 'diverticulitis' implies the presence of both diverticula and inflammation but the latter is often absent in resected specimens of sigmoid colon [37]. This could be explained by resolution of former inflammation but it is likely that the pain and diarrhoea in diverticular disease are produced by the muscle abnormality rather than by any inflammatory change. It is most important when examining surgical or autopsy specimens of diverticular disease to examine every diverticulum for signs of pericolic abscess formation because these can be very small and hidden in fatty tissue.

Haemorrhage

Some degree of overt or occult bleeding is common in diverticular disease. Although in most cases this is continuous with loss of relatively small amounts of blood, it may occasionally be sudden and massive. The cause of the haemorrhage is usually erosion of mucosa inside a diverticulum with exposure of an adjacent artery [19,38] and since diverticula arise at the sites of vascular entry into the colonic wall, the arteries involved may be of considerable size. Sometimes the bleeding derives from vascular granulation tissue either within an infected diverticulum (Fig. 35.8) or at the site of mucosal prolapse at the neck of a diverticulum [21]. It is often stated that massive haemorrhage usually comes from a diverticulum of the right side of the colon [39,40], but in such cases there can be controversy over whether the bleeding arises within the diverticulum itself or from coexisting angiodysplasia [41,42]. Often the amount of inflammation is minimal in patients who have bleeding from diverticula [40] and this makes it all the more difficult to pinpoint the source of the haemorrhage. Rupture of an ectatic vascular channel, which happens to lie at the neck of diverticulum, is a hypothetical possibility that is very difficult to prove or disprove.

Fistulae

The formation of a pericolic abscess and local peritonitis can cause adhesions to the abdominal wall or to organs within the abdominal cavity, with subsequent formation of a fistulous track. Colovesical fistula is the most common [43], but colovaginal, colocolic, coloileal, colocutaneous and coloanal fistulae have all been described. Fistulae may occur as a complication in patients operated on for diverticulitis [44].

Intestinal obstruction

Chronic obstructive symptoms are a common manifestation of diverticular disease because, as described above, there is always some luminal narrowing. Acute intestinal obstruction is rare and seems always to occur in the presence of very extensive inflammation.

Perforation

Free perforation in an infected diverticulum is an uncommon but dangerous complication with a high mortality from generalized peritonitis, usually faecal [36]. Patients being treated with non-steroidal anti-inflammatory drugs (NSAIDs) are particularly vulnerable, probably due to mucosal damage induced by the inhibition of prostanoid synthesis, together with a reduced awareness of warning pain due to the analgesic effect of these drugs. In one study of mode of presentation of patients with diverticular disease in general practice, 19 (61%) of 31 patients taking NSAIDs presented with a perforation or peritonitis, compared with only 8 (13%) of 61 patients not taking NSAIDs [45]. Purulent peritonitis may also follow rupture of a pericolic abscess.

Differential diagnosis

The diagnosis of diverticular disease of the colon, with or without muscle abnormality, is usually obvious. The most important distinctions are from duplication of the colon and from solitary or few diverticula of the caecum and ascending colon which are probably unrelated. When examining surgical specimens of diverticular disease of the sigmoid it is not uncommon to find adenomatous polyps or a small carcinoma hidden between the muscular corrugations. It is sometimes these, rather than the diverticular disease, which are the cause of symptoms, particularly bleeding [46]. On clinical and radiological grounds diverticular disease of the sigmoid colon often mimics Crohn's disease. The induction of lymphoid follicle development in and around the mucosa of diverticula, the presence of fistulae and pericolic abscesses and, particularly, a granulomatous inflammatory reaction within the diverticular segment, can present a diagnostic dilemma [47]. Recent studies have described granulomatous vasculitis within the bowel wall, and small granulomas in the regional lymph nodes, of patients with diverticulitis who did not develop any other features of Crohn's disease on follow-up [48]. Care and critical evaluation of all aspects of the patient's clinical picture are required to avoid inappropriate overdiagnosis of Crohn's disease, therefore [49], and it is questionable whether a diagnosis of Crohn's disease can be made in the absence of inflammatory disease elsewhere in the bowel or in the anus. When the two conditions do coexist, involvement of diverticula by Crohn's disease may result in an increased incidence of diverticulitis [50] and there is often extensive fistula formation.

Aetiology and pathogenesis

Since the diverticula of classical diverticular disease are of pulsion type, at least two factors must be involved in their pathogenesis: raised intraluminal pressure and foci of weakness of the colonic wall. Relevant to this may be a reported increase in both incidence and severity of diverticular disease in obesity [51]. The sites of penetration of blood vessels through the circular muscle coats are undoubtedly predetermined areas of weakness, enhanced by expansion of perivascular adipose tissue in obese individuals, but additional factors must be involved, if only to explain the propensity for involvement of the sigmoid colon. Changes in the connective tissues of the bowel wall influence its tensile strength and elasticity. Defective collagen probably plays a part in the development of diverticula in patients with Marfan's or Ehlers–Danlos syndromes [52,53] and the increasing frequency of diverticular disease with age in Western societies may well be related to the fact that the ageing colon loses its tensile properties, probably due to alterations in the structure and arrangement of collagen molecules [54]. There is also evidence that the thickened colonic wall of diverticular disease has an increased compliance [55].

Many studies have found an increase both in colonic intraluminal pressure [55–57] and in the frequency of colonic contractions [58] in diverticular disease, although others suggest that these changes are confined to those with abdominal symptoms [59]. Simultaneous cineradiology and pressure recordings have shown that the high intraluminal pressures are produced by segmenting, thus converting the affected segment of colon into a series of small compartments [60]. These are partially sealed off from one another by a valvular mechanism produced by alternating and overlapping of the semicircular arcs of thickened circular muscle. Although it is tempting to propose that the muscular thickening of the colonic wall in diverticular disease is a response to increased intraluminal pressure, or a work hypertrophy following repeated contraction, there is no morphological evidence of hypertrophy of individual fibres or of hyperplasia [28,29,56]. The alternative, supported by radiological evidence of a failure of the muscle to elongate causing a permanent state of 'contracture' [61] and the finding of normal colonic pressures in asymptomatic patients [59], is that a primary overactivity of colonic muscle is responsible for the increased intraluminal pressure, occurring intermittently at first but becoming persistent later. One Japanese study has demonstrated increased density of cholinergic (excitatory) nerves in right-sided diverticular disease and reduced nitrergic (inhibitory) nerves. It has been postulated that imbalance of these two elements of the innervation initiates the muscle abnormality in diverticular disease, whether in the sigmoid colon or on the right side of the colon [62]. The thickening of muscle might then be a manifestation of prolonged contraction. Elastosis of the taeniae may be important in maintenance of the muscular thickening, contraction of the elastic fibres producing shortening of the colon and widening of the circular muscle until it eventually becomes corrugated like a concertina [29]. It could even be the primary cause of the muscle abnormality in diverticular disease.

In recent years a number of geographical and population surveys of diverticular disease have indicated the importance of low dietary fibre in its aetiology [63,64], cellulose fibre being particularly protective [65]. Subjects with diverticular disease consume less vegetables, brown bread and potatoes and more meat and dairy products than controls [66]; vegetarians have less than half the expected prevalence of asymptomatic diverticulosis [67]; in Japan an increase in the prevalence of the disease has coincided with a decline in the consumption of dietary fibre [68]; and rats fed a diet low in bran develop colonic diverticula [69]. Dietary fibre derived from plant cell walls binds salt and water within the colon, giving bulky, moist faeces that are easily propelled along the colon by peristalsis. It is postulated that propulsion of the low-volume faeces that result from fibre-deficient diets requires increased muscular effort, leading to muscular thickening, hypersegmentation and increased intraluminal pressure, and ultimately to the formation of diverticula [64]. Clinical studies indicate that symptomatic diverticular disease is improved by a high-fibre diet [70], with a concomitant lowering of sigmoid intraluminal pressure [71] and of the frequency of colonic contractions [58], although this appears to be partly a placebo effect [72].

Although the numerous studies described above have improved our understanding of the pathogenesis of diverticular disease there remain many areas of uncertainty. It seems likely that different mechanisms operate in different patients, the parts played by abnormalities of motility and colonic wall strength varying considerably from case to case. The fact that diverticulosis *per se*, without any morphological evidence of thickened muscle, is commonly seen by pathologists at autopsy and by radiologists in barium enema examinations suggests either that the muscle abnormality in such patients is reversible, the diverticula representing 'scars' of previous episodes of muscular dysfunction, or that the diverticula are the result of a primary weakness of the colonic wall.

Diverticulosis of the right colon

Diverticulosis of the caecum and ascending colon seems to be an entirely different condition from diverticular disease of the sigmoid colon or from generalized diverticulosis. Although it occurs worldwide it is particularly common in Hawaii, Japan and the Orient [12,73,74] where its prevalence overshadows that of sigmoid diverticulosis and appears to be increasing. Right-sided diverticula may be single or few in number—it is uncommon to find more than 15—and affected individuals are younger than those with sigmoid diverticulosis. In Japan solitary diverticula account for about one-third of cases of right-sided diverticulosis [74] but this proportion is much higher in Western countries, where solitary diverticulum of the caecum or ascending colon is not an uncommon incidental finding at laparotomy or autopsy but multiple right-sided diverticulosis is a rarity [75]. Histological examination of the diverticula shows that a few are 'true' diverticula surrounded by attenuated fibres of the colonic muscularis propria, suggesting a congenital maldevelopment, but most appear to be 'false' pulsion-type diverticula composed of mucosal herniations through the muscle coat of the colonic wall. The aetiology of these acquired diverticula is unknown. Thickening of the muscularis propria of the colon, the cardinal feature of sigmoid diverticular disease, is not prominent in right-sided cases but intraluminal pressure studies suggest that abnormal colonic motility might play an important pathogenetic role [76]. It is interesting to note that the adoption of a more Western-type lifestyle in Japan during recent years has been accompanied by an increase in both right-sided and left-sided colonic diverticular disease [74], suggesting that the two conditions may have predisposing factors in common.

Most diverticula of the right colon are asymptomatic, but diverticulitis, which usually mimics acute appendicitis, may lead to haemorrhage, pericolic abscess or peritonitis [73–75] (Fig. 35.9). Some so-called 'solitary ulcers' of the caecum or ascending colon are probably the result of inflammation in or around a solitary diverticulum [77]. A proportion of patients with right-sided diverticulosis suffer from recurrent attacks of right lower quadrant abdominal pain, possibly related to abnormal colonic motility.

The irritable bowel syndrome

Approximately one-half of patients referred to hospital gastroenterology clinics in the UK with symptoms of recurrent abdominal pain or bowel disturbance have no demonstrable pathological abnormality of the intestinal tract despite inten-

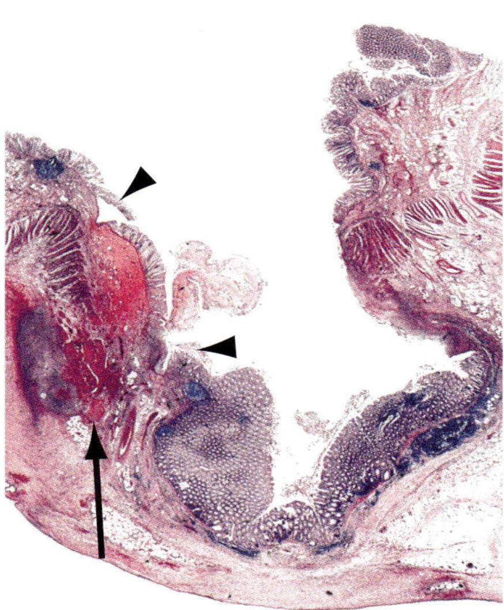

Fig. 35.9 Isolated diverticulum of right colon. There is mucosal ulceration (arrowheads) with early abscess formation in the pericolic fat (arrowed). This may be the pathogenesis of some cases of 'solitary ulcer' of the right colon.

sive investigation. In most of these the clinical features have a sufficiently similar pattern to warrant the recognition of a specific syndrome, called the irritable bowel syndrome [78]. Although it is now recognized that the condition may affect any part of the gastrointestinal tract [79,80] the frequent prominence of large bowel-type symptoms has resulted in the condition being called either 'spastic colon' or even 'mucous colitis' in the past. These symptoms vary from case to case and include abdominal pain, distension, flatulence, urgency, nausea and vomiting, and a spectrum of bowel disturbance from mucous diarrhoea to constipation.

The irritable bowel syndrome affects women more than men, with a maximum incidence in the third and fourth decades of life. By definition, pathological examination of the intestinal tract reveals no abnormality and the aetiology is poorly understood. Nevertheless, many studies have highlighted a high frequency of underlying anxiety or depression in affected patients [78,81] and gastrointestinal symptoms typical of the irritable bowel syndrome are common in those with established depressive illnesses. In many cases the symptoms follow an episode of stress or some other adverse life event provoking an anxiety state [82], while in others the condition may be the result of food intolerance [83] or follows an episode of infective gastroenteritis [78]. Symptomatic improvement following a high-fibre diet and antispasmodic drugs in some patients [84] has suggested to some that abnormalities of intestinal motility play a major role in the pathogenesis. Indeed a number of motor disorders have been identified, but different studies have given conflicting results and to date have failed to establish a consistent abnormality [80]. Other reports have failed to confirm the benefits of a high fibre intake and found that personality factors exerted a much greater influence on the response to treatment and themselves caused alterations of intestinal motility [85,86]. In many patients there is also evidence of an enhanced visceral sensation in that the intestine is unusually sensitive to luminal distension in the irritable bowel syndrome [87]. It has been suggested that interactions between physical factors such as dietary fibre, the patient's underlying personality, and acute stress-inducing life events are involved in the aetiology of the irritable bowel syndrome, and that the varying contributions of these three factors in the individual case should dictate the optimal clinical management [88]. It is relevant that two-thirds of patients benefit from biofeedback therapy and that permanent remission occurs in the majority of these (Kamm, personal communication).

Idiopathic constipation, megacolon and pseudo-obstruction

Disorders of colonic motility resulting in impairment or failure of propulsion of faecal contents are not uncommon and result in a spectrum of clinical effects ranging from chronic constipation to acute functional colonic obstruction, so-called pseudo-obstruction, which may be indistinguishable clinically from mechanical or organic obstruction due to inflammation or neoplasia. Chronic obstruction of the large intestine from any cause may result in total or segmental dilatation of the bowel, a condition which has been termed 'megacolon' or 'megarectum'. In such cases the muscle coats in the affected zone may be hypertrophied or atrophic depending upon the causative agent. When mechanical obstruction has been excluded it has been conventional to consider abnormalities of colonic autonomic nervous innervation in the aetiology of this group of conditions. Hirschsprung's disease, aganglionosis of the distal large intestine, is an important cause that can be confirmed or excluded by rectal biopsy. Although congenital in origin it may not present clinically until adolescence or even adult life [89]. More recently, the application of specialist techniques to the study of colorectal neuronal innervation [90] has allowed other more subtle abnormalities to be recognized. Some cases result from the effects of inflammation, infection, metabolic disorders or toxins on the colonic nerve supply, others are associated with disorders of the central nervous system, including psychiatric illnesses. In a minority a primary myopathy of the colonic smooth muscle may be demonstrable.

Idiopathic constipation

Unexplained constipation is common in Western society, especially in young women [91,92], but its aetiology is very poorly understood. At least two factors appear to be involved: an abnormality of colonic motility which results in slow transit of luminal contents, and a failure of defecation mechanisms; the relative importance of these varies between individual cases. The severity of the symptoms is also variable but in those worst affected there may be no more than one bowel action a week (even with the help of laxatives), abdominal pain, bloating and nausea. Despite this, it is unusual to find dilatation or enlargement of the colon sufficiently marked to warrant the term megacolon. There is a clinical overlap between idiopathic constipation and chronic colonic pseudo-obstruction that is considered below.

In patients with constipation due to slow colonic transit the underlying mechanisms are often obscure. In many there appears to be a functional abnormality of motility but histological studies of colons from patients whose symptoms are sufficiently marked to warrant colonic resection may demonstrate abnormalities of the myenteric plexus with damage or loss of argyrophilic neurones [93,94]. However, it is uncertain whether these changes are primarily responsible for the disordered motility or whether they are consequences of laxative consumption, since these drugs are neurotoxic (see below). Sometimes there is a concomitant increase in Schwann cells [93]. It has been suggested that this may be a result of extrinsic damage to the myenteric plexus, as might occur during pelvic surgery or childbirth, but so-called schwannosis is a common feature in the colonic myenteric plexus, of doubtful significance, and perhaps a phenomenon secondary to the motility disturbance. The finding of reduced numbers of vasoactive intestinal peptide-containing nerve fibres within the circular smooth muscle coat of the colon in four patients with idiopathic constipation [95] is also probably secondary rather than causative. Although a significant proportion of women with severe constipation give a history of previous pregnancy or gynaecological surgery, the intestinal symptoms usually antedate these events and their aetiological significance is at present unclear.

Chronic constipation may be a very disabling condition. The worst-affected patients have responded poorly to pharmacological agents and colectomy has hitherto been the only measure to improve their symptoms. The defecatory disorder that is undoubtedly present in some patients with severe constipation may be the critical initiating factor in many cases. The mechanism is poorly understood but there is some evidence that incoordination of the striated muscle of the pelvic floor leading to contraction rather than relaxation on attempted defecation is an important factor [96]. Defective rectal sensation leading to failure of initiation of defecation mechanisms may also contribute [92]. An important observation is that a significant proportion of patients with idiopathic constipation derive permanent benefit from pelvic biofeedback therapy [97,98], suggesting that in many cases the problem may be functional and lie within the central nervous system. It seems likely that many of the features associated with idiopathic constipation such as disorders of micturition and symptoms of Raynaud's phenomenon [92], may also be the result of malfunctioning central nervous and autonomic reflexes.

Colonic pseudo-obstruction

Colonic pseudo-obstruction describes a clinical syndrome in which the symptoms and signs of colonic obstruction occur in the absence of any recognizable mechanical obstructing lesion. Sometimes other parts of the gastrointestinal tract, notably the small intestine, are also affected, when the term chronic intestinal pseudo-obstruction is used (see p. 267). Colonic pseudo-obstruction may be divided into acute and chronic forms.

Acute colonic pseudo-obstruction

Acute colonic pseudo-obstruction occurs nearly always in elderly, hospitalized, bedridden patients who are suffering from a wide range of conditions including chronic neurological diseases, cardiac failure, chronic alcoholism and malignancy [99]. The term paralytic ileus of the colon has been used for the syndrome and, as with small intestinal ileus, a significant proportion of cases follow abdominal surgery. Symptoms are of rapidly progressive colonic obstruction mimicking acute mechanical obstruction, and perforation, usually of the caecum, may occur in some patients who are not treated by colonoscopic deflation or surgical decompression [100]. In most cases the condition is transient and reversible, and cases managed by colonoscopic deflation usually have no further symptoms, especially if the underlying disease process is also controlled and the patient is mobilized. The aetiology of acute colonic pseudo-obstruction is quite unknown. Postoperative cases may have a similar aetiology to postoperative small intestinal ileus (see p. 267) but in others it seems that chronic immobility somehow leads to an acute functional failure of colonic transit.

Chronic colonic pseudo-obstruction

Chronic colonic pseudo-obstruction is usually manifested by chronic constipation and in many patients this leads to megacolon. Perforation of the colon is extremely rare. Often abnormal colonic motility occurs secondary to an underlying systemic disease, although sometimes there is a primary disorder of the colon itself. The various causes of chronic colonic pseudo-obstruction are listed in Table 35.1. They can be usefully divided into a number of groups.

Disorders of colonic smooth muscle

Disorders of smooth muscle leading to colonic pseudo-obstruction may be inherited or acquired. Inherited visceral myopathy, which may exist as either an autosomal dominant or an autosomal recessive form, often results in motility abnormalities of the whole gastrointestinal tract, especially the small intestine [101,102], but sometimes there is selective

Table 35.1 Causes of chronic colonic pseudo-obstruction and megacolon.

SMOOTH MUSCLE DISORDERS
Primary
Inherited visceral myopathy:
1 autosomal dominant
2 autosomal recessive
Sporadic visceral myopathy
Secondary
Collagen diseases:
1 scleroderma
2 dermatomyositis
Myotonic dystrophy
Progressive muscular dystrophy
Amyloidosis
NEUROLOGICAL DISORDERS
Primary
Inherited disorders:
1 familial visceral neuropathies (autosomal recessive)
2 neurofibromatosis
3 ganglioneuromatosis in multiple endocrine neoplasia type IIb
Developmental disorders:
1 Hirschsprung's disease
2 hypoganglionosis
3 hyperganglionosis (neuronal colonic dysplasia)
Sporadic visceral neuropathy:
1 Shy–Drager syndrome
Secondary
Infective disorders:
1 Chagas' disease
2 cytomegalovirus
Malignant disease (paraneoplastic syndrome):
1 small cell carcinoma of bronchus
Metabolic disorders:
1 diabetes mellitus
2 hypothyroidism
Drug induced:
1 psychotropic drugs (phenothiazines, tricyclic antidepressants, anticholinergic drugs)
2 antineoplastic drugs (vinca alkaloids, daunorubicin)
3 anthraquinone laxatives

involvement of the large bowel [103]. Atrophy of the colonic muscle coats leads to a failure of motility, eventually resulting in a dilated atonic, thin-walled megacolon. Histopathological examination in familial visceral myopathy reveals degeneration of intestinal smooth muscle with nuclear enlargement and hyperchromasia, cytoplasmic vacuolation and a progressive interstitial fibrosis (Fig. 35.10) which culminates in the complete fibrous replacement of the muscular coats [102]. Both muscularis mucosae and muscularis propria may be involved [103]; in the latter the longitudinal muscle coat is often more affected than the circular muscle [101].

Acquired damage to colonic smooth muscle is seen in the collagen diseases including dermatomyositis [203] and scleroderma (systemic sclerosis) [104]. Involvement of the large intestine is particularly common in scleroderma, and symptoms of colonic pseudo-obstruction may even precede other manifestations of the disease. Replacement of the smooth muscle coats of the intestinal wall by collagen and elastic fibres is the main histological abnormality. This occurs patchily at first, but in advanced cases the circular muscle coat becomes obliterated by fibrosis. The taeniae coli are relatively spared. This muscular fibrosis mimics closely that found in familial visceral myopathy (Fig. 35.11), although vacuolar degeneration of the surviving smooth muscle fibres in visceral myopathy is said to be useful in making the distinction histologically [105]. Submucosal fibrosis is often inconspicuous. Examination of the arterial supply to the bowel wall, particularly the marginal vessels, will sometimes show intimal proliferation with elastosis and luminal narrowing. Scattered haemosiderin-laden macrophages in the colonic wall suggest that the changes are at least in part due to ischaemia. Indeed, infarction of the colon may be a presenting manifestation of scleroderma [106]. The patchy fibrosis of the muscle coats accounts for the characteristic macroscopic appearances of colonic scleroderma. Large, multiple sacculations appear which are confined to the antimesenteric border, presumably because the tissues of the mesenteric side continue to give support to the weakened bowel wall, or possibly because the blood supply is more precarious at the antimesenteric border. In some specimens there are no sacculations, only a dilated, thin-walled colon.

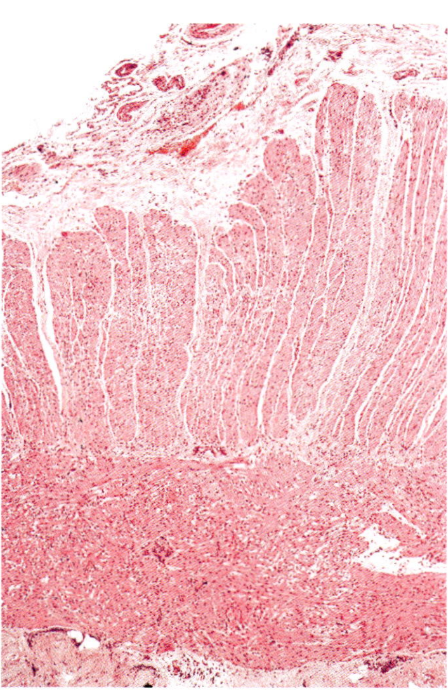

Fig. 35.10 Familial visceral myopathy of autosomal recessive type. There is vacuolar degeneration of myocytes in the longitudinal layer of the muscularis propria. There is patchy fibrosis of the circular muscle layer.

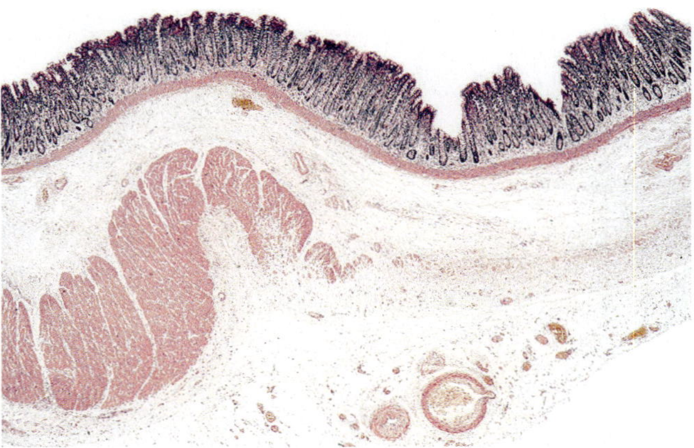

Fig. 35.11 Systemic sclerosis. The histological appearances of the transverse colon in a patient with pseudo-obstruction. There is severe patchy replacement of the muscularis propria by relatively acellular fibrous tissue.

Abnormal colonic motility, especially constipation, is common in patients with myotonic dystrophy [107,108] and progressive muscular dystrophy [109], in whom atrophy of the colonic smooth muscle fibres without fibrosis may be found. There may be a surprising degree of lymphocytic infiltration in the muscularis propria, not to be confused with a myositis. Colonic motor dysfunction also occurs rarely in systemic amyloidosis, possibly due to a combination of smooth muscle infiltration, autonomic neuropathy and vascular insufficiency [110].

Neurological disorders

Chronic colonic pseudo-obstruction may result from disorders of colonic autonomic nervous innervation. These may affect either the intrinsic intramural nerve plexuses or the extramural components of the sympathetic and parasympathetic nervous system. Our knowledge of such disorders has been greatly hampered by difficulty in studying the colonic nervous system in any detail, but more recently the application of special neuropathological techniques has provided important information [90]. Furthermore, the recent recognition that many intrinsic nerves are of 'peptidergic' type will allow further understanding of the pathological processes involved as they are identified by immunocytochemistry [111].

Generally speaking defects of colonic innervation may produce a number of different clinical and pathological effects. Denervation of intestinal smooth muscle usually results in peristaltic activity that is increased in rate but uncoordinated. Although occasionally this causes diarrhoea, it far more commonly results in constipation with colicky abdominal pain due to a failure of colonic transit. The functional obstruction leads to luminal dilatation which, along with the 'overwork' of denervation, stimulates hypertrophy of the colonic smooth muscle [112]. The final result is therefore a dilated megacolon whose wall shows considerable muscular thickening. Not all examples of damaged colonic innervation have this result, however. Some neurological lesions, notably those caused by drugs or toxins, are accompanied by atrophy rather than hypertrophy of smooth muscle, so that they result in megacolon in which the colonic wall is thin, inert and adynamic. In many cases of acquired neuropathic pseudo-obstruction pale-staining ovoid cytoplasmic inclusion bodies are present in scattered myocytes within the muscularis propria [113]. These inconspicuous bodies seem to be markers of denervation, rather than specific products of a degenerative myopathy.

Neurological lesions leading to chronic colonic pseudo-obstruction may be congenital or acquired. By far the most common congenital disorder is classical Hirschsprung's disease in which there is aganglionosis of the large intestine extending proximally from the anorectum over a variable distance. Related developmental abnormalities include aganglionosis of the entire colon, zonal aganglionosis, hypoganglionosis and hyperganglionosis (colonic neuronal dysplasia) although these are not as well characterized as Hirschsprung's disease itself. These conditions are unusual among diseases causing colonic pseudo-obstruction in that they can usually be diagnosed with relative ease by biopsy, without sophisticated neuropathological techniques. They are considered fully with developmental disorders on p. 447 but it is important to remember that a small proportion of cases of Hirschsprung's disease present not in infancy but in adolescence or even adult life when they cause constipation and megacolon [114]. Proliferation of the intramural nerves in both submucosal and myenteric plexuses with the formation of giant ganglia, similar to that of neuronal colonic dysplasia, may occur in neurofibromatosis [115] and in type IIb multiple endocrine neoplasia (medullary thyroid carcinoma, phaeochromocytoma and mucosal neuromas) [116] (Fig. 35.12) and sometimes this is associated with megacolon. Occasionally the process involves the lamina propria to result in mucosal ganglioneuromatosis, which can be recognized in biopsy specimens. A similar mucosal abnormality has been described in association with familial juvenile polyposis [117], although this was not accompanied by symptoms of abnormal colonic motility.

Another rare cause of chronic colonic pseudo-obstruction is familial visceral neuropathy. At least two varieties, both showing probable autosomal recessive inheritance, have been recognized to cause abnormal colonic motility [101], and in both there are associated abnormalities of the central nervous system. The first is characterized by the presence of eosinophilic intranuclear inclusions within the neurones of both myenteric and submucosal plexuses, accompanied by neuronal loss [101,118]. These inclusions, which appear to consist of non-viral filamentous proteins, may also be found in the brain, spinal cord, autonomic ganglia and peripheral nerves, where they are presumed to cause the variety of neurological symptoms that accompanies the intestinal abnormality. The second form of familial visceral neuropathy is associated with mental

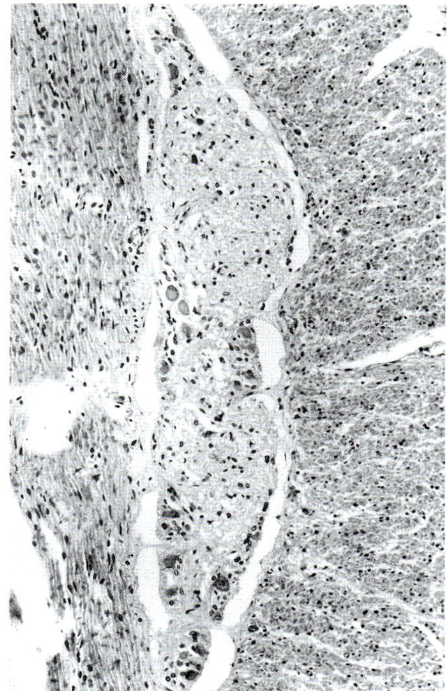

Fig. 35.12 Ganglioneuroma-like expansion of myenteric plexus in the colon of a young woman with multiple endocrine neoplasia type IIb.

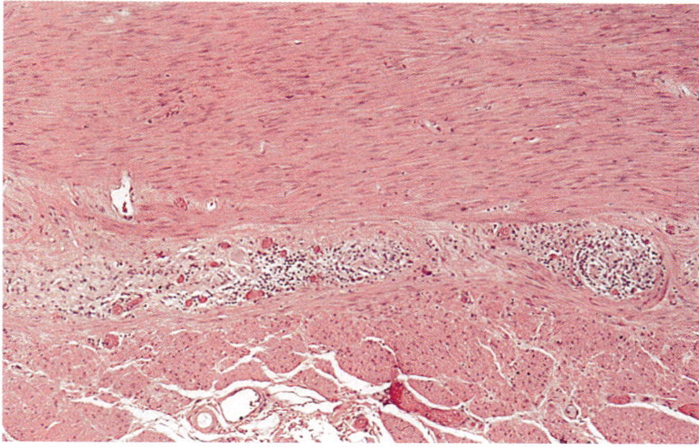

Fig. 35.13 Autonomic plexitis. The colonic myenteric plexus is infiltrated by lymphocytes and plasma cells in this patient with pseudo-obstruction. Many of the neurones show degenerative changes. The condition was idiopathic in this man of 28, who suffered from progressive constipation. However, similar features can be seen in Chagas' disease or as a result of cytomegalovirus or Epstein–Barr virus infection and also as a paraneoplastic effect in, for example, small cell carcinoma of the lung.

retardation and calcification of the basal ganglia [119]. Routine histological staining of the colon fails to demonstrate an abnormality but detailed neuropathological examination shows degeneration of the intramural neurones. Sporadic cases of visceral neuropathy affecting the colon and other parts of the gastrointestinal tract, without extra-intestinal pathology, have also been described rarely [101]. They appear to be degenerative disorders of the intestinal plexuses but their aetiology is unknown.

Acquired disorders of visceral nervous innervation leading to chronic colonic pseudo-obstruction may result in a number of ways. By far the most common cause worldwide is Chagas' disease, infection with the parasite *Trypanosoma cruzi*, which has a specific affinity for the myenteric plexus (see p. 49). Some seven million people, almost entirely in South America, are said to be affected. The inflammatory reaction to the parasite, consisting of lymphocytes and plasma cells, results in destruction of the myenteric plexus with marked neuronal loss, often with Schwann cell hyperplasia. Smooth muscle hypertrophy, a consequence of denervation, is common, as is megacolon [120,121]. A similar inflammatory destruction of the myenteric plexus has been described with cytomegalovirus infection [122], in Epstein–Barr virus infection [123] and also in patients with small cell (oat cell) carcinoma of the lung [99,101,112,124] (Fig. 35.13). In the latter situation it has been postulated that antigens on the neoplastic cells elicit an immunological reaction which cross-reacts with neural tissue in the myenteric plexus. Similar lesions in the posterior root ganglia have been found in other paraneoplastic neurological syndromes.

Autonomic neuronal damage leading to chronic colonic pseudo-obstruction is sometimes part of a more widespread chronic autonomic neuropathy. This is classically seen in the Shy–Drager syndrome, where colonic symptoms are frequently overshadowed by other manifestations of autonomic failure, notably orthostatic hypotension. In this condition the nerve cells both in the myenteric plexus and in the extramural sympathetic chain show a distinctive vacuolar change [112]. Similar colonic symptoms, rarely leading to megacolon, may be found when autonomic neuropathy occurs in metabolic disorders, notably diabetes mellitus [125] and myxoedema [126], although in these conditions the primary pathology usually occurs in the Schwann cells rather than in the neurones themselves [112].

In recent years it has been recognized that drugs may be important causes of damage to the colonic autonomic innervation. Those implicated include psychotropic drugs, especially phenothiazines and tricyclic antidepressants, anticholinergic drugs, and antineoplastic drugs used in cancer chemotherapy, notably the vinca alkaloids and daunorubicin [90]. It has been postulated that the high frequency of severe constipation and megacolon in psychotic patients [127] may be due to the toxic effects of large doses of phenothiazines used in their management [99], and similar problems in patients with Parkinson's disease may be related to the use of anticholinergic drugs.

The condition of cathartic colon, in which the colon is thin, dilated and atonic with marked melanosis coli, was attributed by Smith [128] to a toxic neuropathy of the submucosal and myenteric plexuses induced by chronic ingestion of laxatives, especially of anthraquinone type. However, this has recently been questioned as an entity [129,130]. There is no dispute that these drugs cause melanosis of the colonic mucosa (see p. 635). However, since the original description of the condition, there have been no acceptable reported cases of atonic, dilated colon directly attributable to anthraquinone drugs. It seems likely that the features originally described were the end-stage of one or more neuromuscular problems unrelated to any laxatives the patients may have taken.

With the exception of classical Hirschsprung's disease [131] there have been few studies of the peptidergic nervous system of the colon in disorders of motility. One study has shown decreased numbers of mucosal nerve fibres containing vasoactive intestinal peptide (VIP) and substance P, with a concurrent reduction in endocrine cells containing enteroglucagon and somatostatin, in patients with Chagas' disease but no such changes in autonomic neuropathy of extrinsic origin [132]. There is also a case report of idiopathic megacolon coexisting with enterochromaffin cell hyperplasia [133]—whether this represents a causative or a chance association is uncertain.

Complications

Perforation of the colon is very unusual in idiopathic constipation, pseudo-obstruction and megacolon. Most complications result from faecal overloading or impaction, which frequently leads to non-specific mucosal inflammation, sometimes with crypt abscesses. Occasionally these changes progress to stercoral ulceration, when pain, rectal bleeding and even perforation may then occur (see p. 636). Melanosis is common. Usually it is of slight degree, but if long-term purgatives have been used it can be very conspicuous (see p. 635).

Volvulus

A volvulus is a twisting of the bowel in such a way as to obstruct its lumen; many of the effects are secondary to interruption of the venous return. The classical sites of large bowel volvulus are the caecum and the sigmoid colon, although there are reports of volvulus of the transverse colon [134] and of the splenic flexure [135].

Caecum

Caecal volvulus is a rare cause of intestinal obstruction in the Western World, although it is reportedly more common in India, Africa and Scandinavian countries. The essential predisposing condition is an abnormally mobile caecum [136]. Colonic distension, chronic constipation, previous abdominal surgery and pregnancy may be additional factors. Twisting of the mesentery with obstruction of the blood supply leads to infarction, gangrene or other manifestations of ischaemia (see p. 541).

Sigmoid colon

Sigmoid volvulus is due to twisting of a large redundant sigmoid loop on an elongated mesentery [137]. An uncommon disease in the Western World, it is frequent in countries such as Iran, Africa, India, Scandinavia, Russia and Peru [136,138,139]. It is interesting, and probably relevant, that the condition is rare in those countries where diverticular disease of the colon is common. The geographical distribution has been explained by dietary factors leading to bowel distension—in those countries where volvulus is prevalent the population eats a high-residue or cereal diet which is often taken as one large meal during the day [140]. Sigmoid volvulus in such high-incidence areas is usually seen in those under 50 years of age while in Western countries affected individuals are often elderly, give a history of constipation, and frequently suffer from mental illness [141]. There are also differences in the gross appearances of the distended sigmoid loop between sigmoid volvulus in 'high-risk' areas and that in the West. In the former the affected bowel is long and thin-walled and has a narrow mesentery while in the Western world the sigmoid loop shows marked muscular thickening of its wall and a broader mesentery which contains thick-walled blood vessels and shows fibrous scarring due to repeated attacks of volvulus [142]. Twisting sufficient to cause infarction and gangrene of the bowel wall is rare in the Western type of volvulus but common in high-incidence areas. Paradoxically, the affected segment shows marked faecal loading in low-incidence areas while in countries with a high-residue diet the sigmoid loop is distended, mainly with gas. Melanosis coli is sometimes present if the patient comes from the Western world, and occasionally there is pneumatosis coli in the affected segment [143]. Although most reports stress the importance of diet in the aetiology of sigmoid volvulus, congenital factors, such as a long sigmoid loop, also play a part, as indicated by one report of sigmoid volvulus in three members of a family [144]. Another rarer variety of sigmoid volvulus is so-called ileosigmoid knotting. In this condition, a loop of ileum knots around the base of a sigmoid volvulus in a complex manner, often resulting in gangrene of both bowel loops [145]. This condition is virtually unknown in the Western world but quite well recognized in Africa, Finland and eastern Europe.

Mucosal prolapse and the solitary ulcer syndrome

Prolapse of large intestinal mucosa may be found in a number of situations [146]. It occurs at the margin of a colostomy [147], at the apex of a prolapsing haemorrhoid, alongside any polypoid lesion of the large bowel, and at the margins of colonic diverticula. However, the best recognized site of mucosal prolapse is the anterior wall of the rectum, where it gives rise to the so-called solitary ulcer syndrome [148], a fairly common but poorly recognized benign condition which is important because it may be confused both clinically and histologically with carcinoma of the rectum—we have knowledge of patients in whom such a mistaken diagnosis has led to unnecessary major excision. The name 'solitary ulcer' itself is misleading because sometimes there is more than one ulcer and there seems to be a stage of the disease when no ulceration is present.

Solitary ulcer of the rectum is quite unrelated to so-called solitary ulcer of the small intestine (see p. 353) or right colon (see p. 458). It occurs predominantly in young adults of either sex, who may present with any of the diverse symptoms of anorectal disease. Rectal bleeding is most common and may be severe enough to require transfusion; other symptoms include the passage of mucus, perineal pain and tenesmus. There may be associated complete rectal prolapse. Macroscopically, solitary ulcers are distinctive. They are situated on the anterior or anterolateral walls of the rectum and are usually flat, well demarcated lesions with an irregular shape, often covered by a white slough (Fig. 35.14). They vary in size from 0.5 to 5 cm in diameter. The surrounding mucosa shows a mild proctitis and may appear lumpy. In cases in which no ulcer is present the anterior rectal mucosa shows a localized roughened inflamed area. Although the solitary ulcer syndrome is benign in its behaviour, it is notorious for its chronicity. No treatment is entirely satisfactory and often patients have to adjust to their symptoms.

Biopsy of the abnormal mucosa in solitary ulcer syndrome reveals characteristic appearances [148,149], now recognized to be distinctive, of mucosal prolapse [146]. The earliest and most significant change is a curious obliteration of the lamina propria by fibrosis and smooth muscle fibres extending towards the lumen from a thickened muscularis mucosae (Fig. 35.15). In a tangentially cut biopsy the appearance of mucosal glands surrounded by muscle can give the false impression of invasive carcinoma. Additional features include superficial mucosal erosion, irregularity of the crypts with metaplastic-like changes in the epithelium [150] and depletion of goblet cells. Occasionally the lesion becomes covered by a mass of exuberant granulation tissue to give rise to a 'cap' polyp (see p. 630).

Histochemical stains for mucins show a predominance of sialomucins over the normal sulphomucins [150,151]. When an ulcer is present it is invariably superficial and never penetrates beyond the submucosa. Its floor is covered by necrotic cells overlying organizing granulation tissue. In some cases there is misplacement of mucus-filled glands lined by normal colonic epithelium into the submucosa at the edge of the ulcer, another feature that may be mistaken for adenocarcinoma (Fig. 35.16). This appearance has been described under a variety of names such as 'localized colitis cystica profunda' (not to be confused with the diffuse condition also given this name—see p. 478) [152], hamartomatous inverted polyp of the

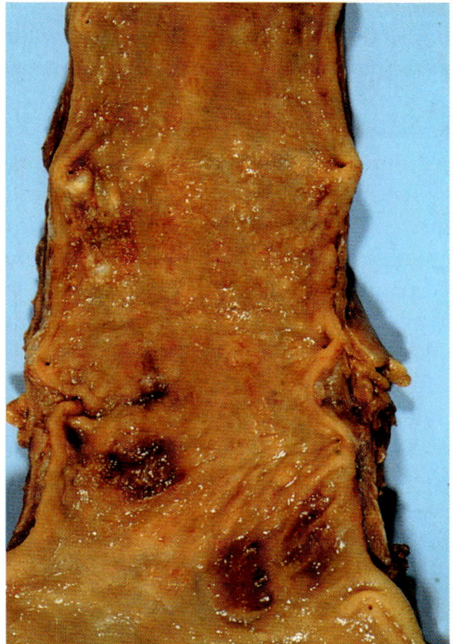

Fig. 35.14 Solitary ulcer of rectum. Despite the name, these lesions are often multiple. They are typically covered by granulation tissue and slough. The ulcers are shallow but have an indurated texture and irregular thickening of mucosa at the edges is a potential cause of clinical confusion with carcinoma.

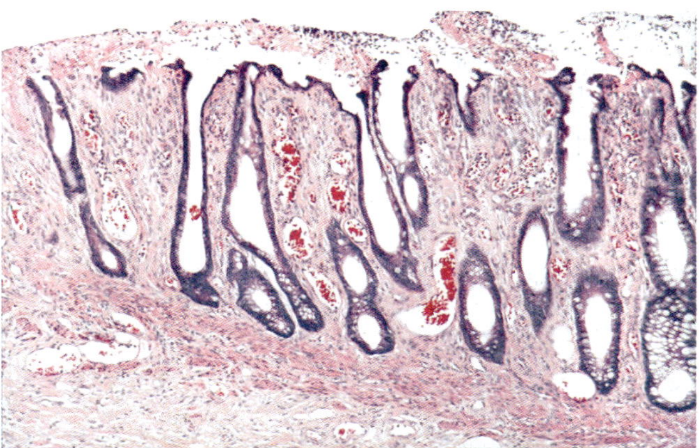

Fig. 35.15 Histology of the edge of a solitary rectal ulcer (proctectomy specimen). There is surface erosion and the crypt epithelium shows regenerative hyperplasia. The lamina propria is fibrosed and contains ectatic blood capillaries. Smooth muscle fibres extend upwards from the muscularis mucosae between the bases of the crypts, which tend to be pinched and pointed.

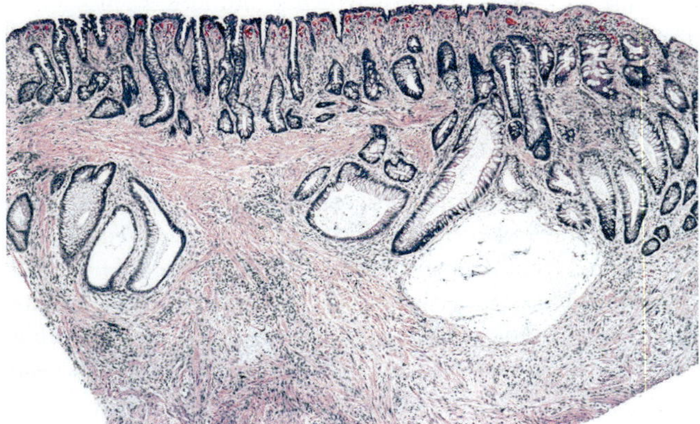

Fig. 35.16 Solitary rectal ulcer syndrome. In this case there is misplacement of mucus-containing glands into the submucosa with the formation of cysts. The appearance is sometimes called 'colitis cystica profunda'.

rectum [153] and enterogenous cyst [154]. Thickening of the media and even fibrinoid necrosis of submucosal blood vessels has been reported in occasional biopsies [146]. Finally, in resection specimens, histological examination may reveal fibrosis of the submucosa and thickening of the muscularis propria [155].

The pathogenesis of the solitary ulcer syndrome has become clearer in recent years. There is now little doubt that mucosal prolapse during excessive straining at stool is the primary abnormality, with superadded trauma and ischaemia eventually leading to ulceration [150]. The excessive straining which results in the mucosal prolapse is seen as an attempted response to overcome an abnormality of the pelvic floor musculature during defecation, notably in the puborectalis muscle and the external anal sphincter which undergo inappropriate contraction rather than relaxation during straining [156]. Repeated trauma of the prolapsing mucosa against the contracting puborectalis muscle and mucosal ischaemia due to the high intrarectal pressures necessary for voiding act synergistically to cause mucosal damage and eventually lead to ulceration [157,158]. Similar prolapse of the anterior rectal mucosa, but usually without ulceration, occurs in the so-called descending perineum syndrome, a condition in which there is 'descent' of the perineum with loss of the normal anorectal angle during straining at stool [159]. There may also be incontinence. Affected patients, women more commonly than men, give a long history of abnormal straining. The descending perineum syndrome differs from the solitary ulcer syndrome in that, instead of overactivity of the puborectalis muscle or of the anal sphincter, there is denervation of the pelvic floor musculature that can often be demonstrated histochemically. This may be due to a traction neuropathy of the pudendal or perineal nerves secondary to the excessive straining, or it may result from damage at childbirth or some other pelvic injury.

Intussusception and complete rectal prolapse

Colonic intussusception is a relatively uncommon condition that is most frequent in the early years of life. In adults it is usually secondary to a benign or malignant tumour that has a polypoid configuration [160,161]; in the neonatal period no cause is usually found while in older children there is frequently a coexisting viral-type illness which may lead to mesenteric lymphadenopathy (see p. 264). There are three main varieties: caecocolic, colocolic and sigmoidorectal. When intussusception occurs it is usually in a distal direction, although retrograde intussusception of the colon has been described [162].

Caecocolic intussusception is very rare, except apparently in West Africa where it is the most common variety of all intussusceptions [163,164]. This West African type has no known cause. Caecocolic intussusception has also been reported following appendicectomy due to oedema and inflammation of the appendix stump [165].

Colocolic and sigmoidorectal intussusception are almost invariably caused by tumours [166]. Among benign lesions lipoma appears to be the most common, but we have seen smooth muscle tumours, adenomatous polyps and villous adenomas causing intussusception. Adenocarcinoma is the usual malignant tumour causing intussusception. Sigmoidorectal intussusception seems to be rarer than the colocolic variety.

Complete rectal prolapse through the anal sphincter is in essence an antegrade intussusception of the rectal wall that usually begins at a circular fold 6–8 cm above the dentate line [167,168]. It is seen mainly in young children (1–3 year olds) and elderly nulliparous women. In children it is usually precipitated by alterations in bowel habit, either diarrhoea or constipation, and resolves without any specific treatment [169]. In elderly women, on the other hand, its aetiology is quite different. Affected patients often give a long history of straining at stool, mucous diarrhoea and anal incontinence, and laxity of the musculature of the pelvic floor and the external anal sphincter are thought to be important predisposing factors. In some patients there is histochemical evidence of denervation of the external sphincter [170]. The condition appears to be related to the descending perineum syndrome (see above) and it would appear that sometimes an initial mucosal prolapse leads first to rectal intussusception (internal procidentia) and later to prolapse of the full thickness of the rectal wall through the anal sphincter to produce complete rectal prolapse.

Trauma

Traumatic perforation of the colon or rectum is caused by knife and bullet wounds as well as blunt trauma to the abdominal wall, pelvis or perineum [171,172]. Large intestinal perforation, especially of the rectosigmoid region, is a well recognized complication of barium enema [173], sigmoidoscopy or colonoscopy [174], and there are rare reports of diathermy for colonoscopic polypectomy leading to explosive rupture of the colon due to the ignition of inflammable gases, chiefly hydrogen, which are produced by the bacterial fermentation of non-absorbed carbohydrates [175]. For this reason mannitol, itself a non-absorbed carbohydrate, is no longer recommended for bowel preparation for colonoscopy if electrosurgery is to be used. Impalement injury to the rectum and perineum is not uncommon, especially in farm labourers, building workers and children [176,177]. Pitchforks, chair legs and iron railings are among the offending objects. A particularly dangerous practice is the so-called 'compressed air joke', in which the nozzle of a compressed air pipe is placed against the area of the buttocks [178]. Pneumatic rupture of the colon results and it is important to realize that the nozzle does not have to touch either the skin or the clothes. The placing of fireworks in the region of the anus can also have dramatic effects and there is one bizarre report of a patient who exploded a firework up his own rear causing a laceration of the rectal wall [179]. More recently there are reports of colonic perforation following seat-belt injury at road traffic accidents [180] and of severe perineal, anal and rectal lacerations following bizarre sexual practices, notably 'fisting', the insertion of a hand, fist or even the whole forearm into the rectum for the purposes of sexual stimulation [181].

There are reports of spontaneous rupture of the colon in adults and children. In the former it appears to be related to constipation, excessive straining at stool and the taking of alkalis [182,183]. The sigmoid colon is the most common site, and perforation of the right colon appears to be rare [184,185]. In children with cystic fibrosis, the meconium plug syndrome (mucoviscidosis, see p. 258) is one of the causes [186]. Gross pneumoperitoneum with extensive surgical emphysema is a rare complication of colonic perforation [187].

Foreign bodies

Most swallowed foreign bodies pass through the gastrointestinal tract without complications, but fish, chicken and meat bones seem to be particularly dangerous [188]. Metallic foreign bodies such as coins, safety pins and nails are relatively harmless. There is experimental evidence that soft, malleable objects are more likely to give rise to complications than hard objects [189]. When foreign bodies are found in surgical specimens or in the faeces they are often surrounded by a globular mass of mucus. We know of one patient who deliberately swallowed an intact razor blade in order to avoid overseas military service. This was passed per rectum 10 days later, completely encased in a mass of jelly-like mucus.

The two main complications caused by foreign bodies are perforations and obstruction, and these are both more common in the small bowel than the colon and rectum. Not infrequently, the foreign body precipitates symptoms by getting stuck in diseased bowel, usually in cases of diverticulitis [190] or carcinoma [191]. Pericolic abscess formation due to foreign body perforation can be the mode of presentation.

Obstruction due to food is not uncommon in the small intestine, but we have never seen this in the large bowel. Calculi of varying types may occasionally become impacted in the colon. These may be gallstones, true enteric stones composed of bile salts or minerals formed within the small intestine when there is stasis (as in diverticula), or false stones such as bezoars or calcified faecoliths [190,192,193]. Faecal masses may become so large and hard that they cause obstruction of the distal large bowel [194].

For those readers with an overdeveloped sense of the ridiculous or a frankly pornographic sense of humour the study of foreign bodies in the rectum can be rewarding. There is an extensive literature which describes a great variety of objects that have been inserted accidentally [195,196] or deliberately [197–200]. If the latter, then the patient is usually either mentally disturbed, a sexual pervert, a smuggler of drugs such as cocaine (a 'back-packer') [201], a victim of assault or occasionally driven to introduce a foreign body in order to obtain relief of severe symptoms referable to the anus or rectum. It is well known that the rectum is occasionally used by psychotic patients for storing personal possessions. The variety of objects inserted can almost be equalled by the ingenious methods that have been devised for their removal [200]. Complications include intestinal obstruction, laceration and pressure necrosis of the bowel wall, and perforation, sometimes with fatal results. The discharge of fetal bones per rectum has been reported on a number of occasions [202].

References

1 Spriggs EI, Marxer OA. Intestinal diverticula. *Q J Med*, 1925; 19: 1.
2 Pemberton JJ, Black BM, Maino CR. Progress in the surgical management of diverticulitis of the sigmoid colon. *Surg Gynecol Obstet*, 1947; 85: 523.
3 Welch CE, Allen AW, Donaldson GA. Appraisal of resection of colon for diverticulitis of sigmoid. *Ann Surg*, 1953; 138: 332.
4 Smith CC, Christenson WR. The incidence of colonic diverticulosis. *Am J Roentgenol*, 1959; 82: 996.
5 Manousos ON, Truelove SC, Lumsden K. Prevalence of colonic diverticulosis in the general population of the Oxford area. *Lancet*, 1967; iii: 762.
6 Eastwood MA, Sanderson J, Pocock SJ, Mitchel WD. Variation in the incidence of diverticular disease within the City of Edinburgh. *Gut*, 1977; 18: 571.
7 Oshsner HC, Bargen JA. Diverticulosis of the large intestine. *Ann Intern Med*, 1935; 9: 282.
8 Kocour EJ. Diverticulosis of the colon; its incidence in 7000 consecutive autopsies with reference to its complications. *Am J Surg*, 1937; 37: 433.

9 Hughes LE. Post-mortem survey of diverticular disease of the colon. Part 1. Diverticulosis and diverticulitis. *Gut*, 1969; 10: 336.

10 Kyle J, Davidson AI. The changing pattern of hospital admission for diverticular disease of the colon. *Br J Surg*, 1975; 62: 537.

11 Parks TG. Natural history of diverticular disease of the colon. *Clin Gastroenterol*, 1975; 4: 53.

12 Mendeloff AI. Thoughts on the epidemiology of diverticular disease. *Clin Gastroenterol*, 1986; 15: 855.

13 Kyle J, Adesola AO, Tinckler LF, de Baeux J. Incidence of diverticulitis. *Scand J Gastroenterol*, 1967; 2: 77.

14 Kohler R. The incidence of colonic diverticulosis in Finland and Sweden. *Acta Chir Scand*, 1963; 126: 148.

15 Kim EH. Hiatus hernia and diverticulosis of the colon. *N Engl J Med*, 1964; 271: 764.

16 Pan C-Z, Liu TH, Chen MZ, Chang HC. Diverticular disease of colon in China: a 60-year retrospective study. *Chinese Med J*, 1984; 97: 391.

17 Segal I, Solomon A, Hunt JA. Emergence of diverticular disease in the urban South African black. *Gastroenterology*, 1977; 72: 215.

18 Levy N, Stermer E, Simon J. The changing epidemiology of diverticular disease in Israel. *Dis Colon Rectum*, 1985; 28: 477.

19 Slack WW. The anatomy, pathology and some clinical features of diverticulosis of the colon. *Br J Surg*, 1962; 50: 185.

20 Watt J, Marcus R. The pathology of diverticulosis of the intertaenial area of the pelvic colon. *J Pathol Bacteriol*, 1964; 88: 97.

21 Morson BC. The muscle abnormality in diverticular disease of the sigmoid colon. *Br J Radiol*, 1963; 36: 385.

22 Hughes LE. Post-mortem survey of diverticular disease of the colon. Part II. The muscle abnormality in the sigmoid colon. *Gut*, 1969; 10: 344.

23 Parks TG. Post-mortem studies of the colon with special reference to diverticular disease. *Proc R Soc Med*, 1968; 61: 932.

24 Williams I. Changing emphasis in diverticular disease of the colon. *Br J Radiol*, 1963; 36: 393.

25 Fleischner FG, Ming SC, Henken EM. Revised concepts on diverticular disease of the colon. *Radiology*, 1964; 83: 859; 84: 599.

26 Williams I. Diverticular disease of the colon without diverticula. *Radiology*, 1967; 89: 401.

27 Cassano C, Torsoli A. Idiopathic muscular strictures of the colon. *Gut*, 1968; 9: 325.

28 Slack WW. Bowel muscle in diverticular disease. *Gut*, 1966; 7: 668.

29 Whiteway J, Morson BC. Elastosis in diverticular disease of the sigmoid colon. *Gut*, 1985; 26: 258.

30 Gore S, Shepherd NA *et al*. Endoscopic crescentic fold disease of the sigmoid colon: the clinical and histopathological spectrum of a distinctive endoscopic appearance. *Int J Colorectal Dis*, 1992; 7: 76.

31 Makapugay LM, Dean PJ. Diverticular disease-associated chronic colitis. *Am J Surg Pathol*, 1996; 20: 94.

32 Peppercorn MA. Drug-responsive chronic segmental colitis associated with diverticula: a clinical syndrome in the elderly. *Am J Gastroenterol*, 1992; 87: 609.

33 Kelly JK. Polypoid prolapsing mucosal folds in diverticular disease. *Am J Surg Pathol*, 1991; 15: 871.

34 Mathus-Vliegen EM, Tytgat GN. Polyp-simulating mucosal prolapse syndrome in (pre-) diverticular disease. *Endoscopy*, 1986; 18: 84.

35 Nakamura S, Kino I *et al*. Inflammatory myoglandular polyps of the colon and rectum. A clinicopathological study of 32 pedunculated polyps, distinct from other types of polyps. *Am J Surg Pathol*, 1992; 16: 772.

36 Hughes LE. Complications of diverticular disease: inflammation, obstruction, and haemorrhage. *Clin Gastroenterol*, 1975; 4: 147.

37 Morson BC. The muscle abnormality in diverticular disease of the colon. *Proc R Soc Med*, 1963; 56: 798.

38 Meyers MA, Alonso DR, Gray GF, Baer JW. Pathogenesis of bleeding diverticulosis. *Gastroenterology*, 1976; 71: 577.

39 Olsen WR. Haemorrhage from diverticular disease of the colon. *Am J Surg*, 1968; 115: 247.

40 Casarella WJ, Kanter IE, Seaman WB. Right-sided colonic diverticula as a cause of acute rectal haemorrhage. *N Engl J Med*, 1972; 286: 450.

41 Boley SJ, DiBiase A, Brandt LJ, Sammartano RJ. Lower intestinal bleeding in the elderly. *Am J Surg*, 1979; 137: 57.

42 Welch CE, Athanasoulis CA, Galdabini JJ. Haemorrhage from the large bowel with special reference to angiodysplasia and diverticular disease. *World J Surg*, 1978; 2: 73.

43 Small WP, Smith AN. Fistula and conditions associated with diverticular disease of the colon. *Clin Gastroenterol*, 1975; 4: 171.

44 Colcock BP, Stahman FD. Fistulas complicating diverticular disease of the sigmoid colon. *Ann Surg*, 1972; 175: 838.

45 Wilson RG, Smith AN *et al*. Complications of diverticular disease and non-steroidal anti-inflammatory drugs: a prospective study. *Br J Surg*, 1990; 77: 1103.

46 Teague RH, Thornton JR, Manning AP, Salmon PR, Read AE. Colonoscopy for investigation of unexplained rectal bleeding. *Lancet*, 1978; i: 1350.

47 Gledhill A, Dixon MF. Crohn's-like reaction in diverticular disease. *Gut*, 1998; 42: 392.

48 Burroughs S, Bowrey DJ, Morris-Stiff GJ, Williams GT. Granulomatous inflammation in sigmoid diverticulitis: two diseases or one? *Histopathology*, 1998; 33: 349.

49 Shepherd NA. Diverticular disease and chronic idiopathic inflammatory bowel disease: associations and masquerades. *Gut*, 1996; 38: 801.

50 Meyers MA, Alonso DR, Morson BC, Bartram C. Pathogenesis of diverticulitis complicating granulomatous colitis. *Gastroenterology*, 1978; 74: 24.

51 Schauer PR, Ramos R *et al*. Virulent diverticular disease in young obese men. *Am J Surg*, 1992; 164: 443.

52 Mielke JE, Becker KL, Gross JB. Diverticulitis of the colon in a young man with Marfan's syndrome. *Gastroenterology*, 1965; 48: 379.

53 Beighton PH, Murdoch JL, Votteler T. Gastrointestinal complications of the Ehlers–Danlos syndrome. *Gut*, 1969; 10: 1004.

54 Smith AN. Colonic muscle in diverticular disease. *Clin Gastroenterol*, 1986; 15: 917.

55 Parks TG, Connell AM. Motility studies in diverticular disease of the colon. *Gut*, 1969; 10: 538.

56 Arfwidsson S. Pathogenesis of multiple diverticula of the sigmoid colon in diverticular disease. *Arch Chir Scand Suppl*, 1964; 342: 5.

57 Painter NS, Truelove SC. The intraluminal pressure patterns in diverticulosis. *Gut*, 1964; 5: 201.
58 Taylor I, Duthie HL. Bran tablets and diverticular disease. *Br Med J*, 1976; 1: 988.
59 Weinreich J, Andersen D. Intraluminal pressure in the sigmoid colon. II. Patients with sigmoid diverticula and related conditions. *Scand J Gastroenterol*, 1976; 11: 581.
60 Painter NS, Truelove SC, Ardran GM, Tuckery M. Segmentation and the localization of intraluminal pressures in the human colon, with special reference to the pathogenesis of colonic diverticula. *Gastroenterology*, 1965; 49: 169.
61 Williams I. Diverticular disease of the colon, a 1968 view. *Gut*, 1968; 9: 498.
62 Tomita R, Tanjoh K *et al*. Physiological studies on nitric oxide in the right sided colon of patients with diverticular disease. *Hepatogastroenterology*, 1999; 46: 2839.
63 Painter NS, Burkitt DP. Diverticular disease of the colon: a deficiency disease of western civilisation. *Br Med J*, 1971; 2: 450.
64 Painter NS, Burkitt DP. Diverticular disease of the colon: a 20th century problem. *Clin Gastroenterol*, 1975; 4: 3.
65 Aldoori WH, Giovannucci EL *et al*. A prospective study of dietary fiber types and symptomatic diverticular disease in men. *J Nutr*, 1998; 128: 714.
66 Manousos O, Day NE, Tzonou A *et al*. Diet and other factors in the aetiology of diverticulosis: an epidemiological study in Greece. *Gut*, 1985; 26: 544.
67 Gear JSS, Ware A, Fursdon P *et al*. Symptomless diverticular disease and intake of dietary fibre. *Lancet*, 1979; 1: 511.
68 Ohi G, Minowa K, Oyama T *et al*. Changes in dietary fiber intake among Japanese in the 20th century: a relationship to the prevalence of diverticular disease. *Am J Clin Nutr*, 1983; 38: 115.
69 Berry CS, Fearn T, Fisher N, Gregory JA, Hardy J. Dietary fibre and prevention of diverticular disease of the colon: evidence from rats. *Lancet*, 1984; 2: 294.
70 Painter NS, Almeida AZ, Colebourne KW. Unprocessed bran in treatment of diverticular disease of the colon. *Br Med J*, 1972; 2: 137.
71 Findlay JM, Smith AN, Mitchell WD, Anderson JB, Eastwood MA. Effect of unprocessed bran on colon function in normal subjects and in diverticular disease. *Lancet*, 1974; 1: 146.
72 Ornstein MH, Littlewood ER, Baird IM, Fowler J, North WRS, Cox AG. Are fibre supplements really necessary in diverticular disease of the colon? A controlled clinical trial. *Br Med J*, 1981; 282: 1353.
73 Peck DA, Labat R, Waite VC. Diverticular disease of the right colon. *Dis Colon Rectum*, 1968; 11: 49.
74 Sugihara K, Muto T, Morioka Y, Asano A, Yamamoto T. Diverticular disease of the colon in Japan. *Dis Colon Rectum*, 1984; 27: 531.
75 Perry PM, Morson BC. Right-sided diverticulosis of the colon. *Br J Surg*, 1971; 58: 902.
76 Sugihara K, Muto T, Morioka Y. Motility study in right-sided diverticular disease of the colon. *Gut*, 1983; 24: 1130.
77 Williams KL. Acute solitary ulcers and acute diverticulitis of the caecum and ascending colon. *Br J Surg*, 1960; 47: 351.
78 Chaudhary NA, Truelove SC. The irritable bowel syndrome. A study of the clinical features, predisposing causes and prognosis in 130 cases. *Q J Med*, 1962; 31: 307.
79 Moriarty KJ, Dawson AM. Functional abdominal pain. Further evidence that the whole gut is affected. *Br Med J*, 1982; 284: 1670.
80 Schuster MM, Whitehead WE. Physiologic insights into irritable bowel syndrome. *Clin Gastroenterol*, 1986; 15: 839.
81 Hislop IG. Psychological significance of the irritable bowel syndrome. *Gut*, 1971; 12: 452.
82 Ford MJ, Miller PMcC, Eastwood J, Eastwood MA. Life events, psychiatric illness and the irritable bowel syndrome. *Gut*, 1987; 28: 160.
83 Bentley SJ, Pearson DJ, Rix KJB. Food hypersensitivity in irritable bowel syndrome. *Lancet*, 1983; ii: 295.
84 Harvey RF, Mauad EC, Brown AM. Prognosis in the irritable bowel syndrome: a 5-year prospective study. *Lancet*, 1987; i: 963.
85 Tucker DM, Sandstead HH, Logan GM *et al*. Dietary fibre and personality factors as determinants of stool output. *Gastroenterology*, 1981; 81: 879.
86 Latimer P, Sarna S, Campbell D, Latimer M, Waterfall W, Daniel EE. Colonic motor and myoelectrical activity: a comparative study of normal subjects, psychoneurotic patients and patients with irritable bowel syndrome. *Gastroenterology*, 1981; 80: 893.
87 Ritchie JA. The irritable bowel syndrome. Part II. Manometric and cineradiographic studies. *Clin Gastroenterol*, 1977; 3: 622.
88 Eastwood MA, Eastwood J, Ford MJ. The irritable bowel syndrome: a disease or a response? *J R Soc Med*, 1987; 80: 219.
89 Barnes PRH, Lennard-Jones JE, Hawley PR, Todd IP. Hirschsprung's disease and idiopathic megacolon in adults and adolescents. *Gut*, 1986; 27: 534.
90 Smith B. *The Neuropathology of the Alimentary Tract*. Williams & Wilkins, Baltimore, 1972.
91 Lane WA. Chronic intestinal stasis. *Br Med J*, 1909; i: 1408.
92 Preston DM, Lennard-Jones JE. Severe chronic constipation of young women: 'idiopathic slow transit constipation'. *Gut*, 1986; 27: 41.
93 Preston DM, Butler MG, Smith B, Lennard-Jones JE. Neuropathology of slow transit constipation. *Gut*, 1983; 24: A997.
94 Krishnamurthy S, Schuffler MD, Rohrmann CA, Pope CE. Severe idiopathic constipation is associated with a distinctive abnormality of the colonic myenteric plexus. *Gastroenterology*, 1985; 88: 26.
95 Koch TR, Carney JA, Go L, Go VLW. Idiopathic chronic constipation is associated with decreased colonic vasoactive intestinal peptide. *Gastroenterology*, 1988; 94: 300.
96 Turnbull GK, Lennard-Jones JE, Bartram CI. Failure of rectal expulsion as a cause of constipation: why fibre and laxatives sometimes fail. *Lancet*, 1986; i: 767.
97 Chiotakakou-Faliakou E, Kamm MA *et al*. Biofeedback provides long-term benefit for patients with intractable, slow and normal transit constipation. *Gut*, 1998; 42: 517.
98 Roy AJ, Emmanuel AV *et al*. Behavioural treatment (biofeedback) for constipation following hysterectomy. *Br J Surg*, 2000; 87: 100.
99 Anuras S, Baker CRF. The colon in the pseudoobstructive syndrome. *Clin Gastroenterol*, 1986; 15: 745.
100 Nivatvongs S, Vermeulen FD, Fang DT. Colonoscopic decompression of acute pseudoobstruction of the colon. *Ann Surg*, 1982; 196: 598.
101 Krishnamurthy S, Schuffler MD. Pathology of neuromuscular disorders of the small intestine and colon. *Gastroenterology*, 1987; 93: 610.
102 Mitros FA, Schuffler MD, Teja K, Anuras S. Pathologic features of familial visceral myopathy. *Hum Pathol*, 1982; 13: 825.

103 Fitzgibbons PL, Chandrasoma PT. Familial visceral myopathy. Evidence of diffuse involvement of intestinal smooth muscle. *Am J Surg Pathol*, 1987; 11: 846.

104 Poirier TJ, Rankin GB. Gastrointestinal manifestations of progressive systemic scleroderma based on a review of 364 cases. *Am J Gastroenterol*, 1972; 58: 30.

105 Schuffler MD, Beegle RG. Progressive systemic sclerosis of the gastrointestinal tract and hereditary hollow visceral myopathy: two distinguishable disorders of intestinal smooth muscle. *Gastroenterology*, 1979; 77: 664.

106 Edwards DAW, Lennard-Jones JE. Diffuse systemic sclerosis presenting as infarction of the colon. *Proc R Soc Med*, 1960; 53: 877.

107 Goldberg HI, Sheft DJ. Esophageal and colon changes in myotonia dystrophica. *Gastroenterology*, 1972; 63: 134.

108 Pruzanski W, Huvos AG. Smooth muscle involvement in primary muscle disease. I. Myotonic dystrophy. *Arch Pathol*, 1967; 83: 229.

109 Huvos AG, Pruzanski W. Smooth muscle involvement in primary muscle disease. II. Progressive muscular dystrophy. *Arch Pathol*, 1967; 82: 234.

110 Gilat T, Spiro HM. Amyloidosis and the gut. *Am J Dig Dis*, 1968; 13: 619.

111 Bishop AE, Ferri G-L, Probert L, Bloom SR, Polak JM. Peptidergic nerves. *Scand J Gastroenterol*, 1982; 17 (Suppl 71): 43.

112 Smith B. The neuropathology of pseudo-obstruction of the intestine. *Scand J Gastroenterol*, 1982; 17 (Suppl 71): 103.

113 Knowles CH, Bennett N, Feakins R, Scott SM, Martin JE. Smooth muscle denervation in humans is associated with inclusion body formation in the gastrointestinal tract. *J Pathol*, 2000; 190 (Suppl S): A3.

114 Barnes PRH, Lennard-Jones JE, Hawley PR, Todd IP. Hirschsprung's disease and idiopathic megacolon in adults and adolescents. *Gut*, 1986; 27: 534.

115 Feinstat T, Tesluk H, Schuffler MD *et al.* Megacolon and neurofibromatosis: a neuronal intestinal dysplasia. *Gastroenterology*, 1984; 86: 1573.

116 Carney JA, Go VLW, Sizemore GW, Hayles AB. Alimentary-tract ganglioneuromatosis: a major component of the syndrome of multiple endocrine neoplasia, Type 2b. *N Engl J Med*, 1976; 295: 1287.

117 Mendelsohn G, Diamond MP. Familial ganglioneuromatous polyposis of the large bowel. *Am J Surg Pathol*, 1984; 8: 515.

118 Schuffler MD, Bird TD, Sumi SM, Cook A. A familial neuronal disease presenting as intestinal pseudoobstruction. *Gastroenterology*, 1978; 75: 889.

119 Cockel R, Hill EE, Rushton DI, Smith B, Hawkins CF. Familial steatorrhoea with calcification of the basal ganglia and mental retardation. *Q J Med*, 1973; 42: 771.

120 Todd IP, Porter NH, Morson BC, Smith B, Friedmann CA, Neal RA. Chagas' disease of the colon and rectum. *Gut*, 1969; 10: 1009.

121 Martins-Campos IV, Tafuri WL. Chagas' enteropathy. *Gut*, 1973; 14: 910.

122 Sonsino E, Mouy R, Foucaud P *et al.* Intestinal pseudoobstruction related to cytomegalovirus infection of myenteric plexus. *N Engl J Med*, 1984; 311: 196.

123 Debinski HS, Kamm MA, Talbot IC, Khan G, Kangro HO, Jeffries DJ. DNA viruses in the pathogenesis of sporadic chronic idiopathic intestinal pseudo-obstruction. *Gut*, 1997; 41: 100.

124 Schuffler MD, Baird HW, Fleming CR *et al.* Intestinal pseudo-obstruction as the presenting manifestation of small cell carcinoma of the lung: a paraneoplastic neuropathy of the gastrointestinal tract. *Ann Intern Med*, 1983; 98: 129.

125 Berenyi MR, Schwartz GS. Megasigmoid syndrome in diabetes and neurologic disease. *Am J Gastroenterol*, 1967; 47: 311.

126 Bacharach T, Evans JR. Enlargement of the colon secondary to hypothyroidism. *Ann Intern Med*, 1957; 47: 121.

127 Watkins GL, Oliver GA, Rosenberg BF. Giant megacolon in the insane. *Ann Surg*, 1961; 153: 409.

128 Smith B. Pathology of cathartic colon. *Proc R Soc Med*, 1972; 65: 288.

129 Gattuso JM, Kamm MA. Adverse effects of drugs used in the management of constipation and diarrhoea. *Drug Saf*, 1994; 10: 47.

130 Muller-Lissner S. What has happened to the cathartic colon? *Gut*, 1996; 39: 486.

131 Tsuto T, Okamura H, Fukui K *et al.* Immunohistochemical investigations of gut hormones in the colon of patients with Hirschsprung's disease. *J Pediatr Surg*, 1985; 20: 266.

132 Long RG, Bishop AE, Barnes AJ *et al.* Neural and hormonal peptides in rectal biopsy specimens from patients with Chagas' disease and chronic autonomic failure. *Lancet*, 1980; i: 559.

133 Lindop GBM. Enterochromaffin cell hyperplasia and megacolon: report of a case. *Gut*, 1983; 24: 575.

134 Eisenstat TE, Raneri AJ, Mason GR. Volvulus of the transverse colon. *Am J Surg*, 1977; 134: 396.

135 Sachidananthan CK, Soehner B. Volvulus of the splenic flexure of the colon. *Dis Colon Rectum*, 1972; 15: 466.

136 Dowling BL, Gunning AJ. Caecal volvulus. *Br J Surg*, 1969; 56: 124.

137 Sutcliffe MML. Volvulus of the sigmoid colon. *Br J Surg*, 1968; 55: 903.

138 Gelfand M. *The Sick African*, 3rd edn. Cape Town: Juta and Co, 1957: 720.

139 Perlmann JJ. Clinical contributions to pathology and surgical treatment of intestinal occlusion. *Arch Klin Chir*, 1925; 137: 245.

140 Delafield RH, Hellreigel K, Meza A, Urteaga O. Sigmoid volvulus. *Rev Gastroenterol*, 1953; 20: 29.

141 Khoury GA, Pickard R, Knight M. Volvulus of the sigmoid colon. *Br J Surg*, 1977; 64: 587.

142 Hughes LE. Sigmoid volvulus. *J R Soc Med*, 1980; 73: 78.

143 Gillon J, Holt S, Sircus W. Pneumatosis coli and sigmoid volvulus: a report of four cases. *Br J Surg*, 1979; 66: 802.

144 Northeast ADR, Dennison AR, Lee EG. Sigmoid volvulus: new thoughts on the epidemiology. *Dis Colon Rectum*, 1984; 27: 260.

145 Shepherd JJ. The epidemiology and clinical presentation of sigmoid volvulus. *Br J Surg*, 1969; 56: 353.

146 DuBoulay CEH, Fairbrother J, Isaacson PG. Mucosal prolapse syndrome—a unifying concept for solitary ulcer syndrome and related disorders. *J Clin Pathol*, 1983; 36: 1264.

147 Rosen Y, Vaillant JG, Yermakov V. Submucosal mucous cysts at a colostomy site: relationship to colitis cystica profunda and report of a case. *Dis Colon Rectum*, 1976; 19: 453.

148 Rutter KRP, Riddell RH. The solitary ulcer syndrome of the rectum. *Clin Gastroenterol*, 1975; 4: 505.

149 Madigan MR, Morson BC. Solitary ulcer of the rectum. *Gut*, 1969; 10: 871.
150 Franzin G, Scarpa A, Dina R, Novelli P. 'Transitional' and hyperplastic-metaplastic mucosa occurring in solitary ulcer of the rectum. *Histopathology*, 1981; 5: 527.
151 Ehsanullah M, Filipe MI, Gazzard B. Morphological and mucus secretion criteria for differential diagnosis of solitary ulcer syndrome and non-specific proctitis. *J Clin Pathol*, 1982; 35: 26.
152 Epstein SE, Ascari WQ, Ablow RC, Seaman WB, Lattes R. Colitis cystica profunda. *Am J Clin Pathol*, 1966; 45: 186.
153 Allen MS. Hamartomatous inverted polyps of the rectum. *Cancer*, 1954; 19: 257.
154 Talerman A. Enterogenous cysts of the rectum. *Br J Surg*, 1971; 58: 643.
155 Kang YS, Kamm MA *et al*. Pathology of the rectal wall in solitary rectal ulcer syndrome and complete rectal prolapse. *Gut*, 1996; 38: 587.
156 Rutter KRP. Electromyographic changes in certain pelvic floor abnormalities. *Proc R Soc Med*, 1974; 67: 53.
157 Womack NR, Williams NS, Holmfield JHM, Morrison JFB. Pressure and prolapse—the cause of solitary rectal ulceration. *Gut*, 1987; 28: 1228.
158 Rutter KRP. Solitary rectal ulcer syndrome. *Proc R Soc Med*, 1975; 68: 22.
159 Parks AG, Porter NH, Hardcastle JD. The syndrome of the descending perineum. *Proc R Soc Med*, 1966; 59: 477.
160 Dick A, Green GJ. Large bowel intussusception in adults. *Br J Radiol*, 1961; 34: 769.
161 Bond MR, Roberts JBM. Intussusception in the adult. *Br J Surg*, 1964; 51: 818.
162 Strange SL. Retrograde intussusception of the colon. *Proc R Soc Med*, 1956; 49: 579.
163 Cole GJ. Caeco-colic intussusception in Ibadan. *Br J Surg*, 1966; 53: 415.
164 Richards RC, Richards RC. Idiopathic caeco-caecal intussusception. *Am J Surg*, 1966; 112: 641.
165 Levis CD. Caeco-colic intussusception following appendicectomy. *Br Med J*, 1958; ii: 550.
166 Davidson JRM. Sigmoido-rectal intussusception. *Aust N Z J Surg*, 1966; 36: 13.
167 Broden B, Snellman B. Procidentia of the rectum studied with cineradiography: a contribution to the discussion of causative mechanisms. *Dis Colon Rectum*, 1968; 11: 330.
168 Ihre T, Seligson U. Intussusception of the rectum—internal procidentia: treatment and results in 90 patients. *Dis Colon Rectum*, 1975; 18: 391.
169 Corman ML. Rectal prolapse in children. *Dis Colon Rectum*, 1985; 28: 535.
170 Parks AG, Swash M, Urich H. Sphincter denervation in anorectal incontinence and rectal prolapse. *Gut*, 1977; 18: 656.
171 Roof WR, Morris GC, DeBakey ME. Management of perforating injuries to the colon in civilian practice. *Am J Surg*, 1960; 99: 641.
172 Claydon C, Martin JD. Trauma to the rectum. *Am Surg*, 1968; 34: 317.
173 Grodsky L. Perforation of the colon and rectum during administration of barium enema. *Dis Colon Rectum*, 1959; 2: 216.
174 Macrae FA, Tan KG, Williams CB. Towards safer colonoscopy: a report on the complications of 5,000 diagnostic or therapeutic colonoscopies. *Gut*, 1983; 24: 376.
175 Bigard MA, Gaucher P, Lasalle C. Fatal colonic explosion during colonoscopic polypectomy. *Gastroenterology*, 1979; 77: 1307.
176 Thomas LP. Impalement of the rectum. *Lancet*, 1953; i: 704.
177 Kaufer N, Shein S, Levowitz BS. Impalement injury of the rectum. *Dis Colon Rectum*, 1967; 10: 394.
178 Comline SC. Pneumatic rupture of the rectum. *Br Med J*, 1952; ii: 745.
179 Butters AG. An unusual rectal injury. *Br Med J*, 1955; i: 602.
180 Shennan J. Seat-belt injuries of the left colon. *Br J Surg*, 1973; 60: 673.
181 Shook LL, Whittle R, Rose EF. Rectal fist insertion. An unusual form of sexual behaviour. *Am J Forensic Med Pathol*, 1985; 6: 319.
182 Berger PL, Shaw RE. Spontaneous rupture of the colon. *Br Med J*, 1961; i: 1422.
183 Dickinson PH, Gilmour J. Spontaneous rupture of the distal large bowel. *Br J Surg*, 1961; 49: 157.
184 Shanon DP. Spontaneous rupture of the ascending colon. *Br J Surg*, 1962; 50: 199.
185 Yeo R. Spontaneous perforation of the caecum. *Postgrad Med J*, 1967; 43: 65.
186 Thomas CS, Brockman SK. Idiopathic perforation of the colon in infancy. *Ann Surg*, 1966; 164: 853.
187 Maw AR. Perforation of the sigmoid colon. *Br J Surg*, 1968; 55: 712.
188 Ashby S, Hunter-Craig D. Foreign body perforation of the gut. *Br J Surg*, 1967; 54: 382.
189 Harjola PT, Scheinin TM. Experimental observations on intestinal obstruction due to foreign bodies. *Acta Chir Scand*, 1963; 126: 144.
190 Pryor JH. Gall-stone obstruction of the sigmoid colon with particular reference to aetiology. *Br J Surg*, 1959; 47: 259.
191 Persky L, Frank ED. Foreign body perforation of the gastrointestinal tract. *N Engl J Med*, 1952; 246: 223.
192 Miller JDR, Costopoulos LB, Holmes CE, Willox GL. Gall stone ileus of the colon. *Br J Radiol*, 1965; 38: 960.
193 Atwell JD, Pollock AV. Intestinal calculi. *Br J Surg*, 1960; 47: 367.
194 Kaufman SA, Karlin H. Faecaloma of the sigmoid flexure. *Dis Colon Rectum*, 1966; 9: 133.
195 Israel GI. An unusual foreign body in the rectum. *Dis Colon Rectum*, 1961; 4: 139.
196 Lowicki EM. Accidental introduction of giant foreign body into the rectum. *Ann Surg*, 1966; 163: 395.
197 Lockhart-Mummery JP. *Diseases of the Rectum and Colon*. London: Ballière, Tindall and Cox, 1937: 377.
198 Vaughn AM, White MS. Foreign body (drinking glass) in the rectum. *JAMA*, 1959; 171: 2307.
199 Fuller RC. Foreign bodies in the rectum and colon. *Dis Colon Rectum*, 1965; 8: 123.
200 Eftaiha M, Hambrick E, Abcarian H. Principles of management of colorectal foreign bodies. *Arch Surg*, 1977; 112: 691.
201 Beerman R, Nunez D *et al*. Radiographic evaluation of the cocaine smuggler. *Gastrointest Radiol*, 1986; 11: 351.
202 Barnett VH. Discharge of foetal bones by the rectum. *Br Med J*, 1951; 2: 1385.
203 Kleckner FS. Dermatomyositis and its manifestations in the gastrointestinal tract. *Am J Gastroenterol*, 1970; 53: 141.

36 Inflammatory disorders of the large intestine

Introduction

Inflammatory disorders are common in the large bowel, sometimes in association with small intestinal disease, but more often as primary pathology of the large intestine. It is usual for a considerable length of the large bowel to be affected, and the diseased mucosa can be visualized and biopsied through various endoscopic manoeuvres, including the rigid proctosigmoidoscope and the flexible sigmoidoscope and colonoscope. Many infective pathological processes of the large intestine are more usually diagnosed by microbiological methods and often do not require histological assessment. Thus bacterial cultures are readily made of faecal material and various parasites can be demonstrated in faeces or mucus on direct microscopy. Nevertheless it is important for pathologists to recognize the histological appearances of these infective colitides, primarily because they can closely mimic the pathology of chronic inflammatory bowel disease. Erroneous treatment with immunosuppressive therapy, for instance in amoebiasis, can have grave consequences for the patient.

So it is important for the histopathologist to be able to differentiate between the histological appearances of infective causes of colitis and those of Crohn's disease and ulcerative colitis. Bacterial infections that mimic chronic inflammatory bowel disease are those, logically, that invade the mucosa. The most common of these are those caused by *Salmonella*, *Shigella* and *Campylobacter*. The pathology of these organisms is often referred to as 'acute self-limiting colitis'. In pathological practice many of the diagnostic difficulties concerning large intestinal inflammatory disorders relate to the distinction between Crohn's disease and ulcerative colitis. To maintain a perspective on the size of this problem, it should be remembered that only in 20–25% of cases of Crohn's disease is the disease limited to the large intestine, although the assessment of the differential diagnosis of chronic inflammatory bowel disease inevitably forms a large part of the workload in a specialized gastrointestinal pathology practice.

Inflammation due to viruses

Although acute gastrointestinal infection is a major cause of morbidity throughout the world and viruses play a leading part in its aetiology, viral infection of the colorectum rarely comes to the attention of the practising histopathologist. In fact, in most acute viral infection of the intestines, the small intestine is the primary seat of infection: for a fuller description of viral infection, the interested reader is referred to Chapter 23. In this chapter, only those viral infections whose cytopathic effects are demonstrable in histopathological sections of colorectal mucosal biopsies will be considered.

Adenoviruses

Adenoviruses are most commonly associated with respiratory infection but they also cause acute diarrhoea, especially in outbreaks in children. For the histopathologist, probably the most important associations are causing lymphoid hyperplasia in the terminal ileum and subsequent intussusception in infants [1], and the common occurrence of the infection in acquired immune deficiency syndrome (AIDS) diarrhoea, the inclusions being readily demonstrable in colorectal epithelium by immunohistochemical techniques [2,3].

Cytomegalovirus (CMV)

The role of this herpes group virus as a primary colonic pathogen is disputed. Infection is usually subclinical and it is uncertain whether the virus can initiate infection [4] or simply prevents healing of established ulcers [5]. Overt CMV disease can develop in patients who are immunologically suppressed, especially in those with AIDS [6,7]. In the colon, infection is associated with ulceration, which may be minute or up to several centimetres across. The ulcers are discrete and punched out with oedematous margins. There is a well established relationship, for instance, with chronic inflammatory bowel disease, CMV being able to secondarily involve the inflamed mucosa, and it may also initiate a relapse of the disease. CMV infection is more common, as a secondary infection, in patients with ulcerative colitis than Crohn's disease [8,10]. If primary disease does exist, it seems most likely to be in those patients where the organisms are associated with a vasculitis [4,6], although a self-limiting colitis in immunocompetent individuals has been described [9,11].

The diagnosis of CMV infection depends on demonstrating the characteristic nuclear inclusions within macrophages or in capillary endothelial cells (Fig. 36.1). The inclusion is dark and amphophilic but pinkish-red with a Giemsa stain. These inclusions are easily overlooked and the diagnosis should be borne in mind when confronted by large atypical cells in the floor of an ulcer. Immunohistochemical staining with anticytomegalovirus antibody demonstrates clear staining of the inclusions and is a very useful routine stain in patients in whom no definite or occasional smudgy doubtful inclusions are seen on haematoxylin and eosin (H&E) staining.

Herpes simplex virus

This DNA virus can cause a proctitis restricted to the distal 10 cm of the rectum. It is a consequence of unprotected anal intercourse and oral–faecal contact [12]. It is therefore more common in homosexuals and immunosuppressed individuals, including patients with AIDS. Anal fissures may coexist with herpes proctitis [12]. The rectal mucosa may be friable and ulcerated. On microscopy the rectal mucosa shows multinucleate giant cells, intranuclear inclusions and a perivascular

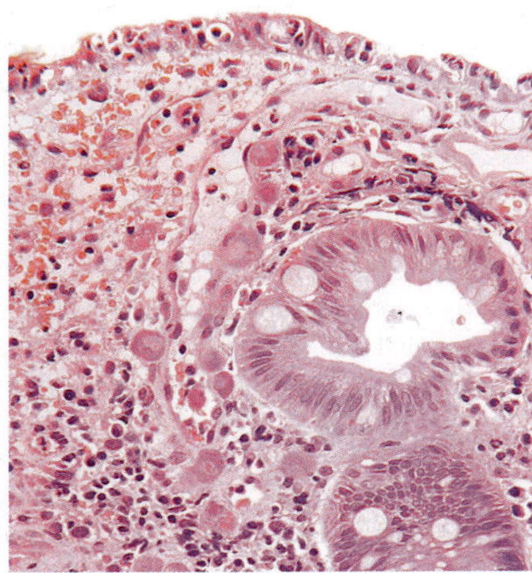

Fig. 36.1 Rectal mucosal biopsy from a patient who happens to have chronic ulcerative colitis, showing multiple cytomegalovirus inclusions within vascular endothelial cells and some within the lamina propria.

lymphocytic infiltrate [13]. Immunohistochemical staining is useful to confirm the diagnosis.

HIV and AIDS in the large intestine

Although enterocolic infection with human immunodeficiency virus (HIV) and AIDS has been covered in the corresponding chapter on the small intestine (see p. 274), some comments on the disease are appropriate. Notwithstanding the success of antiviral therapy, notably HAART (highly active antiretroviral therapy) in controlling the disease and its complications [13,14], the complications of AIDS are still regularly seen by the histopathologist analysing biopsies of the colorectum. HIV infection itself is associated with a characteristic enhanced apoptosis [15]. Such increased apoptotic activity is often closely associated with intraepithelial T lymphocytes and is typically prominent in crypt bases [2,15]. The features are similar to those seen in graft-versus-host disease. Despite these changes, the colorectal epithelial cells usually appear morphologically and morphometrically normal.

It is the infective complications of HIV infection, especially AIDS, that most often come to the attention of the practising histopathologist. Whilst the individual infections will be dealt with in the appropriate sections, it is important to note that evidence of viral infection (particularly CMV, herpes simplex virus and adenovirus), bacterial infection (including sexually transmitted bacteria, bacteria causing bacillary colitis and atypical mycobacterial infection), protozoal infection and infections caused by larger organisms may all be seen as a colorectal complication of AIDS [3]. Furthermore multiplicity of infections is a characteristic feature of AIDS. Identification of one opportunistic infection should always alert the pathologist to the possibility of identifying other organisms in biopsy and resection material [16].

Bacterial infection

Shigellosis

All four shigella species (*Shigella dysenteriae*, *S. flexneri*, *S. boydii* and *S. sonnei*) are pathogenic and only a small number of organisms are required as an infecting dose. Epidemics of bacillary dysentery are a major problem in many Third World countries where there is an association with a high population density as well as conditions of bad sanitation, poor personal hygiene and contaminated food. Shigellosis is seen more commonly in AIDS patients where the condition may behave somewhat differently from that in the non-immunocompromised host. Along with salmonella and campylobacter, shigella may be more difficult to eradicate in the AIDS patient and may result in bacteraemia. Due to the higher recurrence rate in AIDS patients they may require long-term treatment.

The *Shigella* bacterium is a non-motile Gram-negative bacillus. Person-to-person transmission and ingestion of infected food and water are responsible for the infection. *S. sonnei* will generally cause a much more severe colitis than the others and the mildest colitis is usually seen with *S. dysenteriae*. Toxins are released in the bowel lumen and there is bacterial invasion of colonic mucosa, both of which contribute to shigellosis. The organism's virulence depends on its ability to invade cells [18]. A toxin is produced and a cross-reactivity exists between this toxin and toxins of certain *Escherichia coli* species, salmonella strains and *Vibrio cholerae*. The toxin and the Shiga-like toxin of these other bacteria probably have a role in the pathogenesis of diarrhoea [19, 59]. The *Shigella* cytotoxin reduces protein synthesis in the mucosal epithelial cells, whilst an endotoxin causes mitochondrial damage leading to cell death and formation of ulcers. Further absorption of the endotoxin leads to thrombosis of small vessels with consequent haemorrhage and ischaemia causing further epithelial damage. Consequently transmural inflammation may be seen [18]. The inflammation is most severe in the rectum and sigmoid colon, but colonoscopy may disclose a pancolitis [19,20] and occasionally the terminal ileum can be involved. The affected mucosa shows friability, adherent mucopurulent exudate and occasionally aphthoid ulcers. Deep ulceration of the colon has been demonstrated radiologically in severe infection [21], but normally inflammation is superficial and perforation rare. The regional lymph nodes are usually enlarged.

Histologically, the initial inflammation is seen in the lymphoid follicles of the mucosa, which breaks down to form ulcers. It has been shown that in experimental peroral infection in the guinea pig, dysenteric bacilli penetrate the intact epithelium of the intestine and pass through the mucous membrane in a matter of a few hours [22]. Inflammatory changes follow and include the formation of crypt abscesses, focal haemorrhages and goblet cell depletion. The inflammatory response diminishes from the surface down through the mucosa with virtually no reaction in the submucosa [20]. Electron microscopic studies on rectal biopsy material have failed to reveal any specific change which might differentiate shigellosis from other inflammatory disorders of the large intestine [21,22]. The colorectal biopsy appearances in shigellosis are similar to those of other bacterial infections of the large intestine, notably salmonellosis and campylobacter infection (see p. 476). The histology in human rectal biopsy material has a notable resemblance to that reported for experimental shigellosis in Rhesus monkeys [23].

Salmonella colitis

Food poisoning by *Salmonella* organisms is a common problem in the UK [24,25]. *S. typhi, paratyphi, argona, javiana* and *oranienburg* all may cause salmonella gastroenteritis [26]. *S. enteritidis* has been increasing as a cause of food poisoning in recent years, usually from infected eggs and poultry [27]. Whereas the organisms *S. typhi* and *S. paratyphi* cause septicaemic illnesses, salmonella infection of food poisoning type (salmonellosis) is generally confined to the gastrointestinal tract. In some patients this results in vomiting and profuse watery diarrhoea, usually with colicky periumbilical abdominal pains suggesting predominantly gastric and small intestinal involvement. In others, dysenteric features such as frequent small-volume bloody motions, tenesmus and tenderness of the sigmoid colon are present. The appreciation of colonic involvement and its frequency in salmonellosis has gained acceptance over the last two decades [25,28,29].

The pathology of salmonella colitis has been appreciated from necropsy and biopsy studies. Fatal infection is mostly a disease of the young or elderly [30]. A postmortem series of 68 children who died with salmonella enteritis, mostly under 1 year of age and many with nutritional deficiencies, showed bowel lesions in 46 cases with colitis more prominent than enteritis [31]. In another autopsy study of nine patients, despite fatalities, the lack of gross abnormalities with only minimal mucosal reddening is emphasized [30]. Others have described more severe abnormalities with gross oedema and transverse ulceration. The left colon was most affected in these series [32–34], but we have also seen predominantly right-sided disease. In these autopsy studies, the histology was of a subtle diffuse colitis with prominent crypt abscesses and crypt epithelial damage [30]. Signs of healing were frequent. Superficial mucosal necrosis is common, with haemorrhage and occasional fibrin thrombi [29].

In clinical practice, the colonoscopic appearances are of mucosal hyperaemia, friability and inflammation, which may be patchy or diffuse. It is important to remember salmonellosis as a cause of patchy inflammation at colonoscopy: it should not be expected always to be a diffuse colitis. The biopsy pathology of the rectal mucosa in salmonella infection [32,35] is described along with the other forms of infective colitis below (see p. 476).

The concurrence of salmonellosis and chronic idiopathic inflammatory bowel disease suggests that this association is not a rarity and it can present problems in diagnosis and management [33,34]. The appearances in rectal biopsies in such patients are of inflammatory bowel disease with active inflammation [35]. It is probable that, in ulcerative colitis and Crohn's disease, there is a predisposition to a supervening salmonella infection and this would be more likely to occur with prolonged steroid therapy [38]. The possibility that some of these cases, in which no antecedent bowel disturbance was present, represent ulcerative postdysenteric colitis [36–38] seems less likely as, in countries where bacillary dysentery is prevalent, this is very unusual. In contrast, persistent diarrhoea with or without ulceration of the colon is not uncommon in amoebic dysentery [39,40]. It is now possible to analyse food by polymerase chain reaction (PCR) to detect both salmonella and shigella.

Rectal mucosal prolapse in association with massive diarrhoea may sometimes occur. Appendicitis or ileitis may be seen, complicated occasionally by toxic megacolon and/or perforation. Patients with salmonellosis may develop extraintestinal manifestations, including erythema nodosum and reactive arthropathy. Infection with *Salmonella* may be particularly problematic in those with HIV infection or with sickle cell disease.

Campylobacter colitis

Until recently, campylobacter species could not be grown from the stool and did not rank as a significant cause of gastroenteritis [41,42]. Since then, following the development of a suitable stool culture media, the bacterium has moved from relative obscurity to being recognized as one of the most common causes of acute bacterial diarrhoea [42,43]. *Campylobacter* are Gram-negative spiral bacilli, which were previously (until 1964) classified as *Vibrio* spp. [44]. Initial isolations from humans suggested primary disease in the small intestine [45,46], but more recently evidence of a colitis has been definitively demonstrated with changes characteristic of infective proctocolitis seen in colorectal biopsies [47,48] (see p. 476). Infection may occur from person to person but is more usually acquired from food, water or domestic pets [49]. Abdominal pain is a prominent clinical symptom that may result in admission to a surgical ward and subsequent unwarranted surgery [47]. Indeed the organism can induce an appendicitis [46]. Ileocaecal disease, focal Crohn's-like colonic involvement or diffuse disease have all been described at colonoscopy [47]. The pathogenesis of the diarrhoea is not clear, for it has not been definitely established whether the organism is toxigenic and/or invasive [49,50]. Clinically both a small bowel secretory component and an invasive colonic phase seem likely.

Enteroinvasive *Escherichia coli* diarrhoea

This group of *E. coli* is closely related to *Shigella* spp. Dysentery is produced by destruction of the epithelium in the colon with ulceration and blood, mucus and pus in the stools. Mucosal attachment and plasmids are involved in the pathogenesis [51,52]. Other *E. coli* causing small intestinal disease are considered elsewhere (see pp. 276–7).

Enteropathogenic *E. coli*

Haemorrhagic colitis usually results from verotoxin-producing *E. coli* (VTEC), now known as Shiga toxin-producing *E. coli* [53–57]. There are two common and distinct cytotoxins: Shiga-like toxin T and Shiga-like toxin II. Enterohaemorrhagic *E. coli* adhere to the luminal surface, as they do in animals when they elaborate a toxin prior to absorption of the toxin. The absorption of the toxin, as in shigellosis, interferes with protein synthesis and results in epithelial and endothelial damage [57,60]. The cellular insult is not limited to the bowel. The endothelium of the kidneys is also damaged to produce haemolytic–uraemic syndrome and thrombotic thrombocytopenic purpura, resulting from the failure of secretion of anticoagulant substances from the damaged vascular endothelial cells, leading to thrombosis in small blood vessels. Unsurprisingly, given these pathogenetic mechanisms at play, the bowel may show a close histopathological resemblance to ischaemic colitis.

The incidence of *E. coli* infection is highest in the summer. *E. coli* 0157 (E0157) can survive in water and may consequently be associated with water-borne outbreaks. It is also recognized to occur in hamburgers and other processed beef. *E. coli* in such processed meat is more sensitive to heat than other bacteria but may survive for long periods in extreme cold conditions, even in the domestic freezer [58]. For this reason, thorough cooking of hamburgers is exceptionally important since a minced beef product may carry *E. coli* in the centre of the product where it will be less likely to be destroyed during cooking.

The incubation period of the colitis is 3–4 days, whilst the infective diarrhoea usually lasts for 2–9 days. Asymptomatic infections may occur, as may a milder form of the disease. The immunocompromised, the very young and the very elderly are more susceptible to haemolytic–uraemic syndrome (HUS) [57] and thrombocytopenic purpura (TTP), following E0157 infection. The progression of the syndrome to HUS and TTP does not seem to be influenced by antibiotic therapy.

The clinical differential diagnosis includes ischaemic colitis, pseudomembranous colitis, chronic inflammatory bowel disease and occasionally acute appendicitis, if the disease is predominantly a right-sided colitis or ileocolitis. Colonoscopy may reveal a normal-looking mucosa with oozing of blood, or it may reveal pseudomembrane formation, thereby mimicking pseudomembranous or ischaemic colitis. Patchy erosions ulceration may be seen in the right side of the colon. In children more commonly the entire colon is involved.

The histopathological appearances are fundamentally those of infective colitis (see below), but mucosal haemorrhage and intravascular platelet thrombi are sometimes conspicuous [58,59]. Since the changes are distinctly patchy, multiple biopsies are helpful in achieving the diagnosis but the severity of the histological changes may relate poorly to the severity of the illness. The focal nature of the change is a useful distinguishing feature in the differential diagnosis between E0157 infection and acute ulcerative colitis.

Clostridial infections

Clostridial species are especially implicated in inflammatory and necrotizing disease in the small intestine (see Chapter 21). *Clostridium difficile* causes pseudomembranous colitis (see p. 516) as well as cases of sporadic diarrhoea. The enterotoxigenic varieties of *C. perfringens* are implicated in pig-bel and may cause infective colitis [61–63]. Pig-bel is a form of small bowel ulceration usually seen after gorging on undercooked pork in Papua New Guinea [61]. Pig-bel has been reported to affect the colon as well as the small bowel and may even be seen in vegetarians [64]. *C. septicum* is the putative pathogen in neutropenic colitis (see p. 522).

The biopsy diagnosis of infective colitis

As few patients come to surgery for this condition, the histopathologist is usually asked to make the diagnosis of infective proctocolitis on biopsy material. Perhaps the most critical factor in this assessment is the timing of the biopsy, for the typical changes of infective colitis are usually only seen early in the course of the infection [65,66]. In the majority of cases, the changes begin to resolve or assume a more chronic picture after about 7–10 days: It then becomes harder to distinguish infective colitis from other forms of inflammatory bowel disease [67–70].

In the typical biopsy, the initial impression at low magnification is of a mucosa widened by oedema and an inflammatory infiltrate, the latter appearing like sprinkled salt grains across the lamina propria [67,71–75] (Figs 36.2–36.4). Focal clusters of polymorphs are present throughout the biopsy, often adjacent to dilated capillaries or alongside crypts. Pericryptal haemorrhage may be striking at low power [74]. A characteristic strongly in favour of infective disease is the presence of polymorphs within the epithelium of the crypts but not yet in great numbers within the crypt lumen. This appearance, the incipient crypt abscess or 'cryptitis' (Fig. 36.3), is in contrast to the true crypt abscess, which does occur in infective colitis but is much more prevalent in active chronic ulcerative colitis and Crohn's disease [67,74,75]. The epithelium associated with these intraepithelial polymorphs may be degenerate

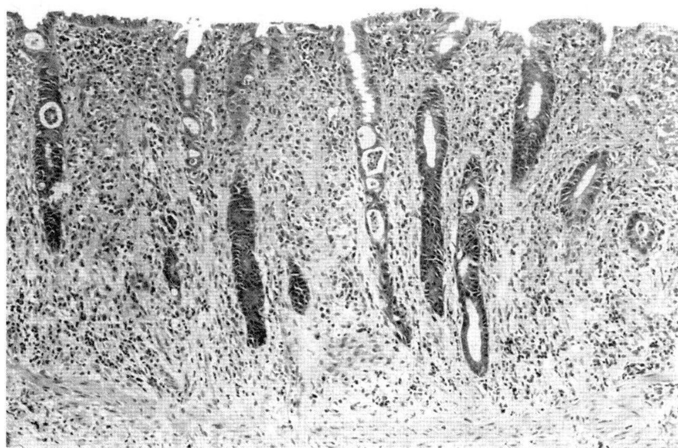

Fig. 36.2 Infective colitis illustrating the regular crypt alignment, but many are degenerate and show intraluminal polymorphs gathered in a beaded appearance along their length (string of pearls sign).

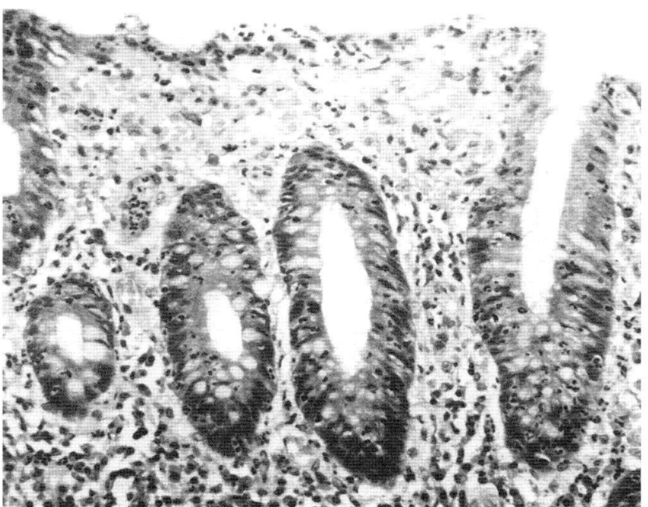

Fig. 36.3 Infective colitis: large numbers of polymorphs are caught up between the crypt epithelial cells (incipient crypt abscesses), which is a characteristic feature of infective colitis.

or may be gathered into small projecting tufts between individual crypts.

One further characteristic feature of infective colitis is that the acute inflammatory changes are distinctly patchy across the biopsy. The absolute number of plasma cells and lymphocytes within the lamina propria may well be increased but this is partially masked by the oedema. It is the dominance of the polymorphonuclear neutrophils over the chronic inflammatory cell infiltrate, especially plasma cells, that is of key diagnostic importance when making the distinction between infection and other causes of proctocolitis. The crypt pattern remains regular, except in severe shigellosis [73], but the superficial crypt epithelium shows reactive and degenerative changes along with numerous neutrophils [73,74]. There is mucin depletion and the individual crypt epithelial cells appear flattened. This is reflected in dilatation of the superficial half of many of the crypts. In some, this area may degenerate completely. This abnormality of crypt outline forms a conspicuous feature at the initial examination of the biopsy (Fig. 36.4). The term 'crypt withering' has been suggested for this appearance (although this feature is also a characteristic change in subacute ischaemic colitis). Epithelial bridges may be present across the crypt lumens giving an additional feature known as the 'string of pearls' sign [32]. Other abnormalities in the histopathology of infective colitis are less specific. Luminal pus is frequent and margination of polymorphs is prominent within congested capillaries.

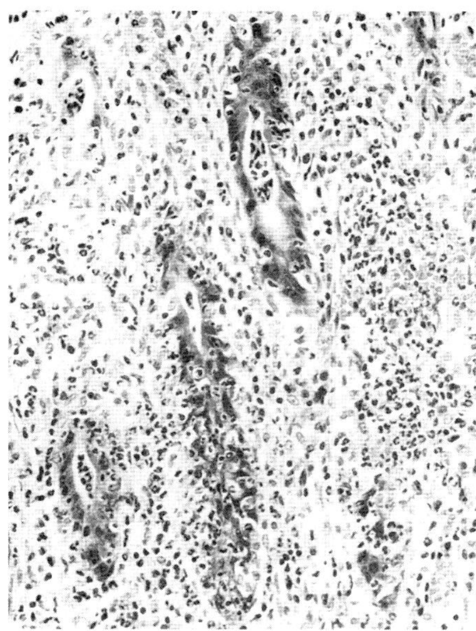

Fig. 36.4 Infective colitis. In this rectal biopsy crypt 'withering' with destruction by polymorphs is seen. The lamina propria contains mostly polymorphs and little increase in chronic inflammatory cells.

This descriptive account of infective colitis represents the characteristic pattern, and as mentioned earlier, is common only early in the disease [32]. Interobserver variability between histopathologists is considerable in the reporting of biopsies showing acute self-limiting colitis [74]. There have been attempts to identify simple, objective criteria for the histological diagnosis of acute colitis 1–10 weeks after onset [74]. However, such methods, involving cell counting, are difficult to incorporate into routine diagnostic practice. One study of biopsies taken from 1 to 10 weeks after onset of diarrhoea identified that those without significant inflammation, with irritable bowel syndrome, had a concentration of lamina propria cells in the upper third of the lamina propria, whilst increased lamina propria acute inflammatory cell numbers in the upper and middle third correlated well with infective colitis. In chronic inflammatory bowel disease, there was increased lamina propria cellularity in the lower third of the lamina propria, usually known as a basal plasmacytosis [67].

Not all biopsies in infective colitis, even if taken early in the disease and with positive cultures, show the typical features [72]. Some biopsies may simply appear oedematous or even normal, although unless colonoscopy is undertaken, more characteristic lesions elsewhere in the colon cannot be excluded [74]. The main value of a biopsy in infective disease is in those cases that are culture negative [72]. Here, in the presence of characteristic histology, a confident diagnosis can be made. It is also important that such patients are not misdiagnosed as having ulcerative colitis or Crohn's disease. Where there is doubt about the diagnosis, a follow-up biopsy between 6 and 8 weeks later is often helpful. In the majority of cases of infection, the histological appearances will have reverted to normal. This should not be the case in ulcerative colitis. It must be pointed out that in some series a small number of biopsies from patients with clinical infective disease may have biopsies interpreted as more like Crohn's disease or ulcerative colitis [48,74–79].

The complications of infective colitis

The complications of acute bacillary dysentery include myocarditis, splenitis, liver abscess and effusions into the joints, but these are only found in severe infections, usually with *Shigella*, which produces a powerful exotoxin [59,60]. Acute bacillary dysentery can be followed by a chronic state in which organisms remain in the bowel and ulceration of the intestine persists. Alternatively, the initial inflammation may have been so severe that, despite healing, permanent structural changes are found. These include the appearances known as colitis cystica profunda in which mucous retention cysts are found in the submucosa [80], presumably derived from epithelium misplaced during the acute stage of the disease. This must be distinguished from colitis cystica superficialis which is an entirely different condition seen occasionally in children dying from debilitating disease such as leukaemia, pellagra and tropical sprue [81], but has been seen by us in one case of *S. flexneri* and to a lesser degree by others [87].

'Postdysenteric colitis' was a term introduced to describe persistent inflammation and irritability of the bowel following attacks of both bacillary and amoebic dysentery, more commonly the latter [36–38,82]. The original infecting organism is often no longer present. There are three forms: the non-ulcerative which is really a problem of abnormal intestinal motility; the ulcerative which responds to antibacterial or anti-amoebic treatment; and the ulcerative which fails to respond to therapy and may be related to ulcerative colitis. Cases have been described in which there is destruction of the deep muscle layers of the colon by fibrosis and the formation of strictures [39].

There has been much controversy in the past over the relationship between bacillary dysentery and ulcerative colitis. The prevailing view is that ulcerative colitis is a separate condition, although occasionally it may be precipitated by an attack of acute infective colitis. Indeed in one series up to one-quarter of patients experienced the first attack of chronic inflammatory bowel disease after tropical exposure and a clinical illness indistinguishable from infective enterocolitis [78]. The problem of distinguishing the pathology of bacillary dysentery from ulcerative colitis in surgical specimens does not usually arise, although it may be an important issue in rectal biopsies. Fulminant colitis can occasionally arise during the course of an infection and lead to a colectomy [82,83]. The diagnosis then depends on recognizing any mucosal features of infection against the background of the changes of fulminant disease (see p. 492).

Tuberculosis

Tuberculosis of the gastrointestinal tract, whether primary or secondary, usually involves the terminal ileum, caecum and appendix [84–87]. Involvement of the colon and rectum is less common, even in countries where intestinal tuberculosis is frequent [87], though there are reports from India [84,86], Israel [87], Iraq [88] and South Africa [89,90]. It is rare in Britain [91] and the US [92–94], and is almost always secondary: we have seen few acceptable examples of primary tuberculosis of the distal large bowel, though it is documented [95–100].

The clinical and therapeutic implications of a diagnosis of intestinal tuberculosis are so important to the patient that great care must be taken to make a clear distinction from other conditions, which give a similar histological reaction. In the Western world the differential diagnosis from Crohn's disease is the most important [98]. The most common macroscopic appearance is in the form of sharply defined ulceration with an excavated base covered by a slough. The ulcers may be multiple but are usually few in number. The surrounding bowel is thickened and indurated. Fat wrapping is not usually seen in tuberculosis, and may therefore be a helpful distinguishing feature from Crohn's disease [99]. Miliary tubercles may be seen both on the mucosal and serosal surfaces. Such an appearance is unusual in Crohn's disease, which involves a large length of bowel with more superficial ulceration and/or a cobblestone pattern.

The microscopic distinction between Crohn's disease and tuberculosis is discussed on pp. 279 and 296. Colonoscopic examination and biopsy is proving more and more useful for making the diagnosis [99–101]. In such biopsy work, the diagnostic yield is increased by taking large numbers of biopsies [99]. Special stains for organisms should be performed whenever tuberculosis is seriously considered for they can be seen even in the absence of granulomas [99]. Generally speaking, the diagnosis of intestinal tuberculosis should not be accepted without demonstration of the characteristic caseating tubercles or the presence of tubercle bacilli in histological sections along with culture. Although intestinal tuberculosis was, until recently, an unusual diagnosis in the UK and western Europe, there is some evidence of a modest resurgence of the disease, matching the large increase in cases of pulmonary tuberculosis seen in these countries in the last 10 years. Nevertheless the disease remains unusual in patients born and resident in the UK and then it is likely to be secondary to open pulmonary tuberculosis. Even now, most cases seen in the British Isles are found in immigrants, from Asian countries in particular.

Yersinia enterocolitica colitis

Besides causing an ileocolitis (see p. 278), *Yersinia enterocolitica* can be a frequent cause of colitis. Perversely, up to 25% of stool culture-positive individuals may be asymptomatic [102]. Canada, Scandinavia, Belgium and Germany have a high incidence of the disease and it is increasing in the UK [103–105]. It may be found in bulk tank milk [106]. It is generally a self-limiting disease or one easily amenable to antibiotics. There are case reports of gut perforation, pancreatitis and a presentation with diverticulitis [107–111]. *Y. enterocolitica* infection can also be associated with a wide range of autoimmune problems and systemic illness that include myocarditis, arthritis and erythema nodosum [111].

There have been several colonoscopic accounts of the colitis of *Y. enterocolitica* [109,110]. In general there is widespread patchy disease which in half the cases may spare the lower sigmoid and rectum, making rectal biopsy unreliable [110]. Punched-out or aphthoid ulcers are characteristic [111]. In one series, despite positive stool culture and abdominal symptoms, 50% had a normal colonoscopic examination and biopsy [109]. Microscopy is usually that of a focal non-specific inflammation, which disappears with clinical recovery [110]. Granulomas are not usually a feature of *Y. enterocolitica* colitis.

Sexually transmitted infective diseases in the large intestine

The increasing freedom of sexual expression in the last few decades has presented the gastroenterologist with a large array of sexually transmitted diseases [112–114]. This is seen predominantly in the homosexual population where the anorectum is involved in sexual acts. Apart from the well established sexually transmitted infections such as gonorrhoea and syphilis, it is now appreciated that several gastrointestinal pathogens can be transmitted in this manner, including *Salmonella* spp. and *Campylobacter* spp. These infections have been collectively grouped together as the gay bowel syndrome [113]. Many of the common pathogens seen in the large intestine of non-immunosuppressed patients also occur in the immunosuppressed, and as mentioned above many of them will have much more severe consequences in these patients. In AIDS patients without specific infection, diarrhoea may be related to increased apoptotic activity within the crypt epithelial cells, a picture resembling graft-versus-host disease [112] (see p. 474).

Gonorrhoea

Rectal gonorrhoea is virtually always acquired by homosexual contact in the male but, in the female, up to 30% of cases are the result of spread from the vagina [116]. Although older papers describe severe histological abnormality, the more recent literature emphasizes how often rectal gonorrhoea is present with normal sigmoidoscopic and histological examination [117–119]. Indeed a third or more of cases are asymptomatic. The differences between past and more recent reports may relate to the presence of other pathogens in the older literature, written in an era of less than adequate microbiological facilities. Rectal gonorrhoea has been considered to be an independent risk factor for HIV infection [120]. It has been proposed that gonorrhoea produces an inflamed rectal mucosa with compromised epithelial integrity, which predisposes an individual to subsequent HIV infection [120].

In a large series, 84% of cases of rectal gonorrhoea had a normal proctoscopic appearance and 68% a normal rectal biopsy [118]. In the majority with an abnormal biopsy, there was a mild to moderate increase in lymphocytes and plasma cells within the lamina propria. Crypt architecture remained normal. Only 5% showed acute inflammatory cells in the lamina propria with migration into the crypt and surface epithelium in a manner resembling the pattern associated with more common bacterial enteropathogens. Detection of *Neisseria gonorrhoeae* is best carried out by direct culture or via a smear preparation from the mucosal surface. A rectal biopsy is simply an aid and does not provide a diagnostic appearance.

Syphilis

The primary lesion of syphilis occurs at the site of infection. The majority of large intestinal cases are in homosexual or bisexual males and seen as chancres at the anal margin or in the anal canal. However, lesions may occur in the rectum and these can mimic a carcinoma, solitary ulcer, polyp or fistula [121–123]. Biopsy of a syphilitic lesion is characterized by large numbers of plasma cells and proliferating capillaries lined by prominent endothelial cells. Organisms can be demonstrated by silver stains or by using an immunofluorescence antibody [124].

In secondary syphilis a proctitis may be present. In some cases the histological appearance can resemble that of a typical bacterial infection [125] and small granulomas have also been documented. The inflammatory abnormalities in the biopsies of patients with syphilis can be more florid than those in patients with gonorrhoeal infection [125].

Lymphogranuloma venereum

The L1, L2 and L3 immunotypes of *Chlamydia trachomatis*, an obligate intracellular bacterium, cause this condition. Synonyms include lymphogranuloma inguinale, lymphopathia venereum, climatic bubo and Nicolas–Favre disease. It is important to distinguish it from granuloma venereum and Crohn's disease. In the past, the disease was considered one of tropical and subtropical countries [126], being rare in the UK. However, with better methods of diagnosis available it is realized that infection is not uncommon in the homosexual population in Western countries. The diagnosis of lymphogranuloma venereum can be made by a direct demonstration on tissue sections using monoclonal antibodies [127] or by serological detection of changing antibody levels to particular immunotypes.

The primary infection is transmitted by sexual contact. Males tend to develop a lesion on the genitalia, followed by a suppurative inflammatory reaction in the inguinal gland (buboes) which does not usually result in rectal involvement, whereas females usually develop rectal and colonic lesions, presumably as the result of lymphatic spread from the vagina. When lymphogranuloma of the rectum occurs in males, it is invariably the result of homosexual practices and it is possible that, in females, rectal coitus may sometimes cause it. Accidental non-venereal infection has been reported in juveniles.

Lymphogranuloma venereum of the rectum and colon presents in two phases [128]: an initial distal, subacute proctocolitis; followed by a chronic stage with the formation of a stricture, usually in the rectum. Like other venereal diseases the acute phase seldom causes severe problems. It can be asymptomatic or present as mild or chronic diarrhoea due to a distal proctitis. Rectal biopsy shows an acute proctitis with neutrophils, plasma cells and lymphocytes infiltrating the mucosa. Crypt abscesses and occasional granulomas may be present, the latter related to damaged crypts. The picture may be confused with Crohn's disease or other causes of acute infectious proctocolitis. The distinction, however, seldom poses a clinical problem.

The pathology of the chronic phase of proctocolitis has been documented by sigmoidoscopic and radiological methods [126,129]. The rectal mucosa is granular, nodular and oedematous with rigidity of the underlying tissues. Mild abnormality may extend up as far as the transverse colon and a pancolitis has been documented [130]. The most constant and severe changes are in the rectum. There is therefore a definite right to left gradient, and severe macroscopic disease in the right colon is very unlikely to be due to lymphogranuloma venereum [130]. Distally there may be associated perianal abscesses and fistulae.

Strictures of the rectum [114,131] are usually tubular with an abrupt line of demarcation from the non-involved bowel above. The wall of the rectum is thickened and rigid with a severely ulcerated mucosa, with that mucosa surviving appearing polypoid and haemorrhagic. There is severe stenosis of the lumen, which may be contracted down to a diameter as small as 1 cm. The perirectal tissues may also show fibrosis and there is much scarring of the anus, often with a characteristic bridging of the perianal skin. So-called burnt-out strictures are not uncommon. In these, the rectum is stenosed but the mucosa is smooth and intact.

Microscopically, there is a non-specific inflammatory reaction with infiltration by lymphocytes and plasma cells together with much fibrosis. The intensity of scarring, which is often transmural, is greater than in Crohn's disease and neural hyperplasia is common. The formation of epithelioid cell granulomas is rare in the chronic form of the disease although it is well recognized in inguinal lymph nodes in the acute stage. Inflammation diminishes proximal to the sigmoid colon and when present is limited to the mucosa [126].

The pathologist's diagnostic problem is to distinguish the appearances of lymphogranuloma venereum from Crohn's disease. The gradient of disease from left to right side is opposite to that in most cases of Crohn's disease. On microscopy, transmural fibrosis favours lymphogranuloma venereum and the lymphocytic infiltrate is seldom as packeted as that in Crohn's colitis [131]. Although some have shown that antibodies to a lymphogranuloma venereum strain are present in 69% of patients with Crohn's disease [132], subsequent studies have failed to substantiate this relationship [133].

The incidence of carcinoma in lymphogranulomatous strictures of the rectum is not high [134] (Fig. 36.5); both adenocarcinoma and squamous cell carcinoma are described and we have seen three patients with squamous cell carcinoma arising in long-standing stricture of the rectum due to lymphogranuloma venereum. In all cases there was extensive involvement of the rectum and anal canal [135]. The biopsy diagnosis can be difficult because the squamous mucosa of the anal canal tends to grow up over the ulcerated rectum giving rise to appearances which may be mistaken for malignancy.

Chlamydia trachomatis proctitis

The non-lymphogranuloma venereum immunotypes of *Chlamydia trachomatis* are mainly confined to infections of the genitourinary system but can cause mild proctitis on occasions [136]. Focal collections of polymorphs occur in the lamina propria in what is a non-specific inflammatory picture. The diagnosis should be sought in the correct clinical setting [137].

Infections due to other specific bacteria

Intestinal spirochaetosis

Rectal, colonic and occasionally appendiceal mucosa can be colonized by rows of spiral organisms embedded in the epithelial cell border [138,139]. These organisms appear as a

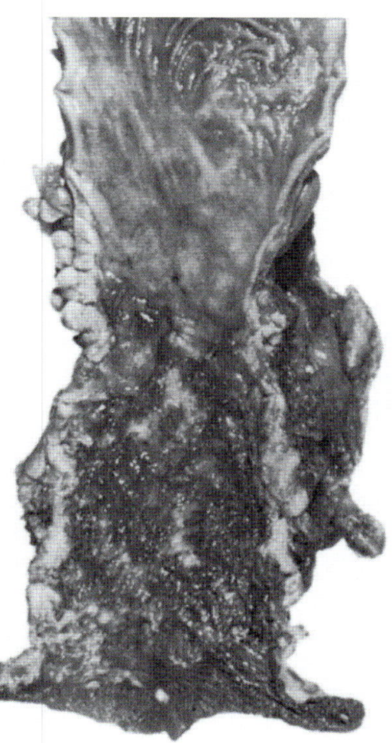

Fig. 36.5 Squamous cell carcinoma arising in a longstanding stricture of the rectum caused by lymphogranuloma inguinale.

violaceous hue on the luminal aspect of the cell when stained routinely with H&E (Fig. 36.6), but the periodic acid–Schiff (PAS) reagent or Warthin–Starry method emphasizes the bacterial colonization of the mucosal surface. The organisms can be found in about 5% of colorectal biopsies from patients attending gastroenterology clinics [138,140] but in up to 36% of biopsies from homosexuals [141]. The taxonomy of the organism has been disputed but *Brachyspira aalborgi* is now generally accepted [142]. Other groups of spirochaetes similar to those found in the pig intestine have also been isolated from human stool [143].

These epithelial spirochaetes are not normally associated with any morphological abnormalities. However, there are a few reports of spirochaetes within epithelial cells [144] and subepithelial macrophages and the number of IgE-containing plasma cells within the lamina propria may be raised [145]. Degranulation of mast cells has also been demonstrated. The pathogenic role of these spirochaetes remains contentious, with most opinion favouring the view that they are not of pathological significance [140]. However, some patients with diarrhoea in whom spirochaetosis was the only abnormal finding have been cured by a course of antibiotics, notably metronidazole, that eliminated the organisms [145,146].

The electron microscopic appearances of the infestation are characteristic but this is not necessary for the diagnosis. Re-

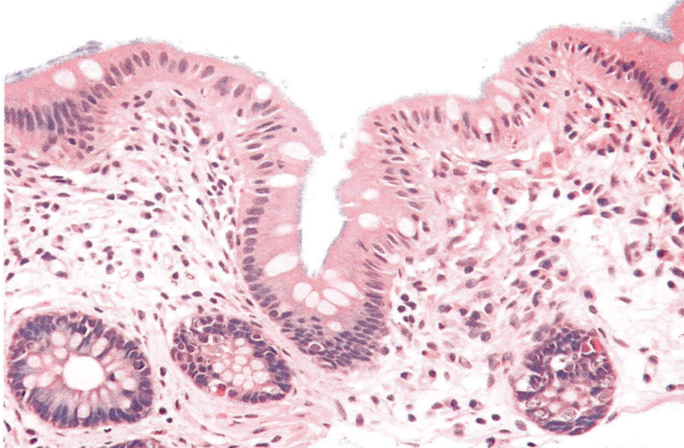

Fig. 36.6 Intestinal spirochaetosis. There is patchy colonization of the luminal surface of the epithelial cells by a single haematoxyphilic layer of spirochaetes.

viewing the slides under oil will reveal the morphology of the spirochaetes. On occasion the infestation can be confused with a slightly thick glycocalyx, especially when the haematoxylin stain is especially heavy or uses certain haematoxylin types (e.g. Harris' haematoxylin) that will stain mucus. The diffuse nature of the infestation contrasts with that of the mucin staining, which is distinctly patchy.

Actinomycosis

The appendix (see Chapter 30) and ileocaecal region (Chapter 21) are the most common sites of actinomycosis within the abdominal cavity [147]. Caused by the Gram-positive filamentous bacterium, *Actinomyces israelii*, the disease is rare in the colon [148–152] but rather more common in the rectum [150] where it is usually associated with anal fistulae. We have seen one example of actinomycosis in the rectum without associated fistulae [150]. This presented as an induration of the rectum without mucosal ulceration and the diagnosis was made by rectal biopsy in which colonies of actinomyces were found. There are two varieties of rectal involvement: one in which the disease is primary in the rectum, and the other due to spread from the ileocaecal region. Actinomycosis should be considered in the differential diagnosis of smooth submucosal strictures of the rectum.

It is likely that actinomycosis is invasive only when the intestinal wall has been breached by some other condition such as diverticulitis or trauma [152]. We have seen colonies of actinomyces in the pericolic abscesses of diverticular disease but it is extremely rare for these to provoke much inflammatory reaction. Granulomas forming at the suture line after anterior resection of the sigmoid colon and rectum may contain actinomyces [153], but it is unusual for this to lead to pericolic abscess formation, fibrosis or stenosis of the anastomosis. Intra-abdominal actinomycosis is also associated with use of the intrauterine contraceptive device [154].

Aeromonas infection

Aeromonas hydrophila, a Gram-negative bacillus, may cause proctocolitis in HIV-infected patients. It is also a cause of colorectal infection in both adults and children without HIV. Culture from the tissues will reveal many organisms. There is considerable necrosis in the base of large ulcers.

Inflammation due to fungi

There is no doubt that, as with lesions in the oesophagus and stomach, fungi can secondarily infect primary ulcerating lesions of rectum and colon. There are case reports of primary infection with mucormycosis [155], cryptococcosis [156] and histoplasmosis. *Histoplasma* is the organism most likely to involve the gut and can mimic Crohn's disease [157] or cause perforation [158]. It may also involve the intestines as a complication of AIDS. Most cases of fungal infection of the bowel are unsuspected and the diagnosis relies on identifying the fungus in the histological section. The majority of cases occur as part of disseminated disease or in immunologically suppressed individuals [159]. In the colon fungal infection may mimic ulcerative colitis or present as a mass.

Disseminated histoplasmosis predominantly affects immune-compromised patients but is fairly infrequent in AIDS patients outside endemic areas for histoplasmosis, such as the valleys of the Mississippi and Ohio rivers and central and South America. Macrophages containing the fungus are usually present in large numbers in mesenteric lymph nodes, liver, spleen and bone marrow. There are occasional reports of histoplasmosis confined to the colon [158]. Such colorectal histoplasmosis may mimic chronic inflammatory bowel disease or may complicate inflammatory bowel disease.

Protozoal infection

Amoebiasis

Amoebiasis is a primary infection of the large intestine caused by the protozoon *Entamoeba histolytica*. The organism's normal habitat is in the crypts of the caecum and ascending colon [39,160]. It is worldwide in its distribution, though more prevalent in the tropics than in temperate climates. Acute vegetative forms, the trophozoites, are present in the large bowel in sufferers from the disease: these are passed in the stools, encyst into a more resistant form and may survive in food and fluid vehicles to be reingested. The cysts survive the gastric acid pH and the capsule of the cyst is digested in the small intestine with the release of four trophozoites that then colonize the right colon. Here their lysosomal enzymes damage the mucosa releasing red blood cells, which they ingest. The spread of amoebiasis is by faecal–oral contamination, usually of uncooked foods, such as salads and contaminated water supplies. It is a disease associated with poor hygiene and therefore commoner in underdeveloped countries. In Western countries, patients usually give a history of foreign travel but this is not invariable [161], and in such cases there may readily be confusion with other inflammatory conditions such as diverticulitis [162] and ulcerative colitis [163,164].

Infection is also now accepted as one of the sexually transmitted diseases [160,165] but not all forms of *E. histolytica* are pathogenic. Virulence correlates with the position of a phosphoglucomutase band on starched gel electrophoresis of cultured *E. histolytica*. Some 22 different patterns, zymodene types, are recognized and only nine have been associated with tissue invasiveness [166,167]. It cannot be automatically assumed, therefore, because cysts are identified in the stool of a patient, that amoebiasis is the correct diagnosis. Furthermore, asymptomatic carriage of virulent zymodene types is recognized. Such patients usually have positive amoebic serology in contrast to those carrying the non-virulent forms [169]. Identifying trophozoites with ingested red blood cells is indicative of tissue invasion and pathogenicity. In the homosexual population there is dispute as to whether identifying amoebic cysts in the presence of proctitis always signifies infection that requires treatment [168,169]. In a study from India, cyst carriage eradication was noted to occur spontaneously [168]. In addition, homosexuals can also harbour other species of non-pathogenic amoebae such as *E. hartmanni* and *E. coli*.

Macroscopic appearances

The earliest lesions of amoebic colitis are small, yellow elevations of the mucosal surface containing semifluid necrotic material infected with the parasite. When these lesions rupture into the lumen the amoebae continue to proliferate, undermining the adjacent intact mucous membrane to leave a discrete oval ulcer with overhanging edges (Fig. 36.7a) and extending into the submucosa.

Amoebic ulcers are most frequent in the caecum, ascending colon and rectum, but may be scattered throughout the large intestine, and are especially numerous in the region of the flexures. Diffuse amoebic colitis involving the entire large bowel is the most dangerous form of disease. In surgical specimens the ulcers are oval in shape, but tend to lie with their long axis transversely across the bowel. They are flat, without induration of the underlying bowel wall, and have a characteristic hyperaemic edge. Amoebic colitis is one of the causes of flask-shaped ulcers, with overhanging mucosa at the edges and deep ulceration of the submucosa. Ragged, yellowish-white membranes cover the floor of the ulcer, especially in severe cases. In severe cases, the ulceration becomes confluent, leaving isolated patches of intact, hyperaemic mucosa among ex-

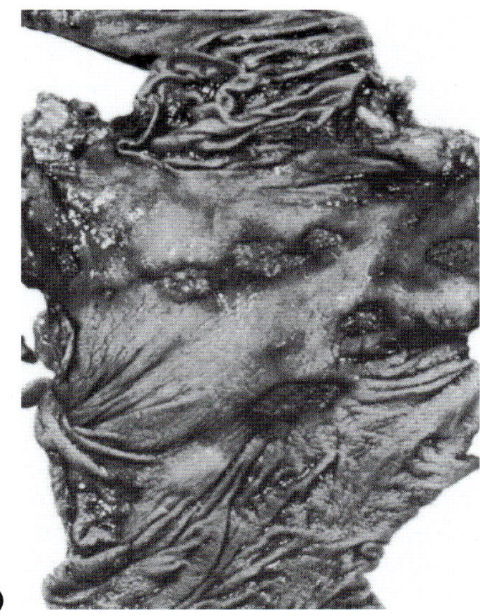

(a)

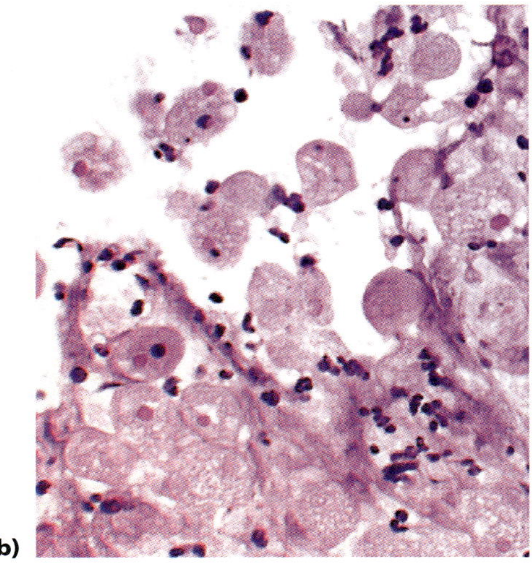

(b)

Fig. 36.7 Amoebiasis. (a) Multiple amoebic ulcers of the caecum and ascending colon. Note the haemorrhagic mucosa around the ulcers. (b) Multiple amoebae are seen on the surface: they have prominent nuclear karyosomes and contain engulfed erythrocytes.

tensive areas of necrosis. Extensive inflammatory polyposis has been demonstrated as a complication of amoebic colitis and this may be a source of confusion with inflammatory bowel disease [170]. We have seen examples of amoebic infection isolated in the appendix and presenting clinically as acute appendicitis.

Microscopic appearances

The inflammatory reaction of amoebic colitis is found around the ulcers, and in severe cases passes right through the bowel wall. There is oedema, vascular congestion and infiltration with leucocytes, especially eosinophils. Amoebae are found on or just beneath the surface of the ulcers (Fig. 36.7b), particularly beneath the overhanging margin, but in severe cases they accompany the inflammatory reaction into the bowel wall and may be seen within blood vessels. They are readily recognized in H&E preparations by their round contour and large size relative to other cells. The PAS reaction can be a useful method for demonstrating them more vividly in histological preparations, especially when formalin fixation has been delayed. Counterstaining with Martius yellow effectively delineates the ingested red cells [171].

The diagnosis of amoebic colitis may be made by finding cysts or active forms of *Entamoeba histolytica* in the stools, in scrapings from the surface of rectal ulcers or in rectal biopsies. With the appreciation of the existence of the numerous non-pathogenic zymodene forms, it is important to identify trophozoites with ingested red blood cells. The stools must be unformed in order to achieve this, as only cysts can be found in formed stools [169]. Colorectal biopsies should be taken from the edge of an ulcer, because the amoebae are usually to be found there, lying within a pool of mucus protected by the overhanging edge. If no biopsy material is obtained it is worth blocking out the aspirated mucus [169]. Despite extensive sectioning, amoebae may only be identified in up to 50% of biopsy material [170]. Amoebae are easily recognized as large round cells with small, dark nuclei. The proportion of cytoplasm to nucleus is greater than in other cells and this will often contain ingested red blood corpuscles, which differentiates *E. histolytica* from *E. coli* and other non-pathogenic intestinal amoebae.

Several stages in the development of the classical flask-shaped ulcer have been described [172,173,174]. Initially, in a biopsy, there is non-specific inflammation with small groups of neutrophil polymorphs near the surface, oedema and congestion, a picture similar to that early in many bacterial infections. Subsequently, focal areas of the mucosa become thinned and depressed followed by surface ulceration. The ulcers are covered by basophilic debris in which the organisms can be seen. Polymorphs are prominent in the mucosa but not crypt abscesses. In the most severe cases there is marked tissue necrosis and the mucosa is replaced by a thick amorphous grey-blue exudate. Organisms may be seen within this but not inflammatory cells. These are confined to the mucosa on either side. At all stages only the demonstration of amoebae allows the diagnosis to be made, but a thick acellular basophilic slough with adjacent mucosal changes similar to those seen in bacterial infections may raise suspicions of the diagnosis.

Complications

These are local, the result of migration of amoebae through the bowel wall or adjacent structures, and systemic, following amoebic invasion of blood vessels. Local complications are partly caused by secondary bacterial infection. However, the progress of mucosal disease through transmural invasion to colonic infarction and perforation can be clinically insignificant, with patients often presenting late and in extremis [175]. Toxic megacolon may occur [82] and there can be invasion of the perianal skin with the formation of extensive granulomatous lesions [176]. Likewise, amoebic ulceration of the abdominal wall may occur around colostomy openings and following the drainage of pericolic and appendiceal abscesses. In cutaneous amoebiasis, the causative organisms can be recovered from the surface of the lesion. Other complications include polyarthritis [177], postdysenteric colitis [36–38] and haemorrhage [39].

A mass-like lesion, the so-called amoeboma, is a recognized late complication of amoebic colitis [178]. This can develop months or many years after the original infection. It is a chronic form of the disease in which localized secondary infection and fibrosis lead to the formation of a tumour-like mass, which may be mistaken for carcinoma or diverticulitis. Amoebomas are usually single and involve a short segment of colon. They are commonest in the right colon and rectum [178,179], and are rarely seen in the transverse colon [170]. Internal fistulae between loops of affected bowel seem to be very rare [173]. In surgical specimens there is pronounced stenosis of the lumen, the result of intramural and extramural inflammation with fibrosis and abscess formation. Both cysts and active forms of *Entamoeba histolytica* can usually be found in the affected tissues, though in very chronic cases, these may be absent.

The most serious complication of amoebic colitis is invasion of blood vessels within the bowel wall, subsequent spread of amoebae to the liver in the portal bloodstream and the development of amoebic hepatitis or amoebic liver abscess. In amoebic hepatitis there is a non-specific inflammatory reaction in the portal tracts without necrosis or abscess formation. Amoebae are not found. In amoebic liver abscess small zones of necrosis of the parenchyma enlarge and coalesce to form cavities filled with sterile pus. A zone of hyperaemia surrounds the lesions, which are often in the right lobe. Bleeding occurs into the abscess, the contents of which become a dark reddish-brown colour and have been likened to anchovy sauce. Microscopically the abscess is an area of necrosis of liver parenchyma in which amoebae may be found, although in very chronic cases they may be absent. Such an abscess may progress to a chronic state, become encapsulated with fibrous tissue and undergo calcification. It can rupture into the peritoneal cavity, through the diaphragm and into the pleural cavity causing amoebic empyema. Spread to the brain and kidneys may result from invasion of the bloodstream.

Cryptosporidiosis

The protozoon *Cryptosporidium*, and the related *Isospora belli*, is a recognized cause of diarrhoea in the immunocompromised, and crytposporidiosis is the commonest infective cause of diarrhoea in UK patients with AIDS [180,181–183]. However, as well as in immunocompromised patients [183], it is also documented in previously healthy individuals [184], both children and adults, and is a recognized as a cause of traveller's diarrhoea [184]. *Cryptosporidium parvum* is the only type of the genus known to infect humans. The primary site of infection by cryptosporidia is the upper small bowel and the interested reader is referred elsewhere for a fuller account of the infection (see p. 284). Notwithstanding its primary site of infection, the disease is most often diagnosed microbiologically in stool samples and colorectal biopsies may demonstrate the protozoa adherent to the surface of colorectal epithelium on the surface of the mucosa and within crypts. Here they appear as uniform haematoxyphilic dots. Electron microscopy reveals the characteristic forms of the organism's life cycle.

AIDS patients are unable to clear the organism, clearance being the usual defence mechanism in immunocompetent individuals, and the infection in AIDS patients will persist for the rest of the patient's life, unless eradicated by appropriate treatment. Such infection is usually seen in patients with CD4 counts of less than 100. Cryptosporidiosis is often seen in association with other pathogens in the gut, particularly *Giardia*, microsporidia and CMV.

Microsporidiosis

Microsporidia are spore-forming intracellular protozoa which may cause encephalitis as well as enterocolitis. They are found as pathogens in birds, fish and some mammals. They are found more commonly in HIV-infected patients. Subtyping requires expertise and electron microscopy. Although these organisms may be seen as intracellular parasites of the colorectal epithelium in AIDS patients [141,185–188], a fuller account may be found on p. 285. At the time of colonoscopy, few if any abnormalities have been ascribed to the infestation, although, if the terminal ileum is entered, there may be some villous abnormalities seen.

Balantidiasis

Balantidium coli is a large, ciliated protozoon, which causes changes in the colon and rectum similar to those seen in amoebic colitis [189,190]. Tissue diagnosis depends on recognizing organisms within histological sections.

Chagas' disease (intestinal trypanosomiasis)

The colopathy resulting from chronic infection with South American trypanosomiasis, caused by *Trypanosoma cruzi*, results in neuromuscular pathology of the colon and rectum, including colomegaly, neuropathy, loss of myenteric ganglia and muscle hypertrophy. It is dealt with in Chapter 35.

Helminthic infection

Helminthic infection most commonly occurs in the small intestine and, apart from schistosomiasis, primary infection of the colorectum is not often observed by the practising histopathologist: it is much more common in the small intestine (see pp. 286–8). Occasional cases of hyperinfestation with strongyloidiasis are seen in the large bowel, especially in immunocompromised hosts.

Schistosomiasis

Infestation of the large intestine is most commonly caused by *Schistosoma mansoni* [191] and *S. japonicum* [192]. *S. haematobium* is found in the bladder and only rarely involves the intestine [193]. *S. mansoni* is endemic in African and central South American countries, including the Caribbean islands. *S. japonicum* is found in Japan, China and the Philippine Islands and the countries of south-east Asia. *S. haematobium* is found in Africa, particularly Egypt, and in countries of the near Middle East.

Infection occurs in humans while wading or bathing in water contaminated with the larval stage of the worm, the cercaria. This penetrates the skin and enters venules, from whence it is carried through the heart and systemic circulation to the liver where the cercariae mature to form adult worms. These migrate to the mesenteric veins, and particularly the submucosal vessels of the gut, where they lay their ova. The latter pass through the intestine into the faeces. The cycle is completed in water contaminated with faeces containing eggs. The latter hatch out, liberating larvae which are ingested by the intermediate host, the snail within which the second larval stage of cercariae develop and eventually emerge in a free-swimming form.

The pathological changes in schistosomiasis are essentially the result of an inflammatory reaction to the eggs in the tissues of the intestinal wall. The severity of the action depends on host immunity and the infecting dose. Lesions are most common in the rectum and left colon and are then nearly always due to *S. mansoni*. On the right side of the colon and the appendix, *S. japonicum* is more common and *S. haematobium* is only rarely responsible for disease [194].

In the early stages there is an acute proctitis and colitis accompanied by oedema, haemorrhage and discharge of eggs into the bowel lumen. There then follows a state of chronic infection, which leads to a great variety of morphological appearances. Localized or diffuse ulceration, strictures due to extensive granulomatous inflammation, pericolic masses and polyposis are the main types. Schistosomal localized or diffuse polyposis, due to the chronic inflammation of the infestation, may be confused with other types, including the inflammatory polyposis caused by ulcerative colitis and familial adenomatous polyposis.

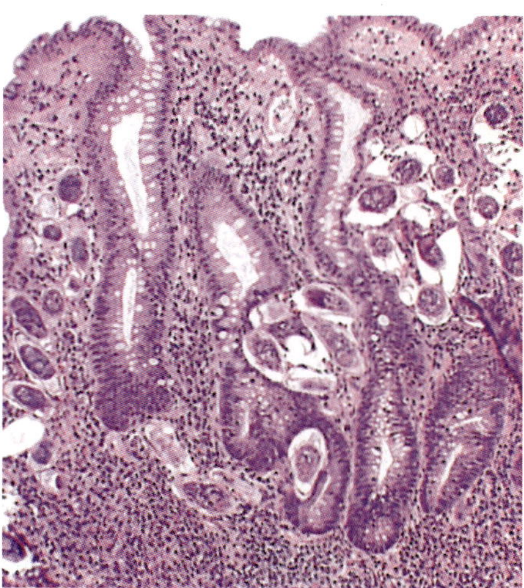

Fig. 36.8 Rectal biopsy with multiple schistosome eggs within the lamina propria.

The microscopic appearances of schistosomiasis are characteristic (Fig. 36.8). The eggs are surrounded by epithelioid cell histiocytes and giant cells. Outside these there is infiltration by leucocytes, mainly eosinophils, and proliferation of fibroblasts. In chronic cases, a characteristic concentric fibrosis develops around the granuloma. Not infrequently, eggs may be embedded in tissue without any surrounding inflammatory reaction. The eggs of *S. mansoni* are oval and possess a lateral spine. In *S. haematobium* the egg has a terminal spine but is much the same size and shape. The lateral spine of *S. japonicum* is smaller than that of *S. mansoni* and the egg is more spherical.

The diagnosis of schistosomiasis is made by finding the schistosomal granulomas in rectal biopsies [192,195]. Because old, effete ova may invoke no inflammatory response, it is worthwhile examining multiple levels of any biopsy from a patient in whom schistosomiasis is suspected. A Ziehl–Neelsen stain is useful as the chitinous coats of the ova of *S. mansoni* stain red.

There is an increased incidence of carcinoma of the large bowel in patients with chronic schistosomal infection [196,197]. Dysplasia probably precedes the development of carcinoma in a fashion similar to ulcerative colitis.

Ulcerative colitis

Ulcerative colitis is a chronic inflammatory bowel disease (IBD) of the large intestine, which effectively always begins in the rectum. It may spread proximally to involve the whole large intestine, although the changes are nearly always more chronic and severe in the distal large intestine. It is a disease characterized by periods of exacerbation and remission. Less commonly there is continuous low-grade activity, a single attack or fulminant disease with dilatation. Involvement of the terminal ileum can occur in total colitis, in continuity with disease in the colon, but this has comparatively little importance from the point of view of pathology and treatment.

Of critical importance in the counterdistinction from the other major form of chronic inflammatory bowel disease affecting the colorectum, Crohn's disease, ulcerative colitis is primarily an inflammatory condition of the mucosa although in cases of fulminant disease, deeper layers of the bowel wall are involved. The inflammation is of exudative and vascular type and generally unproductive of granulation tissue or fibrosis. The appearance of the bowel depends much on the severity and length of history of disease. Operation is usually performed for chronic extensive colitis involving at least the rectum and left side of the colon, so that the study of surgical specimens gives the picture of the more severe forms only. The great majority of patients with this disease have milder and less extensive forms of ulcerative colitis (disease restricted to the rectum, so-called ulcerative proctitis, is the commonest manifestation of the disease), and much has been learnt from the study of colonoscopic biopsies.

Ulcerative colitis is classically diffuse in its distribution. However, not all the diseased bowel need be in a similar state of activity and this can create a false impression of segmental involvement. The other exceptions to the continuous nature of the disease are the appendiceal 'skip lesion' of ulcerative colitis [198–203] and the more recently described caecal patch lesion [204]. It appears unlikely that the appendiceal 'skip lesion' is due to medical therapy. One study found that appendiceal involvement is rare in total colitis and more common as a skip lesion in patients with distal colitis [203]. Both of these focal lesions in the proximal large intestine are rare and the caecal patch lesion is difficult to diagnose on the basis of colonoscopic biopsies. Focality of inflammatory activity can also be occasioned by treatment, especially local steroid therapy, by enema, in the rectum [205]. It is important for pathologists to recognize that in a small number of cases the colorectal mucosa, especially the rectal mucosa, can return to normality after treatment of classical ulcerative colitis [206–208].

Aetiology and pathogenesis

The aetiology of ulcerative colitis remains unknown, despite extensive research over many years into likely causes, such as infection, diet and environmental factors, primary immunological defects, abnormalities of mucin, genetic defects and psychomotor disorders. Abnormalities have been detected in several of these different areas of research. The pathogenesis of the disease is ultimately likely to encompass a genetic factor in association with the action of external agents and altered host immunology.

Epidemiological factors

The peak age incidence for either sex on first attendance is in the third decade. However, very young children can be affected [209,210], and there are also first-time presentations in the elderly [211] in whom the anatomical distribution of the disease may be different [225]. The disease is common in most communities of Anglo-Saxon origin in north-western Europe, North America and New Zealand with incidence figures between 58 and 105 per 100 000 of the population. Prevalence figures for Scandinavia reach over 100 per 100 000 of the population [212,213]. The disease shares many epidemiological similarities with Crohn's disease and is uncommon in eastern Europe, southern Europe and the Third World. However, the epidemiological data from the Third World are difficult to interpret due to a high incidence of infection.

Generally the incidence is reported to be stable or gradually rising [212,214], although there are isolated marked rises in some stable well documented communities [213,215]. There is a higher incidence of ulcerative colitis in towns and urban communities compared with rural societies [17]. In the Western world in countries where ulcerative colitis and Crohn's disease are common, the incidence appears stable, although it is rising in countries where it was previously unknown or rare. This may represent increased awareness or diagnostic expertise. The incidence of Crohn's disease is rising in children, probably for similar reasons, although other factors have been proposed, including infection by *Mycobacterium paratuberculosis* [216,217] and MMR vaccination [218]. The latter is of doubtful significance: it is covered more fully elsewhere (see p. 289). In nearly all studies, the Jewish population has a greater incidence of ulcerative colitis than other groupings [219–221], and family members are at an increased risk of developing inflammatory bowel disease of either major type [219–221].

Genetics

A genetic factor is probable as siblings and first-degree relatives of patients with ulcerative colitis carry an increased risk of developing not only ulcerative colitis but also Crohn's disease. Furthermore, the relatives of patients with Crohn's disease have an increased risk of developing ulcerative colitis, calculated to be about eightfold [222]. The search for human leucocyte antigen (HLA) markers of susceptibility in ulcerative colitis has been proceeding for some time [223] but a statistical approach involving a survey of current world literature suggests that patients with HLA-1327 and BW35 carry an increased risk [224].

Genes conveying susceptibility to IBD were suggested at the turn of the century [221]. For many years the evidence that susceptibility to IBD is genetically determined remained largely circumstantial. Family studies have suggested a genetic factor [220,224]. McConnell reported a high prevalence of Crohn's disease and ulcerative colitis among relatives of IBD patients. Of 522 patients with Crohn's disease, 187 (35.2%) were found to have an affected family member, of which 87 (16.7%) were first-degree relatives [221]. The equivalent frequency in the group with ulcerative colitis was 20 out of a total of 171 patients (11.7%) [221]. More recently, Satsangi found that 41 of 317 (13%) patients with Crohn's disease had a positive family history of IBD [222]. A positive family history of IBD seems to be the single most important factor determining an individual's risk of developing inflammatory bowel disease, although both family studies and twin studies indicate a stronger genetic effect for Crohn's disease than for ulcerative colitis. The greatest risk is in those with a monozygotic twin with Crohn's disease or those who have two affected parents. The risk of getting IBD if two parents are affected is in the region of 30–40% [224]. Even in other relatives, however, the risk of getting IBD with a positive family history is greater than other known risk factors such as smoking, diet, social class and others. Mixed pedigrees of families with both Crohn's disease and ulcerative colitis have been recognized for some time. Kirsner reported that of 103 families with more than one case of IBD, 31 families contained both Crohn's disease and ulcerative colitis patients [226]. Two UK studies have also demonstrated similar findings [221,227]. Relatives of patients with Crohn's disease are at increased risk of both Crohn's disease and (albeit to a much lesser extent) ulcerative colitis. Likewise, the family of an individual with ulcerative colitis are at increased risk of both ulcerative colitis and Crohn's disease. There are a number of other clues that the two forms of IBD may share some genetic determinants, particularly when considering ulcerative colitis and the subset of patients with Crohn's disease confined to the large intestine. These include the identification of monozygotic twins, one with ulcerative colitis and the other with Crohn's disease (3% in one study), the existence of indeterminate colitis, found in up to 10% of cases of IBD, in which the clinical and pathological features do not distinguish between ulcerative colitis and Crohn's disease, and the sharing of immunological markers such as perinuclear antineutrophil cytoplasmic antibody (p-ANCA) [228,229].

Reproducible work has now indicated the presence of IBD-associated genes on regions of chromosomes 12 and 16. The data supporting these chromosomal regions for IBD susceptibility are shown in Table 36.1. More recently a further susceptibility gene, *NOD2*, located on chromosome 16, has been shown to be important in Crohn's disease inheritance. *NOD2* is the first susceptibility gene for Crohn's disease to be identified in a reproducible manner [230–232].These novel data support the notion that Crohn's disease represents an abnormal immune response to enteric bacteria in genetically susceptible individuals. Thirty-five polymorphisms of the *NOD* gene have been identified [232]. It remains uncertain how many of these are associated with Crohn's disease susceptibility. Three are known to have a definite association at present and these may allow genetic classification of disease. Future work may establish whether or not there is a particular *NOD2* polymorphism which is associated with a particular phenotype or perhaps with other Crohn's-like diseases such as gastrointestinal tuberculosis and Behçet's disease [232].

Table 36.1 Worldwide linkage data for the inflammatory bowel disease candidate regions on chromosomes 12 and 16 ([234] reproduced with permission).

Centre	Chromosome 12 linkage (MLS)	Chromosome 16 linkage (MLS)
Oxford	4.11	2.25
Paris	NS	3.2
Los Angeles	2.7	2.5
Pittsburgh	2.75	NS
Chicago/Baltimore	NS	2.5
Toronto	0.3	0.2
Canberra	0.6	6.3
New York	2.08	0.9
Leuven	NS	NS
Axys Pharmaceuticals	1.8	1.7

MLS, maximum lod score; NS, not significant.

Microbiological agents and other environmental factors

The search for a microbial cause for ulcerative colitis has been inconclusive but has produced fewer false trails than similar work on Crohn's disease [235,236]. The approaches have been either to try to identify infective agents in the stool and mucosa or to demonstrate raised antibody titres to particular organisms in patients' sera. The difficulty is to establish whether an abnormality, when present, is the primary defect or simply a secondary phenomenon. Patients with ulcerative colitis have raised antibody titres to a lipopolysaccharide extract of *Escherichia coli* 014, an antibody common to most Enterobacteria [237,238]. This antibody cross-reacts with goblet cell antigen in colonic epithelium [176]. Similar antibodies are raised in first-degree female relatives who have an undamaged mucosa [239,240]. The sharing of antigens between the large intestine and intestinal bacteria has also proved the basis of methods for inducing experimental colitis in animals [176,241].

As well as *E. coli*, raised antibody titres have been demonstrated to certain Bacteroides spp., *Eubacterium*, *Peptococcus* and *Mycobacterium kansasii* antigens [242,243]. Such raised titres may not be specific, as patients with ulcerative colitis have high titres to a large number of non-cross-reacting *Escherichia coli* antigens suggesting that the serological abnormalities are epiphenomena [244]. All may result because antigens have easy access across a damaged mucosa or because there is stimulation of cross-reacting B cells. Bacterial investigation of the stools and of the mucosa-associated flora in ulcerative colitis patients have also produced variable results.

Some have identified increased numbers of coliform organisms whilst others have found no significant alteration in these flora [245–248]. *E. coli* spp. present in patients with ulcerative colitis have increased adhesive qualities compared to a control population [249]. Cell wall-deficient variants [249] of several bacterial species have been found in colonic tissues including agents which, on electron microscopy, resemble *M. kansasii*.

None of the common enteropathogens are consistently associated with ulcerative colitis but many of these infections may herald the onset of disease or precipitate a relapse. In one study almost one-quarter of patients with an attack of 'colitis' following a recent visit to a tropical environment were shown to have developed ulcerative colitis [77]. The onset of the disease was presumably initiated by an infection or a significant change in colonic flora. For instance, the presence of *Clostridium difficile* may have a role in the relapse of colitis in patients receiving antibiotics [115].

Bowel wall filtrates from patients with ulcerative colitis have a cytopathic effect on tissue cell lines and this had been thought to implicate a viral aetiology [250]. However, claims that this effect has been passaged and that the virus has been demonstrated by electron microscopy have been proven incorrect: it has been shown either that these effects are artefactual due to contaminants or that the viruses have been present in control tissues [251]. Thus, although colitic tissue filtrates may contain a cytotoxin, there is no proof that it is a virus [252]. A further approach has been the inoculation of tissue filtrates into animals at different sites in an attempt to identify a transmissible agent. This has usually been into the bowel wall or the footpad. Yet again, conflicting results have emerged [252–255]. Overall the animal transmission work, the attempts to isolate a causative bacterium or virus and the serological evidence for an infective agent have yielded tantalizing results but have not yet identified an acceptable causative agent.

Depletion of goblet cell mucin is a characteristic feature of ulcerative colitis and mucus has an important role in preserving the integrity of the colonic mucosa against trauma and bacterial attack. A further line of investigation into the aetiology and pathogenesis of ulcerative colitis has been to study this colonic mucus. No primary abnormality of colonic mucus has been found: several components of colonic mucin have been identified [256] and a reduction in one type found in ulcerative colitis, even in cases in remission. This might have important implications for the pathogenesis of the disease. Studies on the sialated and sulphated mucin content of mucosa have demonstrated a decrease in sulphomucins. The changes in mucin pattern are not related to alteration in bacterial faecal degradation enzymes or to any differential susceptibility of mucus in ulcerative colitis to desialylation or desulphation [257,258]. It is therefore of relevance that, amongst the wealth of epidemiological data on inflammatory bowel disease, it has become apparent that non-smokers are more susceptible to ulcerative colitis than smokers. This could be linked to the finding that the colonic mucosa of smokers demonstrates increased glycoprotein synthesis, compared to non-smokers, which would help maintain the protective colonic mucosal barrier [259–261].

Helicobacters have been isolated from human faeces and in animal models they can cause IBD-like disease. In an immunodeficient mice model, *H. hepaticus* has been shown to induce an ulcerative colitis-like disease, with colonic inflammation and epithelial necrosis [262]. *H. hepaticus* does not seem to be essential for colitis in other knockout models [263] and the relevance of this animal model to human ulcerative colitis is not yet known. *H. pylori* serology has been studied in patients and controls [264]. IgG antibodies have been found in 52% of controls and in 22% of Crohn's disease and ulcerative colitis patients. Patients treated with sulphasalazine rarely had IgG antibody prevalence: this raises the question that sulphasalazine may have an anti-*Helicobacter* effect. One study used the ^{13}C urea breath test to detect *H. pylori*, and found little difference between IBD patients and controls [265]. On the evidence available, *H. pylori* does not seem to have a role in the cause of chronic inflammatory bowel disease in humans. However, it remains possible, but not proven, that other *Helicobacter* species may have a role in colonic inflammation. An epidemiological study from Sweden of 300 cases of Crohn's disease diagnosed before the age of 30 years, noted that these affected patients tended to be born in the 3-month periods following five epidemics of measles during the 10-year period [266]. No increase was seen in ulcerative colitis. In a subsequent study, reviewing the maternity records of 25 000 babies, these workers identified four mothers who had had measles during pregnancy: three of the four children had developed severe Crohn's disease [267]. The three cases showed the presence of the measles virus antigen by immunogold electron microscopy. The authors concluded that exposure to measles virus *in utero* or in the perinatal period inferred an increased risk of Crohn's disease. A further study based on the UK population suggested that the risk might also apply to children vaccinated against measles [268]. The epidemiological studies linking measles virus and measles vaccination to Crohn's disease and other diseases (notably autism) have been criticized on the grounds of reporting and recall bias, incompleteness of data collection and small numbers. Other investigators have ascertained many more cases of women exposed to measles during pregnancy whose offspring have not developed Crohn's disease. Immunohistochemical evidence has indicated that the measles protein apparently demonstrated in the human tissues is of human, and not viral, origin: the current conclusion is that there is no specificity to the association between measles exposure and subsequent Crohn's disease [269,270].

Granulomatous Crohn's disease resembles intestinal tuberculosis, both clinically and in its mucosal pathology, whilst *M. paratuberculosis* causes an enterocolitis in cattle, known as Johne's disease, although this has little histological similarity to human intestinal tuberculosis or Crohn's disease. Isolating mycobacteria from IBD tissue has been very difficult, perhaps because these fastidious organisms are extremely difficult to culture. In recent years, researchers have turned to the much more sensitive and specific technique of DNA amplification. *M. paratuberculosis* has been demonstrated in Crohn's disease tissue and less so in ulcerative colitis tissue [271]. However, no consistent results have yet been found to support the notion that this bacterium is specifically involved in the pathogenesis of either form of IBD, particularly Crohn's disease. The clinical data that immunosuppressive treatment of IBD is usually beneficial, even in those with profound immunosuppression [272], would suggest that mycobacterial infection is unlikely to cause IBD.

Immunology

To explain the aetiology of ulcerative colitis and the basis for its pathogenesis by an immunological defect is an attractive thesis, which has resulted in a plethora of complex and contentious findings [273]. The basic difficulties are twofold. The first is to exclude the possibility that any abnormality detected is not simply a technical artefact, for much immunological methodology is complex and involves, by necessity, *in vitro* studies. The second is to establish that the observation is of primary and not secondary importance, for many of the reported defects only correlate with disease activity. Amongst the earliest suggestions was that the disease was due to a primary allergy to cow's milk [274,275], based on the finding of serum antibodies to milk proteins in patients with ulcerative colitis. However, this was not confirmed in subsequent work using a different methodology [239]. These investigations are a good example of false trails and the problems of immunological technique.

All limbs of the immune system have been investigated in ulcerative colitis and no consistent antecedent abnormalities in humoral or cell-mediated immunity have been demonstrated. Circulating immunoglobulin levels can be normal or raised and there is evidence for alteration in complement turnover and activation [240]. There is probably no major defect in circulating B- and T-cell populations and, although there are accounts of diminished immunoregulatory function [276], they are probably all secondary to disease activity [277]. However, these might yet have a role in the pathogenesis of the disease. Of particular interest, and related to the prevalence of humoral antibodies to gut bacteria, is the observation that circulating lymphocytes in ulcerative colitis are cytotoxic to colonic epithelial cells. This effect is blocked by lipopolysaccharide extract from *E. coli* 0119:1314 which, in turn, can activate cytotoxicity amongst normal lymphocytes [278,279]. Similar cytotoxicity can be demonstrated in the population of mucosal lymphocytes from patients with ulcerative colitis but these first need to be armed by an antibody [279].

Two populations of lymphocytes exist in the mucosa, those within the epithelium and those of the lamina propria. The intraepithelial cells are mostly T suppressor cells and those in the lamina propria T helper cells [280]. In ulcerative colitis there is an increased number of antigen-presenting cells in the mucosa [281]. The large number of polymorphs in the mucosa in active ulcerative colitis, manifest by numerous crypt abscesses, may be the response to mucosal damage from lymphokines released by activated lymphocytes. Polymorphs may also be attracted by the increased production of leucotriene B4 found in the mucosa in inflammatory bowel disease [282]. This is a powerful chemotactic agent, the product of one pathway of arachidonic acid metabolism.

There is increased B-cell activity in the mucosa in ulcerative colitis with alteration in the ratios of IgA and IgG and in IgG-containing cells [283]. Some investigators claim to have demonstrated increased numbers of IgE-containing plasma cells [284,285]. There is evidence, however, that those patients with distal bowel disease and raised numbers of IgE-containing plasma cells in the mucosa represent a distinct group with allergic proctitis [286]. Besides the indices of humoral and cellular immunity already mentioned, the mucosa contains increased numbers of mast cells and eosinophils, which might be markers of the type I immediate hypersensitivity reaction [284]. These features are, however, not specific to this pattern of immune response.

There have been many attempts to produce experimental colitis in animals, using immunological manipulation [287]. The injection of antibody/antigen complexes into rabbits after rectal irritation by formalin produces an acute colitis and this can become chronic by previously sensitizing the animal to common enterobacterial Kunin antigen [288,289]. The fact that previous sensitization converts an acute disease to a chronic picture may well have relevance to the human situation where infection can precipitate or cause relapse of ulcerative colitis. Colitis has also been induced in rabbits via a cell-mediated mechanism [290] as well as by chemical means using carrageenan [291]. This model has been shown to depend on the presence of at least some of the gut flora, as prior antibiotic treatment prevents disease and germ-free animals are also unaffected [292].

One of the strongest and most consistent observations concerning the aetiopathogenesis of chronic inflammatory bowel disease is that previous appendicectomy protects patients from developing ulcerative colitis [293,294]. This relationship is thought to have an immune basis because the appendix is an important antigen-presenting site in the gut.

Macroscopic appearances in surgical specimens

Observation of the external appearance reveals certain important features. The serosa is intact and retains its normal shiny surface though there is considerable congestion and dilatation of blood vessels. The only exception to this is in acute fulminating disease when involvement of the full thickness of the bowel wall with or without perforation causes acute inflammatory serosal changes. The regional lymph nodes are sometimes enlarged, but do not contain granulomas in non-diverted ulcerative colitis. The length of the colon and rectum is reduced. Often the shortening is a very striking feature producing a grossly contracted bowel with obliteration of the sigmoid loop. This shortening is due to a muscular abnormality and is most obvious in the distal colon and rectum. Fibrosis makes little contribution and is largely lacking as a feature of the inflammatory response in colitis. It is noteworthy that the shortening of the colon is sometimes reversible [295]. The contraction is accompanied by a reduction in the transverse calibre, which is particularly marked in the distal large bowel. In the rectum it accounts for the increase in the sacrorectal distance, which is an important sign in the radiographic diagnosis of ulcerative colitis.

Involvement of the terminal ileum in ulcerative colitis is often not seen on external examination, but severe involvement can be associated with a tendency to dilatation, with rigidity and muscular thickening of the bowel wall. Accurate assessment of the extent of involvement of the large bowel at laparotomy is difficult because of the diffuse nature of the mucosal changes and the fact that early or slight involvement cannot be felt by the operator. Radiography is more accurate, but even this tends to underestimate the extent of disease.

On opening a surgical specimen of ulcerative colitis fresh from the operating theatre, the first notable feature is the amount of blood present on the mucosal surface. This is a reflection of a great increase in the capacity of the vascular bed and may be of importance in the pathogenesis of the disease, justifying the use of the French terminology *rectocolite hémorrhagique*. The mucosa has a granular or velvety surface appearance and is extremely friable (Figs 36.9 and 36.10). In active disease it can be readily scraped off, laying bare the deep muscle coats, which are otherwise unaffected except in fulminant colitis (Fig. 36.11). The earliest form of macroscopically recognizable mucosal architectural damage is erosion. Full-thickness ulceration of the mucosa is usually patchy but any intact intervening mucosa is always diseased. The ulceration may have a linear distribution, especially in the colon where it is related to the line of attachment of the taeniae coli (Fig. 36.9).

(a)

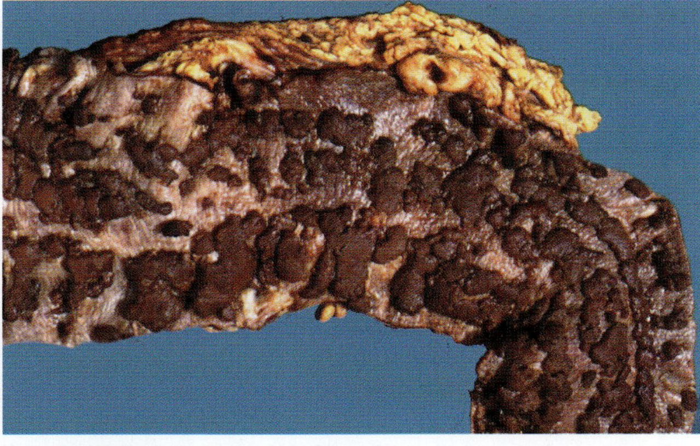

(b)

Fig. 36.9 Severe ulcerative colitis. (a) Active disease involves the majority of the large bowel in a diffuse, continuous fashion from the rectum to the mid ascending colon. (b) There is widespread ulceration that tends to be linear, interspersed with residual islands of dark, granular, haemorrhagic mucosa.

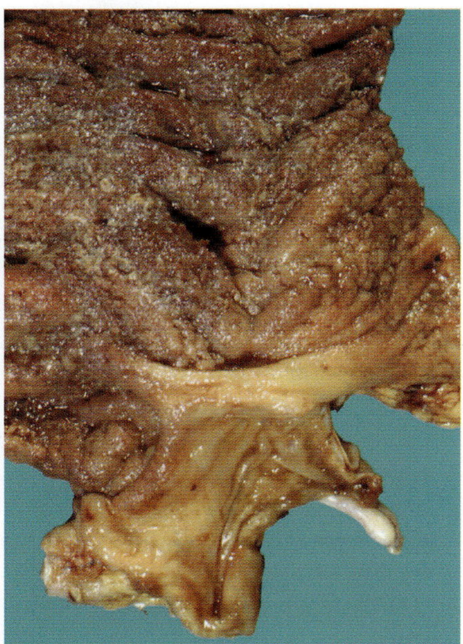

Fig. 36.10 Active ulcerative colitis affecting the right side of the colon. The mucosa of the caecum and ascending colon is diffusely inflamed with a uniform, granular, velvety appearance. This extends up to the ileocaecal valve: the mucosa of the terminal ileum is unaffected.

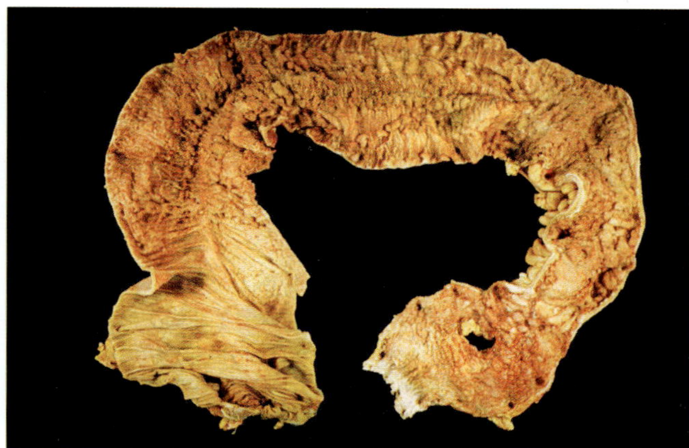

Fig. 36.11 Fulminant ulcerative colitis with toxic dilatation. The transverse colon is particularly dilated and shows deep ulceration with residual mucosal islands. Many inflammatory polyps are seen in the left side of the colon.

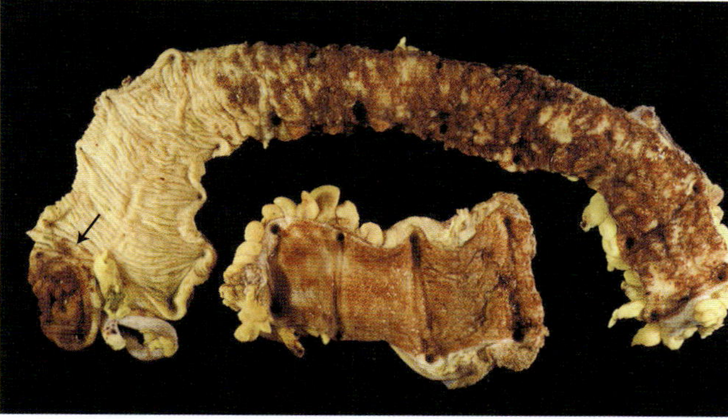

Fig. 36.12 Active ulcerative colitis. This specimen shows the colon (above) and the separated rectum (below). There is severe diffuse left-sided disease with a sharp cut off in the mid transverse colon. Within the caecum there is a round disc-like area of discontinuous active disease (arrow), a so-called caecal patch lesion.

It must be emphasized that the inflammatory changes in ulcerative colitis are continuous (except in the two acceptable focal lesions of ulcerative colitis described previously: the appendiceal 'skip lesion' [198–203] and the caecal patch lesion [206] (Fig. 36.12)). However, severely affected areas may sometimes be separated by patches of less obviously involved mucosa, as not all regions of the bowel show equal activity.

The mucosal changes of ulcerative colitis involve the rectum in the first place (idiopathic chronic ulcerative proctitis) and may remain localized or may spread proximally in continuity until a larger part of or the entire large bowel may be involved. Attempts have been made to explain the extent of colitis; by implication, genetics may be important in deciding the extent of disease. Anatomical variations in arterial supply to the colon are, we believe, a less likely explanation [296].

True ulcerative colitis with a sigmoidoscopically and histologically normal rectum probably never occurs: in occasional cases the rectal mucosa may look endoscopically normal but will show signs of disease when examined microscopically [297]. This picture of rectal sparing can be misleading and can also be produced by healing in response to local steroid enemas. It is best termed *relative rectal sparing* rather than true rectal sparing. On occasion, relative rectal sparing may occur in some patients with ulcerative colitis in the absence of rectal instillation of anti-inflammatory drugs. In general the severity of the mucosal changes in surgical specimens is usually greatest in the distal large bowel and tends to diminish proximally. Even in total colitis, the disease is usually more severe in the left colon and rectum (Fig. 36.11). Macroscopically, the proximal limit of the disease shows an abrupt transition from disease to normal mucosa but a gradual change is more usually seen histologically. Clearly the exact mucosal appearances will depend on the stage of activity at the time of resection.

One of the significant features of ulcerative colitis is the relative lack of fibrosis. It is essentially an exudative type of inflammation which, even in very chronic cases, does not provoke the formation of granulation tissue with fibrosis. There may be an increase in the amount of collagen in the superficial submucosa, particularly of the rectum in some patients, but this is quantitatively very small even when there is a long history of severe disease. Rarely strictures occur on the basis of hyperplasia of the muscularis mucosae [298]. If true fibrous strictures are present in a colon showing diffuse inflammation, the diagnosis of Crohn's disease, rather than ulcerative colitis, should be considered. Alternatively stricture formation can be the result of coexistent diverticular disease or of malignant change.

Polyps in ulcerative colitis

Polypoid change in ulcerative colitis is common, being present in from 12 to 20% of cases and more commonly associated with bouts of previous severe disease [299,300]. The term 'pseudopolyp' has been used to describe these postinflammatory polyps. We believe this to be a poor term and think that 'inflammatory polyp' is a better expression as it indicates the way in which the polyps are formed. They are the result of full-thickness ulceration of the mucosa with undermining of adjacent intact mucosa, which is relatively raised up so that it projects into the lumen (Fig. 36.11). These inflammatory polyps or mucosal tags may be present in large numbers and adopt bizarre shapes. They adhere to one another to form mucosal bridges across the lumen. If healing takes place, the polyps remain as evidence of past disease, so-called colitis polyposa (Fig. 36.13). The polyposis of ulcerative colitis is more prominent in the colon than the rectum and may be seen proximal to the area of active disease. Benign inflammatory polyps rarely become dysplastic.

Adenomas can occur in ulcerative colitis as in the rest of the population. The distinction from a dysplasia-associated lesion

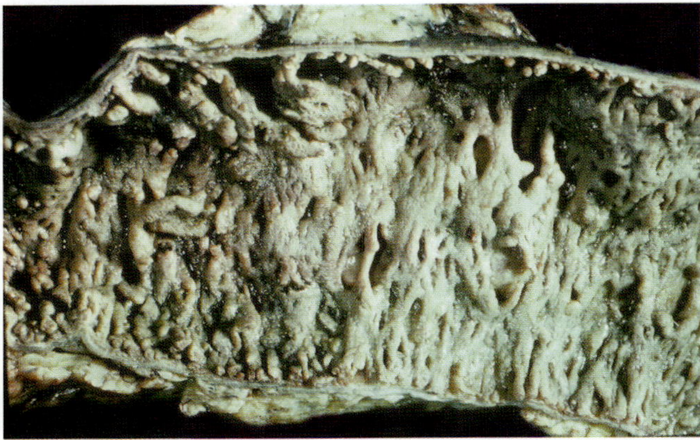

Fig. 36.13 Inactive ulcerative colitis. Re-epithelialization following previous ulceration in the descending colon has given rise to a most irregular mucosal surface with innumerable inflammatory polyps and tags.

or mass (DALM) in ulcerative colitis can be difficult, but can be of critical importance for the management and prognosis of individual patients. Adenomas can be straightforward to diagnose in ulcerative colitis if they occur in the adenoma age group, in non-colitic mucosa, especially on the right side of the colon and are pedunculated. If they are sessile and within the area of colitis, the distinction can be much more difficult. In the younger age group such lesions are more likely to represent DALMs. Biopsies from adjacent flat mucosa are sometimes helpful when they show dysplasia, suggesting a field change and thereby helping to substantiate the diagnosis of a DALM. The pattern of dysplasia may sometimes be different in that the nuclear distribution in dysplastic epithelium in DALMs is more random than the consistent basally orientated nuclear distribution usually seen in adenomas [301–303].

Ileal involvement in ulcerative colitis

When the terminal ileum is involved, the mucosal changes are similar to those seen in the colon. They are always in continuity with disease in the large bowel and are associated with a rigid dilated and incompetent ileocaecal valve. Although the expression 'backwash ileitis' is not necessarily accurate, because there is, as yet, no evidence that ileal disease is the result of such a mechanism, it is in common usage. Ileitis is found in about 10% of colectomy specimens for ulcerative colitis, the extent of involvement varying from 5 to 25 cm, but is only very rarely longer. It is extremely rare for prestomal ileitis to occur following colectomy and ileostomy and this may be a fatal complication. It is probable that it is not due to the ulcerative colitis but is a complication of the ileostomy operation [304]. Ulcers are scattered throughout the ileum and jejunum. The intervening mucosa is normal or oedematous. The ulcers readily perforate, giving rise to peritonitis and the formation of faecal fistulae.

Inflammation of the ileum also occurs in pelvic ileal reservoirs with an adaptive colonic phenotypic change of the mucosa to produce a picture similar to the original colitis and in the ileum proximal to the pouch (prepouch ileitis). For a full account of all the small intestinal manifestations of chronic ulcerative colitis, the interested reader is referred elsewhere (see p. 305).

Fulminant colitis

Some 5–13% of all patients with ulcerative colitis have a fulminating episode [305,306], either as a first attack or in an acute relapse, and in a proportion the colon may be resected as an emergency measure (Fig. 36.11). In our experience, as in those of others [307,308], the appearances are then distinctive. A segment of large bowel, almost invariably the transverse colon, becomes acutely dilated, so-called toxic megacolon, and all coats including the muscle are markedly thinned. The intestine has the consistency of wet blotting paper and there is extensive mucosal ulceration with surviving islands of mucosa showing intense congestion. Single or multiple perforations of the thinned bowel, either spontaneous or produced at the time of operation, were common previously but no colitic should be allowed to reach this state in the 21st century. A major contribution to reducing mortality in ulcerative colitis was made by Dr Sidney Truelove over 40 years ago [309]. His approach to timely surgery in the sick colitic patient depended on an accurate co-operation and collaboration between physician and surgeon, coupled with reproducible criteria for assessing the severity of disease activity [309,310].

In fulminant colitis there is frequently a fibrinous or fibrinopurulent exudate on the peritoneal surface. The caecum and ascending colon are not invariably involved [311]. Furthermore, the lower sigmoid and rectum may be macroscopically spared and so mislead the examining sigmoidoscopist [297,312]. In fulminant ulcerative colitis there is evidence of inflammation beyond the mucosa, unlike what is normally seen in ulcerative colitis. However, the pattern of this inflammation is important. In fulminant ulcerative colitis, the active inflammation extends into the muscularis propria in a diffuse pattern. This is quite different from the focal lymphoid aggregates and follicles, which are seen in a transmural distribution in Crohn's disease. The myenteric plexus is not directly affected and the colonic dilatation might be due to a primary toxic atrophy of muscle cells [306,313].

The fulminant stage is one in which a diagnosis of indeterminate colitis may be appropriate if the histological features do not allow a positive distinction between ulcerative colitis and Crohn's disease [314]. It should also be appreciated that fulminant colitis can occur during the course of the many causes of colitis and the intensity and distribution of ulceration is similar in all, often making it difficult to make a macroscopic diagnosis in this phase of the disease [315]. In those cases of fulminant colitis where the histological features do not allow the original cause of the colitis to be determined, all other clinical, radiological, endoscopic and histological material should be reviewed. It is important to obtain pretreatment as well as post-treatment biopsies, since post-treatment changes may be misleadingly patchy. The length of history may be helpful: if long, the colitis is unlikely to be due to infection. Stool culture may also be helpful. If there has been a colectomy, with the rectum left *in situ*, and an ileostomy formed, the ensuing histological changes in the diverted rectum may be helpful. The crypt architecture is likely to be normal in most cases of infective proctocolitis but abnormal in ulcerative colitis. The overwhelmingly helpful feature in this situation is the difference in response to diversion shown by Crohn's disease and ulcerative proctocolitis patients. Diversion of the faecal stream in ulcerative colitis will result in severe changes of diversion superimposed on ulcerative colitis, whereas in diversion of Crohn's proctocolitis, there is usually remission of the inflammatory changes [316,317]. Diversion-related changes are usually well established within 3 months [318].

Appendiceal involvement

The appendix is involved in about 75% of total colectomy specimens performed for ulcerative colitis. This may be continuous or as a skip lesion [200–203]. Such a 'skip lesion', although apparently suggestive of Crohn's disease, should not be regarded as a contraindication to pouch surgery. This mucosal appendicitis does not lead to acute suppurative appendicitis because the inflammation remains confined to the mucosa with a histological appearance identical to that seen in ulcerative colitis in the colon and rectum [198].

Ulcerative proctitis

Localized non-specific inflammation of the rectal mucosa can be caused by a great variety of circumstances such as mucosal prolapse, trauma, suppositories, radiation, antibiotic therapy, piles, persistent diarrhoea, Crohn's disease and, in more recent years, increasing numbers of infectious agents, the latter having particular importance in the homosexual population. When these causes have been excluded, one is left with an idiopathic pattern of distal disease [319] for which there are many synonyms, including proctosigmoiditis, idiopathic proctitis, non-specific proctitis, lymphoid follicular proctitis (see below) and ulcerative proctitis.

The precise extent of the disease should be determined by flexible sigmoidoscopy and biopsy, for it is found that endoscopically normal mucosa may be histologically inflamed [320]. Approximately 10% of these cases of distal inflammatory disease will develop more extensive ulcerative proctocolitis [315], whereas 15% will have recurrent bouts of active disease and 75% will enter permanent remission. Extension of disease usually occurs within 2 years and seldom after 5 years [319]. There is some evidence that distal disease may predominate in an elderly population [225]. The symptoms from severe proctitis may be disabling as a result of defecatory frequency and urgency. Chronic ulcerative proctitis may sometimes be remarkably resistant to medical therapy, including 5-aminosalicylic acid, steroids, immunosuppressive agents and arsenic. A considerable number of patients with only rectal involvement, seen in a specialized IBD practice, may benefit greatly from restorative proctocolectomy [321].

Microscopic appearances

The chronic and intermittent nature of ulcerative colitis with periods of exacerbation and remissions makes it convenient to divide the appearances into active disease, resolving disease and disease in remission.

Active colitis

In active colitis, one of the most striking features is the diffuse inflammatory cell infiltrate involving crypts and lamina propria along with congestion and dilatation of the capillary blood vessels. The vascular changes account for the bleeding tendency experienced during endoscopic examination. The mucosa appears thickened and the surface epithelium takes on an undulating or low villiform appearance (Fig. 36.14). The muscularis propria and serosa remain free of inflammation except in fulminating colitis.

An early feature of the histology of ulcerative colitis is the formation of crypt abscesses in the mucosa. It must be emphasized that they are not specific to ulcerative colitis, for they occur in a great variety of other intestinal inflammatory conditions including simple appendicitis, Crohn's disease and infective colitis. They are, however, particularly conspicuous in active ulcerative colitis and tend to identify the acute phase. The crypt abscess may be the result of secondary infection of an already damaged mucosa. There is an accumulation of polymorphonuclear leucocytes, mucus and organisms derived from the faeces within the crypts, probably the result of blocking of the crypt outlet (Fig. 36.15). The small microabscess thus created expands and either bursts into the lumen of the bowel, elaborating pus into the faeces, or spreads into the loose tissue of the submucosa. It is significant that polymorphonuclear leucocytes are preponderant within the lumen of the crypts in ulcerative colitis whilst, unlike in infective colitis, comparatively small numbers are seen migrating between the epithelial cells. This can be a helpful feature in the differentiation of ulcerative colitis from infective proctocolitis.

Crypt abscesses play an important role in the mechanism of mucosal ulceration and in the formation of inflammatory polyps. When they burst into the loose submucosal tissues, there is a tendency to spread longitudinally beneath the mucous membrane, which sloughs off leaving an ulcer (Figs 36.17 & 36.18). The mucosal margins of these ulcerated areas are further undermined and are relatively raised up to form poly-

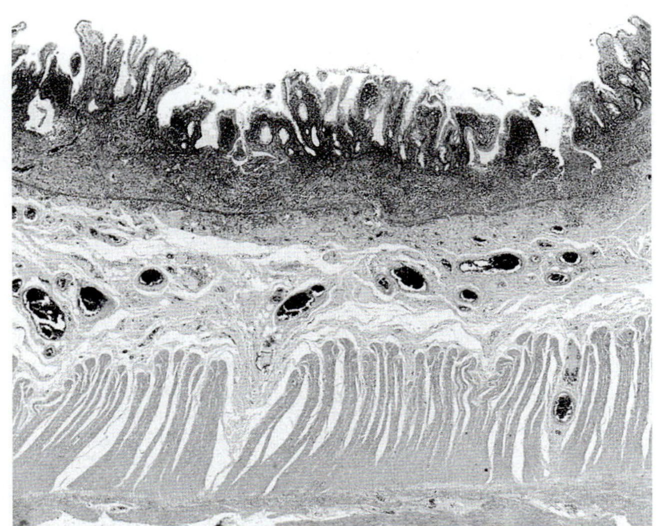

(a)

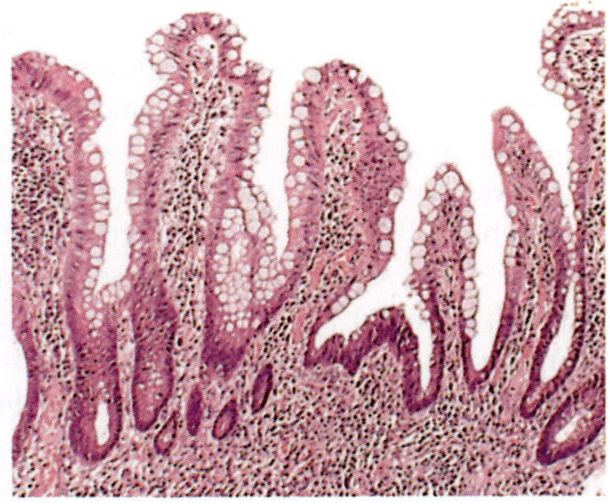

(b)

Fig. 36.14 (a) Active ulcerative colitis emphasizing the mucosal nature of the disease, all the damage and inflammation being limited to this layer of the bowel wall. (b) After prolonged active disease the mucosa can adopt a villiform pattern.

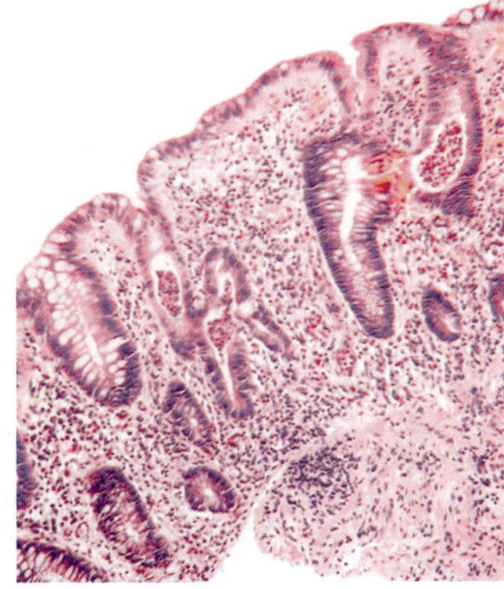

Fig. 36.15 Active ulcerative colitis. There is crypt architectural distortion with variation in intercrypt spacing and a diffuse increase in acute and chronic inflammatory cells. Neutrophil polymorphs infiltrate the crypt epithelium to form crypt abscesses.

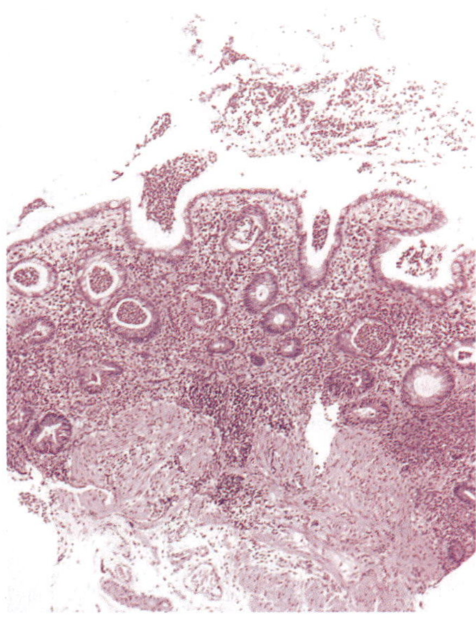

Fig. 36.16 Active ulcerative colitis. There is severe active chronic inflammation with crypt abscesses, early crypt rupture, pus on the luminal surface and incipient erosion. The architecture is distorted and the crypt epithelium is attenuated with goblet cell depletion.

poid tags of mucous membrane projecting into the lumen. These mucosal tags or inflammatory polyps can be short or extremely long [322].

The inflammatory damage to the crypts produces a variety of degenerative and regenerative changes in the crypt epithelium. There is loss of goblet cells (Fig. 36.16), often with enlargement and hyperchromatism of nuclei of the absorptive cells. Such changes must not be mistaken for dysplasia (see below). Paneth cells which, apart from in the right colon, are absent from the rest of the large bowel, appear in the crypt epithelium [323], but are most common in long-established disease. Their significance is not clear but there is evidence that they may be involved in regulating the gut flora [324] and they can be particularly numerous in those patients with long-standing colitis who develop malignant change [325]. Although increased numbers of endocrine cells may also be seen in the base of the crypts, because the latter are often larger than normal in ulcerative colitis, the absolute numbers of these cells is probably not increased [326].

The damage to the crypts (Fig. 36.17) produces crypt architectural distortion and incomplete regeneration results in crypt branching and shortening. Persistent mucosal architectural abnormalities are characteristic of chronic ulcerative colitis but transient irregularities may be observed in

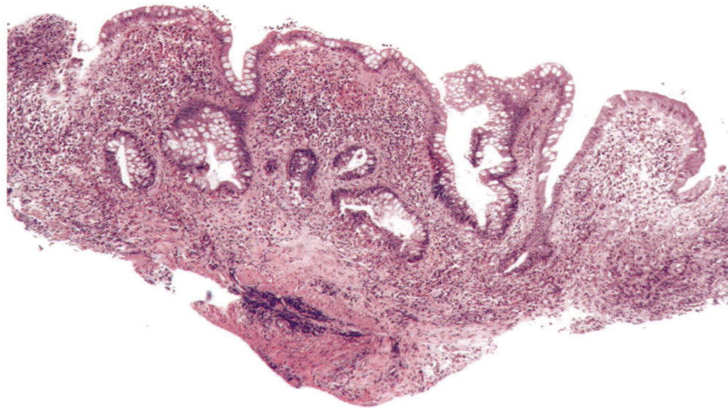

Fig. 36.17 Resolving ulcerative colitis. The fading inflammatory infiltrate is becoming somewhat patchy and only focal acute inflammation remains. The goblet cell population is recovering. Regenerative epithelial hyperplasia is seen in the bases of crypts, which themselves show marked distortion.

regenerating mucosa from many causes. A particular problem in the differential diagnosis of inflammatory bowel disease is the giant cell reaction and poorly formed granulomas in relation to crypt damage and liberated mucin. These granulomas usually contain mucin and/or neutrophils. So-called cryptolytic granulomas present difficulty in that they may be seen in Crohn's disease [327] but also in other forms of colitis [328], most notably in the colitis associated with diverticular disease [329]. Such a feature needs careful assessment, as genuine basally orientated sarcoid-type granulomas do not occur in undiverted ulcerative colitis. In diverted ulcerative colitis, several types of granuloma may be seen in all sites in the bowel wall and in draining lymph nodes [330].

In active colitis, accompanying the changes in the crypts and surface epithelium, there is a heavy diffuse infiltrate of inflammatory cells in the lamina propria. These include neutrophils, lymphocytes, plasma cells, eosinophils and mast cells. Studies of immunoglobulin-containing plasma cells in ulcerative colitis demonstrate an increase in the major forms of IgA, IgG and IgM [281]. The increase correlates with disease activity and the rise of IgG- and IgM-containing cells is proportionally more than for IgA-containing cells [331]. There remains dispute as to whether the demonstration of an increase in IgE-containing plasma cells delineates a specific group of ulcerative colitics whose disease has an allergic basis [285,286].

In some cases of ulcerative colitis, large numbers of eosinophils may be seen in the lamina propria. This infiltrate has been the subject of much study in attempts to correlate it with clinical outcome, but there have been no consistent results [331]. The same conclusion has to be made about mast cell numbers [331,334,335] although difficulties in techniques for demonstrating degranulated mast cells complicate the issue. In long-standing disease, hyperplasia of mucosal basal lymphoid follicles becomes a prominent feature, particularly in the rectum [336], but transmural inflammation in the form of lymphoid aggregates, characteristic of Crohn's disease, is never seen in untreated ulcerative colitis although it is a feature of the diverted rectum in ulcerative colitis [330].

Some authors have described vascular lesions of polyarteritis type in submucosal vessels in ulcerative colitis, but these have not been a feature of our own material [336a]. Inflammation within blood vessels may be seen close to ulcerated areas but this is usually a secondary feature. Granulomatous vasculitis, the preserve of Crohn's disease [336b], has only been described in ulcerative colitis in association with diversion [336c]. The assessment of disease activity in chronic inflammatory bowel disease is usually by clinical and endoscopic criteria in routine practice. The only exception is in the histological contribution to the diagnosis of pouchitis. The importance of routine, repeated biopsy examination in chronic inflammatory bowel disease is to reconfirm the diagnosis, to exclude concurrent infection and to assess for the presence of dysplasia. Histological scoring of disease activity in ulcerative colitis and Crohn's disease is usually confined to therapeutic trials of new drugs. Several *ad hoc* scoring systems have been devised for this purpose. Most are not evidence-based or tested for their reproducibility. Most are based on the presence and site of neutrophil polymorphs and the amount of crypt and epithelial destruction caused by them.

Whilst Truelove, in Oxford, devised the first recorded method relating to the amount of polymorph infiltrate and epithelial damage, the scoring system introduced by Riley and colleagues remains popular [336d]. This system, and modifications of it, has been used to show that a mild activity score (occasional small groups of neutrophils in the lamina propria) correlate with early relapse after cessation of treatment. This may be argued as the only clinically useful reason for considering the use of scoring in routine clinical practice. In reality it would, however, merely be a way of prompting the reporting pathologist to look for neutrophil groups in the lamina propria, an important part of the descriptive microscopy report. More recently a histological scoring system, which has been tested for its reproducibility, has been published [337]. This represents a great advance in standardization and comparison of results of therapeutic trials.

Active colitis—fulminant phase

Ulcerative colitis is primarily a disease of the mucosa and inflammation does not extend beyond the sub-mucosal layer except in acute fulminating disease. In this form there is a characteristic transmural inflammation (Fig. 36.18). Extensive loss of mucosa occurs and any surviving mucous membrane shows intense vascular congestion and oedema but with a relatively mild inflammatory cell response. In areas of mucosal ulceration, the submucosal tissues largely disappear laying bare the deep muscle coats which may be covered by only a thin layer of very vascular granulation tissue. The fibres of the muscularis propria are separated by oedematous exudate becoming stretched and thinned. At many points this proceeds

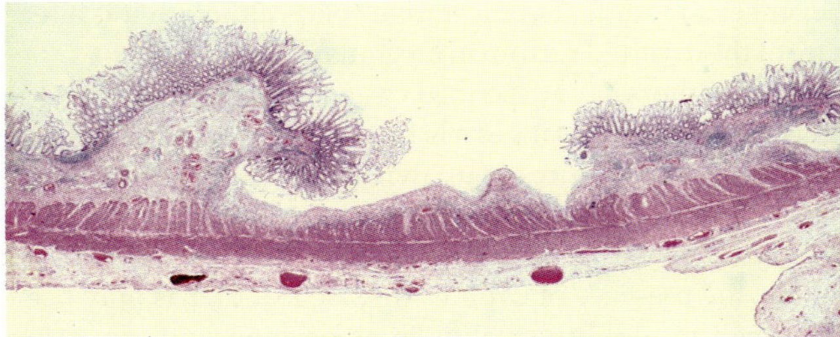

Fig. 36.18 Histology of fulminant colitis with toxic dilatation. There is extensive, deep ulceration into the muscularis propria and the surviving mucosa is undermined giving a polypoid appearance.

to incipient or complete perforation. This damage to muscle may cause a regular pattern of longitudinal splitting of the muscle coat initially resembling the fissuring of Crohn's disease. Such an appearance must therefore be carefully evaluated in the context of other changes.

Resolving colitis

The relapses and remissions of ulcerative colitis imply that inflammation may resolve spontaneously. Furthermore, resolution can occur at different rates in different anatomical areas of the colon. This can give a false impression of segmental disease, not only macroscopically but also microscopically [205,207,338]. With resolution of disease, the numbers of inflammatory cells of all types begin to diminish and their distribution becomes uneven. The goblet cell population returns towards normal and, depending on the severity of the attack, the crypt architecture will show evidence of damage. Some crypts may appear short, others branched.

Quiescent colitis

Varying degrees of crypt atrophy and distortion are the hallmarks of quiescent disease. Shortfall of the crypt with regard to the muscularis mucosae and crypt loss are convenient ways of assessing this atrophy and the lamina propria may show an unusual 'empty' appearance (Fig. 36.19). On the other hand, there may be lymphoid hyperplasia in the rectum (Fig. 36.20). Crypts are normally present in the large bowel mucosa at a frequency of six per millimetre in a biopsy, which includes muscularis mucosae. In a biopsy without muscularis mucosae, the mucosa may be stretched out and appear atrophic when it is not. Oedema may also cause mimicry of crypt atrophy; this may follow administration of bowel preparation fluids, especially older hyperosmolar solutions [339].

Whilst most patients have some residual changes of previous damage (crypt distortion, atrophy, Paneth cell metaplasia) it has become increasingly recognized that a group of ulcerative colitis patients may show complete resolution with no evidence of previous disease [205–207]. This must always raise

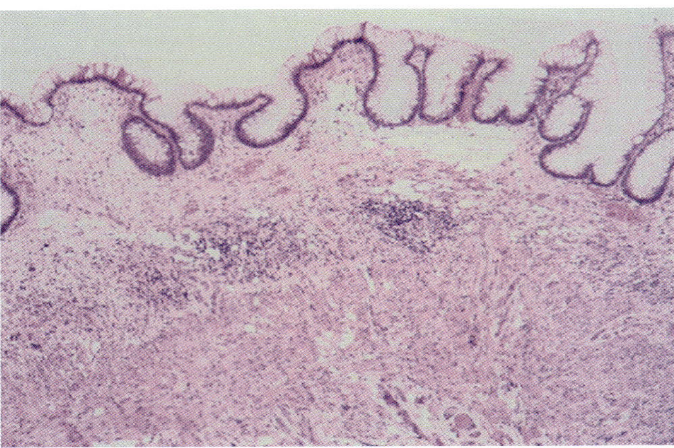

Fig. 36.19 Ulcerative colitis in remission. The crypts are atrophic, branched, and shortened such that they do not reach the thickened muscularis mucosae. Mononuclear cells are sparse in the lamina propria, giving it an 'empty' appearance.

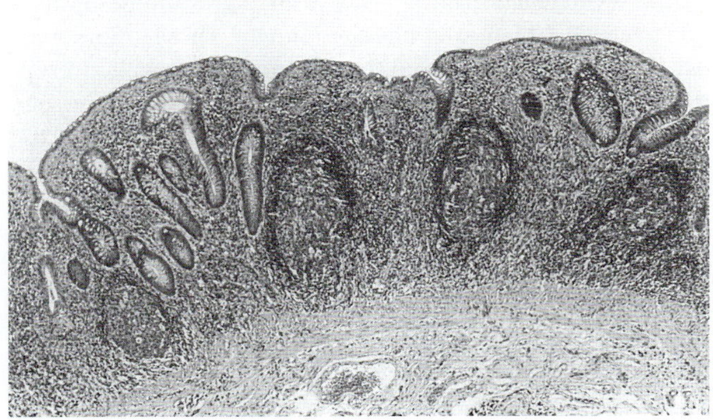

Fig. 36.20 Inactive ulcerative colitis in a rectal biopsy. Large numbers of lymphoid follicles are seen with a background of chronic inflammatory cells and crypt distortion. This appearance is sometimes termed 'lymphoid follicular proctitis'.

the question as to whether the original diagnosis was really ulcerative colitis or an infective colitis and a careful review of all clinical data and histological material is warranted. After such review there remains a patient group with genuine ulcerative colitis, with collateral evidence for such a diagnosis, including coexistent primary sclerosing cholangitis, who undoubtedly show evidence of complete mucosal recovery.

The condition of the patient group with histological evidence of ulcerative colitis with crypt architectural distortion but with normal radiology and colonoscopy has been termed 'minimal change colitis' [340]. This should not be confused with microscopic colitis, since there is crypt architectural distortion, which is not a feature of microscopic colitis. Minimal change colitis may be seen after treatment or at presentation, and indeed may never develop endoscopically recognizable changes, although some authors claim that minor vascular abnormalities may be seen at colonoscopy. It is not clear why some patients will show quite florid atrophy, yet in others the mucosa returns to a state close to normality.

Inflammatory polyps can occur, though they reflect more a phase of healing following a bout of severe disease rather than being, by necessity, a sign of chronicity. Occasionally thickening of the muscularis mucosae is seen, but a characteristic finding in ulcerative colitis, especially in rectal biopsies, is the double muscularis mucosae [341]. The upper layer is thought to be a new layer of smooth muscle, possibly derived from the pericryptal fibroblasts. This may lead to diagnostic confusion on examination of a mucosal biopsy, for inflammatory changes may be misinterpreted as extending beneath the muscularis mucosae if only the superficial neomuscularis mucosae is included. Mucosal inflammation will then be erroneously thought to be within the submucosa, potentially leading to a misdiagnosis of Crohn's disease.

The rectum in ulcerative proctocolitis following ileorectal anastomosis

The macroscopic and histological changes in the rectum following ileorectal anastomosis are no different from those in the rectum in continuity with an inflamed colon. Biopsies from the anastomosis may be misinterpreted as small bowel metaplasia. It is crucial that the pathologist is made aware of the previous operation of ileorectal anastomosis, when presented with a biopsy from this area. The dysplasia and carcinoma risk in this circumstance relates to the original disease extent: in total or extensive colitis it will be as high as if the whole colon were still present. The pathological changes of inflammation are quite different from those in the diverted rectum in ulcerative colitis.

The effects of drugs on the macroscopic and microscopic appearances of ulcerative colitis

It is possible that many of the difficulties concerning the classification of chronic inflammatory bowel disease on mucosal biopsies may arise because of the effects of drug therapy. Furthermore, the difficulties are compounded by variations in the distribution of disease when modified by drug therapy, underpinning the importance of assessing multiple colonoscopic biopsies, from multiple sites, in the accurate diagnosis of chronic inflammatory bowel disease [207,208].

Cyclosporin has been recently introduced as an effective drug in the treatment of severe ulcerative colitis otherwise unresponsive to conventional medical therapy [342,343]. It has been recognized to have important consequences for the histopathologist and may lead to misdiagnosis of dysplasia [344]. The changes induced by cyclosporin are villiform mucosal regeneration and epithelial regenerative changes which are severe with marked nuclear enlargement, sometimes extending to the mucosal surface, but usually with plentiful eosinophilic cytoplasm. Perhaps the most helpful feature is that the 'pseudodysplasia' induced by cyclosporin is strikingly diffuse, with many and sometimes all crypts showing similar changes, in a way not usually associated with ulcerative colitis-associated dysplasia. Despite this, it is very important that the clinician alerts the pathologist to the fact that the patient has been on cyclosporin and that the pathologist is cautious not to overdiagnose dysplasia in this circumstance.

Dysplasia and malignancy in ulcerative colitis

Carcinoma of the large intestine is an accepted complication of ulcerative colitis. At maximum risk are those with total or extensive colitis, those with a history of at least 8 years and probably those with an early age of onset [345,346], though this latter feature is disputed [347]. These are imprecise generalizations, for cancer is well documented in colitics with only limited left-sided disease [348] and in whom the history is less than 5 years [349]. However, they do form the basis of a practical approach to cancer surveillance programmes. Cancer in colitis accounts for less than 1% of deaths from large bowel malignancies and, within the colitic population, approximately 3–5% will eventually develop a carcinoma [350]. There is also geographical variation in the occurrence of cancer in colitis as the incidence of this complication is lower in Israel and central Europe than in western European countries [351,352].

Calculating the risk of cancer in the population of ulcerative colitics is complex. A variety of figures are quoted that depend on how the patient cohorts have been assembled, including referred patients (cancer being the referring reason), non-symptomatic patients (cancer as an incidental finding at surgery) and interval patients (cancer diagnosed at least 1 year after referral). For example, considering all three groups mentioned, the constant cumulative risk is 17-fold, but if interval patients are considered alone, there is only a sixfold increase. In a group with an unknown referral bias and extensive colitis, the risk is 5% at 10 years, more than 20% at 20 years and over 40% at 25 years [353–355]. However, in carefully defined cohorts of primary referrals using standardized morbidity ratios, rather lower figures emerge. Patients with extensive colitis had a 19-fold increase in risk compared to the general population, whilst those with left-sided disease had a fourfold increase. Cumulative risks were 7.2% at 20 years and 16.5% at 30 years. Individuals are at greatest risk of developing cancer around the age of 50 years, regardless of age of onset. Those patients with extensive colitis may turn out to have a genetic predisposition to colorectal cancer [347].

Having defined the type of patient with ulcerative colitis most susceptible to malignant change, the management of the individual patient remains a formidable problem. Prophylactic proctocolectomy for all patients with total colitis and a history of symptoms exceeding 10 years would certainly result in major surgery being performed for patients who are never going to develop carcinoma. There are difficulties in persuading a patient who has spent many years becoming adjusted to a lifestyle with the disease that a major operation, with permanent ileostomy, is necessary. Moreover, some patients developing carcinoma in colitis have few symptoms, and are in remarkably good general health. Panproctocolectomy carries a mortality and morbidity, which must be taken into account. On the other hand, there is sufficient risk to health and life other than cancer in some long-standing colitics on medical treatment alone to make colectomy attractive as a definitive solution.

The prognosis of cancer in colitis is probably no worse than in the general population, providing similar stages are compared [355,356,357]. With the appreciation of the significance of dysplasia in colonoscopic and rectal biopsy material [357a], a more rational approach to the problem of cancer and colitis is possible [355–360].

Features in surgical specimens

There are three features that distinguish cancer in colitis from ordinary intestinal cancer. First, the tumours are often multiple, which is to be expected in view of the widespread precancerous dysplastic change (see below). Reports from St Mark's Hospital (London, UK) have previously suggested that cancers are more common on the left side and rectum [361,362], but there is a referral bias at this hospital in favour of rectal disease. Surveys from elsewhere suggest there is little difference in the distribution of cancer between colitics and non-colitics [363,364].

The second feature is that cancer in colitis is often flat and infiltrating with an ill-defined edge and can sometimes be felt more easily than seen. In many ways, it resembles the macroscopic pathology of carcinoma of the stomach rather than ordinary carcinoma of the colon. Thirdly, there is a higher incidence of high-grade and mucinous carcinomas than in ordinary colorectal cancer. In non-colitic cancers, it is now known that right-sided mucinous tumours have a better prognosis than left-sided mucinous tumours. Whether this distinction holds in ulcerative colitis is not yet known. It is essential that many sections from all parts of a colectomy specimen are examined in the search for small cancers and dysplasia in flat mucosa, which cannot be seen by the naked eye, though carcinoma, in contrast to dysplasia, is rare in completely flat mucosa [365,366]. However, such flat cancers may be seen in a retained rectum in ulcerative colitis, where unexpected carcinomas are found within the proctectomy specimen, which were not identified on endoscopic or histological examination of mucosal biopsies.

Macroscopic features of dysplasia in ulcerative colitis

Dysplasia in the non-colitic is virtually always polypoid apart from in flat adenomas [364,365] and is the basis of the adenoma–carcinoma sequence [362]. As such, the tubular or villous adenoma is an easily recognized lesion endoscopically and surgically. Dysplasia in the colitic is rarely polypoid and, like cancer in colitis, is most often marked by plaques or a velvety/chamois leather-like mucosal appearance (Fig. 36.21). Such lesions are referred to as dysplasia-associated lesions or masses (DALMs) [365] and have important implications. Notwithstanding the occurrence of these DALMs, the dysplastic mucosa in ulcerative colitis may be entirely flat [366]. The ill-defined nature of the dysplastic lesion makes it difficult for the colonoscopist to select areas for targeted biopsy. It has been calculated that the likelihood of a cancer arising without a visible lesion is 2%, whereas 28% of non-cancer-associated dysplasia is undetected macroscopically [367]. The presence of a macroscopic lesion (DALM) has considerable management implications, for such lesions are commonly the sites of carcinoma even though only low-grade dysplasia may be present in a superficial mucosal biopsy [368]. Thus the finding of a DALM should lead to consideration of panproctocolectomy: the accurate distinction of such lesions from true adenomas cannot be overemphasized as the latter lesions may be adequately treated by local excision.

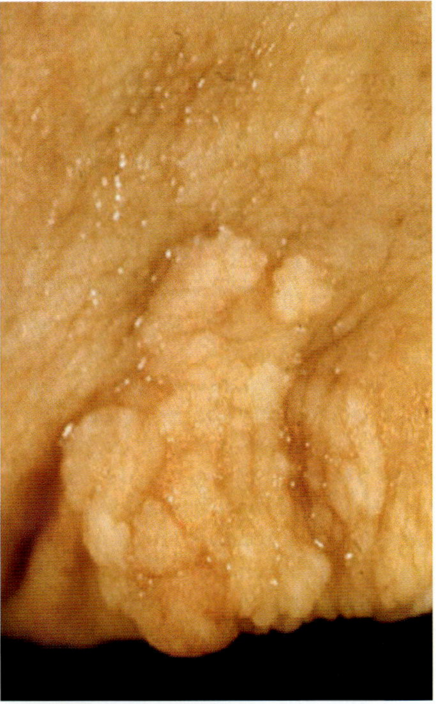

Fig. 36.21 The plaque-like appearance of an area of raised dysplasia (DALM) in chronic ulcerative colitis.

Microscopic features of dysplasia in ulcerative colitis

There are three situations in which dysplasia is seen histologically in ulcerative colitis: raised dysplasia (Figs 36.22 and 36.23), flat dysplasia (Fig. 36.24) and dysplasia occurring in an incidental adenoma. Confusingly, the dysplasia associated with a raised mucosa has been called 'adenomatous' because it assumes a histological pattern like that seen in villous adenomas. We believe that such terminology has the propensity to confuse because it fails to clarify the critical difference between epithelial dysplasia *due to* ulcerative colitis and that occurring *incidentally* in adenomas in the colon and rectum. Characteristically DALM-associated dysplasia most often adopts this low villous pattern (Fig. 36.22) rather than a tubular type of proliferation, but in either case manifests itself as a velvety or nodular macroscopic appearance.

The cytological and architectural criteria for dysplasia in colitis are similar to those applied to other glandular epithelia. It must be emphasized that while cytological changes in the crypt epithelium are a *sine qua non* for the diagnosis of dysplasia, the two most important changes required to make a diagnosis of dysplasia are more architectural in nature. As already indicated, a villiform architecture is characteristic. However, we believe that the most important feature for the diagnosis of dysplasia, wherever it is seen in the gastrointestinal tract, is the failure of maturation from crypt base to surface. This *loss of basal-luminal differentiation axis* should be regarded as the most useful criterion for the establishment of the presence of dysplasia in ulcerative colitis (Figs 36.23a and 36.24).

Cytologically there is variation of epithelial nuclear position causing the appearance of stratification of cells within the crypts. Nuclear chromatin is coarse and results in hyperchromatism. Mitoses are increased and finding them in the upper third of the crypt is a warning sign to search for other features of dysplasia. Failure of crypt maturation is evidenced by the finding of less differentiated cells seen high up, with their accompanying nuclear abnormalities, and goblet cells reduced. Mucin may be limited to the cell apices or be seen on the basal side of the nucleus—so-called dystrophic/inverted goblet cells (Fig. 36.23b). There is, however, a pattern of dysplasia where the nuclear changes are limited to the lower two thirds of the crypts and are accompanied by increased p53 expression in this part of the crypt [369]. These lesions may be accompanied by well differentiated adenocarcinoma [356,370]. These are often difficult lesions to diagnose and, in our opinion, any diagnosis of dysplasia which is considered in the presence of nuclear maturation towards the surface of the

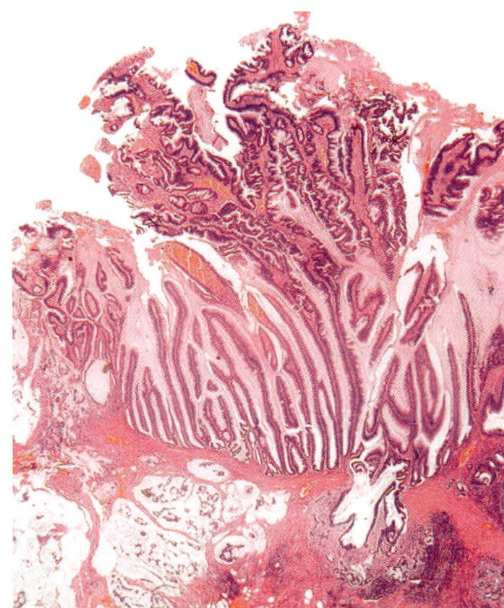

Fig. 36.22 Villiform high grade dysplasia in ulcerative colitis with an underlying invasive mucinous adenocarcinoma in the submucosa.

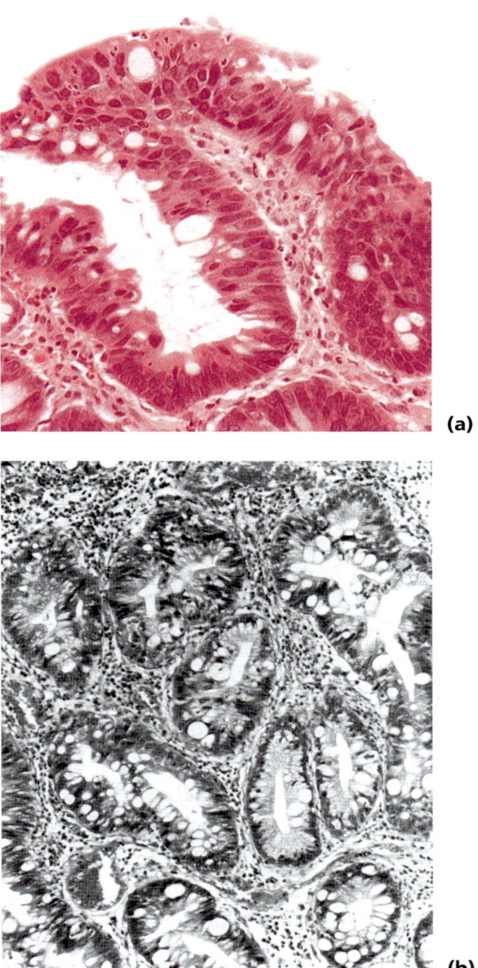

Fig. 36.23 High grade dysplasia in ulcerative colitis. (a) There is failure of maturation and dysplastic cells with multilayered pleomorphic nuclei extending onto the luminal surface. (b) There is irregular budding of the dysplastic crypts, which show nuclear stratification and dystrophic (misplaced) goblet cells whose normal polarity is lost.

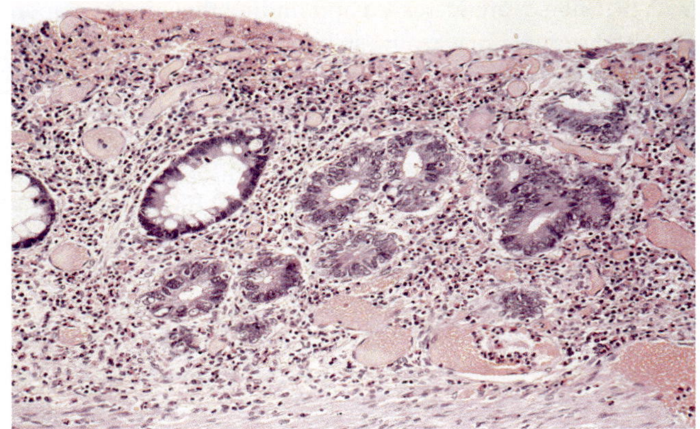

(a)

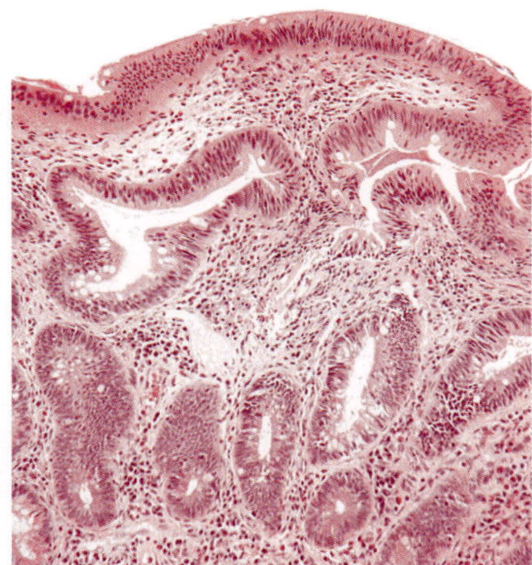

(b)

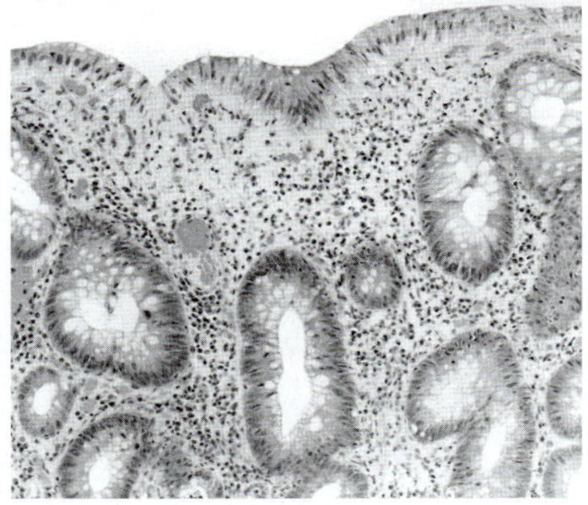

(c)

Fig. 36.24 Dysplasia in flat mucosa. (a) High grade dysplasia affecting all parts of the crypt uniformly (right). (b) Low grade dysplasia with multilayering of enlarged nuclei extending on to the surface. (c) Indefinite for dysplasia. There is only minor nuclear stratification and crowding with little nuclear pleomorphism and some surface maturation.

crypt should be referred to a pathologist with a recognized interest in dysplasia in inflammatory bowel disease for a further opinion.

The main architectural abnormalities often result in a thickened mucosa, produced either by elongation of the crypts to give a villous pattern or by budding in a more adenomatous fashion [370]. These changes may be superimposed on the already distorted architecture to be found in long-standing ulcerative colitis. They may be limited to only a few crypts or parts of crypts. In biopsy work unless more than four crypts are involved it is probably not wise to issue an unequivocal report of dysplasia [367].

Unfortunately, none of the cytological or architectural features are unique to dysplasia and each can be seen in isolation in inflamed or regenerating epithelium. Extreme caution is necessary before a diagnosis of dysplasia can be made in active disease or in the presence of florid regeneration [367], especially after cyclosporin therapy [344]. In active colitis, the heavy inflammatory infiltrate is a warning sign to interpret epithelial changes with caution. The resolving and regenerating phase of active disease, when inflammation is less obvious, causes the greatest interpretative problems. Epithelial cells are of variable shape, often cuboidal or low columnar in morphology, and nuclei are enlarged, often vesicular with prominent nucleoli. Loss of polarity gives some degree of pseudostratification, but the cell numbers are not increased and the epithelium does not appear crowded. The architecture is distorted, flattened over a healing ulcer, but often irregularly villiform increasing the difficulty in making a distinction from dysplasia.

Some changes more specific to dysplasia in flat mucosa have been described. These include proliferation of enlarged darkly staining cells arranged in a line along the whole length of the crypts and accompanied by eosinophilic cytoplasm, with absent goblet cells (Fig. 36.24a). This type of dysplasia often gives rise to a very poorly differentiated type of carcinoma in colitis. Sometimes the dysplastic cells become vacuolated, stain poorly with a mucin stain and resemble the clear cell type of carcinoma of the stomach and colorectum. Finally, a variety known as pancellular dysplasia has large hyperchromatic nuclei with loss of polarity and affects all cell lines including Paneth cells, argentaffin and goblet cells.

Although distinction between sporadic adenomas and DALM lesions of ulcerative colitis has been discussed previously (see 'Polyps in ulcerative colitis' above), it is as well to reaffirm some of the important histological differentiating features at this stage. These are listed in Table 36.2. In practice these criteria are often difficult to apply. In our practices, we also find immunohistochemistry of some use; a p53 positive, bcl-2-negative phenotype favours DALM, whilst a sporadic adenoma more often shows the reverse: p53 negative and bcl-2 positive [369,373,374].

A further problem posed in chronic ulcerative colitis is the distinction between regenerative hyperplasia and dysplasia within inflammatory polyps complicating ulcerative colitis (see Polyps in ulcerative colitis above). Fortunately, dysplasia in inflammatory polyps is distinctly unusual [322]. An important concept for the colonoscopist is that no polypoid lesion in ulcerative colitis should be biopsied or removed in isolation; it

Table 36.2 Biopsy classification of dysplasia in inflammatory bowel disease ([387] reproduced with permission).

	Adenoma		Dysplasia in IBD		
Feature	**Low**	**High**	**Low**	**High**	**Repair in IBD**
Inflammation	–	–	–	–	++
Cytological features					
Cells					
flattened-low cuboidal cells	–	–	–	–/+	++
high columnar cells	+	+	+	+	–
dystrophic goblet cells	?	?	+	+	–
abnormal mucin secretion	+	+	+	+	–/+
mucin depletion	+/–	+	+	+	+
Nuclei					
enlargement (elongation) of nuclei	+	++	+	++	–/+
crowding of nuclei	+	++	+	++	–/+
stratification of nuclei	–/+	++	–/+	++	–/+
hyperchromatism	–/+	+	–/+	+	–/+
coarse chromatin	–	++	–	++	–/+
polymorphism	–	++	–	++	–
loss of polarity	–	+	–	++	–
rounded–vesicular nuclei	–	+	–	++	+/–
prominent nuclei	–	+	–	+	–/+
frequent mitoses	+/–	+	+/–	++	+/–
abnormal location of mitoses	+	++	+	+	–
Glandular architecture					
lengthening of crypts	+	+	+	+	–
enlargement of crypts	+	+	+	+	–/+
branching of crypts	+	++	+	++	–/+
bridging and budding of crypts	–	++	+	++	+
back-to-back orientation of crypts	–	++	+	++	–
increased number of crypts	+	++	+	++	–
Villiform surface	–	+	+	+	–/+

–, absent; +, present; ++, common.

must always be accompanied by biopsies from flat mucosa: these will aid the pathologist in making the distinction between regenerative hyperplasia and dysplasia.

The classification of dysplasia

The need to classify dysplasia is based on the belief that increasingly severe degrees of dysplasia have increasing malignant potential [367]. This concept is by no means absolute, both in general terms, and in ulcerative colitis in particular. Thus it is apparent that macroscopically raised lesions with changes limited to low-grade dysplasia may yet show an associated cancer [365]. Nevertheless, the classification of dysplasia high or low grade forms the basis of the clinical management and cancer surveillance programmes [375–382].

The classification is subjective and is into two grades, low and high, with the term 'indefinite' used to cover equivocal appearances [367] (see Table 36.2). Limiting the number of definitive categories to two rather than three aids management of individual patients and makes classification less subject to the vagaries of pathological diagnosis and interobserver variation. In low-grade dysplasia at least some of the features outlined earlier must be recognized. The architecture can be villiform as in adenomatous polyps, or small groups of crypts may be enlarged with moderate nuclear pleomorphism, hyperchromatism and loss of polarity (Fig. 36.24b). A serrated outline can give an appearance akin to metaplastic polyps [367]. In high-grade dysplasia, there is usually architectural abnormality and the cytological changes are marked. There is often cribriform crypt branching with back-to-back crowding of glands. The most severely dysplastic area determines the final grade.

The necessity for an *indefinite for dysplasia* category (Fig. 36.24c) emphasizes the limitations of light microscopy and routine staining in the diagnosis of dysplasia. We believe that this category is one of some importance in the management of chronic ulcerative colitis. The use of the term does not infer that the pathologist is being indefinite but rather that there are changes present in colorectal biopsy or biopsies that could represent dysplasia but that accompanying features (most usually florid inflammation) serve to make the distinction between inflammatory/regenerative changes and true dysplasia impossible to make. Thus the category may be applied when any one or a small number of features of genuine dysplasia are seen but in insufficient amounts to warrant a confident opinion.

It is reasonable to make a diagnosis of *indefinite for dysplasia* in three predominant circumstances. Firstly, there may be small foci of possible dysplasia, say, in less than four crypts [367]. Such microscopic foci demand further assessment by colonoscopy and extensive biopsy, including the site of the site where the biopsy in question derived, to establish whether dysplasia is really present. Second is the problem area of biopsy orientation. The most important diagnostic criterion for dysplasia is failure of maturation of the abnormal cytological changes towards the surface. If the biopsy is tangentially orientated, then full and accurate assessment may not be possible, even after reorientation of the biopsy in the wax block: *indefinite for dysplasia* would be an appropriate diagnosis in this situation with a recommendation for early further colonoscopy and multiple biopsies. Thirdly, and most importantly, cytological changes in the presence of severe active inflammation may be particularly florid and demand the designation of *indefinite for dysplasia*. Treatment for active ulcerative colitis may induce remission of the disease, with diminution of the cytological changes associated with active inflammation. Thus further colonoscopy and multiple biopsies, after this treatment, may allow a clear distinction between regenerative and dysplastic changes to be made.

With the diagnosis of dysplasia, and the implications carried by the diagnosis of high-grade dysplasia, there are inevitably problems of intra- and interobserver variation. These problems mostly arise with the low-grade and indefinite categories [367,379,383,384]. However, the classification has been demonstrated to be reliable [384] amongst general histopathologists, with back-to-back glandular crowding, villous architecture, hyperchromasia and nuclear stratification being the features most readily appreciated. It is unusual for high-grade dysplasia not to be recognized [384], and the conditional probability for a diagnosis of dysplasia versus no dysplasia has been shown to be 0.759. This means that the chance of one histopathologist, randomly chosen, agreeing with a first pathologist who has diagnosed dysplasia is 75% [382]. It has to be accepted that these interobserver studies have been performed outside the clinical arena. It is a general belief, supported by clinical studies, that the pathological assessment of dysplasia in ulcerative colitis, in surveillance programmes, works well in practice but remains one that demands very close co-operation and collaboration between pathologist and clinician [387,388].

The implications of dysplasia in ulcerative colitis

Series of clinicopathological, surgical and endoscopic studies have shown that dysplasia is a suitable marker for cancer surveillance, and when high grade, especially in concert with an endoscopic mass or lesion, is an indicator that radical surgery should be considered [380,381,388]. When an endoscopic lesion is present, about 65% of patients will already have a carcinoma (Fig. 36.22) [388]. In flat mucosa showing dysplasia with no endoscopic lesion visible, the likelihood of carcinoma is much less [365,368,375,377]. Undoubtedly cancer can develop in the absence of dysplasia and not every patient with high-grade dysplasia necessarily progresses to cancer. Dysplasia can also be limited to just one focus well removed from a cancer.

The chances of detecting dysplasia in a colonoscopic surveillance programme depend on its extent and the extent of mucosal sampling. A review of the many series has shown that the maximum diagnostic yield of cancer based on finding high-grade dysplasia is 62% [392]. The likelihood of a rectal biopsy showing high-grade dysplasia when a cancer was subsequently resected has been shown to be between 73% and 87%. This gives a sensitivity of high-grade dysplasia for cancer using rectal biopsy of approximately 50% and a positive predictive value of just below 50% [392]. However, within any one series, all grades of dysplasia with and without carcinomas are documented.

Patients with long-standing ulcerative colitis are usually part of a cancer surveillance programme and subject to annual colonoscopy, or at a minimum, annual targeted multiple rectal biopsies. With a correctly planned programme, the risk of missing a cancer before it becomes incurable is low [392]. Because dysplasia is relatively unusual and the diagnosis of dysplasia not an easy histopathological task, it is important for pathologists to ensure particular safeguards in their reporting procedures.

The diagnosis of high-grade dysplasia, in flat mucosa or in a DALM, with its concomitant risk of cancer, calls for the immediate consideration of a proctocolectomy. This decision is a clinicopathological one and the pathologist should attempt to confirm the diagnosis in one of the following ways.

1 Documentation of high-grade dysplasia in other biopsies taken during the same examination.

2 Documentation of high-grade dysplasia in the same area at a repeat examination.

3 Confirmation of the diagnosis by another interested pathologist or, perhaps, expert gastrointestinal pathologist.

4 Distinction of DALM from adenoma, by finding dysplasia in flat mucosa, or by using supportive immunohistochemical techniques (see above).

Clinical management following a diagnosis of low-grade dysplasia is less certain. Essentially the pathologist should follow the same safeguards. In flat mucosa, low-grade dysplasia can safely be observed by colonoscopic surveillance with extensive biopsies of the entire colon within close time frames. Certainly initially colonoscopy should be repeated at 3–6 months. Should such close surveillance fail to reveal any further dysplasia, then the time between colonoscopic surveillance can be extended. However, in the presence of a macroscopic lesion (DALM), even if only low-grade dysplasia is detected, panproctocolectomy should be seriously considered [365], as a cancer is already likely to be present within that lesion [393,394].

Management of neoplasia complicating ulcerative colitis

Panproctocolectomy is the correct treatment for cancer complicating colitis, whatever the site of the primary tumour. This is essential because the entire mucosa of the colon and rectum is cancer prone. The only exception is when distant metastases have already occurred, in which case a more limited or palliative operation such as total colectomy and/or ileorectal anastomosis can be justified. In the past, some surgeons have managed ulcerative colitis by total colectomy and ileorectal anastomosis as a definitive operation. This does not cure the inflammation in the surviving rectum, which remains at risk from the development of carcinoma if the history of the disease extends beyond 10 years [375,376]. This is not now a recommended surgical operation for the treatment of ulcerative colitis without metastatic disease, but there remain patients who have had this operation; they must be part of a surveillance programme because of the risk of neoplasia in the remaining rectum.

Despite the presence of high-grade dysplasia, between 30% and 50% of patients will not have a cancer on resection [376,377]. Rather than errors of judgement, such cases are the foundation of cancer prevention and should be regarded as a success in any surveillance programme. However, as mentioned, not all cases of dysplasia necessarily progress to cancer. Until improved markers of malignant potential are developed, a small number of patients will continue to undergo potentially unnecessary major surgery.

Whether restorative proctocolectomy (ileal pouch surgery) is appropriate depends on the site of the carcinoma. In lower third tumours of the rectum, this is not usually an option but for middle third and higher, most surgeons would consider it. Patients with carcinoma or high-grade dysplasia in their colectomy specimen are at high risk (25%) of developing high-grade dysplasia or adenocarcinoma within the columnar cuff of the anal canal [395]. The pouch–anal anastomosis is therefore often performed in the circumstance using a hand-sewn technique with mucosectomy [396]. An alternative is to perform the more usual stapled anastomosis and to survey the columnar cuff [397] and to perform a mucosectomy at a later time if dysplasia develops [395]. The advantages of a stapled anastomosis are ease of surgery and reduced risk of incontinence in the future.

Other complications of chronic ulcerative colitis

Liver pathology

The liver is often affected in ulcerative colitis and liver function tests are frequently abnormal with the commonest being a raised alkaline phosphatase. The incidence of liver disease depends on the severity and extent of the colitis, but significant liver problems occur in between 5 and 8% of patients [398,399]. Involvement of the liver may either be coincidental or have a more direct relationship to the colitis. Fatty change and viral hepatitis are examples of the former. The chronic nature of ulcerative colitis, and the exposure of the patient to injections, infusions and a hospital environment all increase the susceptibility of the patient to viral infection. Nutritional and absorptive problems contribute to fatty infiltration. Sclerosing cholangitis, pericholangitis, cirrhosis, cholangiocarcinoma and chronic active hepatitis are the major complications related more directly to the colitis. Occasionally granulomas and amyloidosis may be found [399–401].

Pericholangitis and primary sclerosing cholangitis are both diseases of the biliary tract seen most commonly in association with total ulcerative colitis [402–404]. Indeed 70% of patients with sclerosing cholangitis are found to have ulcerative colitis. Pericholangitis affects small ducts and sclerosing cholangitis the larger ducts but both conditions are now considered part of the same disease process and progression from small to large duct involvement has been demonstrated [405]. The basic pathology includes varying degrees of periductular fibrosis and cholangitis, along with portal tract enlargement leading on to piecemeal necrosis and eventually biliary cirrhosis [406]. Increased copper can be demonstrated in periportal positions. Ductular disease may present before the colitis and colectomy does not protect the patient from its progression. The disease can also occur in the absence of colitis, suggesting the two conditions might share a common cause or factor.

Cholangiocarcinoma (adenocarcinoma of the bile duct epithelium) is probably the most serious hepatic complication associated with ulcerative colitis. The incidence is 0.4–1.4% [407] and it may develop years after a panproctocolectomy [408]. The tumour may be relatively slow growing and, if jaundice can be relieved, survival is surprisingly long. Cirrhosis occurs in up to 5% of patients, usually in those with severe and total colitis; it may arise on the basis of long-term autoimmune-type chronic hepatitis [409,410].

Other extraintestinal manifestations of chronic ulcerative colitis

There are a large number of extraintestinal manifestations of ulcerative colitis [410,418]. These include arthritis, ankylosing spondylitis, pyoderma gangrenosum, erythema nodosum, pericarditis, uveitis and episcleritis [410]. Amyloidosis is a rare complication [400,401] as many original reports are believed to have been cases of Crohn's disease [401]. Complications may also be the result of therapy. Of the commonly used drugs, both steroids and sulfasalazine have well documented side-effects.

Crohn's disease of the large intestine

The pathology of Crohn's disease and its aetiopathogenesis, its complications and its management have been fully described in Chapter 21 (p. 288). The pathological appearances of colorectal Crohn's disease are fundamentally the same as those in the small intestine, and are therefore described more briefly here.

Lockhart-Mummery and Morson described Crohn's colitis in 1960, when they distinguished its macroscopic and histological features from ulcerative colitis [411,412]. Crohn's colitis usually presents with diarrhoea, rectal bleeding or perianal disease; recurrent abdominal pain and intestinal obstruction are much less conspicuous than in small bowel disease. Anal and perianal disease, including oedematous skin tags, cavitating ulcers, fissures, fistulae, abscesses and anal canal strictures (see Chapter 43) may occur in 75% of patients with colonic Crohn's disease at some time during the course of their illness; such manifestations are more common during severe attacks when the colon is extensively involved. They are also associated with other extraintestinal manifestations [400].

Large bowel Crohn's disease may coexist with small intestinal disease, when it is most commonly manifested as involvement of the terminal ileum and the right side of the colon [403], or it may be limited to the colon, a situation found in some 15–30% of patients. Unlike Crohn's disease in the small bowel, where there is often a clear demarcation between diseased and non-diseased intestine, the transition between affected and unaffected areas in the colon is usually less clear cut. Colonic Crohn's disease has three major patterns of distribution: a diffuse colitis that may be difficult to distinguish from ulcerative colitis macroscopically, stricturing disease, and Crohn's proctitis. These patterns may coexist or change from one to another during the course of a patient's illness. It is important to remember that the rectum is macroscopically normal in 50% of cases of Crohn's colitis.

Macroscopic appearances

The serosa of the bowel is often hyperaemic and erythematous with a slightly dusky blue appearance due to vascular congestion, and there may be a covering of inflammatory exudate. There may be dense fibrous adhesions to other loops of bowel or other intra-abdominal organs. Fat wrapping may be difficult to assess within the colon but is usually present and of course this will not be assessable in the lower part of the rectum which is entirely surrounded by fat normally.

The pathological hallmark of colonic Crohn's disease in the large bowel, as in the small intestine, is discontinuous, patchy, or focal disease and this is seen most obviously from the mucosal aspect. Accordingly, ulceration may vary within a single specimen from deep serpiginous fissuring ulcers (Fig. 36.25) to tiny aphthoid ulcers surrounded by normal or mildly oedematous bowel (Fig. 36.26). Such aphthoid ulcers are thought to represent the earliest manifestations of Crohn's disease and appear to start as erosions of mucosa overlying lymphoid follicles. Larger ulcers are usually discrete with oedematous, overhanging, slightly violaceous edges and they are often stellate in outline [411–413,416,417]. Other examples have a more linear 'tramline' appearance with two roughly parallel lines of discrete ulceration running along the length of the colon, often, but not always, related to the point of mesocolic vascular entry into the bowel wall. After ulcer healing tramline indentations of the mucosal surface frequently remain. Cobblestoning of the mucosal surface of the colon, resulting from areas of marked oedema of the mucosa and submucosa separated by crevices that represent narrow fissuring ulcers (Fig. 36.25), is rarely as conspicuous as in the small bowel and is not unique to Crohn's disease, being sometimes seen in ischaemia. Fistulae are found in up to 60% of patients, whereas overt perforation of active colonic Crohn's disease is uncommon. This probably reflects the fact that the inflammatory process penetrates the tissue planes slowly and causes loops of inflamed bowel to adhere to one another, effectively walling off any perforation or abscess that may have formed. Fistulae, perforations and abscesses form from the base of the fissuring ulcers, where there is extension of the inflammatory process into the serosa and adjacent structures.

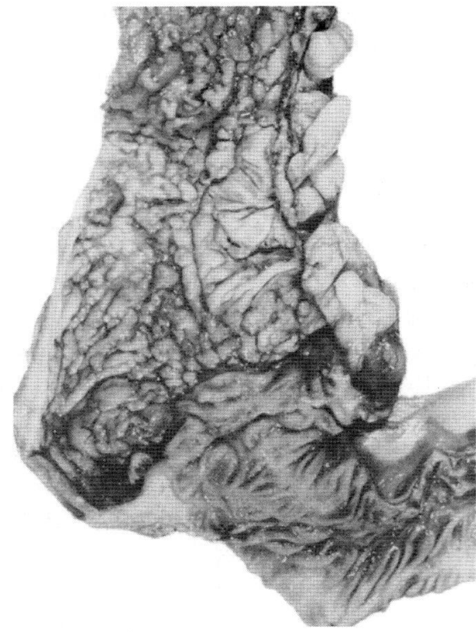

Fig. 36.25 Crohn's disease of the colon. The terminal ileum is normal but there is a typical cobblestone appearance in the caecum and ascending colon.

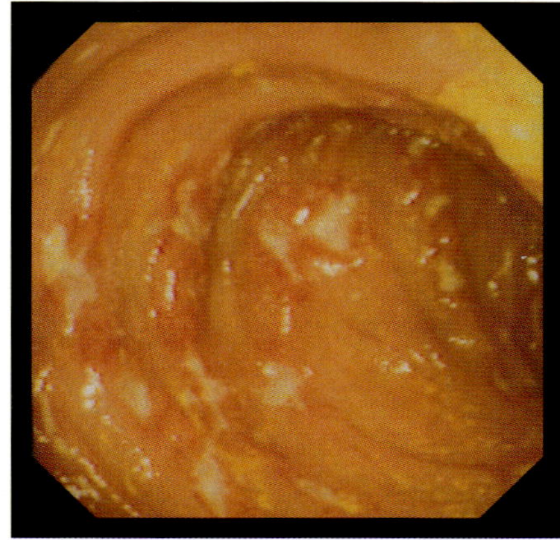

(a)

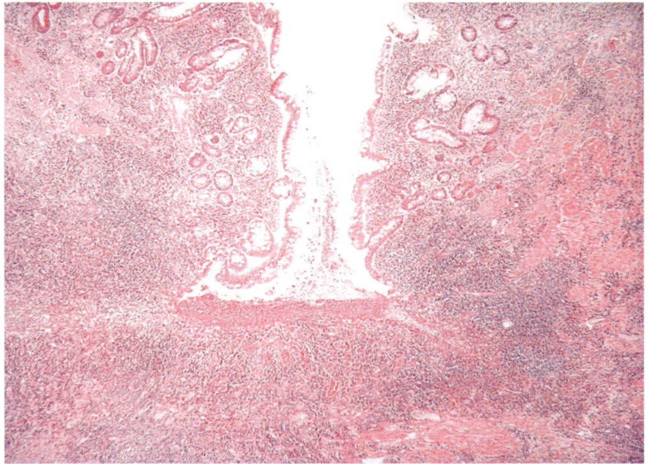

(b)

Fig. 36.26 (a) Endoscopic appearance of multiple aphthoid ulcers in Crohn's disease. (b) Histology of an aphthoid ulcer with ulcer slough overlying a lymphoid follicle surrounded by mucosa with focal crypt architectural distortion and patchy chronic inflammation.

Colonic strictures in Crohn's disease, as those in the small bowel, usually result from transmural inflammation, fibrosis and fibromuscular proliferation. They have no particular macroscopic distinguishing features from those due to ischaemia, chronic infective disorders and drug-induced strictures (see below), but they may serve in the distinction from ulcerative colitis, in which they are very uncommon. On the other hand, diffuse colonic involvement with Crohn's disease, while uncommon, can be difficult to distinguish macroscopically from ulcerative colitis. Useful pointers towards Crohn's disease include rectal sparing and the presence of anal or perianal inflammation. Mucosal pseudopolyps (inflammatory polyps) may be seen in Crohn's disease, sometimes adopting giant proportions up to 5 cm in maximum dimension [414,415]. Tall, narrow filiform polyps may also be seen. A particular feature of some cases of Crohn's disease is the presence of a 'sentinel' inflammatory polyp on the proximal side of an ulcerated stricture.

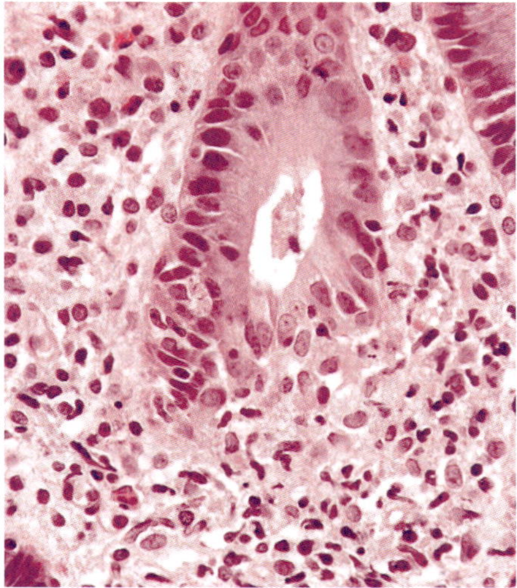

Fig. 36.27 Crohn's disease with a cryptolytic microgranuloma.

Microscopic appearances

The diagnosis of Crohn's disease is usually made by a combination of clinical, endoscopic, radiological, operative and pathological findings. It is an important, lifelong diagnosis for the patient and should not be made lightly. The pathological diagnosis is usually easier on the resected specimen than in a mucosal biopsy [416,417]; both are considered briefly here.

Mucosal biopsy appearances of Crohn's disease

The most typical histological feature of Crohn's disease in mucosal biopsies is patchy active chronic inflammation. The mucosa contains an infiltrate of lymphocytes, plasma cells and macrophages that varies from place to place, even within a small biopsy, both vertically and longitudinally in the mucosa, but it is especially noticeable when multiple biopsies are examined from the same patient, either synchronously or metachronously [419–422]. In deep biopsies it may be seen to extend into the submucosa, where its density may be proportionately greater than in the mucosa. Sometimes the infiltrate contains eosinophils or mast cells, but the most useful diagnostic finding is the presence of aggregates of eosinophilic macrophages (microgranulomas) (Fig. 36.27) or full-blown non-caseating epithelioid granulomas.

Active disease is manifested by the presence of neutrophil polymorphs, and typically these are also seen to have a patchy or focal distribution, such that apparently single crypts, or even segments of crypts, may be acutely inflamed while their neighbours are apparently unaffected [68] (Fig. 36.28). This so-called focal active colitis in a background of patchy chronic inflammation is highly characteristic of Crohn's disease, but it must be distinguished from 'isolated' focal active colitis (when there is no background chronic inflammation), which can be found in a number of other conditions (see p. 519) [427,428].

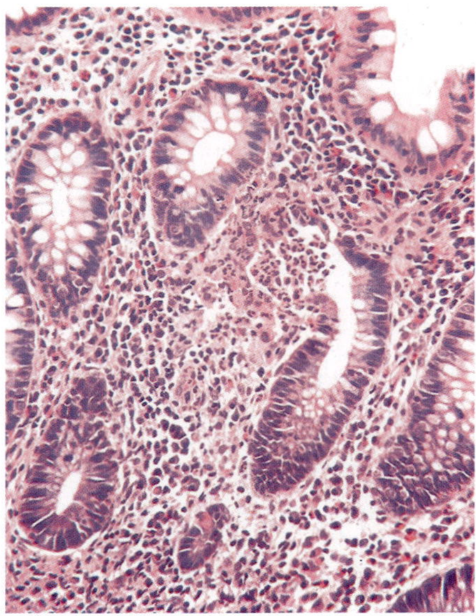

Fig. 36.28 Crohn's disease. Focal acute and chronic inflammation destroying part of a single crypt while leaving the remainder of that crypt and the adjacent crypts unaffected.

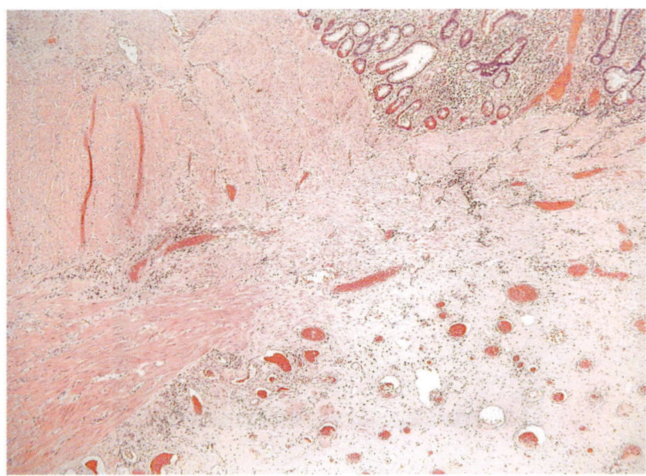

Fig. 36.29 Connective tissue changes throughout all layers of the bowel in Crohn's disease. There is muscularization of the submucosa and neuromuscular hyperplasia in the muscularis propria. Perineural chronic inflammation is also noted in the myenteric plexus.

Migration of neutrophils into crypt lumina may result in crypt abscess formation, and rupture of inflamed crypts releases mucus into the surrounding lamina propria. As described above in ulcerative colitis, this can sometimes result in pericryptal aggregates of macrophages and it is important to recognize these for what they are and not attribute to them the same diagnostic relevance as 'proper' granulomas and microgranulomas [424–426]. In some biopsies of Crohn's colitis the acute inflammation is more diffuse, especially when the disease is highly active with ulceration, and in these cases the pattern can be indistinguishable from ulcerative colitis. Nevertheless, the inflammation often fails to induce marked mucous (goblet cell) depletion and the crypt architecture is often surprisingly preserved. In long-standing cases the epithelium may show metaplasia, with the appearance of either Paneth cells or pseudopyloric metaplasia (ulcer-associated cell lineage) [423], although the latter is less common in colonic Crohn's disease than in the small bowel [429].

Resection specimens

In the majority of resection specimens the most striking histological feature is ulceration that characteristically takes the form of deep, knife-like fissures that are lined by ulcer slough and surrounded by inflammatory granulation tissue. These extend into and often through the colonic wall to form fistulae, to terminate in an extramural abscess, or to communicate with other fissuring ulcers extending laterally to produce a complex network of sinuses and fistulae. In other cases there may be more widespread mucosal ulceration with large, deep, but still discrete, mucosal defects with overhanging oedematous edges. Despite the severity of the ulceration, it is often remarkable that in Crohn's disease the mucosa within a few millimetres may be virtually normal. On the other hand, the very earliest lesions, the so-called aphthoid ulcers, result from superficial erosion over reactive mucosal lymphoid follicles. Ulcer healing in Crohn's disease may result in entrapment or misplacement of epithelium from the mucosa into the deeper layers of the bowel wall, usually with some accompanying lamina propria. This may give rise to intramural mucus-filled cysts (colitis cystica profunda) and confusion with carcinoma must obviously be resisted.

The patchiness of the inflammation that is the histological hallmark of Crohn's disease, described above in mucosal biopsies, extends throughout the full thickness of the bowel wall (Fig. 36.26) where it is manifested as round or ovoid lymphoid aggregates that may measure up to a few millimetres in diameter. These may be found in all layers of the bowel wall, but they are most obvious in the submucosa and when they line up along the outer aspect of the muscularis propria to form a 'Crohn's rosary' [206]. Associated with the transmural inflammation is gross bowel wall thickening, involving all the layers, with oedema and fibrosis being especially prominent in the submucosa. Lymphangiectasia is also a common feature, which is best appreciated in the submucosa and subserosa. Intramural epithelioid granulomas are seen in 50% of cases of Crohn's colitis. They too may be present at all layers through the bowel wall and in the regional lymph nodes, although they are generally inconspicuous in the lymph nodes unless numerous within the bowel wall. They are commonly found alongside blood vessels, and especially adjacent to lymphatics, and sometimes there may be a full-blown granulomatous lymphangitis, phlebitis or even arteritis.

Connective tissue changes of Crohn's disease (Fig. 36.29) affecting all layers of the bowel wall [417,430,431] include thickening and disruption of the muscularis mucosae, fibrosis and focal muscularization of the submucosa, fibrous scarring of the muscularis propria, and marked neuronal hyperplasia of the intramural and extramural nerve fibres [430,431]. Perineural chronic inflammation may be seen in the submucosal (Meissner's) plexus, as well as in the myenteric (Auerbach's) plexus.

Cases are described in which the histological features of Crohn's disease are limited to the mucosa and the submucosa [435]. These have been termed 'superficial Crohn's disease' and are very rare in our experience.

The differential diagnosis of Crohn's disease and ulcerative colitis

In this section we are mainly concerned with the important differentiation between colorectal Crohn's disease and chronic ulcerative colitis, the two main forms of chronic inflammatory bowel disease. This account will therefore concentrate on the means at the disposal of the diagnostic pathologist of differentiating these conditions, as such a distinction has important management implications for the patient.

Firstly, it should be stated clearly that it is occasionally impossible on pathological evidence alone to make an accurate and confident distinction between these two disorders. This is particularly the case in acute fulminant disease [206]. However, even in long-term disease which has been subject to innumerable colonoscopic biopsies the distinction may still not be possible. It is therefore imperative for the pathologist to retain an open mind and not be overly concerned about the use of labels such as 'equivocal chronic inflammatory bowel disease' in the situation of chronic inflammatory bowel disease treated medically and subject to multiple colonoscopically derived biopsies and 'indeterminate colitis' after definitive surgery.

Macroscopic differences from ulcerative colitis

The distinction between ulcerative colitis and large intestinal Crohn's disease can, in many cases, be made solely on the macroscopic pathology. The ease with which this can be achieved does depend on the way the surgical specimen has been prepared. It is important that the fresh colectomy specimen is promptly fixed in formalin solution in a way that preserves the pathological anatomy and in particular allows close inspection of the mucosal surface.

In Table 36.3, 11 main differences in the macroscopic pathology of these two diseases are demonstrated. It must be emphasized that these differences are not definitive and in some cases there is considerable overlap.

The comparative macroscopic pathology of ulcerative colitis and large intestinal Crohn's disease can be summarized as follows.

1 Ulcerative colitis is an inflammatory disease, primarily of the mucosa of the colon and rectum. It spreads from the rectum in continuity to involve part or the whole of the large intestine. In contrast, Crohn's disease is nearly always a discontinuous process. Commonly, there are diseased areas widely separated by normal tissue. Even with extensive involvement, there are usually small patches of uninvolved bowel. A segmental colitis with histologically normal bowel on either side is most unlikely to represent ulcerative colitis [433–435], although after treatment macroscopic patchiness may be apparent.

2 The rectum is always involved in ulcerative colitis. It must be emphasized that sigmoidoscopy alone is not enough to determine this, for occasionally a diseased mucosa may be found histologically when the sigmoidoscopic appearances reveal no abnormality. The rectum may also be involved in Crohn's disease, but the presence of a colitis with a normal rectum is highly suggestive of Crohn's disease. In a minority of cases of ulcerative colitis, the mucosal changes in the rectum can be minimal and easily overlooked.

3 The terminal ileum is involved in only 10% of colectomy

Table 36.3 Macroscopic differences in the pathology of ulcerative colitis and Crohn's disease in the large intestine.

Ulcerative colitis	Crohn's disease
Disease in continuity	Disease discontinuous
Rectum almost always involved	Rectum normal in 50%
Terminal ileum involved in 10%	Terminal ileum involved in 30%
Granular and ulcerated mucosa (no fissuring)	Discretely ulcerated mucosa; cobblestone appearance; fissuring
Often intensely vascular	Vascularity seldom pronounced
Normal serosa (except in acute fulminating colitis)	Serositis common
Muscular shortening of colon;fibrous strictures very rare	Shortening due to fibrosis; fibrous strictures common
Never spontaneous fistulae	Enterocutaneous or intestinal fistulae in 10%
Inflammatory polyposis common and extensive	Inflammatory polyposis less prominent and less extensive
Malignant change well recognized	Malignant change rare
Anal lesions in less than 25%; acute fissures, excoriation and rectovaginal fistula	Anal lesions in 75%; anal fistulae (often multiple); anal ulceration or chronic fissure; oedematous anal tags

specimens for ulcerative colitis. Often this involvement is for a very short distance, but uncommonly it may affect as much as 25 cm of the most distal ileum. Involvement is much more common in Crohn's disease.

4 In ulcerative colitis there is a granular haemorrhagic appearance of the mucosa, sometimes with patchy superficial ulceration but without fissuring. The appearance is in marked contrast with Crohn's disease, which shows a thickened wall, stenosis of the lumen and serpiginous mucosal ulceration, often with a cobblestone appearance and the presence of fissures (Fig. 36.25). Discontinuous disease may be present, a feature that is not usually seen in ulcerative colitis. An impression of discontinuous disease in ulcerative colitis may be given if one area of the mucosa is less active than others or in specific situations such as the caecal patch lesion (see above).

5 Fresh operation specimens of ulcerative colitis are often intensely vascular and congested, especially in very active disease. Vascularity is not a prominent feature of Crohn's disease, in which oedema is a better index of activity.

6 Inspection of the serosal surface of a colectomy specimen with ulcerative colitis will show normal shiny peritoneum, except in fulminating disease with toxic megacolon. Serositis, with or without granuloma formation, is a regular feature of Crohn's disease. Fat wrapping may also be seen in Crohn's disease of the colon, but it may be more difficult to evaluate in the colon compared with the small intestine.

7 In ulcerative colitis, there is a striking shortening of the large intestine. This is never due to fibrosis but is the result of a muscle abnormality, which is sometimes reversible and also accounts for the loss of the haustral pattern, such a valuable sign in the radiographic diagnosis. If a true stricture is present in chronic ulcerative colitis, then it is malignant until proven otherwise, but may alternatively be due to coexistent diverticular disease. Crohn's disease characteristically produces fibrous strictures.

8 Spontaneous internal or enterocutaneous fistulae are a feature of Crohn's disease and never occur in ulcerative colitis. They are caused by a fissure penetrating right through the bowel wall and causing a serosal reaction which then leads to adherence to neighbouring bowel or adjacent structures such as bladder or the anterior abdominal wall. For the same reason, chronic pericolic abscess formation only occurs in Crohn's disease.

9 Extensive inflammatory polyposis in the form of mucosal tags is common in colectomy specimens of ulcerative colitis and involves the colon more than the rectum. In Crohn's disease polyposis is a less prominent [431] and extensive feature, although cobblestoning in Crohn's disease can mimic the presence of multiple polyps.

10 Malignant change is a well established feature of ulcerative colitis. There is an increased risk of malignancy throughout the gastrointestinal tract in Crohn's disease [436] but it is low and cancer surveillance for the detection of dysplasia is certainly not universally recommended.

11 Anal lesions are much commoner in Crohn's disease than in ulcerative colitis. In the latter there may be acute superficial ulceration of the anal canal and excoriation of the skin around the anus, but chronic lesions such as fistulae, ulceration and oedematous anal tags are characteristic of Crohn's disease. In operative specimens, extensive perianal and perirectal chronic inflammation is seen in Crohn's disease but in ulcerative colitis the inflammation is more superficial.

Microscopic differences from ulcerative colitis

When analysing a resection specimen of the colon and/or rectum removed for chronic inflammatory bowel disease, sections should be taken from all parts of the colectomy specimen, especially from those areas which may be most productive of the important microscopic signs of fissuring ulceration and transmural inflammation. Lymph nodes should be extensively sampled, especially those draining areas of active disease, for microscopic examination in order to detect epithelioid cell granulomas. Eleven principal microscopic differences between these two diseases are given in Table 36.4 and are summarized as follows.

1 Ulcerative colitis is essentially a superficial inflammation of the mucosa of the rectum and colon with involvement of the submucosal layer only in the presence of full-thickness mucosal ulceration. Even in very chronic long-standing cases, the muscularis propria and serosa remain free of inflammatory infiltration. The exception is in fulminant colitis and toxic megacolon when the intense inflammatory reaction causes separation and splitting of the muscle fibres of the muscularis propria with eventual perforation through the greatly thinned bowel wall. In contrast, Crohn's disease is a transmural inflammation spreading throughout the bowel wall.

2 In ulcerative colitis the width of the submucosal layer is normal or reduced whereas it is characteristically widened in Crohn's disease to a variable extent by oedema, fibrosis and inflammatory cell infiltration. There are other submucosal signs such as lymphangiectasia, neuronal hyperplasia and vascular changes, all of which are features of Crohn's disease and are not seen in ulcerative colitis.

3 Intense congestion and dilatation of the blood supply to the bowel wall (particularly capillaries and veins) is more prominent in the submucosa in ulcerative colitis, particularly with very active disease; it is not conspicuous in Crohn's disease.

4 Focal hyperplasia of lymphoid tissue is restricted to the base of the mucosa and the superficial submucosa in ulcerative colitis and is most common in the rectum. In Crohn's disease such focal collections of lymphocytic cells are characteristically distributed across the bowel wall, particularly in the submucosa and just outside the muscularis propria where they present as a 'Crohn's rosary'. They may be found quite some way out in the pericolic fat. This *transmural inflammation in the form of lymphoid aggregates* is one of the most

Table 36.4 Microscopic differences in the pathology of ulcerative colitis and Crohn's disease of the large intestine.

Ulcerative colitis	Crohn's disease
Mucosal and submucosal inflammation (except in acute fulminating colitis)	Patchy transmural inflammation
Width of submucosa normal or reduced	Width of submucosa normal or increased
Often intense vascularity; little oedema	Vascularity seldom prominent; oedema marked
Focal lymphoid hyperplasia restricted to the mucosa and superficial submucosa	Focal lymphoid hyperplasia (lymphoid aggregates) in mucosa, submucosa, serosa and pericolic tissues
'Crypt abscesses' very common	'Crypt abscesses' fewer in number
Mucus secretion grossly impaired	Mucus secretion slightly impaired
Paneth cell metaplasia common	Paneth cell metaplasia rare
Epithelial cell granulomas absent from bowel and lymph nodes	Epithelial cell granulomas in 60–70% in bowel and lymph nodes
'Fissuring' absent	'Fissuring' very common
Precancerous epithelial change occurs	Precancerous change uncommon
Anal lesions—non-specific inflammation	Anal lesions; epithelial cell granulomas often present

distinctive and specific features of Crohn's disease in both large and small intestine.

5 Crypt abscesses are not specific for ulcerative colitis: they can be found in a wide variety of inflammations of gut, including simple appendicitis, infective colitis, adjacent to inflamed tumours and in Crohn's disease. However, they are a particularly common feature of ulcerative colitis because of the great extent of mucosal inflammation.

6 In ulcerative colitis there is much epithelial destruction with goblet cell depletion and a corresponding impairment in the amount of mucin secretion. In Crohn's disease areas of involved gut will often retain what is an almost normal population of goblet cells despite considerable adjacent inflammation. It is a useful histological sign which can be detected in H&E sections as well as with special stains.

7 The cycles of epithelial destruction and repair in ulcerative colitis may lead to Paneth cell metaplasia, especially in very long-standing disease. Paneth cell metaplasia is less conspicuous in Crohn's disease.

8 Granulomas are found in at least 50% of Crohn's colitis resections. They consist of collections of epithelioid cells and giant cells of Langhans type without any central caseation. They may be found anywhere in the affected bowel wall as well as in the regional lymphatic glands. Their numbers vary greatly from specimens in which they are very sparse indeed to others in which they are abundant. In about 30–40% of cases of Crohn's disease, no granulomas can be found. They are not usually found in the regional lymph glands without also being present in the bowel wall. Classical basally orientated well formed epithelioid cell granulomas are not a feature of chronic ulcerative colitis. However, giant cells and histiocytes, in aggregation, may be seen in association with damaged crypts in ulcerative colitis and a careful evaluation of such appearances is necessary.

9 Fissuring ulceration is the most important sign of Crohn's disease and can be found in most cases if looked for carefully. Fissures appear as knife-like linear ulcers, which are lined by a layer of necrotic inflammatory cells surrounded by granulation tissue. They may also appear in histological sections as intramural or submucosal abscesses but their shape depends on the way that the section has been cut. They are not a feature of chronic ulcerative colitis.

10 Dysplasia is much more common in ulcerative colitis: it is described but is very rare in Crohn's disease. The main impact of ulcerative colitis is on the mucosa of the large bowel leading to repeated cycles of diffuse epithelial destruction and repair, which may at least partly explain the proneness to malignant change. In contrast, the intestinal epithelium is relatively unaffected by this process in Crohn's disease.

11 Epithelioid cell granulomas can also be found in the anal lesions of Crohn's disease, sometimes widely involving the tissues of the perianal region. They are never found in the perianal region in ulcerative colitis.

Indeterminate colitis

When all of the distinguishing features between ulcerative colitis and Crohn's disease have been considered, there will still be approximately 10% of specimens of inflammatory bowel disease in which the diagnosis remains in doubt [314]. It has been stated that these difficulties in differential diagnosis are due either to the overlapping histological features of the two diseases or to the fact that ulcerative colitis and Crohn's disease represent ends of the spectrum of one disease [207,208,433–435,437]. However, a thorough study of cases in which there was just such a diagnostic dilemma has clarified the problem to a certain extent.

The term 'colitis indeterminate' (now referred to as 'indeterminate colitis') was coined to describe those operative specimens, representing about 10% of the total, that do not conform to the standard macroscopic and microscopic features of ulcerative colitis and Crohn's disease [314,437] (Figs 36.30 & 36.31). However, they do conform to a recognizable clinical and pathological pattern. Mostly, the difficult cases are examples

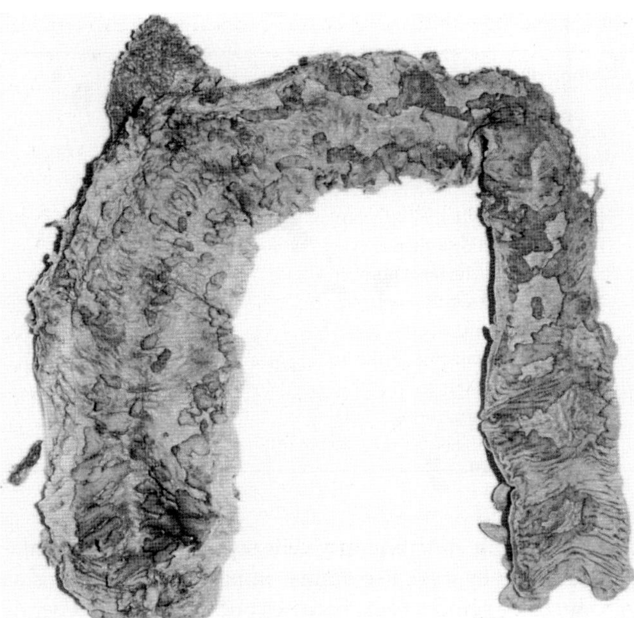

Fig. 36.30 Colitis indeterminate. There is extensive ulceration predominant on the right side of the colon with discontinuous ulceration on the left, features that are typical of neither ulcerative colitis nor Crohn's disease.

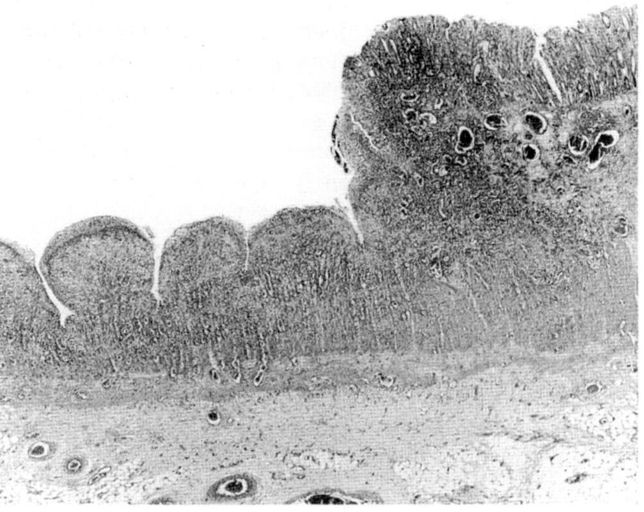

Fig. 36.31 Extensive ulceration, parallel fissures, transmural inflammation and relatively preserved mucosa (to the right of the field) are features observed in colitis indeterminate.

of extensive acute and severe colitis, often with some degree of dilatation of the colon. In this state, the maximal overlap of the pathology of Crohn's disease and ulcerative colitis is present and discriminating attributes are few or unreliable. For example, relative rectal sparing is an accepted feature of many cases of Crohn's disease of the large bowel, yet this can be seen in fulminant ulcerative colitis mainly because the predominant impact of the disease is seen in the more proximal colon, especially the transverse colon. This accentuates relative sparing of the lower left colon and rectum. The healing effect of steroid enemas is another factor responsible for such appearances. Another misleading appearance is the discontinuous ulceration caused by the unusually variable intensity of the inflammation in fulminant ulcerative colitis. The minor histological changes in intact mucosa between ulcerated areas suggests previous inflammation which has resolved and may be the only clue that genuine skip lesions are not present.

Fissuring ulceration is an accepted parameter of Crohn's disease, but is occasionally seen in very acute ulcerative colitis. However, the quality of the fissuring is different. The fissures in acute colitis are clefts, sparsely lined by inflammatory cells, whereas in Crohn's disease they tend to be serpiginous and covered by granulation tissue. Transmural inflammation with myocytolysis of the muscularis propria can occur in both types of non-specific inflammatory bowel disease and is common to toxic megacolon of any cause.

It must be accepted that the examination of the surgical specimen alone may not reveal sufficient discriminating criteria for a diagnosis of ulcerative colitis or Crohn's disease and thus the designation of indeterminate colitis is appropriate. Clues to the correct diagnosis may be found in the study of preoperative or postoperative rectal and colonic biopsies and, of course, in the subsequent progress of the disease which may in later surgical material reveal diagnostic criteria. The importance of establishing a sequential record of rectal and colonic biopsy appearances in all cases of non-specific inflammatory bowel disease cannot be overemphasized. The terminology indeterminate colitis is essentially a temporary classification until such a time that further clinical and pathological criteria become available to establish a diagnosis of either Crohn's disease or ulcerative colitis. In our experience careful follow-up eventually provides this evidence in most cases. In particular, follow-up of the diverted rectum may be helpful. Crohn's disease tends to recover with diversion [438,440,441,441a], whereas ulcerative colitis tends to develop more marked inflammation [441].

It has become particularly important to differentiate between colonic Crohn's disease and ulcerative colitis since the advent of restorative proctocolectomy (pelvic ileal reservoir surgery) [442–444]. The long-term results of pelvic ileal reservoir construction in patient groups with indeterminate colitis show that those who subsequently develop Crohn's disease usually have a poor outcome, whereas the majority, probably in excess of 80% of patients with a diagnosis of indeterminate colitis, have an outcome similar to that of pouch patients with ulcerative colitis [443], although one study has suggested a 19% failure rate for pouches in indeterminate colitis as opposed to 8% failure in the ulcerative colitis group [443]. A further study from Canada has reported a 95% success rate for pouches in ulcerative colitis and an 81% success rate for pouches in cases of indeterminate colitis [445]. In comparing ulcerative colitis patients with those with a diagnosis of indeterminate colitis, at the time of total colectomy, there appear to be clear-cut differences in rates of pelvic sepsis and perineal complications and patients and surgeons need to be warned of this potential problem in the indeterminate colitis patient group [446].

Synchronous and metachronous Crohn's disease and ulcerative colitis

There are rare reports, some not entirely convincing, that Crohn's disease and ulcerative colitis can occur in the same patient simultaneously [447,448]. Whilst we are aware of the very occasional case where the colorectum has shown the classical pathology of ulcerative colitis with the small bowel showing unequivocal features of Crohn's disease, we believe that extreme caution is appropriate before concluding that Crohn's disease and ulcerative colitis are synchronously coexistent in the same patient. Most of these cases will represent only Crohn's disease. We, and others, have certainly seen metachronous ulcerative colitis and Crohn's disease, the former usually occurring first with the patient later developing small intestinal Crohn's disease [449].

The role of upper gastrointestinal biopsies in differentiating Crohn's disease from ulcerative colitis

Focal active gastritis and focal active duodenitis, in the absence of *Helicobacter pylori*, can be demonstrated in up to 40% of cases of Crohn's disease where the endoscopic appearances are normal. This may provide additional helpful information in distinguishing Crohn's disease from ulcerative colitis. However, studies have shown evidence of focal active gastritis in ulcerative colitis patients and the duodenum may also show active inflammation in ulcerative colitis. In one study, 12% of ulcerative colitis patients showed a chronic active gastritis [450]. The topic of inflammatory change in the mucosa of the stomach and duodenum in both Crohn's disease and ulcerative colitis is dealt with more extensively in the appropriate section (see Chapters 12 and 21).

Inflammatory polyposis in inflammatory bowel disease

There is a variety of florid (giant) inflammatory polyposis of the colorectum, which occurs in both major types of chronic inflammatory bowel disease but is much commoner in ulcerative colitis [414]. In such cases the mucosa is replaced by a thick polypoid mass of mucosal fronds. This type of polyposis has a macroscopic appearance like that of seaweed or even spaghetti. Sometimes the polyps are remarkably thin and filiform and they may have a curious resemblance to worms. The polyposis is often segmental or focal and may completely fill the lumen of the colon, producing obstructive symptoms (Fig. 36.32). Ulceration is conspicuous by its absence on macroscopic inspection and adjacent flat mucosa can appear quite normal. The appropriate histological diagnosis should be sought by ignoring the polyposis and searching for the ordinary discriminating criteria between ulcerative colitis and Crohn's disease. If there is no ulceration or transmural inflammation and the disease is confined to the polypoid mucosa then a diagnosis of ulcerative colitis is more likely. Faeces tend to become trapped within the maze of mucosal fronds and this can cause local inflammation. The pathogenesis of this inflammatory polyposis reflects previous severe ulceration [322,414].

Diverticular disease and chronic inflammatory bowel disease of the large intestine

The pathology of Crohn's disease can sometimes be superimposed upon that of diverticular disease of the sigmoid colon [332]. Likewise the changes of diverticular disease can be seen occasionally in colectomy specimens removed for diffuse ulcerative colitis [333]. When the pathologist is examining surgical specimens of diverticulitis he or she should be alert for the presence of any macroscopic or microscopic criteria for either type of non-specific inflammatory bowel disease. In some

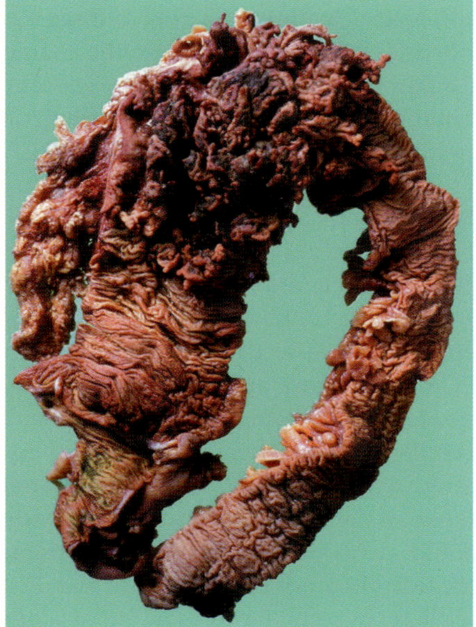

Fig. 36.32 'Giant' inflammatory polyposis in ulcerative colitis. There is a huge exophytic mass composed of irregular haemorrhagic mucosal fronds that is filling the transverse colon. The proximal and distal mucosa is relatively unaffected but showed histological features of inactive ulcerative colitis.

cases of diverticulitis the mucosa between the diverticula may be normal. In other cases there may be a diffuse or a localized sigmoid colitis associated with diverticular disease. There are reports of a limited segmental sigmoid colitis where inflammation of the luminal mucosa between diverticula is present, apparently unassociated with concomitant Crohn's disease or ulcerative colitis [452–454]. Mechanical damage to the redundant mucosa, a feature of diverticular disease, may account for this. The disease may present as diffuse segmental colitis or as a crescentic fold disease; in the latter, at colonoscopy, there are crescents of erythematous mucosa on mucosal folds. The histological appearances may be of normal mucosa, mucosal prolapse or features resembling chronic inflammatory bowel disease.

To differentiate this diverticular colitis (now the preferred designation) from both types of chronic inflammatory bowel disease requires sound clinicopathological correlation. Biopsies from the rectum will help to exclude ulcerative colitis if they are histologically normal. The situation is very much complicated by the fact that a small number of cases of diverticular colitis, without evidence of rectal involvement, will evolve into classical ulcerative colitis [453–455].

Whilst there is this intriguing relationship between diverticular colitis and ulcerative colitis, there is considerable potential for pathological diagnostic confusion between complicated diverticular disease and Crohn's disease. Such perplexity is more usually encountered in the resected sigmoid colon than in biopsies. For transmural inflammation in the form of lymphoid aggregates may be seen in complicated diverticular disease, and granulomatous inflammation, with granulomatous vasculitis and other characteristic pathological, and radiological features of Crohn's disease, have also been described [451,456,457]. However, the character of the transmural inflammation, such a distinctive feature of Crohn's disease, is subtly different in complicated diverticular disease compared with that seen in Crohn's disease. In Crohn's disease it is a true transmural inflammation, whereas in diverticulitis, the lymphoid aggregates radiate out around the inflamed diverticulum.

Whilst there are therefore considerable grounds for mimicry of both ulcerative colitis and Crohn's disease by complicated diverticular disease, diverticular disease, ulcerative colitis and Crohn's disease are all relatively common, especially in the elderly, and it is manifest that diverticular disease and chronic inflammatory bowel disease may coexist. Nevertheless, ulcerative colitis or Crohn's disease, apparently occurring in isolation in the sigmoid colon affected by diverticular disease, should always be regarded with extreme caution. Evidence for inflammatory bowel disease should always be sought elsewhere, in rectal biopsies in the case of ulcerative colitis and by comprehensive clinical, biochemical, radiological and endoscopic investigation in the case of Crohn's disease.

Other granulomatous pathology in the large intestine

Reports of sarcoidosis [458] of the colorectum should be treated with caution, if isolated to the intestine, for these are more likely to be examples of segmental Crohn's disease or intestinal tuberculosis. A similar histological appearance can also be seen as a local reaction to malignant disease [459]. Involvement of the large bowel in sarcoidosis is extremely rare and is usually clinically silent [460,461].

Biopsy in the differential diagnosis of chronic inflammatory bowel disease and infective proctocolitis

In a biopsy with inflamed colorectal mucosa, the most common differential diagnoses to consider are chronic inflammatory bowel disease, both ulcerative colitis and Crohn's disease, and infective colitis. However, there are many other conditions which may mimic these entities: appreciation of clinical context, especially age and previous treatment, be it medical or surgical, cannot be overemphasized as many such iatrogenic pathological entities, and numerous other conditions, can closely mimic chronic inflammatory bowel disease. Ischaemia, for example, is a consideration in the elderly, but not in a teenager. Recent antibiotics or recent travel may also direct attention to the relevant clinical diagnosis. The correct classification of chronic inflammatory bowel disease clearly has important long-term implications for the patient. Classification is bedevilled by the problem that there is no single histological feature that is invariably present in any one condition and invariably absent from the others. Thus even a granuloma, though it may help to exclude chronic ulcerative colitis, does not necessarily imply a diagnosis of Crohn's disease, for it may indicate an infective granulomatous pathology.

The diagnostic problems in biopsy work usually centre on the active phases of the various forms of inflammatory bowel disease and the resolving phase of ulcerative colitis. In remission, the architectural distortion so typical of chronic ulcerative colitis seldom causes diagnostic confusion. Crypt architectural distortion, a villiform surface, goblet cell depletion, prominent crypt abscesses and a diffuse, predominantly plasma cell, infiltrate of the lamina propria, point strongly to a diagnosis of ulcerative colitis. By contrast, in infective proctocolitis, the crypts remain aligned but some degree of crypt degeneration is seen (Fig. 36.33). Polymorphs are the most conspicuous inflammatory cell, migrating in a characteristic way between the crypt epithelial cells to produce a cryptitis, and also seen clustered in the lamina propria. There is frequently obvious mucosal oedema and the plasma cell infiltrate is light to moderate. In general the diagnosis of infective

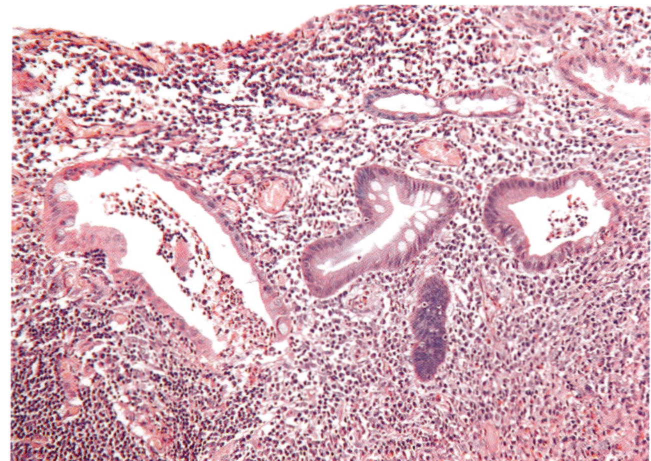

(a)

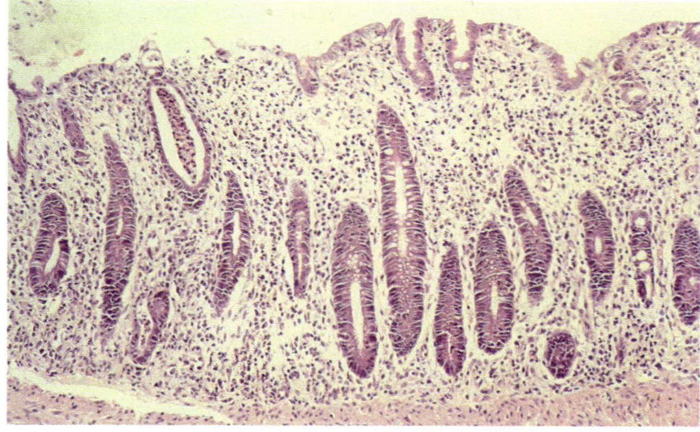

(b)

Fig. 36.33 (a) Active chronic ulcerative colitis (UC) and (b) acute infective colitis. Important differences are in the crypt architecture (distorted in UC, preserved in infective colitis) and in the content of the lamina propria (oedema and predominantly acute inflammation in infective colitis, heavy diffuse acute and chronic inflammation in UC).

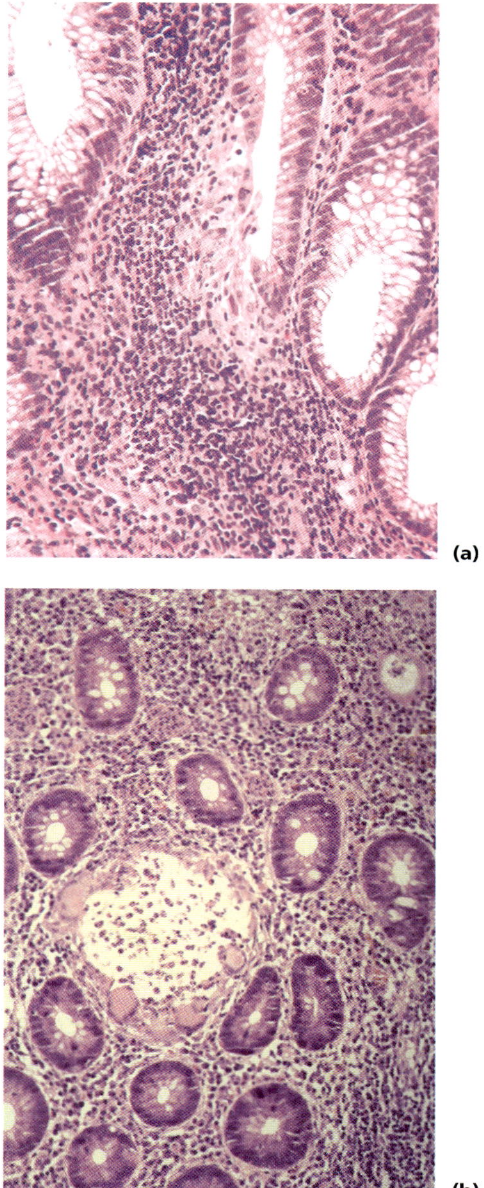

(a)

(b)

Fig. 36.34 (a) A cryptolytic granuloma that appears to be destroying part of a crypt in a segmental manner in Crohn's disease. (b) Foreign body-type giant cells surround mucus at the site of a ruptured crypt in a patient with ulcerative colitis.

proctocolitis is suggested by appreciating that there is an absence of the features that characterize Crohn's disease and ulcerative colitis [32], most notably by assessment of the acute to chronic inflammatory cell ratio.

Whilst granulomas are undeniably useful in the diagnosis of Crohn's disease, their identification is neither entirely specific nor particularly sensitive for that diagnosis. They are only present in 25–28% of biopsy material in Crohn's disease. Granulomas may occur in *Campylobacter* colitis, *Chlamydia* proctitis, yersiniosis and of course tuberculosis [84,96]. There has to be careful interpretation of mucosal giant cells associated with an ill-defined clustering of inflammatory cells and histiocytes formed secondarily and adjacent to damaged crypts (Fig. 36.34). These can be seen in ulcerative colitis.

In Crohn's disease, in the face of a moderate inflammatory cell infiltrate, the crypts remain aligned with little mucin depletion. This infiltrate is often patchy and basal lymphoid aggregates are a useful sign. Neutrophils may form crypt abscesses but their numbers seldom match those seen in ulcerative colitis or infection. Microgranulomas [462,463], focal collections of inflammatory cells including histiocytes but not crypt related, are a useful pointer to Crohn's disease. In the absence of granulomas, patchy chronic inflammation on a background of regular crypt architecture favours Crohn's disease, as does observing inflammatory cells in the submucosa. A pitfall is the biopsy appearance of a patient with resolving ulcerative colitis. Here the goblet cell population is recovering, the acute inflammatory infiltrate diminished and the distribution of plasma cells and lymphocytes often patchy. Considerable reliance must be placed on crypt distortion with the caveat that this can be irregular in areas of healing ulceration of whatever aetiology. The presence of crypt irregularity has been shown to be reliable in several studies militating against a diagnosis of infection [464–469]. In severe *Shigella* dysentery, however, extensive crypt distortion is well described [20,22]. This may indicate that *Shigella* can be an exception or that in severe colitis the value of architectural damage as a distinguishing attribute is less valid.

Both ulcerative colitis and Crohn's disease may present in a similar way to infective colitis or be precipitated by it [33]. A problem facing the pathologist is to know how often the biopsy of these two conditions may mimic infection or vice versa. Reports suggest that between 7 and 30% of biopsies from patients who are culture positive or carry a confident clinical diagnosis of infective colitis can have a biopsy more in keeping with ulcerative colitis or Crohn's disease [35,92,439]. Figures for the converse, patients with Crohn's disease or ulcerative colitis but with biopsies resembling infection, are around 5–7%. However, because the mucosal appearances in infective colitis and ulcerative colitis vary with the time from the onset of disease, especially in the cases of infection and ulcerative colitis, such figures must be viewed with caution. Emphasis is laid on the value of the study of sequential biopsies to solve these diagnostic dilemmas.

Special stains are of little value in this important differential diagnosis. A change in goblet cell mucin pattern from predominantly sulphomucin to sialomucin is common to both ulcerative colitis and Crohn's disease and simply reflects disease activity [256,258]. In an individual biopsy the distribution of immunoglobulin-containing plasma cells is of no help [483] though there is a suggestion that the plasma cell IgG : IgM ratio is permanently raised in Crohn's disease [470,471] and the plasma cell IgG : IgM and IgG : IgA ratios remain low in infection [470].

Colonoscopic biopsies

The widespread use of colonoscopic examination allows the assessment of the distribution of pathology in the colon and rectum [472] and reduces the sampling error inherent in a single biopsy. The distinguishing histological attributes of the patterns of inflammatory bowel disease are no different in a colonoscopic biopsy from those in a rectal biopsy. A series of diffusely inflamed colonoscopic biopsies throughout the left colon and a normal right colon favour the diagnosis of ulcerative colitis even though the rectal biopsy might have been equivocal. On the other hand, variation in the intensity of inflammation between biopsy sites and within individual biopsies suggests Crohn's disease, even if there are no specific microscopic features seen. Indeed it is this focal and patchy active inflammation that is, in biopsies, one of the most useful pathological findings in colonoscopic biopsies. Patients with the common causes of infective proctocolitis seldom require colonoscopy, but the biopsies are usually uniformly inflamed with the characteristics described earlier [439].

Colonoscopic patterns of inflammation will be altered by treatment as not all areas of the colon need respond equally. The rectum following local steroid enemas may appear relatively spared, perhaps suggesting Crohn's disease. Of considerable diagnostic importance is the colonoscopist's account of the macroscopic pathology. This can be diagnostic even when the biopsies may be considered non-specific. An accuracy of 89% has been claimed for colonoscopic examination in distinguishing Crohn's disease from ulcerative colitis, with most difficulty occurring in cases of severe inflammatory activity, as one might expect [472]. By contrast it must be remembered that biopsies may be abnormal when colonoscopy appears normal. Published interobserver variation studies in the diagnostic utility of multiple colonoscopic biopsies in IBD are rare. A recent study shows poor agreement but does suggest that some of the features used by experts may be taught to non-experts [420].

Sequential biopsy is an aid to diagnosis, differentiating the varied natural histories of the main forms of inflammatory bowel disease. In infective proctocolitis, the majority of cases return to normal within 2–3 weeks and virtually always within 3 months [439,464,469]. In ulcerative colitis, besides the waxing and waning of the inflammatory infiltrate, permanent crypt architectural damage develops usually over many months. In Crohn's disease, a pattern of exacerbation and remission is not microscopically evident and the crypt alignment remains intact. Therefore, in the clinical context of any individual patient in whom there is difficulty in interpreting the rectal biopsy, a colonoscopic series and subsequent follow-up biopsies are invaluable and usually result in a definitive diagnosis.

Drug-induced proctocolitis

Drugs are important causes of colonic inflammation. Apart from the antibiotic-associated colitides described below, a wide range of other drugs may either directly cause inflammation in pre-existing normal large bowel mucosa or activate chronic inflammatory bowel disease that has previously been in remission. When drugs produce colitides in their own right, the pattern of inflammation is variable. Occasionally the microscopic appearances are sufficiently characteristic to allow the histopathologist to suggest the likely aetiology but more often they are much less specific, encompassing those of acute self-limiting colitis, microscopic colitis (see below), or idiopathic chronic inflammatory bowel disease.

Non-steroidal anti-inflammatory drugs and proctocolitis

It is now well established that consumption of non-steroidal anti-inflammatory drugs (NSAIDs) may result in the reactivation of bowel inflammation in individuals known to have idiopathic chronic inflammatory bowel disease, especially ulcerative colitis [473]. However, in some patients this group of drugs has also been implicated as initiating ulcerative colitis, in that there is sometimes a clear association between therapy and the onset of the disease. In both of these scenarios the histological appearances of colorectal biopsies are usually indistinguishable from those in ulcerative colitis patients where there is no drug history, although occasionally some of the features described below that are more particularly linked with NSAIDs may also be found.

The most useful histological feature in distinguishing NSAID-related colitis from non-specific colitis in mucosal biopsies is an increase in apoptotic bodies in the crypt epithelium where, in normal circumstances, they are hardly ever seen [474]. Sometimes they may also be prominent in the lymphocytes and mononuclear cells of the superficial lamina propria. This increased apoptotic activity may result in accumulation of a lipofuscin pigment and some degree of melanosis coli [475]. There is often a generalized increase in chronic inflammatory cells in the lamina propria, and there may also be a striking eosinophil leucocyte infiltrate, increased intraepithelial T lymphocytes, or thickening of the subepithelial collagen plate, resulting in a picture resembling eosinophilic colitis, lymphocytic colitis or collagenous colitis, respectively (see below). Accordingly, in all cases of colitis which do not easily fit a typical histological pattern, the pathologist should consider the possibility of an NSAID-induced colitis, and especially in cases of microscopic colitis with unusual histological features including a triumvirate of mucosal eosinophilia, epithelial cell apoptosis and surface intraepithelial lymphocytosis [476].

NSAIDs may also cause isolated ulcers in the right side of the colon, which may mimic Crohn's disease or give rise to bleeding or perforation. They may also be responsible for diaphragm disease in the colon, which is identical to diaphragm disease in the small bowel [477,478] (see p. 299). When used as suppositories, NSAIDs may give rise to a localized proctitis, ulceration of the rectum resembling solitary rectal ulcer, and rectal strictures [479,480].

While NSAIDs are probably the commonest cause of drug-induced colitis in the UK other drugs may also be involved, as described below.

Colitis related to heavy metal therapy

The colitides associated with heavy metal therapy are exceptionally uncommon. It is, however, important to be aware of them since they may have severe consequences. Gold, mercury, silver and arsenic may all cause colitis [481–483]. Gold is the commonest of these in clinical practice because it is often used for the treatment of intractable rheumatoid arthritis, and while gold-induced colitis is uncommon, it was sufficiently severe to result in death in 42% [483] of cases in one series. Macroscopically (or endoscopically) the picture is of multiple petechial haemorrhages [484], focal ulceration, or an appearance suggesting pseudomembranous colitis [485]. Toxic megacolon may develop. Histologically there is diffuse chronic mucosal inflammation rich in eosinophils [484], usually with relative preservation of crypt architecture, apart from occasional crypt dropout. The mechanism of gold-induced colitis is not clear, but may be either a direct toxic effect or a hypersensitivity reaction [484].

Colitis related to chemotherapeutic agents

Chemotherapy is designed to have an effect on cells in mitosis in order to be useful in tumour treatment. The agents used also affect other mitotically active cells including colonocytes. Cell death compromises normal mucosal protection mechanisms leading to inflammation and ulceration. The commonest drug responsible is 5-fluorouracil, which is used as part of the chemotherapy for colorectal cancer. Mucosal effects may be seen at about 4 days after the start of treatment. There is a marked increase in apoptosis [474], the crypt epithelium becomes degenerate with markedly atypical pyknotic and karyorrhectic nuclei, and there may be superficial mucosal necrosis. Epithelial restitution and ulcer healing may result in enlarged nuclei with bizarre morphology and hyperplastic, disorganized and cystically dilated crypts [486, 487].

Drug-induced ischaemic colitis

Ischaemic colitis may be a consequence of therapy with ergotamine for migraine, interleukin-2 and alpha-interferon therapy [488]. It may also be seen with oral contraceptive therapy with oestrogen and progesterone [489] when it can mimic chronic inflammatory bowel disease clinically [490]. Cocaine body packers involved in drug smuggling may also develop ischaemic colitis if the contents of one of their ingested packages should be released into the intestine [491].

Other drugs which occasionally cause colitis

Methyldopa and penicillamine may cause occasional cases of diffuse colitis. Isotretinoin and acyclovir can produce an allergic colitis [475,492,493]. Isotretinoin may also activate idiopathic chronic inflammatory bowel disease [492].

Fibrosing colonopathy in cystic fibrosis

Fibrosing colonopathy is a uncommon condition that affects

children and young adults with cystic fibrosis who take high-dose enteric-coated pancreatic enzyme supplements [494]. Patients present with watery diarrhoea, abdominal distension and anorexia [494,495]. Since the advent of low-dose pancreatic enzyme supplements, cases are much less common. The condition may affect the whole colon or part of it, usually the right side. Macroscopically there is stricturing with superimposed ulceration and the affected bowel may be cobblestoned in appearance. The main histological abnormality is marked submucosal fibrosis with dense mature collagen bands, sometimes with associated haemorrhage. There may also be thickening of the muscularis propria, while the overlying mucosal changes are of non-specific chronic and acute inflammation.

Pseudomembranous colitis and antibiotic-associated diarrhoea and colitis

Terminology

Since the discovery that *Clostridium difficile* and its toxins are the main cause of pseudomembranous colitis [385,496–498], it has become clear that there is a spectrum of clinical and pathological findings interrelating the organism, the pattern of colitis, the presence of diarrhoea and a recent course of antibiotics. Consequently more careful terminology is necessary. Pseudomembranous colitis can be restricted to a pathognomonic colonoscopic, macroscopic and histological picture. Antibiotic-associated colitis refers to patients with diarrhoea following a recent course of antibiotics with histological evidence of colitis that is not pseudomembranous. Antibiotic-associated diarrhoea defines patients with diarrhoea related to a recent course of antibiotics but with no microscopic evidence of mucosal disease [371,372]. Within these definitions *C. difficile* and its toxin is seen in 6% of patients with antibiotic-associated diarrhoea, 38% with antibiotic-associated colitis and 97% of those with pseudomembranous colitis [499,500].

Pseudomembranous colitis

In the modern era, pseudomembranous colitis is regarded as an iatrogenic disease associated with antibiotics and caused by the bacterium *C. difficile* and its associated toxins [385,389,390,501]. However, it was described before antibiotics were discovered [502] and in the preantibiotic period seems to have been mostly a complication of intestinal surgery involving any site in the gastrointestinal tract. Until the discovery of its bacterial aetiology, the pathogenesis of the disease was believed to be ischaemic. In these early reports it is not always possible to separate ischaemic necrosis [503] from the confluent mucosal damage seen in severe cases of pseudomembranous colitis. Unlike the preantibiotic era cases, antibiotic-associated pseudomembranous colitis is largely limited to the colon and rectum although occasionally involvement of the terminal ileum is seen (see p. 277) and the disease has also been described in ileal conduits [504].

Macroscopic appearances

In the established case of pseudomembranous colitis, there are discrete raised indurated creamy-yellow plaques usually from 15 mm in diameter but occasionally up to 2 cm in diameter which are firmly attached to the underlying mucosa (Fig. 36.35) and separated from each other by congested but otherwise normal areas of mucosa. With more extensive involvement, the plaques may coalesce and the necrotic membrane formed may then be indistinguishable from those seen in some cases of ischaemic enterocolitis with superficial infarction. The disease is primarily mucosal and, at laparotomy, surgeons may fail to detect any peritoneal abnormality. However, there can be slight dilatation of the bowel and serosal hyperaemia. Toxic megacolon is a rare occurrence [505], as is perforation [506].

The rectum is frequently but not invariably involved so that in most patients the plaques can be seen and biopsied at proctoscopy and/or sigmoidoscopy [507]. The factors controlling the distribution and growth of the lesions are not known but in patients coming to surgery it is customary to find the major length of the large bowel involved. The examining physicians must, however, be aware that the rectum and sigmoid colon can be spared [508].

Microscopic appearances

The histological picture corresponding to the discrete plaque

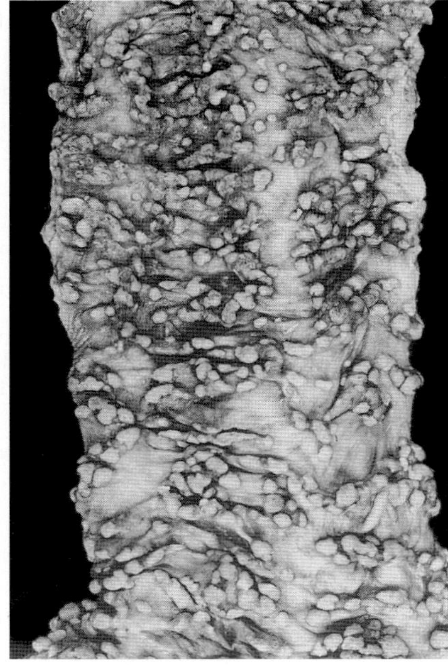

Fig. 36.35 Pseudomembranous colitis illustrating the discrete, raised and indurated mucosal plaques.

is characteristic [496,509]. Each plaque represents a small focus of disrupted crypts (Fig. 36.36a). The base of each crypt often survives, while the superficial two-thirds is dilated and filled with degenerative absorptive cells and goblet cells, liberated mucus, fibrin and acute inflammatory cells. All coalesce to form the yellow plaque visible on the mucosal surface. Although the cellular components of the crypts are lost, their ghost outlines remain. Initially the mucosa between such foci can be normal, be slightly oedematous or show small clusters of polymorphs involving individual crypts and surface epithelium. As the lesions enlarge the crypt destruction becomes more complete so that a stage is reached when a layer of inflammatory slough rests on the muscularis mucosae. At this point of full-thickness mucosal necrosis, the features are no longer diagnostic and merge with other diseases capable

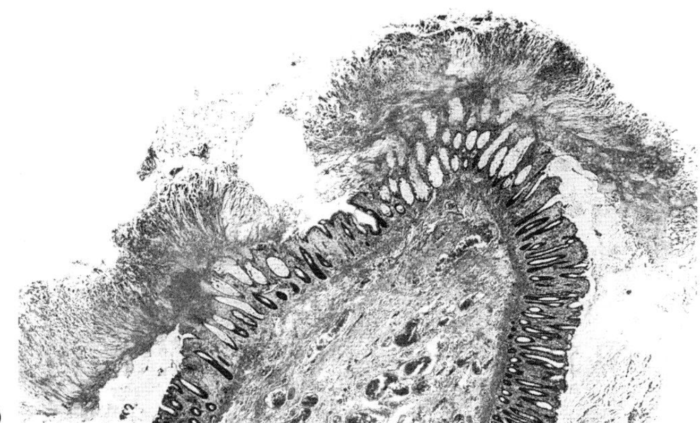

(a)

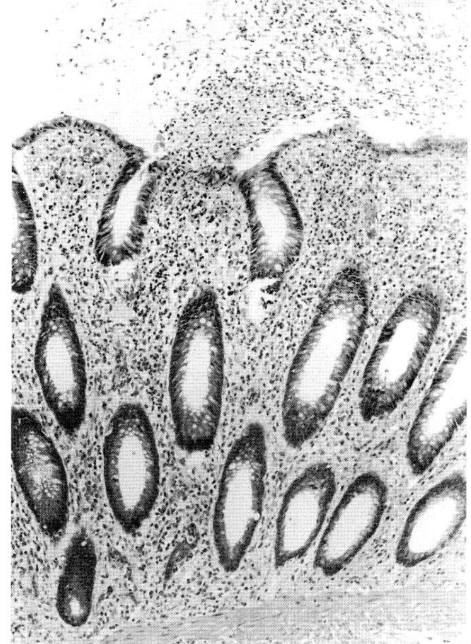

(b)

Fig. 36.36 (a) The typical histological lesions of pseudomembranous colitis showing focal disrupted crypts distended by mucin and polymorphs. (b) A tiny intercryptal erosion with a surface wisp for inflammatory cells characteristic of early pseudomembranous colitis.

of producing complete mucosal necrosis, such as arterial ischaemia.

In the early stages of the development of the typical lesion, and prior to recognizable macroscopic lesions, one may find tiny superficial intercryptal erosions (Fig. 36.36b). Between two crypts the surface epithelium is destroyed and replaced by a wisp of fibrin and acute inflammatory cells. This *summit lesion* [509] represents the earliest stage at which a confident morphological diagnosis can be made. However, it is important to examine the adjacent mucosa, as superficial erosions of the mucosa are a feature of many different types of mucosal pathology, caused by many different aetiological factors. However, they are usually accompanied by changes appropriate to the conditions in question, for example, the solitary ulcer (mucosal prolapse) syndrome in the rectum. Failure to appreciate this may account for lesions of pseudomembranous colitis being described in an unusual clinical setting [510].

The three patterns described—the summit lesion, the focal crypt lesion and the state of confluent mucosal necrosis—represent three stages in the evolution of the pathology, types I, II and III, respectively [596]. In cases coming to colectomy, although all stages can be seen, obviously more extensive necrosis is commoner. Capillary microthrombi are a variable accompaniment to the spectrum, which were at one time felt to be of prime aetiological importance [503]. It cannot be ruled out that toxins of *C. difficile* may mediate mucosal damage via a vascular mechanism, thereby implicating ischaemia in at least part of the pathogenesis. In line with the notion that vascular factors are important in the pathogenesis of pseudomembranous colitis, it is notable that identical histological changes may be seen in multifocal mucosal ischaemia from other causes, especially the small vessel disease produced by 'shower' cholesterol emboli from an atheromatous aortic aneurysm, usually seen after aortic aneurysm surgery.

The role of *Clostridium difficile*

Clostridium difficile can be detected in all but a few isolated reports of pseudomembranous colitis [511,512]. In the majority of these cases there is a strong association with antibiotics but this is not invariable [513–515]. In many cases the disease develops after the course of antibiotic therapy is completed. The relationship between *C. difficile* and the disease is complex and emphasized by the observation that toxigenic organisms are carried by up to 64% of healthy neonates [511] and by a small percentage of adults without any diarrhoea [389,390,516]. It is clear that, following antibiotics, some individuals can harbour the organism and its toxin without developing diarrhoea and that, in others with diarrhoea, the organism, but no toxin can be found. In general, the higher the faecal toxin titres the more likely a membrane is to be found [389,499,517]. It is not clear why some patients after exposure to antibiotics and colonization by *C. difficile* will develop pseudomembranous colitis, yet others only antibiotic-associated diarrhoea. This could be explained by variations in pathogenicity amongst strains of *C. difficile* [500,516].

The organism produces four toxins, the main ones being toxin A, a potent enterotoxin, and toxin B, a cytotoxin [390,516–518]. Both are believed necessary to produce disease and may act synergistically. Toxin B acts systemically on sites initially damaged by local production of toxin A [207]. Both can be present in the absence of disease [511]. Variation in ratios between the toxins and the inhibitory action of other gut flora may account for the wide spectrum of patterns of *C. difficile*-associated colonic disease [371,519]. Indeed in the hamster model, exposure to antibiotics and *C. difficile* is insufficient to cause disease if the animals are caged in sterile conditions. Clearly expression of the disease requires not only the organism but additional susceptibility factors within the bowel lumen or in the colonic mucosa [520]. The organism has been associated with exacerbations of ulcerative colitis and Crohn's disease [165,517] and it has a minor role in cases of sporadic diarrhoea in the community [510].

Antibiotic-associated colitis

In antibiotic-associated colitis, by definition no membrane is present and the three patterns of pseudomembranous colitis are conspicuous by their absence. The disease is specifically a biopsy diagnosis, as such patients do not warrant surgery. However, the mucosa often shows mild changes akin to those seen in infectious proctocolitis [372,510]. Mild focal inflammation of the mucosa is present with clusters of polymorphs and only a minimal increase in plasma cells. The neutrophils are usually superficial and infiltrate the upper halves of the crypts. Tiny microabscesses can be seen in the surface epithelium [372] and the surface epithelial cells can take on a crenated appearance. These might be forerunners to the summit lesions [372].

This picture cannot be considered diagnostic but may form the basis of a helpful clinical suggestion when reporting such a biopsy. It only occurs in a minority of patients with antibiotic-associated colitis, the remainder having minor mucosal inflammatory changes but without any distinctive patterns. A transient right-sided haemorrhagic antibiotic-associated colitis has been described with ampicillin and penicillin [229,372] but no pathological details are documented. This may be related to the haemorrhagic colitis in connection with toxin-producing *E. coli* 0157 : H17.

Antibiotic-associated diarrhoea

In antibiotic-associated diarrhoea, there is no demonstrable mucosal abnormality despite a history of recent antibiotics. Few such patients are subject to a total colonoscopic examination, which is the only sure way to exclude evidence of colonic disease. In only 10–20% of such cases can *C. difficile* be demonstrated. This serves to emphasize that, for the majority of cases of diarrhoea associated with antibiotics, the cause is unknown [385].

Biopsy in the differential diagnosis of *C. difficile*-related pathology

The recognition of the typical type I and type II lesions of pseudomembranous colitis is seldom a problem in the differential diagnosis of inflammatory bowel disorders of the colon and rectum. Care is needed in the interpretation of the type I summit lesion, for similar intercryptal erosions can be seen in the solitary ulcer syndrome and even on the surface of polyps when they have been subject to intraluminal trauma. Looking for the ghost outlines of crypts beneath the inflammatory membrane in the type II pattern of pseudomembranous colitis may help distinction from ischaemic mucosal necrosis. In the latter the adjacent mucosa, if any is present, may often be haemorrhagic or show other ischaemic features. Mucosa adjacent to lesions in pseudomembranous colitis is only mildly abnormal, showing oedema and focal inflammatory cells. A heavy plasma cell infiltrate and crypt irregularity are generally features against a diagnosis of pseudomembranous colitis at any stage.

The biopsy in antibiotic-associated colitis cannot be confidently distinguished from mild changes seen in other forms of infective proctocolitis, though there may be a few morphological clues [372]. In such cases, stool culture and a toxin test are indicated. Deeper levels through the paraffin block may reveal summit lesions and the patient should be carefully questioned about recent antibiotics.

Brainerd diarrhoea

An outbreak of chronic diarrhoea of sudden onset occurred in 122 residents of Brainerd, Minnesota between December 1983 and July 1984 [521]. The disease has a characteristic sudden onset and marked urgency with a secretory diarrhoea, a lack of systemic symptoms and no response to antibiotics. It has been associated with consumption of raw milk, and in another outbreak with water on a ship [522]. Histologically there is a surface intraepithelial lymphocytosis (but not in the crypt epithelium) with no thickening of the subepithelial collagen plate nor crypt distortion [523]. There is no excess of lamina propria cells. This superficial intraepithelial lymphocytosis was demonstrated in 20 out of 22 cases. Three cases had a focal active colitis, and two were completely normal. All cases had normal duodenal mucosal biopsies [523]. Although it is self-limiting and is likely to be of viral aetiology [522], its importance to pathologists is that its histological features are not those usually associated with acute self-limiting colitis and are more like those of lymphocytic colitis.

Focal active colitis

Focal active colitis is a relatively recently recognized histological diagnosis in colorectal biopsies that describes focal crypt infiltration by neutrophil polymorphs in the absence of any other significant microscopic abnormality [427]. It is not an uncommon finding in biopsy practice, and although it can be observed in some biopsies from patients who have Crohn's disease it is in no way specific for that condition and may be found in several other colitides. These include ischaemic colitis, infective colitis and partially treated ulcerative colitis.

One study of 42 cases of focal active colitis in patients with no past history of chronic idiopathic inflammatory bowel disease and no other diagnostic biopsy features [427] found that 19 patients had had an acute self-limiting colitis, four had an antibiotic-associated colitis, two had ischaemic colitis, six had irritable bowel syndrome, and 11 had isolated focal active colitis in the absence of any endoscopic abnormality or of any symptoms. No patient developed chronic idiopathic inflammatory bowel disease on follow-up. It was noted that 20 patients were immunosuppressed and 19 were taking NSAIDs. Another study of 31 cases [428] produced broadly similar findings, with 15 being related to infection and three to ischaemia. Nine were incidental findings in patients being screened for colorectal neoplasia but four patients were found to have Crohn's disease. It would appear, therefore, that many cases of focal active colitis are infective in origin and others may be related to non-steroidal anti-inflammatory drugs or ischaemia. While the lesion should always lead to consideration of the possibility of Crohn's disease, in the absence of any other findings it should not be used to label a patient with this diagnosis.

Irradiation proctocolitis

Patients who have received radiation therapy to the pelvis or abdomen may be subject to bowel injury with subsequent complications which may occur immediately, or at variable times after treatment, even as long as 20–30 years later. The late changes have an ischaemic aetiology consequent to the vascular damage, which is one of the hallmarks of radiation injury [386,524,525]. The radiotherapy is usually for cervical or bladder cancer, and the distal colon and rectum, or the ileocaecal area, are the common sites of damage, these being fixed sites, and in the case of the rectosigmoid area in close proximity to the target organ. Between 1 and 12% of patients may develop complications [386,391]. The complications include proctitis, radionecrotic ulceration with stenosis, intestinal obstruction, internal fistulae, perforation, haemorrhage into the lumen and mucosal inflammation [386,391,526].

The precision of modern radiotherapy means that it is now rare to see the early acute changes in patients treated for cancer elsewhere [527]. However, with the recent advent of short- and long-course preoperative radiotherapy for rectal cancer, the diagnostic histopathologist is now exposed to such acute radiation pathology in sections of rectal mucosa. Occasionally this can have a disturbing appearance due to the cytological atypia of the crypt epithelium (Fig. 36.37). Many a pathologist has made an erroneous diagnosis of diffuse dysplasia or florid viral cytopathic effect on the basis of these changes. Clues to the diagnosis of acute radiotherapy effect, whether in the treatment of rectal cancer or after radiotherapy for cancers elsewhere, are the diffuse nature of the cytological abnormalities, the reduced mitotic activity and, highly characteristically, eosinophil crypt abscesses [527]. These changes may also be seen in the small percentage of patients presenting with proctitis in the first month following radiotherapy [527].

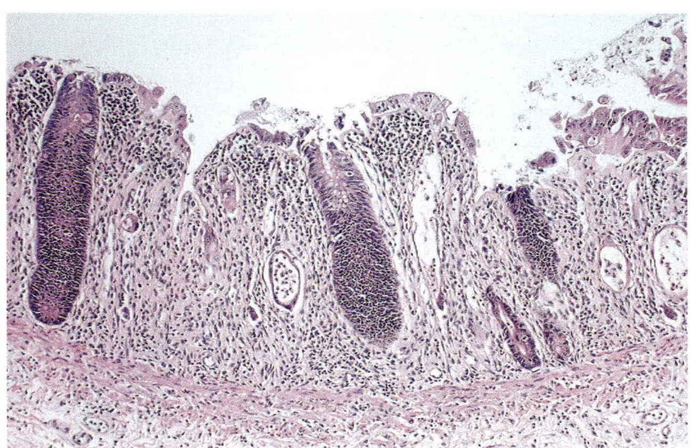
(a)

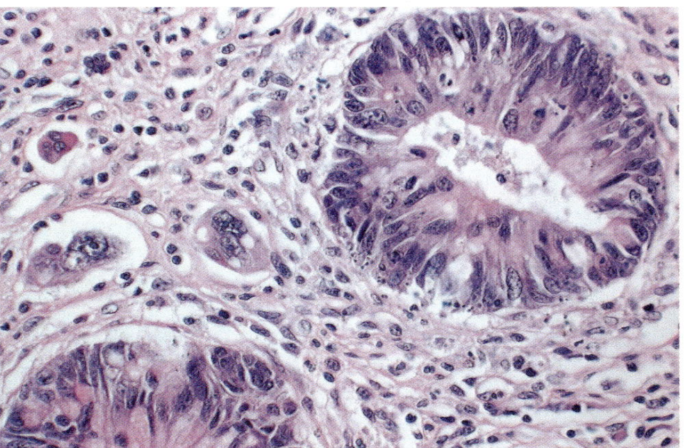
(b)

Fig. 36.37 Acute radiation proctitis. (a) There is mucosal oedema and acute inflammation, but the most noticeable feature at low power is the 'withering' of crypts with cystic dilatation. Surviving crypts are enlarged and show marked regenerative hyperplasia. (b) High power shows residual crypt fragments in the lamina propria marked by groups of isolated pleomorphic, degenerate epithelial cells. Surviving whole crypts show regenerative changes, but also prominent apoptotic bodies.

The majority of patients with chronic radiation proctocolitis present within 3 months to 2 years and the remainder over a much longer period. The macroscopic picture reveals a granular and haemorrhagic mucosa. There may be multiple ulcers covered by yellowish-white slough. Stenosis of the colon is common with serosal fibrosis and adhesions. Perforation is also a common presentation [524].

On microscopic examination, the pathology is most evident in connective tissue and in blood vessels, the brunt being borne by the submucosa. The connective tissue is first oedematous and myxoid before becoming homogenous and eosinophilic [527]. Bizarre fibroblasts are especially characteristic. The blood vessels, especially arteries and arterioles, show varying degrees of intimal fibrosis accompanied by fibrinoid necrosis in some instances and commonly fibrin thrombi [525]. Endothelial cells are prominent and atypical, often alongside intimal foamy macrophages. These latter cells were thought diagnostic of radiation damage at one time [525] but similar cells are one of the hallmarks of the vascular changes in eclampsia in the placental bed [528]. Telangiectasia is common and believed to occur because of the developing rigidity in the connective tissue [525]. Following healing of areas of ulceration permanent damage to the mucosa is manifest by crypt atrophy in conjunction with the features above. This can be appreciated in mucosal biopsies (Fig. 36.38). The vascular changes also occur adjacent to obviously involved bowel. This is important for the surgeon to appreciate when carrying out a resection and also for the pathologist when examining what may appear a normal biopsy.

The long delay in presentation in many cases of radiation proctocolitis reflects the slow development of the vascular changes, but presentation is accelerated in patients with diabetes or hypertension in whom there will be superimposed atherosclerotic vascular disease. Radiation proctitis has occasionally been treated by local instillation of formalin enemas [529,530]. Biopsies after this treatment are usually haemorrhagic and not well preserved; it is difficult to identify consistent changes.

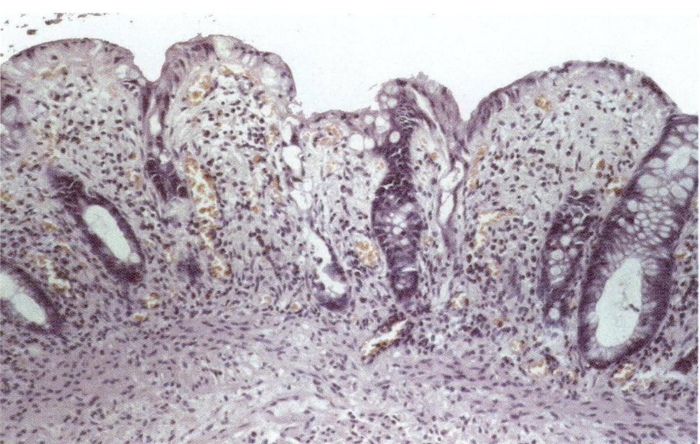

Fig. 36.38 Chronic radiation change with mild crypt architectural distortion, lamina propria fibrosis, vascular ectasia, and focal crypt 'withering'.

Diversion proctocolitis

Pathological changes peculiar to defunctioning of the whole or part of the large intestine, by ileostomy or colostomy, to divert the faecal stream were first described in an earlier edition of this very textbook. However, the term 'diversion colitis' was coined by Glotzer [531]. The inflammation may mimic that of chronic inflammatory bowel disease [532] but crypt distortion is usually absent [533]. The pathological changes may resolve following restoration of faecal stream [533,534]. Amelioration of the pathological changes has also been shown after butyrate enemas, suggesting that this condition is a result of reduction of butyrate, a fatty acid critical for colonic epithelial cell proliferation, due to a lack of intraluminal bacteria [534]. However, the only controlled trial of butyrate therapy for diversion proctocolitis did not show a consistent response [535] and increased numbers of nitrate-producing bacteria have been suggested as a cause for the inflammation in diversion proctocolitis [536].

Before the development of colectomy and ileostomy, usually for inflammatory bowel disease, it was customary to perform caecostomy alone, and such patients were sometimes left with a defunctioned bowel for many years. Such patients have allowed the comprehensive study of diversion proctocolitis. With increasing time, the bowel contracts down more and more until its lumen is as small as 1 cm in diameter [318] The mucosa is granular in appearance due to the distinctive lymphoid follicular hyperplasia and apthoid ulceration that occurs in diversion proctocolitis (Fig. 36.39) [537–539]. There is also diffuse chronic inflammation in the lamina propria. Some authors have referred to this as 'diversion reaction' [540], restricting the use of the term 'diversion proctocolitis' for those cases with ulceration and acute inflammation in conjunction with lymphoid follicular hyperplasia and diffuse mucosal chronic inflammation. The important feature of diversion proctocolitis is the relative lack of crypt architectural distortion; this allows its distinction, often, from chronic inflammatory bowel disease [542]. In diversion disease, the submucosa and serosa contain an excess of adipose tissue and the muscularis propria is thickened.

The prediversion condition of the large intestine is important in determining the outcome after diversion. Diverting the faecal stream from pre-existing normal large bowel mucosa, as in diverticular disease, carcinoma or Hirschsprung's disease, results in the endoscopic and histological changes of diversion proctocolitis as described above. However, if the bowel has been previously involved by Crohn's disease, the inflammation is characteristically ameliorated by diversion of the faecal stream [440,441,541,542]. Conversely, in ulcerative colitis patients, in whom the rectum is diverted as part of the three-

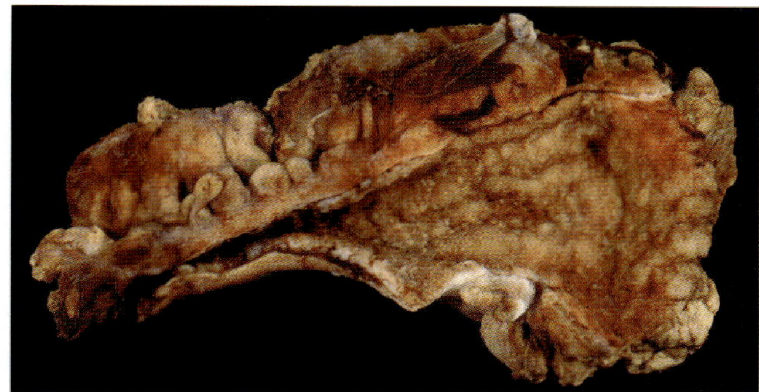
(a)

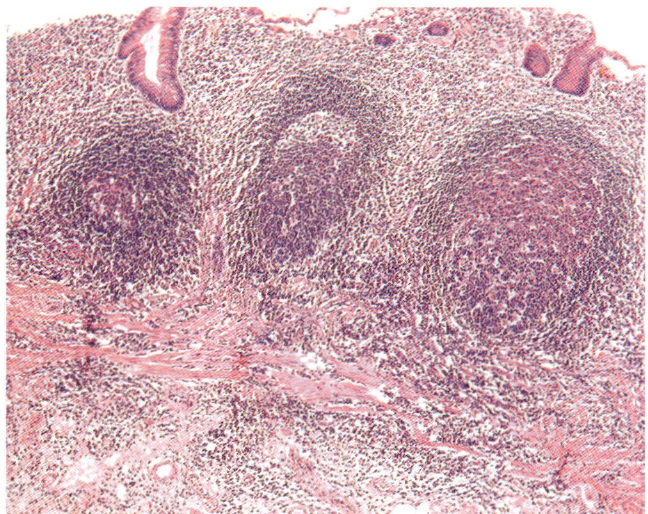
(b)

Fig. 36.39 Diverted rectum from a patient with ulcerative colitis. (a) Macroscopically the mucosa shows focal ulceration and a diffuse granular or nodular appearance due to lymphoid follicular hyperplasia, confirmed histologically. (b) The crypt architecture is distorted due to the co-existing ulcerative colitis; it is not a feature of 'pure' diversion colitis.

stage ileal pouch procedure, the superimposition of diversion changes upon those of ulcerative proctitis tends to exacerbate the inflammatory changes [533,542]. Furthermore, in such a diverted rectum, the combination of ulcerative colitis and diversion-induced pathology, possibly with additional ischaemic changes induced by surgery, incites additional pathological changes including transmural inflammation (often in the form of lymphoid aggregates), fissuring ulceration and microgranulomas (including within draining lymph nodes), such that the pathology closely mimics Crohn's disease [330]. It could be the ischaemic component of the pathology which produces an appearance like that of pseudomembranous proctocolitis [330].

It should be emphasized that the effects of surgery, particularly diversion, may produce perplexing histological appearances. We strongly advocate that a diagnosis of ulcerative colitis or indeterminate colitis must never be changed to Crohn's disease based solely on the pathological assessment of the diverted rectum [330,533]. All pathological material, particularly that of the original colectomy, should be reviewed, along with all available clinical, radiological and endoscopic information [541].

Whilst diversion in the rectum of ulcerative colitis shows these dramatic pathological appearances, the histological appearances of diverted Crohn's disease typically show 'burnt-out disease' with fibrosis and a lack of active inflammation. Granulomas become effete and hyalinized. Probably a reflection of the age and relative inactivity of the granulomatous pathology is the distinctive presence of Schaumann bodies (which are an unusual feature in Crohn's colitis) within these granulomas [437]. Microcarcinoids have also been reported in the diverted rectum in ulcerative colitis [543].

In summary, diversion proctocolitis can provide perplexing histological appearances that closely mimic inflammatory bowel disease of both types, in specific situations. It is clearly important not to make an unwarranted diagnosis of Crohn's disease or ulcerative colitis in previously diverted large intestine. It is clear that the inflammation associated with diversion subsides when bowel continuity is restored [532,533] or in some cases with the instillation of butyrate enemas [534,535].

Necrotizing colitis

A gangrenous process involving patches of colon has been described and attributed to infection with *Clostridium welchii* [544–546]. However, it is difficult to know whether this is simply acute ischaemia with tissue necrosis followed by secondary invasion by *C. welchii* from the faeces. The literature contains a confusing host of conditions encompassing terms such as necrotizing enterocolitis [544], haemorrhagic enterocolitis [547] and phlegmonous enterocolitis in which it is difficult to separate primary, usually clostridial, infections from secondary infection subsequent to ischaemia. The picture is seen in both small and large bowel. The term 'acute intestinal failure' has been coined for this group.

Neonatal necrotizing enterocolitis and the necrotizing enteritis of pig-bel, which may also have specific clostridial associations, are described elsewhere (see p. 277). There remain a number of cases in which the term necrotizing colitis has to be used. There is a variable length of large bowel, which is deeply discoloured black or purple. The mucosa ranges from being frankly gangrenous and covered by a yellow-green membrane (hence the original inclusion of pseudomembranous colitis) to, in mild cases, being simply congested and oedematous. On microscopy, the mucosa has undergone varying degrees of necrosis and haemorrhage. There is submucosal oedema and, depending on severity, the muscle coat shows signs of myocytolysis. Clostridial organisms in the tissue should be sought but, as mentioned, it is difficult to eliminate a primary ischaemic insult especially as most patients will be elderly, postoperative or have a chronic debilitating medical disease.

Neutropenic colitis

This is a segmental necrotizing and ulcerating inflammatory condition affecting the terminal ileum, caecum and ascending colon though it can be more extensive in some cases [550–556]. Clinically it resembles acute appendicitis with abdominal pain and fever. It occurs in patients with neutropenia [555] from a wide variety of causes [553–556,557]. Most cases are believed to be due to invasion by *Clostridium septicum* and the organisms can be demonstrated invading the mucosa and submucosa [546,556,558]. It is interesting that, whilst this organism is not a normal inhabitant of the colon, it is found in the normal appendix. Mucosal damage may be the result of leukaemic infiltration, cytotoxic therapy or haemorrhage in the patient group with thrombocytopenia. Occasionally other clostridia may be implicated [545]. In patients at risk, it is important to be alert for the condition and institute specific therapy. Until more recently the condition usually went undiagnosed and was fatal [560,561].

The affected bowel shows ulceration and necrosis, haemorrhage and pronounced oedema, these features overlapping with ischaemia and the type III pattern of pseudomembranous colitis. In some cases ulceration is minimal with submucosal oedema and patchy necrosis of the muscularis being predominant [552]. In preserved areas of mucosa, crypt degeneration reminiscent of infection may be seen but with no acute inflammatory cell accompaniment.

Neonatal necrotizing enterocolitis

Neonatal necrotizing enterocolitis is a disease of premature infants occurring during neonatal intensive care in over 90% of cases. It happens most often in the first 2 weeks of life and after enteric feeding has commenced. The hallmark of the diagnosis is the radiological demonstration of pneumatosis intestinalis [557]. The terminal ileum and ascending colon are the most common sites but the entire gastrointestinal tract may be involved [557–559]. The bowel is congested and thickened due to oedema and the presence of gas-filled cysts. With time it becomes necrotic, covered by fibrinous exudate. There is often perforation. The mucosa may be intact and have a cobblestone appearance due to the gas cysts, but usually it is necrotic and covered by a membrane.

Microscopy shows submucosal gas-filled cysts, vascular congestion, oedema and a variable inflammatory infiltrate in the mucosa and submucosa. The inflammatory component may appear relatively minor in the face of such extensive mucosal necrosis [557]. Small vessel thrombosis can be seen and giant cells may line the gas-filled cysts [557]. Gas-filled cysts are not always apparent [561] and, in their absence, the pathology simply merges into the group of conditions collectively known as the necrotizing enterocolopathies. Whether such cases have a different aetiology is not currently known. The role for bacteria has, for many years, been proposed as at least one component of the disease, but as with other varieties of necrotizing bowel disease, whether this role is primary or secondary remains a conundrum. Indeed, one bacterium may initiate damage only later to be overgrown by opportunistic flora. A wide range of organisms, including viruses, have been implicated in causing neonatal necrotizing enterocolitis, but clostridia have usually been implicated, in particular *Clostridium butyricum* [562], *C. perfringens* and *C. difficile*. This is because of the similarities of the disease to other clostridial enterotoxaemias in animals and adult humans, namely pig-bel, neutropenic enterocolitis and pseudomembranous colitis.

Microscopic colitis

This term refers to a group of patients with long-standing chronic diarrhoea, normal colonoscopy and microscopic chronic inflammation [563–565]. There may be rectal sparing in up to 30% of cases [476]. Increasingly the term incorporates a broad spectrum of pathological appearances within the context of the characteristic clinical presentation (chronic watery, bloodless diarrhoea of unknown aetiology) and a normal (or near-normal) colonoscopic appearance. Whilst originally the term was allocated to a patient group with non-specific histological appearances [567–570], now the term is used to encompass other more specific histological conditions, most notably collagenous colitis and lymphocytic colitis. The term can also be used to denote a group of idiosyncratic reactive colopathies, especially drug reactions, in which there may be non-specific histological features or there may be changes more specific to drug reactions such as a prominent eosinophil infiltrate in the lamina propria, pronounced apoptotic activity or modest melanosis coli.

In the patient group originally described as having 'microscopic colitis', colonoscopic biopsies show a modest increase in plasma cells and lymphocytes throughout the colon with or without some neutrophils. There is no crypt distortion. There are none of the typical features of ulcerative colitis, Crohn's disease or infection. It must be reaffirmed that the diagnosis can only be suggested in the correct clinical context of chronic watery, bloodless diarrhoea of unknown aetiology, accompanied by a total low-grade colitis with normal crypt architecture. Laxative abuse [571] must be carefully excluded in such patients. Pathophysiological studies [572] have shown a depressed colonic absorption of water and altered sodium, chloride and bicarbonate exchange. There remains considerable dispute as to whether this condition is a definite entity or simply part of the spectrum of collagenous colitis and lymphocytic colitis. The latter may develop after a prolonged period of non-specific colitis and it shows a similar pattern of altered absorption [572]. It seems likely that all three entities are related because a review of the original cases diagnosed as microscopic colitis has revealed focal thickening of the subepithelial collagen plate as seen in collagenous colitis [573–575]. None of these conditions should be confused with the entity of minimal change colitis, which is a pattern of mild colitis with crypt distortion seen within the spectrum of Crohn's disease and ulcerative colitis.

Lymphocytic colitis

The characteristic symptom of lymphocytic colitis is chronic watery diarrhoea that may be continuous or intermittent. It may have a sudden explosive onset and may persist for many years. The watery diarrhoea is thought to result from decreased water absorption in some patients [549,552,570] whereas in others it may be related to bile acid malabsorption [576,577]. Crampy abdominal pain and weight loss can occasionally occur, but they are not typical. Some patients also show features of malabsorption, and the condition may be associated with a lymphocytic enteritis that may or may not respond to gluten withdrawal [575–582] or with tropical sprue [583,584]. Conversely, about 40% of coeliac disease patients have increased intraepithelial lymphocytes in the large bowel mucosa, although this is generally much less marked than in lymphocytic colitis. Lymphocytic colitis is also associated with collagenous colitis (see below) and with lymphocytic gastritis (see p. 120) [578]. It affects individuals of a wide age range, including children, and occurs equally in men and women [549,566,580,585]. A seronegative non-destructive arthritis is seen in some, raising the possibility that the condition may be related to a systemic immunological disturbance or to therapeutic agents such as NSAIDs.

The diagnostic hallmark of lymphocytic colitis is a diffuse increase in intraepithelial lymphocytes (T cells) in excess of 20 per 100 epithelial cells [565] (Fig. 36.40). There is also diffuse lamina propria chronic inflammation with increased lymphocytes and plasma cells and sometimes prominent eosinophils and/or mast cells. Neutrophils may also be seen in the lamina propria, usually in small numbers, but they rarely invade the crypt epithelium. The surface epithelium may be degenerate, and sometimes becomes detached from the underlying lamina propria, a feature also seen in collagenous colitis. Unlike collagenous colitis, there is no thickening of the subepithelial collagen plate and the disease is usually relatively diffusely distributed throughout the colonic mucosa. Paneth cell metaplasia may be seen and does not imply chronic idiopathic inflammatory bowel disease. It is important to realize that the intraepithelial lymphocytosis of lymphocytic colitis is diffuse and not focal. Focal intraepithelial lymphocytosis may be seen in Crohn's disease, in some mucosal polyps and in diverticular disease [476].

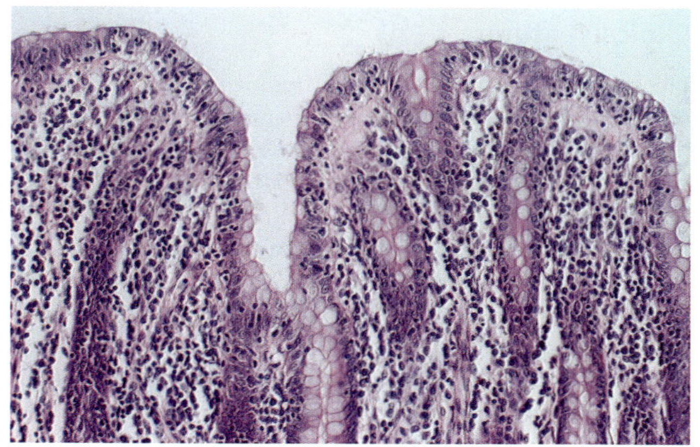
(a)

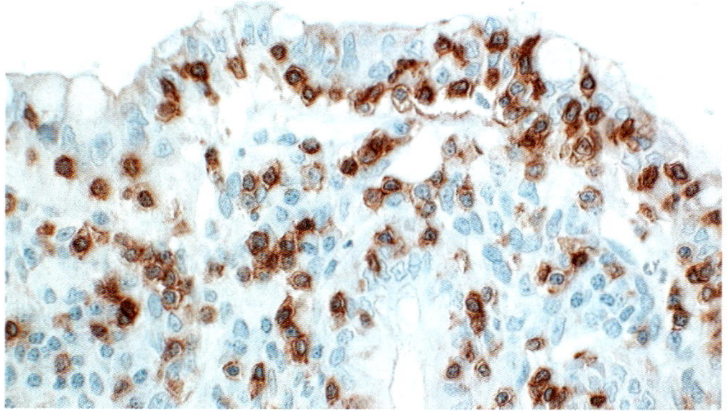
(b)

Fig. 36.40 Lymphocytic colitis. (a) There is diffuse chronic mucosal inflammation and a normal crypt architecture. (b) Intraepithelial lymphocytes are markedly increased and are shown to be T-cells by CD3 immunostaining.

A recently published large series found that in most patients lymphocytic colitis is an isolated condition whose clinical course is benign and self-limiting—after a mean period of 38 months' follow-up the watery diarrhoea had resolved in 25 out of 27 cases, the histological changes had returned to normal in all but three of these, and none progressed to collagenous colitis [549,578,585]. Whether any form of medical therapy influences outcome is uncertain.

Collagenous colitis

Lindstrom is credited with the first description of the entity in 1976 [563]. The diagnosis can only be made from histological analysis of colonoscopic biopsies and other investigations are usually unhelpful. No case, as far as we are aware, has come to colectomy. However, in some cases, which fail to respond to medical treatment, diversion of the faecal stream has been successful.

Clinical features

The patients are predominantly women, the sex ratio of women to men being at least 4 : 1. Persistent chronic watery, bloodless diarrhoea, often severe enough to present with incontinence, is an invariable symptom. The length of history is variable, from weeks up to 20 years in some cases [476,564]. Laboratory investigations and barium studies are usually unhelpful. Occasionally the white count and blood viscosity are raised. Barium enema shows none of the features associated with the more common forms of inflammatory bowel disease, generally being normal apart from individual cases with minor abnormalities [573]. Similarly sigmoidoscopy and colonoscopy are normal [476] or, at most, showing minor non-specific abnormalities such as alteration of the vascular pattern or slight mucosal friability. There may be some association with rheumatoid arthritis and thyroid disease such that a link with autoimmunity has been suggested [566]. Despite the often long history and the frequency of bowel action, with up to 20 stools per day being recorded [566], patients suffer few complications provided there is adequate fluid balance during the exacerbations of diarrhoea.

Pathology

It is only from a rectal or colonic biopsy that the diagnosis can be made. The majority of cases show involvement of the rectum [685], but this is not invariable [476,566] for up to 30% have rectal sparing, with normal rectal biopsies. Colonoscopic biopsies are necessary for complete investigation, as the transverse and proximal colon are most likely to show the changes of the disease and are also the areas most likely to be maximally involved. The diagnosis depends on demonstrating a thickened collagen band immediately beneath the surface colonic or rectal epithelium [586–588] (Fig. 36.41). The accompanying changes are variable but are usually those of a mild colitis, the mucosa being infiltrated by small numbers of inflammatory cells and occasionally giant cells [589]. There may be an infiltrate of intraepithelial lymphocytes without crypt damage and, in our experience, as well as others, this can predate the appearance of a collagen band [588].

Beneath the surface epithelium in a normal colonic or rectal biopsy are a basal lamina and a thin band of collagen. Before making the diagnosis of collagenous colitis, the thickness of the normal collagen band must be appreciated and any increase in thickness assessed only on a well orientated specimen. The normal subepithelial collagen plate is 3–7 μm thick [573] and varies according to site, increasing slightly from right to left colon [586]. It has been shown to be 3 μm thick when measured in an autopsy population of otherwise healthy people involved in fatal road traffic accidents [575]. In 4% of this series of 457 patients, it was greater than 10 μm but only in those with a thickness of over 15 μm was there diarrhoea. In the literature there is a wide range of thickness

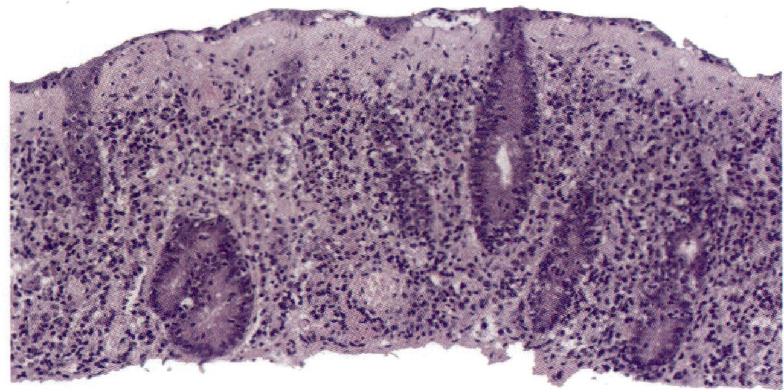
(a)

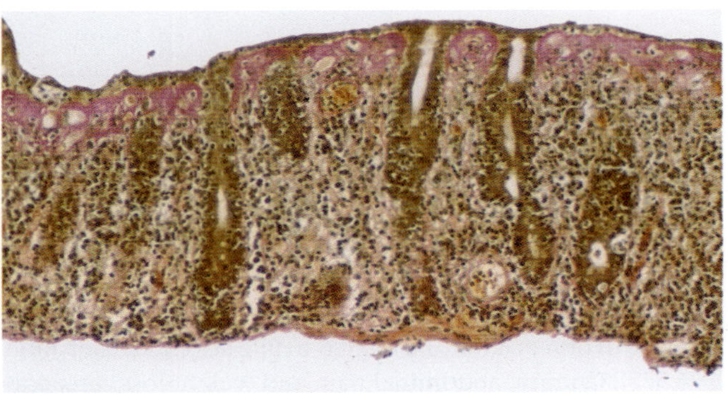
(b)

Fig. 36.41 Collagenous colitis. (a) There is diffuse chronic inflammation and eosinophilic thickening of the subepithelial collagen plate, (b) confirmed by van Gieson staining for collagen. Focal separation of the surface epithelium from the underlying connective tissue is a common feature in this condition.

associated with collagenous colitis from 10 to 70 μm [578]. Because the collagen thickness has been found to vary both in the time course of the disease [578] and by biopsy site, it is important to take the average of several measurements along any one biopsy and to study several biopsies. Only by these procedures can a confident diagnosis be made. There are documented examples of an abnormal band developing over several years [578], which means that sequential biopsies are also an important part of the diagnostic procedures in prolonged unexplained intermittent diarrhoea. It is also important to appreciate that the band may be present at times when diarrhoea is absent.

The collagen band does not normally extend downwards alongside the crypts. That it is collagen should always be confirmed by any of the standard collagen stains, for superficial oedema of the lamina propria and amyloidosis may give rise to similar appearances. The band is birefringent under polarized light and stains pale pink using the PAS reagent. The mucosal inflammatory infiltrate that accompanies the abnormal band does not have any characteristic features but, whatever the aetiology of the band, there is a background element of colitis. In occasional cases this inflammatory cell infiltrate may be particularly florid and associated with a marked neutrophil polymorph infiltrate. This form of severe collagenous colitis is usually associated with surface epithelial degeneration and superficial erosions. It is usually these severe forms of collagenous colitis that are associated with the modest colonoscopic abnormalities that have been described in the disease, especially in the more proximal colon.

The collagenous nature of this subepithelial band when studied with the electron microscope has been confirmed [573]. Collagen typing has been carried out in a few cases and the band has been shown to be mostly type III and some type I [573]. This is a pattern derived from fibroblasts and supports the concept that the abnormality originates in the pericryptal fibroblasts.

Pathogenesis

It was initially postulated that the thick collagen band interfered with water absorption. However, in one case the diarrhoea was shown to be secretory in nature with a net secretion of fluid and electrolytes into the lumen [572]. It was suggested the anionic secretion could be prostaglandin mediated. This in turn was switched on by mucosal hypoxia from the collagenous diffusional barrier. Nearly all workers turn to the pericryptal fibroblast as the source of the increased collagen. This fibroblast is the cell responsible for normal subepithelial collagen production: it may be demonstrated by a specific monoclonal antibody [588].

Abnormal amounts of subepithelial collagen have been found in metaplastic polyps [476,590–592] and such polyps are believed to result from quantitative, but not qualitative, changes in maturation. They are hypermature and such a state might apply to the pericryptal fibroblast sheath in collagenous colitis. The other main theory for the pathogenesis of collagenous colitis is an inflammatory one. This does not necessarily exclude involvement of the pericryptal fibroblasts at some stage. As previously mentioned, there are documented cases of an established colitis preceding the development of the abnormal collagen band by 1–2 years, suggesting a primary inflammatory pathology as the initial event. This is supported by the interrelationship between lymphocytic colitis and collagenous colitis with cases of the former evolving into the latter. However, no other recognized forms of chronic inflammatory disease of the colorectum, such as ulcerative colitis, infective colitis and Crohn's disease have been observed to develop a collagen band. Considering other diseases, a band of collagen is occasionally seen in the jejunum in coeliac disease in the entity known as collagenous sprue. Apart from two cases with associated villous atrophy [578] no firm connection with small bowel abnormalities, in particular collagenous sprue [541] has been established for collagenous colitis. Abnormal collagen plates can be found in patients with adenocarcinoma [592], megacolon, polyps and diverticular disease. Some cases of microscopic colitis, including cases of collagenous and lymphocytic colitis, are related to NSAID therapy.

At present the aetiology of collagenous colitis is unknown and its specificity has been questioned [569]. Nevertheless, in our experience, it has such individual clinical and pathological features that we would unequivocally regard the disease as a specific entity. More recently, a variant of microscopic colitis has been described wherein there is persistent watery bloodless diarrhoea, normal colonoscopy and diffuse mucosal chronic inflammation with normal crypt architecture but characterized by multinucleate giant cells [589]. Whether this is a specific entity is yet to be determined. Finally, it is worth reaffirming that several of these subtypes of 'microscopic colitis' may be closely associated with drug therapy [476,585].

Phlegmonous colitis

This rare form of inflammatory disease of the intestines is manifest mainly as a cellulitis of the submucosa that can affect any region of the gastrointestinal tract. It is rare, but when it occurs, it is commoner in the stomach than at other sites [593]. The serosal aspect of the bowel is congested and the affected length slightly thickened. The mucosa is usually intact with thickened mucosal folds and there is obvious submucosal oedema and expansion. Histology reveals an intense diffuse infiltrate of neutrophils in the oedematous submucosa spread throughout the involved segment [391]. There is variable spillover of the inflammation into the muscle coat and mucosa. The latter is usually intact but may show focal ulceration or haemorrhage. A Gram stain may demonstrate organisms in the submucosa. Cases have shown Gram-negative rods, Gram-positive rods and rarely Gram-positive cocci. The involved segment is of variable length but the whole small and large intestine is occasionally affected.

Although a variety of organisms have been grown from the blood which include pneumococci, group B β-haemolytic streptococci and *Escherichia coli*, the focus of infection is often not found and the route by which the organism comes to preferentially involve the submucosa is also unknown.

Transient colitis and acute self-limiting colitis

The term 'transient colitis' was coined to delineate a group of patients who suffer a single attack of relatively mild colitis of short duration clinically believed to be infective but with negative stool cultures. The biopsy diagnosis of a single attack of proctitis or proctocolitis, in the absence of positive bacteriology or specific histological features to suggest chronic inflammatory bowel disease, is a frequent problem in pathological practice. The microscopic picture in a biopsy is similar to that of culture-positive infective colitis but does include some with a picture more in favour of Crohn's disease or ulcerative colitis. It also includes biopsies from patients with unexplained spontaneously resolving diarrhoea in which the biopsy, although inflamed, cannot be categorized further. Only a prolonged follow-up period can confidently exclude Crohn's disease or ulcerative colitis. Even so, there are patients who have had single attacks of ulcerative colitis or proctitis. However, it is likely that many such cases in the past may have been genuine infections prior to the recognition of *Salmonella* [32] and *Campylobacter* colitis [41].

The term 'acute self-limiting colitis' is a term favoured in American studies and describes a patient with signs and symptoms of infectious diarrhoea with a corresponding biopsy picture [76]. Both culture-positive and culture-negative cases are included. It is therefore a broader term than transient colitis. Rectal biopsies taken from healthy volunteers in countries with a high background incidence of infective diarrhoea may show increased inflammatory cells in the lamina propria and structural abnormalities at electron microscopy. This tropical colopathy has been compared to similar findings in the small intestine in such areas [594].

Obstructive colitis

The term 'obstructive colitis' denotes the occurrence of inflammation and ulceration proximal to a complete or partial obstruction, usually carcinoma or an inflammatory stricture due to diverticular disease or Crohn's disease. It is usually separated from the site of obstruction by a segment of normal mucosa, often in excess of 10 cm. The condition may closely mimic chronic inflammatory bowel disease, with the diffuse nature of the involvement and predominant mucosal pathology perhaps suggesting ulcerative colitis whilst the focal nature of the disease, with a segment of normal mucosa beyond it, is reminiscent of Crohn's disease [595]. A similar change may be seen in the colonic pseudo-obstruction in Ogilvie's syndrome, a complication of pregnancy, in which the colon becomes grossly dilated, especially the caecum and/or ascending colon, often leading to perforation. Rarely obstructive pathology, with similar macroscopic and microscopic pathology, is seen in the small intestine (see p. 308).

References

1 Nicolas JC, Ingrand D, Fortier B, Bricout F. A one-year virological survey of acute intussusception in childhood. *J Med Virol*, 1982; 9: 267.

2 Francis N. Light and electron microscopic appearances of pathological changes in HIV gut infection. *Baillieres Clin Gastroenterol*, 1990; 4: 495.

3 Blanshard C, Francis N, Gazzard BG. Investigation of chronic diarrhoea in acquired immunodeficiency syndrome. A prospective study of 155 patients. *Gut*, 1996; 39: 824.

4 Foucar E, Mukai K, Sutherland DE, Van Buen CT. Colon ulceration in lethal cytomegalovirus infection. *Am J Clin Pathol*, 1981; 76: 788.

5 Goodman ZD, Boitnott JK, Yardley JH. Perforation of the colon associated with cytomegalovirus infection. *Dig Dis Sci*, 1979; 24: 376.

6 Meisalman MS, Cello JP, Margaretten W. Cytomegalovirus colitis: report of the clinical endoscopic and pathologic findings in two patients with acquired immune deficiency syndrome. *Gastroenterology*, 1985; 88: 171.

7 Frager DH, Frager JD, Wolf EL *et al*. Cytomegalovirus colitis in acquired immune deficiency syndrome: radiologic spectrum. *Gastrointest Radiol*, 1986; 11: 241.

8 Cooper HS, Raffenberger EC, Jones L. Cytomegalovirus inclusions in patients with ulcerative colitis and toxic dilatation requiring colonic resection. *Gastroenterology*, 1977; 72: 1253.

9 Surawicz CM, Myerson D. Self-limited cytomegalovirus in immunocompetent individuals. *Gastroenterology*, 1988; 94: 194.

10 Hunt NAC, Jewell DP, Mortensen NJMcC, Warren BF. Cytomegalovirus infection complicating ulcerative colitis. *CPD Bull Cell Pathol*, 1999; 1: 72.

11 Rompalo AM. Diagnosis and treatment of sexually acquired proctitis and proctocolitis: an update. *Clin Infect Dis*, 1999; 28: S84.

12 Goodell S, Quinn TS, Mkotichian E, Schuffler MD, Holmes KK, Corey L. Herpes simplex virus proctitis in homosexual men. *N Engl J Med*, 1983; 308: 868.

13 Kotter DP, Gaetz HP, Lange M, Klein EB, Holt PR. Enteropathy associated with acquired immunodeficiency syndrome. *Ann Intern Med*, 1984; 101: 421.

14 Nelson JA, Wiley CA, Reynolds-Kohler C, Reese CA, Margaretten W, Levy JA. Human immunodeficiency virus detected in bowel epithelium from patients with gastrointestinal symptoms. *Lancet*, 1988; i: 259.

15 Kotler DP, Weaver SC, Terzakis JA. Ultrastructural features of epithelial cell degeneration in rectal crypts of patients with AIDS. *Am J Surg Pathol*, 1986; 10: 531.

16 Francis N. Infectious complications of HIV disease: a selective review. *Curr Diag Pathol*, 1994; 1: 142.

17 Monk M, Mendeloff AI, Siegel CL, Lilienfeld A. An epidemiological study of ulcerative colitis and regional enteritis among adults in Baltimore—II Social and demographic factors. *Gastroenterology*, 1969; 56: 847.

18 Donoghue-Rolfe A, Keusch GT, Edson, C, Thorley-Lawson, D, Jacewicz, M. Pathogenesis of *Shigella* diarrhoea. *J Exp Med*, 1984; 160: 1767.

19 Speelman P, Kabir I, Islam M. Distribution and spread of colonic lesions in shigellosis. A colonoscopic study. *J Infect Dis*, 1984; 150: 899.

20 McElfatrick RA, Wurtzebach LR. Collar-button ulcers of the colon in a case of shigellosis. *Gastroenterology*, 1973; 65: 303.

21 Takeuchi A, Sprinz H, Labrec EH, Formal SB. Experimental bacillary dysentery. An electron microscopic study of the response of the intestinal mucosa to bacterial invasion. *Am J Pathol*, 1965; 47: 1011.

22 Gonzalez-Licea A, Yardley JH. A comparative ultrastructural study of the mucosa in idiopathic ulcerative colitis, shigellosis and other human colonic diseases. *Bull Johns Hopkins Hosp*, 1966; 118: 444.

23 Rout WR, Formal SB, Giannella RA, Dammin GJ. Pathophysiology of *Shigella* diarrhoea in the Rhesus monkey: intestinal transport, morphological and bacteriological studies. *Gastroenterology*, 1975; 68: 270.

24 Christie AB. Salmonellosis. *Br J Hosp Med*, 1971; 5: 331.

25 Mandal B, Mani V. Colonic involvement in salmonellosis. *Lancet*, 1976; ii: 901.

26 McGovern VJ, Slavutin LJ. Pathology of *Salmonella* colitis. *Am J Surg Pathol*, 1979; 3: 483.

27 Boyd JF. Pathology of the alimentary tract in *Salmonella typhimurium* food poisoning. *Gut*, 1985; 26: 935.
28 Appelbaum PC, Scragg J, Schonland MM. Colonic involvement in salmonellosis. *Lancet*, 1976; ii: 102.
29 Boyd JF. *Salmonella typhimurium*, colitis and pancreatitis. *Lancet*, 1969; ii: 901.
30 Axon ATR, Poole D. Salmonellosis presenting with cholera-like diarrhoea. *Lancet*, 1973; i: 745.
31 Radsel-Medvescek A, Zargi R, Acko M, Zajc–Satler J. Colonic involvement in salmonellosis. *Lancet*, 1977; i: 601.
32 Day DW, Mandal BK, Morson BC. The rectal biopsy appearances in *Salmonella* colitis. *Histopathology*, 1978; 2: 117.
33 Dronfield MW, Fletcher J, Langman MJS. Coincident *Salmonella* infections and ulcerative colitis: problems of recognition and management. *Br Med J*, 1974; i: 99.
34 Mandal BK. Ulcerative colitis and acute *Salmonella* infection. *Br Med J*, 1974; i: 326.
35 Black PH, Kunz LJ, Swartz MN. Salmonellosis—a review of some unusual aspects. *N Engl J Med*, 1960; 262: 864.
36 Stewart GT. Post-dysenteric colitis. *Br Med J*, 1950; i: 405.
37 Powell SJ, Wilmot AJ. Ulcerative post-dysenteric colitis. *Gut*, 1966; 7: 438.
38 Fung WP, Monteiro EH, Ang HB, Kho KM, Lee SK. Ulcerative post-dysenteric colitis. *Am J Gastroenterol*, 1972; 57: 341.
39 Patterson M, Schoppe L. The presentations of amoebiasis. *Med Clin North Am*, 1982; 66 (3): 689.
40 Harries J. Amoebiasis: a review. *J R Soc Med*, 1982; 75: 190.
41 Rettig PJ. *Campylobacter* infections in human beings. *J Paediatr*, 1979; 94: 855.
42 Cadranel S, Rodesch P, Butzler JP, Dekeyser P. Enteritis due to 'related *Vibrio*' in children. *Am J Dis Child*, 1973; 126: 152.
43 Price AB, Jewkes J, Sanderson PJ. Acute diarrhoea. *Campylobacter* colitis and the role of rectal biopsy. *J Clin Pathol*, 1979; 32: 990.
44 Lambert ME, Schofield PF, Ironside AG, Mandal BK. *Campylobacter* colitis. *Br Med J*, 1979; i: 857.
45 Blaiser MJ, Laforce FM, Wilson NA, Wang WLL. Reservoirs for human campylobacteriosis. *J Infect Dis*, 1980; 141: 665.
46 Megraud F, Tachoire C, Latrille J, Bondonny JM. Appendicitis due to *Campylobacter jejuni*. *Br Med J*, 1982; 285: 1165.
47 Loss RW Jr, Mangla JC, Pereira M. *Campylobacter* colitis presenting as inflammatory bowel disease with segmental colonic ulcerations. *Gastroenterology*, 1980; 79: 138.
48 Blaser MJ, Parsons RB, Wang WL. Acute colitis caused by *Campylobacter fetus* spp. *jejuni*. *Gastroenterology*, 1980; 78: 448.
49 Gubina M, Zajc-Satler J, Dragas AZ, Zeleznilc Z, Mehle J. Enterotoxin activity of campylobacter species. In: Newell DG, ed. *Campylobacter: Epidemiology, Pathogenesis and Biochemistry*. Lancaster: MTP Press Ltd, 1982: 188.
50 Firehammer B, Myers LL. Experimental *Campylobacter jejuni* infections in calves and lambs. In: Newell DG, ed. *Campylobacter: Epidemiology, Pathogenesis and Biochemistry*. Lancaster: MTP Press Ltd, 1982: 168.
51 Candy DCA, McNeish AS. Human *Escherichia coli* diarrhoea. *Arch Dis Child*, 1984; 59: 395.
52 Riley LW, Remis RS, Helgerson SD *et al*. Hemorrhagic colitis associated with a rare *Escherichia coli* serotype. *N Engl J Med*, 1983; 308: 681.
53 Pai CH, Gordon R, Sims HV, Bryan LB. Sporadic cases of haemorrhagic colitis associated with *Escherichia coli* 0157:H7. *Ann Intern Med*, 1984; 101: 738.
54 Smith HR, Rowe B, Gross RJ, Fry NK, Scotland SH. Haemorrhagic colitis and verocytoxin-producing *Escherichia coli* in England and Wales. *Lancet*, 1987; i: 1062.
55 Morrison DM, Tyrell DLJ, Jewell LD. Colonic biopsy in verotoxin-induced haemorrhagic colitis and thrombotic thrombocytopenic purpura (TTP). *Am J Clin Pathol*, 1986; 86: 108.
56 Kelly JK, Pai CK, Jadusingh IH, MacInnis ML, Shaffer EA, Hershfield NB. The histopathology of rectosigmoid biopsies from adults with bloody diarrhoea due to verotoxin-producing *Escherichia coli*. *Am J Clin Pathol*, 1987; 88: 78.
57 Richardson SE, Kamali MA, Becker LE, Smith CR. The histopathology of the hemolytic uremic syndrome associated with verotoxin-producing *Escherichia coli* infections. *Hum Pathol*, 1988; 19: 1102.
58 Doyle MP, Schoeni JL. Survival and growth characteristics of *Escherichia coli* associated with hemorrhagic colitis. *Appl Environ Microbiol*, 1984; 48: 855.
59 Tesh VI, O'Brien AD. The pathogenetic mechanisms of Shiga toxin and the Shiga like toxins. *Mol Microbiol*, 1991; 5: 1817.
60 Van Heyningen WE, Gladstone GP. The neurotoxin of *Shigella shigae*. 1. Production, purification and properties of the toxin. *Br J Exp Pathol*, 1953; 34: 202, 221 & 230.
61 Mural TG, Walker PD. The Pigbel story of Papua New Guinea. *Trans R Soc Trop Med Hyg*, 1991; 85: 119.
62 Borriello SP, Larson HE, Welch A, Barclay F, Stringer MF, Bartholomew BA. Enterotoxigenic *Clostridium perfringens*: a possible cause of antibiotic-associated diarrhoea. *Lancet*, 1984; i: 305.
63 Borriello SP. Newly described clostridial diseases of the gastrointestinal tract: *Clostridium perfringens* enterotoxin-associated diarrhoea and neutropenic enterocolitis due to *Clostridium septicum*. In: Borriello SP, ed. *Clostridia in Gastrointestinal Disease*. Boca Raton, Florida: CRC Press Inc, 1985: 223.
64 Farrant JM, Traill Z, Conlon C *et al*. Pigbel-like syndrome in a vegetarian in Oxford. *Gut*, 1996; 39: 336.
65 Kumar NB, Norstrant TT, Appelman HD. The histopathologic spectrum of acute self-limiting colitis (acute infectious-type colitis). *Am J Surg Pathol*, 1982; 6: 523.
66 Talbot IC, Price AB. Infective colitis. In: *Biopsy Pathology of Colorectal Disease*. London: Chapman & Hall, 1987: 81.
67 Surawicz CM. The role of rectal biopsy in infectious colitis. *Am J Surg Pathol*, 1968; 12 (Suppl. 1): 82.
68 Tanaka M, Riddell RH, Saito H, Soma Y, Hidaka H, Kudo H. Morphological criteria applicable to biopsy specimens for effective distinction of inflammatory bowel disease from other forms of colitis and of Crohn's disease from ulcerative colitis. *Scand J Gastroenterol*, 1999; 34: 55.
69 Lessells AM, Beck JS, Burnett RA *et al*. Observer variability in the histopathological reporting of abnormal rectal biopsy specimens. *J Clin Pathol*, 1994; 47: 48.
70 Jenkins D, Goodall A, Scott BB. Simple objective criteria for diagnosis of causes of acute diarrhoea on rectal biopsy. *J Clin Pathol*, 1997; 50: 580.
71 Choudari CP, Mathan M, Rajan DP, Raghavan R, Mathan VI. A correlative study of etiology, clinical features and rectal mucosal pathology in adults with acute infectious diarrhoea in Southern India. *Pathology*, 1985; 17: 443.
72 Allison MC, Hamilton-Dutoit SJ, Dhillon AP, Pounder RE. The value of rectal biopsy in distinguishing self-limiting colitis from early inflammatory bowel disease. *Q J Med*, 1987; 65: 985.
73 Anand BS, Malhotra V, Bhattacharya SK *et al*. Rectal histology in acute bacillary dysentery. *Gastroenterology*, 1986; 90: 654.
74 Surawicz CM, Belie L. Rectal biopsy helps to distinguish acute self-limited colitis from idiopathic inflammatory bowel disease. *Gastroenterology*, 1984; 86: 104.
75 Dickinson RT, Gilmour HM, McClelland DBL. Rectal biopsy in patients presenting to an infectious diseases unit with diarrhoeal disease. *Gut*, 1979; 20: 141.

76 Koplan JP, Fineberg HV, Ferraro MJB, Rosenberg M. Value of stool cultures. *Lancet*, 1980; ii: 413.
77 Harries AD, Myers B, Cook GC. Inflammatory bowel disease: a common cause of bloody diarrhoea in visitors to the tropics. *Br Med J*, 1985; 291: 1686.
78 Mandal BK, Schofield PF, Morson BC. A clinicopathological study of acute colitis: the dilemma of transient colitis syndrome. *Scand J Gastroenterol*, 1982; 17: 865.
79 Willoughby CP, Piris J, Truelove SC. *Campylobacter* colitis. *J Clin Pathol*, 1979; 32: 986.
80 Goodall HB, Sinclair ISR. Colitis cystica profunda. *J Pathol Bacteriol*, 1957; 73: 33.
81 Denton J. The pathology of pellagra. *Am J Trop Med*, 1925; 5: 173.
82 Luvuno FM, Mtshali Z, Baker LW. Toxic dilatation complicating fulminating amoebic colitis. *Br J Surg*, 1982; 69: 56.
83 Anderson JB, Tanner AH, Brodribb AJM. Toxic megacolon due to *Campylobacter* colitis. *Int J Colorectal Dis*, 1986; 1: 58.
84 Ukil AC. Early diagnosis and treatment of intestinal tuberculosis. *Indian Med Gaz*, 1942; 77: 613.
85 Anscombe AR, Keddie NC, Schofield PF. Caecal tuberculosis. *Gut*, 1967; 8: 337.
86 Tandon HD, Prakash A, Rao VB, Prakash O, Nair SK. Ulceroconstrictive disorders of the intestine in Northern India: a pathological study. *Indian J Med Res*, 1966; 54: 129.
87 Gefel A, Pruzanski W, Altman R. The clinical picture and rare variants of primary gastro-intestinal tuberculosis. *Gastroenterol Basel*, 1963; 99: 359.
88 Hamandi WJ, Thamer MA. Tuberculosis of the bowel in Iraq. A study of 86 cases. *Dis Colon Rectum*, 1965; 8: 158.
89 Dinner M. Tuberculosis of the gastrointestinal tract in the non-white population of the Transvaal. *S Afr J Surg*, 1965; 3: 97.
90 Schuurmans-Stekhoven JHA. Tuberculous enterocolitis. *S Afr Med J*, 1965; 39: 1199.
91 Hawley PR, Wolfe HRI, Fullerton JM. Hypertrophic tuberculosis of the rectum. *Gut*, 1968; 9: 461.
92 Walker-Davis J. Hyperplastic tuberculosis of the rectum. *Am J Surg*, 1957; 93: 490.
93 Rhoades ER, Klein LJ, Welsh JD. A case of probable tuberculosis of the distal colon. *Gastroenterology*, 1960; 38: 654.
94 Need RL, Behnke RH. Tuberculous ulcers of the distal colon. *Am Rev Resp Dis*, 1963; 88: 69.
95 Chaudary A, Gupta MS. Colorectal tuberculosis. *Dis Colon Rectum*, 1986; 29: 738.
96 Klimach OE, Ormerod LP. Gastrointestinal tuberculosis: a retrospective review of 109 cases in a District General Hospital. *Q J Med*, 1985; 56: 569.
97 Kwiniemi H, Ristkari S, Ramo J. Tuberculosis of the large bowel. *Acta Chir Scand*, 1984; 150: 345.
98 Ehsannulah M, Isaacs A, Filipe MI, Gazzard BG. Tuberculosis presenting as inflammatory bowel disease. *Dis Colon Rectum*, 1984; 27: 134.
99 Franklin G, Mohapatra M, Perillo RP. Colonic tuberculosis diagnosed by colonoscopic biopsy. *Gastroenterology*, 1979; 76: 362.
100 Koo J, Ho J, Ong GB. The value of colonoscopy in the diagnosis of ileocaecal tuberculosis. *Endoscopy*, 1982; 14: 48.
101 Radhakrishnan S, Nakib BA, Sheikh H, Menon N. The value of colonoscopy in schistosomal, tuberculous and amoebic colitis. *Dis Colon Rectum*, 1986; 29: 891.
102 Snyder JD, Christenson E, Feldman RA. Human *Yersinia enterocolitica* infection in Wisconsin. *Am J Med*, 1982; 72: 768.
103 Weir WRC. *Yersinia* infection. *Curr Opin Gastroenterol*, 1985; 1: 135.
104 Editorial. Yersiniosis today. *Lancet*, 1984; i: 84.
105 Vantrappen G, Agg HO, Ponette E, Geboes K, Bertrand PH. *Yersinia* enteritis and enterocolitis: gastroenterological aspects. *Gastroenterology*, 1977; 72: 220.
106 Corer TL, Aber RC. *Yersinia enterocolitica*. *N Engl J Med* 1989; 321: 16.
107 Leino R, Granfors K, Havia T, Heinonen R, Lampinen M, Towanen A. Yersiniosis as a gastrointestinal disease. *Scand J Infect Dis*, 1987; 19: 63.
108 Rabinovitz M, Stremple JF, Wells KE, Store BG. *Yersinia enterocolitica* infection complicated by intestinal perforation. *Arch Intern Med*, 1987; 147: 1662.
109 Simmonds SD, Noble MA, Freeman HJ. Gastrointestinal features of culture-positive *Yersinia enterocolitica* infection. *Gastroenterology*, 1987; 92: 112.
110 Rutgeerts P, Geboes K, Ponette E, Coremans G, Vantrappen G. Acute infective colitis caused by endemic pathogens in Western Europe: endoscopic features. *Endoscopy*, 1982; 14: 212.
111 O'Loughlin EV, Humphreys G, Dunn I *et al*. Clinical, morphological and biochemical alterations in acute intestinal yersiniosis. *Pediatr Res*, 1986; 20: 602.
112 Hawe P. Fibrous stricture of the rectum due to lymphogranuloma venereum. *Proc R Soc Med*, 1951; 44: 426.
113 Kazal HL, Sohn N, Carrasco JI, Robilotti JG, Delanev WE. The gay bowel syndrome: clinicopathologic correlation in 260 cases. *Ann Clin Lab Sci*, 1976; 6: 184.
114 Weller IVD. The gay bowel. *Gut*, 1985; 26: 869.
115 Greenfield C, Ramirez JRA, Pounder RE *et al*. *Clostridium difficile* and inflammatory bowel disease. *Gut*, 1983; 24: 713.
116 Nicol CS. Some aspects of gonorrhoea in the female with special reference to infection of the rectum. *Br J Ven Dis*, 1948; 24: 26.
117 Kilpatrick ZM. Gonorrhoeal proctitis. *N Engl J Med*, 1972; 287: 967.
118 McMillan A, Gilmour HM, Slatford K, McNeillage GJC. Proctitis in homosexual men. *Br J Ven Dis*, 1983; 59: 260.
119 Klein EJ, Fisher LS, Chow AW. Anorectal gonococcal infection. *Ann Intern Med*, 1977; 86: 340.
120 McMillan A, McNeillage GJC, Gilmour HM, Lee FD. Histology of rectal gonorrhoea in men, with a note on anorectal infection with *Neisseria meningitidis*. *J Clin Pathol*, 1983; 36: 511.
121 Wells BT, Kierland RR, Jackman RJ. Rectal chancre. Report of a case. *Am Med Assoc Arch Derm*, 1959; 79: 719.
122 Marino AWM. Proctologic lesions observed in male homosexuals. *Dis Colon Rectum*, 1964; 7: 121.
123 Smith D. Infectious syphilis of the rectum. Report of a case. *Dis Colon Rectum*, 1965; 8: 57.
124 Quinn TC, Lukehart SA, Goodell S, Mkrtrichiam E, Shuffler MD, Holmes KC. Rectal mass caused by *Treponema pallidum*: confirmation by immunofluorescent staining. *Gastroenterology*, 1982; 82: 135.
125 McMillan A, Lee FD. Sigmoidoscopic and microscopic appearance of the rectal mucosa in homosexual men. *Gut*, 1981; 22: 1035.
126 Saad EA, de Gouveia OF, Filho PD, Teixeira D, Pereira AA, Erthal A. Ano-rectal-colonic lymphogranuloma venereum. *Gastroenterol Basel*, 1962; 97: 89.
127 Klotz SA, Drutz DJ, Tam MR, Reed KH. Hemorrhagic proctitis due to lymphogranuloma venereum serogroup LZ. Diagnosis by fluorescent monoclonal antibody. *N Engl J Med*, 1983; 308: 1563.
128 Annamunthodo H. Rectal lymphogranuloma venereum in Jamaica. *Ann R Coll Surg*, 1961; 29: 141.
129 Annamunthodo H, Marryatt J. Barium studies in intestinal lymphogranuloma venereum. *Br J Radiol*, 1961; 34: 53.
130 de la Monte S, Hutchins GM. Follicular proctitis and neuromatous hyperplasia with lymphogranuloma venereum. *Hum Pathol*, 1985; 16: 1025.

131 Miles RPM. Rectal lymphogranuloma venereum. *Br J Surg*, 1957; 45: 180.

132 Schuller JL, Picket-van Ulsen J, Veeken IVD, Michel MF, Stolz E. Antibodies against chlamydia of lymphogranuloma-venereum type in Crohn's disease. *Lancet*, 1979; i: 19.

133 Swarbrick ET, Price HL, Kingham JGC, Blackshaw AJ, Griffiths PD. Chlamydia, cytomegalovirus and yersinia in inflammatory bowel disease. *Lancet*, 1979; 2: 11.

134 Levin I, Romano S, Steinberg M, Welsh RA. Lymphogranuloma venereum: rectal stricture and carcinoma. *Dis Colon Rectum*, 1964; 7: 129.

135 Morson BC. Anorectal venereal disease. *Proc R Soc Med*, 1964; 57: 179.

136 Quinn TC, Goodell SE, Mkrtrichian E *et al*. *Chlamydia trachomatis* proctitis. *N Engl J Med*, 1981; 305: 195.

137 Munday PE, Dawson SG, Johnson AP *et al*. A microbiological study of non-gonococcal proctitis in passive male homosexuals. *Postgrad Med J*, 1981; 57: 705.

138 Nielsen RH, Orholm M, Pedersen JO, Hovind-Hougen K, Teglbjaerg PS, Thaysen EH. Colorectal spirochaetosis: clinical significance of the infestation. *Gastroenterology*, 1983; 85: 62.

139 Nielsen RH, Lundbeck FA, Teglbjaerg PS, Ginnerup P, Hoving-Hougen K. Intestinal spirochaetosis of the vermiform appendix. *Gastroenterology*, 1985; 88: 971.

140 Lee FD, Kraszewski A, Gordon J, Howie JGR, McSeveney D, Harland N. Intestinal spirochaetosis. *Gut*, 1971; 12: 126.

141 Conew LA, Woodard DR, Potts BE, Byrd RG, Alexander RM, Last MD. An update on the acquired immunodeficiency syndrome (AIDS). *Dis Colon Rectum*, 1986; 29: 60.

142 Hovind-Hougen K, Birch-Anderson A, Nielson RH *et al*. Intestinal spirochaetosis: morphological characterisation and cultivation of *Brachyspira aalbergi*, gen., nov. sp. nov. *J Clin Microbiol*, 1982; 16: 1127.

143 Tompkins DS, Foulkes SJ, Godwin PGR, West AP. Isolation and characterisation of intestinal spirochaetes. *J Clin Pathol*, 1986; 39: 535.

144 Antonalcopoulas G, Newman J, Wilkinson M. Intestinal spirochaetosis: an electron microscopic study in an unusual case. *Histopathology*, 1982; 6: 477.

145 Gebbers J-O, Ferguson DJP, Mason C, Kelly P, Jewell DP. Spirochaetosis of the human rectum associated with an intraepithelial mast cell and IgE plasma cell response. *Gut*, 1987; 28: 588.

146 Douglas JG, Crucioli V. Spirochaetosis: a remediable cause of diarrhoea and rectal bleeding? *Br Med J*, 1981; 283: 1362.

147 Mahant TS, Kohli PK, Mathur RJM, Bhushurmath SR, Wig JD, Kaushik SP. Actinomycosis caecum. *Digestion*, 1983; 27: 53.

148 James AW, Phelps AH. Actinomycosis of the colon. *Can J Surg*, 1977; 20: 150.

149 MacHaffie RA, Zaayer RL, Saichek H, Sciortino AL. Unusual case of actinomycosis manifested as abdominal wall abscess. *Gastroenterology*, 1957; 33: 830.

150 Morson BC. Primary actinomycosis of the rectum. *Proc R Soc Med*, 1961; 54: 723.

151 Miller AG. Actinomycosis of the colon: case report. *Dis Colon Rectum*, 1964; 7: 207.

152 Klaaberg KE, Kronborg O, Olsen H. Enterocutaneous fistulisation due to actimycosis odontolyticus. *Dis Colon Rectum*, 1985; 28: 526.

153 Whitaker BL. Actinomycetes in biopsy material obtained from suture line granulomata following resection of the rectum. *Br J Surg*, 1964; 51: 445.

154 Asuncion CM, Cinti DC, Hawkins HB. Abdominal manifestations of actinomycosis in IUD users. *J Clin Gastroenterol*, 1984; 6: 343.

155 de Foe E. Mucormycosis of the colon. *Am J Roentgenol*, 1961; 86: 86.

156 Unat EK, Pars B, Kosyak JP. A case of cryptococcosis of the colon. *Br Med J*, 1960; ii: 1501.

157 Alberti-Flor JJ, Granda A. Ileocaecal histoplasmosis mimicking Crohn's disease in a patient with Job's syndrome. *Digestion*, 1986; 33: 176.

158 Lee SH, Barnes WG, Hodges GR, Dixon A. Perforated granulomatous colitis caused by *Histoplasma capsulatum*. *Dis Colon Rectum*, 1985; 28: 171.

159 Capell MS, Mandell W, Grimes MM, Neu HC. Gastrointestinal histoplasmosis. *Dig Dis Sci*, 1988; 33: 353.

160 Goldmeier D, Sargeaunt PG, Price AB *et al*. Is *Entamoeba histolytica* in homosexual men a pathogen? *Lancet*, 1986; i: 641a.

161 Morton TC, Neale RA, Sage M. Indigenous amoebiasis in Britain. *Lancet*, 1951; i: 766.

162 McAllister TA. Diagnosis of amoebic colitis on routine biopsies from the rectum and sigmoid colon. *Br Med J*, 1962; i: 362.

163 Tucker PC, Webster PD, Kilpatrick ZM. Amoebic colitis mistaken for inflammatory bowel disease. *Arch Intern Med*, 1975; 135: 681.

164 Berkovitz D, Bernstein LH. Colonic pseudopolyps in association with amoebic colitis. *Gastroenterology*, 1975; 68: 786.

165 McMillan A, Gilmour HM, McNeillage GJC, Scott GR. Amoebiasis in homosexual men. *Gut*, 1984; 25: 356.

166 Editorial. Is that amoeba harmful or not? *Lancet*, 1985; i: 732.

167 Sargeaunt PG, Williams JE, Green JD. The differentiation of invasive and non-invasive *Entamoeba histolytica* by isoenzyme electrophoresis. *Trans R Soc Trop Med Hyg*, 1978; 72: 519.

168 Nanda R, Baveja U, Anand BS. *Entamoeba histolytica* cyst passers: clinical features and outcome in untreated subjects. *Lancet*, 1984; ii: 301.

169 Alvarez-Fuertez G, Pelaez M, Velasco AG. Paraffin inclusion of rectal mucus for diagnosis of amoebiasis. Preliminary results. *Dis Colon Rectum*, 1963; 6: 172.

170 Prathap IC, Gilman R. The histopathology of acute intestinal amoebiasis. *Am J Pathol*, 1970; 60: 229.

171 Hulman G, Taylor LA. PAS/Martius yellow technique for demonstrating *Entamoeba histolytica*. *J Med Lab Sci*, 1987; 44: 396.

172 Hadley GP, Mickel RE. Fulminating amoebic colitis in infants and children. *J R Coll Surg Edinb*, 1984; 29: 370.

173 Adams EB, MacLeod IN. Invasive amoebiasis: 1. Amoebic dysentery and its complications. *Medicine*, 1977; 56: 325.

174 Pittman FE, Hennigar GR. Sigmoidoscopic and colonic mucosal biopsy finding in amoebic colitis. *Arch Pathol*, 1974; 97: 155.

175 Cade D, Webster GD. Amoebic perforation of the intestine in children. *Br J Surg*, 1974; 61: 159.

176 Perlmann P, Hammarstrom S, Lagercrantz R, Campbell D. Autoantibodies to colon in rat and human ulcerative colitis: cross reactivity with *Escherichia coli* 0:14 antigen. *Proc Soc Exp Biol Med*, 1967; 125: 975.

177 Rappaport EM, Rossein AX, Rosenblum LA. Arthritis due to intestinal amoebiasis. *Ann Intern Med*, 1951; 34: 1224.

178 Rominger JM, Shah AN. Ameboma of the rectum. *Gastrointest Endosc*, 1979; 25: 71.

179 Gabriel WB. A case of amoebic ulceration of the rectum and anus. *Proc R Soc Med*, 1939; 32: 902.

180 Casemore DP, Sands RL, Curry A. Cryptosporidium species a 'new' human pathogen. *J Clin Pathol*, 1985; 38: 1321.

181 Current WL, Reese NC, Ernst JV, Bailey WS, Heyman MB, Weinstein WM. Human cryptosporidiosis in immunocompe-

tent and immunodeficient persons. Studies of an outbreak and experimental transmission. *N Engl J Med*, 1983; 308: 1252.
182 Soave R, Danner RL, Honig CL *et al*. Cryptosporidiosis in homosexual men. *Ann Intern Med*, 1984; 100: 504.
183 Fletcher A, Sims TA, Talbot IC. Cryptosporidial enteritis without general or selective immune deficiency. *Br Med J*, 1982; 285: 22.
184 Jokipii L, Polyola S, Jokipii AMM. Cryptosporidium: a frequent finding in patients with gastrointestinal symptoms. *Lancet*, 1983; ii: 358.
185 Cook GC. Opportunistic parasitic infections associated with the acquired immune deficiency syndrome (AIDS): parasitology, clinical presentation, diagnosis and management. *Q J Med*, 1987; 65: 967.
186 Dworkin B, Wormser GP, Rosenthal WS *et al*. Gastrointestinal manifestations of the acquired immunodeficiency syndrome: a review of 22 cases. *Am J Gastroenterol*, 1985; 80: 774.
187 Modigliani R, Bories C, Le Charpentier Y *et al*. Diarrhoea and malabsorption in acquired immunodeficiency syndrome: a study of four cases with special emphasis on opportunistic protozoal infestations. *Gut*, 1985; 26: 179.
188 De Hovitz JA, Pape JW, Boncy M, Johnson WD. Clinical manifestations and therapy of *Isospora belli* infection in patients with the acquired immunodeficiency syndrome. *N Engl J Med*, 1986; 315: 87.
189 McCarey AG. Balantidiasis in South Persia. *Br Med J*, 1952; i: 629.
190 Baskerville L, Ahmed Y, Ramchand S. Balantidium colitis: report of a case. *Am J Dig Dis*, 1970; 15: 727.
191 Prata A. *Schistosomiasis mansoni*. *Clin Gastroenterol*, 1978; 7 (1): 49.
192 Warren KS. *Schistosomiasis japonica*. *Clin Gastroenterol*, 1978; 7 (1): 77.
193 Azar JE, Schraibman IG, Pitchford RJ. Some observations on *Schistosoma haematobium* in the human rectum and sigmoid. *Trans R Soc Trop Med Hyg*, 1958; 52: 562.
194 Gelfand M, Hammar B. Acute intestinal obstruction from a granuloma due to *Schistosoma haematobium* in the large intestine. *Trans R Soc Trop Med Hyg*, 1966; 60: 231.
195 Kruatrachue M, Bhaibulaya MN, Harinasuta C. Evaluation of rectal biopsy as a diagnostic method in *Schistosoma japonicum* in man in Thailand. *Ann Trop Medical Parasitol*, 1964; 58: 276.
196 Ming-Chai C, Jen-Chun H, Pei Yu C *et al*. Pathogenesis of carcinoma of the colon and rectum in *Schistosomiasis japonica*. A study of 90 cases. *Chin Med*, 1965; 184: 513.
197 Ming-Chaff C, Pei YuC, Chi-Yuan C *et al*. Colorectal cancer in schistosomiasis. *Lancet*, 1981; i: 971.
198 Davison AM, Dixon MF. The appendix as a 'skip lesion' in ulcerative colitis. *Histopathology*, 1990; 16: 93.
199 Hewavisenthi SJ, Deen KI. An appendiceal skip lesion in ulcerative colitis. *Ceylon Med J*, 1998; 43: 244.
200 Groisman GM, George J, Harpaz N. Ulcerative appendicitis in universal and non universal ulcerative colitis. *Mod Pathol*, 1994; 7: 322.
201 Cohen T, Pfeffer RB, Valensi Q. 'Ulcerative appendicitis' occurring as a skip lesion in chronic ulcerative colitis; report of a case. *Am J Gastroenterol*, 1974; 62: 151.
202 Channer JL, Smith JHF. 'Skip' lesions in ulcerative colitis. *Histopathology*, 1990; 17: 286.
203 Yang SSK, Jung HY, Kang GH *et al*. Appendiceal orifice inflammation as a skip lesion in ulcerative colitis: an analysis in relation to medical therapy and disease extent. *Gastrointest Endosc*, 1999; 49: 743.
204 D'Haens G, Geboes K, Peeters M, Baert F, Ectors N, Rutgeerts P. Patchy caecal inflammation associated with distal ulcerative colitis: a prospective endoscopic study. *Am J Gastroenterol*, 1997; 92: 1275.
205 Levine TS, Tzardi M, Mitchell S, Sowter C, Price AB. Diagnostic difficulty arising from rectal recovery in ulcerative colitis. *J Clin Pathol*, 1997; 50: 354.
206 Tanaka M, Riddell RH. The pathological diagnosis and differential diagnosis of Crohn's disease. *Hepatogastroenterology*, 1990; 37: 18.
207 Kleer CG, Appelman HD. Ulcerative colitis: patterns of involvement in colorectal biopsies and changes with time. *Am J Surg Pathol*, 1998; 22: 983.
208 Kim B, Barnett JL, Kleer CG Appelman HD. Endoscopic and histological patchiness in treated ulcerative colitis. *Am J Gastroenterol*, 1999; 94: 3258.
209 Coll I, Stevenson DL. Case of infantile ulcerative colitis. *Br Med J*, 1958; ii: 952.
210 Mir-Madjlessi SH, Michener WM, Farmer RG. Course and prognosis of idiopathic ulcerative proctosigmoiditis in young patients. *J Pediatr Gastroenterol Nutr*, 1986; 5: 570.
211 Brocklehurst JC. Colonic disease in the elderly. *Clin Gastroenterol*, 1985; 14 (4): 725.
212 Mayberry JF. Some aspects of the epidemiology of ulcerative colitis. *Gut*, 1985; 26: 968.
213 Binder V, Both H, Hansen PK, Hendriksen C, Kreiner S, Torp-Pederson K. Incidence and prevalence of ulcerative colitis and Crohn's disease in the County of Copenhagen, 1962–1978. *Gastroenterology*, 1982; 83: 563.
214 Calkins BM, Lilienfeld AM, Garland C, Mendeloff AI. 1984; Trends in incidence rates of ulcerative colitis and Crohn's disease. *Dig Dis Sci*, 29: 913.
215 Kirsner JB, Shorter RG. Recent developments in non-specific inflammatory bowel disease. *N Engl J Med*, 1982; 306: 837.
216 Hermon-Taylor J. Protagonist. *Mycobacterium avium* subspecies *paratuberculosis* is a cause of Crohn's disease. *Gut*, 2001; 49: 755.
217 White SA, Nassau E, Burnham R, Stanford JL, Lennard-Jones JE. Further evidence for a mycobacterial aetiology of Crohn's disease. *Gut*, 1978; 19: A443.
218 Montgomery SM, Morris DL, Pounder RE, Wakefield AJ. Measles vaccination and inflammatory bowel disease. *Lancet*, 1997; 350; 1774.
219 Mayberry JF, Rhodes J, Newcombe JG. Familial prevalence of inflammatory bowel disease in relatives of patients with Crohn's disease. *Br Med J*, 1980; 280: 84.
220 McConnell RB. Genetic factors. In: Brooke BN, Wilkinson AW, eds. *Inflammatory Disease of the Bowel*. London: Pitman Medical, 1980: 8.
221 Lewkonia RM, McConnell RB. Familial inflammatory bowel disease: hereditary or environment. *Gut*, 1976; 17: 235.
222 Satsangi J, Rosenberg WMC, Jewell DP. The prevalence of inflammatory bowel disease in relatives of patients with Crohn's disease. *Eur J Gastroenterol Hepatol*, 1994; 6: 413.
223 Biemond I, Burnham WR, Amaro JD, Langman MJS. HLA-A and -B antigens in inflammatory bowel disease. *Gut*, 1986; 27: 934.
224 Parkes M, Satsangi J. Genetic factors. In: Jewell DP, Mortensen NJMcC, Warren BF, eds. *Challenges in Inflammatory Bowel Disease*. Oxford: Blackwell Science, 2001.
225 Zimmerman J, Gavish D, Rachmilewitz D. Early and late onset ulcerative colitis: distinct clinical features. *J Clin Gastroenterol*, 1985; 7: 492.
226 Kirsner JB. Genetic aspects of inflammatory bowel disease. *Clin Gastroenterol*, 1973; 2: 557.
227 Probert CSJ, Jayanthi V, Hughes AO *et al*. Prevalence and family

risk of ulcerative colitis and Crohn's disease: an epidemiological study among Europeans and South Asians in Leicestershire. *Gut*, 1993; 34: 1547.

228 Hertervig E, Wieslander J, Johansson C *et al*. Anti-neutrophil cytoplasmic antibodies in chronic inflammatory bowel disease. *Scand J Gastroenterol*, 1995; 30: 693.

229 Duerr RH, Targan SR, Landers CJ *et al*. Anti-neutrophil cytoplasmic antibodies in ulcerative colitis: comparison with other colitides/diarrhoeal illnesses. *Gastroenterology*, 1992; 100: 1590.

230 Hugot JP, Chamaillard M, Zouali H *et al*. Association of Nod 2 leucine rich repeat variants with susceptibility to Crohn's disease. *Nature*, 2001; 411: 599.

231 Ogura Y, Bonen D, Inohara N *et al*. A frameshift mutation in Nod 2 associated with susceptibility to Crohn's disease. *Nature*, 2001; 411: 603.

232 McGovern DP, Van Heel DA, Ahmad T, Jewell DP. *NOD 2* (*CARD 15*), the first susceptibility gene for Crohn's disease. *Gut*, 2001; 49: 752.

233 Toffler RB, Pingould EG, Burrell MI. Acute colitis related to penicillin and penicillin derivatives. *Lancet*, 1978; ii: 707.

234 Jewell DP, Mortensen NJ, Warren BF, eds. *Challenges in Inflammatory Bowel Disease*. Oxford: Blackwell Science, 2001.

235 Beeken WL. Transmissible agents in inflammatory bowel disease. *Med Clin North Am*, 1980; 64 (6): 1021.

236 Cave D, Kirsner JB, McClaren L *et al*. Infectious agents in inflammatory bowel disease (IBD), a status report. *Gastroenterology*, 1980; 78: 1185.

237 Thayer WR Jr, Brown M, Sangree MH, Katz J, Hersh T. *Escherichia coli* 0:14 and colon hemagglutinating antibodies in inflammatory bowel disease. *Gastroenterology*, 1969; 57: 311.

238 Carlsson HE, Lagercrantz R, Perlmann P. Immunological studies in ulcerative colitis. VIII. Antibodies to colon antigens in patients with ulcerative colitis, Crohn's disease and other diseases. *Scand J Gastroenterol*, 1977; 12: 707.

239 Hodgson HJF, Potter BJ, Jewell DP. Immune complexes in ulcerative colitis and Crohn's disease. *Clin Exp Immunol*, 1977; 29: 187.

240 Potter BJ, Brown DJC, Watson A, Jewell DP. Complement inhibitors and immunoconglutinins in ulcerative colitis and Crohn's disease. *Gut*, 1980; 21: 1030.

241 Lagercrantz R, Perlmann P, Hammarstrom S. Immunological studies in ulcerative colitis. V. Family studies. *Gastroenterology*, 1971; 60: 381.

242 Perlmann P, Hammarstrom S, Lagercrantz R. Immunological features of idiopathic ulcerative colitis and Crohn's disease. *Gastroenterology*, 1973; 5: 17.

243 Asherson GL, Holborrow PJ. Auto-antibody production in rabbits. VII. Auto-antibodies to gut by the injection of bacteria. *Immunology*, 1966; 10: 16.

244 Brown WR, Lee E. Radioimmunological measurements of bacterial antibodies 11. Human serum antibodies reactive with *Bacteroides fragilis* and *Enterococcus* in gastrointestinal and immunological disorders. *Gastroenterology*, 1974; 66: 145.

245 Tabaqchali S, O'Donoghue DP, Bettelheim KA. *Escherichia coli* antibodies in patients with inflammatory bowel disease. *Gut*, 1978; 19: 108.

246 Gorbach SL, Nahas L, Plaut AG, Weinstein L, Patterson JF, Levitan R. Studies of intestinal microflora. V. Fecal microbial ecology in ulcerative colitis and regional enteritis: relationship to severity of disease and chemotherapy. *Gastroenterology*, 1968; 54: 575.

247 Keighley MRB, Arabi Y, Dimock F, Burdon DW, Allan RN, Alexander-Williams J. Influence of inflammatory bowel disease on intestinal microflora. *Gut*, 1978; 19: 1099.

248 Dickinson RJ, Varian SA, Axon ATR, Cooke EM. Increased incidence of faecal coliforms with *in vitro* adhesive and invasive properties in patients with ulcerative colitis. *Gut*, 1980; 21: 787.

249 Belsham MR, Darwish R, Watson WC, Sullivan SN. Bacterial L forms in inflammatory bowel disease. *Gastroenterology*, 1980; 78: 1139.

250 Gitnick GL, Rosen VJ, Arthur MH, Hertweck SA. Evidence for the isolation of a new virus from ulcerative colitis patients. Comparison with virus derived from Crohn's disease. *Dig Dis Sci*, 1979; 24: 609.

251 Yoshimura HH, Estes MK, Graham DY. Search for evidence of a viral aetiology for inflammatory bowel disease. *Gut*, 1984; 25: 347.

252 McLaren LC, Gitnick G. Ulcerative colitis and Crohn's disease tissue cytotoxins. *Gastroenterology*, 1982; 82: 1381.

253 Cave DR, Mitchell DN, Brooke BN. Evidence of agent transmissible from ulcerative colitis tissue. *Lancet*, 1976; i: 1311.

254 Cave D. Aetiology: transmissable agents. In: Allan RN, Keighley MRB, Alexander-Williams J, Hawkins C, eds. *Inflammatory Bowel Disease*. Edinburgh: Churchill Livingstone, 1983: 343.

255 Thayer WR. Executive summary of the AGA-NFIC sponsored workshop on infectious agents in inflammatory bowel disease. *Dig Dis Sci*, 1979; 24: 781.

256 Podolsky D, Isselbacher KJ. Glycoprotein composition of colonic mucosa. Specific alteration in ulcerative colitis. *Gastroenterology*, 1984; 87: 991.

257 Ehsanullah M, Filipe MI, Gazzard B. Mucin secretion in inflammatory bowel disease: correlation with disease activity and dysplasia. *Gut*, 1982; 23: 485.

258 Rhodes JM, Black RR, Gallimore R, Savage A. Histochemical demonstration of desialation and desulphation of normal and inflammatory bowel disease rectal mucus by faecal extracts. *Gut*, 1985; 26: 1312.

259 Logan RFA, Edmond M, Somerville KW, Langman MJS. Smoking and ulcerative colitis. *Br Med J*, 1984; 288: 751.

260 Vessey M, Jewell D, Smith A, Yeates D, McPherson K. Chronic inflammatory bowel disease, cigarette smoking, and use of oral contraceptives: findings in a large cohort of women of childbearing age. *Br Med J*, 1986; 292: 1101.

261 Cope GF, Heatley RV, Kelleher J. Smoking and colonic mucus in ulcerative colitis. *Br Med J*, 1986; 293: 481.

262 Cahill RJ, Foltz CJ, Fox JG *et al*. Inflammatory bowel disease: an immunity-mediated condition triggered by bacterial infection with *Helicobacter hepaticus*. *Infect Immun*, 1997; 65: 3126.

263 Sellon RK, Tonkonogy S, Schultz M *et al*. Resident enteric bacteria are necessary for development of spontaneous colitis and immune system activation in interleukin 10 deficient mice. *Infect Immun*, 1998; 66: 5224.

264 El-Omar E, Penman I, Cruickshank G *et al*. Low prevalence of *Helicobacter pylori* in inflammatory bowel disease: association with sulfasalazine. *Gut*, 1994; 35: 1385.

265 Sousa LS, Santos AM, Macedo TC *et al*. Prevalence of *Helicobacter pylori* infection in inflammatory bowel disease—a controlled study. *Gut* 1996; 39: A238.

266 Ekbom A, Zack M, Adami HO. Perinatal measles infection and subsequent Crohn's disease. *Lancet*, 1994; 344: 508.

267 Ekbom A, Dasak P, Kraaz W, Wakefield AJ. Crohn's disease after in-utero measles exposure. *Lancet*, 1996; 348: 515.

268 Thompson NP, Montgomery SM, Pounder RE, Wakefield AJ. Is measles vaccination a risk factor for inflammatory bowel disease? *Lancet*, 1995; 345: 1071.

269 Metcalf J. Is measles infection associated with Crohn's disease? *Br Med J*, 1998; 316: 166.

270 Iizuka M, Chiba M, Yukawa M *et al*. Immunohistochemical

analysis of the distribution of measles related antigen in the intestinal mucosa in inflammatory bowel disease. *Gut*, 2000; 46: 163.

271 Sanderson JD, Moss MT, Tizard MIV, Hermon-Taylor J. *Mycobacterium paratuberculosis* DNA in Crohn's disease tissue. *Gut*, 1992; 33: 890.

272 James SP. Remission of Crohn's disease after human immunodeficiency virus infection. *Gastroenterology*, 1988; 95: 1667.

273 Jewell DP, Rhodes JM. Immunology of ulcerative colitis. In: Allen RN, Keighley MRB, Alexander-Williams J, Hawkins C, eds. *Inflammatory Bowel Disease*. Edinburgh: Churchill Livingstone, 1983: 155.

274 Truelove SC. Ulcerative colitis produced by milk. *Br Med J*, 1961; i: 154.

275 Jewell DP, Truelove SC. Circulating antibodies to cow's milk proteins in ulcerative colitis. *Gut*, 1972; 13: 796.

276 Auer IO, Roder A, Frohlich J. Immune status in Crohn's disease. VI. Immunoregulation elevated by multiple, distinct T-suppressor cell assay of lymphocyte proliferation, and by enumeration of immunoregulatory T-lymphocyte subsets. *Gastroenterology*, 1984; 86: 1531.

277 Shorter RG, Cardoza MR, Spencer RJ, Huizenga KA. Further studies of *in vitro* cytotoxicity of lymphocytes for colonic epithelial cells. *Gastroenterology*, 1969; 57: 30.

278 Shorter RG, Cardoza MR, Remine SG, Spencer RJ, Huizenga KA. Modification of *in vitro* cytotoxicity of lymphocytes from patients with chronic ulcerative colitis or granulomatous colitis for allogeneic epithelial cells. *Gastroenterology*, 1970; 58: 692.

279 Shorter RG, McGill DB, Bahn RC. Cytotoxicity of mononuclear cells for autologous colonic epithelial cells in colonic disease. *Gastroenterology*, 1984; 86: 13.

280 Selby WS, Janossy G, Bofill M, Jewell DP. Intestinal lymphocyte subpopulations in inflammatory bowel disease—an analysis by immunohistological and cell isolation techniques. *Gut*, 1984; 25: 32.

281 Wilders MM, Drexhage HA, Kolye M, Verspaget HW, Meuwissen SGM. Veiled cells in chronic idiopathic inflammatory bowel disease. *Clin Exp Immunol*, 1984; 55: 377.

282 Sharon P, Stenson WF. Enhanced synthesis of leukotriene B4 by colonic mucosa in inflammatory bowel disease. *Gastroenterology*, 1984; 86: 453.

283 van Spreeuwal JP, Meyer CJLM, Rosekrans PCM, Lindeman J. Immunoglobulin-containing cells in gastrointestinal pathology—diagnostic applications. In: Sommers SC, Rosen RP, Fechner RE, eds. *Pathology Annual*. Connecticut: Appleton-Century Crofts, 1986: 295.

284 Lloyd G, Green FW, Fox H, Mani V, Turnberg L. Mast cells and inununoglobulin E in inflammatory bowel disease. *Gut*, 1975; 16: 861.

285 O'Donoghue DP, Kumar P. Rectal IgE in inflammatory bowel disease. *Gut*, 1979; 20: 149.

286 Rosekrans PCM, Meijer CJLM, Van Der Wal AM, Lindeman J. Allergic proctitis, a clinical and immunopathological entity. *Gut*, 1980; 21: 1017.

287 MacPherson B, Pfeiffer CJ. Experimental colitis. *Digestion*, 1976; 14: 424.

288 Hodgson HJF, Potter BJ, Skinner J, Jewell DP. Immune complex-mediated colitis in rabbits. An experimental model. *Gut*, 1978; 19: 225.

289 Mee AS, McLaughlin JE, Hodgson HJF, Jewell DP. Chronic immune colitis in rabbits. *Gut*, 1979; 20: 1.

290 Rabin BS, Roger SJ. A cell mediated immune model of inflammatory bowel disease in the rabbit. *Gastroenterology*, 1978; 75: 29.

291 Watt J, Marcus R. Carrageenan-induced ulceration of the large intestine in the guinea pig. *Gut*, 1971; 12: 164.

292 Onderdonk AB, Bartlett JG. Bacterial studies of experimental ulcerative colitis. *Am J Clin Nutr*, 1979; 32: 258.

293 Mizoguchi A, Mizoguchi E, Chiba C, Bhan A. Role of appendicectomy in the development of inflammatory bowel disease in TCR-A mutant mice. *J Exp Med*, 1996; 184: 707.

294 Sandler R. Appendicectomy and ulcerative colitis. *Lancet*, 1998; 352: 1797.

295 Kirsner JB, Palmer WL. Klotz reversibility in ulcerative colitis. *Radiology*, 1951; 57: 1.

296 Hamilton MI, Dick R, Crawford L, Thompson NP, Pounder RE, Wakefield AJ. Is proximal demarcation of ulcerative colitis determined by the territory of the inferior mesenteric artery? *Lancet*, 1995; 345: 688.

297 Spiliadis CA, Lennard-Jones JE. Ulcerative colitis with relative sparing of the rectum: clinical features, histology and prognosis. *Dis Colon Rectum*, 1987; 30: 334.

298 Goulston SJM, McGovern VJ. The nature of benign strictures in ulcerative colitis. *N Engl J Med*, 1969; 281: 290.

299 Jalan KN, Sircus W, Walker RJ, McManus JPA, Prescott RJ, Card WI. Pseudopolyposis in ulcerative colitis. *Lancet*, 1969; 2: 555.

300 Kelly JK, Gabos S. The pathogenesis of inflammatory polyps. *Dis Colon Rectum*, 1987; 30: 251.

301 Mueller E, Vieth M, Stolte M, Mueller I. The differentiation of true adenomas from colitis-associated dysplasia in ulcerative colitis: a comparative immunohistochemical study. *Hum Pathol*, 1999; 30: 898.

302 Stolte M, Schneider A. Differential diagnosis of adenomas and dysplasias in patients with ulcerative colitis. In: Tytgat GNJ, Bartelsman JFWM, Van Deventer SJH, eds. *Inflammatory Bowel Diseases*. Dordrecht: Kluwer Academic Publishers, 1995: 133.

303 Torres C, Antonioli D, Odze RD. Polypoid dysplasia and adenomas in inflammatory bowel disease: a clinical, pathologic, and follow-up study of 89 polyps from 59 patients. *Am J Surg Pathol*, 1998; 22: 275.

304 Thayer WR, Spiro HM. Ileitis after ileostomy: prestomal ileitis. *Gastroenterology*, 1962; 42: 547.

305 Fazio VW. Toxic megacolon in ulcerative colitis and Crohn's colitis. *Clin Gastroenterol*, 1980; 9 (2): 389.

306 Lumb GR, Protheroe RHB, Ramsay GS. Ulcerative colitis with dilatation of the colon. *Br J Surg*, 1955; 43: 182.

307 Roth JLA, Valdes-Dapena A, Stein GN, Bockus HL. Toxic megacolon in ulcerative colitis. *Gastroenterology*, 1959; 37: 239.

308 Lennard-Jones JE, Vivian AB. Fulminating ulcerative colitis. Recent experience and management. *Br J Med*, 1960; ii: 96.

309 Truelove SC, Witts LJ. Cortisone in ulcerative colitis. *Br Med J*, 1955; 1: 1041.

310 Travis SPL, Farrant JM, Ricketts C *et al.* Predicting outcome in severe ulcerative colitis. *Gut*, 1996; 38: 905.

311 Lumb GR, Protheroe RHB. Ulcerative colitis: a pathologic study of 152 surgical specimens. *Gastroenterology*, 1958; 34: 381.

312 Burnham WR, Ansell ID, Langman MJ. Normal sigmoidoscopic findings in severe ulcerative colitis, an important and common occurrence. *Gut*, 1980; 21: A460.

313 Sampson PA, Walker FC. Dilatation of the colon in ulcerative colitis. *Br J Med*, 1961; ii: 1119.

314 Price AB. Overlap in the spectrum of non-specific inflammatory bowel disease—'colitis-indeterminate'. *J Clin Pathol*, 1978; 31: 567.

315 Ritchie JK, Powell-Tuck J, Lennard-Jones JE. Clinical outcome of first ten years of ulcerative colitis and proctitis. *Lancet*, 1978; i: 1140.

316 Edwards CM, George BD, Warren BF. Diversion colitis: new light through old windows. *Histopathology*, 1999; 35: 86.

317 Edwards CM, George BD, Jewell DP, Warren BF, Mortensen NJMcC, Kettlewell MGW. Role of a defunctioning stoma in the management of large bowel Crohn's disease. *Br J Surg*, 2000; 87: 1063.

318 Roe AM, Warren BF, Brodribb AJ, Brown C. Diversion colitis and involution of the defunctioned anorectum. *Gut*, 1993; 34: 382.

319 Farmer RG. Non-specific ulcerative proctitis. *Gastroenterol Clin North Am*, 1987; 16: 157.

320 Das KM, Morecki R, Nair P. Berkowitz idiopathic proctitis. 1. The morphology of proximal colonic mucosa and its clinical significance. *Am J Dig Dis*, 1977; 22: 524.

321 Samaresekera DN, Stebbing JF, Kettlewell MGW, Jewell DP, Mortensen NJMcC. Outcome of restorative proctocolectomy with ileal reservoir for ulcerative colitis: comparison of distal colitis with more proximal disease. *Gut*, 1996; 30: 574.

322 Kelly JK, Langevin JM, Price LM, Hershfield NB, Share S, Blustein P. Giant and symptomatic inflammatory polyps of the colon in idiopathic inflammatory bowel disease. *Am J Surg Pathol*, 1986; 10: 420.

323 Watson AJ, Roy AD. Paneth cells in the large intestine in ulcerative colitis. *J Pathol Bacteriol*, 1960; 80: 309.

324 Elmes ME, Stanton MR, Howells CHL, Lowe GH. Relation between the mucosal flora and Paneth cell population of human jejunum and ileum. *J Clin Pathol*, 1984; 37: 1272.

325 Morson BC, Pang L. Rectal biopsy as an aid to cancer control in ulcerative colitis. *Gut*, 1967; 8: 423.

326 Gledhill A, Enticott ME, Howe S. Variation in the argyrophil cell population of the rectum in ulcerative colitis and adenocarcinoma. *J Pathol*, 1986; 149: 287.

327 Lee FD, Maguire C, Obeidat W *et al.* Importance of cryptolytic lesions and pericryptal granulomas in inflammatory bowel disease. *J Clin Pathol*, 1997; 50: 148.

328 Warren BF, Price AB, Shepherd NA, Williams GT. Importance of cryptolytic lesions and pericryptal granulomas in inflammatory bowel disease. *J Clin Pathol*, 1997; 50: 880.

329 Burroughs SH, Bowrey DJ, Morris-Stiff GJ, Williams GT. Granulomatous inflammation in sigmoid diverticulitis: two diseases or one? *Histopathology*, 1998; 33: 349.

330 Warren BF, Shepherd NA, Bartolo DCC, Bradfield JWB. Pathology of the defunctioned rectum in ulcerative colitis. *Gut*, 1993; 34: 514.

331 Sarin SK, Malhotra V, sen Gupta S, Karol A, Anand BS, Gaur SK. Significance of eosinophil and mast cell counts in rectal mucosa in ulcerative colitis. A prospective controlled study. *Dig Dis Sci*, 1987; 32: 363.

332 Schmidt GT, Lennard-Jones JE, Morson BC, Young A. Crohn's disease of the colon and its distinction from diverticulitis. *Gut*, 1968; 9: 7.

333 Sladen GE, Filipe MI. Is segmental colitis a complication of diverticular disease. *Dis Col Rectum*, 1984; 27: 513.

334 Rosekrans PCM, Meijer CJLM, Van Der Wal AM, Cornelisse CJ, Lindeman J. Immunoglobulin containing cells in inflammatory bowel disease of the colon: a morphometric and immunohistochemical study. *Gut*, 1980; 21: 941.

335 Heatley RV, James PD. Eosinophils in rectal mucosa. A simple method of predicting the outcome of ulcerative proctitis. *Gut*, 1978; 20: 787.

336 Flejou JF, Potet F, Bogomoletz WV *et al.* Lymphoid follicular proctitis: a condition different from ulcerative proctitis. *Dig Dis Sci*, 1988; 33: 314.

336a Warren S, Sommers SC. Pathogenesis of ulcerative colitis. *Am J Pathol*, 1949; 25: 657.

336b Wakefield AJ, Sankey EA, Dhillon AP *et al.* Granulomatous vasculitis in Crohn's disease. *Gastroenterology*, 1991; 100: 1279.

336c Rice AJ, Abbott CR, Mapstone NM. Granulomatous vasculitis in diversion proctocolitis. *Histopathology*, 1999; 34: 276.

336d Riley SA, Mani V, Goodman MJ, Dutt S, Herd ME. Microscopic activity in ulcerative colitis: what does it mean? *Gut*, 1991; 32: 174.

337 Geboes K, Riddell RH, Ost A, Jensfeldt B, Persson T, Lofberg R. A reproducible grading scale for histological assessment of inflammation in ulcerative colitis. *Gut*, 2000; 47: 404.

338 Bernstein CN, Shanahan F, Anton PA, Weinstein WM. Patchiness of mucosal inflammation in treated ulcerative colitis: a prospective study. *Gastrointest Endosc*, 1995; 42: 232.

339 Teague RH, Manning AP. Preparation of the large bowel for colonoscopy. *J Int Med Res*, 1977; 5: 374.

340 Elliott PR, Williams CB, Lennard-Jones JE *et al.* Colonoscopic diagnosis of minimal change colitis in patients with a normal sigmoidoscopy and normal air contrast barium enema. *Lancet*, 1982; 1: 650.

341 Soundy VC, Davies SE, Warren BF. The double muscularis mucosae in ulcerative colitis: is it all new? *Histopathology*, 1998; 32: 484.

342 Lichtiger S, Present DH, Kombluth A *et al.* Cyclosporine in severe ulcerative colitis refractory to steroid therapy. *N Engl J Med*, 1994; 330: 1841.

343 Hyde G, Thillainayagam AV, Jewell DP. Intravenous cyclosporin as rescue therapy in severe ulcerative colitis: time for a reappraisal? *Eur J Gastroenterol Hepatol*, 1998; 10: 411.

344 Hyde G, Warren BF, Jewell DP. Pathology of cyclosporin induced changes in ulcerative colitis. *Colorectal Dis*, 2002; in press.

345 Baker W, Glass R, Ritchie J, Aylett S. Cancer of the rectum following colectomy and ileorectal anastomosis for ulcerative colitis. *Br J Surg*, 1978; 65: 862.

346 Lennard-Jones JE, Morson BC, Ritchie JK, Williams CB. Cancer surveillance in ulcerative colitis. Experience over 15 years. *Lancet*, 1983; ii: 149.

347 Gyde SN, Prior P, Allan RN *et al.* Colorectal cancer in ulcerative colitis: a cohort study of primary referrals from three centres. *Gut*, 1988; 29: 206.

348 Geller SA, Janowitz HD, Aufses AH. Cancer in universal and left-sided ulcerative colitis: factors determining risk. *Gastroenterology*, 1979; 77: 290.

349 Allen DC, Biggart JD, Pyper PC. Large bowel mucosal dysplasia and carcinoma in ulcerative colitis. *J Clin Pathol*, 1985; 38: 30.

350 Mottet NK. Histopathologic spectrum of regional enteritis and ulcerive colitis. In: *Major Problems in Pathology*. Philadelphia: W.B. Saunders, 1971: 220.

351 Gilat T, Fireman Z, Grossman A *et al.* Colorectal cancer in patients with ulcerative colitis. *Gastroenterology*, 1988; 94: 870.

352 Maratka Z, Nedbal J, Kocianova J, Havelka J, Kudrmann J, Hendl J. Incidence of colorectal cancer in proctocolitis: a retrospective study of 959 cases over 40 years. *Gut*, 1985; 26: 43.

353 de Dombal FT, Watts JMcK, Watkinson G, Goligher JC. Local complications of ulcerative colitis: stricture, pseudopolyposis and carcinoma of colon and rectum. *Br J Med*, 1966; 1: 1442.

354 Devroede G, Taylor WF, Saver WG, Jackman RJ, Stickler GB. Cancer risk and life expectancy of children with ulcerative colitis. *N Engl J Med*, 1971; 285: 17.

355 MacDermott RP. Review of clinical aspects of cancer of the colon in patients with ulcerative colitis. *Dig Dis Sci*, 1985; 12: 1145.

356 Jones HW, Grogono J, Hoare AM. Surveillance in ulcerative colitis: burdens and benefits. *Gut*, 1988; 29: 325.

357 Hinton JM. Risk of malignant change in ulcerative colitis. *Gut*, 1966; 7: 427.

357a Collins RH, Feldman M, Fordtran JS. Colon cancer, dysplasia and surveillance in patients with ulcerative colitis. *N Engl J Med*, 1987; 316: 1654.

358 Manning AP, Bulgim OR, Dixon MF, Axon ATR. Screening by colonoscopy for colonic epithelial dysplasia in inflammatory bowel disease. *Gut*, 1987; 28: 1489.

359 Lennard-Jones JE. Compliance, cost and common sense limit cancer control in colitis. *Gut*, 1986; 27: 1403.

360 Fozard JBJ, Dixon MF. Colonoscopic surveillance in ulcerative colitis—dysplasia through the looking glass. *Gut*, 1989; 30: 285.

361 Butt JH, Konishi F, Morson BC, Lennard-Jones JE, Ritchie JK. Macroscopic lesions in dysplasia and carcinoma complicating ulcerative colitis. *Dig Dis Sci*, 1983; 28: 18.

362 Muto T, Bussey HJR, Morson BC. The evolution of cancer of the colon and rectum. *Cancer*, 1975; 36: 2251.

363 Slater G, Greenstein AJ, Gelernt I, Kreel I, Bauer J, Aufses H. Distribution of colorectal cancer in patients with and without ulcerative colitis. *Am J Surg*, 1985; 149: 780.

364 Granquist S, Gabrielsson N, Sundelin P, Thorgeirsson T. Precancerous lesions in the mucosa in ulcerative colitis. A radiographic, endoscopic and histopathologic study. *Scand J Gastroenterol*, 1980; 15: 289.

365 Blackstone MO, Riddell RH, Rogers BHG, Levin B. Dysplasia associated lesion or mass (DALM) detected by colonoscopy in longstanding ulcerative colitis: an indication for colectomy. *Gastroenterology*, 1981; 80: 366.

366 Lennard-Jones JE, Morson BC, Ritchie JK, Shove DC, Williams CB. Cancer in colitis: assessment of the individual risk by clinical and histological criteria. *Gastroenterology*, 1977; 73: 1280.

367 Riddell RH, Goldman H, Ransohoff DF *et al*. Dysplasia in inflammatory bowel disease: standardised classification with provisional clinical applications. *Hum Pathol*, 1983; 4: 931.

368 Talbot IC, Price AB. Dysplasia in inflammatory bowel disease. In: *Biopsy Pathology in Colorectal Disease*. London: Chapman & Hall, 1987: 149.

369 Noffsinger AE, Belli JM, Miller MA, Fenoglio-Preiser CM. A unique basal pattern of p53 expression in ulcerative colitis in association with mutation in the p53 gene. *Histopathology*, 2001; 39: 482.

370 Manning AP, Bulgim OR, Dixon MF, Axon ATR. Screening by colonoscopy for colonic epithelial dysplasia in inflammatory bowel disease. *Gut*, 1987; 28: 1489.

371 Welkon CJ, Long SS. *Clostridium difficile* in patients with cystic fibrosis. *Am J Dis Child*, 1985; 139: 805.

372 Lishman AH, Al-Jumaili IJ, Record CO. Spectrum of antibiotic-associated diarrhoea. *Gut*, 1981; 22: 34.

373 Hao XP, Ilyas M, Talbot IC. Expression of Bcl-2 and p53 in the colorectal adenoma–carcinoma sequence. *Pathobiology*, 1997; 65: 26.

374 Schneider A, Stolte M. Differential diagnosis of adenomas and dysplastic lesions in patients with ulcerative colitis. *Z Gastroenterol*, 1993; 31: 653.

375 Brostrom O, Lofberg R, Ost A, Reichard H. Cancer surveillance of patients with long standing ulcerative colitis: a clinical, endoscopical and histological study. *Gut*, 1986; 27: 1408.

376 Rosenstock E, Farmer RG, Petras R, Surak MV, Rankin GB, Sullivan BH. Surveillance for colonic carcinoma in ulcerative colitis. *Gastroenterology*, 1985; 89: 1342.

377 Butt JH, Price AB, Williams CB. Dysplasia and cancer in ulcerative colitis. In: Allen RN, Keighley MRB, Alexander-Williams J, Hawkins C, eds. *Inflammatory Bowel Disease*. Edinburgh: Churchill Livingstone, 1983: 140.

378 Riddell RH, Morson BC. Value of sigmoidoscopy and biopsy in detection of carcinoma and premalignant change in ulcerative colitis. *Gut*, 1979; 20: 575.

379 Ranshoff DF, Riddell RH, Levin B. Ulcerative colitis and colon cancer. Problems in assessing the diagnostic usefulness of mucosal dysplasia. *Dis Colon Rectum*, 1985; 28: 383.

380 Kewenter J, Hulten L, Ahren C. The occurrence of severe epithelial dysplasia and its bearing on treatment of long-standing ulcerative colitis. *Ann Surg*, 1982; 195: 209.

381 de Dombal FT, Softley A. Cancer and inflammatory bowel disease—changing perspectives. In: de Dombal FT, Myran J, Bouchier IAD, Watkinson G, eds. *Inflammatory Bowel Disease, Some International Data and Reflections*. Oxford: Oxford University Press, 1985: 247.

382 Biasco G, Migholi M, Di Febo G, Rossini FP, Grigioni WF, Barbara L. Cancer and dysplasia in ulcerative colitis: preliminary report of a prospective study. *Ital J Gastroenterol*, 1984; 16: 212.

383 Dixon MF, Brown LJR, Gilmour HM *et al*. Observer variation in the assessment of dysplasia in ulcerative colitis. *Histopathology*, 1988; 13: 385.

384 Eaden JA, Abrams K, McKay EH, Denley H, Mayberry J. Inter-observer variation between general and specialist gastrointestinal pathologists when grading dysplasia in ulcerative colitis. *J Pathol*, 2001; 194: 152.

385 Bartlett JG, Chang TW, Gurwith M, Gorbach SL, Onderdonk AB. Antibiotic-associated pseudomembranous colitis due to toxin-producing clostridia. *N Engl J Med*, 1978; 298: 531.

386 Schofield PF, Holden D, Carr ND. Bowel disease after radiotherapy. *J R Soc Med*, 1983; 76: 463.

387 Geboes, K. How is dysplasia recognised? In Jewell, DP, Warren BF, Mortensen, NJ, eds. *Challenges in Inflammatory Bowel Disease*. Oxford: Blackwell Science, 2001.

388 Collins RH, Feldman M, Fordtran JS. Colon cancer, dysplasia and surveillance in patients with ulcerative colitis. *N Engl J Med*, 1987; 316: 1654.

389 Gerding DN, Olsen MM, Peterson LR *et al*. *Clostridium difficile*-associated diarrhoea and colitis in adults. A prospective case-controlled epidemiologic study. *Arch Intern Med*, 1986; 146: 95.

390 Taylor NS, Thorne GM, Bartlett JG. Comparison of two toxins produced by *Clostridium difficile*. *Infect Immun*, 1981; 34: 1036.

391 Berthrong M, Fajardo LF. Radiation injury in surgical pathology. Part II, Alimentary tract. *Am J Surg Pathol*, 1981; 5: 153.

392 Lennard-Jones JE, Morson BC, Ritchie JK, Shove DC, Williams CB. Cancer in colitis: assessment of the individual risk by clinical and histological criteria. *Gastroenterology*, 1977; 73: 1280.

393 Dobbins WD. Editorial: current status of pre-cancer lesions in ulcerative colitis. *Gastroenterology*, 1977; 73: 1431.

394 Yardley JH, Bayless TM, Diamond MP. Cancer in ulcerative colitis. *Gastroenterology*, 1979; 76: 221.

395 Ziv Y, Fazio VW, Sirimarco MT, Lavery IC, Goldblum JR, Petras RE. Incidence, risk factors and treatment of dysplasia in the anal transitional zone after ileal pouch–anal anastomosis. *Dis Colon Rectum*, 1994; 37: 1281.

396 Parks AG, Nicholls RJ. Proctocolectomy without ileostomy for ulcerative colitis. *Br Med J*, 1978; 2: 85.

397 Thompson-Fawcett MW, Rust NA, Warren BF, Mortensen NJ. Aneuploidy and columnar cuff surveillance after stapled ileal pouch–anal anastomosis in ulcerative colitis. *Dis Colon Rectum*, 2000; 43: 408.

398 Dew MJ, Thompson H, Allan RN. The spectrum of hepatic dysfunction in inflammatory bowel disease. *Q J Med*, 1979; 48: 113.

399 Perrett AD, Higgins G, Johnston HH, Massarella GR, Truelove SC, Wright R. The liver in ulcerative colitis. *Q J Med*, 1971; 40: 211.

400 Rand JA, Brandt LJ, Baker NH, Lynch J. Ulcerative colitis complicated by amyloid. *Am J Gastroenterol*, 1980; 74: 185.

401 Shorvon PJ. Amyloidosis and inflammatory bowel disease. *Am J Dig Dis*, 1977; 20: 209.

402 Chapman RWG, Marborgh BAM, Rhodes JM *et al*. Primary sclerosing cholangitis: a review of its clinical features, cholangiography and hepatic histology. *Gut*, 1980; 21: 870.

403 Meuwissen SGM, Feltkamp-Vroom T, de la Riviere AB, Von Dem Borne AEG Kr, Tytgat GN. Analysis of the lymphoplasmacytic infiltrate in Crohn's disease with special reference to identification of lymphocyte subpopulations. *Gut*, 1976; 17: 770.

404 Ludwig J, Larusso NF, Wiesner RE. Primary sclerosing cholangitis. In: Peters RL, Craig JR, eds. *Liver Pathology*. Edinburgh: Churchill Livingstone, 1986: 193.

405 Wee A, Ludwig J. Pericholangitis in chronic ulcerative colitis. Primary sclerosing cholangitis of small bile ducts. *Ann Intern Med*, 1985; 102: 581.

406 Barbatis C, Grases P, Shepherd HA *et al*. Histological features of sclerosing cholangitis in patients with chronic ulcerative colitis. *J Clin Pathol*, 1985; 38: 778.

407 Mir-Madjlessis SH, Farmer RG, Sivak MV. Bile duct carcinoma in patients with ulcerative colitis. Relationship to sclerosing cholangitis: report of six cases and review of the literature. *Dig Dis Sci*, 1987; 32: 145.

408 Ritchie JK, Allan RN, Macartney J, Thompson H, Hawley PR, Cooke WT. Biliary tract carcinoma associated with ulcerative colitis. *Q J Med*, 1974; 43: 263.

409 Olsson R, Hulten L. Concurrence of ulcerative colitis and chronic active hepatitis. Clinical courses and results of colectomy. *Scand J Gastroenterol*, 1975; 10: 331.

410 Mayer L, Janowitz HD. Extra-intestinal manifestations of ulcerative colitis including reference to Crohn's disease. In: Allan RN, Keighley MRB, Alexander-Williams J, Hawkins C, eds. *Inflammatory Bowel Disease*. Edinburgh: Churchill Livingstone, 1983: 121.

411 Lockhart-Mummery HE, Morson BC. Crohn's disease (regional enteritis) of the large intestine and its distinction from ulcerative colitis. *Gut*, 1960; 1: 87.

412 Cornes JS, Stecher M. Primary Crohn's disease of the colon and rectum. *Gut*, 1961; 2: 189.

413 Kent TH, Ammon RK, Denbesten L. Differentiation of ulcerative colitis and regional enteritis. *Arch Pathol*, 1970; 89: 20.

414 Joffe N. Localized giant pseudopolyposis secondary to ulcerative or granulomatous colitis. *Clin Radiol*, 1977; 28: 609.

415 Buchanan WM, Fyee AHB. Giant pseudopolyposis in granulomatous colitis. *J Pathol*, 1979; 127: 51.

416 Morson BC. Histopathology of Crohn's disease. *Proc R Soc Med*, 1968; 61: 79.

417 Lockhart-Mummery HE, Morson BC. Crohn's disease of the large intestine. *Gut*, 1964; 5: 493.

418 Greenstein AJ, Janowitz HD, Sachar DB. The extra-intestinal complications of Crohn's disease and ulcerative colitis: a study of 700 patients. *Medicine*, 1976; 55: 401.

419 Jenkins D, Balsitis M, Gallivan S *et al*. Guideline for the initial biopsy diagnosis of suspected chronic idiopathic inflammatory bowel disease. The British Society of Gastroenterology, initiative. *J Clin Pathol*, 1997; 50: 93.

420 Bentley E, Jenkins D, Campbell FC, Warren BF, Riddell RH. How could pathologists improve the initial diagnosis of colitis? Evidence from an international workshop. *J Clin Pathol* in press.

421 Riddell RH. Pathology of idiopathic inflammatory bowel disease. In: Kirsner JB, Shorter RG, eds. *Inflammatory Bowel Disease*. Philadelphia: Lea & Febiger, 1988.

422 Haggitt RC. The differential diagnosis of idiopathic inflammatory bowel disease. In: Norris HT, ed. *Pathology of the Colon, Small Intestine and Anus*. New York: Churchill Livingstone, 1983: 21.

423 Hanby AM, Wright NA. The ulcer-associated cell lineage: the gastrointestinal repair kit? *J Pathol*, 1993; 171: 3.

424 Rotterdam H, Korelitz BI, Sommers SC. Microgranulomas in grossly normal rectal mucosa in Crohn's disease. *Am J Clin Pathol*, 1977; 67: 550.

425 Cook MG, Dixon MF. An analysis of the reliability of detection and diagnostic value of various pathological features in Crohn's disease and ulcerative colitis. *Gut*, 1973; 14: 255.

426 Schmitz-Moormann P, Pittner PM, Sangmeister M. Probability of detecting a granuloma in colorectal biopsy of Crohn's disease. *Pathol Res Pract*, 1984; 178: 227.

427 Greenson JK, Stern RA, Carpenter SL, Barnett JL. The clinical significance of focal active colitis. *Hum Pathol*, 1997; 29: 729.

428 Volk EE, Shapiro BD, Easley KA, Goldblum JR. The clinical significance of a biopsy based diagnosis of focal active colitis: a clinicopathologic study of 31 cases. *Mod Pathol*, 1998; 11: 789.

429 Longman RJ, Warren BF. Is the colonic reparative cell lineage yet to be discovered? *Gut*, 2000; 47: 307.

430 Borley NR, Mortensen NJ, Kettlewell MG, George BD, Jewell DP, Warren BF. Connective tissue changes in ileal Crohn's disease: relationship to disease phenotype and ulcer associated cell lineage. *Dis Colon Rectum*, 2001; 44: 388.

431 Borley NR, Mortensen NJ, Jewell DP, Warren BF. The relationship between inflammatory and serosal connective tissue changes in ileal Crohn's disease: evidence for a possible causative link. *J Pathol*, 2000; 190: 196.

432 McQuillan A, Appelman H. Superficial Crohn's disease: a study of 10 patients. *Surg Pathol*, 1989; 2: 3.

433 Kent TH, Ammon RK, Denbesten L. Differentiation of ulcerative colitis and regional enteritis. *Arch Pathol*, 1970; 89: 20.

434 Margulis AR, Goldbert HI, Lawson TL *et al*. The overlapping spectrum of ulcerative colitis and granulomatous colitis: a roentgenographic–pathological study. *Am J Roentgenol Radium Ther Nucl Med*, 1971; 113: 325.

435 Lewin K, Swales JD. Granulomatous colitis and atypical ulcerative colitis. *Gastroenterology*, 1966; 59: 211.

436 Gyde SN, Prior P, Macartney JC, Thompson H, Waterhouse JAH, Allan RN. Malignancy in Crohn's disease. *Gut*, 1980; 21: 1024.

437 Lee KS, Medline A, Shockey S. Indeterminate colitis in the spectrum of inflammatory bowel disease. *Arch Pathol Lab Med*, 1979; 193: 173.

438 Harper PH, Truelove SC, Lee EC, Kettlewell MG, Jewell DP. Split ileostomy and ileocolostomy for Crohn's disease of the colon and ulcerative colitis. A 20 year survey. *Gut*, 1983; 24: 106.

439 Surawicz MC. Diagnosing colitis. Biopsy is best. *Gastroenterology*, 1987; 92: 538.

440 Winslet MC, Andrews H, Allan RN, Keighley MRB. Faecal diversion in the management of Crohn's disease of the colon. *Dis Colon Rectum*, 1993; 36: 757.

441 Edwards CM, George BD, Warren BF. Diversion colitis—new light through old windows. *Histopathology*, 1999; 35: 86.

441a Warren BF, Shepherd NA. The role of pathology in pelvic ileal reservoir surgery. *Int J Colorectal Dis*, 1992; 7: 68.

442 Geboes K. Crohn's disease, ulcerative colitis or indeterminate colitis—how important is it to differentiate? *Acta Gastroenterol Belg*, 2001; 64: 197.

443 Yu CS, Pemberton JH, Larson D. Ileal pouch–anal anastomosis in patients with indeterminate colitis. *Dis Colon Rectum*, 2000; 43: 1487.

444 McIntyre PB, Pemberton JH, Wolff BG, Dozois RR, Beart RWJ. Indeterminate colitis. Long-term outcome in patients after ileal pouch–anal anastomosis. *Dis Colon Rectum*, 1995; 38: 51.

445 Atkinson KG, Owen DA, Wankling G. Restorative proctocolectomy and indeterminate colitis. *Am J Surg*, 1994; 167: 516.
446 Koltun WA, Schoetz DJJR, Roberts PL, Murray JJ, Coller JA, Veidenheimer MC. Indeterminate colitis predisposes to perineal complications after ileal pouch–anal anastomosis. *Dis Colon Rectum*, 1991; 34: 857.
447 White CL, Hamilton SR, Diamond MP, Cameron JL. Crohn's disease and ulcerative colitis in the same patient. *Gut*, 1983; 24: 587.
448 Ever S, Spadaccini C, Walker P, Ansel H, Schwartz M, Sumner HW. Simultaneous ulcerative colitis and Crohn's disease. *Am J Gastroenterol*, 1980; 73: 345.
449 Dwarakanath AD, Nash J, Rhodes JM. 'Conversion' from ulcerative colitis to Crohn's disease associated with corticosteroid treatment. *Gut*, 1994; 35: 1141.
450 Parente F, Cucino C, Bollani S *et al*. Focal gastric inflammatory infiltrates in inflammatory bowel disease: prevalence, immunohistochemical characteristics and diagnostic role. *Am J Gastroenterol*, 2000; 95: 705.
451 Meyers AA, Alonso DR, Morson BC, Bartram C. Pathogenesis of diverticulitis complicating granulomatous colitis. *Gastroenterology*, 1978; 74: 24.
452 Van Rosendaal GM, Andersen MA. Segmental colitis complicating diverticular disease. *Can J Gastroenterol*, 1996; 10: 361.
453 Gore S, Shepherd NA, Wilkinson SP. Endoscopic crescentic fold disease of the sigmoid colon: the clinical and histopathological spectrum of a distinctive endoscopic appearance. *Int J Colorectal Dis*, 1992; 7: 76.
454 Magapugay LM, Dean PJ. Diverticular disease-associated chronic colitis. *Am J Surg Pathol*, 1996; 20: 94.
455 Periera MC. Diverticular disease-associated colitis: progression to severe chronic ulcerative colitis after sigmoid surgery. *Gastrointest Endosc*, 2000; 51: 379.
456 Gledhill A, Dixon MF. Crohn's like reaction in diverticular disease. *Gut*, 1998; 42: 392.
457 Shepherd NA. Diverticular disease and chronic idiopathic inflammatory bowel disease: associations and masquerades. *Gut*, 1996; 38: 801.
458 Gourevitch A, Cunningham IJ. Sarcoidosis of the sigmoid colon. *Postgrad Med J*, 1959; 35: 689.
459 Gregorie HB Jr, Otherson HB Jr, Moore McKP Jr. The significance of sarcoid-like lesions with malignant neoplasms. *Am J Surg*, 1962; 104: 477.
460 Tobi M, Kobrin I, Ariel I. Rectal involvement in sarcoidosis. *Dis Colon Rectum*, 1982; 25: 491.
461 Gould SR, Handley AJ, Barnado DE. Rectal and gastric involvement in a case of sarcoidosis. *Gut*, 1973; 14: 971.
462 Petri M, Poulsen SS, Christensen K, Jamum S. The incidence of granulomas in serial sections of rectal biopsies from patients with Crohn's disease. *Acta Pathol Microbiol Immunol Scand [A]*, 1982; 90: 145.
463 Rotterdam H, Korelitz BI, Sommers SC. Microgranulomas in grossly normal rectal mucosa in Crohn's disease. *Am J Clin Pathol*, 1977; 67: 550.
464 Nostrant TT, Kumar NB, Appelman HD. Histopathology differentiates acute self-limited colitis from ulcerative colitis. *Gastroenterology*, 1987; 92: 319.
465 Green FMY, Fox H. The distribution of mucosal antibodies in the bowel of patients with Crohn's disease. *Gut*, 1975; 16: 125.
466 Editorial. Which type of colitis? *Lancet*, 1988; 1: 336.
467 Talbot IC, Price AB. Infective colitis. In: *Biopsy Pathology of Colorectal Disease*. London: Chapman Hall, 1987: 81.
468 Surawicz CM. The role of rectal biopsy in infectious colitis. *Am J Surg Pathol*, 1968; 12 (Suppl 1): 82.
469 Surawicz CM, Belic L. Rectal biopsy helps to distinguish acute self-limited colitis from idiopathic inflammatory bowel disease. *Gastroenterology*, 1984; 86: 104.
470 van Spreeuwel JP, Lindeman J, Meyer CJLM. A quantitative study of immunoglobulin containing cells in the differential diagnosis of acute colitis. *J Clin Pathol*, 1985; 38: 774.
471 Skinner JM, Whitehead R. The plasma cells in inflammatory disease of the colon: a quantitative study. *J Clin Pathol*, 1974; 27: 643.
472 Pera A, Bellando P, Caldera D *et al*. Colonoscopy in inflammatory bowel disease. Diagnostic accuracy and proposal of an endoscopic score. *Gastroenterology*, 1987; 92: 181.
473 Kaufmann HJ, Taubin HL. Non steroidal anti-inflammatory drugs activate quiescent chronic inflammatory bowel disease. *Ann Intern Med*, 1987; 107: 513.
474 Lee FD. Importance of apoptosis in the histopathology of drug related lesions in the large intestine. *J Clin Pathol*, 1993; 46: 118.
475 Byers RJ, Marsh P, Parkinson D, Haboubi NY. Melanosis coli is associated with an increase in colonic epithelial apoptosis and not with laxative use. *Histopathology*, 1997; 30: 160.
476 Warren BF, Edwards CM, Travis SPL. Commentary. 'Microscopic colitis'; classification and terminology. *Histopathology*, 2002; 40: 374.
477 Robinson MHE, Wheatley T, Leach IH. Non steroidal anti-inflammatory drug induced colonic stricture: an unusual cause of colonic obstruction and perforation. *Dig Dis Sci*, 1995; 40: 2.
478 Fellows IW, Clarke JMF, Roberts PF. Non steroidal anti-inflammatory drug induced jejunal and colonic diaphragm disease: a report of two cases. *Gut*, 1992; 33: 1424.
479 Gizzi G, Villani V, Grandi GM *et al*. Anorectal lesions in patients taking suppositories containing nonsteroidal anti-inflammatory drugs (NSAIDs). *Endoscopy*, 1990; 22: 146.
480 Levy N, Gaspar E. Rectal bleeding and indomethacin suppositories. *Lancet*, 1975; 1: 577.
481 Fam AG, Paton TW, Shamess CJ, Lewis AJ. Fulminant colitis complicating gold therapy. *J Rheumatol*, 1980; 7: 479.
482 Szpak MW, Johnson RC, Brady CE *et al*. Gold induced enterocolitis. *Gastroenterology*, 1979; 76: 1257.
483 Wong V, Wyatt J, Lewis F, Howdle P. Gold induced enterocolitis complicated by cytomegalovirus infection: a previously unrecognised association. *Gut* 1993; 34: 1002.
484 Jackson CW, Haboubi NY, Whorwell PJ, Schofield PF. Gold induced enterocolitis. *Gut*, 1986; 27: 452.
485 Reinhart WH, Kappeler M, Halter F. Severe pseudomembranous and ulcerative colitis during gold therapy. *Endoscopy*, 1983; 17: 70.
486 Floch MH, Hellman L. The effect of 5 fluorouracil in rectal mucosa. *Gastroenterology*, 1965; 48: 430.
487 Miller SS, Muggia AL, Spiro HM. Colonic histological changes induced by 5 fluorouracil. *Gastroenterology*, 1962; 43: 391.
488 Sparano JA, Dutcher JP, Kaleya R *et al*. Colonic ischaemia complicating immunotherapy with interleukin 2 and interferon alpha. *Cancer*, 1991; 68: 1538.
489 Deana DG, Dean PJ. Reversible ischaemic colitis in young women associated with oral contraceptive use. *Am J Surg Pathol*, 1995; 19: 454.
490 Tedesco FJ, Volpicelli NA, Moore FS. Estrogen and progesterone associated colitis: a disorder with clinical and endoscopic features mimicking Crohn's colitis. *Gastrointest Endosc*, 1982; 28: 274.
491 Nalbundian H, Sketh N, Dietrich R *et al*. Intestinal ischaemia caused by cocaine ingestion: report of two cases. *Surgery*, 1985; 97: 374.
492 Martin P, Manley PN, Depew WT. Isotretinoin associated proctosigmoiditis. *Gastroenterology*, 1987; 93: 606.

493 Moshkowitz M, Konikoff FM, Arbert N *et al*. Acyclovir associated colitis. *Am J Gastroenterol*, 1993; 83: 2110.
494 Pawel BR, de Chadarevian JP, Franco ME. The pathology of fibrosing colonopathy of cystic fibrosis: a study of 12 cases and review of the literature. *Hum Pathol*, 1997; 28: 395.
495 Ramsden WH, Moya EF, Littlewood JM. Colonic wall thickness, pancreatic enzyme dose and type of preparation in cystic fibrosis. *Arch Dis Childhood*, 1998; 79: 339.
496 Price AB, Davies DR. Pseudomembranous colitis. *J Clin Pathol*, 1970; 30: 1.
497 Price AB. Pseudomembranous colitis. In: Wright R, ed. *Recent Advances in Gastrointestinal Pathology*. London: W.B. Saunders, 1980: 151.
498 Bartlett JG, Moon N, Chang TW, Taylor N, Onderdonk AB. Role of *Clostridium difficile* in antibiotic-associated pseudomembranous colitis. *Gastroenterology*, 1978; 75: 778.
499 Burdon DW, George RH, Mogg GAG *et al*. Faecal toxin and severity of antibiotic-associated pseudomembranous colitis. *J Clin Pathol*, 1981; 34: 548.
500 Borriello SP, Ketley JM, Mitchell TJ *et al*. *Clostridium difficile*—a spectrum of virulence and analysis of putative determinants in the hamster model of antibiotic-associated colitis. *J Med Microbiol*, 1987; 24: 53.
501 Larson HE, Price AB. Pseudomembranous colitis: presence of clostridial toxin. *Lancet*, 1977; ii: 1312.
502 Penner A, Bernheim AI. Acute post-operative enterocolitis. *Arch Pathol*, 1939; 27: 996.
503 Whitehead R. Ischaemic enterocolitis: an expression of the intravascular coagulation syndrome. *Gut*, 1971; 12: 912.
504 Shortland JR, Spencer RC, Williams JL. Pseudomembranous colitis associated with changes in an ileal conduit. *J Clin Pathol*, 1983; 36: 1184.
505 Cone JB, Wetzel W. Toxic megacolon secondary to pseudomembranous colitis. *Dis Colon Rectum*, 1982; 25: 478.
506 Snooks SJ, Hughes A, Horsburgh AG. Perforated colon complicating pseudomembranous colitis. *Br J Surg*, 1984; 71: 291.
507 Seppala K, Hjelt L, Sipponon P. Colonoscopy in the diagnosis of antibiotic-associated colitis. A prospective study. *Scand J Gastroenterol*, 1981; 16: 465.
508 Tedesco FJ, Corless JK, Brownstein RE. Rectal sparing in antibiotic-associated pseudomembranous colitis: a prospective study. *Gastroenterology*, 1982; 83: 1259.
509 Price AB. Histopathology of clostridial gut disease in man. In: Borriello SP, ed. *Clostridia in Gastrointestinal Disease*. Boca Raton, Florida: CRC Press, 1985: 177.
510 Price AB, Day DW. Pseudomembranous and infective colitis. In: Anthony PP, MacSween RNM, eds. *Recent Advances in Histopathology* 11. Edinburgh: Churchill Livingstone, 1981: 99.
511 Holst E, Helin I, Mardh PA. Recovery of *Clostridium difficile* from children. *Scand J InfectDis*, 1981; 13: 41.
512 Dickinson RJ, Rampling A, Wight DGD. Spontaneous pseudomembranous colitis not associated with *Clostridium difficile*. *J Infect*, 1985; 10: 252.
513 Cundy T, Trafford JA, Thom BT, Somerville PG. *Clostridium difficile* and non-antibiotic associated colitis. *Lancet*, 1980; ii: 595.
514 Rocca JM, Hecker R, Pieterse A, Rich GE, Rowland R. *Clostridium difficile* colitis. *Aust N Z J Med*, 1984; 14: 606.
515 Wald A, Mendelow H, Bartlett JG. Non-antibiotic associated pseudomembranous colitis due to toxin producing clostridia. *Ann Intern Med*, 1980; 92: 798.
516 Wren B, Heard SR, Tabacqchali S. Association between production of toxins A and B and types of *Clostridium difficile*. *J Clin Pathol*, 1987; 40: 1397.
517 Meyers S, Mayer L, Boltone E, Desmond E, Janowitz HD. Occurrence of *Clostridium difficile* toxin during the course of inflammatory bowel disease. *Gastroenterology*, 1981; 80: 697.
518 Sullivan NM, Pellett S, Wilkins TD. Purification and characterisation of toxin A and B of *Clostridium difficile*. *Infect Immun*, 1982; 35: 1032.
519 Larson HE, Price AB, Borriello SP. Epidemiology of experimental enterocolitis due to *Clostridium difficile*. *J Infect Dis*, 1980; 142: 408.
520 Keighley MRB, Burdon DW, Alexander-Williams J *et al*. Diarrhoea and pseudomembranous colitis after gastrointestinal operations. A prospective study. *Lancet*, 1978; ii: 1165.
521 Osterholm MT, MacDonald KL, White KE *et al*. An outbreak of a newly recognised chronic diarrhoea syndrome associated with raw milk consumption. *JAMA*, 1986; 256: 484.
522 Mintz ED, Weber JT, Guris D *et al*. An outbreak of Brainerd diarrhoea among travellers to the Galapagos Islands. *J Infect Dis*, 1998; 177: 1041.
523 Bryant DA, Mintz ED, Puhr ND, Griffin PM, Petras RE. Colonic intraepithelial lymphocytosis associated with an epidemic of chronic diarrhoea. *Am J Surg Pathol*, 1996; 20: 1102.
524 Perkins DE, Spjut HE. Intestinal stenosis following radiation therapy. A roentgenologic–pathologic study. *Am J Roentgenol Radium Ther Nucl Med*, 1962; 88: 953.
525 Hasleton PS, Carr N, Schofield PF. Vascular changes in radiation bowel disease. *Histopathology*, 1985; 9: 517.
526 Decosse JJ, Rhodes RS, Wentz WB, Reagan JW, Dwoken HJ, Holden WD. The natural history and management of radiation induced injury of the gastrointestinal tract. *Ann Surg*, 1969; 170: 369.
527 Gelfand MD, Tepper M, Katz LA, Binder HJ, Yesner R, Floch MH. Acute irradiation proctitis in man. Development of eosinophilic abscesses. *Gastroenterology*, 1968; 54: 49.
528 McFadyean IR, Price AB, Giersson RT. The relation of birthweight to histological appearances in vessels of the placental bed. *Br J Obstet Gynaecol*, 1986; 93: 476.
529 Counter SF, Froese DP, Hart MJ. Prospective evaluation of formalin therapy for radiation proctitis. *Am J Surg*, 1999; 177: 396.
530 Pikarsky AJ, Belin B, Efron J, Weiss EG, Nogueras JJ, Wexner SD. Complications following formalin installation in the treatment of radiation induced proctitis. *Int J Colorectal Dis*, 2000; 15: 96.
531 Glotzer DJ, Glick ME, Goldman H. Proctitis and colitis following diversion of the faecal stream. *Gastroenterology*, 1981; 80: 438.
532 Geraghty JM, Talbot IC. Diversion colitis: histological features in the colon and rectum after defunctioning colostomy. *Gut*, 1991; 32: 1020.
533 Warren BF, Shepherd NA. Diversion proctocolitis. *Histopathology*, 1992; 21: 91.
534 Harig JH, Soergel KH, Komorowski RA, Wood CM. Treatment of diversion colitis with short-chain fatty acid irrigation. *N Engl J Med*, 1989; 320: 23.
535 Guillemot F, Colombel JF, Neut C *et al*. Treatment of diversion colitis by short chain fatty acids. Prospective and double blind study. *Dis Colon Rectum*, 1991; 34: 861.
536 Neut C, Guillemot F, Colombel JF *et al*. Nitrate reducing bacteria in diversion colitis: a clue to inflammation? *Dig Dis Sci*, 1997; 42: 2577.
537 Yeong ML, Bethwaite PB, Prasad J, Isbister WH. Lymphoid follicular hyperplasia—a distinctive feature of diversion colitis. *Histopathology*, 1991; 19: 55.
538 Lusk LB, Reichen J, Levine JS. Apthous ulceration in diversion colitis. *Gastroenterology*, 1984; 87: 1171.
539 Murray FE, O'Brien MJ, Birkett DH, Kennedy SM, Lamont TJ.

Diversion colitis. Pathologic findings in a resected sigmoid colon and rectum. *Gastroenterology*, 1987; 93: 1404.
540 Haque S, Eisen RN, West AB. The morphologic features of diversion colitis: studies of a paediatric population with no other disease of the intestinal mucosa. *Hum Pathol*, 1993; 24: 211.
541 Korelitz BI, Cheskin LJ, Sohn N, Sommer SC. The fate of the rectal segment after diversion of the fecal stream in Crohn's disease: its implications for surgical management. *J Clin Gastroenterol*, 1985; 7: 37.
542 Harper PH, Lee EC, Kettlewell MGW, Bennett MK, Jewell DP. Role of the faecal stream in the maintenance of Crohn's colitis. *Gut*, 1985; 26: 279.
543 Griffiths AP, Dixon MF. Microcarcinoids and diversion colitis in a colon defunctioned for 18 years. Report of a case. *Dis Colon Rectum*, 1992; 35: 685.
544 Killinback MJ, Lloyd Williams K. Necrotizing colitis. *Br J Surg*, 1962; 49: 175.
545 Wade DS, Nara HR, Douglas HO. Neutropenic enterocolitis—clinical diagnosis and treatment. *Cancer* 1992; 69: 17.
546 Newbold KM, Lord MG, Bagun TP. Role of clostridial organisms in neutropenic enterocolitis. *J Clin Pathol*, 1987; 40: 471.
547 Kay AW, Richards RL, Watson AJ. Acute necrotizing (pseudomembranous) enterocolitis. *Br J Surg*, 1958; 46: 45.
548 Williams LF, Anastasia LF, Hasiokis CA, Bosniak MA, Byrne JJ. Non-occlusive mesenteric infarction. *Am J Surg*, 1967; 114: 374.
549 Mullhaupt B, Guller U, Anabitarte M, Guller R, Fried M. Lymphocytic colitis: clinical presentation and long term course. *Gut*, 1998; 43: 629.
550 Taylor JT, Dodds WJ, Gonys JE, Komorowski RA. Typhlitis in adults. *Gastrointest Radiol*, 1985; 10: 363.
551 Alt B, Glass N, Sollinger H. Neutropenic enterocolitis in adults. *Am J Surg*, 1985; 149: 405.
552 Kies MS, Luedke DW, Boyd JF, McCue MJ. Neutropenic enterocolitis. *Cancer*, 1979; 43: 730.
553 Moir DH, Bale PM. Necropsy findings in childhood leukemia emphasizing neutropenic enterocolitis and cerebral calcification. *Pathology*, 1976; 8: 247.
554 Mulholland MW, Delaney JP. Neutropenic colitis and aplastic anaemia. *Ann Surg*, 1983; 197: 81.
555 King A, Rampling A, Wight DGD, Warren RE. Neutropenic enterocolitis due to *Clostridium septicu*m infection. *J Clin Pathol*, 1984; 37: 335.
556 Rifkin GD. Neutropenic enterocolitis and *Clostridium septicum* infection in patients with agranulocytosis. *Arch Intern Med*, 1980; 140: 834.
557 Santulli TV, Schullinger JN, Heird WC *et al.* Acute necrotising enterocolitis in infancy: a review of 64 cases. *Pediatrics*, 1975; 55: 376.
558 Kleigman RM, Fanaroff AA. Neonatal necrotising enterocolitis, a nine year experience. 1. Epidemiology and uncommon observations. *Am J Dis Child*, 1981; 135: 603.
559 Kleigman RM, Fanaroff AA. Neonatal necrotising enterocolitis, a nine year experience. 2. Outcome assessment. *Am J Dis Child*, 1981; 135: 608.
560 Rosen Y, Woon OKH. Phlegmonous enterocolitis. *Am J Dig Dis*, 1978; 23: 248.
561 Kleigman RM, Fanaroff AA. Neonatal necrotising enterocolitis in the absence of pneumatosis intestinalis. *Am J Dis Child*, 1982; 136: 618.
562 Howard FM, Flynn DM, Bradley JM, Noone P, Szawattcowski M. Outbreak of necrotising enterocolitis caused by *Clostridium butyricum*. *Lancet*, 1977; ii: 1099.
563 Lindstrom CG. 'Collagenous colitis' with watery diarrhoea—a new entity? *Pathol Eur*, 1976; 11: 87.
564 Bogomoletz WV. Collagenous colitis: a clinicopathological review. *Surv Dig Dis*, 1983; 1: 19.
565 Kingham JGC, Levison DA, Ball JA, Dawson AM. Microscopic colitis—a case of chronic watery diarrhoea. *Br Med J*, 1982; 285: 1601.
566 Bohr J, Tysk C, Jarnerot G. Microscopic colitis. *Medicine*, 1998; 26:93.
567 Jessurun J, Yardley JH, Lee EL, Vendrell DD, Schiller LR, Fordtran JS. Microscopic and collagenous colitis: different names for the same condition? *Gastroenterology*, 1986; 91: 1583.
568 Bogomoletz WV, Adnet JJ, Birembaut P, Feydy P, Dupont P. Collagenous colitis: an unrecognised entity. *Gut*, 1980; 21: 164.
569 Williams GT, Rhodes J. Collagenous colitis: disease or diversion. *Br Med J*, 1987; 294: 855.
570 Lazenby AJ, Yardley JH, Giardello FM, Jessurlen J, Bayless T. Lymphocytic ('microscopic') colitis: a comparative histopathologic study with particular reference to collagenous colitis. *Hum Pathol*, 1989; 20: 18.
571 Read NW, Krejs GJ, Read MG *et al.* Chronic diarrhoea of unknown origin. *Gastroenterology*, 1980; 78: 264.
572 Rask-Madsen J, Grove O, Hansen MGJ, Bulchave K, H-Nielsen R. Colonic transport of water and electrolytes in a patient with secretory diarrhoea due to collagenous colitis. *Dig Dis Sci*, 1983; 28: 1141.
573 Fausa O, Foerster A, Hovig T. Collagenous colitis. A clinical histological and ultrastructural study. *Scand J Gastroenterol*, 1985; 20 (Suppl 107): 8.
574 Farah DA, Mills PR, Lee FD, McLay A, Russell RI. Collagenous colitis: possible response to sulfasalazine and local steroid therapy. *Gastroenterology*, 1985; 88: 792.
575 Gledhill A, Cole FM. Significance of basement membrane thickening in the human colon. *Gut*, 1984; 25: 1085.
576 Bossart R, Henry K, Booth CC, Doe WF. Subepithelial collagen in intestinal malabsorption. *Gut*, 1975; 16: 18.
577 Rampton DS, Baithum SI. Is microscopic colitis due to bile salt malabsorption? *Dis Colon Rectum*, 1987; 30: 950.
578 Christ AD, Meier R, Bauerfeind P, Wegmann W, Gyr K. Simultaneous lymphocytic gastritis and lymphocytic colitis, with development of collagenous colitis. *Schweiz Med Wochenscr*, 1993; 123: 1487.
579 Saul SH. The watery diarrhoea–colitis syndrome. A review of collagenous and microscopic/lymphocytic colitis. *Int J Surg Pathol*, 1993; 1: 65.
580 Bo-Linn GW, Vendrell DD, Lee E, Fordtran JS. An evaluation of the significance of microscopic colitis in patients with chronic diarrhoea. *Clin Invest*, 1985; 75: 1559.
581 Hamilton I, Sanders S, Hopwood D, Bouchier IAD. Collagenous colitis associated with small bowel villous atrophy. 1986; 27: 1394.
582 Bogomoletz WV. Collagenous, microscopic and lymphocytic colitis: an evolving concept. *Virchows Arch A Pathol Anat*, 1994; 424: 573.
583 Fine KD, Lee EL, Meyer RL. Colonic histopathology in untreated celiac sprue or refractory sprue: is it lymphocytic colitis or colonic lymphocytosis? *Hum Pathol*, 1998; 29: 1433.
584 Dubois RN, Lazenby AAJ, Yardley JH *et al.* Lymphocytic enterocolitis in patients with 'refractory sprue'. *JAMA*, 1989; 262: 935.
585 Fraser AG, Warren BF, Chandrapala R, Jewell DP. Microscopic colitis: a clinical and pathological review. *Scand J Gastroenterol*, in press.
586 Jessurun J, Yardley JH, Guardello FM, Hamilton SR, Bayless TM. Chronic colitis with thickening of the subepithelial collagen layer (collagenous colitis). *Hum Pathol*, 1987; 18: 839.

587 Teglbjaerg PS, Thaysen EH, Jensen HH. Development of collagenous colitis in sequential biopsy specimens. *Gastroenterology*, 1984; 87: 703.

588 Hwang WS, Kelly JK, Shaffer E, Hershfield NB. Collagenous colitis: a disease of pericryptal fibroblast sheath? *J Pathol*, 1986; 149: 33.

589 Librecht L, Ectors N, Staels F, Geboes K. Microscopic colitis with giant cells. *Histopathology*, 2002; 40: 335.

590 Richman PI, Tilly R, Jass JR, Bodmer WF. Colonic pericrypt sheath cells: characterization of cell type with new monoclonal antibodies. *J Clin Pathol*, 1987; 40: 593.

591 Pascal RR, Kaye GI, Lane N. Colonic pericryptal fibroblast sheath: replication, migration and cytodifferentiation of a mesenchymal cell system in adult tissue. *Gastroenterology*, 1986; 54: 835.

592 Kaye GI, Fenoglis CM, Pascal RR, Lane N. Comparative electron microscopic features of normal hyperplastic and adenomatous human colonic epithelium. *Gastroenterology*, 1973; 64: 926.

593 Blei ED, Abrahams C. Diffuse phlegmonous gastroenterocolitis in a patient with an infected peritoneojugular venous shunt. *Gastroenterology*, 1983; 84: 636.

594 Mathan MM, Mathan VI. Rectal mucosal morphologic abnormalities in normal subjects in Southern India: a tropical colopathy. *Gut*, 1985; 26: 710.

595 Levine TS, Price AB. Obstructive enterocolitis: a clinicopathological discussion. *Histopathology*, 1994; 25: 57.

37 Vascular disorders of the large intestine

Anatomy

The colon is supplied by both the superior mesenteric and the inferior mesenteric arteries. The latter artery becomes the superior rectal (haemorrhoidal) artery when it crosses the pelvic brim. It supplies most of the rectum, bifurcating into left and right branches which pass downwards on either side of the mesorectum. The middle and inferior rectal (haemorrhoidal) arteries, derived from the internal iliac and pudendal arteries, respectively, contribute to the blood supply of the lower rectum. Two important anastomotic links exist between the inferior and superior mesenteric arteries which, following occlusion of one of the major vessels, have a role in maintaining the viability of the bowel. The marginal artery is an arterial arcade situated along the mesocolic surface of the entire colon, connecting the main branches of the inferior and superior mesenteric vessels. The second anastomotic link is the 'arc of Riolan' between the left colic artery and the middle colic artery. The splenic flexure is potentially a vulnerable region, being at the junction of the main distribution zones of the superior and inferior mesenteric vessels. However, injection studies suggest that there is not consistently a 'watershed' at this point and an analysis of cases reveals more lower left-sided ischaemic colitis than disease at the splenic flexure [1,2]. Venous return is to the portal system. The internal rectal plexus outside the rectal wall communicates via the superior and inferior rectal veins with the portal and systemic venous systems, respectively. Portosystemic anastomoses are present around the lower rectum and anus.

Causes of ischaemic colitis

Ischaemic injury to the large bowel can be the result of either arterial or venous impairment. The aetiology and pathogenesis are very similar to those affecting the small bowel and are listed in Table 23.1 and discussed in Chapter 23.

The inferior mesenteric artery, like its superior counterpart, is liable to atheromatous narrowing, especially at its origin from the aorta, and the same factors of gradual arterial occlusion, more acute blockage and hypotension, which can cause ischaemia in the small intestine, are equally applicable in the large. Venous thrombosis or obstruction also have similar effects and ischaemic lesions in the large bowel, whether full thickness, with gangrene, or less extensive, with predominantly mucosal damage and subsequent stricture formation, bear a striking similarity to those seen in the small bowel.

As with small intestinal ischaemia, in up to 30% of cases no vascular lesion is evident. Thus, ischaemic colitis can occur purely as a result of shock [3], in marathon runners [4], or may sometimes be truly idiopathic.

In those cases in which no cause is immediately apparent, it is important to remember that drugs can be responsible for ischaemic colitis. Most frequent causes among these are non-steroidal anti-inflammatory drugs, which tend to affect the right side of the colon more than the left and, in addition to flat ulcers, can cause diaphragm-like strictures [5]. Other drugs shown to cause ischaemic colitis are cocaine [6,7], pseudoephedrine [8] widely used in patent cough medicines, and 5-hydroxytryptamine agonists used in the treatment of migraine, such as sumatriptan [9].

Nomenclature

The aetiology of ischaemia and its rate of onset determine the pathology of ischaemic colitis just as in the small bowel. The spectrum ranges from infarction and gangrene [10] to fleeting transient episodes [11,12]. Between these two is a slow-onset pattern, usually chronic and progressing to a stricture. In the past, phrases such as 'haemorrhagic necrotizing colitis' or enterocolitis have been used to describe acute intestinal ischaemia (p. 519). For the pathologist, ischaemic colitis remains a useful term as it clearly demarcates the aetiology from inflammatory bowel disease. It can be qualified by terms reflecting severity and duration of the ischaemic episode [13]. In the acute ischaemic conditions a major aetiological problem is the role of bacteria, in particular clostridial species. Ischaemic mucosa is more susceptible to secondary invasion by such organisms. On the other hand *Clostridium difficile* is the primary agent in pseudomembranous colitis [14,15]. This conflict remains to be resolved in such conditions as necrotizing enteritis (p. 277) and neonatal necrotizing enterocolitis (p. 352). A milder form of colitis in infancy, associated with overgrowth of enteric bacteria, has been termed 'ecchymotic colitis' [16].

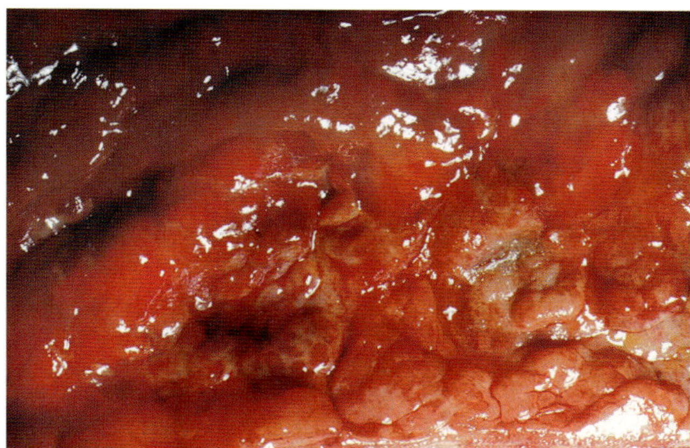

Fig. 37.1 Acute ischaemic necrosis (infarction) of the colon. The mucosa is deeply congested and thrown into coarse cobblestone-like folds due to submucosal oedema and haemorrhage. This gives the radiological sign of 'thumbprinting'.

Ischaemic lesions

The reaction of the colon to ischaemia can be divided into three phases [1]: acute, with haemorrhage and necrosis [2]; reparative, with granulation tissue formation and fibrosis; and [3] residual pathology, with ischaemic stricture and chronic complications [2]. The same morphological classification can also be applied to ischaemic disease of the small intestine (see Chapter 23).

The location and extent of ischaemic lesions in the colon are a reflection of the anatomy and physiology of the blood supply. It is not generally realized that, compared to the small bowel, the colon has a relatively poor blood supply and this is particularly true of the left side. The importance of the anastomotic vessels between the superior and inferior mesenteric vessels has already been mentioned (p. 540). In a review of over 1000 cases of ischaemic colitis, the distribution was right colon 8%, transverse colon 15%, splenic flexure 23%, descending colon 27%, sigmoid colon 23% and rectum 4% [17]. Rectal involvement is being recognized with increasing frequency [17–20], can result in gross appearances resembling carcinoma [21] and can occur after aortic surgery [22]. There are a few case reports of caecal ischaemia [23], and right-sided disease was reported in 25% of one series of ischaemic colitis [24]. It must be remembered that combined involvement of small and large intestine is not infrequent [25,26]. The susceptibility of the colon to ischaemia can be demonstrated at autopsy when careful microscopic examination often reveals early mucosal lesions, many of which are agonal in nature.

Macroscopic appearance

Compared with the small bowel, the appearances of infarction of the colon vary according to the length of history prior to examination either of a surgical specimen or at autopsy. In the early stages the bowel is dilated and darkly congested with red, oedematous mucosa [10] (Fig. 37.1). The wall is friable and is usually thinner than normal. Mucosal ulceration can be superficial only, but is sometimes deep and typically linear in distribution. Sometimes ulceration is confluent and extensive. The lumen is filled with altered blood and there is an inflammatory peritoneal reaction, sometimes with frank perforation. Inflammatory polyposis due to undermining ulceration of mucosa with the formation of mucosal tags is not uncommon. The whole appearance can mimic that seen in fulminating ulcerative colitis with toxic megacolon. When infarction of the colon involves only part of the thickness of the wall, mucosal necrosis may give rise to a shaggy white or grey membrane loosely adherent to the surface. This is the basis of the confusion with pseudomembranous colitis. In some cases patches of gangrene are present due to complete necrosis of the tissues of the bowel wall—so-called necrotizing colitis (see p. 519). Similar segmental lesions occur in the small bowel [27].

In patients who survive an episode of infarction for some days or longer, then signs of resolution will appear. The bowel wall becomes thicker, contracted and indurated. The very dark appearance is replaced by signs of revascularization. These changes fade imperceptibly into the stage of ischaemic stricture. With the formation of a stricture and the disappearance of any acute changes the macroscopic picture may be less specifically ischaemic and may resemble Crohn's disease.

The vascular supply to the bowel wall should always be examined for evidence of thrombosis or anatomical abnormality of a main vessel, remembering that an occlusion may not be demonstrable in 20–32% of cases [2,28]. At autopsy the abdominal aorta and origins of the main mesenteric vessels should be inspected for evidence of thromboses [29].

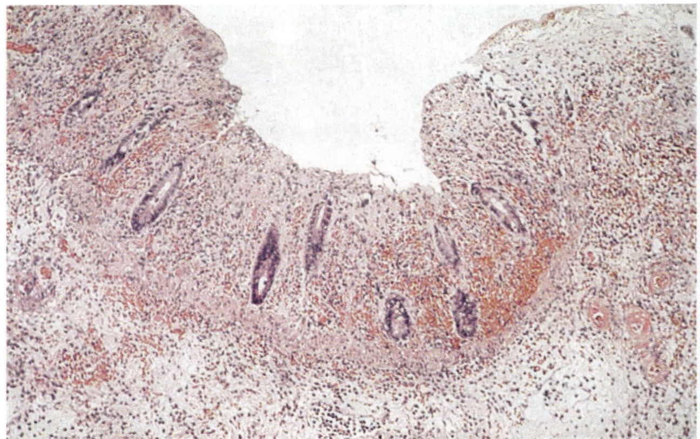

Fig. 37.2 Acute colonic ischaemia, showing dissolution of the upper parts of the crypts, with an impression that those remaining are 'bursting' (e.g. right of field). The lamina propria contains haemorrhagic acute inflammtory exudate.

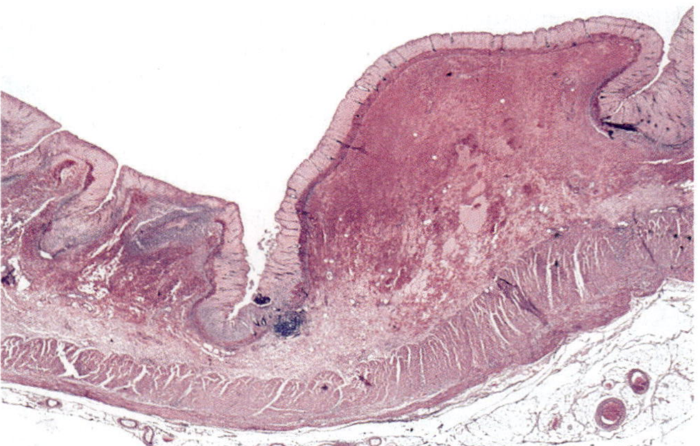

Fig. 37.3 Acute colonic ischaemia, with mucosal necrosis (pale zone), prominent submucosal oedema and haemorrhage.

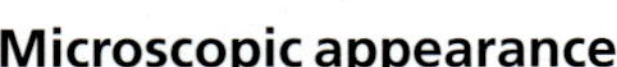

Microscopic appearance

Acute ischaemia

The microscopic pathology of infarcted colon is distinctive and may be readily distinguished from acute ulcerative colitis and other inflammatory bowel diseases. There is haemorrhage into the mucosa and sometimes the submucosa, with oedema and necrosis. The mucosal crypts often appear to be 'bursting' and are covered with a surface deposit of fibrin and necrotic tissue (Fig. 37.2). In severe cases only a shadowy outline of the normal histology remains. Gram stains will often reveal colonies of bacteria, particularly *Clostridia*, in the mucosa and submucosa.

There is only a moderate leucocytic infiltration during the early stages, but this increases later and is accompanied by sloughing with mucosal ulceration. Fibrin thrombi within mucosal and submucosal capillaries are particularly characteristic [10,30]. Frequently, following ischaemic ulceration, there is an acute endophlebitis of veins draining the ulcerated areas, within the submucosa and bowel wall (Fig. 37.3). This may even extend along the veins to involve the extramural mesenteric veins, in the manner of a pyelophlebitis. It has been suggested that such a picture can arise *de novo*, and be the *cause* rather than the effect of ischaemic ulceration (see below) but this can be very difficult to confirm in an individual case.

In many examples of acute ischaemic disease of the colon the histological changes are confined to the mucosa and submucosa. This is usually patchy with intact normal intervening mucosa which is raised up by submucosal oedema or haemorrhage (Fig. 37.3). This gives a cobblestone appearance which accounts for the diagnostic 'thumbprinting' radiological sign. It would appear that the muscularis propria is relatively resistant to the effects of acute deprivation of blood. However, as in early small intestinal ischaemia, the muscle fibres can show impaired staining and loss of nuclei.

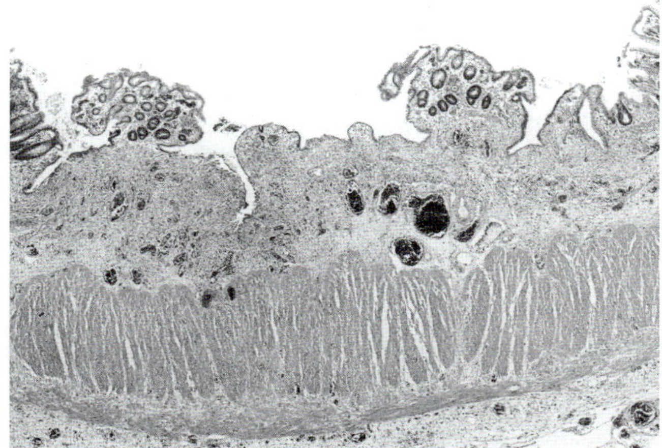

Fig. 37.4 Fissuring ulceration with submucosal granulation tissue in ischaemic colitis. Re-epithelialization is occurring on the surface.

Reparative phase

The effects of acute ischaemia are followed by subacute and chronic inflammation with the formation of granulation tissue and a mixed population of acute and chronic inflammatory cells. Capillary proliferation, macrophage activity and fibroblast production complete the picture until the mucosal epithelium begins to regenerate. Microscopic fissures may lead down to or into the muscularis propria at points of deeper anoxic damage (Fig. 37.4). Entrapped particles of foreign material may provoke a giant cell reaction. The granulation tissue reaction is generally exuberant and, in conjunction with the residual islands of inflamed and sometimes hyperplastic mucosal glands, presents a pattern mimicking Crohn's disease or active fulminant ulcerative colitis. Eosinophil leucocytes and iron pigment-laden histiocytes are a variable element. The presence of iron-positive granules in histiocytes reflects previous haemorrhage in the submucosa and mucosa and is important in differentiating ischaemia from inflammatory bowel disease. Epithelial cell regeneration is visible at the margin of the mucosal ulcers in the form of young cells growing in a thin sheet over the bed of inflamed granulation tissue or mingling with the fibrin, leucocyte exudate and the population of lymphocytes and histiocytes on the gut luminal surface. Bacteria can sometimes be demonstrated at the mucosal surface but rarely penetrate deep tissues unless gangrene is present. The regenerating epithelium can show such florid hyperplastic changes that, to the unwary, confusion with dysplasia is possible [31].

Ischaemic strictures

Most cases of severe and extensive infarction of the colon never reach the stage of stricture because the small intestine is also involved and the patient dies of shock. Because of this, most ischaemic strictures treated by surgical excision are relatively short. They are uncommon in the right colon and are rare in the rectum. They occur relatively frequently in the left colon, at the 'watershed 'of the blood supply between the territories of the superior and inferior mesenteric arteries, although, as mentioned above [1,17], they may not be as specifically located at the splenic flexure as has been alleged. Ischaemic colitis in general, as mentioned earlier, predominates in the descending and sigmoid colon. The strictures may be tubular or fusiform (Fig. 37.5) and in some there is striking sacculation of the gut wall (Fig. 37.6). In all cases there is obvious fibrosis which may extend deeply into the pericolic tissue. The submucosa is characteristically widened and filled with white granulation tissue (Fig. 37.7). Mucosal ulceration tends to be patchy. The differential diagnosis from segmental Crohn's disease of the colon may be difficult prior to microscopic examination. The principal histological features of ischaemic stricture (Figs 37.8a,b) are seen in all layers of the bowel wall. The mucosa shows patchy atrophy and irregularity of crypts, typical of healed ulceration. There may be persisting ulceration, lined by granulation tissue packed with dilated capillaries. There is splaying of the fibres and fibrosis of the muscularis mucosae. The submucosal layer is initially widened and filled with oedematous granulation tissue, with conspicuous fibroblasts and a sprinkling of chronic inflammatory cells, including lymphocytes, eosinophils and plasma cells. As the healing progresses, the submucosa becomes less cellular, denser and thinner. Fibrous tissue extends downwards between the fasciculi of the inner part of the circular muscle, which become attenuated and separated (Fig. 37.8c). At the edge of ulcerated areas epithelial regeneration is present with columnar epithelium beginning to grow over the surface (Fig. 37.8a). Neighbouring intact mucosa is not always normal but shows patchy atrophy and irregularity of crypts, suggestive of healing with incomplete restitution. Macrophages containing haemosiderin pigment are sometimes a prominent feature of the cellular infiltrate and, when present, are of considerable diagnostic help. The submucosal arterioles tend to be thick walled and tortuous. There is often prominent fibrinoid necrosis in the walls of submucosal

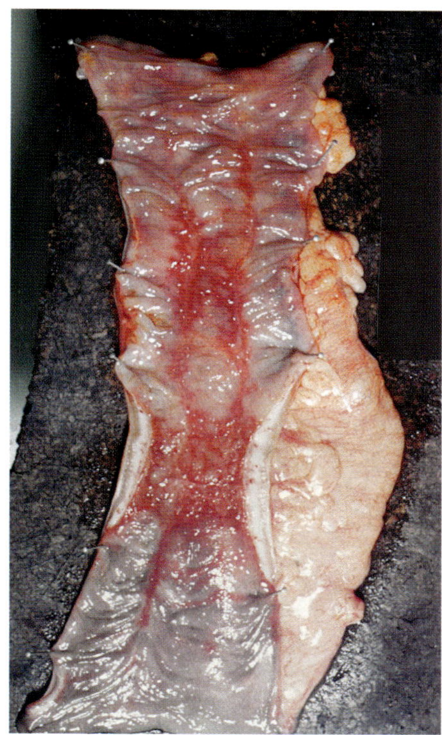

Fig. 37.5 Fusiform ischaemic stricture of descending colon. The submucosa at the site of the stricture is thickened by white fibrous tissue. There is longitudinal linear ulceration of the mucosa above and below the stricture, together with cobblestone-like thickening of folds due to submucosal oedema.

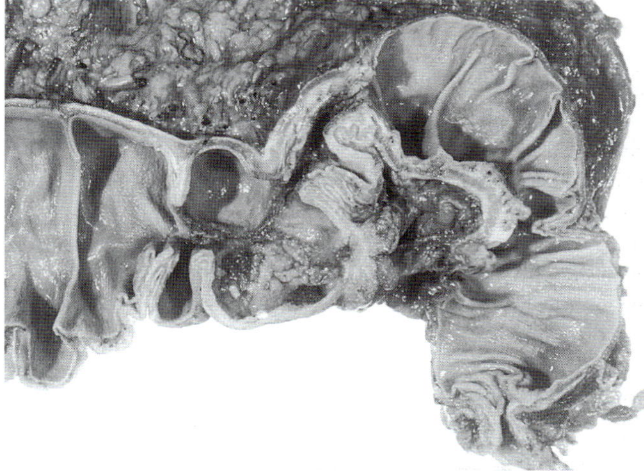

Fig. 37.6 Ischaemic stricture of splenic flexure of colon. There is stenosis with sacculation and linear mucosal ulceration.

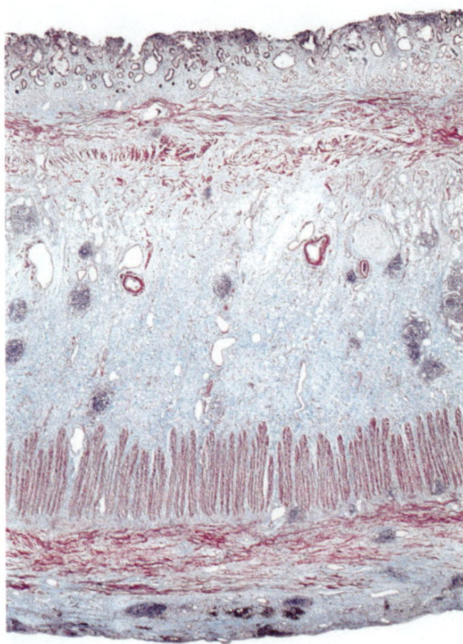

Fig. 37.7 Longitudinal section from an ischaemic colonic stricture, showing widening of the submucosa by oedema (with granulation tissue formation).

vessels near the surface of the ulcerated bowel but this is probably due to proximity to the reparative inflammatory process rather than a primary arteritis. The muscularis propria in ischaemic stricture is relatively spared but may show patchy fibrosis with replacement and separation of its fibres by granulation tissue (Fig. 37.8b) identical and continuous with that seen in the submucosal layer. The inflammatory process also involves the serosa and pericolic tissues but this is always patchy.

The histological picture at this stage of ischaemic colitis strongly resembles the appearances in the healing phase of myocardial ischaemia, and is distinct from the microscopic pathology of idiopathic proctocolitis or Crohn's disease. Transmural hyperplasia of lymphoid tissue, intramural fissuring and sarcoid granulomas are conspicuously absent. Crypt abscesses are only occasionally seen. Conversely, haemosiderin-laden macrophages have not been noted in the inflammatory infiltrate of proctocolitis or Crohn's disease.

Ischaemic colitis has been produced in animals, and it is interesting that the histology of the lesions resembles those in human disease with certain species differences [32].

Transient or evanescent ischaemic colitis

Apart from full-thickness infarction of the colon with gangrene and perforation or superficial infarction with healing and later stricture formation, there is also a transient or reversible form of ischaemia [33,34]. In a typical case there is a short illness characterized by cramping abdominal pain and diarrhoea with minimal to moderate rectal bleeding and with radiological features of ischaemia which quickly revert to normal. Although the diagnosis is usually clinical, the pathologist may obtain material either when the disease involves the rectum or sigmoid colon [12], or from colonoscopy if more proximal disease is present [35,36]. Sequential biopsies show features of acute haemorrhagic necrosis of the mucosa with a subsequent return to normal or to a regenerative mucosal pattern (Fig. 37.9) [12,35]. Transient or prodromal episodes may be a part of chronic ischaemia in the patients described by Marston who have major vessel stenosis [37]. Somewhat confusingly, the term 'transient colitis' has also been used as a synonym for 'acute self-limited colitis' to describe patients with the clinical picture of infective colitis but who are culture negative [38] (p. 525). Thus, such a diagnostic classification needs qualification by the words 'ischaemic' or 'infective' to denote the likely aetiology. Transient ischaemic disease may also be part of the pathological picture produced by the contraceptive pill [39].

Obstructive colitis

Obstructive colitis occurs proximal to 1–5% of obstructing colorectal lesions [17]. The obstruction is most frequently either a tumour or diverticular disease [40], but any disturbance of motility can be responsible. Thus, obstructive colitis occurs proximal to the affected segment in Hirschsprung's disease, in pseudo-obstruction, whether idiopathic or due to other conditions, in constipation, especially when faeces become impacted [41], and as an effect of certain drugs which impair motility, such as chlorpromazine [42]. It is important to remember that distal active ulcerative colitis interrupts normal peristalsis, leading to a form of pseudo-obstruction. This will cause mild diffuse chronic inflammation in the proximal colon which may mislead the pathologist to overinterpret the extent of the ulcerative colitis. However, inflammation in the latter circumstance is rarely severe, with only occasional scattered crypt abscesses and no ulceration. In contrast, obstructive colitis secondary to the other causes listed above often leads to deep punched-out and longitudinal linear ulcers covered by fibrinopurulent material with congestion and haemorrhage of adjacent mucosa which can be elevated due to submucosal oedema. Perforation sometimes occurs [40,41]. Occasionally, especially in neonates and the elderly, there is a severe necrotizing colitis. This is more fully described under the heading 'Necrotizing enterocolitis' in Chapter 23. In nearly all cases described the colitis has been proximal to the obstruction and separated from it by a short zone of relatively normal mucosa. The histology is essentially the same as for the earlier stages of ischaemic bowel disease and in severe cases can be that of 'indeterminate colitis' (see p. 509). The bowel may be massively distended [40] and perforation can occur [41]. It has been sug-

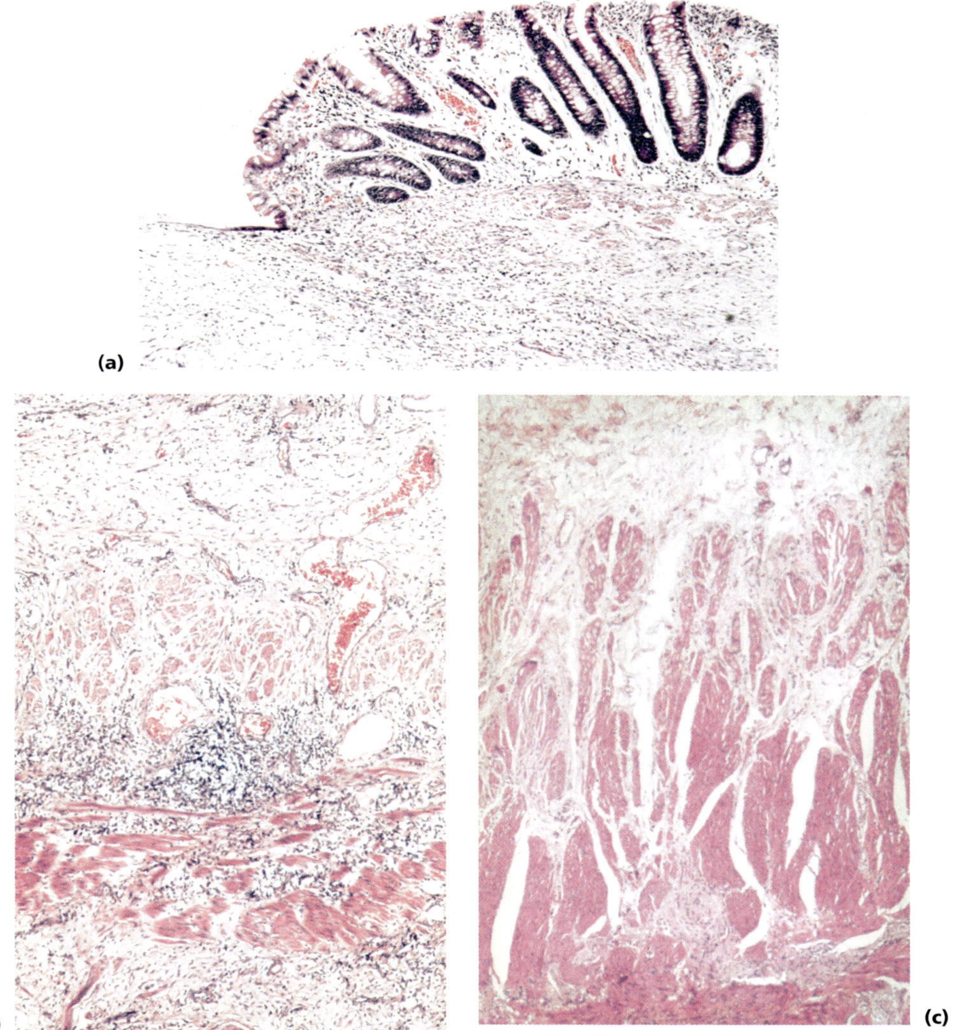

Fig. 37.8 (a) Histology of ischaemic colitis. Regenerating epithelium is growing over the edge of ulcerated mucosa. The submucosa is filled with granulation tissue. (b) Ischaemic colitis. The bundles of the muscularis propria are separated by young fibrous tissue. Note the chronic inflammatory cell infiltrate, most prominent in the region of the myenteric plexus, more loosely arranged than in Crohn's disease and unlike ulcerative colitis. (c) Healing phase of ischaemic colitis. There is maturation of the fibrous tissue which separates the fascicles of the muscularis propria.

gested [43] that a rise in intraluminal pressure related to the obstruction results in a fall in the intramural blood flow with resulting ischaemic necrosis. Many of the cases reported are on the right side which is to be expected as segments of colon with the largest diameter have the greatest mural tension, this acting to occlude mucosal circulation [44]. When this factor is added to others, such as stagnation of faecal material, proliferation of luminal flora, perhaps hypermobility and straining to overcome the obstruction, it is surprising that ischaemic bowel disease and colorectal carcinoma do not occur together more commonly. However, obstructive colitis does manifest itself more frquently in the elderly, who may also have a background of generalized atherosclerosis and cardiac insufficiency. It is obviously important to distinguish the ischaemic picture of obstructive colitis and antecedent carcinoma from malignant change in ulcerative colitis.

Endoscopic features and biopsy

The endoscopic features depend on the stage of ischaemia. In acute ischaemia the mucosa appears swollen and bluish purple with contact bleeding [36]. There may be focal left-sided ulceration. When a stricture is present it may be difficult to distinguish the appearances from Crohn's disease, especially if no adjacent mucosal abnormalities are present [40].

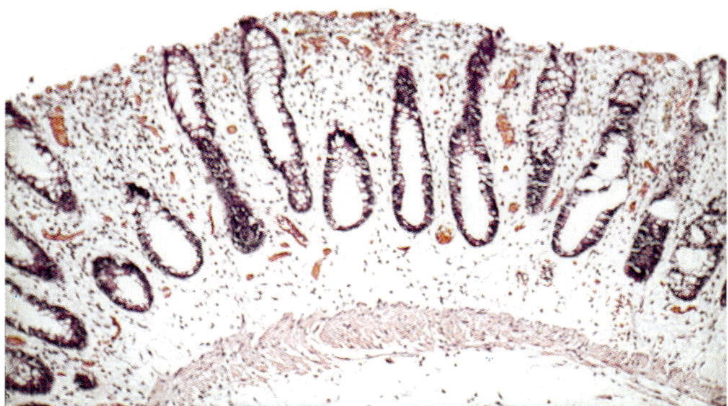

Fig. 37.9 A colonoscopic biopsy from a patient with a self-limiting episode of ischaemic colitis, showing oedema and some haemorrhage but with little inflammation. The crypt epithelium is regenerating.

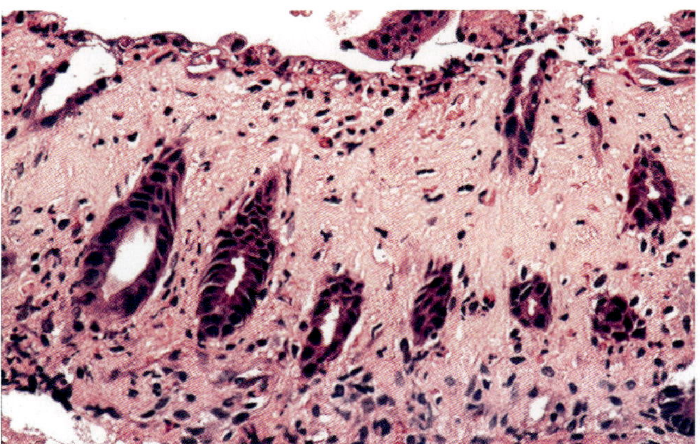

Fig. 37.10 Ischaemic colitis in a woman of 50 with abdominal pain and blood mixed with the stool. Barium enema showed thumbprinting in the region of the splenic flexure. On colonoscopy there was linear ulceration at the splenic flexure. This biopsy of splenic flexure mucosa shows degenerative damage to the epithelium of the surface with 'withering' of the crypts. The luminal half of the lamina propria is eosinophilic partly due to collagen but partly due to fibrin. This should not be confused with the discrete abnormal collagen band seen in collagenous colitis.

In chronic ischaemic proctitis white mucosal scars can be detected at sigmoidoscopy [18].

Biopsy is seldom carried out or warranted in acute gangrenous ischaemia, being more usual in non-resolving disease and in evanescent colitis [12]. Characteristic of such less severe disease is the damage to the superficial half of the mucosa (Fig. 37.10) [25]. The epithelial cells appear flattened or degenerate and there can be complete loss of occasional crypts (Fig. 37.11). The more severe the ischaemia the greater will be the crypt loss. The lamina propria takes on a dense eosinophilic quality. Inflammatory cells are present in small numbers compared to ulcerative colitis and Crohn's disease, whilst any submucosa present can appear oedematous.

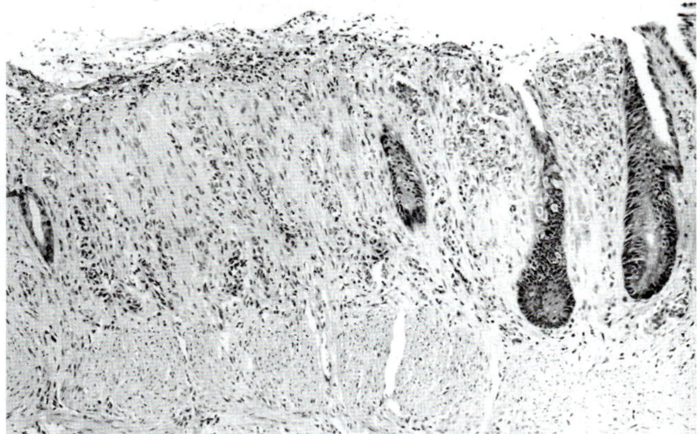

Fig. 37.11 In this colonic mucosal biopsy there is advanced ischaemic damage, with cellular fibrous tissue within the lamina propria as well as loss of crypts.

Biopsy during the recovering phases of ischaemia will show regenerative hyperplasia of the crypts. They can be distorted and, depending on the initial severity, present a varying picture of crypt atrophy. Fibrosis of the lamina propria is to be expected with healing. There is little inflammation but iron-laden macrophages are a characteristic feature.

The diagnosis is relatively straightforward when an arteritis or vascular occlusion is found, providing the latter is primary. Thus, it must be seen well away from any area of ulceration. Occluded vessels in the base of an ulcer are more usually a secondary event.

The differential diagnosis of the acute ischaemic biopsy is from pseudomembranous colitis, infection and collagenous colitis. If there is severe mucosal necrosis a distinction from the type III lesion of pseudomembranous colitis may not be possible (p. 517). Although there is damage to the superficial half of the crypts in both the early lesions of pseudomembranous colitis and ischaemia, in the latter they look thinned and degenerate rather than distended by mucinous debris as in the former. The degenerative look to the upper half of the crypts in ischaemia (Fig. 37.10a) can also resemble the crypt 'withering' characteristic of infective colitis (p. 478). However, the accompanying inflammatory changes in infection are very different. Occasionally the eosinophilia of the lamina propria, particularly in those cases of ischaemic colitis in which there is conspicuous inflammatory cell infiltration, may cause confusion with collagenous colitis. A stain for collagen and the characteristic history of collagenous colitis (p. 523) resolve the problem.

In the biopsy of chronic ischaemia the crypt irregularity of healed ulceration may suggest ulcerative colitis, and from a stricture the fibrosis present can resemble Crohn's disease. Iron-laden macrophages are not seen in either of these two conditions and mucosal fibrosis, as opposed to submucosal fibrosis, is unlike Crohn's disease. Colonoscopy with biopsies demonstrating the distribution of the disease will show the diagnostic differences.

Many of the characteristic features of chronic ischaemic damage in the mucosa are to be seen in the mucosal prolapse syndrome (p. 464) and mucosal ischaemia undoubtedly occurs when mucosa prolapses, due to mechanical stress on small blood vessels.

Angiodysplasia

This vascular malformation has been claimed to be the most common cause of bleeding in the elderly [45], though, as with many sweeping statements of this nature, other workers disagree [46]. The controversy on incidence also applies to autopsy investigations with an incidence range of from 2% [47,48] up to 50% [48,49]. An angiodysplasia is best defined as an ectasia of normal pre-existing colonic submucosal veins with or without ectasia of the overlying mucosal capillaries. The contour of the mucosa is seldom altered and there is no associated clinical syndrome as there can be with telangiectasias. The lesions are commonest in the right colon [50,51] where over 70% are found [46], though in some series a more even left-sided spread has been noted [52,53]. Occasionally they are found in the small intestine and stomach. Not all lesions bleed and in one colonoscopic series they were an incidental finding in 79% of cases [53]. They can be multiple in 10–50% of cases [52,54].

The diagnosis is made by angiography, at endoscopy or on histological examination. Radionucleotide scanning may prove to be more sensitive than angiography as it can detect bleeding of rates of 0.1 mL/min, angiography requiring 0.5 mL/min [48]. The endoscopist sees prominent bright vessels radiating from a raised cherry-red central point, or a localized 7–10-mm blush of dilated superficial vessels [46]. They are friable to touch and bleed easily in contrast to 'cosmetic angiodysplasias' which are 3–6-mm red blot lesions on the mucosa that do not bleed on touch and are of no significance [46].

Macroscopically, under the dissecting microscope the normal mucosal honeycomb vascular pattern is replaced by clusters of tortuous vessels resembling a coral reef [48,55]. These ectatic mucosal capillaries communicate with enlarged submucosal veins and venules. It is the latter that are believed to be the primary and constant abnormality. However, because of the wide range in size and tortuosity of submucosal vessels [1,48], it is unwise to make the diagnosis of angiodysplasia in the absence of mucosal abnormalities [48,55]. The mucosa can present a spectrum of change from just one or two ectatic capillaries to crypts pushed apart by large numbers (Fig. 37.12) [48,56].

The pathological diagnosis is difficult both in a biopsy and in a surgical resection. In biopsy work the abnormal submucosal veins may not be sampled and the number of ectatic mucosal capillaries is variable. They also are frequently disrupted in the biopsy process. Consequently, biopsy fails to substantiate the diagnosis in up to 50% of cases [48,57].

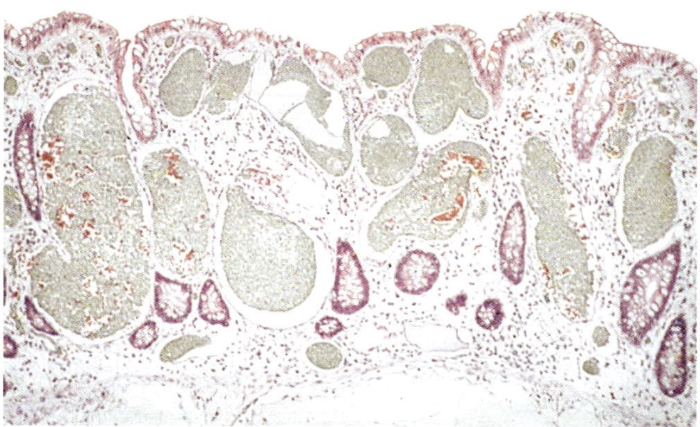

Fig. 37.12 Angiodysplasia of the colon, with abnormal vessels in the mucosa and submucosa. This is a section of a colon following arterial perfusion of an aqueous suspension of barium sulphate before fixation.

In the surgical specimen the lesions are tiny and fixation causes additional shrinkage. The cases are often surgical emergencies done at night and the bowel is well fixed by the time the pathologist inspects it next day. For a reasonable chance of identifying any angiodysplasia the bowel needs to be received fresh and unopened. The major vessels can then be sought and injected with contrast media such as barium sulphate, with or without warm gelatine solution [55]. Still unopened, the bowel should be rinsed out, then distended with formalin and fixed for 48 hours. At this stage it can be X-rayed. Only then is it opened and the mucosa inspected for lesions. Another radiograph is often helpful at this stage. If difficulty is still present the specimen can be rendered transparent using dehydration procedures [58] and examined under the dissecting microscope. An alternative method, using transillumination to examine mucosa stripped away from the deeper layers of the fixed bowel wall [59], has been claimed to avoid the need to perform vascular perfusion, but we have found it to be of only limited value.

Angiodysplasias are considered degenerative lesions [45]. They are believed to result from chronic low-grade obstruction of the submucosal veins where they traverse the muscularis propria. This occurs over a time scale of many years until the submucosal veins become dilated and tortuous. The resulting back-pressure causes further dilatation of the mucosal vessels draining into the veins. The predeliction of angiodysplasias for the right colon is due to the tension on the right side being greater than in other segments. According to Laplace's principle, the tension in the wall for a given intraluminal pressure is highest in the segment with the greatest diameter, i.e. the right colon.

Most patients with angiodysplasia are over the age of 60, but there are some well documented cases in younger patients [53,60]. Aortic stenosis may be associated with angiodysplasia [45] but is unlikely to be causally related. It seems more likely that patients with angiodysplasia will bleed if aortic stenosis is present.

Other primary vascular lesions

The majority of these conditions are considered in Chapter 23. When the colon is involved the pathology is similar to that seen in the small intestine. Polyarteritis nodosa, systemic lupus erythematosus, Wegener's granulomatosis, Behçet's disease and idiopathic enterocolic lymphocytic phlebitis are worthy of special mention here.

Polyarteritis nodosa

Segmental involvement of the colon in polyarteritis nodosa is rare but may occur as a manifestation of generalized disease or as an isolated lesion apparently confined to the bowel. The diagnosis can be made on sigmoidoscopy and we have had experience of one case of sigmoid involvement in which a rectal biopsy revealed the characteristic histology in the arterioles of the submucosal layer. A subsequent resection of the sigmoid colon was performed and the specimen showed patchy mucosal ulceration and gangrene with a curious peach-like colour of the intervening intact mucosa. The pericolic fatty tissue was indurated and microscopic examination revealed extensive fat necrosis. In other aspects, the histology was typical. Polyarteritis nodosa presenting with perforation of the colon has been reported [61].

Systemic lupus erythematosus

In addition to occasionally causing ischaemic colitis, systemic lupus erythematosus has been linked with a severe ischaemic proctitis [62].

ANCA-associated vasculitides, including Wegener's granulomatosis

In a review of six patients with Wegener's granulomatosis who developed ischaemic colitis, specific vasculitic features were seen in mucosal biopsies of three patients. Four perforations occurred and surgical intervention was required six times [63]. Other anti-neutrophil cytoplasmic antigen (ANCA)-associated vasculitides [64] such as Churg–Strauss syndrome have been reported to cause perforating colonic as well as enteric ulceration [65].

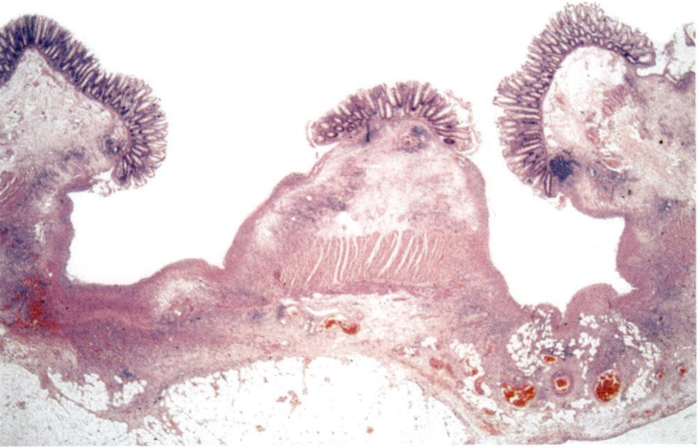

Fig. 37.13 Colonic ulceration in Behçet's disease. The ulcers are 'punched-out' and can be deep and perforating. There is a characteristic lack of inflammatory or other reaction in the tissue adjacent. This is a section of colon removed from a patient known to have Behçet's disease who presented with an acute abdomen and which was found to have perforated.

Behçet's disease

We have seen a number of patients with Behçet's disease who developed deeply penetrating multiple punched-out colonic ulcers of varying sizes with intervening normal mucosa (Fig. 37.13) [66]. Apart from the ulcers, the mucosa in these cases is normal and shows no features of either ischaemia or idiopathic inflammatory bowel disease.

Idiopathic enterocolic lymphocytic phlebitis

There have been several reports of patients with ischaemic colitis as well as ischaemic enteritis in whom the mesenteric veins show a florid mural inflammatory infiltrate, mainly lymphocytic, with or without associated thrombosis [67–69]. Despite careful documentation, it is uncertain whether this is a primary phlebitis or a secondary phenomenon following idiopathic ischaemic colitis, akin to a pyelophlebitis, such as may occur as a complication of appendicitis. In some cases the endophlebitis is granulomatous in nature [70]. Idiopathic myointimal hyperplasia of mesenteric veins [71,72], a condition in which mucosal veins in an ischaemic segment of large bowel show hyaline mural thickening with luminal occlusion, may be a late reparative stage of enterocolic lymphocytic phlebitis [68].

References

1 Binns JC, Isaacson P. Age-related changes in the colonic blood supply: their relevance to ischaemic colitis. *Gut*, 1978; 19 (5): 384.

2 Alschibaya T, Morson BC. Ischaemic bowel disease. *J Clin Pathol*, 1977; 30 (Suppl 11): 68.

3 Zeitz M. Shock-associated nonocclusive ischemic colitis: a very rare event in young patients after trauma. *Int J Colorectal Dis*, 2001; 16 (1): 58.

4 Lucas W, Schroy PC III. Reversible ischemic colitis in a high endurance athlete. *Am J Gastroenterol*, 1998; 93 (11): 2231.

5 Puspok A, Kiener HP, Oberhuber G. Clinical, endoscopic, and histologic spectrum of nonsteroidal anti-inflammatory drug-induced lesions in the colon. *Dis Colon Rectum*, 2000; 43 (5): 685.

6 Niazi M, Kondru A, Levy J, Bloom AA. Spectrum of ischemic colitis in cocaine users. *Dig Dis Sci*, 1997; 42 (7): 1537.

7 Linder JD, Monkemuller KE, Raijman I, Johnson L, Lazenby AJ, Wilcox CM. Cocaine-associated ischemic colitis. *South Med J*, 2000; 93 (9): 909.

8 Dowd J, Bailey D, Moussa K, Nair S, Doyle R, Culpepper-Morgan JA. Ischemic colitis associated with pseudoephedrine: four cases. *Am J Gastroenterol*, 1999; 94 (9): 2430.

9 Knudsen JF, Friedman B, Chen M, Goldwasser JE. Ischemic colitis and sumatriptan use. *Arch Intern Med*, 1998; 158 (17): 1946.

10 McGovern VJ, Goulston SJM. Ischaemic enterocolitis. *Gut*, 1965; 6: 213.

11 Heron HC, Khubchandani IT, Trimpi HD, Sheets JA, Stasik JJ. Evanescent colitis. *Dis Colon Rectum*, 1981; 24 (7): 555.

12 Dawson MA, Schaefer JW. The clinical course of reversible ischemic colitis. Observations on the progression of sigmoidoscopic and histological changes. *Gastroenterology*, 1971; 60 (4): 577.

13 Marston A. Ischaemia. *Clin Gastroenterol*, 1985; 14 (4): 847.

14 Bartlett JG, Chang TW, Gurwith M, Gorbach SL, Onderdonk AB. Antibiotic-associated pseudomembranous colitis due to toxin-producing clostridia. *N Engl J Med*, 1978; 298 (10): 531.

15 Larson HE, Price AB. Pseudomembranous colitis. Presence of clostridial toxin. *Lancet*, 1977; 2 (8052 8053): 1312.

16 Canioni D, Pauliat S, Gaillard JL *et al*. Histopathology and microbiology of isolated rectal bleeding in neonates: the so-called 'ecchymotic colitis'. *Histopathology*, 1997; 30 (5): 472.

17 Reeders JWAJ, Tytgat GNJ, Rosenbusch G, Gratama S. *Ischaemic Colitis*. The Hague: Martinus-Nijhoff, 1984.

18 Devroede G, Vobecky S, Masse S *et al*. Ischemic fecal incontinence and rectal angina. *Gastroenterology*, 1982; 83 (5): 970.

19 Orr G, Jones PF. Ischaemic proctitis followed by stricture. *Br J Surg*, 1982; 69 (7): 433.

20 Bharucha AE, Tremaine WJ, Johnson CD, Batts KP. Ischemic proctosigmoiditis. *Am J Gastroenterol*, 1996; 91 (11): 2305.

21 Jeck T, Sulser H, Heer M. Local ischemia causes carcinoma-like changes of the rectum. *Dis Colon Rectum*, 1996; 39 (9): 1026.

22 Jaeger HJ, Mathias KD, Gissler HM, Neumann G, Walther LD. Rectum and sigmoid colon necrosis due to cholesterol embolization after implantation of an aortic stent-graft. *J Vasc Interv Radiol*, 1999; 10 (6): 751.

23 Schuler JG, Hudlin MM. Cecal necrosis: infrequent variant of ischemic colitis. Report of five cases. *Dis Colon Rectum*, 2000; 43 (5): 708.

24 Arnott ID, Ghosh S, Ferguson A. The spectrum of ischaemic colitis. *Eur J Gastroenterol Hepatol*, 1999; 11 (3): 295.

25 Whitehead R. The pathology of intestinal ischaemia. *Clin Gastroenterol*, 1972; 1: 613.

26 Whitehead R. The pathology of ischemia of the intestines. *Pathol Annu*, 1976; 11: 1.

27 Welch TP, Sumitswan S. Acute segmental ischaemic enteritis in Thailand. *Br J Surg*, 1975; 62 (9): 716.

28 Renton CJC. Non-occlusive intestinal infarction. *Clin Gastroenterol*, 1972; 1: 655.

29 Croft RJ, Menon GP, Marston A. Does 'intestinal angina' exist? A critical study of obstructed visceral arteries. *Br J Surg*, 1981; 68 (5): 316.

30 Brandt LJ, Gomery P, Mitsudo SM, Chandler P, Boley SJ. Disseminated intravascular coagulation in nonocclusive mesenteric ischemia: the lack of specificity of fibrin thrombi in intestinal infarction. *Gastroenterology*, 1976; 71 (6): 954.

31 Zhang S, Ashraf M, Schinella R. Ischemic colitis with atypical reactive changes that mimic dysplasia (pseudodysplasia). *Arch Pathol Lab Med*, 2001; 125 (2): 224.

32 Marston A. Laboratory studies of intestinal ischaemia. In: Marston A, ed. *Vascular Disease of the Gut: Pathophysiology, Recognition and Management*. London: Edward Arnold, 1986: 30.

33 Boley SJ, Schwartz S, Lash J, Sternhill V. Reversible vascular occlusion of the colon. *Surg Gynecol Obstet*, 1963; 116: 53.

34 Marston A, Pheils MT, Thomas ML, Morson BC. Ischaemic colitis. *Gut*, 1966; 7 (1): 1.

35 McNeill C, Green G, Bannayan G, Weser E. Ischemic colitis diagnosed by early colonscopy. *Gastrointest Endosc*, 1974; 20 (3): 124.

36 Scowcroft CW, Sanowski RA, Kozarek RA. Colonoscopy in ischemic colitis. *Gastrointest Endosc*, 1981; 27 (3): 156.

37 Marston A, Clarke JM, Garcia Garcia J, Miller AL. Intestinal function and intestinal blood supply: a 20 year surgical study. *Gut*, 1985; 26 (7): 656.

38 Mandal BK, Schofield PF, Morson BC. A clinicopathological study of acute colitis: the dilemma of transient colitis syndrome. *Scand J Gastroenterol*, 1982; 17 (7): 865.

39 Deana DG, Dean PJ. Reversible ischemic colitis in young women. Association with oral contraceptive use. *Am J Surg Pathol*, 1995; 19 (4): 454.

40 Gratama S, Smedts F, Whitehead R. Obstructive colitis: an analysis of 50 cases and a review of the literature. [Review] [30 references] *Pathology*, 1995; 27 (4): 324.

41 Gekas P, Schuster MM. Stercoral perforation of the colon: case report and review of the literature. *Gastroenterology*, 1981; 80 (5 Part 1): 1054.

42 Hay AM. Association between chlorpromazine therapy and necrotizing colitis: report of a case. *Dis Colon Rectum*, 1978; 21 (5): 380.

43 Feldman PS. Ulcerative disease of the colon proximal to partially obstructive lesions: report of two cases and review of the literature. *Dis Colon Rectum*, 1975; 18 (7): 601.

44 Levine TS, Price AB. Obstructive enterocolitis: a clinicopathological discussion. *Histopathology*, 1994; 25 (1): 57.

45 Boley SJ, Sammartano R, Adams A, DiBiase A, Kleinhaus S, Sprayregen S. On the nature and etiology of vascular ectasias of the colon. Degenerative lesions of aging. *Gastroenterology*, 1977; 72 (4 Part 1): 650.

46 Danesh BJ, Spiliadis C, Williams CB, Zambartas CM. Angiodysplasia—an uncommon cause of colonic bleeding: colonoscopic evaluation of 1,050 patients with rectal bleeding and anaemia. *Int J Colorectal Dis*, 1987; 2 (4): 218.

47 Baer JW, Ryan S. Analysis of cecal vasculature in the search for vascular malformations. *Am J Roentgenol*, 1976; 126 (2): 394.
48 Price AB. Angiodysplasia of the colon. *Int J Colorectal Dis*, 1986; 1 (2): 121.
49 Sabanathan S, Nag SB. Angiodysplasia of the colon: a post-mortem study. *J R Coll Surg Edinb*, 1982; 27 (5): 285.
50 Meyer CT, Troncale FJ, Galloway S, Sheahan DG. Arteriovenous malformations of the bowel: an analysis of 22 cases and a review of the literature. *Medicine (Baltimore)*, 1981; 60 (1): 36.
51 Richter JM, Hedberg SE, Athanasoulis CA, Schapiro RH. Angiodysplasia. Clinical presentation and colonoscopic diagnosis. *Dig Dis Sci*, 1984; 29 (6): 481.
52 Smith GF, Ellyson JH, Parks SN *et al*. Angiodysplasia of the colon. A review of 17 cases. *Arch Surg*, 1984; 119 (5): 532.
53 Hochter W, Weingart J, Kuhner W, Frimberger E, Ottenjann R. Angiodysplasia in the colon and rectum. Endoscopic morphology, localisation and frequency. *Endoscopy*, 1985; 17 (5): 182.
54 Tedesco FJ, Griffin JW Jr, Khan AQ. Vascular ectasia of the colon: clinical, colonoscopic, and radiographic features. *J Clin Gastroenterol*, 1980; 2 (3): 233.
55 Pounder DJ, Rowland R, Pieterse AS, Freeman R, Hunter R. Angiodysplasias of the colon. *J Clin Pathol*, 1982; 35 (8): 824.
56 Mitsudo SM, Boley SJ, Brandt LJ, Montefusco CM, Sammartano RJ. Vascular ectasias of the right colon in the elderly: a distinct pathologic entity. *Hum Pathol*, 1979; 10 (5): 585.
57 Stamm B, Heer M, Buhler H, Ammann R. Mucosal biopsy of vascular ectasia (angiodysplasia) of the large bowel detected during routine colonoscopic examination. *Histopathology*, 1985; 9 (6): 639.
58 Reynolds DG. Injection techniques in the study of intestinal vasculature under normal conditions and in ulcerative colitis. In: Boley SJ, Schwartz SS, Williams LF, eds. *Vascular Disorders of the Intestine*. New York: Appleton-Century Crofts, 1971: 383.
59 Thelmo WL, Vetrano JA, Wibowo A, DiMaio TM, Cruz-Vetrano WP, Kim DS. Angiodysplasia of colon revisited: pathologic demonstration without the use of intravascular injection technique. *Hum Pathol*, 1992; 23 (1): 37.
60 Allison DJ, Hemingway AP. Angiodysplasia: does old age begin at nineteen? *Lancet*, 1981; 2: 979.
61 Burke AP, Sobin LH, Virmani R. Localized vasculitis of the gastrointestinal tract. *Am J Surg Pathol*, 1995; 19 (3): 338.
62 Reissman P, Weiss EG, Teoh TA, Lucas FV, Wexner SD. Gangrenous ischemic colitis of the rectum: a rare complication of systemic lupus erythematosus. *Am J Gastroenterol*, 1994; 89 (12): 2234.
63 Storesund B, Gran JT, Koldingsnes W. Severe intestinal involvement in Wegener's granulomatosis: report of two cases and review of the literature [see comments]. [Review] [10 references] *Br J Rheumatol*, 1998; 37 (4): 387.
64 Gross WL. Systemic necrotizing vasculitis. [Review] [89 references] *Bailliéres Clin Rheumatol*, 1997; 11 (2): 259.
65 Kurita M, Niwa Y, Hamada E *et al*. Churg–Strauss syndrome (allergic granulomatous angiitis) with multiple perforating ulcers of the small intestine, multiple ulcers of the colon, and mononeuritis multiplex. *J Gastroenterol*, 1994; 29 (2): 208.
66 Leonard N, Palazzo J, Jameson J, Denman AM, Talbot IC, Price AB. Behçet's colitis has distinctive pathological features. *Int J Surg Pathol*, 1998; 6 (1): 1.
67 Flaherty MJ, Lie JT, Haggitt RC. Mesenteric inflammatory veno-occlusive disease. A seldom recognized cause of intestinal ischemia. *Am J Surg Pathol*, 1994; 18 (8): 779.
68 Saraga E, Bouzourenne H. Enterocolic (lymphocytic) phlebitis: a rare cause of intestinal ischemic necrosis: a series of six patients and review of the literature. *Am J Surg Pathol*, 2000; 24 (6): 824.
69 Tuppy H, Haidenthaler A, Schandalik R, Oberhuber G. Idiopathic enterocolic lymphocytic phlebitis: a rare cause of ischemic colitis. *Mod Pathol*, 2000; 13 (8): 897.
70 Martinet O, Reis ED, Joseph JM, Saraga E, Gillet TM. Isolated granulomatous phlebitis: rare cause of ischemic necrosis of the colon: report of a case. *Dis Colon Rectum*, 2000; 43 (11): 1601.
71 Abu-Alfa AK, Ayer U, West AB. Mucosal biopsy findings and venous abnormalities in idiopathic myointimal hyperplasia of the mesenteric veins. *Am J Surg Pathol*, 1996; 20 (10): 1271.
72 Savoie LM, Abrams AV. Refractory proctosigmoiditis caused by myointimal hyperplasia of mesenteric veins: report of a case. *Dis Colon Rectum*, 1999; 42 (8): 1093.

38 Epithelial tumours of the large intestine

In this edition, colorectal adenoma and adenocarcinoma have been integrated into a single chapter to emphasize the continuous spectrum of neoplasia represented by these lesions. Nevertheless, it is necessary to consider adenoma and adenocarcinoma separately with respect to epidemiology, classical pathology and clinical management. Additionally, polyps that have in the past been classified as non-neoplastic may contain clonal genetic changes and have neoplastic potential (see Chapter 40).

Most colorectal adenomas present as a protuberant mass or polyp. They must be differentiated from other types of epithelial polyp listed in Table 38.1 and described in Chapter 40. In Table 38.1, epithelial polyps are classified according to the pathological process that is believed to underlie their genesis. Adenomas are benign neoplasms but have malignant potential. Hyperplastic polyps have also been described as metaplastic polyps and hypermature polyps. This multiplicity of terms indicates that the precise nature of the hyperplastic polyp remains unclear. Less frequent are the epithelial hamartomas or malformations as represented by juvenile and Peutz–Jeghers polyps. Inflammatory stimuli give rise to a range of inflammatory polyps. Lymphoid polyps (not strictly epithelial) may be included under this category (Chapter 39).

Historically, the adenoma has been considered as the most important type of epithelial polyp in the colorectum. In addition to its clinical relevance as a precancerous lesion, the adenoma provides the researcher with a model of early neoplastic change that has contributed to our understanding of the mechanisms of colorectal carcinogenesis. Epidemiological research provides insight into disease aetiology. However, since national registries exist for cancer but not adenoma, population-based studies have focused on risk factors for colorectal cancer. They provide some insight into aetiology, but will not explain the initiation of an adenoma or why some individuals develop multiple adenomas. Apart from environmental factors, different genetic (hereditary) factors will operate at key points along the neoplastic pathway. The hereditary syndromes familial adenomatous polyposis (FAP) and hereditary non-polyposis colorectal cancer (HNPCC) would be extreme

Table 38.1 Histological classification of epithelial polyps of the colorectum.

Mechanism	Type	Polyposis syndrome
Unknown	Hyperplastic (metaplastic)	Hyperplastic polyposis
Neoplasia	Adenoma: tubular tubulovillous villous	Familial adenomatous polyposis (classical and attenuated) 'Multiple adenoma syndrome'
	Serrated adenoma	Serrated adenomatous or hyperplastic polyposis
Hamartoma	Juvenile	Juvenile polyposis
	Unnamed	Cowden and Bannayan–Ruvalcaba–Riley syndromes
	Peutz–Jeghers	Peutz–Jeghers syndrome
Inflammation	Inflammatory	Inflammatory polyposis

examples of an overriding genetic influence; less penetrant polygenic factors will also be implicated.

The field of molecular genetics has moved with great speed and continues to gather pace. It has been stated that colorectal cancer is the most thoroughly understood solid tumour in terms of its molecular biology. This may be correct, but there is still much to learn. Any attempt to provide a detailed overview of this topic would be rapidly undermined by the emergence of new and important insights. This chapter will adopt a synthetic approach, emphasizing principles rather than detail with respect to aetiology, pathogenesis and applications of molecular technology. This will be complemented by an evidence-based approach to the practical management of colorectal neoplasia.

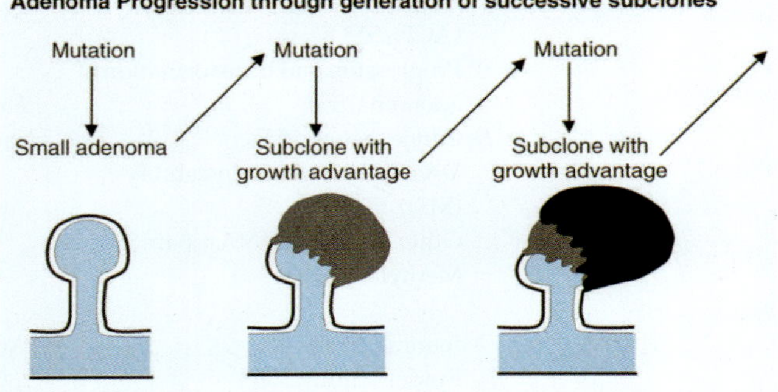

Fig. 38.1 Multistep generation of subclones within a colorectal polypoid neoplasm.

The pathogenesis of colorectal neoplasia: morphological and molecular correlations

Two areas of study explain much of the understanding that now exists in relation to the evolution of colorectal neoplasia. The first is the model provided by the adenoma–carcinoma concept and supported by clinical, pathological and epidemiological data collated over several decades [1]. The second relates to the hereditary bowel cancer syndromes. Uncovering the molecular basis of the syndromes familial adenomatous polyposis (FAP) and hereditary non-polyposis colorectal cancer (HNPCC) led to the discovery of important cancer genes. These genes are implicated in sporadic as well as familial colorectal cancer, and also in extracolonic malignancies. These fundamental insights could not have occurred without the prior clinical and pathological characterization of the syndromes.

Clonality and multistep progression of colorectal neoplasia

The demonstration of specific mutations in cancer genes within DNA extracted from adenomas establishes the clonal nature of these lesions [2]. Neoplastic progression occurs as a stepwise process, governed by the successive generation of subclones with a growth advantage [3]. Each step is caused by a genetic change implicating a cancer gene so that the development of subclones is accompanied by an accumulating mutational burden (Fig. 38.1). The nature, order and timing of the mutational steps will not be the same for each adenoma, although some cancer genes are more likely to be implicated as early and others as late events [2]. The existence of a hereditary or germline mutation in the adenomatous polyposis coli (*APC*) gene means, of course, that this mutation is the inevitable first step in the generation of each adenoma in a subject with FAP. This fact is likely to influence the nature, order and timing of the additional steps. For example, there is evidence that inactivation of the second (wild-type) *APC* allele initiates the development of adenomas in FAP [4]. Inactivation of both *APC* alleles has been observed in small adenomas from subjects with FAP [5]. Subsequently, the vast majority of adenomas remain small for many years and only a very small proportion finally becomes malignant. In sporadic adenomas, by contrast, *APC* mutations may occur at a later stage, since they have been associated with the development of villous change and high-grade dysplasia [6] or the onset of malignancy [7].

Familial adenomatous polyposis (FAP) as a model for early neoplastic change

In this autosomal dominant condition (discussed in more detail on p. 567), affected subjects develop hundreds if not thousands of adenomas [8]. In addition to the visible adenomas are smaller microadenomas including unicryptal adenomas. This condition provides an opportunity to study the earliest stages in the evolution of adenoma. This is not merely of theoretical interest, since the earlier stages in the neoplastic process may be the most amenable to preventative strategies.

There are two major theories on the early evolution of adenomas in FAP that are difficult to reconcile. The first is based on cell kinetic studies and the second on meticulous microreconstruction studies. The cell kinetic studies have given rise to the concept of hyperproliferation as the earliest lesion, whereas microreconstruction studies identify the unicryptal adenoma as the first step.

Hyperproliferation

This has been studied in subjects with sporadic neoplasms, other lesions or risk factors, and in experimental animals. However much of the pioneering work of Lipkin and Deschner was based on colorectal mucosal samples from members of polyposis families, using incorporation of thymidine ^{3}H in short-term culture experiments [9]. In normal crypts, uptake is limited to cells of the lower compartment. In phase 1 lesions, the proliferative zone remains in the lower compartment, but some cycling cells are detected in the upper compartment [9]. In phase 2 lesions, there is a major redistribution of cycling cells into the upper crypt and surface epithelium and this proliferation finally becomes a defined neoplastic lesion or adenoma [10]. There are a number of conceptual difficulties with this model. It has been emphasized that the phase 1 lesion is not a diffuse mucosal change, but occurs in patches [10]. However the size and number of these patches has not been defined. Nor has the progression phase 1 → phase 2 → adenoma been shown to occur as a dynamic continuum.

The development of non-radioactive approaches (bromodeoxyuridine) and monoclonal antibodies to cell cycle products has greatly facilitated cell kinetic research. Several studies have failed to reproduce the findings of Lipkin and Deschner in subjects either with FAP or at increased risk for colorectal cancer for other reasons [11–13]. The existence of the phase 1 lesion as a patch has transformed into the concept of a pancolorectal, diffuse field hyperproliferation [14]. In FAP subtle proliferative changes within normal-appearing mucosa may be shown when quantitative data are subjected to statistical analysis [15]. These subtle changes may be influenced by a variety of factors including anatomical site, gender, age, diet, diurnal variation, disease states, bowel preparation and the proximity of various lesions [16–19]. There is also considerable variation from crypt to crypt, necessitating assessment of around 20 perfectly orientated crypts [20]. One study found no proliferative alteration equivalent to the phase 2 lesion of Lipkin and Deschner in normal-appearing mucosa from subjects with FAP [15]. Presumably the phase 2 lesion is a microadenoma and would therefore have been distinguished from normal mucosa [21].

It is likely that subtle proliferative abnormalities can be demonstrated in the normal-appearing colorectal mucosa of subjects with FAP [15], presumably as a consequence of deficient APC protein. Other changes have been described, including increased crypt fission [22] and decreased apoptosis in the upper crypt and surface epithelium that could be reversed by the administration of a COX-2 inhibitor [23]. The principal use of cell kinetic research has been as an endpoint in chemoprevention studies, in both humans and animals. However, since hyperproliferation has not been shown to be a clinically useful marker of cancer risk, its value as a surrogate endpoint must be viewed with scepticism.

Microadenomas

Unlike lesions defined exclusively on the basis of cell kinetic indices, microadenomas are distinct entities characterized by a combination of morphological, genetic and cell kinetic changes. The earliest microadenoma is the unicryptal adenoma. Microreconstruction studies indicate that the unicryptal adenoma begins as a small bud or outgrowth (literally a new growth) from the side of an apparently normal crypt [22,24]. This bud forms a tubule which moves upwards with the normal migration of the crypt column until it hangs down from the surface epithelium. The neoplastic tubule is usually shorter than its normal counterpart but undergoes fission to produce an oligocryptal adenoma. Growth that is expansile leads to the formation of a polyp. However, neoplastic crypts may show a more horizontal growth pattern, spreading between and around normal crypts [25]. Such adenomas are often flat or depressed, but may subsequently become polypoid as their size increases [26]. There is also evidence that growth of FAP adenomas may be achieved by the mingling of two or more clones giving rise to a polyclonal lesion [27].

It has been debated whether inactivation of the second *APC* allele is an obligatory event for the initiation of adenomas in FAP [28]. Certainly such inactivation occurs early, appears to be obligatory in a mouse model for FAP [29], and is sufficient to explain adenoma growth [4,30].

Morphogenesis of early sporadic neoplasia and aberrant crypt foci (ACF)

As noted above, the inheritance of an *APC* germline mutation may drive or determine a particular sequence of steps in the process of neoplasia. Whilst applying to most if not all the adenomas developing in subjects with FAP, this does not necessarily mean that sporadic neoplasms will evolve through an identical pathway of morphogenesis. Experimental studies involving the administration of carcinogens to animals produce so-called aberrant crypt foci [31]. These may be visualized through low-power examination (*en face*) of the surface epithelium stained with methylene blue dye. Similar lesions may be identified in human colonic mucosa from subjects without FAP. Histological examination of these small foci reveals some to be microadenomas, but the proportion varies in different studies [32,33]. Probably no more than 5% show morphological changes typical of a microadenoma [33]. Others will be early hyperplastic polyps. However, a significant proportion cannot be classified. These show crypt branching and widening, but lack cytological changes indicative of either neoplasia or the crypt serration of a hyperplastic polyp [34]. Interestingly, these hyperplastic foci appear to be clonal and to show mutations in the oncogene K-*ras* [33,34]. The detection of such lesions in subjects without FAP is laborious and only small numbers of definite microadenomas have been subjected to molecular analysis. Microadenomas differ from the non-neoplastic hyperplastic foci by the presence of *APC* mutations [33]. It has therefore been suggested that *APC* mutations initiate the growth of sporadic adenomas as well as adenomas in FAP. Conversely, focal hyperplastic lesions showing K-*ras* mutations may not progress further [33]. These preliminary data do not exclude the possibility of genetic pathways beginning other than with an *APC* mutation. It has been suggested that the discrete phase 1 hyperproliferative lesions of Lipkin and Deschner are equivalent to the non-neoplastic focal hyperplasias [35]. If true and if (as suggested above) phase 2 lesions are microadenomas, this would bring about a simple unification of cell kinetic, genetic and morphological classifications.

The notion that all adenomas must be polypoid is no longer accepted. Flat and depressed adenomas are now well recognized [36,37]. However, the flat adenoma is not always a distinct biological entity. Flatness may merely be a reflection of small size and a lack of mucosal redundancy and prolapse [26]. Conversely, a horizontal or spreading character to the proliferation of neoplastic tubules (as opposed to an upwards and expansile pattern of growth) may lead to the development of a biologically distinct flat or depressed lesion [25]. Interestingly, flat adenomas lack K-*ras* mutations [34,38], which are common within polypoid adenomas [39]. This genetic finding supports the view that flat and polypoid adenomas represent divergent pathways of neoplastic evolution [40].

Progression and transformation of adenoma

The well known model developed by Fearon and Vogelstein [41] integrates molecular insights (loss or mutation of the tumour suppressor genes *APC*, *TP53* and *DCC* and mutation of K-*ras*) with the evolution of adenoma and transition to carcinoma and has stimulated considerable research activity and interest. The classification of adenomas within the model of Fearon and Vogelstein was based not on conventional criteria such as grade of dysplasia or size but on groups that included tubular adenomas from subjects with FAP (class I) and larger sporadic adenomas containing (class III) or not containing (class II) foci of adenocarcinoma [2]. Polyposis and non-polyposis adenomas cannot necessarily be bracketed into a neoplastic continuum. The model does not heed the villous adenoma–mucinous adenocarcinoma sequence in which *TP53* mutations are infrequent [42,43], nor the existence of flat adenomas and *'de novo'* carcinoma in which K-*ras* mutations are infrequent [38,44–46]. Furthermore, neoplasia developing in a background of DNA microsatellite instability occurs through a distinct pathway implicating mutations in *TGF-βRII* receptor [47], *IGF2R* [48] and *BAX* [49].

The sequential development of increasingly aggressive subclones is not the only mechanism underlying neoplastic progression. Adenoma growth is poorly understood, but must implicate crypt fission and the horizontal spread of neoplastic tubules [25]. These processes are likely to be influenced by luminal promoting agents such as bile acids [50] as well as the loss of endogenous growth control mechanisms. Conceivably, adenomatous epithelium may show an abnormal sensitivity to luminal factors that cause minor hyperproliferation in normal mucosa. This would explain the association between diffuse mucosal hyperproliferation and large but not small adenomas [51].

The magnitude of the mutational burden required to bring about malignant transformation is large. Each cell within a malignant subclone will have accumulated multiple mutations. Cancer is an improbable event. Although about 5% of inhabitants of a high-risk country will develop colorectal cancer, only one out of many millions of colorectal epithelial cells gives rise to a malignant neoplasm. Nevertheless, the probability of malignant conversion increases with the generation of each new subclone with a selective growth advantage. The generation of an adenoma is accompanied by the spatial reorganization of the proliferative compartment. Instead of being sequestered within the crypt base, proliferative cells accumulate superficially where they are exposed directly to luminal carcinogens and promoting influences. Expansion of the neoplastic clone through growth further increases the size of the target population. The occurrence of certain mutations will increase the probability of additional mutations. For example, p53 halts the cell cycle and thereby provides a cell with the opportunity to repair genetic damage; inactivation of *TP53* will have the opposite effect [52]. The accumulation of genetic damage may occur at the level of DNA or at a chromosomal level through disruption of cell cycle checkpoint mechanisms [53]. Aneuploidy and loss of tumour suppressor genes are hallmarks of chromoso-

Table 38.2 Genetic changes in colorectal cancer.

Genetic alteration	MSS*	MSI-L*	MSI-H*	References
Mutation				
APC	+++	+++	+	[75–77]
K-*ras*	++	+++	+	[75,78]
TP53	+++	+++	+	[76,79]
TGFβRII	+	+	+++	[47]
IGF2R	–	–	+	[80]
BAX	–	–	++	[49]
caspase-5	–	–	+	[81]
CDX-2	–	–	+	[82]
BCL-10	–	–	+	[83]
E2F-4	–	–	+	[84,85]
Loss of heterozygosity				
5p (*APC*)	+++	++	–	[75,78]
17p (*TP53*)	+++	+++	–	[75,78]
18q (*DCC* or *SMAD4* or *MADR2*)	+++	+++	–	[75,78]
Methylation	+	+++	+++	[86–88]

* Critical review reinforces the distinctive molecular profile of cancers with a high frequency of microsatellite instability (MSI-H) compared with those that are microsatellite stable (MSS) or have a low frequency of microsatellite instability (MSI-L). Separate consideration of sporadic MSI-H cancers and HNPCC cancers may further emphasize the distinction between sporadic MSI-H cancers and other types. For discussion see text.

mal instability whereas diploidy and DNA microsatellite instability are biomarkers of DNA instability.

The final step of conversion of adenoma to adenocarcinoma must be a rate-limiting step since adenomas are relatively numerous in comparison to carcinomas. Furthermore, this step is accompanied by a multiplicity of phenotypic changes implicating enzymes in metabolic pathways [54], increased telomerase activity [55], growth factors promoting stromal proliferation and angiogenesis [56–58], proteolytic enzymes facilitating local invasion [59–61], numerous changes to secretory and membrane-associated glycoproteins [62], alterations in cell adhesion molecules [63] as well as the development of aneuploidy [64].

Cancer genes

The term 'cancer gene' is a misnomer; both oncogenes and tumour suppressor genes are involved in maintaining normal cellular functions. The mutational activation of proto-oncogenes leads to increased and unregulated growth [2,65,66]. The loss of tumour suppressor genes leads to the breakdown of a variety of cell functions including DNA repair, intercellular adhesion and recognition, cell cycle control and multiple signalling pathways implicated in cell regulation [2,67–74] (Table 38.2).

Oncogenes are dominantly acting, mutation of one allele being sufficient to bring about a transforming event. Although several oncogenes have been implicated in the pathogenesis of colorectal cancer, distinction should be made between those activated through a mutation and those that are secondarily up-regulated. K-*ras* is one of the more frequently mutated oncogenes [2,65], whereas *c-myc* is expressed through dysregulation of the wnt signalling pathway [89]. Tumour suppressor genes are recessive in their action; both alleles must be inactivated before there is a full oncogenic effect. However, inactivation of one may bring about a partial effect, subsequently augmented by inactivation of the second allele. The abnormal or mutated gene product may combine with and neutralize the normal product, giving rise to a dominant negative effect [90]. This could explain why a constitutionally deleted *APC* gene may be less harmful than a constitutionally mutated one [91].

Tumour suppressor genes implicated in the initiation of neoplasia have been described as 'gatekeepers', 'caretakers' and 'landscapers' [92]. *APC* controlling proliferation through the wnt signalling pathway is a gatekeeper, the DNA mismatch repair genes are caretakers, while genes acting more indirectly, for example through initiating hamartomatous maldevelopment, are landscapers.

Inactivation of the first tumour suppressor allele is usually through a mutation (inherited or acquired). The second allele may also be mutated, but loss of the allele through a mitotic error such as non-disjunction is frequent. Indeed, loss of heterozygosity (LOH) has provided important insight into the chromosomal location of tumour suppressor genes [93]. Many of the tumour suppressor genes implicated in the pathogenesis of colorectal cancer have been cloned, though additional tumour suppressor genes (Table 38.2) await discovery [94].

Colorectal cancers show consistent LOH for chromosomes 1p [95], 8p [96–98], 14q [99], 17q [99] and 22q [100,101]. Other tumour suppressor genes are likely to be located on these chromosomes.

The mechanism of allele inactivation and the precise location of mutations are relevant to cancer aetiology. Some genetic changes will be spontaneous, chance events. Others will be linked to specific environmental mutagens. Germline *APC* mutations will generally be spontaneous. Acquired, somatic *APC* mutations do not show the same distribution as germline mutations, though overlap is seen [102]. Identification of somatic mutational hotspots should facilitate the characterization of environmental mutagens.

DNA microsatellite instability (MSI)

Microsatellites are non-encoding regions within the genome comprising repetitive tracts of DNA. Most of the marker tracts employed to demonstrate linkage or loss of heterozygosity (see Chapter 2) have been either mononucleotide (e.g. AAAA, etc.) or dinucleotide (e.g. CACACA, etc.) runs. Such repetitive runs are especially prone to mismatch errors during DNA replication. DNA replication errors are normally repaired by a system of DNA mismatch repair proteins implicated in the aetiology of hereditary non-polyposis colorectal cancer (HNPCC) (see p. 570). DNA repair will not occur if the repair mechanism is disrupted. The demonstration of DNA bandshifts or mutations in tumour-derived DNA (that are not present in germline DNA) serves as a biomarker for DNA instability and occurs in HNPCC neoplasms and up to 30% of sporadic colorectal cancers. When bandshifts can be demonstrated in at least 40% of a panel of microsatellite markers, cancers are classified as MSI-high (MSI-H) cancers. Lower frequencies of instability identify MSI-low (MSI-L) cancers while the majority will be microsatellite stable (MSS) [103]. Differences between MSI-H and MSI-L are not merely quantitative. Instability is rarely found in mononucleotide markers in MSI-L cancers whereas mononucleotide markers are sensitive for MSI-H. Furthermore, coding sequences comprising short repetitive mononucleotide runs occur in certain genes and are susceptible to mutation only in MSI-H cancers (listed in Table 38.2).

MSI-H cancers show a significantly reduced frequency of *APC*, K-*ras* and *p53* mutation; loss of heterozygosity or allelic imbalance at 5q, 17p and 18q is very uncommon [75–77,79,104,105]. Since these genetic alterations are implicated in the initiation and progression of adenomas, a different spectrum of mutations must occur in the precursors of MSI-H cancers. MSI-H can rarely be demonstrated in adenomas (other than those occurring in HNPCC). By contrast, MSI-H and loss of expression of the DNA mismatch repair gene *hMLH1* occurs relatively frequently in the dysplastic components of mixed hyperplastic polyps/adenomas and in serrated adenomas [106,107]. Serrated polyps are likely to be the precursors of a defined subset of colorectal cancers, particularly those showing DNA MSI.

Other defects in DNA repair

A recent report described a kindred in which inherited defects of a gene (*MYH*) involved in another type of DNA repair, namely base excision repair of mutations caused by reactive oxygen species, were associated with multiple colorectal adenomas and carcinoma [108]. As would be predicted from the DNA repair defect, the large bowel tumours showed a very high frequency of inactivating somatic mutations of the *APC* gene that were G:C → T:A transversions.

Methylation

Both hypomethylation and hypermethylation of DNA have been linked to colorectal carcinogenesis, though the causes of defective methylation are unknown. Methylation of DNA occurs at CpG sites, particularly when these are clustered into islands [87]. The promoter regions of certain genes are CpG island rich and methylation will lead to gene silencing. Two patterns of methylation have been described. Type A is associated with ageing and implicates genes in normal colorectal mucosa as well as cancers. Type C methylation is limited to genes within cancerous tissues [88]. Some of the type C genes that are methylated are tumour suppressor genes, a notable example being the DNA mismatch repair gene *hMLH1* [88]. This explains, at least in part, the association of the CpG island methylator phenotype (CIMP) with sporadic colorectal cancer showing high-level DNA microsatellite instability (MSI-H) [86]. Additional genes inactivated by methylation in colorectal cancer are *p16* [86], $p14^{ARF}$ [109], *COX-2* [110], oestrogen receptor (*ER*) [111], *HPP1* encoding a transmembrane protein [112,113] and the DNA repair gene O^6 methylguanine DNA methyltransferase (*MGMT*) [114]. The association between methylation of *MGMT* and K-*ras* mutation [114] links *MGMT* to the MSI-L pathway in which there is a high frequency of K-*ras* mutation [75,78]. Methylation may therefore be added to mutation and allele loss as a mechanism for inactivating tumour suppressor genes.

Adenoma

Epidemiology

Population-based data on adenomas are lacking. Colonoscopy is usually indicated by symptoms or signs of colorectal disease such as bleeding or the discovery of adenomas in the rectum. Such a colonoscopic series would be biased through selection and therefore lacking in epidemiological value. An alternative approach entails the meticulous examination of the colon and rectum at autopsy. Because the peak age of mortality varies with different diseases (some of which may be linked negatively or positively with pathogenesis of adenoma) and because patients dying of cancer tend not to be autopsied, even this approach will not exclude bias. However, these studies are a source of important information and have shown that conclusions based upon material taken from surgical files are unreliable. Autopsy surveys indicate that adenomas are evenly distributed throughout the colon with a predilection, if any, for the ascending colon [115–118]. One study has shown that adenomas are more frequent at the opposite ends of the colon [119]. The distribution appears to be age dependent. In younger subjects the left colon and rectum are favoured, but with increasing years the right colon becomes the site of predilection [119–123]. Adenomas are uncommon before the age of 30, but occur with increasing frequency as progressively older cohorts are examined. However, in a large radiological survey the prevalence plateaued beyond the seventh decade [120]. Adenoma frequency is less age dependent than carcinoma frequency [123].

Several studies have shown that adenomas are more prevalent in populations from high-risk areas for colorectal cancer [123–126], but exceptions to this rule have been recorded [119,127]. These exceptions are interesting because they suggest that factors responsible for adenoma and carcinoma formation overlap but are not identical. Observations relating to sex differences offer further support for this idea. Adenomas are more common in males in all regions of the colon [117,126], whereas the sex ratio for cancer outside the rectum is 1 : 1 and may even favour females. Interestingly, adenomas in the right colon have been noted to show more severe dysplasia in females [128,129]. Others describe adenomas in the sigmoid colon and rectum as being larger [123] and more likely to show severe dysplasia in females [128,129]. It would appear that females are less likely to produce adenomas but, once formed, adenomas are more likely to progress to malignancy [123]. In analysing the distribution and pathology of adenomas it is important to stratify these lesions by age, sex and site.

Case-control studies have shown that subjects with adenomas only and subjects with colorectal cancer share similar lifestyle risk factors including diet (fibre, fat and calcium intake), alcohol consumption and use of non-steroidal anti-inflammatory drugs [130–132].

Macroscopic appearances

Small adenomas are usually sessile and slightly redder than the surrounding mucosa (Fig. 38.2). With increasing size adenomas usually become pedunculated, and the head becomes a darker red and is broken into lobules with intercommunicating clefts. This darkening is due to a combination of increased vascularity and the different light-scattering properties of neoplastic (mucin-depleted) epithelium. Large adenomas may be sessile and either flat (rarely), slightly elevated or protuberant. The villous adenoma presents typically as a protuberant soft and often friable sessile mass with a shaggy or velvety surface (Fig. 38.3). However, some villous adenomas are small and pedunculated and conversely tubular adenomas may be large and sessile (Fig. 38.4). Intermediate forms are also encountered. The categorization of adenomas according to their macroscopic appearance is important as it may influence surgical treatment. Sessile adenomas are often less well circumscribed than pedunculated adenomas; because their limits are difficult to define, they have a greater tendency to recur following local excision. Occasionally, adenomas are flat or depressed with a surface that is granular and slightly redder than surrounding normal mucosa.

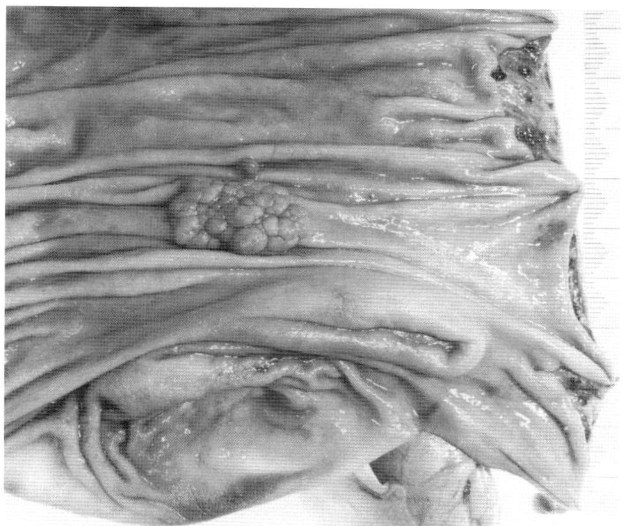

Fig. 38.2 Sessile adenoma in the ascending colon illustrating the typical lobulated surface configuration.

The prevalence of adenomas stratified by size cannot be ascertained from surgical records since these are biased by case selection. Autopsy studies reveal that the average size is a little over 0.5 cm. Even this will be an inflated figure, because the smaller an adenoma, the more likely it is to be overlooked or lost through autolysis. Microadenomas formed of single or small numbers of crypts are invisible. The size of adenomas is also influenced by the country of origin [133] and sex [128,129] of the population under study. At the other end of the scale are the museum specimens in which sizes of up to 15 cm across or involving the entire bowel circumference may be encountered. Such cases are very infrequent.

Microscopic appearances

Based on their microscopic architecture, adenomas are classified as tubular (Fig. 38.5), tubulovillous (Fig. 38.6) and villous (Fig. 38.7) [134]. These terms replace the older nomenclature of adenomatous polyp, papillary adenoma and villous papilloma. The older terms are unsatisfactory not only because of

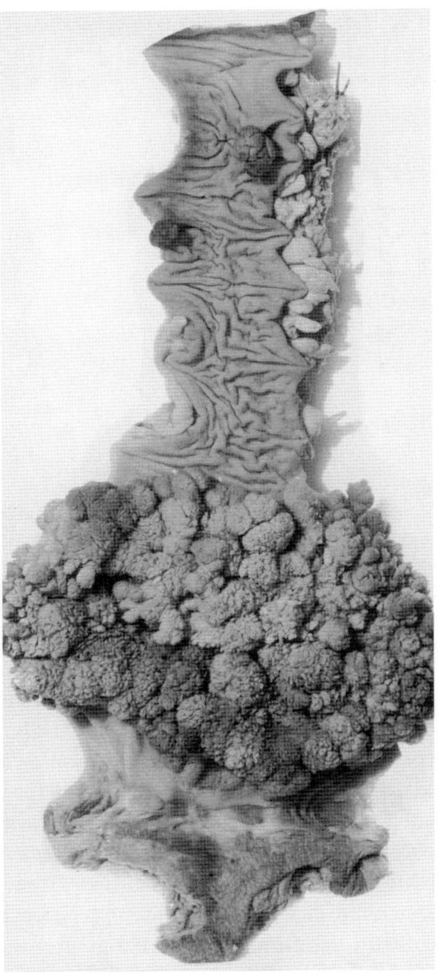

Fig. 38.3 Large villous adenoma of the lower rectum and two tubular adenomas of the sigmoid colon.

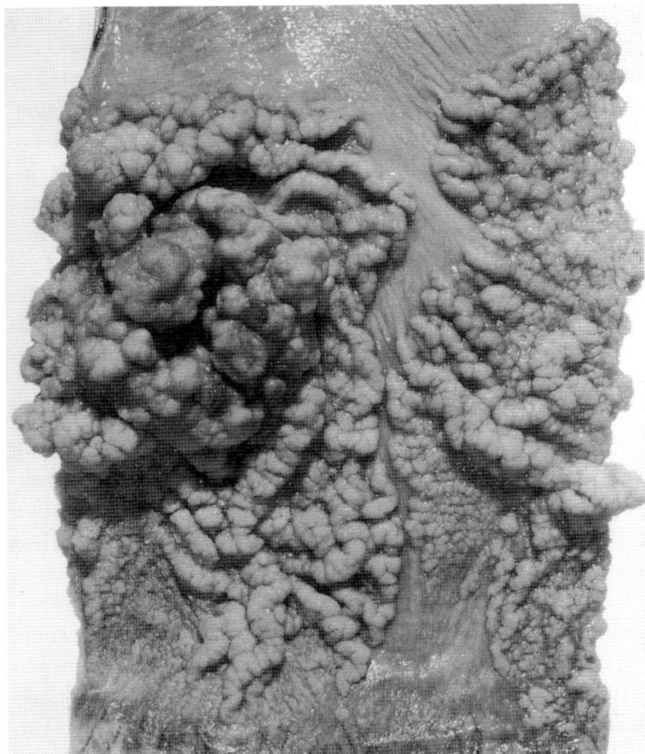

Fig. 38.4 Large sessile tubular adenoma in the upper rectum. The limits of the growth are defined with difficulty.

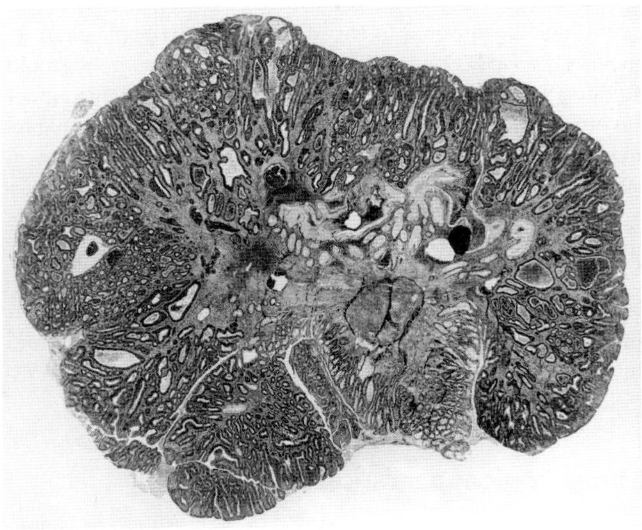

Fig. 38.5 Tubular adenoma on a stalk.

their cumbersome phrasing but because they obscure the essential unity of the concept of adenoma. Furthermore, a series of adenomas will show a spectrum of morphology, with the architectural subclassification being somewhat subjective. Some tubulovillous and villous adenomas may be related histogenetically to hyperplastic polyps and not to tubular adenomas [135] (see 'Serrated adenoma' on p. 562). It has been suggested that a tubular or villous adenoma should include approximately 80% of the appropriate architectural configuration; where the majority component is clearly less than 80%, the intermediate term tubulovillous is invoked. The relative frequency of the three types will depend on the care taken in sampling. However, there is widespread agreement that tubular adenomas are the most common subtype. In surgical material approximately 10% of adenomas are villous, but in autopsy studies only 1% of adenomas are tubulovillous or villous [126].

Tubular adenomas consist of closely packed, branching tubules, separated by varying amounts of lamina propria (Fig. 38.5). The tubules may be relatively regular or show considerable irregularity with much branching, budding and infolding. Tubules may show focal cystic dilatation, leading to secondary infection and haemorrhage in the substance of the

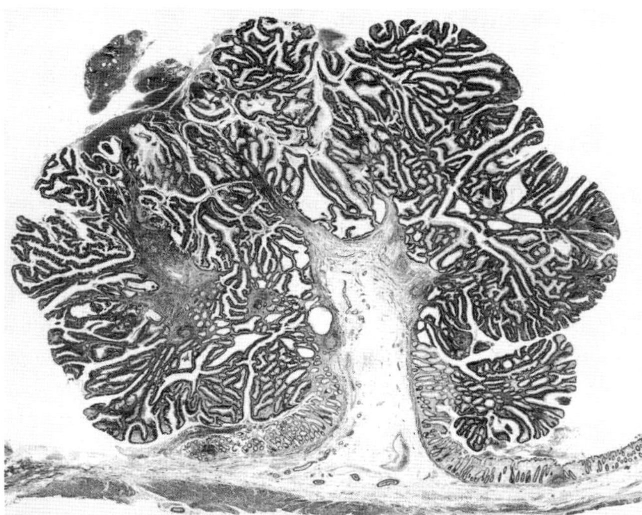

Fig. 38.6 Tubulovillous adenoma.

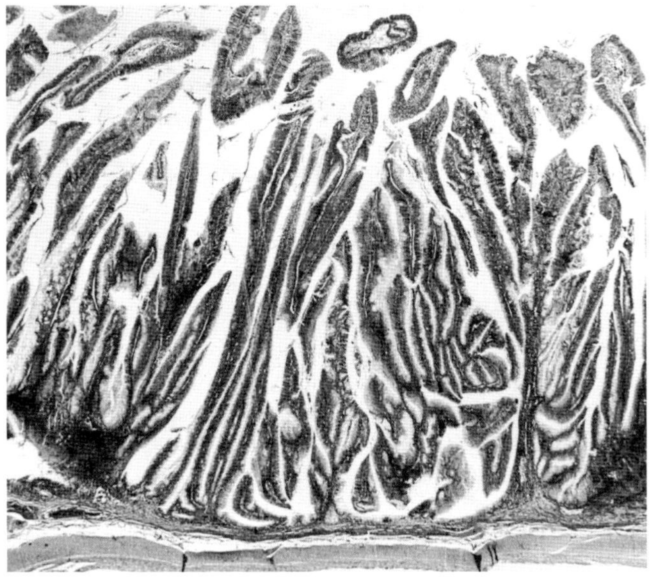

Fig. 38.7 Villous adenoma.

tumour. The stalk of the pedunculated adenoma is composed of normal mucosa and submucosa. Microreconstruction studies show that the term villous adenoma is in fact a misnomer. The perception of a villus is an artefact resulting from the two-dimensional view of a mucosal surface that is in fact thrown into folds or folia. In addition, the shaggy projections of a villous adenoma seen macroscopically and the delicate folia seen microscopically are of quite different orders of magnitude. Inspection of the surface of the adenoma with a dissecting microscope provides better insight into the underlying architecture [136]. Each folium consists of a core of lamina propria covered by a sheet of epithelial cells. Between the folia the epithelium rests upon the muscularis mucosae (Fig. 38.7).

Adenomas show abnormalities of architecture, cytology and differentiation that are encompassed by the term dysplasia [137]. All adenomas are, by definition, dysplastic. The changes may deviate minimally from normal (mild or low-grade dysplasia) through to appearances that approximate to carcinoma *in situ*. The term carcinoma *in situ* is often avoided in histopathological reporting as alarm engendered by its use may precipitate unnecessarily radical surgery. The criteria used for grading dysplasia and carcinoma are different. This is supported by an analysis of the distribution of aneuploid DNA content in a series of adenomas (mild dysplasia 4%, moderate dysplasia 18%, severe dysplasia 36%). Whereas aneuploidy increases in step with dysplasia, it occurs with the same high frequency in graded carcinomas (well differentiated 63%, moderately differentiated 64%, poorly differentiated 63%) [64]. This association between aneuploidy and grade of dysplasia [64,138] validates the concept of grading despite the subjective nature of the exercise.

The most reliable features for assessing the grade of dysplasia are tissue architecture, nuclear changes and cytoplasmic differentiation. In mild dysplasia nuclei are slightly enlarged, elongated, hyperchromatic, crowded and pseudostratified, but polarity is well preserved (Fig. 38.8a). The tubules are regular, though closely apposed, and show branching. Cytoplasmic maturation is slightly curtailed. In moderate dysplasia nuclei are further enlarged, less elongated and show focal loss of polarity (Fig. 38.8b). Mitoses are more numerous. In severe dysplasia nuclear polarity is just discerned or lost. The nuclei are greatly enlarged, round or ovoid and contain prominent nucleoli (Fig. 38.8c). Mitoses are numerous. Cytoplasm is usually basophilic and undifferentiated. Tubules show irregular or complex branching and budding [137].

Most adenomas show mild epithelial dysplasia. The prevalence of severe dysplasia depends on the manner in which adenomas are collected. Data based upon endoscopy records will inflate the frequency of severe dysplasia. Severe dysplasia is found in about 2% of adenomas collected by the meticulous examination of surgical or autopsy specimens [126]. Severe dysplasia is more common in the left colon than in the right colon [137] and is more prevalent in populations at high risk for colorectal cancer [133]. The frequency of severe dysplasia increases with the size of the adenoma and is highest in villous adenomas [1].

Both Paneth cells and endocrine cells [139] can be scattered in a haphazard manner throughout adenomas. In normal tissues and non-neoplastic polyps, these cells are polarized toward the crypt base.

Squamous metaplasia is occasionally seen in adenomas [140,141]. Larger adenomas may show areas of small intestinal metaplastic epithelium comprising mainly eosinophilic enterocyte-like cells, with reduced numbers of goblet cells. The

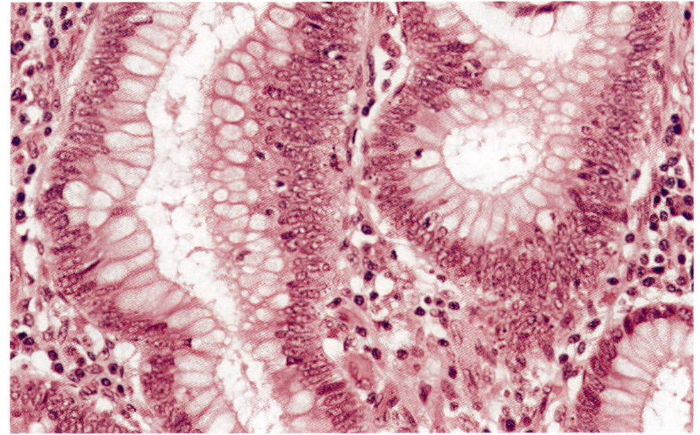

(a)

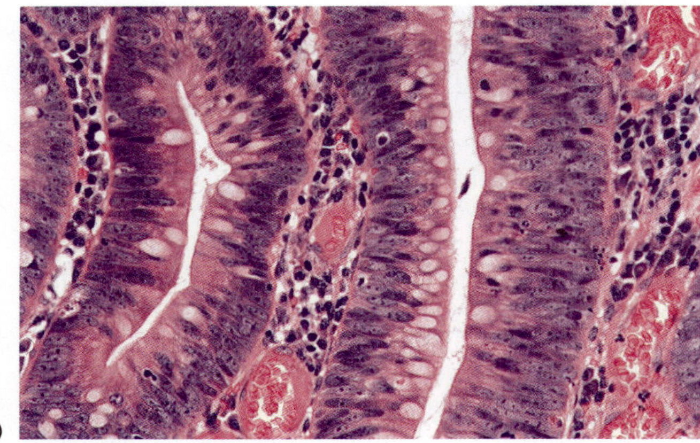

(b)

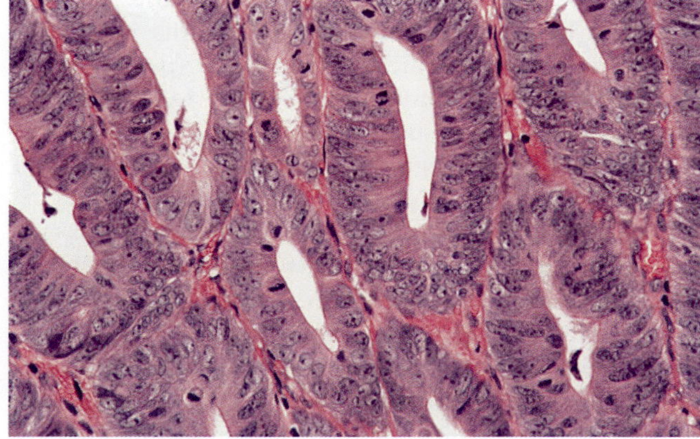

(c)

Fig. 38.8 Mild (a), moderate (b) and severe (c) adenomatous dysplasia.

goblet cell mucin resembles that of small intestine, being mild PAS positive [142].

Special investigations

Chromosome and DNA studies

Direct chromosome analysis requires the isolation of cells in mitosis and is time-consuming. For this reason few studies have been published on the karyotype of adenomas [143]. Tubular adenomas showing low-grade dysplasia usually reveal an entirely normal karyotype [144,145]. However, high-resolution methods have shown consistent karyotypic abnormalities involving 1p32–36 [146]. Trisomies and other more abnormal karyotypes have been described in tubular adenomas showing severe dysplasia [147] and in villous adenomas [147,148]. Cytogenetic studies have been augmented by the introduction of fluorescent *in situ* hybridization (FISH). Cytochemical techniques for the study of DNA content include the microdensitometric analysis of, for example, Feulgen-stained sections and the flow cytometric analysis of cellular or nuclear suspensions stained with a fluorescent dye such as propidium iodide [64]. The latter technique may be successfully applied to fixed, paraffin-embedded tissue. Although flow cytometry is not as sensitive as direct chromosome analysis it facilitates the rapid analysis of many thousands of cells from a large series of cases. Such studies have shown the incidence of aneuploidy is very much lower for adenoma than for carcinoma [64,138,149]. Flow karyotyping bridges the gap between flow cytometry and direct chromosome analysis. Comparative genomic hybridization is time-consuming but is extremely sensitive for allelic imbalance [150].

Enzyme biochemistry and histochemistry

The enzyme profiles of normal colorectal epithelium and carcinoma differ and it might be supposed that the adenomatous profile would fall somewhere in between these extremes. NAD and NADP diaphorases are either normal or increased in carcinomatous epithelium whereas other oxidative enzymes of the citric acid cycle and respiratory chain (succinic dehydrogenase, cytochrome oxidase) show reduced activity [54,151]. NAD and NADP diaphorases represent pathways for the oxidation of NADH and NADPH through a flavoprotein. The preservation or augmentation of such systems would facilitate the glycolytic and pentose phosphate pathways that generate NADH and NADPH and are known to be active in neoplastic tissues [152]. These findings are linked with the switch from aerobic to anaerobic metabolism that occurs in malignant states. Also associated with colorectal malignancy is the reduced activity of hydrolytic enzymes including esterase, acid phosphatase and ATPase [151,153]. In tubular adenomas, oxidative enzyme activities, represented by succinic dehydrogenase, cytochrome oxidase and NAD and NADP diaphorases, either show little alteration from normal or change in a direction opposite to carcinoma. For example, succinic dehydrogenase may show increased activity and NADP diaphorase reduced activity [54,151]. However, in areas of severe dysplasia, succinic dehydrogenase is reduced, as in carcinoma, and NAPD diaphorase is increased [151,153]. Villous adenomas show an enzyme profile similar to carcinoma [153]. Hydrolytic enzymes including acid phosphatase and esterase show, like carcinoma, reduced activity in both tubular and villous adenomas [151,153]. Biochemical and histochemical studies of enzymes from the glycolytic and pentose phosphate pathway show, like carcinoma, an increase in activity. Glucose 6-phosphate and lactate dehydrogenase activities are increased in large adenomas [154] and a higher activity of lactate dehydrogenase has been associated with severe dysplasia [154]. In summary, whilst the enzymology of high-grade dysplasia may be similar to carcinoma, the enzyme profiles of low-grade tubular adenomas may sometimes deviate minimally from normal or in a direction opposite to carcinoma.

Carbohydrate histochemistry

Mucins secreted by adenomas and normal colorectal mucosa differ in quality and quantity. Mucins are secretory glycoproteins made of chains of sugars attached to polypeptide backbone [155]. Staining reactions (whether demonstrated by routine mucin histochemical methods, lectin histochemistry or immunohistochemistry employing antibodies to specific sugar sequences) are usually determined by the nature and arrangement of the peripheral sugars. In normal colorectal goblet cell mucins, the peripheral sugars are mainly represented by sialic acid and two neutral sugars: N-acetyl galactosamine and (in the right colon) fucose. The acidity of large bowel mucus is determined by the presence of sulphate groups as well as by sialic acid. Normal large bowel sialic acid occurs in an O-acetylated form in the majority of individuals, rendering it resistant to digestion by neuraminidase and PAS unreactive [156]. Changes in sialic acid structure, notably loss of O-acetyl group, are accompanied by increased sensitivity to neuraminidase, increased PAS reactivity and altered antigenicity, for example rendering the structure sialosyl-Tn non-cryptic [157]. Such modifications have been described in adenomas [62,142,158], but are not specific markers of neoplastic transformation [159]. Adenomatous mucus also shows alterations in blood group antigen expression [160–163] and lectin binding affinities [163,164]. Many of these changes are not due to alteration in goblet cell mucin (MUC2) but are explained by up-regulation of non-secretory membrane-associated glycoproteins (MUC1) [165].

Taken overall, mucin histochemical studies support the adenoma–carcinoma concept, with adenomas having staining patterns intermediate between normal and cancer [163,164,166–168]. Some histochemical reactions may be progressively altered with increasing epithelial dysplasia, including the expression of sugar sequences with an affinity for peanut lectin [164]. Other modifications may only appear with the advent of severe dysplasia or cancer. Sialic acid alterations would fall into the latter category [142,169]. Likewise, in familial adenomatous polyposis, glycosyltransferase activity is increased in cancerous tissue but adenomatous epithelium does not differ from normal [170].

Mucin core protein expression

Tubular adenomas show loss of MUC2 but increased MUC1 expression with increasing grades of dysplasia [171]. Villosity may be associated with increased expression of secretory mucin. This may include inappropriate expression of gastric mucin (e.g. MUC5AC) as well as intestinal goblet cell mucin MUC2 [172].

Immunoglobulin A (IgA) secretory system

IgA is synthesized by plasma cells within the lamina propria and exported into the bowel lumen. Epithelial cell translocation of IgA is facilitated by the carrier molecule secretory component (SC). SC is a glycoprotein synthesized by the columnar cells of the intestinal mucosa. Dimeric IgA is received by the carrier molecule at the basolateral cell membrane and transported to the cell apex within a vesicle [173]. Increasing dysplasia within adenomas is accompanied by reduced immunocytochemical staining for SC and IgA [174]. This example of maturation arrest is comparable to the loss of mucus production by goblet cells. Loss of staining for SC could also be explained by a change in the direction of cytoplasmic differentiation (metaplasia) towards mucin synthesis.

Tumour antigens

The fact that certain fetal products can be expressed by tumours is well known. However, careful study of fetal antigens has so far failed to disclose examples that are both tissue and tumour specific. For example, carcinoembryonic antigen (CEA) is found in fetal colon and colorectal cancer, but small amounts are also secreted by normal colorectum [175], by heterologous adult tissues including small intestine [176] and by a variety of extracolonic neoplasms. In addition, increased expression of CEA is seen within non-neoplastic lesions such as actively inflamed colitic mucosa [177] and hyperplastic (metaplastic) polyps [178]. The same lack of specificity applies to a family of tumour antigens that is closely related to CEA and to a rapidly growing list of newer tumour markers to which monoclonal antibodies have been raised [158,179,180]. Adenomas show increased expression of many of these products, notably sialosyl-Le^x [180] and sialosyl-Tn [158] as well as CEA [168,181].

Polyamines and ornithine decarboxylase

The polyamines putrescine, spermidine and spermine are small cationic molecules that play an important role in cell proliferation and differentiation [182]. This effect may be mediated by the stabilization of polynucleotides through stereospecific interactions with DNA. Polyamine biosynthetic enzymes are among the most rapidly induced enzymes within the cell. The primary precursors of polyamines are ornithine and methionine. Ornithine decarboxylase is the rate-limiting enzyme in polyamine synthesis [183] and has the shortest half-life of any known mammalian enzyme [184]. Induction of the enzyme ornithine decarboxylase appears to be the final common pathway for a wide range of tumour promoters. Animal studies have shown that both bile salts [185] and dietary fat [186] will increase colonic ornithine decarboxylase activity. Inhibition of ornithine decarboxylase by difluoromethylornithine will prevent the formation of experimental colonic neoplasms [186,187].

Adenomas and carcinomas of the human large bowel have levels of ornithine decarboxylase three times that of normal, and polyamine levels are doubled [188]. Another polyamine metabolite, N-acetylspermidine, shows a more selective association with colorectal cancer with levels five times as high as both adenoma and normal [189]. Polyamines are metabolized by oxidative enzymes and the products of this breakdown inhibit cell growth and promote terminal maturation [190]. There is evidence to suggest that raised levels of colonic ornithine decarboxylase are found in the colonic mucosa of clinically normal family members who carry the genotype of familial adenomatous polyposis [191]. However, this has not been confirmed by others and the effect could be explained by contamination with microadenomas. Paradoxically, reduced ornithine decarboxylase activity has been demonstrated in the normal-appearing mucosa of patients with sporadic colorectal adenoma or carcinoma [192].

Semithin and ultrastructural studies

The fine structure of adenoma has been interpreted in the light of the normal epithelial cell population of the colorectum [193]. This includes undifferentiated cells, differentiating cells, fully differentiated cells and exhausted or senescent cells [194]. Undifferentiated cells lack cytoplasmic clues as to their ultimate direction of differentiation, but are not equivalent to stem cells. They are located in the lower third of the crypt. The nucleocytoplasmic ratio is high, nuclei are vesicular with one or more prominent nucleoli and chromatin is finally dispersed (euchromatin). The cytoplasm shows early evidence of maturation, containing a Golgi apparatus, a few secretory vacuoles, mitochondria, small amounts of rough endoplasmic recticulum, polysomes and free ribosomes. Further differentiation is accompanied by divergence into one of the principal end-cells: endocrine, columnar and goblet cells [195,196]. Goblet cells, endocrine cells and Paneth cells (limited to proximal colon) achieve full maturation within the lower zone of the crypt. However, the columnar cell acquires its final specialization upon leaving the crypt to reach the surface epithelium. Crypt columnar cells are compressed between goblet cells, show secretory or transport vesicles within the apical cytoplasm and lack a well developed microvillous brush border. Surface columnar cells are characterized by cytoplasmic expansion, loss of vacuolation and a well developed microvillous brush border.

In adenomas there is a failure of cytoplasmic maturation. Undifferentiated and differentiating cells are found throughout the crypt and within surface epithelium [193,194]. Secretory vacuoles become prominent within the apical cytoplasm of columnar cells and some may contain electron-dense material [197,198]. Such electron-dense bodies were described by Birbeck and Dukes in adenomas from patients with familial adenomatous polyposis [199]. Histochemical studies on semithin sections have shown that the electron-dense material is a glycoprotein [200]. The glycoprotein is likely to include MUC1. Membrane-associated MUC1 is associated with the apical membrane of normal crypt base columnar cells and MUC1 expression is increased in adenomas [171]. Normal crypt columnar cells from the left colon contain electron-lucent vacuoles, whereas right-sided columnar cells secrete electron-dense material [201]. Larger, cytoplasmic bodies within adenomatous epithelium may represent phagocytosed apoptotic debris [202]. Columnar cells predominate in tubular adenomas, whereas villous adenomas may secrete abundant mucus. The mucus-secreting cells of villous adenomas express the core mucin protein MUC2 that is specific to the goblet cell lineage [203,204].

Serrated adenoma

In the first detailed report on serrated adenoma [205], the original diagnoses for lesions subsequently classified as serrated adenoma included hyperplastic polyp, serrated adenoma and adenoma. Criteria for diagnosing serrated adenoma remain imprecise, no doubt due to the lack of clinical imperative. A pragmatic approach is to label a serrated polyp as an adenoma (for management purposes) if it contains dysplastic epithelium. Through such lumping nothing will be learned of the aetiology, pathogenesis, natural history or clinical significance of the serrated pathway.

Contenders for the diagnosis of serrated adenoma include:

1 large hyperplastic polyps, particularly when multiple and occurring in the proximal colon [206];

2 hyperplastic polyps including foci of dysplasia;

3 large hyperplastic polyps with enterocytic (eosinophilic) change [207];

4 admixed polyps, partly hyperplastic and partly traditional adenoma;

5 admixed polyps, partly hyperplastic and partly serrated adenoma;

6 'classical' serrated adenoma, unequivocally adenomatous but showing a serrated configuration;

7 tubulovillous or villous adenoma with slight or focal serration; and

8 dysplastic epithelium with serration, abundant eosinophilic cytoplasm and enlarged vesicular nuclei containing prominent nucleoli.

The size and heterogeneity of this list illustrates the difficulty in diagnosing serrated adenoma. Nevertheless, the principal problem lies not with the morphological complexity but in the initial recognition of only three types of serrated polyp: hyperplastic polyp, admixed polyp and serrated adenoma, and the suggestion that these are distinct and readily distinguished [205]. At the molecular level, even the traditional hyperplastic polyp may show characteristics typical of a neoplasm (p. 624). The following account will be based on reports of 'classical' serrated adenoma, but it is likely that serrated polyps are related histogenetically and represent a continuum [106,107].

Macroscopic appearances

Serrated adenomas are usually between 5 and 20 mm in diameter, sessile and either protuberant or flat. They resemble a tubulovillous adenoma when protuberant. Magnification of the surface topography may show star-shaped or asteroid crypt openings reminiscent of the hyperplastic polyp [208].

Microscopic appearances

Classical goblet cells are reduced in number as in hyperplastic polyps. Columnar cells are characterized by an eosinophilic cytoplasm (Fig. 38.9). An apical secretory theca may be obvious in H&E sections. No theca is seen in columnar cells with dark eosinophilic cytoplasm. In such cases enterocytic differentiation may be evident, as demonstrated by the presence of a well developed brush border [207]. Endocrine cells are absent, whereas they are scattered in the crypt base of hyperplastic polyps. There is often a complex villous and tubular architecture. The tubules are branched and arranged haphazardly, sometimes horizontally. Bud-like microacini are frequent. Nuclei are crowded, elongated and pseudostratified but the nucleocytoplasmic ratio is usually low and there is little pleomorphism. The proliferative compartment remains in the lower crypt region as in normal mucosa and hyperplastic polyps but unlike traditional adenomas. Nevertheless, mitoses and cell cycle-associated proteins may be demonstrated in an abnormally superficial location. Criteria for grading have not been established but conventional cytological alterations including nuclear enlargement and nucleolar enlargement will be indicative of a higher grade of neoplasia.

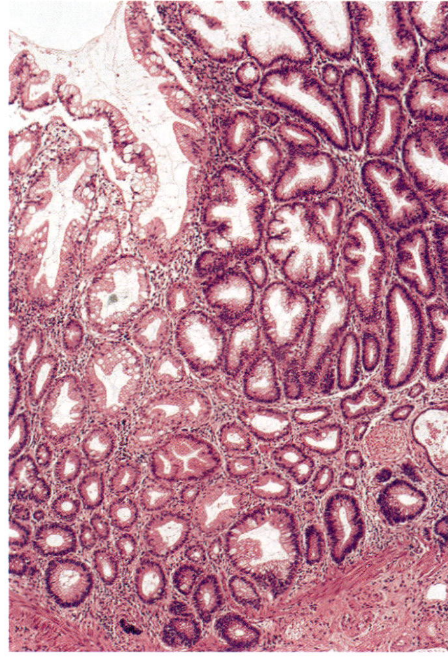

Fig. 38.9 Serrated adenoma arising in hyperplastic polyp.

Special investigations

Two principal biomarkers for the serrated pathway have emerged. Characteristic of the full serrated spectrum is the increased expression of secretory mucin including not only goblet cell mucin MUC2 but also gastric foveolar mucin MUC5AC. These are expressed by the columnar cells as well as cells with a classical goblet morphology. By contrast MUC4, a transmembrane glycoprotein expressed by columnar cells in normal mucosa, is down-regulated. The second biomarker is DNA microsatellite instability (MSI) (p. 556). Present infrequently and to a low level (MSI-L) in typical hyperplastic polyps, MSI-L is a relatively frequent finding in the hyperplastic component of mixed polyps [106]. Transitions to MSI-H coincide with dysplastic change and are associated with loss of expression of the DNA mismatch repair gene *hMLH1* [107]. The involvement of serrated polyps in MSI pathways of colorectal neoplasia has been noted above. However, morphological and molecular pathways do not fall within non-overlapping categories. The traditional adenoma–carcinoma sequence applies not only to the MSS or suppressor pathway but also to the MSI or mutator pathway in the context of HNPCC (p. 570). Serrated polyps are the likely precursors of sporadic MSI-H cancers but may also evolve into MSI-L and MSS cancers [107].

Adenoma–carcinoma sequence and *de novo* carcinoma

The evidence that adenomas can develop into carcinomas is largely circumstantial but nevertheless convincing. The arguments are summarized below.

1 Adenomas are six times as common in surgical specimens of colorectal cancer than in length-, age- and sex-matched colorectal specimens from patients without cancer [209].

2 Metachronous carcinomas are twice as likely to arise in patients with carcinoma and adenoma(s) in the original specimen than in patients with carcinoma alone. This illustrates the risk associated with the presence of multiple adenomas [210].

3 In patients with synchronous carcinomas additional adenomas are found in 75% of specimens [211].

4 Patients treated for large, villous or severely dysplastic adenomas, particularly when multiple, are more likely to develop carcinomas in the future [212].

5 Focal carcinoma may be observed in adenomas (Fig. 38.10), and conversely residual adenoma is often present in surgical specimens of colorectal cancer [1,213] (Fig. 38.11). The latter finding is more common in early cases limited to the bowel wall than in more advanced tumours [214]. Residual adenoma is also more common in second (smaller) synchronous carcinomas. These observations may be explained by the progressive destruction of the adenoma as the carcinoma increases in size.

6 Adenomas occur at an earlier age than carcinomas [215]. This is most clearly evidenced in patients with familial adenomatous polyposis and is supported by the findings of population screening programmes.

7 Adenomas are larger and more numerous in high-risk groups (those with a strong family history of colorectal cancer) [216] and high-risk populations [126,133].

8 A series of adenomas will show all grades of dysplasia ranging from slight deviations from normal through to changes amounting to carcinoma *in situ* [1,137]. Increasing dysplasia is accompanied by an increasing incidence of DNA aneuploidy [64], an important feature of neoplastic transformation. Dysplasia is also accompanied by a progressive increase in genetic changes implicating oncogenes and tumour suppressor genes [2].

9 In an uncontrolled study, removal of adenomas reduced the incidence of cancer in the 'clean' segment [217].

10 Adenoma cells can be transformed into carcinoma cells *in vitro* [218].

Few can doubt that adenomas have an increased propensity for malignant invasion as compared to normal mucosa. It is a fact, however, that adenomas are common lesions and the great majority will fail to become malignant in the course of a typical lifespan [219]. Additionally, removal of between two and three times as many adenomas in the test groups of large randomized controlled population screening studies has led to no reduction in cancer incidence. The reduced mortality in the groups undergoing faecal occult blood testing is explained by the detection of cancer at a relatively early stage [220].

The preceding observations demand critical consideration of the actual proportion of carcinomas that arises within a preexisting adenoma. The generally held view in the West has been that the great majority of cancers arise within an adenoma. Publications purporting to demonstrate *'de novo'* carcinoma are open to various interpretations. It should be recalled that adenomas may on rare occasions be flat or even depressed, presenting essentially as dysplasia within flat mucosa [36,37] (Fig. 38.12). In the West, dysplasia confined to the mucosa is not diagnosed as carcinoma (however severe) and in the face of this rule the *'de novo'* theory is a conceptual impossibility. Some illustrations of *'de novo'* carcinoma may represent early cancers that have destroyed a small adenoma [221] (Fig. 38.13). Others show severe dysplasia only [222], and some examples could even be interpreted as satellite lymphatic spread from a primary cancer to adjacent mucosa

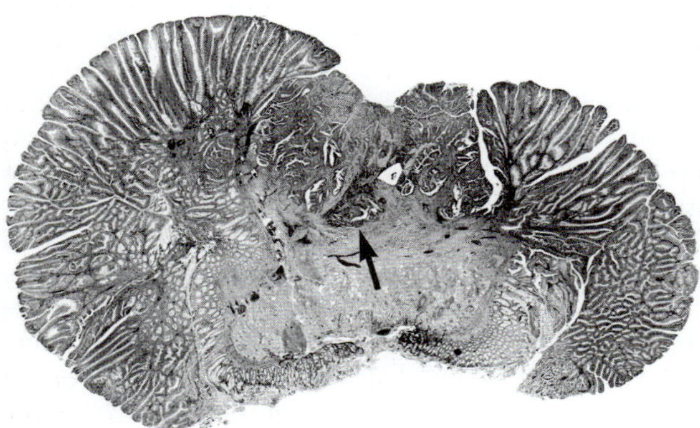

Fig. 38.10 Tubulovillous adenoma with a central focus of invasion by adenocarcinoma (arrowed) across the muscularis mucosae into the stalk.

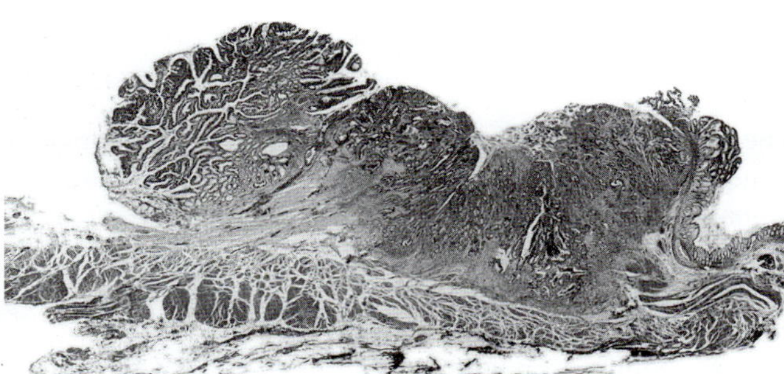

Fig. 38.11 Adenocarcinoma of the colon with residual adenomatous tissue at its edge.

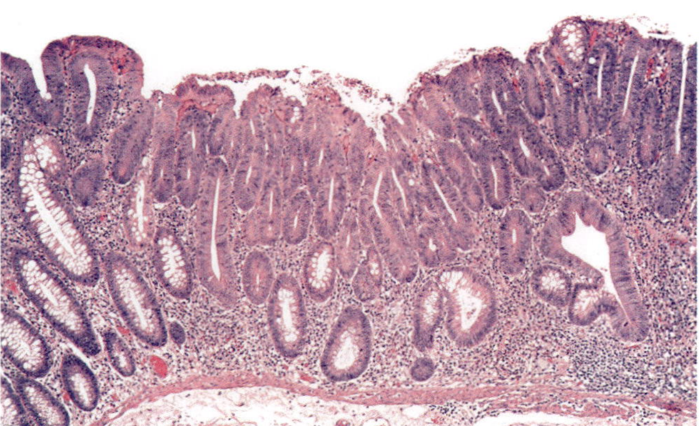

Fig. 38.12 Flat tubular adenoma.

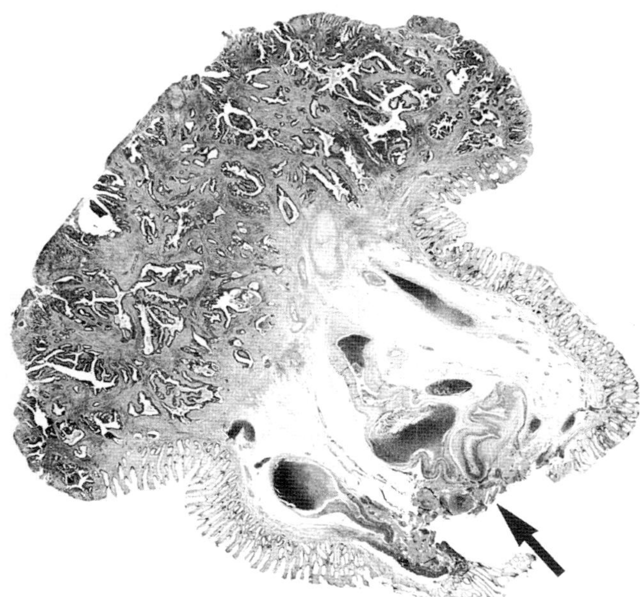

Fig. 38.13 Polypoid adenocarcinoma of the colon. There is no residual adenoma. The margin of local excision (arrowed) features eosinophilic coagulative necrosis due to diathermy burn.

[223]. Nevertheless, recent studies support the view that *'de novo'* cancer and *'classical'* cancer represent divergent evolutionary pathways [40,224]. *'De novo'* cancers show a non-polypoid, superficially spreading growth pattern and possibly a more aggressive course [225–227]. They lack K-*ras* mutations [38,46,228] and do not express goblet cell lineage-specific MUC2 mucin [203]. The origin of a substantial proportion of cancers from small flat lesions with high malignant potential would explain the lack of impact of polypectomy upon cancer incidence.

Malignant potential of adenomas

Morphological features that determine the malignant potential of an adenoma are size, growth pattern and grade of dysplasia. The risk of developing metachronous neoplasia is highest for those with large adenomas with a villous component and is further increased in subjects with multiple adenomas [212].

Size

Several studies have shown that the malignant potential is increased in large adenomas compared to small adenomas [229–231]. The experience at St Mark's Hospital [1] suggests that the prevalence of cancer in adenomas under 1 cm in size is only about 1%, in those between 1 and 2 cm in diameter it is about 10%, and in those over 2 cm in diameter there is nearly a 50% malignancy rate. Sixty per cent of all adenomas in this selected series were small (under 1 cm in diameter), 23% were 1–2 cm in size and only 17% were over 2 cm in diameter. This suggests that as adenomas grow, and there is direct evidence that they can [232,233], so does the risk of cancer increase. However, small adenomas do become malignant and if the figures given above were applied to the general population, the proportion of cancers arising in adenomas less than 1 cm in diameter would be about 5%.

Histological type

The classification of adenomas into those with a predominantly tubular pattern, those with a mainly villous pattern and those with a mixture of tubular and villous areas (tubulovillous adenoma) has shown that in general, the adenoma with a villous pattern has a higher malignant potential than one with a tubular pattern. Thus, in the St Mark's material the malignancy rate for tubular adenomas is about 5% but rises to 40% in villous adenomas. The rate of the intermediate or tubulovillous type (22%) suggests that these tumours behave more like villous than tubular adenomas. The subdivision of adenomas on the basis of their growth pattern is both subjective and dependent on sampling. A retrospective histological review of adenomas [232] found focal villous change in 6% of solitary tumours but in a prospective study using a dissecting microscope and multiple histological sections this figure rose to 35%, reaching 75% in solitary lesions larger than 1 cm in diameter. The frequency with which a villous growth pattern is found increases with the size of the tumour and this points to the possibility that as adenomas grow, there is an increasing tendency for them to adopt a villous type of structure [233]. However, small pedunculated villous adenomas and large sessile tubular adenomas do occur. The factors controlling the growth pattern of adenomas are unknown. *APC* mutations have been associated with villosity in sporadic adenomas [6]. Villosity is often found in HNPCC adenomas [234–236].

The malignant potential of adenomas has been calculated on the basis of their size and histological type and these show that the very common tubular adenoma, under 1 cm in diameter, has a very low malignant potential (1%), whereas the small villous tumour, which is rare, has a 10% malignancy rate. Tubulovillous adenomas of this size have a malignant potential of about 4%. In those tumours between 1 and 2 cm in diameter there is no significant variation in the malignancy rate with histological type, but in polyps over 2 cm in diameter the malignant potential is significantly greater for tumours with a villous component than for tubular adenomas.

It has never been denied that villous tumours may and often do develop malignant change (Fig. 38.14). Earlier controversy centred on tubular adenomas, with some authors stating that they invariably become malignant and others maintaining that they never or very rarely do so [237–240]. The recognition of a spectrum of histological appearances and the appreciation of the importance of size in the malignant potential of adeno-

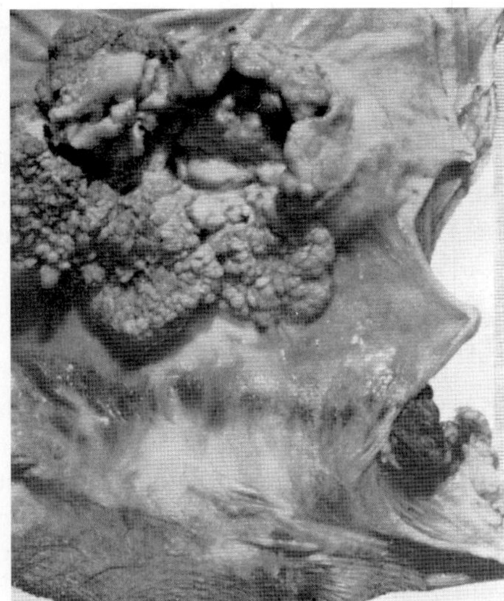

Fig. 38.14 Ulcerating carcinoma of rectum above (above) in continuity with sessile villous adenoma below.

mas brings relativity to this old argument. Although histological type is very important in the assessment of malignant potential it does seem that size has the paramount place [230]. One reason why villous adenomas have a much greater cancer rate than tubular adenomas could simply be that they are usually much larger tumours. However, a study of the cytological appearances in the three histological types of adenoma emphasizes the importance of the degree of epithelial dysplasia and explains why even small villous tumours have a 10 times greater malignant potential than tubular adenomas of the same size [1]. Villosity is associated with HNPCC adenomas and with the serrated neoplasms (p. 562), pathways implicating DNA microsatellite instability and associated with a high risk of malignancy.

Epithelial dysplasia

The grading of adenomas into those showing mild, moderate or severe dysplasia has shown that, irrespective of histological growth pattern, their malignant potential increases with increasing degrees of dysplasia. Small adenomas under 1 cm in diameter, which make up the majority of adenomas, usually show mild dysplasia only and have a very low malignant potential. The malignancy rate rises to 27% if severe dysplasia is present, but this is rare in a polyp of this size. A similar relationship is seen in adenomas 1–2 cm in diameter, those with mild dysplasia having a low malignant potential whereas those with moderate and severe dysplasia are increasingly likely to contain invasive carcinoma. In adenomas over 2 cm in size, the malignancy rate is high but shows little relation to the degree of dysplasia.

Although the trend observed for size and malignant change is considerably greater than the trend for dysplasia and malignancy, there are reasons to suspect that, at the biological level, dysplasia is the most selective marker of increased malignant potential. It should be remembered that the assessment of dysplasia is subjective and prone to sampling error. Furthermore, the most dysplastic area within a malignant adenoma is likely to have been destroyed. In a series of 269 adenomas, aneuploidy was found to correlate with both size and grade of dysplasia but was unrelated to architectural type [64].

Number of adenomas

Is the patient with one or more colorectal adenomas at increased risk of developing cancer subsequently? It would seem that an increased risk of developing metachronous cancer (and adenoma) is primarily related to the number of previously diagnosed adenomas [241,242]. Size was found to be of marginal relevance, but only after 15 years' follow-up [240]. Grade of dysplasia and architectural type appeared to be lacking in any prognostic significance [240]. Rather different findings emerged in a more recent estimate of the risk of developing metachronous cancer [212]. In a large group of subjects treated for sigmoidoscopically detected adenomas, but not followed up, the risk of developing colonic cancer (as compared with the general population) for those with large or villous adenomas was significantly increased (standardized incidence ratio 3.6). This increased to 6.6 with the addition of multiplicity. However, small tubular adenomas were not associated with an increase in risk, even when multiple [212].

Natural history of the adenoma–carcinoma sequence

Given that adenomas may, under certain circumstances, develop malignant change, how long does it take for this to occur? Opportunities to follow this progression occur infrequently since polyps are usually removed upon their discovery. However, observations on this sequence have been made in two clinical situations: first, in a small number of patients who had a benign tumour and refused operation or failed to re-attend after initial diagnosis and who subsequently developed a carcinoma at the same site [1]; and secondly, in patients with familial adenomatous polyposis [243,244].

Observations like these are useful in that they confirm that some adenomas never develop malignant change, whilst in those that do the sequence evolves over a long period, although this is probably very variable. Together with studies of metachronous cancer rates and age distribution curves, they suggest that the adenoma–carcinoma sequence rarely evolves over less than 5 years and often fails to occur at all in a normal adult lifespan. More evidence in support of this general concept comes from the study of familial adenomatous polyposis, in which progression to cancer can be measured in decades. However, in some conditions, for example HNPCC, the adenoma–carcinoma sequence is accelerated [245,246].

Pseudocarcinomatous invasion in adenomas

The presence of benign adenomatous epithelium deep to the muscularis mucosae of adenomas has been described as adenomatous polyp with submucosal cysts [247], pseudocarcinomatous invasion [248] and epithelial misplacement in adenomatous polyps [249]. Tangential sections through the irregular glandular base of an adenoma may produce the appearance of isolated islands of epithelium artefactually [237] but in this case they are superficial to the muscularis mucosae. In one study of a large series of adenomas [247] 2.4% showed the criteria of pseudoinvasion.

Characteristic of this condition is the presence of gland-like structures in the submucosa showing the same degree of dysplasia as the epithelium of the head of the adenoma and in continuity with it across the line of the muscularis mucosae (Fig. 38.15). The cytological characteristics of malignancy are lacking. Submucosal glandular tissue is well circumscribed, and individual glands are surrounded by lamina propria without the desmoplastic reaction to the epithelial cells which is usual in invasive carcinoma. In the majority of cases, deposits of haemosiderin pigment around the submucosal glands are present and areas of recent haemorrhage are also common (Fig. 38.16). Although haemosiderin is often seen in the head of typical adenomas it is unusual in the underlying submucosa or in the neighbourhood of early invasive carcinoma. Sometimes there is marked branching and proliferation of the muscularis mucosae. Pseudoinvasion is particularly associated with larger tumours and in those with a long stalk. It is seen most commonly in adenomas of the sigmoid colon, the site of greatest muscular activity in the large bowel. Together with the histological appearance this suggests that the misplacement of epithelium is secondary to haemorrhage due to repeated twisting of the stalk of an adenoma. Follow-up studies on these patients have shown no evidence of recurrence or metastasis, confirming their benign behaviour. The recognition of pseudoinvasion is important not only in the treatment of individual patients but also in the critical evaluation of the malignant transformation of adenomas.

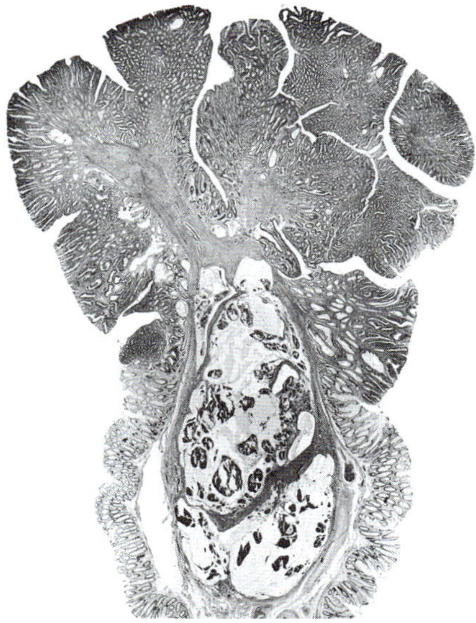

Fig. 38.15 Pseudocarcinomatous invasion into the stalk of a tubular adenoma.

Familial adenomatous polyposis (FAP)

(Familial adenomatous polyposis is also known as familial polyposis coli or adenomatous polyposis coli (APC). N.B. The gene was named *APC* because the abbreviation FAP had been applied previously to another genetic disorder.)

In this condition hundreds if not thousands of adenomas develop throughout the colon and rectum; the risk that one or more of these will become malignant is 100%. The tendency to form numerous adenomas is inherited on an autosomal dominant basis. The disorder affects about 1 in 10 000, 25% being new mutations [250]. The polyposis gene is located on the long arm of chromosome 5 [28,251–253]. Although the abnormal gene is present within all cells, the morphological sequelae are focal and limited to certain organs, notably (but not exclusively) the large bowel. Loss or mutation of the normal allele is required for the initiation of an adenoma [4]. The genetics underlying the morphogenesis of adenomas have been described at the beginning of this chapter, emphasizing the importance of the *APC* gene in the initiation of colorectal neoplasia.

Adenomas usually appear by the second decade of life. Later development may occur, particularly in attenuated forms of the condition [254,255]. The average number of tumours in the colon and rectum is of the order of about 1000, most patients having between 500 and 2500. The locus of the germline mutation influences the number of adenomas and also the incidence of extracolonic complications. Exon 15 mu-

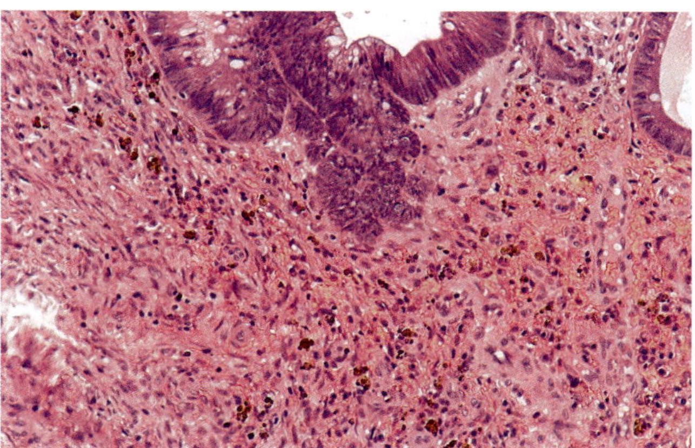

Fig. 38.16 Pseudocarcinomatous invasion in the stalk of an adenoma. The adjacent connective tissue contains deposits of haemosiderin pigment.

tations are common and associated with severe forms of the disease [256]. The figure of 100 adenomas has been suggested as a convenient lower limit [8]. Less than 100 adenomas may be seen at the early stages of the disease and would be diagnostic in the child of an affected parent. FAP is now understood to occur in an attenuated form [254,255]. Adenomas are often few in number, tend to be right sided and may be flat. The development of cancer is delayed with respect to classical FAP [254,255]. Mutations are typically within exons 3 and 4 or the 3′ end of exon 15 [257].

The most usual symptoms are a tendency towards increasing bowel motions that later become associated with the passage of mucus and blood. Adenomas are probably present for at least 10 years before symptoms arise. The average age at diagnosis of polyposis in propositus (new) cases is about 35 years. By this time the increasing severity of the symptoms is usually due to colorectal cancer (present in two-thirds of propositus cases). As would be expected from the presence of very large numbers of adenomas, synchronous carcinomas of the colon and rectum are not uncommon and nearly one-half of polyposis patients with malignant disease have more than one carcinoma.

Inspection of a colectomy specimen removed for FAP will show numerous polyps of diminishing size which gradually become less pedunculated until they are represented by small sessile nodules on the mucosal surface (Fig. 38.17). Some may be so tiny as to be indistinguishable from slight irregularities in the mucous membrane on naked-eye observation (Fig. 38.18). Microscopic examination, however, will disclose these earlier stages of adenomas until they are no more than small collections of intramucosal tubules (Fig. 38.19) or even single neoplastic tubules.

Adenoma–carcinoma sequence

In addition to revealing the early stages in the formation of adenomas, a study of polyposis also adds to our knowledge of the natural history of adenomas. The age distribution at the time of diagnosis of the disease in propositus cases has been known for some time and in the St Mark's Hospital series the mean age is 26–28 years for polyposis patients without associated carcinoma and 39.2 years when cancer is also present. For call-up members of the families found to have polyposis the respective figures are 23.7 years and 33.0 years. In both groups it appears that the adenomas of polyposis exist on average for about 10 years before malignancy appears. Unfortunately, it is not possible to say how long it is before individual adenomas become malignant, but the range must be wide. There are certainly considerable differences in the growth rate of the adenomas as judged by the observation of the retained rectum in patients who have undergone colectomy and ileorectal anastomosis or in patients who have refused or postponed treatment. The increase in size of the polyps may be almost imperceptible over a period of years, or occasionally a tumour may rapidly enlarge and acquire clinical significance within a year or two.

Fig. 38.17 Familial adenomatous polyposis.

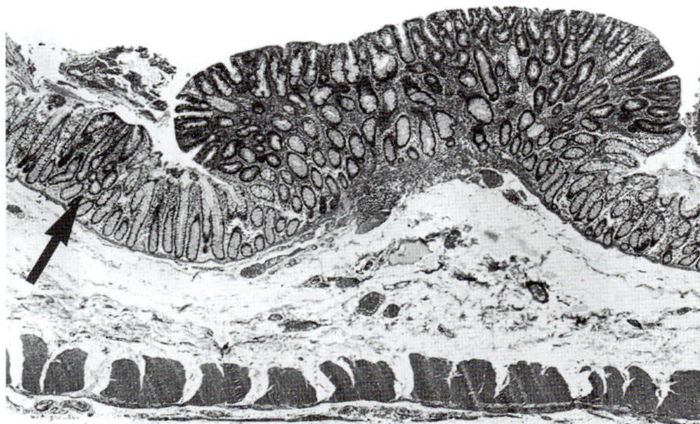

Fig. 38.18 Small tubular adenoma in familial adenomatous polyposis. To the left there is a microadenoma (arrowed) which is not big enough to be visible by surface inspection.

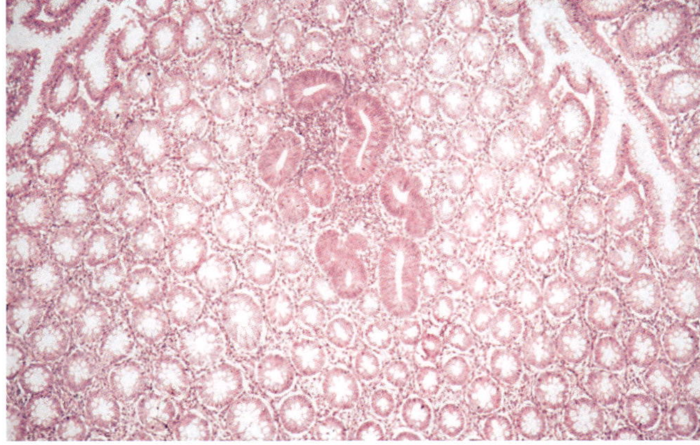

Fig. 38.19 Microadenoma in familial adenomatous polyposis. The mucosa has been sectioned horizontally.

Table 38.3 Length of the precancerous phase in familial adenomatous polyposis.

Period in years	Number of patients observed	Number surviving period without cancer	Number developing cancer in period	Percentage developing cancer
0–5	65	59	6	9.2
5–10	45	35	10	22.2
10–15	23	16	7	30.4
15–20	12	8	4	33.3
20–25	7	4	3	42.6
25–30	3	1	2	66.6
30–35	1	–	1	100.0

The relationship between adenomas and cancer can be studied in polyposis in another way. Some patients have not been treated because they refused operation and some in past years received limited surgery only. By observing when cancer appears in these patients it is possible to gain some idea of the length of the precancerous phase. Sixty-five such patients in the St Mark's Hospital Register were observed over varying periods of time and the results are recorded in Table 38.3. Clearly, the longer adenomas are present in the large intestine the more likely it is that malignancy will supervene. If the period is 5 years only the incidence of cancer is about 10%, but after 20 years the figure is in the region of 50% and it continues to rise steadily after that time. This is in keeping with clinical experience with the propositus cases. On the other hand, it is important to note that large numbers of adenomas can be present for considerable periods of time without cancer appearing, confirming that in general there is a long precancerous phase during which the lesions remain benign and during which cancer prevention methods may be applied.

Cancer prevention

Cancer prevention in FAP is dependent on treating the patient's adenomas before these have undergone malignant change. This in turn is dependent on diagnosing the disease at an early stage. The best way to achieve this is to prepare a complete family pedigree immediately the propositus case is diagnosed. All siblings of the propositus case are suspect and should be examined as soon as possible. It is usually easy to identify which patient has passed on the defective gene and his or her siblings should be examined. All children of any parent with polyposis have a 50:50 chance of inheriting the disease. It is usual to begin sigmoidoscopic examinations at the age of 14 years and, if these are negative, to repeat the examination at 2-year intervals. This policy of intercepting the progress of the disease at the earliest possible age has had the effect of reducing the initial incidence of intestinal cancer from 66% in propositus cases to 7.5% in the group of polyposis patients called up for examination because they were known to be at risk [8]. Now that the polyposis gene has been cloned [252,253], it has become possible to identify affected family members by screening for the family-specific mutation and offering predictive testing [258].

FAP may be treated by total proctocolectomy and either ileostomy or the construction of a neorectum (ileoanal pouch), when all risk of future large bowel cancer is removed. Alternatively, total colectomy and ileorectal anastomosis allows normal function of the bowel, but with a risk of further adenomas and possibly carcinomas appearing in the retained rectum. This risk is minimized by periodic examinations, usually every 6 months, of the rectum and the destruction of any adenomas by excision or diathermy. The St Mark's Hospital records include 174 patients treated by colectomy and ileorectal anastomosis up to the end of 1984, of whom 11 subsequently developed rectal cancer; three of these patients have died as a result of this complication whereas the others are alive and well. Analysis by an actuarial method gives an estimate of the cumulative risk of rectal cancer over a period of 25 years following colectomy of 13% [259]. However, more extended follow-up has disclosed increasing cancer risk beyond the age of 50 years [260]. This reduction in the incidence of rectal cancer has been achieved by the removal of adenomas, thus giving further evidence of the essential part played by adenomas in the evolution of cancer as well as indicating a way in which prevention of intestinal cancer may also be applied in the general population.

FAP is an important model for the study of the relationship of adenoma and adenocarcinoma of the large intestine. It provides an opportunity to observe the early stages in the formation of adenoma, the adenoma–carcinoma sequence and the length of the precancerous phase, and to suggest a possible form of control of intestinal cancer. It also provides a model for testing novel chemopreventive strategies, notably the administration of non-steroidal anti-inflammatory drugs acting through the inhibition of COX-2 [23].

Extracolonic manifestations

Familial adenomatous polyposis may be associated with various extracolonic lesions [261]. Gardner reported a syndrome consisting of adenomatosis coli, multiple epidermal cysts and soft tissue tumours of the skin [262]. The syndrome has been modified by Gardner and others as more examples of extracolonic manifestations have been recorded. These include osteomas of the entire skeleton [263], abdominal and intra-abdominal fibromatosis (desmoid tumours) [264,265], dental abnormalities [266], adenomas of the small intestine, periampullary region of the duodenum and stomach [267–273], carcinoma of the duodenal bulb [274] and periampullary region [275], biliary neoplasia [276], fundic gland polyps in the stomach [270], a histologically distinctive variant of papillary carcinoma of the thyroid [277], tumours of the central nervous system [278], multiple endocrine neoplasia type IIb [279], adrenal tumours [280], hepatoblastoma [281] and congenital hypertrophy of retinal epithelium (CHRPE) [282]. Not only are the colorectal adenomas of familial adenomatous polyposis and Gardner's syndrome indistinguishable, but subclinical osteomas of the mandible have been described in patients with otherwise typical polyposis [283]. It is now clear that FAP and Gardner's syndrome are one and the same condition. The presence of extracolonic manifestations is at least in part influenced by the precise site of the *APC* mutation [282]. However, the possibility of modifying genetic influences cannot be excluded [284]. Whilst the relatively conservative operation of colectomy and ileorectal anastomosis successfully removes the risk of colorectal cancer, an increasing number of patients are dying of the extracolonic manifestations, notably intra-abdominal fibromatosis and carcinoma of the periampullary region. This emphasizes the fact that FAP is in reality a multisystem disease.

Turcot's syndrome

A familial disorder characterized by the association of intestinal neoplasia and malignant tumours of the central nervous system (CNS) has been termed Turcot's syndrome [278]. The association between CNS tumours and FAP is well established, most tumours being medulloblastomas [285]. Subjects with hereditary non-polyposis colorectal cancer also show an increased incidence of CNS tumours, primarily high-grade gliomas [285,286]. There is also evidence for recessive inheritance of Turcot's syndrome caused by compound heterozygous mutations within the DNA mismatch repair gene *PMS2* [287].

Hereditary non-polyposis colorectal cancer (HNPCC)

(HNPCC is also known as Lynch syndrome or hereditary mismatch repair deficiency syndrome (HMRDS).)

The demonstration of linkage [288,289] and subsequent cloning of genes responsible for this condition [70–74], establishes HNPCC as a precancerous autosomal dominant disorder ranking in clinical importance with FAP. It is discussed at this juncture to facilitate comparison with FAP and to emphasize the role of adenoma in the pathogenesis of cancer. Furthermore, the genetic defect is known to influence adenoma progression [245,290–292]. Warthin encountered a large HNPCC family (family G) in the 19th century, subsequently revisited by Lynch. Lynch recognized similar families, and with his coworkers established the following clinical and pathological features: autosomal dominant inheritance, early onset of malignancy, multiple colorectal cancers, increased risk of extracolonic cancers (particularly endometrial), predilection of cancer for the proximal colon and relative reduction of cancer aggressiveness [293–297]. Adenomas were infrequent and Lynch emphasized the absence of premonitory features. Despite the fact that the syndrome is at least as common as FAP and would require similar strategies of cancer prevention, few polyposis registries took up the challenge. It is interesting, in retrospect, to reflect on why the observations of Warthin and Lynch were largely ignored for so many decades. Prior to the establishment in Finland of research into the clinical features, genetics, epidemiology, pathology and screening of HNPCC [298–302], publications on the topic had been generated by Lynch almost exclusively. The separation of families into those with (Lynch I) and without (Lynch II) extracolonic cancers may have little clinical validity [303]. Nevertheless, some colon-specific families may be explained by modifying genetic factors causing early-onset disease in this anatomical location [304]. Others may be explained by an as yet unknown genetic mechanism.

Adenoma–carcinoma sequence

Non-polyposis colorectal cancer families were known to St Mark's Hospital by the 1970s [305]. Adenomas occurred with increased frequency, this being correlated with the number of affected family members [305]. These observations were linked with Veale's suggestion that adenomas could be inherited on an autosomal recessive basis [306]. The suggestion by Lynch that cancer could be inherited on an autosomal dominant basis without involving the stage of adenoma could not be reconciled with the St Mark's viewpoint. As is often the case in such matters, the opposing views had to be reconciled before the truth could emerge. Adenomas began to be described in surgical specimens from subjects with HNPCC as well as in at-risk family members undergoing colonoscopy [234,235,246,300,307]. These were not numerous but developed at an early age and were distinguished by large size, villosity and severity of epithelial dysplasia. The infrequency of adenomas and their sporadic-type anatomical distribution led to the suggestion that the inherited genetic abnormality was not responsible for initiation but accelerated adenoma growth and increased the likelihood of malignant transformation [235].

HNPCC is caused by a germline mutation affecting one of a family of DNA mismatch repair genes (*hMLH1, hMSH2, hMSH6, hPMS1, hPMS2*) [70–74,308]. The genes *hMLH1* and *hMSH2* are implicated in most HNPCC families. Homologous genes are found in bacteria and yeast [309]. Loss of DNA repair proficiency follows inactivation of the second or wild-type allele [310]. This leads to the development of numerous DNA replication errors (RERs), described also as microsatellite instability (MSI) or the mutator phenotype. Oncogenesis results from the mutational inactivation of additional genes implicated in the regulation of growth and differentiation. Genes mutated in adenomas include *TGFβRII, IGF2R, BAX, MSH3* and *MSH6* [47,292]. A family with a germline mutation of *TGFβRII* has been documented [311]. This differed from HNPCC on clinical and pathological criteria and neoplasms did not show DNA microsatellite instability. Another family has been reported with inherited defects of DNA base excision repair [108] (as opposed to mismatch repair): affected individuals had multiple (about 50) adenomas—more than in HNPCC but less than in FAP.

Although virtually all cancers from subjects with HNPCC are MSI-H, adenomas may be MSI-H (the majority), MSI-L or MSS [292]. MSI-H adenomas tend to show severe dysplasia or early cancer [290–292]. Immunohistochemically demonstrated loss of expression of a DNA mismatch repair gene (congruent with the germline mutation) occurs in virtually all HNPCC adenomas regardless of microsatellite status [292]. It is likely that the passage from MSS to MSI-L to MSI-H depends upon the mutation of additional mismatch repair genes ('mutators'), including *hMSH3* and *hMSH6* [292].

Carcinoma in HNPCC

The right-sided predilection and increased tendency to multiplicity is now well documented [312]. Patients are less likely to have lymph node or distant metastases at presentation, even when cancers diagnosed through screening are excluded [312,313]. On histology there is a higher frequency of mucinous and poorly differentiated cancers [312–314]. These adverse prognostic features are offset by the cancers being well circumscribed with a pushing margin. Furthermore a pronounced lymphocytic reaction is typical, except in mucinous cancers. The lymphocytes are intraepithelial (tumour infiltrating), peritumoural or arranged in nodular aggregates deep to the tumour (Crohn's-like). Diffuse invasion, perineural invasion and venous invasion are infrequent [312,314].

There is an increased incidence of cancer in various extracolonic sites: endometrium, ovary, stomach, pancreas, small intestine, lymphoma, renal pelvis, ureter and central nervous system [286,295,296,315]. The increased risk of brain tumour is common to both FAP and HNPCC, though the former tend to be medulloblastomas and the latter high-grade gliomas [285,286]. These probably account for the so-called syndrome of Turcot [285] (p. 570). There is also an increased incidence of cutaneous neoplasia, including sebaceous adenoma and carcinoma [295]. The diagnosis of Muir–Torre syndrome was made in an individual shown 10 years later to be a member of a very large HNPCC family [316]. Muir–Torre syndrome is probably synonymous with HNPCC [296,316,317].

Cancer prevention in HNPCC

As in FAP, cancer prevention is best achieved through the facility of a registry. A family history should be obtained from all subjects with colorectal cancer, noting age at onset and site of all malignancies. The finding of three affected first-degree relatives with colorectal cancer, spanning at least two generations and with at least one of these developing cancer below the age of 50 (Amsterdam criteria) has provided a useful definition [318]. However, genuine families do not always fulfil these criteria. The presence of DNA microsatellite instability and/or immunohistochemically demonstrated loss of a DNA mismatch repair protein confirms the diagnosis. Not all families meeting the above criteria show evidence of a mismatch repair defect [313], indicating the existence of alternative forms of hereditary predisposition to colorectal cancer.

Known affected and at-risk family members require colonoscopic screening from the third decade onwards. Ideally this should be annual screening, at least from the age of 35 years [245]. Screening aims to detect and remove adenomas before they become malignant. The carcinoma : adenoma ratio is high and interval cancers occur despite frequent screening [319]. This fits with the tendency for adenomas to show an increased likelihood of malignant conversion [235]. Many centres advocate screening programmes for extracolonic sites, notably endometrium and ovary [315].

The advent of genetic testing means that screening can be limited to carriers of a mutation [320]. Prophylactic colectomy is likely to become an option for some gene carriers. However, it must be hoped that chemoprevention will be shown to reduce the risk of cancer in the future.

Adenocarcinoma

Cancer of the colon and rectum is one of the more common forms of malignant disease [321]. The mortality rate in the UK is second only to lung cancer for males and breast cancer for females. In the following account, the colon and rectum are considered together since the pathology of adenocarcinoma in these regions of the large intestine is essentially the same. However, there is growing evidence that cancer of the right and left colon are epidemiologically and pathogenetically distinct and this will be given due consideration.

Epidemiology

A striking variation in the frequency of colorectal cancer is seen in different geographical areas [321]. The disease is especially common in North America, northern Europe and Australasia, and is rare in Asia and particularly uncommon in (sub-Saharan) Africa. Worldwide, the average incidence rate for colon cancer in males is 16.6 per 100 000 and for females 14.7 per 100 000. For rectal cancer the average incidence rates are 11.9 per 100 000 in males and 7.7 per 100 000 among females. The greatest variation between low- and high-risk areas is seen for colon cancer in males (60-fold). This figure could be inflated by under-registration. When registries with reasonably reliable data are considered only, the variation becomes about 10-fold. Up to fivefold variations in incidence rates for colon cancer in females are recorded in different Scottish local authority districts. Colon cancer is especially frequent in the north of Scotland.

Site-related data must be regarded as generally unreliable for the purposes of comparing international mortality rates. Nevertheless, interesting time trends for combined colon and rectal cancer mortality are apparent and appear to form a pattern. In countries where the rates were initially low, such as Japan, substantial increases have been observed. Where rates were moderately high at the outset, small increases have occurred. However, in countries where rates were initially very high, gradual falls in mortality have been noted with time [321]. In New Zealand the incidence of colorectal cancer has continued to rise in older subjects, but has fallen in those below 50 years [322].

Relation between anatomical site and epidemiology

There are reasons for and against considering the colon and rectum as a single organ. On the one hand, good correlations between cancer incidence rates for both sites are found when different populations are compared [321]. Cancers of rectum and colon share similar precancerous lesions and conditions as well as histopathological appearances and modes of spread. One must accept also that different criteria are used for defining the anatomical limits of the rectum and many tumours arise at the rectosigmoid junction itself. This raises questions as to the reliability of information recorded in death certificates. On the other hand, important sex differences exist between cancer of the colon and rectum. Up to the age of 55 cancer of the colon is more common in women and thereafter becomes slightly more common in men [323]. In high-risk areas the incidence of right-sided colon cancer may be higher in females of all ages [321,322]. In contrast, rectal cancer is found with equal frequency in both sexes up to the age of 55, but then becomes more common in males [322,323]. By the age of 65 it is nearly twice as common in males and a fourfold difference has been recorded by the age of 80 [324].

There are additional reasons for distinguishing between left- and right-sided cancers. Normal epithelium from left and right colon differs in terms of composition of mucus and expression of blood group antigens (see Chapter 33). The ascending colon and distal colon and rectum are further distinguished by their dissimilar functions. Proximal cancers are more likely to be diploid and show DNA microsatellite instability and other genetic differences [325–327]. There are certainly grounds for suggesting that the weighting of factors implicated in the aetiology of colorectal cancer could be influenced by site or even subsite.

Time-trend studies in high-risk areas for colorectal cancer usually demonstrate gradually falling incidence rates. However, separate consideration of the right and left colon shows that the fall in left-sided cancers is not necessarily accompanied by a fall in the incidence of right-sided cancers. Indeed, several studies now have described increasing incidence rates for right-sided cancers [328,329]. Most of these tumours arise in the region of the ileocaecal valve and lower ascending colon; the true caecum is a rare site for cancer. Five circumstances have been highlighted in which the risk of cancer of the right colon appears to be increased selectively: female sex, previous cholecystectomy—especially in women, a low blood cholesterol prior to surgery, nulliparity and following hormone therapy for prostatic cancer [330]. A common denominator might be altered patterns of bile acid metabolism affecting either the amount or composition of enterohepatically circulating bile acids. The amount or type of bile acid entering the right colon may be especially relevant to carcinogenesis at this site, whereas the faecal concentration of bile acids in the left colon will be modified by other dietary factors such as fibre content. Selenium deficiency has been proposed as an alternative hypothesis to explain the increasing incidence of right-sided cancers [331]. Finally, genetic factors operate in the small but important group of right-sided cancers associated with HNPCC.

Age and sex

Cancer of the colon and rectum usually presents in the seventh decade and worldwide incidence rates show the disease (rectal cancer in particular) to be more common in males. However, it is unsatisfactory to consider age and sex in isolation from each other or from geography, anatomical site within large intestine and trends with time.

In low-risk (developing) areas the average age at diagnosis is about 50 years [332]. However, a relatively small percentage of such populations will reach the 'cancer age' found in the industrial countries. Cancers within low-risk areas or low-risk populations show an unusually high incidence of high-grade and mucinous types [333,334], even when allowance is made for the fact that the incidence of high-grade carcinoma of the colon and rectum decreases with increasing age. Over-representation of HNPCC would be one explanation for this observation. The incidence of metastatic involvement of lymph nodes in resected specimens of colorectal cancer also decreases with advancing years [335].

Probably the youngest reported patient with a genuine carcinoma of the colon was a 9-month-old female infant [336]. Most published cases of intestinal cancer in young persons occur between 10 and 15 years of age and there seems to be a very high incidence of mucinous and signet ring cell carcinomas among them [337]. A proportion of these may carry germline mutations in one of the DNA mismatch repair genes, responsible for the condition HNPCC (see p. 570) [338]. It is important to distinguish cancer of the colon and rectum from juvenile polyps, which can mimic invasive carcinoma if there is much associated necrosis and secondary infection.

Aetiology

Multiple factors are involved in the aetiology of colorectal cancer just as multiple steps are implicated in its pathogenesis. It is likely that both environmental and constitutional factors are interwoven within the aetiology and that the precise composition of factors varies from one individual to another [339]. Thus, neither one factor nor one set of factors will underlie the aetiology of all cases of colorectal cancer. Cancer is ultimately a disorder at the level of the gene. The initiated state may in some instances be constitutional, due, for example, to the inheritance of a mutated tumour suppressor gene. This has been shown to apply to FAP (see p. 567) and HNPCC (p. 570). Alternatively, initiation may be acquired through either a spontaneous mutation or the action of an environmental mutagen. Further mutations and promotional influences will operate within the stepwise process leading to the formation of a malignant neoplasm [2]. This is described in more detail on p. 552.

Environmental factors

The considerable geographical variation in the incidence of colorectal cancer underlies the importance of environmental factors in the aetiology of the disease. This variation does not appear to be related to racial differences, as migrants from low- to high-risk areas acquire the pattern of incidence appropriate to their adopted country [340–342]. The attention of epidemiologists and experimentalists has focused mainly upon diet. Blame has been placed upon the excess consumption of meat and animal fat [343], refined carbohydrate [337,338] and beer [344] at the expense of fibre [345], fruit and vegetables [346,347] and trace elements [331]. It is likely that the various dietary hypotheses are interrelated and that a summation of factors is ultimately responsible for the provision of a carcinogenic microenvironment.

It has been suggested that carcinogens might be produced by the action of bacteria upon a substrate within the large intestine [348]. Diet could influence both the concentration of the substrate and the composition and metabolic activity of the bowel flora. Some workers have considered these substrates to be bile acids [349–351]. The liver synthesizes two bile acids (cholic and chenodeoxycholic) and these are secreted as conjugates with glycine or taurine. The major metabolites produced by the action of the bacterial flora of the large intestine are the products of deconjugation and 7-dehydroxylation: deoxycholic and lithocholic acid. Other metabolites are produced and detected within human faeces [50]. There is evidence that bile acids act as tumour promoters. Surgical and dietary manipulations that increase the faecal bile acid concentration increase also the yield of colorectal cancers in animal experiments [352]. *In vitro* microbial mutagenicity tests such as the Ames test have shown that bile acids are not mutagenic, but indicate deoxycholic and lithocholic acid to be comutagens. Thus, mixtures of bile acids and known mutagens give rise to more mutations than the mutagen alone [353]. Yet faecal samples have been shown to contain mutagens and such mutagenic activity is most pronounced in population groups at high risk of colorectal cancer [354]. A mutagenic lipid compound has been identified (fecapentaene). This mutagen is produced in the colon by anaerobic bacteria and its synthesis is stimulated by a high concentration of faecal bile acids [355]. Bile has been implicated in the aetiology of periampullary adenomas in subjects with FAP [356]. It has also been suggested that the composition of FAP bile differs from that of normal subjects, causing it to be more mutagenic [356].

Faecal bile acid levels have been measured in high- and low-risk populations [354]. This epidemiological approach has been utilized by several groups and supports the role for bile acids in large bowel carcinogenesis [357]. It has been suggested that increased consumption of meat and hence animal fat would account for the high levels of faecal bowel acids detected in high-risk populations [343]. The manner in which meat is cooked may be critical. Frying meat at high temperatures generates carcinogenic heterocyclic amines of which one of the most abundant and well investigated is 2-amino-1-methyl-6-phenylimidazo (4,5-6) pyridine (PhIP) [358]. There is a close relationship between *per capita* meat intake and colorectal cancer incidence in various populations [359,360]. Seventh Day Adventists who consume little or no meat show a relatively low rate of colorectal cancer as compared to their fellow Americans [361]. However, a survey of dietary variations within Seventh Day Adventists showed no relationship between meat consumption and large bowel cancer [362]. New Zealand Maori have a high intake of fat and protein, yet the incidence of colorectal cancer is low in this group [363]. It is relevant also that dietary manipulation has failed to influence the bacterial flora of the large intestine [364]. Case-control studies (in which each patient with colorectal cancer is matched to a 'normal' control) have usually failed to support a link between either meat intake or faecal bile acid levels and colorectal cancer [339]. It is important that patients with colorectal cancer are carefully selected for such studies. Patients with cancer may have modified their diet and the presence of liver metastases could influence bile acid metabolism. It has been argued that the failure of case-control studies to support dietary and/or the faecal bile acid hypothesis may reflect the confounding influences of other important factors (both environmental and genetic) in the aetiology of large bowel cancer [339].

In 1971 Burkitt suggested that the high-fibre diet of the South African Bantu might protect this population from colorectal cancer by increasing the speed of intestinal transit [345]. This would reduce the exposure of the gut to carcinogens. At the same time carcinogens would be diluted by the greater bulk of the stool. The link between fibre, transit time and colorectal cancer has never been substantiated. Nevertheless, the dilutional effect of a bulkier stool remains an attractively simple hypothesis, although experimental models have produced conflicting findings [365]. Alternative roles for fibre have been proposed. 'Fibre' comprises cellulose and hemicellulose derived from plant cell walls. These materials, together with dietary starch that has escaped digestion within the small intestine, are fermented by microorganisms within the right colon. The products of this process include acetic acid, propionic acid and butyric acid. These short-chain fatty acids serve as the principal sources of energy for colorectal epithelium and it is conceivable that a deficiency of these nutrients might compromise the metabolic integrity of colonocytes [366].

The products of fermentation lead to acidification of the stool. Several population studies have demonstrated an association between colorectal cancer and stool pH, a low pH appearing to be protective [367]. An underlying mechanism for this phenomenon may be the decreased 7-hydroxylation of bile acids by bacteria [368]. The yield of dimethylhydrazine-induced tumours in rats was reduced when stools were acidified by the consumption of lactulose and/or sodium sulphate [367]. The ability of fibre to bind and neutralize mutagenic compounds has been demonstrated *in vitro* [347]. Interestingly, this ability varies considerably according to the source of the fibre [347]. A diet rich in protective plant fibre could explain the low incidence of colorectal cancer in certain groups, such as Maori [347].

The use of fibre as a dietary intervention in randomized controlled trials showed no influence over the natural history of colorectal adenoma [369,370]. The preventative effects of fibre may act at the stage of adenoma–carcinoma transition but it is also possible that the clinical importance of adenoma as a premalignant lesion has been exaggerated.

The promoting effects of faecal bile acids are thought to be due to cytotoxic injury leading to regeneration with accompanying increased cell turnover [371]. Ionized fatty acids of dietary origin will also irritate colonic epithelium; a high-fat diet might therefore be linked in a more direct way with colorectal carcinogenesis [372]. Similarly, dietary cholesterol has been proposed as a direct tumour promoter [373]. In the presence of calcium ions the toxic effects of ionized fatty acids and faecal bile acids would be abolished through their conversion to insoluble calcium soaps [372]. Abnormal patterns of cellular proliferation in individuals at high risk for colorectal cancer disappeared when their diets were supplemented with calcium carbonate [16,374]. However, most long-term studies have failed to reproduce this finding [375].

The hypotheses regarding dietary fat, fibre and calcium should not be viewed in isolation, but are linked through a final common pathway, namely the promoting effects of faecal bile acids. However, other dietary hypotheses have been proposed. One case-control study emphasizes the promotional importance of a high calorific intake in the form of refined carbohydrate as well as fat [376]. A high intake of refined carbohydrate may be associated with the development of colorectal adenomas [377]. Conversely, calorific restriction inhibits tumour formation in animals. Cruciferous vegetables may exert a direct protective influence [346], perhaps through the induction of aryl-hydrocarbon hydroxylase by indoles. This enzyme assists in the neutralization of noxious chemicals within the gastrointestinal tract and other surfaces exposed to the environment [378]. Selenium, a rare trace element, reduces the incidence and progression of cancer in animals exposed to carcinogens [379,380]. Low blood selenium levels have been correlated with a reduced activity of glutathione peroxidase. Failure to remove peroxidase may lead to oxidative damage of DNA. Dietary deficiency of selenium has been linked to the increasing incidence of right-sided colonic cancer [331]. However, a prospective study failed to demonstrate an increased risk of colorectal cancer in patients with low selenium levels [381]. The association of colorectal cancer with alcohol consumption, particularly beer, is well founded [344]. Smoking is now implicated also, particularly in the aetiology of adenoma [382–385]. There is growing evidence in support of a protective role for aspirin [386,387].

Endogenous factors

Although adenomas are more common in males than females, adenomas in females are likely to be larger [119] and show a greater incidence of severe dysplasia in some [124] though not all surveys [181]. These observations suggest that either the hormonal environment [388] or the expression of hormone receptors [389] could be influencing the progression of the adenoma–carcinoma sequence. Oestrogens might also exert an indirect action through their effect upon lipid and bile acid metabolism [390]. These observations also explain the similar incidence of cancer but not adenoma in males and females, implying that adenomas in females are more likely to become malignant [123]. Subjects with acromegaly are at increased risk of developing colorectal adenomas [391]. Endocrine cells are well represented within adenomas [139] and the trophic effects of local hormone production may be implicated in the progression of neoplasia. Other epithelial cell products could operate on an autocrine basis to promote growth [392–394].

Such growth factors might also explain the epithelial hyperplasia seen in the mucosa bordering colorectal cancer (transitional mucosa).

Genetic factors

Cancer is now understood to be a genetic disease brought about by the stepwise accumulation of somatic mutations. General principles are provided at the commencement of this chapter. The term 'genetic' does not necessarily imply that cancer is hereditary. Indeed, most of the genetic changes are acquired at the somatic level and are not constitutional or germline. Nevertheless, some mutations acquired as somatic steps may also be inherited. An important example would be the inheritance of a mutation in the *APC* gene, the tumour suppressor gene implicated in the autosomal dominant disorder familial adenomatous polyposis (p. 567). A second example would be the inheritance of a mutated DNA mismatch repair (MMR) gene responsible for the autosomal dominant disorder hereditary non-polyposis colorectal cancer (HNPCC) or Lynch syndrome [70] (p. 570). However, whereas the *APC* gene is thought to be implicated in the pathogenesis of the majority of sporadic large bowel cancers, MMR genes are implicated in only about 15% of sporadic malignancies. Like their hereditary counterparts, sporadic MMR-deficient cancers are characterized by the presence of DNA microsatellite instability (DNA replication errors) and a predilection for the proximal colon [327,395,396].

The demonstration of DNA microsatellite instability within a large bowel cancer invites the following question: does the subject carry a germline mutation or is this a sporadic cancer showing the mutator phenotype? Individuals with a germline mutation are more likely to be young and/or have a positive family history of colorectal cancer [338]. Additionally, whereas cancers in affected members of HNPCC families show evidence of abnormal DNA repair in a high proportion of microsatellite loci, sporadic cancers are bimodally distributed with respect to MSI status [395]. Cancers characterized by a low proportion of unstable loci (MSI-L) are unlikely to be from subjects with HNPCC. Sporadic MSI-H cancers are uncommon in subjects below the age of 60 years. The mechanism underlying a sporadic mismatch repair defect is methylation of the promoter region of *hMLH1* [397]. Methylation assays should help to distinguish sporadic from familial MSI-H cancers in the future. Methylation is clearly an important epigenetic mechanism underlying the aetiology of a subset of colorectal cancers (p. 548). The controlling factors are unknown but genetic influences are likely to be implicated.

Polyposis syndromes other than FAP are associated with an increased risk of colorectal cancer. These include juvenile polyposis (p. 668) and two less ill-understood syndromes: hyperplastic polyposis [398] (p. 626) and mixed polyposis [399] (p. 627). A locus on chromosome 15q has been linked to a syndrome of hereditary colorectal adenoma and carcinoma in which small numbers of adenomas and serrated polyps occur [400]. The genes responsible for these disorders may turn out to be implicated in sporadic colorectal cancer. Turcot's syndrome may not be a distinct entity. Most Turcot families turn out to have either FAP or HNPCC [285]. Similarly, the Muir–Torre syndrome (combining colorectal cancer and other external malignancies with multiple cutaneous neoplasms, notably of sebaceous glands) appears to be synonymous with HNPCC [316]. The *APC* I1307K mutation occurring in Ashkenazi Jews results in a short mononucleotide repeat that in turn is susceptible to truncating mutation. The resulting phenotype is an increased frequency of adenoma and carcinoma in affected families [401]. Germline mutation of *TGFβRII* and *MYH* have also been described as rare causes of familial colorectal cancer [108,311].

When all the above are excluded, including attenuated FAP (p. 567), there still appears to be evidence of an inherited basis to colorectal cancer. For example, the literature includes references to 'adenoma families' [402–404], and 'late-onset familial colorectal cancer' [405]. Common to many of the descriptions are: a family history suggestive of an autosomal dominant gene; more adenomas than the general population but not excessive numbers; adenomas often large and villous; cancers mainly in the left colon and rectum; onset of malignancy later than in HNPCC; and absence of tumour DNA microsatellite instability [404–406].

Genetic factors need not necessarily operate exclusively at the somatic level within the tumour genome. They could also influence intermediary metabolism, either through failing to detoxify potential mutagens or through enhanced synthesis of initiating or promoting compounds. Given the fact that acetylation is involved in the metabolism of arylamine carcinogens, interest has been generated in the observation that fast acetylators are at increased risk of developing colorectal cancer [407,408], though these results have not been reproduced in all populations [409]. As phenotype may be altered by disease status, it is preferable to consider genotype. Studies of N-acetyl transferase 2 (*NAT2*) have shown no relation between genotype and colorectal neoplasia [410], whereas particular *NAT1* alleles may influence cancer risk [411]. It has been stated that genetic effects are confounding with respect to the role of environmental agents in population and case-control studies [339]. The converse would be correct also. Indeed, the fast acetylator effect is observed primarily in high-risk populations in which an abnormal diet-related metabolite would be acetylated at an enhanced rate when the same factor does not feature in the low-risk diet.

The glutathione S-transferases detoxify carcinogens including the epoxides of polycyclic aromatic hydrocarbons [410]. The glutathione S-transferase null genotype has been associated with an increased risk of colorectal cancer [412–414]. The protective effects of leafy vegetables may be mediated by folate, in turn influencing methyl availability. Hypomethylation of DNA occurs as an early step in colorectal carcinogenesis and may be a factor in chromosomal instability [415]. Polymorphisms of methylenetetrahydrofolate reductase influence the activity of the enzyme but, paradoxically, individuals with the less active form of the enzyme were at lower risk for colorectal cancer in two studies [416,417]. Apolipoprotein E (ApoE) regulates cholesterol metabolism. Individuals with the ε4 allele absorb a greater percentage of their luminal cholesterol. This allele was less common in individuals with proximal colorectal cancers [418]. The cytochromes P450 (*CYP1A1* and *CYP2D6*) are implicated in the conversion of polycyclic aromatic hydrocarbons to their DNA binding carcinogenic forms [410]. Homozygosity for the MspI mutant genotype of *CYP1A1* has been associated with colorectal cancer [419].

The attempts to unravel the complex interactions of gene and environment in the aetiology of colorectal cancer have been based upon simplistic assumptions in relatively small case-control studies with no allowance for the fact that colorectal cancer may be a heterogeneous disease following a number of independent morphogenetic pathways. Future studies will need to be much larger and more detailed, heeding the genetic profiles of tumours as well as the innumerable interactions between host polymorphisms and dietary factors.

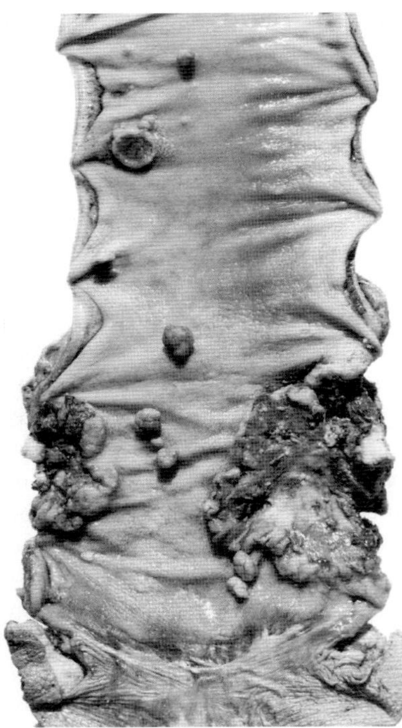

Fig. 38.20 The adenoma carcinoma sequence. There is a large ulcerating carcinoma in the lower rectum surrounded by multiple small adenomas. About 10 cm above the main carcinoma is a small ulcerating cancer.

Histogenesis of colorectal cancer

The dysplasia–carcinoma sequence may be regarded as a morphological counterpart to the multistep concept of carcinogenesis. The usual presentation of dysplasia is in the form of an adenoma; the adenoma–carcinoma sequence is considered on pp. 556–67 together with a discussion of serrated adenoma, flat adenoma and *'de novo'* carcinoma. The origin of colorectal cancer within the dome epithelium overlying gut-associated lymphoid tissue has been documented [420]. Dysplasia occurs in other clinical contexts associated with an increased risk of colorectal cancer including ulcerative colitis (p. 497), in other forms of chronic inflammatory bowel disease such as schistosomiasis [421] and Crohn's disease [422], in patients with juvenile polyposis (see p. 628), and at the site of ureterosigmoidostomy (see p. 630). An increased risk of gastrointestinal cancer may accompany the Peutz–Jeghers syndrome through the advent of dysplasia (see p. 629). Radiation-induced adenocarcinoma of the large bowel is well documented. Patients have usually been treated for cancer of the uterine cervix [423]. Both adenoma and carcinoma have been described in women who as teenagers were exposed to a single large dose of pelvic radiation in the sterilization programme carried out in the Auschwitz concentration camp in 1943 [424].

Multiple neoplasms

Multiple neoplasms of the large intestine are found with remarkable frequency in surgical specimens (Fig. 38.20). In one survey multiple tumours, adenomas or carcinomas, were present synchronously in 20% of patients [1]. The incidence of synchronous adenoma has been reported as 35% [209] and 36% [425]. A proportion of patients with a solitary adenoma or carcinoma will subsequently present with one or more additional neoplasms. The high incidence of multiple neoplasia has important clinical implications. When a single tumour is discovered the whole of the large intestine must be examined, preferably by colonoscopy if this is available, to exclude the presence of synchronous tumours. The indications and timing of follow-up examinations are matters for which it is more difficult to offer precise guidelines. However, the need is greatest for those patients who present with multiple tumours and who continue to produce crops of adenomas. It is of interest that patients with colorectal cancer and synchronous adenomas show improved survival rates as compared with patients without adenomas [426]. This appears to be true even when cases are matched for stage [426]. The recently recognized attenuated form of FAP will account for some examples of multiple neoplasia [254]. However, most subjects with multiple neoplasms will not be members of such families. Different hereditary factors may account for descriptions of 'adenoma families' [406]. Cancer multiplicity occurs in subjects with cancers showing high levels of DNA microsatellite instability (MSI-H) [105,427,428]. This applies whether the cancers are familial (HNPCC) or sporadic. It is unusual to observe multiple adenomas in either situation [234], though some subjects with multiple sporadic MSI-H cancers have multiple hyperplastic polyps, mixed polyps and serrated adenomas as well as traditional adenomas [107].

The incidence of synchronous carcinoma within the large intestine ranges from 2.8% to 8.0% [210,429–434]. In a St Mark's hospital series 3.2% had multiple synchronous large bowel cancers and a further 1.7% of the original group of patients were subsequently found to have a second intestinal cancer. It was noted that 75% of those with multiple synchronous cancers also had adenomas; the corresponding figure for patients with metachronous cancers was 60% [429]. The figure of 1.7% with metachronous cancer underestimates the theoretical risk, since some patients will die prematurely, interrupting the natural course of events, and it is conceivable that the original resection might have removed a fertile field for metachronous growths.

There is a general trend for the incidence of multiple cancers to rise as the number of adenomas increases. Whereas in patients in whom there was evidence of only one adenoma being present the incidence of multiple cancer was less than 2%, the figure for those with more than five adenomas rose to over 30%. It has also been shown in microscopic studies that there is evidence of residual adenoma in about 15% of sporadic cancers occurring singly [244]. If, however, multiple cancers from non-FAP patients are examined in the same way, the proportion in which adenomatous tissue can be found at the periphery of the cancer rises to 27% [429]. In cancers of the colorectum associated with FAP there is an even higher proportion, at 36.2% [8]. Plainly, specimens with multiple synchronous cancers will include a large proportion that are both symptomless and early and in which the search for residual adenoma is likely to be fruitful.

Early colorectal cancer

This term does not describe a specific stage in the histogenesis of colorectal cancer, nor does it represent a distinct clinicopathological entity. The concept of early malignancy serves to identify cancers that are curable and is analogous to the Japanese use of the term 'early gastric cancer'. Neoplasms of the colon and rectum probably have no potential for lymph node metastasis until they have invaded across the line of the muscularis mucosae into the submucosal layer. This may be explained by the relative paucity of lymphatics within colorectal mucosa [435]. As long as neoplastic cells are confined within the mucosa, the nomenclature 'adenoma' or 'dysplasia' is appropriate. Intramucosal neoplasia in the stomach may be associated with lymphatic metastasis. This may reflect the rich lymphatic supply to the gastric mucosa, particularly when affected by intestinal metaplasia. Whatever the reasons for the limited propensity for lymphatic spread in the large intestine, the fact may be exploited to the benefit of the patient who can be spared both the stigma of a diagnosis of cancer and needlessly radical surgery. In particular, the removal of early cancer in the lower rectum by transrectal endoscopic mucosectomy will obviate the need for rectal excision and a permanent colostomy. The term 'early colorectal cancer' is best restricted to cancer extending into but not beyond the submucosa. In cases of early rectal cancer so defined, the incidence of associated lymph node metastasis is 4%, providing poorly differentiated cancers are excluded [214]. Poorly differentiated cancers are in any event unlikely to present as early growths. Once growth extends into the muscularis propria, the risk of lymph node metastasis is about 12% [214]. This figure has remained unchanged at St Mark's hospital for decades. It is difficult to explain the reports of higher rates of nodal metastasis for rectal cancer confined to the bowel wall [436]. With spread in continuity beyond the muscularis propria into the pericolic or perirectal tissues, the figure is greatly increased to 60%. These facts have been used to show that local excision has an important role to play in the treatment of early rectal cancer [437].

Early colorectal cancer presents in three distinct ways: (i) malignant adenoma/polypoid carcinoma; (ii) focus of malignancy in a large sessile adenoma; and (iii) small ulcerating cancer.

Malignant adenoma ('polyp') and polypoid carcinoma

Malignant adenoma and polypoid carcinoma may be conceived as a spectrum ranging from adenoma with a microscopic focus of cancer to polypoid cancer with no adenomatous remnant. Pedunculated tumours should always be removed as a total excisional biopsy that includes both the head and a length of stalk. Step-sections must be taken through the whole tumour to detect the presence of invasion across the muscularis mucosae and the completeness of local excision [438] (Fig. 38.21).

It is generally agreed that malignant colorectal polyps can be managed safely by simple polypectomy provided that certain management protocols are adhered to strictly. The most important factors are completeness of excision and grade of malignancy [439–442]. Additional surgery is required if the cancer is inadequately excised or is poorly differentiated. Demonstration of venous [443] or lymphatic invasion [442] has been shown to influence prognosis adversely by some authors, though others have not shown venous invasion to affect outcome independently of grade and completeness of excision [441,442,444] The assessment of vessel invasion is not always straightforward. However, it would be unwise to ignore unequivocal tumour embolus within an endothelial-lined space.

The definition of completeness of excision varies from study to study. Some insist on a clearance margin of 1 mm [442] or 2 mm [441], whereas the St Mark's practice has been based upon a considered impression backed up by the opinion of the endoscopist. Insistence on a particular clearance distance probably accounts for the low proportion of polyps with favourable histology in some series, for example 26% [442] and 36% [441] versus 77% at St Mark's Hospital [439].

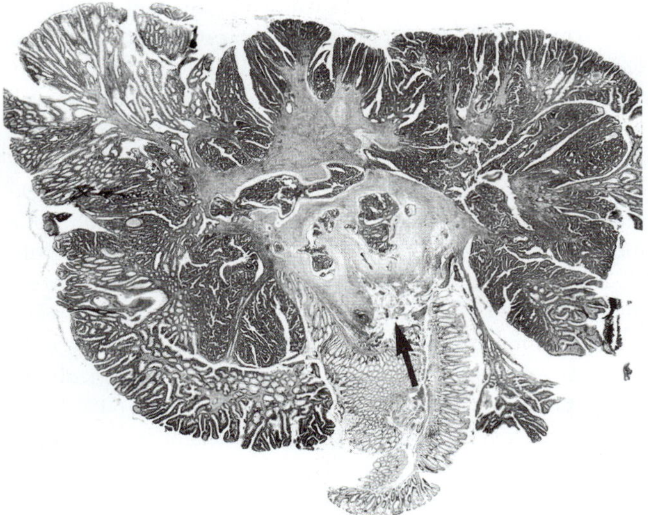

Fig. 38.21 Tubulovillous adenoma. In the central part of the photograph there is invasion of the stalk by well differentiated adenocarcinoma which extends close to the limit of excision as judged by the presence of a diathermy mark (arrowed).

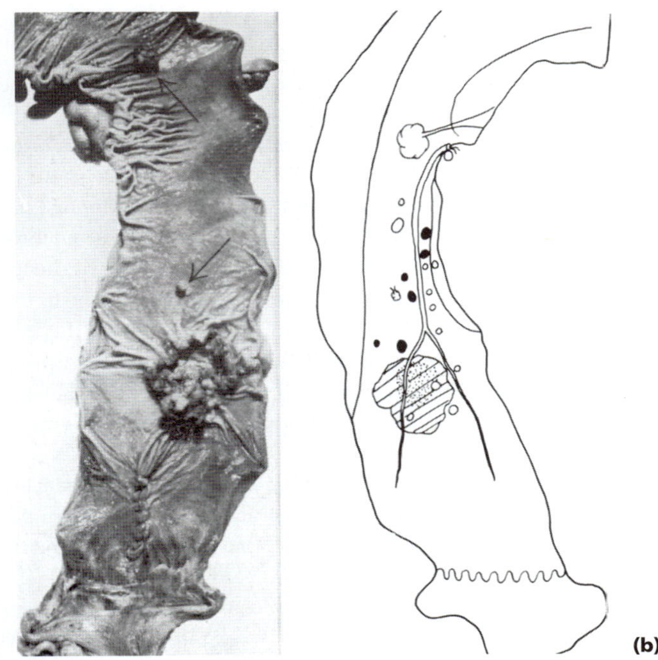

Fig. 38.22 (a) Ulcerated adenocarcinoma of rectum with associated benign adenomas (arrowed). (b) Chart to illustrate lymph node spread.

The decision whether to undertake further surgery depends not only on histology, but also on the site of the lesion and the age and health of the patient.

Focal carcinoma in a large sessile adenoma

This form of early malignancy is usually diagnosed when careful examination is made of a sessile growth that has been removed as a total excisional biopsy by submucous resection. The lesion should be pinned out onto a cork mat and attention must be given to the surgical margins and the careful examination of multiple blocks. Criteria for histological assessment are identical to those for malignant adenomas [439]. Some believe that the absence of a stalk plays a major role in the clinical outcome of local excision. This debate has to some extent been resolved by a study that carefully classifies malignant adenomas according to the level of spread: (i) within head; (ii) within neck; (iii) within stalk; and (iv) within submucosa of the underlying bowel wall [445]. Malignant change within a sessile adenoma must always be grouped in the last category. The clinical outcome for polypoid and sessile growths showing spread into underlying submucosa does not appear to differ [445].

Small ulcerating cancers

Local excision is occasionally undertaken for small, mobile ulcerating cancers (Fig. 38.20) of the lower rectum to spare the patient from rectal excision and a permanent colostomy. The cancer and rim of bowel wall may be removed as a disc. Excellent results are achieved when a strict policy, based upon clinical and histopathological criteria, is adopted [446,447]. In this study the indications for further surgery were incomplete excision, poor differentiation or extension of the growth beyond the rectal wall.

Macroscopic appearances

Up to 40% of all large bowel cancers occur in the rectum and rectosigmoid area. The sigmoid colon accounts for a further 25%. Of the remaining bowel, the ascending colon is a site of predilection and it would appear that the incidence of cancer in the right colon is increasing, especially in high-risk areas for colorectal cancer (see p. 572). However, this could be in part an age-related phenomenon compounded by the greater use of flexible endoscopy in elderly subjects.

Most cancers of the colon and rectum are ulcerating tumours with raised everted edges (Fig. 38.22). Ulcerating tumours may involve the bowel circumference to produce stenosis and obstruction. Some growths may be circumferential yet show little evidence of ulceration. Such annular growths have been called 'string carcinoma', since the effect is that of a string tied tightly around the bowel wall. In spite of their small size these tumours often produce severe stenosis with dilatation of the proximal bowel. String carcinomas occur with greatest frequency in the transverse and descending colon. Symptoms of obstruction are usually late in onset for proximal cancers because the fluid faeces pass easily through the constriction. Protuberant types are less frequent and are

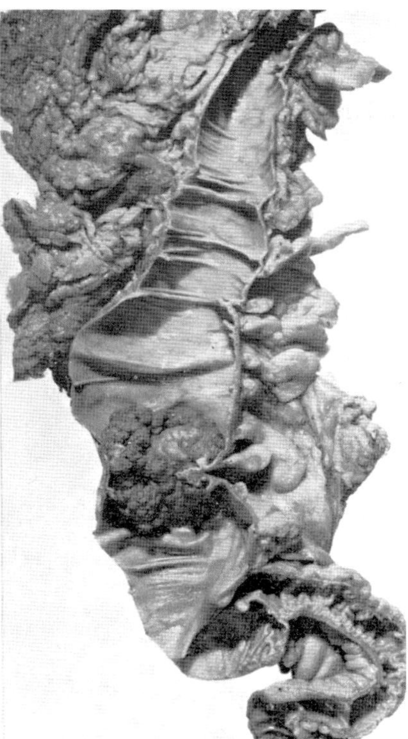

Fig. 38.23 Polypoid adenocarcinoma of ascending colon.

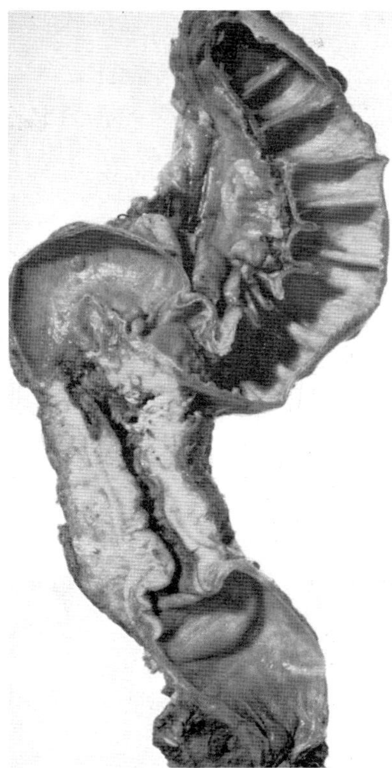

Fig. 38.24 Extensive infiltrating adenocarcinoma of rectum.

often of a relatively low grade of malignancy (Fig. 38.23). The ascending colon is a site of predilection. Some of these tumours have a papillary surface configuration. About 10% of colorectal cancers will show a mucoid appearance on the cut surface of the tumour due to the secretion of abundant mucus by the tumour cells. Most cancers of the colon and rectum remain relatively small and well circumscribed compared to gastric carcinoma. Moreover, they rarely show much submucous or intramural spread beyond their macroscopic borders. This characteristic is important in the consideration of surgical treatment. The diffusely infiltrating scirrhous type of carcinoma which is typically seen in the stomach as 'linitis plastica' is very rarely seen in the large bowel [448] (Fig. 38.24). When it does occur it is more likely to be a secondary manifestation of an occult carcinoma of the stomach than a true primary of the colon or rectum.

Microscopic appearances

The majority of colorectal cancers are adenocarcinomas in which tubular differentiation is easily discerned. The grade of differentiation is gauged mainly on architectural features (Fig. 38.25). In about 20% of cases tubules are either highly irregular or unformed; such tumours are graded as poorly differentiated [449]. When tubules are regular and the cytological appearances recall adenomatous epithelium, tumours are termed well differentiated (20% of cases). Just as the majority of colorectal cancers are relatively well circumscribed at the macroscopic level, so do the majority reveal a relatively well circumscribed invasive margin at the microscopic level. Only a minority (20–25%) can be considered to show diffuse infiltration characterized by extensive permeation and dissection of normal structures (smooth muscle or fat). In addition, an inflammatory response is usually lacking. A grading system which heeds tubule configuration, advancing margin and lymphocytic infiltration has been advocated [449]. Scattered Paneth cells and cells containing argentaffin or argyrophil granules are not an unusual feature but are usually few in number. When endocrine cells are numerous, the designation 'composite carcinoma–carcinoid' has been suggested [450].

Mucinous tumours account for 10% of carcinomas of the large intestine. The term mucinous is reserved for cases secreting a 'substantial' amount of mucus that is easily appreciated on gross inspection of the cut surface of the tumour and occupies more than 50% of the area of histological sections. Two main types are encountered. In the first, glands are distended with mucus and may be disrupted so that mucus enters the interstitial tissues. The glands may be remarkably well differentiated. Such tumours often arise in villous adenomas [451,452], in villous dysplasia in ulcerative colitis [453] and in anorectal fistulae [454]. In the second, highly irregular tubules, chains, laciform strands or clumps of cells are surrounded by mucin lakes (Fig. 38.26). This type occurs, like signet ring cell

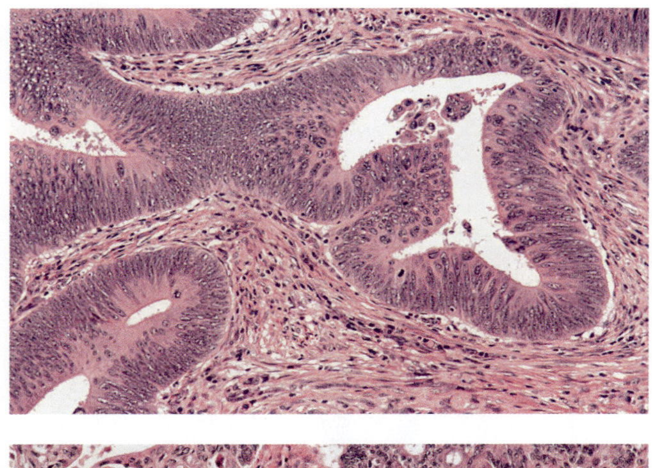
(a)

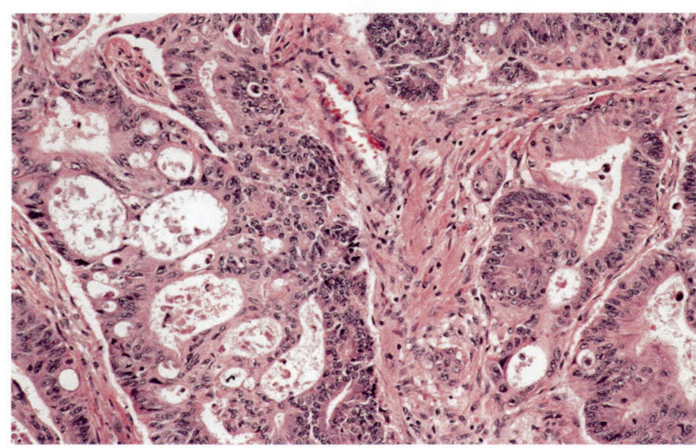
(b)

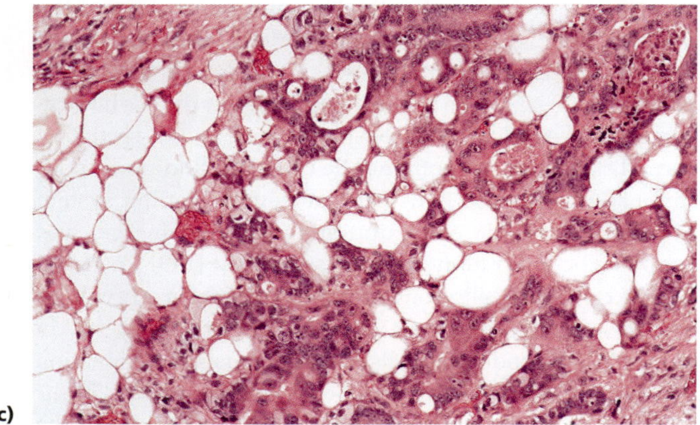
(c)

Fig. 38.25 (a) Well differentiated, (b) moderately differentiated and (c) poorly differentiated adenocarcinoma.

carcinoma, in young individuals and is more frequent in low-risk populations for colorectal cancer [334,452]. Mucinous adenocarcinoma occurs with increased frequency in HNPCC but is more obviously over-represented and likely to be poorly differentiated amongst sporadic MSI-H cancers [313,455]. Assessment of the grade of differentiation may be difficult when the malignant epithelium is disrupted by mucus.

There is general agreement that mucinous carcinomas, especially those occurring in the rectum, are associated with

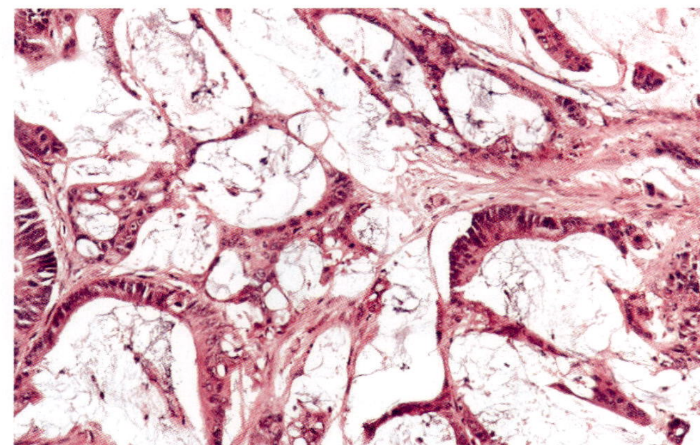

Fig. 38.26 Mucinous adenocarcinoma of rectum.

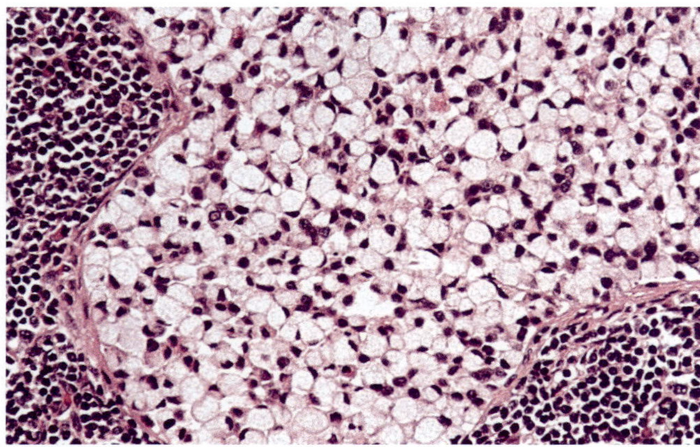

Fig. 38.27 Signet ring cell carcinoma infiltrating lymph node sinus.

a relatively poor prognosis [452,453,456]. In a series of rectal cancers studied at St Mark's Hospital the censored 5-year survival rates for non-mucinous and mucinous adenocarcinoma of the rectum were 62% and 53%, respectively. However, in the presence of other pathological variables, the division into mucinous and non-mucinous types did not contribute independent prognostic information [452]. A notable feature of mucinous carcinomas is the relative lack of a lymphocytic infiltrate [452]. This might be linked to their aggressive behaviour and may be due to the immunosuppressive effects of mucus [457], or to the lack of expression of human leucocyte antigen (HLA) Class I antigens [458].

Unlike their left-sided and rectal counterparts, mucinous cancers of the proximal colon are generally diploid, show high levels of DNA microsatellite instability, lack mutation or loss of *TP53* and are associated with a favourable prognosis [105,327,459]. It is no longer acceptable to group mucinous cancers of the colorectum as though they represented a distinct clinicopathological entity. Tumours composed only of signet ring cells (Fig. 38.27) are rare and most will turn out to be metastases from a gastric primary. Primary signet ring cell carcinoma accounts for less than 1% of cancers of the large bowel

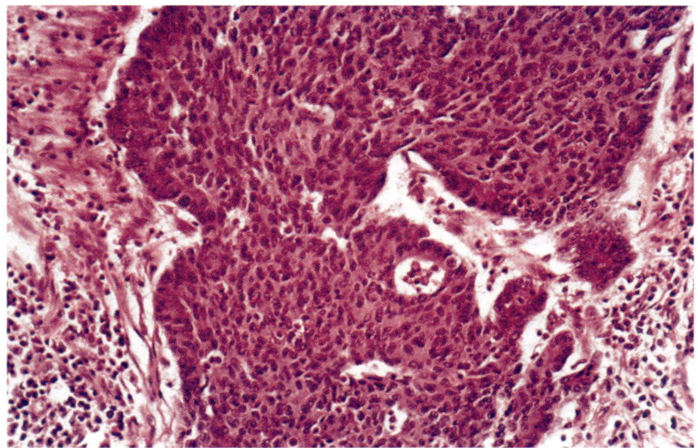

Fig. 38.28 Undifferentiated carcinoma of large bowel.

in high-risk countries. The prognosis is poor [452], though improved survival is described in well circumscribed or exophytic forms of signet ring cell carcinoma [460]. Such well behaving signet ring cell carcinomas are likely to be MSI-H. Linitis plastica-type cancers (with or without signet ring cells) are particularly aggressive [448].

Undifferentiated carcinoma of the large bowel encompasses two quite distinct entities, both of which are rare. In the first, the tumour shows a solid pattern of cells with vesicular nuclei and prominent nucleoli (Fig. 38.28). The cells are often large, but medium and small types occur also. Some areas may show a fascicular pattern, bands of spindle-shaped cells and incomplete acinar differentiation [461]. The latter finding together with the immunocytochemical demonstration of cytoplasmic secretory component [462] and scattered endocrine cells attests to the fact that these tumours are variants of adenocarcinoma. This impression may be confirmed by the demonstration of carcinoembryonic antigen, small amounts of mucus and mucus antigens and specific epithelial cytokeratins. A lack of marked nuclear pleomorphism, a circumscribed invasive margin and sometimes a pronounced peritumoural lymphocytic infiltrate are concordant with a relatively good prognosis which belies the somewhat ominous designation 'undifferentiated'. Cancers of this type (sometimes described as 'medullary') are often MSI-H and may be either familial (HNPCC) or sporadic [105,312,463]. Not only do these tumours form solid clumps of cells, but the peripheral cells often show a darkly staining eosinophilic cytoplasm. This may impart a superficial likeness to a carcinoid tumour. However, the larger cell size, greater degree of nuclear pleomorphism and mitotic activity of the undifferentiated carcinoma should prevent such a mistaken diagnosis. Large cell neuroendocrine carcinoma is another differential diagnosis. The latter will be distinguished by the ribbon-like cellular arrangements, small acini and palisaded clumps. A combination of adequate tissue sampling as well as histochemical and immunocytochemical staining should resolve any diagnostic difficulties.

The second undifferentiated carcinoma is the small cell (neuroendocrine) type [464–466]. In terms of its histology, cytology, ultrastructure and aggressive behaviour this tumour is indistinguishable from its pulmonary counterpart (oat cell carcinoma). Membrane-bound dense-core granules have been demonstrated at the electron microscopic level and tumour cells may express neurofilaments, neurone-specific enolase and chromogranin A [466].

Clear cell adenocarcinoma of the colon and rectum is rare [467,468]. In such cases, tubules are lined by clear cells with some resemblance to carcinoma of the kidney. Similar tumours are seen in the stomach. Other unusual variants include hepatoid [469], embryonal carcinoma-like [470], rhabdoid [471,472] and sarcomatoid carcinoma [473]. Areas of squamous metaplasia in otherwise ordinary adenocarcinomas must be distinguished from genuine adenosquamous carcinoma. Calcification of psammomatous type is occasionally seen in mucus or in areas of tumour necrosis. It can occur in metastatic deposits as well as in the primary growth. Ossification is very rare and is seen within adenocarcinomatous tubules as well as among areas of necrosis and lakes of mucin [474]. There is no evidence that the presence of calcification or ossification affects prognosis.

Biopsy interpretation of carcinoma

The aim of endoscopic biopsy is to confirm a clinical or radiological diagnosis of malignancy, to identify the histological type and lastly to assess the grade of malignancy. The surgeon requires confirmation of the clinical diagnosis even when the presentation is typical of malignancy. Oleogranuloma and solitary ulcer syndrome may simulate carcinoma clinically, and failure to achieve biopsy diagnosis could lead to unnecessary excision of the rectum. Surgery may also be inappropriate for secondary deposits, lymphoma and other radiosensitive tumours. Information about the likely behaviour of a malignant tumour may be proved by histological grading. With this information the surgeon may be in a better position to make a decision about operability and type of surgical procedure. For example, in the case of a large fixed mass at laparotomy, removal is more likely to be attempted if it is known that the growth is of a low grade of malignancy and that fixation could be due to inflammation and fibrosis rather than invasion by carcinoma. However, a small sample obtained by endoscopic biopsy may not be representative of the growth as a whole. Dukes found 80% of resected tumours to be more poorly differentiated than the original biopsy [475]. Restorative operations on the rectum for cure are contraindicated when the growth is of a high grade of malignancy. This is because only a narrow distal resection margin is achieved with restorative surgery by low anterior resection and the risk of pelvic recurrence is high. Ulceration and inflammation affecting the superficial part of a tumour may lead to distortion of crypts that could be mistaken for poor differentiation, especially when the biopsy is small and crushed. Such factors may account for the poor levels of interobserver agreement in biopsy grading [476].

The diagnosis of carcinoma in rectal biopsy should not be made unless there is unequivocal evidence of invasion by malignant cells. Tumour that has crossed the line of the muscularis mucosae is clearly invasive and radical surgical treatment is usually indicated except for selected early colorectal cancers. Invasive adenocarcinoma is also recognizable by its accompanying desmoplastic reaction. A cautious approach to the histological diagnosis of carcinoma is important because the appearances of superficial and small, crushed biopsies of benign adenomas can closely mimic malignancy.

Histochemistry of adenocarcinoma

Epithelial mucins

The most well documented carbohydrates are the polysaccharide chains forming glycoproteins and glycolipids (glycoconjugates). Cell membrane glycoproteins and glycolipids play an important role in cell–cell recognition and interaction and act as receptors for hormones, growth factors, adhesion molecules, foreign antigens and other ligands. Aspects of malignant behaviour are likely to be explained by structural defects in cell membrane glycoconjugates. The core protein of an apical membrane-associated mucin expressed principally by crypt base cells is encoded by *MUC1*. A high proportion of colorectal cancers shows marked up-regulation of *MUC1* [165,457]. Secretory glycoproteins are macromolecules known commonly as mucins. The core protein of goblet cell mucin is encoded by *MUC2* in the main [477].

Although secretory and cell membrane glycoproteins serve different functions, their constituent polysaccharide sequences overlap [155,457]. Histochemical reactivity is largely governed by the terminal sugar sequences and in the normal large bowel these are represented mainly by sialic acid, N-acetyl galactosamine (GalNAc) and fucose [150,154]. When fucose predominates in secretory glycoproteins the product will be detected as a 'neutral' mucin by conventional mucin histochemistry. When sialic acid is present the mucin will be classified as a 'sialomucin' even though fucose and other neutral sugars are represented also. Finally, sulphate esterification of sugars may occur. Again a 'sulphomucin' may include sialic acid and/or fucose amongst the terminal sugar residues. The view that mucous cells secrete either neutral mucus, sialomucin or sulphomucin, as though these were separate and distinct macromolecules, is an oversimplification. In the normal colon, and more especially in the left colon and rectum, the ratio of terminal sialic acid to fucose is high [478,479]. Secretory material within colorectal cancer shows an alteration of this ratio in favour of fucose [478–480]. This is appreciated by the increased diastase–PAS staining of cancer mucin as compared to normal goblet cell mucin. However, cancer 'mucin' has a dual nature. Most cancers express up-regulated MUC1 (a membrane-associated glycoprotein) carrying 'cancer-associated' carbohydrate structures including Lewis^y (Le^y), Le^x, sialylated Le^x (SLe^x), STn, Tn and T antigen [165,457]. Mucinous cancers manufacture genuine secretory mucin derived from cells of goblet lineage (MUC2). Sialic acid associated with MUC2 loses O-acetyl groups in colorectal cancer and is strongly PAS positive [62].

The well known binding affinities of lectins for sugars and disaccharides have been exploited in studies of cancer-associated changes in glyconjugate structure. Reduced expression of GalNAc is demonstrated by *Dolichos biflorus* agglutinin (DBA) [481]. *Ulex europaeus* agglutin-1 (UEA-1) binds to fucose and therefore to the fucose-rich goblet cell mucin of the right colon [163]. Up-regulation of MUC1 (carrying fucose-rich carbohydrate structures) accounts for the increased UEA-1 binding, particularly evident in cancers of the left colon and rectum [457]. Loss of terminal sugars in cancer mucus exposes peanut lectin binding disaccharide sequences [482]. Binding by peanut lectin is increased when sialic acid is removed by prior digestion with neuraminidase. As noted above, sialic acid in the normal colon is usually O-acetylated and resistant to neuraminidase digestion, but cancer-associated sialic acid (being non-O-acetylated) is susceptible to the action of this enzyme [62]. When differences between normal tissues and cancer are exaggerated by prior neuraminidase digestion, this simply reflects the differential susceptibility of sialic acid moieties to this enzyme. The expression within cancers of sialylated tumour markers such as STn, SLe^x and SLe^a does not arise through their neosynthesis. These blood group substances are constituents of normal goblet cell mucin, but the fact that sialic acid is O-acetylated in normal goblet cell mucin (MUC2) renders the structures cryptic [157,481,483].

Glycoproteins synthesized by cancer arising in the left colon and rectum may show neoexpression of blood group substances. Normal goblet cells of the right colon express the blood group substances A, B, H and Le^b according to blood group and secretor status of the individual. The right colon expresses Le^b in secretors only. The classification of blood group carbohydrate sequences is determined by the structure of the polysaccharide backbone [155]. The type I chain family includes H1, Le^b, Le^a and SLe^a. The type II chain counterparts are H2, Le^y, Le^x and SLe^x. Monoclonal antibodies against these blood group antigens [155,161,484–488], against closely related di- and trifucosylated variants [489] and against the core sugar sequences (T, Tn and STn) have demonstrated a bewildering range of changes within cancer mucin. Some of the blood group substance neoexpression results merely from sialic acid modifications giving altered immunoreactivity to the structures STn, SLe^x and SLe^a (which are constitutively expressed in normal colorectal goblet cell mucin) [157,481,483]. Up-regulation of MUC1 could underlie the increased expression of type II blood group substances such as Le^x and Le^y [165,457]. The traditionally held view that cancer mucin arises through defective glycosylation of goblet cell mucin appears to have receded.

Colorectal cancers showing high levels of DNA microsatellite instability (MSI-H) are more likely to be mucinous. This is reflected in their frequent up-regulation not only of MUC2 but also of gastric mucin (M1 or MUC5AC) [455]. The same mucinous phenotype is encountered in serrated polyps and villous adenomas of the colorectum [172].

Tumour antigens

Colorectal cancers may express antigens that are normally associated with embryonic or fetal tissues. These have been referred to as tumour markers, but none is specific to large bowel cancer. They may be detected in trace amounts in adult colon or in other adult tissues or in other tumours. The emergence of fetal antigens is presumably the result of the depression of genes that are switched off in the course of normal development. The list includes carcinoembryonic antigen [175,490], alpha-fetoprotein [179,470], human chorionic gonadotrophin [491], human placental alkaline phosphatase [179], M1 antigens (gastric mucin MUC5AC) [492] and blood group substances (see above). The expression of these markers is lost or reduced in the course of development, only to reappear in neoplasms of the large bowel. Carcinoembryonic antigen (CEA) is present in trace amounts in normal colorectal mucosa [175]. Polyclonal antisera and some monoclonal antibodies raised against CEA cross-react with a family of related molecules, now thought to play a role in cell adhesion [63,493]. CEA finds its main use in serum assessment for the detection of advanced cancer and recurrent tumour, and in radioimmunolocalization.

Antigens expressed by heterologous adult tissues may make an inappropriate appearance in colorectal cancer. The list includes small intestinal mucin antigen (SIMA) [494,495], small intestinal brush border hydrolases [496,497], epithelial membrane antigen [498] and the related human milk fat globule glycoprotein [499]. The latter are both membrane-associated glycoproteins with a MUC1 protein backbone [457].

Differentiation antigens

This term may be applied to any cell product that appears during the normal process of maturation and lineage specialization. The persistence of such markers may serve to identify the tissue of origin of a particular tumour. Antibodies against cytokeratin are especially useful in the identification of epithelial neoplasms [500]. Although cytokeratin is expressed in neoplastic tissues, the fine structural organization of the cytoskeleton is broken down [501]. Loss of differentiation antigens may be used to demonstrate maturation arrest, but loss could also be due to defective synthesis, rapid degradation or export or a change in the direction of differentiation (as occurs in metaplasia). Secretory component has an important role to play in the cellular translocation of dimeric IgA. Several investigators have demonstrated a relationship between poor tumour differentiation and reduced or absent expression of secretory component [174,177].

Fundamental to the development of tissue differentiation is the expanding family of cell adhesion molecules [502], including E-cadherin (epithelial cell to epithelial cell) [503], integrins (epithelial cell to extracellular matrix proteins) [504,505], members of the immunoglobulin supergene family [63], selectins [506] and CD44 [507,508]. Loss or abnormal expression of these molecules underlies the breakdown of differentiation occurring in colorectal and other neoplasms [63,502]. CD44 variants have been implicated in the acquisition of the metastatic phenotype [507,508].

Transitional mucosa

Mucosa bordering colorectal cancer (transitional mucosa) comprises elongated, branched crypts lined by a tall columnar epithelium [509]. Goblet cells stain blue with the high iron diamine–alcian blue technique whereas normal colorectal goblet cells give a brown colour [510]. This difference is probably brought about as much by hypersialylation as by the loss of sulphate esters [159]. Some investigators state that goblet cell sialomucins in transitional mucosa are deficient in O-acetyl substituents and more susceptible to digestion by neuraminidase [511,512]. However, it is now clear that considerable sialomucin heterogeneity occurs in the general population and transitional mucosa is unlikely to show important differences from normal mucosa in terms of its sialic acid content [480,513,514]. There is general agreement that neutral sugars are not increased at the expense of sialic acid in transitional mucosa, in contrast to the mucins of colorectal cancer [479,480,513]. The columnar cells in transitional mucosa appear to be immature at the ultrastructural level and show increased vesiculation of the apical cytoplasm [515]. Sulphated glycoproteins have been detected in these 'intermediate' cells [516]. Other functional changes have been described, including reduced expression of secretory component [177], increased expression of carcinoembryonic [177] and M1 antigens [492] and SIMA [517], and inappropriate expression of blood group antigens [485]. Mucosa with similar appearance has been described in a variety of contexts unrelated to cancer and few continue to regard the change as precancerous [518,519]. Transitional mucosa is not observed adjacent to small adenomas but becomes apparent in the vicinity of larger growths [520]. It may also be associated with non-epithelial and metastatic tumours [521]. It would appear that transitional mucosa accompanies rather than precedes the evolution of large bowel cancer [495]. In false-negative endoscopic biopsies for colorectal cancer, the identification of transitional mucosa may serve to warn that the tumour was missed. The presence of transitional mucosa at the resection margins of operation specimens for colorectal cancer may predict local recurrence and long-term survival [522], but this is unlikely to be an independent effect.

Histological grade and other prognostic factors

Histological grading of cancer may be broadly defined as the attempt to measure tumour aggressiveness. Even though the exercise is subjective, Dukes and Bussey [335] were able to demonstrate a close relationship between grade of tumour and a number of variables including extent of local spread, number of lymph node metastases, venous invasion and prognosis. In a series of 2097 operable rectal cancers 19.4%, 60.4% and 20.2% were of low-, average- and high-grade malignancy, respectively. The corrected 5-year survival rates were 77.3%, 60.6% and 28.9%, respectively. In spite of these impressive figures, Dukes was not a grading enthusiast. He regarded the exercise as a measure of the 'pace' of growth. A fast pace would increase the likelihood of a tumour being at an advanced stage at the time of resection and stage was therefore the final determinant of prognosis. In a paper giving details of a four-grade system, Dukes stated that it was the arrangement of the cells rather than the number of undifferentiated cells that determined the grade [523]. He subsequently adopted the now familiar three-grade system, but never explained how the transition was made. This may in part account for the current lack of uniformity in the grading of colorectal cancer. In a trial involving 22 centres, the percentage of cancers considered to be well differentiated ranged from 3% to 93% [524].

Low-grade or well differentiated tumours are composed of regular tubules lined by columnar epithelium. Nuclei are uniform in size and shape and cellular polarity is usually discerned with ease. There is a distinct resemblance to adenomatous epithelium. Average-grade or moderately differentiated cases are formed of regular or slightly irregular tubules and cellular polarity is only just discerned or lost. In poorly differentiated or high-grade tumours, tubules are highly irregular or absent altogether. In place of tubules are single cells, small clumps (Fig. 38.25) or larger sheets of undifferentiated cells. Distortion of architecture may occur near an ulcerated surface or at the invasive margin; this should be ignored. Tumours are often heterogeneous and one should form an opinion on the most poorly differentiated area [449]. A microacinar morphology is associated with a poor prognosis but does not appear to be an independent factor [525].

It is unclear whether grading makes an independent contribution to survival prediction in the presence of other pathological variables. One can attempt to answer this question by submitting survival data to multivariate analysis, but the care taken in the collection of data will vary within and between centres. If staging is performed suboptimally, then grading may assume undeserved importance. Some surveys have shown that grading does influence outcome independently [526–528]. In a study from St Mark's Hospital the grade-related variables which retained some independent influence upon survival in the presence of stage-related variables were the character of the invasive margin (expanding or infiltrating) and lymphocytic infiltration, but not tumour differentiation [449].

The extensive range of histochemical techniques described in the preceding section (p. 582) provides an important opportunity for grading tumours on the basis of their functional characterization as opposed to the traditional exclusive reliance upon static morphology. In addition to the differentiation antigens (including so-called tumour antigens) documented above, the prognostic significance of histocompatibility antigens (HLA-A, -B, -C and -DR), proteolytic enzymes, tumour angiogenesis [58], tumour DNA content, proliferative activity, nucleolar organizer regions, tumour suppressor gene allele loss, oncogene mutation, enhanced oncoprotein expression and DNA microsatellite instability has been the subject of an ever-increasing number of publications (Table 38.4). It is fair to state, however, that the majority of molecular prognostic markers add little useful or independent prognostic information.

In the normal mucosa important interactions occur between epithelium and the lymphoid population of the lamina propria. One effector arm of this co-operation is the epithelial translocation of dimeric IgA into the bowel lumen. This is achieved through a carrier molecule called secretory component which may be regarded as a columnar cell differentiation antigen. Loss of staining for secretory component is not only closely associated with grade of differentiation [174,177] but correlates with survival [529]. However, the survival advantage could only be demonstrated when tumours with heterogeneous expression were excluded from the analysis. Furthermore, the survival benefit of secretory component positivity is lacking in independent value.

A pronounced peritumoural lymphocytic infiltrate confers an important and independent survival advantage [575]. This might signify the successful limitation of growth by a host response mounted against a tumour showing conjoint expression of major histocompatibility Class I antigens (as in normal epithelium) and tumour-associated neoantigens. However, the distinctive lymphocytic mantle seen at the invasive margin in up to 25% of colorectal cancers sometimes resembles the normal lamina propria [575]. The presence of such a structure may merely indicate the persistence of the normal interactive network involving intestinal epithelium and mucosa-associated lymphoid tissue. This would in turn signal a high level of functional differentiation. Although the peritumoural lymphocytic population may be activated [576,577], through the presentation of tumour antigens and increased expression of Class II (HLA-DR) determinants [578], there is little evidence that such activation culminates as an important lymphocyte-mediated cytodestruction. Cytotoxic lymphocyte failure may be explained by a fas ligand counterattack causing lymphocyte apoptosis [579]. Class II status is not related to either stage or grade [580], though HLA-DR expression has been associated with improved survival [532]. It has been postulated that defective natural killer cell function may be related to an increased metastatic potential [580–582]. In this regard, sialosyl-

Table 38.4 Prognostic factors in colorectal cancer.

Prognostic factors	References
Differentiation markers	
Secretory component	[529,530]
MUC1	[457]
Sialosyl-Tn	[531]
HLA-A, -B, -C and -DR	[532–534]
Laminin	[535]
Integrins	[504]
E-cadherin	[536]
Carcinoembryonic antigen	[537]
CD44	[507,508]
Urokinase	[59,61]
Cathepsin B	[538]
Gelatinase B (MMP-9)	[539,540]
Collagenase	[60]
Nuclear parameters	
DNA ploidy	[541]
S-phase fraction	[541]
Proliferation markers	[542,543]
Nucleolar organizer regions (AgNOR)	[544,545]
Thymidylate synthase	[546]
Mutation	
K-*ras*	[547,548]
TP53	[549,550]
Oncoprotein expression	
myc	[551,552]
p53	[43,553–559]
bcl-2	[66,558,560]
Rb	[561,562]
Nm23	[563–565]
mdr	[543]
mdm-2	[566]
p27	[567]
Allele loss	
17p (TP53)	[100,568–570]
17q	[99]
18q	[100,568,571,572]
22q	[100,101]
Rb	[571]
8p	[97]
DNA microsatellite instability	[395,573,574]

Tn expression by MUC2-type mucin has been shown to inhibit natural killer cell function [583]. Tumours expressing MUC1 may show augmented cytotoxic T-cell function [584]. Peritumoural and tumour-infiltrating lymphocytes occur in increased numbers in tumours showing DNA microsatellite instability [105,312], but are less conspicuous when these tumours are mucinous.

In well differentiated adenocarcinoma, CEA is expressed in a polar manner along the apical cell membrane. Ultrastructural studies have demonstrated CEA within the microvillous glycocalyx [175]. This distribution characterizes normal colorectal columnar epithelium. In moderately differentiated cancers polarity is lost and inappropriate expression occurs along the basolateral membrane [175,537,585]. This relocation may be accompanied by staining of the surrounding stroma and is associated with raised plasma CEA levels [585]. Stromal staining for CEA is said to predict both venous and lymphatic invasion [585]. Poorly differentiated cancers show variable patterns of CEA expression ranging from negative to intensely positive cytoplasmic staining [177,586]. CEA has been subjected to detailed immunohistochemical investigation, but the various staining patterns have not been shown to be useful in predicting survival. The expression of additional tumour markers has been correlated with survival; 10.6% of cancers uniformly positive for gastrointestinal cancer-associated antigen (GICA) were relatively aggressive in their behaviour, but the adverse effect upon survival did not achieve statistical significance when cases were stratified according to stage [587]. Expression of sialosyl-Tn [531] and MUC1 [457] decreases prospects of cure.

Tumour products intimately related to invasion and growth might be expected to predict survival more accurately. It is now appreciated that penetration of the basement membrane is not a prerequisite for malignant invasion. Some cancers may invade with their basement membrane intact [535]. The absence of a basement membrane represents a failure of the malignant epithelium to maintain this structure. Laminin, a glycoprotein, is an important component of the basement membrane. Absence of laminin correlates with distant spread and poor survival rates [535]. Proteolytic enzymes are implicated in malignant invasion. Increased activity of cathepsin B has been described in colorectal cancers that have spread in continuity beyond the bowel wall [588]. The plasminogen activator urokinase augments malignant invasion [589,590]. The ability of a cancer to metastasize may depend on the acquisition of autostimulatory activity through the uncontrolled synthesis of growth factors or increased expression of growth factor receptors [393,394,591,592].

The term aneuploid describes cell populations in which chromosomal numbers deviate from 46 or its multiples. Direct chromosome analysis is time-consuming, but DNA microdensitometry and flow cytometry allow the DNA content of a large number of cells to be measured rapidly [541,593–596]. Flow cytometry is less sensitive than direct karyotyping and a small increase or decrease in the number of chromosomes will not necessarily be resolved. Thus a DNA diploid population may be chromosomally aneuploid. Nuclear suspensions can be prepared from either frozen or formalin-fixed, paraffin-embedded tissue and analysed by flow cytometry [597]. In an unselected series of 203 operable rectal cancers from St Mark's Hospital, 64% were shown to include an aneuploid population [598]. This figure is within the published range, but the range is fairly wide, indicating technical variability. Abnormal DNA content or aneuploidy has an adverse effect upon survival. *TP53* mutation or allele loss often precedes the development of aneuploidy [599]. The magnitude of the independent contribution of ploidy to prediction of survival can be measured. It appears to provide an independent but small effect in the presence of traditional pathological variables [594,596]. However, this is largely explained by the good prognosis of MSI-H cancers which are usually diploid (see below).

The prognostic significance of nuclear and molecular abnormalities has been and continues to be the subject of intense investigation. In general, initial positive findings have been followed by negative or more sober reflections. Table 38.4 lists nuclear and molecular factors that have been linked to prognosis. Of particular importance is the mechanism underlying genetic instability as this explains many additional prognostic findings. Cancers showing high levels of DNA microsatellite instability (MSI-H) have a good prognosis that is independent of stage [573,574]. The same cancers lack many of the molecular characteristics associated with an adverse outcome including aneuploidy, mutation of *TP53* and allele loss at 17p and 18q (Table 38.2). Since many molecular markers are surrogates for the mechanism driving either DNA or chromosomal instability, prognostic studies should always characterize and stratify cancers according to microsatellite status. MSI-H cancers may show an increased response to adjuvant therapy with 5-fluorouracil [600,601]. However, further research is required to confirm a clinically useful predictive role for microsatellite status and this should consider HNPCC versus sporadic MSI-H colorectal cancer separately.

Relation of spread to prognosis

The important routes of spread for colorectal cancer are local, lymphatic, venous and transcoelomic. Pathological staging systems are constructed from two of these variables: extent of local invasion and lymphatic spread. However, there are differing views on the best method of assembling pathological data into a system of classification (Table 38.5).

These controversies are not of paramount importance. Very much more important is the quality of the data generated by the pathologist. Dissection, histological examination and recording of data should be performed with meticulous care [606,607]. Providing this is achieved, the pathologist will provide an important contribution towards any form of staging classification.

Local spread

Limitations of the neoplasm to mucosa, submucosa or muscularis propria should be recorded. While a diagnosis of mucosal carcinoma is made rarely in the West, mucosal carcinoma may be an appropriate diagnosis in ulcerative colitis or in the case of poorly differentiated or signet ring cell carcinoma. A recent American Joint Committee on Cancer recommendation is for TIN (intraepithelial neoplasia) to be subdivided into TIE (intraepithelial) and TIM (intramucosal) carcinoma [605].

Table 38.5 Staging of colorectal cancer.

	Dukes [475]	Dukes & Bussey [335]	Astler-Coller [602]	ACPS [603]	TNM [604,605]
Direct spread					
Mucosa	–	–	A	A1	Tis (TIE and TIM)*
Submucosa	A	A	B1	A2	T1 (a or b)†
Muscle coat	A	A	B1	A3	T2
Beyond muscle	B	B	B2	B1	T3
Involving adjacent organs	B	B	B2	B1	T4A
Transperitoneal (free surface)	B	B	B2	B2	T4B
Lymph node spread					
None	(A/B)	(A/B)	(A/B1/B2)	(A/B/D)	N0
1–3	C	C1	C1/C2‡	C1	N1
> 3	C	C1	C1/C2‡	C1	N2
Apical node	C	C2	C1/C2‡	C2	N1/N2
Residual local tumour (transection of tumour)	–§	–§	–	D1	R1**
Distant spread	–§	–§	–	D2	M1††

*TIE, intraepithelial; TIM, intramucosal.

†a, no lymphatic/venous invasion; b, lymphatic/venous invasion.

‡C1, direct spread confined to wall; C2, spread beyond muscle coat.

§Absent, curative; present, palliative.

**R0, no residual tumour; R1, microscopic residual disease; R2, macroscopic residual disease.

††M0, no distant spread; M1, distant spread.

The outer border of the muscularis propria is an easily recognized and important anatomical landmark. Prospects for cure are reduced and lymph node metastases occur with greater frequency when tumour has spread beyond the bowel wall so defined. Some parts of the bowel are invested by peritoneum. When considering spread of cancer the outer edge of the muscularis propria determines whether spread is within or beyond the bowel wall, not the peritoneal layer. In a series of operable rectal cancers confined to the bowel wall, the cumulative probability of survival at 5 years was 97.7%, regardless of the presence of lymph node metastases [449]. Dukes classified invasion beyond the rectal wall into slight, moderate and extensive [475] and showed that this exercise, albeit subjective, held important prognostic significance [335]. The extent of extramural spread, and in particular involvement of the non-peritonealized circumferential resection margin, is highly predictive of local recurrence as well as survival, especially in rectal cancer. Techniques for measuring spread beyond the bowel wall as well as surgical clearance at the deep or circumferential margin of excision have been described and it is essential that pathologists employ these to assess these very important prognostic factors [608,609]. Incomplete excision may be due not only to extensive local spread in continuity, but to lymph node metastases or discrete nodules of tumour at the deep surgical margin. Surgical factors are of great importance. In rectal cancer, sharp mesorectal dissection outside the plane of the mesorectal fascia propria reduces the incidence of local recurrence [610]. The proximal margin of a specimen is very rarely involved by tumour. The distal margin may occasionally be involved in low anterior resections of rectum, especially when the tumour is of high-grade malignancy or shows extensive vascular permeation. Tumours showing extensive spread may involve adjacent structures or organs including prostrate, bladder, uterus and bony pelvis.

Lymphatic spread

Lymph node metastasis occurs as a progressive process with carcinoma spreading in anatomical sequence from node to node. When spread to the regional lymph nodes occurs, lymph flow can be blocked and so-called retrograde lymphatic metastasis may then arise [611]. This is only apparent in advanced cancer and is associated with a very poor prognosis.

The presence of lymph node metastases in an operation specimen of colon or rectal cancer (Dukes C cases) greatly worsens prognosis. In a series of 2037 operable rectal cancers, the corrected 5-year survival rate was reduced to 32.0% for lymph node-positive cases as compared to 83.7% for cases without lymph node metastases (Dukes A and B cases) [335]. The prognosis also varies with the number of involved lymph nodes. For one, two to five, six to 10 and more than 10 affected nodes the 5-year survival rates were 63.6%, 36.1%, 21.9% and 2.1%, respectively [335]. This observation has been reaffirmed [449,612,613] and illustrates the importance of meticulous lymph node dissection. Reports should indicate the number of nodes harvested and the number with metastases. A nodule of tumour without residual lymph node should be regarded as a replaced node if it is 3 mm in diameter or more [614]. The presence of smaller tumour nodules is associated with an adverse outcome [615]. The use of cytokeratin immunohistochemistry and RT-PCR-based approaches to identify lymph node micrometastases has been advocated [616–621]. It is likely that micrometastases would confer an adverse outcome but with a small independent effect, if any, in the presence of meticulously reported routine prognostic features.

Spread to inguinal lymph nodes occurs in rectal cancer. In the St Mark's Hospital series of operation specimens only 2% of all rectal cancers showed involvement of inguinal nodes, but if cancers of the lower third of the rectum were taken alone the figure rose to 7%. Inguinal node involvement rarely occurs in the absence of haemorrhoidal node metastasis.

Lymph node reactions including enlargement, follicular and parafollicular hyperplasia and sinus histiocytosis as well as the number of lymph nodes retrieved indicate host resistance and an improved prospect for survival [622,623]. A survival advantage has been recorded for Dukes C cases when affected nodes show reactive changes [624]. Lymph node-positive cases in which distant spread is confined to the bowel wall also show an improved survival [625].

Venous spread

Careful sectioning of a specimen of colorectal cancer may reveal invasion of large extramural veins by tumour. It would seem as though the tumour, having found a path of least resistance, has sent a root-like process along the lumen of the vessel. Histological examination shows venous invasion to be a frequent finding, but prognosis is appreciably worsened only when large extramural veins are affected [626]. The 5-year survival rate is then reduced from 55% to 30%. However, venous invasion did not influence prognosis independently of other pathological variables in patients undergoing curative surgery for rectal cancer [449].

For every 100 patients with operable large bowel cancer, approximately 50 will be cured, 10 will die with pelvic recurrence, five will die with lymphatic spread, but 35 will die with blood-borne metastases. It is unclear whether blood-borne metastases emanate from single clonogenic tumour cells shed into the circulation or from larger embolic clumps that have separated from tongues of tumour growing within veins. The demonstration of tumour cells within veins is not a reliable sign of coexisting metastatic spread to distant organs. Blood-borne spread is determined by factors other than the ability to invade veins. The liver is by far the most frequently involved organ (77%), the lungs (15%), bones (5%) [627] and brain being next in order of frequency [628,629]. It is likely that a cascade system operates, with metastases first developing in the liver, next in the lungs and finally in other sites [630]. There is no evidence that the distribution of liver metastases is determined by the location of the primary growth within the large bowel [631]. The spleen [632], kidneys, pancreas, adrenals, breast, thyroid and skin [633] are rarely involved. One report suggests that the incidence of ovarian metastases from primary carcinoma of the colon may be higher than is usually appreciated [634]. It may be mistaken for primary mucinous adenocarcinoma. The presence of necrosis suggests a colorectal origin. Immunostaining for cytokeratin 7 (CK7) (positive in ovarian cancer) and cytokeratin 20 (positive in colorectal cancer) is a useful technique for making the distinction. Metastasis to the penis has been reported on a number of occasions [635]. There is an unusual case report of a metastasis in the nail bed of a finger from carcinoma of the rectum which presented as a paronychia [636].

Peritoneal involvement

The greater part of the colon and the anterior wall of the upper rectum are invested by the serosal membrane. This comprises a sheet of connective tissue containing blood vessels and lymphatics, an elastic lamina and finally a thin sheet of flattened mesothelial cells, the peritoneum. As stated above, a tumour is defined as having spread beyond the bowel wall when it has breached the muscularis propria and invades the serosal connective tissue. However, it is most unlikely that transcoelomic spread will occur until there is ulceration, either microscopic or macroscopic, through the peritoneum [637]. Fortunately, the peritoneum is a most effective barrier to direct spread. It is not uncommon to observe intact peritoneum tightly stretched over the underlying growth. Once malignant cells have passed through the peritoneal membrane, they can be disseminated in the abdominal cavity [637]. Transperitoneal spread is an independent adverse prognostic factor in cancer of the colon [638] and upper rectum [637]. Poorly differentiated carcinomas produce multiple deposits, whereas well differentiated carcinomas are more likely to produce solitary or few metastases. These can appear in any part of the abdominal cavity as well as in operation wounds. The ovary is a site of predilection for transcoelomic spread from colonic carcinomas. Sometimes it can be difficult, if not impossible, to distinguish between primary and secondary adenocarcinoma in the ovary when a primary tumour of the colon is also present [639]. In the TNM system, T4 cases should be divided into those invading adjacent organs (T4A) and those with tumour deposits on the free peritoneal surface (T4B) [605].

About one in 10 patients who have had surgical resection for carcinoma of the colon subsequently develop peritoneal deposits. This can be anticipated by the detection of transperitoneal spread in operation specimens [638], but it may be difficult to detect, both macroscopically and microscopically, when it occurs in the clefts between appendices epiloicae.

Implantation

There is no doubt that cancer of the large bowel can give rise to implantation metastases [640]. Large numbers of exfoliated malignant cells may be found within operation specimens and at a distance from their source; these retain the capacity to divide and form experimental tumours in animals [641]. Implantation could occur within the lumen of the bowel or outside it, usually as a result of peritoneal involvement or surgical manipulation. Implantation metastasis from carcinoma of the colon and rectum has been described in anal fistulae and wounds (usually surgical) at the anus. There are reports of implantation onto the raw surface of the anal canal after haemorrhoidectomy from an unsuspected carcinoma of the colon [642,643]. Most recurrences in abdominal incisions, around colostomies and in the perineum after excision of the rectum for cancer are likely to be the result of implantation from the peritoneal surface of the growth or via the surgeon's hands whilst he or she is manipulating the growing edge of the carcinoma. From a surgical point of view, so-called suture-line recurrence is the most important variety of implantation metastasis today [644,645]. This can occur as the result of implantation of malignant cells from the bowel lumen onto the raw surface of the bowel after intestinal anastomosis. Alternatively, it may arise when free malignant cells from inside or outside the bowel are trapped within the suture line. Many suture-line recurrences are due to inadequate resection of the primary growth, particularly when there has been extensive and diffusely infiltrating local spread or retrograde lymphatic spread [646]. In experimental cancer in animals, growths have been shown to occur preferentially at anastomotic sites. It would seem that the creation of an anastomosis acts as a promoting factor, but there is no direct evidence that such a mechanism could give rise to metachronous neoplasia in humans.

Pelvic recurrence

The incidence of regrowth of carcinoma in the pelvis after excision of the rectum is about 10% [647]. This mostly occurs with carcinomas of the lower (extraperitoneal) rectum, because this is encased by the narrowing pelvic funnel which makes adequate surgical removal of the primary tumour difficult. Pelvic recurrence is most common in rectal cancers with lymph node metastases, in those which have extensive local spread in continuity and in tumours of a high grade of malignancy.

Staging and prognosis of colorectal cancer

Pathological staging for operable cancer of the large bowel offers some guide to prognosis and allows patients in trials of, for example, operative technique or adjuvant therapy to be stratified into comparable groups. The Dukes classification

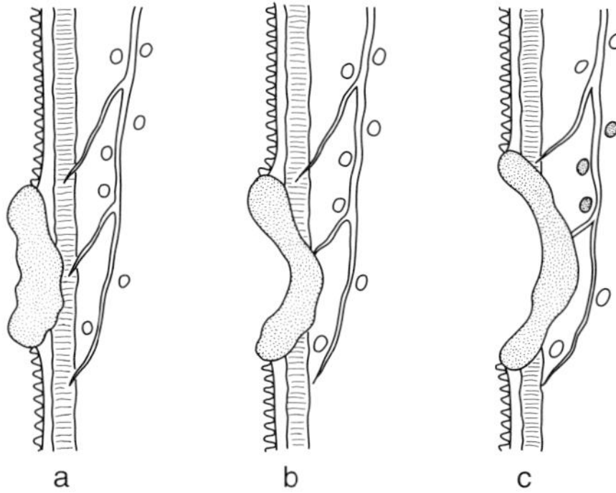

Fig. 38.29 Dukes classification of rectal carcinoma. For explanation see text.

[475] was introduced at St Mark's Hospital in 1928 and is now accepted all over the world as a valuable guide to prognosis (Fig. 38.29). The Dukes A case (15% of all operated patients) is one in which the intestinal cancer has spread through muscularis mucosae into the tissues of the bowel wall, but not beyond the muscularis propria, and there are no lymph node metastases. Corrected 5-year survival is virtually 100%. A Dukes B case (35% of all operated patients) is one in which the growth has spread beyond the muscularis propria into the pericolic or perirectal tissues in continuity, but without forming lymph node metastases. About 75% of Dukes B patients will be cured of their disease. Once the lymph nodes are involved (Dukes C case) the prognosis becomes poor, with only about 35% of patients surviving 5 years. About 50% of all operated cancers are in this stage. There is evidence that Dukes C patients in whom the growth is confined to the bowel have a better prognosis [625], but only about 5% of C cases fall into this category.

Although Dukes appreciated the importance of distinguishing between radical (curative) and palliative (non-curative) operations, his classification of rectal cancer was based on the pathological study of both curative and non-curative operations. It is important to subject all surgical specimens to meticulous examination, but most would agree that curative and non-curative operations should be separated for the purpose of prognostication and patient stratification [648]. An operation is defined as non-curative if there is evidence of distant spread or incomplete surgical removal of the primary growth. Histological confirmation should be obtained whenever this is feasible. Even more important is microscopic assessment of involvement of the non-peritonealized circumferential surgical resection margin following apparently curative resections, especially in rectal cancer, because this is highly predictive of local recurrence and a more powerful prognostic factor than Dukes stage [649]. Piecemeal, as opposed to *en bloc*, removal of the tumour and bowel perforation (carrying the risk of extramural dissemination of viable cancer cells) similarly compromise the chance of cure. The most widely used staging system is that recommended by the Union International Contre Cancer (UICC) or TNM-based system. UICC/TNM stages I, II and III equate to (curative) Dukes A, B and C, whereas stage IV indicates distant spread [614].

Table 38.6 Four prognostic groups for rectal carcinoma [606].

Total score	Prognostic group	Corrected 5-year survival (%)
0–1	I	94
2	II	83
3	III	56
4–5	IV	27

Approximately 50% of patients undergoing 'curative' surgery will eventually succumb with recurrent disease. The usual explanation will be the presence of occult hepatic metastasis at the time of surgery [650]. The ideal prognostic classification for patients undergoing curative surgery should distinguish between those who are cured and those with occult residual disease. This ideal has been approached by identifying variables which have an important and independent influence upon survival. In one prognostic model, these features were the number of involved lymph nodes, extent of direct spread, character of invasive margin and presence of a peritumoural lymphocytic infiltrate [651]. In the prognostic classification derived from this model, unfavourable findings including positive lymph nodes, spread beyond muscularis propria, diffuse infiltration and lack of peritumoural lymphocytic infiltrate are each assigned a score of 1. If there are more than four positive lymph nodes, this variable attracts a score of 2 [651]. The total score for an individual specimen will be in the range of 0–5. This range is collapsed into four prognostic groups as shown in Table 38.6.

Complications

Intestinal obstruction is the most common complication of carcinoma of the large bowel. It has an unfavourable effect upon prognosis after surgical treatment, which is probably due to the fact that obstruction is often associated with relatively advanced disease [652]. Free perforation is uncommon and indicates an unfavourable prognosis also, not only because of immediate peritonitis, but because of escape and dissemination of malignant cells into the abdominal cavity. Penetration of the wall of the colon by carcinoma is sometimes associated with the development of a pericolic abscess. Internal fistula is very rare. Intussusception of the colon in adults is more often due to carcinoma than benign tumours or other causes [653]. Acute appendicitis can be precipitated by proximal large bowel growths causing back-pressure on the caecum with obstruction of the lumen of the appendix [654]. Colonic ulceration proximal to obstructing carcinomas is due to associated ischaemic colitis and is important because it has to be distinguished from cancer arising in ulcerative colitis [655].

Non-metastatic cutaneous manifestations of cancer of the colon and the rectum such as acanthosis nigricans and dermatomyositis are infrequent [656]. Carcinomas of the lower rectum are often accompanied by secondary haemorrhoids. This is important because haemorrhoids may be the presenting sign and superficial examination may not reveal the carcinoma above them, with consequent delay in diagnosis. It is imperative that every patient presenting with haemorrhoids has a full clinical examination to exclude coexisting carcinoma or other neoplasm.

Rare or unexpected associations with colorectal cancer have been described. In a series of patients with Barrett's oesophagus aged 64 years or older, 38% were found to have colorectal cancer [657], but this association has not been confirmed [658]. A case of caecal carcinoma has been reported in a patient with collagenous colitis [659]. There are several descriptions of gastrointestinal malignancy in association with Cronkhite–Canada syndrome, particularly from Japan [660].

Pathological changes following radiotherapy

Radiotherapy or chemoradiotherapy is often used preoperatively in subjects with rectal cancer staged as T3 or T4 by endorectal ultrasonography and magnetic resonance imaging. The clinical aims are to reduce the frequency of local recurrence, increase the rate of operability, increase the frequency of anterior resection over abdominoperineal excision and improve overall survival [661]. Responsiveness to preoperative radiotherapy varies from case to case. Radiosensitivity depends on the intact state of the apoptotic pathway controlled by p53 and $p21^{WAF1}$; patients with wild-type p53 are more likely to be radioresponsive [662]. Histological changes in rectal cancers treated by preoperative radiotherapy include tumour necrosis, stromal fibrosis and granulomatous reactions. Infiltrating lymphocytes disappear and the configuration of the advancing border is obscured. In cases with complete tumour destruction, signs of previous tumour may include pools of mucin and foci of calcification. Proctitis cystica profunda, a complication of radiotherapy, should be distinguished from well differentiated mucinous adenocarcinoma. Lymph nodes are often difficult to find and the total yield will be reduced in size as well as number. Radiation changes in the adjacent mucosa should be distinguished from inflammatory bowel disease [661].

Endocrine cell or carcinoid tumours

Endocrine cell neoplasms of the large intestine are uncommon, accounting for less than 1% of all colorectal neoplasms, but about 30% of all endocrine cell tumours of the gastrointestinal tract [663]. Most arise in the rectum, while colonic endocrine cell neoplasms are concentrated in the right colon and caecum.

Right-sided endocrine cell tumours usually present as bulky polypoid or ulcerating masses that are macroscopically indistinguishable from carcinomas; many will have already metastasized to regional lymph nodes and distant sites [664]. The great majority are EC-cell carcinoids similar to those arising in the ileum and appendix (see pp. 367 and 420) and are composed of solid clumps or islands of uniform cells with eosinophilic granular cytoplasm that is argentaffin and argyrophil and stains for 5-hydroxytryptamine. The larger, overtly malignant varieties show mitotic activity and necrosis. However, an associated carcinoid syndrome is uncommon, even in the presence of liver metastases. Right hemicolectomy is warranted for all but small superficial lesions that can be completely excised endoscopically; an overall 5-year survival rate of only 23% has been reported [663].

Rectal endocrine tumours present in two macroscopic forms [665]. The usual finding is that of a small nodule less than 1 cm in diameter and discovered fortuitously. The cut surface is pink or tan. These can be safely treated by local excision, provided that removal is complete. Less commonly, the tumour presents as a large growth that has often metastasized. Three histological patterns are encountered, of which the ribbon type is the most common. The ribbons comprise two or more layers of cells arranged along a delicate core of vascular connective tissue (Fig. 38.30). The ribbons may be straight, convoluted or interlacing. The next most common pattern is a mixed classical and tubular type, with the tubular component often being the more conspicuous (Fig. 38.31). Rectal endocrine tumours are mostly L-cell tumours that are argyrophil but not argentaffin [665]. They show variable immunostaining for chromogranin A but more consistent staining for chromogranin B and synaptophysin. Many are positive for prostatic acid phosphatase, but not prostatic-specific antigen [666]. They coexpress a range of enteroglucagons or glicentin-related peptides, including glucagon-29, glucagon-37, glicentin,

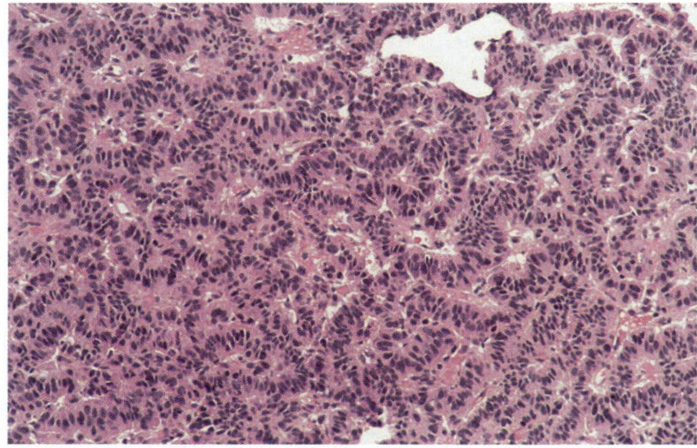

Fig. 38.30 Endocrine tumour of rectum with ribbon pattern.

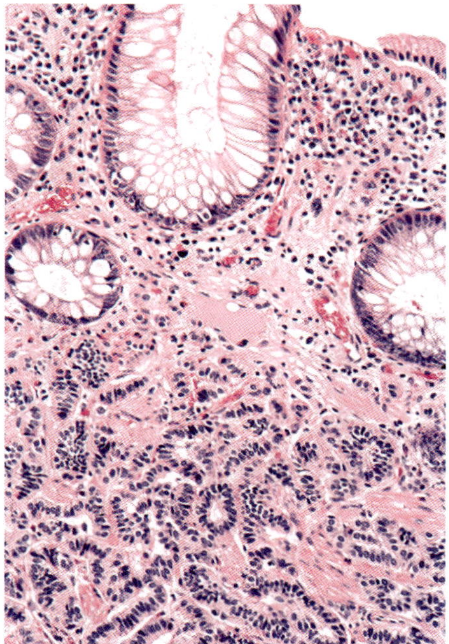

Fig. 38.31 Histology of a rectal endocrine tumour with a mixed pattern; there is a desmoplastic stromal reaction.

proglucagon cryptic fragments, PYY, PP and pro-PP icosapeptide, and regularly contain minor populations of serotonin, substance P, somatostatin, insulin, enkephalin, β-endorphin, neurotensin, α-hCG and motilin-containing cells [667]. A single tumour may secrete several different hormones. Features of rectal endocrine tumours that indicate malignancy include size greater than 2 cm, vascular invasion, spread into and beyond the muscularis propria, nuclear pleomorphism, high mitotic activity and necrosis: lymph node metastases are recorded in 60–80% of such cases [666,668]. On the other hand, well differentiated tumours measuring less than 1 cm that are confined to the mucosa or submucosa and show none of these 'atypical' histological features virtually never metastasize and can be safely treated by local excision.

It is not always a simple matter to distinguish malignant endocrine tumours from adenocarcinomas that have either adopted a 'carcinoid-like' growth pattern or contain a conspicuous population of endocrine cells. An example of the latter is the so-called goblet cell carcinoid which has been described in the colon [669] as well as the appendix. The small cell undifferentiated carcinoma ('oat cell') may be placed at the most malignant end of the endocrine spectrum. That such difficulties of classification should arise is not surprising in the light of the fact that endocrine cells and other epithelial cells arise from a common stem cell. It is of interest that an association exists between colorectal endocrine neoplasia and both synchronous (including contiguous) and metachronous epithelial neoplasia [665]. Endocrine cell hyperplasia and neoplasia has been recorded in patients with long-standing ulcerative colitis, with [670] and without [671] synchronous dysplasia and cancer. These observations indicate the sharing of aetiological factors in the processes of endocrine and non-endocrine epithelial neoplasia.

Rare forms of colorectal cancer

Squamous cell carcinoma

Primary squamous cell carcinoma of the colon and rectum does occur, but is excessively rare [672–674]. Before such a condition can be accepted as genuine, care must be taken to exclude metastatic tumour presenting as a primary growth. This is most likely to come from the cervix. Squamous carcinoma of the rectum complicating chronic ulcerative colitis has been reported on a number of occasions [675]. Indeed, although it would appear to account for only 1–2% of all cancers complicating ulcerative colitis, this represents a relative incidence 50–100 times greater than in the general population. However, there may be difficulty in deciding whether such a tumour is primarily arising from rectal mucosa or whether it is really an upward extension of a carcinoma of the anal canal. Squamous cell carcinomas of the anal canal often arise above the dentate line and spread preferentially upwards, giving the false impression of a primary rectal tumour. There are rare but well documented reports of basaloid squamous cell carcinoma arising proximal to the anorectal region [676,677].

Squamous cell carcinomas of the large bowel could arise in four ways. Firstly, the genetic defect causing stem cell transformation could result in concomitant squamous differentiation. Secondly, chronic inflammation, radiation or some other stimulus could lead to squamous metaplasia of columnar epithelium (see below). Thirdly, squamous carcinoma could arise in metaplastic foci that are sometimes found in adenomas [135]. The presence of congenital squamous heterotopias would be the fourth explanation. The demonstration of normal or dysplastic squamous epithelium in the immediate vicinity of a squamous carcinoma [672,674] lends support to the second and fourth hypotheses. Squamous cell carcinomas appear to be comparable to adenocarcinoma in terms of their clinical behaviour.

Adenosquamous carcinoma

This is a tumour in which both adenocarcinomatous and squamous carcinomatous elements are present, but are separate although contiguous, thus making a distinction from the much commoner squamous metaplasia in an adenocarcinoma [134]. Either histological type may predominate. Intercellular bridges and keratin should be demonstrated in the squamous part. This tumour is rare but can be found in all parts of the large bowel, although our experience is that it is seen mostly in the right colon and rectum. These tumours may behave in an aggressive manner and the squamous component may have the greater metastatic potential [678].

Carcinosarcoma

There is one report of a carcinosarcoma of the colon [679].

Secondary carcinoma

The stomach is probably the most common source of both solitary and multiple secondary carcinomatous deposits in the colon and rectum. These may present as single or multiple strictures mimicking primary colorectal cancer and even Crohn's disease or ulcerative colitis. The latter is simulated when there is widespread and diffuse mural spread of malignant cells giving rise to a shortened, tubular colon on radiological examination. Symptoms may be referable to the colon only, and the primary disease in the stomach may be difficult to demonstrate, even at laparotomy. Metastases from carcinoma of the breast [680,681] are not uncommon and again, the colorectal involvement may be the source of the patient's main complaint, together with either a past history of breast cancer or an undetected lump in the breast. Involvement of the rectum by carcinoma of the prostate is unusual and it is even more uncommon for prostatic carcinoma to present with signs and symptoms of rectal disease in the absence of, or overshadowing, urinary symptoms. In such cases the rectal disease presents as a stricture, anterior rectal ulcer or anterior submucous mass [682,683]. The pathologist must always be alert for the possibility of secondary carcinoma or endometriosis when studying large bowel biopsies in which the appearances of the tumour are unusual or unlike ordinary colorectal cancer. Among other commoner sources of secondary colorectal cancer are the ovary, kidney [684], cervix [685,686] and lung.

Squamous metaplasia of the rectum

It is doubtful whether squamous metaplasia of previously normal rectal mucosa has been described. On the other hand, minor degrees of upgrowth by squamous epithelium of the anal canal over ulcerated rectal mucosa in continuity are quite common in prolapsing haemorrhoids and involve only a small area of the mucosa of the lower rectum. Two examples of very extensive upgrowth of squamous epithelium have been described [687,688], and a third case has been seen at St Mark's Hospital. Malignant change to squamous cell carcinoma occurred in one of these [688]. In the remaining two examples the extension by squamous epithelium was in continuity with the squamous mucosa of the anal canal and there was evidence of self-induced trauma, primarily involving the anterior anorectal wall.

References

1 Muto T, Bussey HJR, Morson BC. The evolution of cancer of the rectum. *Cancer*, 1975; 36: 2251.

2 Vogelstein B, Fearon ER, Hamilton SR *et al*. Genetic alterations during colorectal tumor development. *N Engl J Med*, 1988; 319: 525.

3 Shibata D, Schaeffer J, Li Z-H, Capella G, Perucho M. Genetic heterogeneity of the c-K-ras locus in colorectal adenomas but not in adenocarcinomas. *J Natl Cancer Inst*, 1993; 85: 1058.

4 Levy DB, Smith KJ, Beazebarclay Y *et al*. Inactivation of both APC alleles in human and mouse tumors. *Cancer Res*, 1994; 54: 5953.

5 Ichii S, Horii A, Nakatsuru S *et al*. Inactivation of both APC alleles in an early stage of colon adenomas in a patient with familial adenomatous polyposis (FAP). *Hum Mol Genet*, 1992; 1: 387.

6 De Benedetti L, Sciallero S, Gismondi V *et al*. Association of APC gene mutations and histological characteristics of colorectal adenomas. *Cancer Res*, 1994; 54: 3553.

7 Zauber NP, Sabbath-Solitare M, Marotta SP, Bishop DT. K-ras mutation and loss of heterozygosity of the adenomatous polyposis coli gene in patients with colorectal adenomas with in situ carcinoma. *Cancer*, 1999; 86: 31.

8 Bussey HJR. *Familial Polyposis Coli*. Baltimore: Johns Hopkins University Press, 1975.

9 Deschner EE, Lipkin M. Proliferative patterns in colonic mucosa in familial polyposis. *Cancer*, 1975; 35: 413.

10 Lipkin M. Phase 1 and phase 2 proliferative lesions of colonic epithelial cells in disease leading to colonic cancer. *Cancer*, 1974; 34: 878.

11 Nakamura S, Kino L, Baba S. Nuclear DNA content of isolated crypts of background colonic mucosa from patients with familial adenomatous polyposis and sporadic colorectal cancer. *Gut*, 1993; 34: 1240.

12 Nakamura S, Goto J, Kitayama Y, Sheffield JP, Talbot IC. Flow cytometric analysis of DNA synthetic phase fraction of the normal appearing colonic mucosa in patients with colorectal neoplasms. *Gut*, 1995; 37: 398.

13 Wong AJ, Kohn GJ, Schwartz HJ, Ruebner BH, Lawson MJ. Colorectal cancer and noncancer patients have similar labeling indices by microscopy and computed image analysis. *Hum Pathol*, 1995; 26: 1329.

14 Terpstra OT, van Blankenstein M, Dees J, Eilers GAM. Abnormal pattern of cell proliferation in the entire colonic mucosa of patients with colon adenoma or cancer. *Gastroenterology*, 1987; 92: 704.

15 Mills SJ, Shepherd NA, Hall PA *et al*. Proliferative compartment deregulation in the non-neoplastic colonic epithelium of familial adenomatous polyposis. *Gut*, 1995; 36: 391.

16 Lipkin M, Newmark H. Effect of added dietary calcium on colonic epithelial-cell proliferation in subjects at high risk for familial colonic cancer. *N Engl J Med*, 1985; 313: 1381.

17 Potten CS, Kellett M, Rew DA, Roberts SA. Proliferation in human gastrointestinal epithelium using bromodeoxyuridine in vivo: data for different sites, proximity to a tumour, and polyposis coli. *Gut*, 1992; 33: 524.

18 Cats A, Kleibeuker JH, Kuipers F *et al*. Changes in rectal epithelial cell proliferation and intestinal bile acids after subtotal

colectomy in familial adenomatous polyposis. *Cancer Res*, 1992; 52: 3552.

19 Roncucci L, Ponz de Leong M, Scalmati A *et al*. The influence of age on colonic epithelial cell proliferation. *Cancer*, 1988; 62: 2373.

20 Macrae FA, Kilias D, Sharpe K *et al*. Rectal epithelial cell proliferation: comparison of errors of measurement with inter-subject variance. *J Cell Biochem*, 1994; 19: 84.

21 Jass JR. Evolution of hereditary bowel cancer. *Mutat Res*, 1993; 290: 13.

22 Wasan HS, Park H-S, Liu KC *et al*. APC in the regulation of intestinal crypt fission. *J Pathol*, 1998; 185: 246.

23 Keller JJ, Offerhaus GJA, Polak M *et al*. Rectal epithelial apoptosis in familial adenomatous polyposis patients treated with sulindac. *Gut*, 1999; 45: 822.

24 Nakamura S, Kino I. Morphogenesis of minute adenomas in familial polyposis coli. *J Natl Cancer Inst*, 1984; 73: 41.

25 Kubota O, Kino I, Nakamura S-I. A morphometrical analysis of minute depressed adenomas in familial polyposis coli. *Pathol Int*, 1994; 44: 200.

26 Kubota O, Kino I. Minute adenomas of the depressed type in familial adenomatous polyposis of the colon. A pathway to ordinary polypoid adenomas. *Cancer*, 1993; 72: 1159.

27 Novelli MR, Williamson JA, Tomlinson IPM *et al*. Polyclonal origin of colonic adenomas in an XO/XY patient with FAP. *Science*, 1996; 272: 1187.

28 Bodmer WF, Bailey CJ, Bodmer J *et al*. Localization of the gene for familial adenomatous polyposis on chromosome 5. *Nature*, 1987; 328: 614.

29 Oshima M, Oshima H, Kitagawa K *et al*. Loss of Apc heterozygosity and abnormal tissue building in nascent intestinal polyps in mice carrying a truncated Apc gene. *Proc Natl Acad Sci USA*, 1995; 92: 4482.

30 Lamlum H, Papadopoulou A, Ilyas M *et al*. APC mutations are sufficient for the growth of early colorectal adenomas. *Proc Natl Acad Sci USA*, 2000; 97: 2225.

31 Bird RP, McLellan EA, Bruce WR. Aberrant crypts, putative precancerous lesions, in the study of the role of diet in the aetiology of colon cancer. *Cancer Surv*, 1989; 8: 189.

32 Roncucci L, Stamp D, Medline A, Cullen JB, Bruce WR. Identification and quantification of aberrant crypt foci and microadenomas in the human colon. *Hum Pathol*, 1991; 22: 287.

33 Jen J, Powell SM, Papadopoulos N *et al*. Molecular determinants of dysplasia in colorectal lesions. *Cancer Res*, 1994; 54: 5523.

34 Minamoto T, Ronai Z, Yamashita N *et al*. Detection of Ki-ras mutation in non-neoplastic mucosa of Japanese patients with colorectal cancers. *Int J Oncol*, 1994; 4: 397.

35 Otori K, Sugiyama K, Hasebe T, Fukushima S, Esumi H. Emergence of adenomatous aberrant crypt foci (ACF) from hyperplastic ACF with concomitant increase in cell proliferation. *Cancer Res*, 1995; 55: 4743.

36 Muto T, Kamiya J, Sawada T *et al*. Small flat adenoma of the large bowel with special reference to its clinicopathological features. *Dis Colon Rectum*, 1985; 28: 847.

37 Kuramoto S, Ihara O, Sakai S *et al*. Depressed adenoma in the large intestine. Endoscopic features. *Dis Colon Rectum*, 1990; 33: 108.

38 Yamagata S, Muto T, Uchida Y *et al*. Lower incidence of K-*ras* codon 12 mutation in flat colorectal adenomas than in polypoid adenomas. *Jpn J Cancer Res*, 1994; 85: 147.

39 McLellan EA, Owen RA, Stepniewska KA, Sheffield JP, Lemoine NR. High frequency of K-ras mutations in sporadic colorectal adenomas. *Gut*, 1993; 34: 392.

40 Jass JR. Colorectal adenoma progression and genetic change: is there a link? *Ann Med*, 1994; 27: 301.

41 Fearon ER, Vogelstein B. A genetic model for colorectal tumorigenesis. *Cell*, 1990; 61: 759.

42 Hanski C, Bornhoeft G, Shimoda T *et al*. Expression of p53 protein in invasive colorectal carcinomas of different histologic types. *Cancer*, 1992; 70: 2272.

43 Mulder JWR, Baas IO, Polak MM, Goodman SN, Offerhaus GJA. Evaluation of p53 protein expression as a marker for long-term prognosis in colorectal carcinoma. *Br J Cancer*, 1995; 71: 1257.

44 Aoki T, Takeda S, Yanagisawa A *et al*. APC and p53 mutations in de novo colorectal adenocarcinomas. *Hum Mutat*, 1994; 3: 342.

45 Yukawa M, Fujimori T, Maeda S, Tabuchi M, Nagasako K. Comparative clinicopathological and immunohistochemical study of ras and p53 in flat and polypoid type colorectal tumours. *Gut*, 1994; 35: 1258.

46 Minamoto T, Sawaguchi K, Mai M *et al*. Infrequent K-*ras* activation in superficial-type (flat) colorectal adenomas and adenocarcinomas. *Cancer Res*, 1994; 54: 2841.

47 Markowitz S, Wang J, Myeroff L *et al*. Inactivation of the type II TGF-β receptor in colon cancer cells with microsatellite instability. *Science*, 1995; 268: 1336.

48 Souza RF, Appel R, Yin J *et al*. The insulin-like growth factor II receptor gene is a target of microsatellite instability in human gastrointestinal tumours. *Nat Genet*, 1996; 14: 255.

49 Rampino N, Yamamoto H, Ionov Y *et al*. Somatic frameshift mutations in the *BAX* gene in colon cancers of the microsatellite mutator phenotype. *Science*, 1997; 275: 967.

50 Hill MJ. Bile, bacteria and bowel cancer. *Gut*, 1983; 24: 871.

51 Paganelli GM, Biasco G, Santucci R *et al*. Rectal cell proliferation and colorectal cancer risk level in patients with nonfamilial adenomatous polyps of the large bowel. *Cancer*, 1991; 68: 2451.

52 Lane DP. A death in the life of p53. *Nature*, 1993; 362: 786.

53 Lengauer C, Kinzler KW, Vogelstein B. Genetic instabilities in human cancers. *Nature*, 1998; 396: 643.

54 Wattenberg LW. A histochemical study of five oxidative enzymes in carcinoma of the large intestine in man. *Am J Pathol*, 1959; 35: 113.

55 Chadeneau C, Hay K, Hirte HW, Gallinger S, Bacchetti S. Telomerase activity associated with acquisition of malignancy in human colorectal cancer. *Cancer Res*, 1995; 55: 2533.

56 Skinner SA, Frydman GM, O'Brien PE. Microvascular structure of benign and malignant tumors of the colon in humans. *Dig Dis Sci*, 1995; 40: 373.

57 Bossi P, Viale G, Lee AKC *et al*. Angiogenesis in colorectal tumors: Microvessel quantitation in adenomas and carcinomas with clinicopathological correlations. *Cancer Res*, 1995; 55: 5049.

58 Frank RE, Saclarides TJ, Leurgans S *et al*. Tumor angiogenesis as a predictor of recurrence and survival in patients with node-negative colon cancer. *Ann Surg*, 1995; 222: 695.

59 Mulcahy HE, Duffy MJ, Gibbons D *et al*. Urokinase-type plasminogen activator and outcome in Dukes' B colorectal cancer. *Lancet*, 1994; 344: 583.

60 Hewitt RE, Leach IH, Powe DG *et al*. Distribution of collagenase and tissue inhibitor of metalloproteinases (TIMP) in colorectal tumours. *Int J Cancer*, 1991; 49: 666.

61 Tan K, Powe DG, Gray T, Turner DR, Hewitt RE. Regional variations of urokinase-type plasminogen activator in human colorectal cancer: a quantitative study by image analysis. *Int J Cancer*, 1995; 60: 308.

62 Jass JR, Smith M. Sialic acid and epithelial differentiation in colorectal polyps and cancer—a morphological, mucin and lectin histochemical study. *Pathology*, 1992; 24: 233.

63 Pignatelli M, Vessey CJ. Adhesion molecules: novel molecular tools in tumor pathology. *Hum Pathol*, 1994; 25: 849.

64 Goh HS, Jass JR. DNA content and the adenoma–carcinoma sequence in the colorectum. *J Clin Pathol*, 1986; 39: 387.

65 Bos JL, Fearon ER, Hamilton SR *et al.* Prevalence of *ras* gene mutation in human colorectal cancers. *Nature*, 1987; 327: 293.

66 Bosari S, Moneghini L, Graziani D *et al.* bcl-2 oncoprotein in colorectal hyperplastic polyps, adenomas, and adenocarcinomas. *Hum Pathol*, 1995; 26: 534.

67 Su L-K, Vogelstein B, Kinzler K. Association of the APC tumor suppressor protein with catenins. *Science*, 1993; 262: 1734.

68 Smith KJ, Levy DB, Maupin P *et al.* Wild-type but not mutant APC associates with the microtubule cytoskeleton. *Cancer Res*, 1994; 54: 3672.

69 Cawkwell L, Lewis FA, Quirke P. Frequency of allele loss of DCC, p53, RB1, WT1, NF1, NM23 and APC/MCC in colorectal cancer assayed by fluorescent multiplex polymerase chain reaction. *Br J Cancer*, 1994; 70: 813.

70 Leach FS, Nicolaides NC, Papadopoulos N *et al.* Mutations of a *mut*S homolog in hereditary nonpolyposis colorectal cancer. *Cell*, 1993; 75: 1215.

71 Fishel R, Lescoe MK, Rao MRS *et al.* The human mutator gene homolog MSH2 and its association with hereditary nonpolyposis colon cancer. *Cell*, 1993; 75: 1027.

72 Papadopoulos N, Nicolaides NC, Wei Y-F *et al.* Mutation of a *mutL* homolog in hereditary colon cancer. *Science*, 1994; 263: 1625.

73 Bronner CE, Baker SM, Morrison PT *et al.* Mutation in the DNA mismatch repair gene homologue *hMLH1* is associated with hereditary non-polyposis colon cancer. *Nature*, 1994; 368: 258.

74 Nicolaides NC, Papadopoulos N, Liu B *et al.* Mutations of two PMS homologues in hereditary nonpolyposis colon cancer. *Nature*, 1994; 371: 75.

75 Konishi M, Kikuchi-Yanoshita R, Tanaka K *et al.* Molecular nature of colon tumors in hereditary nonpolyposis colon cancer, familial polyposis, and sporadic colon cancer. *Gastroenterology*, 1996; 111: 307.

76 Salahshor S, Kressner U, Påhlman L *et al.* Colorectal cancer with and without microsatellite instability involves different genes. *Genes Chromosomes Cancer*, 1999; 26: 247.

77 Olschwang S, Hamelin R, Laurent-Puig P *et al.* Alternative genetic pathways in colorectal carcinogenesis. *Proc Natl Acad Sci USA*, 1997; 94: 12122.

78 Jass JR, Biden KG, Cummings M *et al.* Characterisation of a subtype of colorectal cancer combining features of the suppressor and mild mutator pathways. *J Clin Pathol*, 1999; 52: 455.

79 Fujiwara T, Stoker JM, Watanabe T *et al.* Accumulated clonal genetic alterations in familial and sporadic colorectal carcinomas with widespread instability in microsatellite sequences. *Am J Pathol*, 1998; 153: 1063.

80 Souza RF, Lei J, Yin J *et al.* A transforming growth factor-β1 receptor type II mutation occurs in ulcerative colitis-associated and sporadic colorectal neoplasms, but not in gastric or esophageal carcinomas. *Gastroenterology*, 1997; 112: 40.

81 Schwartz S Jr, Yamamoto H, Navarro M *et al.* Frameshift mutations at mononucleotide repeats in *caspase*-5 and other target genes in endometrial and gastrointestinal cancer of the microsatellite mutator phenotype. *Cancer Res*, 1999; 59: 2995.

82 Wicking C, Simms LA, Evans T *et al.* *CDX2*, a human homologue of *Drosophila caudal*, is mutated in both alleles in a replication error positive colorectal cancer. *Oncogene*, 1998; 17: 657.

83 Simms LA, Young J, Wicking C *et al.* The apoptotic regulatory gene, BCL10, is mutated in sporadic mismatch repair deficient colorectal cancers. *Cell Death Differ*, 2000; 7: 236.

84 Souza RF, Yin J, Smolinski KN *et al.* Frequent mutation of the *E2F-4* cell cycle gene in primary human gastrointestinal tumors. *Cancer Res*, 1997; 57: 2350.

85 Ikeda M, Orimo H, Moriyzma H *et al.* Close correlation between mutations of *E2F4* and *hMSH3* genes in colorectal cancers with microsatellite instability. *Cancer Res*, 1998; 58: 594.

86 Ahuja N, Mohan AL, Li Q *et al.* Association between cPG island methylation and microsatellite instability in colorectal cancer. *Cancer Res*, 1997; 57: 3370.

87 Ahuja N, Li Q, Mohna AL, Baylin SB, Issa JP. Aging and DNA methylation in colorectal mucosa and cancer. *Cancer Res*, 1998; 58: 5489.

88 Toyota M, Ahuja N, Ohe-Toyota M *et al.* CpG island methylator phenotype in colorectal cancer. *Proc Natl Acad Sci USA*, 1999; 96: 8681.

89 He TC, Sparks AB, Rago C *et al.* Identification of c-MYC as a target of the APC pathway. *Science*, 1998; 281: 1509.

90 Su L-K, Johnson KA, Smith KJ *et al.* Association between wild-type and mutant APC gene products. *Cancer Res*, 1993; 53: 2728.

91 Cross I, Delhanty J, Chapman P *et al.* An intrachromosomal insertion causing 5q22 deletion and familial adenomatous polyposis coli in two generations. *J Med Genet*, 1992; 29: 175.

92 Kinzler K, Vogelstein B. Landscaping the cancer terrain. *Science*, 1998; 280: 1036.

93 Solomon E, Voss R, Hall V *et al.* Chromosome 5 allele loss in human colorectal carcinomas. *Nature*, 1987; 328: 616.

94 Turley H, Pezzella F, Kocialkowski S *et al.* The distribution of the deleted in colon cancer (DCC) protein in human tissues. *Cancer Res*, 1995; 55: 5628.

95 Leister I, Weith A, Bruderlein S *et al.* Human colorectal cancer: high frequency of deletions at chromosome 1p35. *Cancer Res*, 1990; 50: 7232.

96 Cunningham C, Dunlop MG, Bird CC, Wyllie AH. Deletion analysis of chromosome 8p in sporadic colorectal adenomas. *Br J Cancer*, 1994; 70: 18.

97 Kelemen PR, Yaremko ML, Kim AH *et al.* Loss of heterozygosity in 8p is associated with microinvasion in colorectal carcinoma. *Genes Chromosomes Cancer*, 1994; 11: 195.

98 Yaremko ML, Wasylyshyn ML, Paulus KL, Michelassi F, Westbrook CA. Deletion mapping reveals two regions of chromosome 8 allele loss in colorectal carcinomas. *Genes Chromosomes Cancer*, 1994; 10: 1.

99 Purdie CA, Piris J, Bird CC, Wyllie AH. 17q allele loss is associated with lymph node metastasis in locally aggressive human colorectal cancer. *J Pathol*, 1995; 175: 297.

100 Iino H, Fukayama M, Maeda Y *et al.* Molecular genetics for

clinical management of colorectal carcinoma. *Cancer*, 1993; 73: 1324.

101 Yana I, Kurahashi H, Nakamori S *et al.* Frequent loss of heterozygosity at telomeric loci on 22q in sporadic colorectal cancers. *Int J Cancer*, 1995; 60: 174.

102 Nagase H, Nakamura Y. Mutations of the APC (Adenomatous Polyposis Coli) gene. *Hum Mutat*, 1993; 2: 425.

103 Boland CR, Thibodeau SN, Hamilton SR *et al.* A National Cancer Institute Workshop on microsatellite instability for cancer detection and familial predisposition: development of international criteria for the determination of microsatellite instability in colorectal cancer. *Cancer Res*, 1998; 58: 5248.

104 Heinen CD, Richardson D, White R, Groden J. Microsatellite instability in colorectal adenocarcinoma cell lines that have full-length adenomatous polyposis coli protein. *Cancer Res*, 1995; 55: 4797.

105 Jass JR, Do K-A, Simms LA *et al.* Morphology of sporadic colorectal cancer with DNA replication errors. *Gut*, 1998; 42: 673.

106 Iino H, Jass JR, Simms LA *et al.* DNA microsatellite instability in hyperplastic polyps, serrated adenomas, and mixed polyps: a mild mutator pathway for colorectal cancer? *J Clin Pathol*, 1999; 52: 5.

107 Jass JR, Iino H, Ruszkiewicz A *et al.* Neoplastic progression occurs through mutator pathways in hyperplastic polyposis of the colorectum. *Gut*, 2000; 47: 43.

108 Al-Tassan N, Chmiel NH, Maynard J *et al.* Inherited variants of MYH associated with somatic G:C→T:A mutations in colorectal tumors. *Nat Genet*, 2002; 30: 227.

109 Robertson KD, Jones PA. The human ARF cell cycle regulatory gene promoter is a CpG island which can be silenced by DNA methylation and down-regulated by wild-type p53. *Mol Cell Biol*, 1998; 18: 6457.

110 Toyota M, Shen L, Ohe-Toyota M *et al.* Aberrant methylation of the *Cyclooxygenase 2* CpG island in colorectal tumors. *Cancer Res*, 2000; 60: 4044.

111 Issa J-PJ, Ottaviano YL, Celano P *et al.* Methylation of the oestrogen receptor CpG island links ageing and neoplasia in human colon. *Nat Genet*, 1994; 7: 536.

112 Jass JR, Young J, Leggett BA. Hyperplastic polyps and DNA microsatellite unstable cancers of the colorectum. *Histopathology*, 2000; 37: 295.

113 Young J, Biden KB, Simms LA *et al.* HPP1: a transmembrane protein commanly methylated in colorectal polyps and cancers. *Proc Natl Acad Sci (USA)* 2001; 98: 265.

114 Esteller M, Toyota M, Sanchez-Cespedes M *et al.* Inactivation of the DNA repair gene *O^6-methylguanine-DNA methyltransferase* by promoter hypermethylation is associated with G to A mutations in K-*ras* in colorectal tumorigenesis. *Cancer Res*, 2000; 60: 2368.

115 Correa P. Epidemiology of polyps and cancer. In: Morson BC, ed. *The Pathogenesis of Colorectal Cancer.* Philadelphia: W.B. Saunders, 1978: 126.

116 Stemmermann GN, Yatani R. Diverticulosis and polyps of the large intestine. A necropsy study of Hawaii Japanese. *Cancer*, 1973; 31: 1260.

117 Williams AR, Balasooriya BAW, Day DW. Polyps and cancer of the large bowel: a necropsy study in Liverpool. *Gut*, 1982; 23: 835.

118 Coode PE, Chan KW, Chan YT. Polyps and diverticula of the large intestine: a necropsy survey in Hong Kong. *Gut*, 1985; 26: 1045.

119 Vatn MH, Stalsberg H. The prevalence of polyps of the large intestine in Oslo: an autopsy study. *Cancer*, 1982; 49: 819.

120 Bernstein MA, Feczko PJ, Halpert RD, Simms SM, Ackerman LV. Distribution of colonic polyps: increased incidence of proximal lesions in older patients. *Radiology*, 1985; 155: 35.

121 Eide TJ. The age, sex and site specific occurrence of adenoma and carcinoma of the large intestine within a defined population. *Scand J Gastroenterol*, 1986; 21: 1083.

122 Gerharz C-D, Gabbert H, Krummel F. Age dependent shift to the right in the localisation of colorectal adenomas. *Virchows Arch A*, 1987; 411: 591.

123 Jass JR, Young PJ, Robinson EM. Predictors of presence, multiplicity, size and dysplasia of colorectal adenomas. A necropsy study in New Zealand. *Gut*, 1992; 33: 1508.

124 Correa P, Strong JP, Reif A, Johnson WD. The epidemiology of colorectal polyps. Prevalence in New Orleans and international comparisons. *Cancer*, 1971; 39: 2258.

125 Rickert RR, Auerbach O, Garfinkel L, Hammond EC, Frasca JM. Adenomatous lesions of the large bowel: an autopsy survey. *Cancer*, 1979; 43: 1847.

126 Clark JC, Collan Y, Eide TJ *et al.* Prevalence of polyps in an autopsy series from areas with varying incidence of large-bowel cancer. *Int J Cancer*, 1985; 36: 179.

127 Eide TJ, Stalsberg H. Polyps of the large intestine in northern Norway. *Cancer*, 1978; 42: 2839.

128 Vatn MH, Myren J, Serck-Hanssen A. The distribution of polyps in the large intestine. *Ann Gastroenterol Hepatol*, 1985; 4: 239.

129 Hoff G, Foerster A, Vatn MH, Gjone E. Epidemiology of polyps in the rectum and sigmoid colon. Histological examination of resected polyps. *Scand J Gastroenterol*, 1984; 20: 677.

130 Martínez ME, McPherson RS, Annegers JF, Levin B. Cigarette smoking and alcohol consumption as risk factors for colorectal adenomatous polyps. *J Natl Cancer Inst*, 1995; 87: 274.

131 Martínez ME, McPherson RS, Levin B, Annegers JF. Aspirin and other nonsteroidal anti-inflammatory drugs and risk of colorectal adenomatous polyps among endoscoped individuals. *Cancer Epidemiol Biomarkers Prev*, 1995; 4: 703.

132 Martínez ME, McPherson RS, Annegers JF, Levin B. Association of diet and colorectal adenomatous polyp: dietary fiber, calcium, and total fat. *Epidemiology*, 1996; 7: 264.

133 Konishi F, Muto T, Kamiya J *et al.* Histopathologic comparison of colorectal adenomas in English and Japanese patients. *Dis Colon Rectum*, 1984; 27: 515.

134 Jass JR, Sobin LH. *Histological Typing of Intestinal Tumours. WHO International Classification of Tumours*. Berlin: Springer-Verlag, 1989.

135 Goldman H, Ming S, Hickock DF. Nature and significance of hyperplastic polyps of the human colon. *Arch Pathol*, 1970; 89: 349.

136 Thompson JJ, Enterline HT. The macroscopic appearance of colorectal polyps. *Cancer*, 1981; 48: 151.

137 Konishi F, Morson BC. Pathology of colorectal adenomas. *J Clin Pathol*, 1982; 35: 830.

138 Banner BF, Chacho MS, Roseman DL, Coon JS. Multiparameter flow cytometric analysis of colon polyps. *Am J Clin Pathol*, 1987; 87: 313.

139 van den Ingh HF, van den Broek LJ, Verhofstad AAJ, Bosman FT.

Neuroendocrine cells in colorectal adenomas. *J Pathol*, 1986; 148: 231.

140 Williams GT, Blackshaw AJ, Morson BC. Squamous carcinoma of the colorectum and its genesis. *J Pathol*, 1979; 129: 139.

141 Kontozoglou T. Squamous metaplasia in colonic adenomata: report of two cases. *J Surg Oncol*, 1985; 29: 31.

142 Agawa S, Jass JR. Sialic acid histochemistry and the adenoma–carcinoma sequence in colorectum. *J Clin Pathol*, 1990; 43: 528.

143 Griffin CA, Lazar S, Hamilton SR *et al*. Cytogenetic analysis of intestinal polyps in polyposis syndromes: comparison with sporadic colorectal adenomas. *Cancer Genet Cytogenet*, 1993; 67: 14.

144 Messinetti S, Zelli GP, Marcellino LR, Alcini E. Benign and malignant tumours of the gastrointestinal tract. Chromosome analysis in study and diagnosis. *Cancer*, 1968; 21: 1000.

145 Paraskeva C, Buckle BG, Sheer D, Wigley CB. The isolation and characterization of colorectal epithelial cell lines at different stages in malignant transformation from familial polyposis coli patients. *Int J Cancer*, 1984; 34: 49.

146 Bomme L, Bardi G, Pandis N *et al*. Clonal karyotypic abnormalities in colorectal adenomas: clues to the early genetic events in the adenoma–carcinoma sequence. *Genes Chromosomes Cancer*, 1994; 10: 190.

147 Enterline HT, Arvan DA. Chromosome constitution of adenoma and carcinoma of the colon. *Cancer*, 1967; 20: 1746.

148 Reichman A, Martin P, Levin B. Karyotypic findings in a colonic villous adenoma. *Cancer Genet Cytogenet*, 1982; 7: 51.

149 Quirke P, Fozard JBJ, Dixon MF *et al*. DNA aneuploidy in colorectal adenomas. *Br J Cancer*, 1986; 53: 477.

150 Meijer GA, Hermsen MAJA, Baak JPA *et al*. Progression from colorectal adenoma to carcinoma is associated with non-random chromosomal gains as detected by comparative genomic hybridisation. *J Clin Pathol*, 1998; 51: 901.

151 Nachlas MM, Hannibal MJ. Histochemical observations on the polyp–carcinoma sequence. *Surg Gynecol Obstet*, 1961; 112: 534.

152 Vatn MH, Tjora S, Arva PH, Serck-Hanssen A, Stromme JH. Enzymatic characteristics of tubular adenomas and carcinomas of the large intestine. *Gut*, 1982; 23: 193.

153 Czernobilsky B, Tsou K-C. Adenocarcinoma, adenomas and polyps of the colon. Histochemical study. *Cancer*, 1968; 21: 165.

154 Hoff G, Clausen OPF, Fjordvang H *et al*. Epidemiology of polyps in the rectum and sigmoid colon. Size, enzyme levels, DNA distributions and nuclear diameter in polyps of the large intestine. *Scand J Gastroenterol*, 1985; 20: 983.

155 Hounsell EF, Feizi T. Gastrointestinal mucus. Structures and antigenicities of their carbohydrate chains in health and disease. *Med Biol*, 1982; 60: 227.

156 Sugihara K, Jass JR. Heterogeneity of colorectal goblet cell mucus and its relation to neoplastic disease. *J Pathol*, 1986; 148: 83.

157 Jass JR, Allison LM, Edgar S. Monoclonal antibody TKH2 to the cancer-associated epitope sialosyl Tn shows cross-reactivity with variants of normal colorectal goblet cell mucin. *Pathology*, 1994; 26: 418.

158 Itzkowitz SH, Bloom EJ, Lau T-S, Kim YS. Mucin associated Tn and sialosyl-Tn antigen expression in colorectal polyps. *Gut*, 1992; 33: 518.

159 Jass JR, Roberton AM. Colorectal mucin histochemistry in health and disease: a critical review. *Pathol Int*, 1994; 44: 487.

160 Vowden P, Lowe A, Lennox ES, Bleehen NM. Colonic polyp epithelial ABH blood group isoantigen (BGI) expression related to histological type and size. *Br J Surg*, 1984; 71: 906.

161 Brown A, Ellis IO, Embleton MJ *et al*. Immunohistochemical localization of Y hapten and the structurally related H type-2 blood-group antigen on large-bowel tumours and normal adult tissues. *Int J Cancer*, 1984; 33: 727.

162 Abe K, Hakomori S, Ohshiba S. Differential expression of difucosyl Type 2 chain (Le^y) defined by monoclonal antibody AH6 in different locations of colonic epithelia, various histological types of colonic polyps, and adenocarcinomas. *Cancer Res*, 1986; 46: 2639.

163 Yonezawa S, Nakamura T, Tanaka S, Sato E. Glycoconjugate with *Ulex europaeus* agglutinin-I-binding site in normal mucosa, adenoma and carcinoma of the human large bowel. *J Natl Cancer Inst*, 1977; 69: 777.

164 Boland CR, Montgomery CK, Kim YS. A cancer-associated mucin alteration in benign colonic polyps. *Gastroenterology*, 1982; 82: 664.

165 Ajioka Y, Xing P-X, Hinoda Y, Jass JR. Correlative histochemical study providing evidence for the dual nature of human colorectal cancer mucin. *Histochem J*, 1997; 29: 143.

166 Yuan M, Itzkowitz SH, Ferrell LD *et al*. Expression of lewis^x and sialylated lewis^x antigens in human colorectal polyps. *J Natl Cancer Inst*, 1987; 78: 479.

167 Goldman H, Ming S-C. Mucins in normal and neoplastic gastrointestinal epithelium. Histochemical distribution. *Arch Pathol*, 1968; 85: 580.

168 Greaves P, Filipe MI, Abbas S, Ormerod MG. Sialomucins and carcinoembryonic antigen in the evolution of colorectal cancer. *Histopathology*, 1984; 8: 825.

169 Eide TJ, Nielsen K, Solberg S. Dysplasia in colorectal adenomas related to the presence of O-acetylated sialic mucin and to morphometric measurements. *APMIS*, 1987; 95: 365.

170 Quinlan DC, Davidson A, Watne AL. Dynamics of glycoprotein metabolism with familial polyposis coli-derived colonic epithelial tissue. *Semin Surg Oncol*, 1987; 3: 174.

171 Ajioka Y, Watanabe H, Jass JR. MUC1 and MUC2 mucins in flat and polypoid colorectal adenomas. *J Clin Pathol*, 1997; 50: 417.

172 Biemer-Hüttmann A-E, Walsh MD, McGuckin MA *et al*. Immunohistochemical staining patterns of MUC1, MUC2, MUC4, and MUC5AC mucins in hyperplastic polyps, serrated adenomas, and traditional adenomas of the colorectum. *J Histochem Cytochem*, 1999; 47: 1039.

173 Brandtzaeg P. Transport models for secretory IgA and secretory IgM. *Clin Exp Immunol*, 1981; 44: 221.

174 Isaacson P. Immunoperoxidase study of the secretory immunoglobulin system in colonic neoplasia. *J Clin Pathol*, 1982; 35: 14.

175 Ahnen DJ, Nakane PK, Brown WP. Ultrastructural localization of carcinoembryonic antigen in normal intestine and colon cancer. *Cancer*, 1982; 49: 2077.

176 Isaacson P, Judd MA. Immunohistochemistry of carcinoembryonic antigen in the small intestine. *Cancer*, 1978; 42: 1554.

177 Rognum TO, Elgjo K, Brandtzaeg P, Ørjasaeter H, Bergan A. Plasma carcinoembryonic antigen concentrations and immunohistochemical patterns of epithelial cell marker antigens in patients with large bowel carcinoma. *J Clin Pathol*, 1982; 35: 922.

178 Jass JR, Filipe MI, Abbas E *et al*. A morphologic and histochemical study of metaplastic polyps of the colorectum. *Cancer*, 1984; 53: 510.

179 Skinner JM, Whitehead R. Tumor-associated antigens in polyps and carcinoma of the human large bowel. *Cancer*, 1981; 47: 1241.

180 Yuan M, Itzkowitz SH, Ferrell LD *et al*. Expression of Lewis^x antigens on human colorectal polyps. *J Natl Cancer Inst*, 1982; 28: 479.

181 O'Brien MJ, Winawar SJ, Graham Zauber A *et al*. The National Polyp Study. Patient and polyp characteristics associated with high grade dysplasia in colorectal adenomas. *Gastroenterology*, 1990; 98: 371.

182 Heby O. Role of polyamines in the control of cell proliferation and differentiation. *Differentiation*, 1981; 19: 1.

183 Pegg AE, Williams-Ashman HG. Bio-synthesis of putrescine. In: Morris DR, Marton LJ, eds. *Polyamines in Biology and Medicine*. New York: Marcel Dekker, 1981.

184 Russel DH, Snyder SH. Amine synthesis in the regenerating rat liver: extremely rapid turnover of ornithine decarboxylase. *Mol Pharmacol*, 1969; 5: 253.

185 Takano S, Matsushima M, Erturk E, Bryan GT. Early induction of rat colonic epithelial ornithine and S-adenosyl-L-methionine decarboxylase activities by N-methyl-N-nitro-N-nitrosoguanidine of bile salts. *Cancer Res*, 1984; 44: 3226.

186 Rozhin J, Wilson PS, Bull AW, Nigro D. Ornithine decarboxylase activity in the rat and human colon. *Cancer Res*, 1984; 44: 3226.

187 Kingsnorth A, King WWK, Diekama KA *et al*. Inhibition of ornithine decarboxylase with 2-difluoremethylornithine: reduced incidence of dimethylhydrazine-induced colonic tumors in mice. *Cancer Res*, 1983; 43: 2545.

188 LaMuraglia GM, Lacaine F, Malt RA. High ornithine decarboxylase activity and polyamine levels in human colorectal neoplasia. *Ann Surg*, 1986; 204: 89.

189 Takenoshita S, Matsuzaki S, Nakano G *et al*. Selective elevation of the N-acetylspermidine level in human colorectal adenocarcinomas. *Cancer Res*, 1984; 44: 845.

190 Scalabrino G, Ferioli ME. Polyamines in mammalian tissues. Part I. *Adv Cancer Res*, 1981; 35: 151.

191 Luk GD, Baylin SB. Ornithine decarboxylase as a biologic marker in familial colonic polyposis. *N Engl J Med*, 1984; 311: 80.

192 Moorehead RJ, Hooper M, McKelvey STD. Assessment of ornithine decarboxylase activity—rectal mucosa as a marker for colorectal adenomas and carcinomas. *Br J Surg*, 1987; 74: 364.

193 Imai H, Saito S, Stein AA. Ultrastructure of adenomatous polyps and villous adenomas of the large intestine. *Gastroenterology*, 1965; 48: 188.

194 Kaye GI, Fenoglio CM, Pascal RR, Lane N. Comparative electron microscopic features of normal, hyperplastic and adenomatous human colonic epithelium. *Gastroenterology*, 1973; 64: 926.

195 Cheng H, Leblond CF. Origin, differentiation and renewal of the four main epithelial cell types in the mouse small intestine V. Unitarian theory of the origin of the four epithelial cell types. *Am J Anat*, 1974; 141: 537.

196 Kirkland SC. Clonal origin of columnar, mucous, and endocrine cell lineages in human colorectal epithelium. *Cancer*, 1988; 61: 1359.

197 Mughal S, Filipe MI. Ultrastructural study of the normal mucosa–adenoma–cancer sequence in the development of familial polyposis coli. *J Natl Cancer Inst*, 1978; 60: 753.

198 Mughal S, Filipe MI, Jass JR. A comparative ultrastructural study of hyperplastic and adenomatous polyps, incidental and in association with colorectal cancer. *Cancer*, 1981; 48: 2746.

199 Birbeck MS, Dukes CE. Electron microscopy of rectal neoplasms. *Proc R Soc Med*, 1963; 56: 793.

200 Mughal S, Filipe MI. Histogenesis of malignant transformation in the colonic epithelium. A detailed study on semi-thin sections. *Acta Gastroenterol Belg*, 1978; 41: 215.

201 Shamsuddin AM, Phelps PC, Trump BF. Human large intestinal epithelium: light microscopy, histochemistry and ultrastructure. *Hum Pathol*, 1982; 13: 790.

202 Strater J, Koretz K, Gunthert AR, Moller P. In situ detection of enterocytic apoptosis in normal colonic mucosa and in familial adenomatous polyposis. *Gut*, 1995; 37: 819.

203 Blank M, Klussmann E, Kruger-Krasagakes S *et al*. Expression of MUC2-mucin in colorectal adenomas and carcinomas of different histological types. *Int J Cancer*, 1994; 59: 301.

204 Winterford CM, Walsh MD, Leggett BA, Jass JR. Ultrastructural localization of epithelial mucin core proteins in colorectal tissues. *J Histochem Cytochem*, 1999; 47: 1063.

205 Longacre TA, Fenoglio-Preiser CM. Mixed hyperplastic adenomatous polyps / serrated adenomas. A distinct form of colorectal neoplasia. *Am J Surg Pathol*, 1990; 14: 524.

206 Torlakovic E, Snover DC. Serrated adenomatous polyposis in humans. *Gastroenterology*, 1996; 110: 748.

207 Yokoo H, Usman MI, Wheaton S, Kampmeier PA. Colorectal polyps with extensive absorptive enterocyte differentiation. *Arch Pathol Lab Med*, 1999; 123: 404.

208 Matsumoto T, Mizuno M, Shimuzu M *et al*. Serrated adenoma of the colorectum: colonoscopic and histologic features. *Gastrointest Endosc*, 1999; 49: 736.

209 Eide TJ. Prevalence and morphological features of adenomas of the large intestine in individuals with and without colorectal carcinoma. *Histopathology*, 1986; 10: 111.

210 Bussey HJR, Wallace MH, Morson BC. Metachronous carcinoma of the large intestine and intestinal polyps. *Proc R Soc Med*, 1967; 60: 208.

211 Heald RJ, Lockhart-Mummery HE. The lesion of the second cancer of the large bowel. *Br J Surg*, 1972; 59: 16.

212 Atkin WS, Morson BC, Cuzick J. Long-term risk of colorectal cancer after excision of rectosigmoid adenomas. *N Engl J Med*, 1992; 326: 658.

213 Eide TJ. Remnants of adenomas in colorectal carcinomas. *Cancer*, 1983; 51: 1866.

214 Morson BC. Factors influencing the prognosis of early cancer of the rectum. *Proc R Soc Med*, 1966; 59: 607.

215 Bussey HJR. Age and cancer of the large intestine. *Cancer and Aging*. Thule International Symposia. Stockholm: Nordiska Bokhandelhs Forlag, 1968.

216 Gaglia P, Atkin WS, Whitelaw S *et al*. Variables associated with the risk of colorectal adenomas in asymptomatic patients with a family history of colorectal cancer. *Gut*, 1995; 36: 385.

217 Gilbertson VA, Nelms JM. The prevention of invasive cancer of the rectum. *Cancer*, 1978; 41: 137.

218 Paraskeva C, Hague A, Rooney N *et al*. A single human colonic adenoma cell line can be converted in vitro to both a colorectal adenocarcinoma and a mucinous carcinoma. *Int J Cancer*, 1992; 51: 661.

219 Pollock AM, Quirke P. Adenoma screening and colorectal cancer. The need for screening and polypectomy is unproved. *Br J Med*, 1991; 303: 3.

220 Kronborg O, Fenger C. Clinical evidence for the adenoma–carcinoma sequence. *Eur J Cancer Prev*, 1999; 8: S73.

221 Spratt JSJ, Ackerman LV. Small primary adenocarcinomas of the colon and rectum. *JAMA*, 1962; 179: 337.
222 Desigan G, Wang M, Alberti-Flor J *et al*. *De novo* carcinoma of the rectum: a case report. *Am J Gastroenterol*, 1985; 80: 553.
223 Shamsuddin AKM, Bell HG, Petrucci JV *et al*. Carcinoma *in situ* and microinvasive carcinoma of the colon. *Pathol Res Pract*, 1980; 167: 374.
224 Bedenne L, Faivre J, Boutron MC *et al*. Adenoma–carcinoma sequence or 'de novo' carcinogenesis? *Cancer*, 1992; 69: 883.
225 Shimoda T, Ikegami M, Fujisaki J *et al*. Early colorectal carcinoma with special reference to its development de novo. *Cancer*, 1989; 64: 1138.
226 Minamoto T, Sawaguchi K, Ohta T, Itoh T, Mai M. Superficial-type adenomas and adenocarcinomas of the colon and rectum: a comparative morphological study. *Gastroenterology*, 1994; 106: 1436.
227 Hunt DR, Cherian M. Endoscopic diagnosis of small flat carcinoma of the colon: report of three cases. *Dis Colon Rectum*, 1990; 33: 143.
228 Ando M, Takemura K, Maruyama M. *et al*. Mutations in c-K-ras 2 gene codon 12 during colorectal tumorigenesis in familial adenomatous polyposis. *Gastroenterology*, 1992; 103: 1725.
229 Grinnell RS, Lane N. Benign and malignant adenomatous polyps and papillary adenomas of the colon and rectum. An analysis of 1856 tumours in 1335 patients. *Surgery*, 1958; 106: 519.
230 Enterline HT, Evans GW, Mercado-Lugo R, Miller L, Fitts WT Jr. Malignant potential of adenomas of colon and rectum. *JAMA*, 1962; 179: 322.
231 Silverberg SG. Focally malignant adenomatous polyps of the colon and rectum. *Surg Gynecol Obstet*, 1970; 131: 103.
232 Fung CHK, Goldman H. The incidence and significance of villous change in adenomatous polyps. *Am J Clin Pathol*, 1970; 53: 21.
233 Kaneko M. On pedunculated adenomatous polyps of colon and rectum with particular reference to their malignant potential. *Mt Sinai J Med*, 1972; 39: 103.
234 Jass JR, Stewart SM. Evolution of hereditary non-polyposis colorectal cancer. *Gut*, 1992; 33: 783.
235 Jass JR, Stewart SM, Stewart J, Lane MR. Hereditary non-polyposis colorectal cancer: morphologies, genes and mutations. *Mutat Res*, 1994; 290: 125.
236 Green SE, Bradburn DM, Varma JS, Burn J. Hereditary non-polyposis colorectal cancer. *Int J Colorectal Dis*, 1998; 13: 3.
237 Castleman B, Krickstein HI. Do adenomatous polyps of the colon become malignant? *N Engl J Med*, 1962; 267: 469.
238 Spratt JS Jr, Ackerman LV, Moyer CA. Relationship of polyps of colon to colonic cancer. *Ann Surg*, 1958; 148: 682.
239 Helwig EB. Adenomas and pathogenesis of cancer of the colon and rectum. *Dis Colon Rectum*, 1958; 2: 5.
240 Lescher TC, Dockerty MB, Jackman RJ, Beahrs DH. Histopathology of the larger colonic polyp. *Dis Colon Rectum*, 1967; 10: 118.
241 Kellokumpu I, Husa A. Colorectal adenomas: morphologic features and the risk of developing metachronous adenomas and carcinomas in the colorectum. *Scand J Gastroenterol*, 1987; 22: 833.
242 Morson BC, Bussey HJR. Magnitude of risk for cancer patients with colorectal adenomas. *Br J Surg*, 1985; 72: 23.
243 Morson BC. The evolution of colorectal carcinoma. *Clin Radiol*, 1984; 35: 425.
244 Morson BC. The polyp–cancer sequence in the large bowel. *Proc R Soc Med*, 1974; 67: 451.
245 Lynch HT, Smyrk T, Jass JR. Hereditary nonpolyposis colorectal cancer and colonic adenomas: aggressive adenomas? *Semin Surg Oncol*, 1995; 11: 406.
246 Jass JR. Colorectal adenomas in surgical specimens from subjects with hereditary non-polyposis colorectal cancer. *Histopathology*, 1995; 27: 263.
247 Fechner RE. Adenomatous polyp with submucosal cysts. *Am J Clin Pathol*, 1973; 59: 498.
248 Muto T, Bussey HJR, Morson BC. Pseudocarcinomatous invasion in adenomatous polyps of the colon and rectum. *J Clin Pathol*, 1973; 26: 25.
249 Greene FI. Epithelial misplacement in adenomatous polyps of the colon and rectum. *Cancer*, 1974; 33: 206.
250 Bisgaard ML, Fenger K, Bülow S, Niebuhr E, Mohr J. Familial adenomatous polyposis (FAP). Frequency, penetrance and mutation rate. *Hum Mutat*, 1994; 3: 121.
251 Leppert M, Dobbs M, Scambler P *et al*. The gene for familial polyposis maps to the long arm of chromosome 5. *Science*, 1987; 238: 1411.
252 Kinzler KW, Nilbert MC, Su L-K *et al*. Identification of FAP locus genes from chromosome 5q21. *Science*, 1991; 253: 661.
253 Groden J, Thliveris A, Samowitz W *et al*. Identification and characterization of the familial adenomatous polyposis gene. *Cell*, 1991; 66: 589.
254 Lynch HT, Smyrk T, McGinn T *et al*. Attenuated familial adenomatous polyposis (AFAP). A phenotypically and genotypically distinctive variant of FAP. *Cancer*, 1995; 76: 2427.
255 Leppert M, Burt R, Hughes JP *et al*. Genetic analysis of an inherited predisposition to colon cancer in a family with a variable number of adenomatous polyps. *N Engl J Med*, 1990; 322: 904.
256 Nagase H, Miyoshi Y, Horii A *et al*. Correlation between the location of germ-line mutations in the APC gene and the number of colorectal polyps in familial adenomatous polyposis patients. *Cancer Res*, 1992; 52: 4055.
257 Leggett BA, Young JP, Biden K *et al*. Severe upper gastrointestinal polyposis associated with sparse colonic polyposis in a familial adenomatous polyposis family with an APC mutation at codon 1520. *Gut*, 1997; 41: 518.
258 Van der Luijt R, Meera Khan P, Vasen H *et al*. Rapid detection of translation-terminating mutations at the adenomatous polyposis coli (APC) gene by direct protein truncation test. *Genomics*, 1994; 20: 1.
259 Bussey HJR, Eyers AA, Ritchie SM, Thomson JPS. The rectum in adenomatous polyposis: the St Mark's policy. *Br J Surg*, 1985; 72: 29.
260 Nugent KP, Phillips RKS. Rectal cancer risk in older patients with familial adenomatous polyposis and an ileorectal anastomosis: a cause for concern. *Br J Surg*, 1992; 79: 1204.
261 Cohen SB. Familial polyposis coli and its extracolonic manifestations. *J Med Genet*, 1982; 19: 193.
262 Gardner EJ, Richards RC. Multiple cutaneous and subcutaneous lesions occurring simultaneously with hereditary polyposis and osteomatosis. *Am J Hum Genet*, 1953; 5: 139.
263 Gardner EJ. Follow-up study of a family group exhibiting dominant inheritance for a syndrome including intestinal polyps, osteomas, fibromas and epidermal cysts. *Am J Hum Genet*, 1962; 14: 376.

264 McAdam WAF, Goligher JC. The occurrence of desmoids in patients with familial coli. *Br J Surg*, 1970; 57: 618.

265 Simpson RD, Harrison EG, Mayo CW. Mesenteric fibromatosis in familial polyposis: a variant of Gardner's syndrome. *Cancer*, 1964; 17: 526.

266 Gardner EJ. Gardner's syndrome re-evaluated after twenty years. *Proc Utah Acad*, 1969; 46: 1.

267 Bussey HJR. Extracolonic lesions associated with polyposis coli. *Proc R Soc Med*, 1972; 65: 294.

268 Utsunomiya J, Maki T, Iwama T *et al*. Gastric lesion of familial polyposis coli. *Cancer*, 1974; 34: 745.

269 Ushio K, Sasagawa M, Doi H *et al*. Lesions associated with familial polyposis coli: studies of lesions of the stomach, duodenum, bones and teeth. *Gastrointest Radiol*, 1976; 1: 67.

270 Watanabe H, Enjoji M, Yao T, Ohsata K. Gastric lesions in familial adenomatosis coli. *Hum Pathol*, 1978; 9: 269.

271 Järvinen H, Nyberg M, Peltokallio P. Upper gastrointestinal tract polyps in familial adenomatosis coli. *Gut*, 1983; 24: 333.

272 Sarre RG, Frost AG, Jagelman DG *et al*. Gastric and duodenal polyps in familial adenomatous polyposis: a prospective study of the nature and prevalence of upper gastrointestinal polyps. *Gut*, 1987; 28: 306.

273 Domizio P, Talbot IC, Spigelman AD, Williams CB, Phillips RK. Upper gastrointestinal pathology in familial adenomatous polyposis: results from a prospective study of 102 patients. *J Clin Pathol*, 1990; 43: 738.

274 Itoh H, Iida M, Kuroiwa S, Shigematsu A, Nakayama F. Gardner's syndrome associated with carcinoma of the duodenal bulb: report of a case. *Am J Gastroenterol*, 1985; 80: 248.

275 Sugihara K, Muto T, Kamiya J *et al*. Gardner's syndrome associated with periampullary carcinoma, duodenal and gastric adenomatosis. Report of a case. *Dis Colon Rectum*, 1982; 25: 766.

276 Walsh N, Qizilbash A, Banerjee R, Waugh GA. Biliary neoplasia in Gardner's syndrome. *Arch Pathol Lab Med*, 1987; 111: 76.

277 Harach HR, Williams GT, Williams ED. Familial adenomatous polyposis associated thyroid carcinoma: a distinct type of follicular neoplasia. *Histopathology*, 1994; 25: 549.

278 Turcot J, Despré J-P, St Pierre F. Malignant tumors of the central nervous system associated with familial polyposis of the colon: report of two cases. *Dis Colon Rectum*, 1959; 2: 465.

279 Perkins JT, Blackstone MO, Riddell RH. Adenomatous polyposis coli and multiple endocrine neoplasia type 2b. A pathogenetic relationship. *Cancer*, 1985; 55: 375.

280 Naylor EW, Gardner EJ. Adrenal adenomas in a patient with Gardner's syndrome. *Clin Genet*, 1981; 20: 67.

281 Kingston JE, Herbert A, Draper GJ, Mann JR. Association of hepatoblastoma and polyposis coli. *Arch Dis Child*, 1983; 58: 959.

282 Olschwang S, Tiret A, Laurent-Puig P *et al*. Restriction of ocular fundus lesions to a specific subgroup of APC mutations in adenomatous polyposis coli patients. *Cell*, 1993; 75: 959.

283 Utsunomiya J, Nakamura T. The occult osteomatous changes in the mandible in patients with familial polyposis coli. *Br J Surg*, 1975; 62: 45.

284 Dietrich WF, Lander FS, Smith JS *et al*. Genetic identification of Mom-1, a major modifier locus affecting Min-induced intestinal neoplasia in the mouse. *Cell*, 1993; 75: 631.

285 Hamilton SR, Liu B, Parsons RE *et al*. The molecular basis of Turcot's syndrome. *N Engl J Med*, 1995; 332: 839.

286 Vasen HFA, Sanders EACM, Taal BG *et al*. The risk of brain tumours in hereditary non-polyposis colorectal cancer (HNPCC). *Int J Cancer*, 1996; 65: 422.

287 De Rosa M, Fasano C, Panariello L. *et al*. Evidence for a recessive inheritance of Turcot's syndrome caused by compound heterozygous mutations within the PMS2 gene. *Oncogene*, 2000; 19: 1719.

288 Peltomäki P, Aaltonen LA, Sistonen P *et al*. Genetic mapping of a locus predisposing to human colorectal cancer. *Science*, 1993; 260: 810.

289 Lindblom A, Tannergard P, Werelius B, Nordenskjeld M. Genetic mapping of a second locus predisposing to hereditary non-polyposis colon cancer. *Nat Genet*, 1993; 5: 279.

290 Aaltonen LA, Peltomaki P, Mecklin J-P *et al*. Replication errors in benign and malignant tumours from hereditary nonpolyposis colorectal cancer patients. *Cancer Res*, 1994; 54: 1645.

291 Jacoby RF, Marshall DJ, Kailas S *et al*. Genetic instability associated with adenoma to carcinoma progression in hereditary nonpolyposis colon cancer. *Gastroenterology*, 1995; 109: 73.

292 Iino H, Simms LA, Young J *et al*. DNA microsatellite instability and mismatch repair protein loss in adenomas presenting in hereditary non-polyposis colorectal cancer. *Gut*, 2000; 47: 37.

293 Lynch HT, Lynch PM, Albano WA, Lynch JF. The cancer family syndrome: a status report. *Dis Colon Rectum*, 1981; 24: 311.

294 Lynch HT, Kimberling W, Albano WA *et al*. Hereditary nonpolyposis colorectal cancer (Lynch syndromes I and II). Clinical description of resource. *Cancer*, 1985; 56: 934.

295 Lynch HT, Smyrk TC, Watson P *et al*. Hereditary colorectal cancer. *Semin Oncol*, 1991; 18: 337.

296 Lynch HT, Smyrk TC, Watson P *et al*. Genetics, natural history, tumor spectrum, and pathology of hereditary nonpolyposis colorectal cancer: an updated review. *Gastroenterology*, 1993; 104: 1535.

297 Sankila R, Aaltonen LA, Järvinen HJ, Mecklin J-P. Better survival rates in patients with *MLH1*-associated hereditary colorectal cancer. *Gastroenterology*, 1996; 110: 682.

298 Mecklin J-P, Jarvinen HJ. Clinical features of colorectal carcinoma in cancer family syndrome. *Dis Colon Rectum*, 1986; 29: 160.

299 Mecklin J-P, Jarvinen HJ, Peltokallio P. Cancer family syndrome. Genetic analysis of 22 Finnish kindreds. *Gastroenterology*, 1986; 90: 328.

300 Mecklin J-P, Sipponen P, Jarvinen HJ. Histopathology of colorectal carcinomas and adenomas in cancer family syndrome. *Dis Colon Rectum*, 1986; 29: 849.

301 Mecklin J-P. Frequency of hereditary colorectal carcinoma. *Gastroenterology*, 1987; 93: 1021.

302 Mecklin J-P, Jarvinen HJ, Aukee S, Elomaa I, Karjalainen K. Screening for colorectal carcinoma in cancer family kindreds. *Scand J Gastroenterol*, 1987; 22: 449.

303 Mecklin JP, Jarvinen HJ. Tumour spectrum in cancer family syndrome (hereditary non-polyposis colorectal cancer). *Cancer*, 1991; 68: 1109.

304 Kong S, Amos CI, Luthra R *et al*. Effects of cyclin D1 polymorphism on age of onset of hereditary nonpolyposis colorectal cancer. *Cancer Res*, 2000; 60: 249.

305 Lovett E. Family studies in cancer of the colon and rectum. *Br J Surg*, 1976; 63: 13.

306 Veale AMO. *Intestinal Polyposis*. Cambridge: Cambridge University Press, 1965.

307 Love RR. Adenomas are precursor lesions for malignant growth in non-polyposis hereditary carcinoma of the colon and rectum. *Surg Gynecol Obstet*, 1986; 162: 8.

308 Akiyama Y, Sato H, Yamada T *et al*. Germ-line mutation of the *hMSH6/GTBP* gene in an atypical hereditary nonpolyposis colorectal cancer kindred. *Cancer Res*, 1997; 57: 3920.

309 Strand M, Prolla TA, Liskay RM, Petes T. Destabilisation of tracts of simple repetitive DNA in yeast by mutation affecting DNA mismatch repair. *Nature*, 1993; 365: 274.

310 Parsons R, Li G-M, Longley MJ *et al*. Hypermutability and mismatch repair deficiency in RER+ tumor cells. *Cell*, 1993; 75: 1227.

311 Lu S-L, Kawabata M, Imamura T *et al*. HNPCC associated with germline mutation in the TGF-β type II receptor gene. *Nat Genet*, 1998; 19: 17.

312 Jass JR, Smyrk TC, Stewart SM *et al*. Pathology of hereditary non-polyposis colorectal cancer. *Anticancer Res*, 1994; 14: 1631.

313 Jass JR, Cottier DS, Jeevaratnam P *et al*. Diagnostic use of microsatellite instability in hereditary non-polyposis colorectal cancer. *Lancet*, 1995; 346: 1200.

314 Jass JR. Diagnosis of hereditary non-polyposis colorectal cancer. *Histopathology*, 1998; 32: 491.

315 Vasen HFA, Watson P, Mecklin JP *et al*. The epidemiology of endometrial cancer in hereditary non-polyposis colorectal cancer. *Anticancer Res*, 1994; 14: 1675.

316 Weitzer M, Pokos V, Jeevaratnam P *et al*. Isolated expression of the Muir–Torre phenotype in a member of a family with hereditary non-polyposis colorectal cancer. *Histopathology*, 1995; 27: 573.

317 Hall NR, Williams AT, Murday VA, Newton JA, Bishop DT. Muir–Torre syndrome: a variant of the cancer family syndrome. *J Med Genet*, 1994; 31: 627.

318 Vasen HFA, Mecklin J-P, Khan PM, Lynch HT. The international collaborative group on hereditary non-polyposis colorectal cancer (ICG-HNPCC). *Dis Colon Rectum*, 1991; 34: 424.

319 Vasen HFA, Nagengast FM, Meera Khan P. Interval cancers in hereditary non-polyposis colorectal cancer (Lynch syndrome). *Lancet*, 1995; 345: 1183.

320 Van de Water NS, Jeevaratnam P, Browett PJ *et al*. Direct mutational analysis in a family with hereditary non-polyposis colorectal cancer. *Aust N Z J Med*, 1994; 24: 682.

321 Boyle P, Zaridze DG, Smans M. Descriptive epidemiology of colorectal cancer. *Int J Cancer*, 1985; 36: 9.

322 Jass JR. Subsite distribution and incidence of colorectal cancer in New Zealand 1974–1983. *Dis Colon Rectum*, 1991; 34: 56.

323 Doll R. General epidemiologic considerations in aetiology of colorectal cancer. In: Winawar S, Schottenfeld D, Sherlock P, eds. *Colorectal Cancer: Prevention, Epidemiology and Screening*. New York: Raven Press, 1980: 3.

324 Bussey HJR, Wallace H. In: Dukes CE, ed. *Cancer of the Rectum*. Edinburgh: E & S Livingstone, 1960: 99.

325 Bufil JA. Colorectal cancer: evidence of distinct genetic categories based on proximal or distal tumor location. *Ann Intern Med*, 1990; 113: 779.

326 Delattre O, Olschwang S, Law DJ *et al*. Multiple genetic alterations in distal and proximal colorectal cancer. *Lancet*, 1989; ii: 353.

327 Kim H, Jen J, Vogelstein B, Hamilton SR. Clinical and pathological characteristics of sporadic colorectal carcinomas with DNA replication errors in microsatellite sequences. *Am J Pathol*, 1994; 145: 148.

328 Nomura AMY, Kolonel LN, Hinds MW. Trends in the anatomical distribution of colorectal cancer in Hawaii, 1968–1978. *Dig Dis Sci*, 1979; 26: 1116.

329 Vobecky J, Leduc C, Devroede G. Sex differences in the changing anatomic distribution of colorectal carcinoma. *Cancer*, 1984; 54: 3065.

330 McMichael AJ, Potter JD. Host factors in carcinogenesis: certain bile-acid metabolic profiles that selectively increase the risk of proximal colon cancer. *J Natl Cancer Inst*, 1984; 75: 185.

331 Nelson RL. Is the changing pattern of colorectal cancer caused by selenium deficiency? *Dis Colon Rectum*, 1984; 27: 459.

332 Morson BC. Notes on the pathology of carcinoma of the large intestine. *Natl Cancer Inst Monogr*, 1965; 25: 287.

333 Elmasri SH, Boulos PB. Carcinoma of the large bowel in the Sudan. *Br J Cancer*, 1975; 62: 284.

334 Sutton TD, Jass JR, Eide TJ. Trends in colorectal cancer incidence and histologic findings in Maori and Polynesian residents of New Zealand. *Cancer* 1993; 71: 3839.

335 Dukes CE, Bussey HJR. The spread of cancer and its effect on prognosis. *Br J Cancer*, 1958; 12: 309.

336 Kern WH, William CW. Adenocarcinoma of the colon in a nine-month old infant. Report of a case. *Cancer*, 1958; 11: 855.

337 Recio P, Bussey HJR. The pathology and prognosis of carcinoma of the rectum in the young. *Proc R Soc Med*, 1965; 58: 789.

338 Liu B, Farrington SM, Petersen GM *et al*. Genetic instability occurs in the majority of young patients with colorectal cancer. *Nat Med*, 1995; 1: 348.

339 Hill MJ. Genetic and environmental factors in human colorectal cancer. In: Malt R, Williamson RCN, eds. *Colon Carcinogenesis*. Lancaster: MTP Press, 1982: 73.

340 Haenszel W, Kurihara M. Studies of Japanese migrants. I. Mortality from cancer and other diseases among Japanese in the United States. *J Natl Cancer Inst*, 1968; 40: 44.

341 Correa P, Haenszel W. The epidemiology of large bowel cancer. *Adv Cancer Res*, 1978; 26: 1.

342 McMichael AJ, McCall MG, Hartsthorne JM, Woodings TL. Patterns of gastro-intestinal cancer in European migrants to Australia: the role of dietary change. *Int J Cancer*, 1980; 25: 431.

343 Wynder EL. The epidemiology of large bowel cancer. *Cancer Res*, 1975; 35: 3388.

344 McMichael AJ, Potter AJ, Hetzel BS. Time trends in colo-rectal cancer mortality in relation to food and alcohol consumption: United States, United Kingdom, Australia and New Zealand. *Int J Epidemiol*, 1979; 8: 295.

345 Burkitt DP. Epidemiology of cancer of the colon and rectum. *Cancer*, 1971; 28: 3.

346 Graham S, Dayal H, Swanson M *et al*. Diet in the epidemiology of cancer of the colon and rectum. *J Natl Cancer Inst*, 1978; 61: 709.

347 Ferguson LR, Harris PJ. Studies on the role of specific dietary fibres in protection against colorectal cancer. *Mutat Res*, 1996; 350: 173.

348 Aries VC, Crowther JS, Drasar BS, Hill MJ. Degradation of bile salts by human intestinal bacteria. *Gut*, 1969; 10: 575.

349 Aries VC, Crowther JS, Drasar BS, Hill MJ, Williams REO. Bacteria and the aetiology of cancer of the large bowel. *Gut*, 1969; 10: 334.

350 Hill MJ, Drasar BS, Aries VC *et al*. Bacteria and aetiology of cancer of the large bowel. *Lancet*, 1971; i: 95.

351 Moorehead RJ, Campbell GR, Donaldson JD, McKelvey STD. Re-

lationship between duodenal bile acids and colorectal neoplasia. *Gut*, 1987; 28: 1454.

352 Reddy BS, Narisawa T, Weisburger JH. Effect of diet with high levels of protein and fat on colon carcinogenesis in F344 rats treated with 1,2-dimethylhydrazine. *J Natl Cancer Inst*, 1976; 57: 567.

353 Wilpart M, Mainguet P, Maskens A, Roberfroid M. Mutagenicity of 1,2-dimethylhydrazine towards *Salmonella typhimurium*, co-mutagenic effect of secondary bile acids. *Carcinogenesis*, 1983; 4: 45.

354 Reddy BS, Sharma C, Darby L, Laakso K, Wynder E. Metabolic epidemiology of large bowel cancer: fecal mutagens in high- and low-risk populations for colon cancer, a preliminary report. *Mutat Res*, 1980; 72: 511.

355 Gupta I, Suzuki K, Bruce WR, Krepinski M, Locke FB. A model study of fecapentaenes: mutagens of bacterial origin with alkylating properties. *Science*, 1984; 225: 521.

356 Spigelman AD, Skates DK, Venitt S, Phillips RKS. DNA adducts, detected by 32P-postlabelling in the foregut of patients with familial adenomatous polyposis and in unaffected controls. *Carcinogenesis*, 1991; 12: 1727.

357 Hill MJ. Metabolic epidemiology of large bowel cancer. In: De Cosse D, Sherlock P, eds. *Gastrointestinal Cancer*. Hague: Martinus-Nijhoff, 1981: 187.

358 Oshima M, Oshima H, Tsutsumi M *et al*. Effects of 2-amino-1-methyl-6-phenylimidazo[4,5-b]pyridine on intestinal polyp development in Apc delta 716 knockout mice. *Mol Carcinog*, 1996; 15: 11.

359 Drasar BS, Irving D. Environmental factors and cancer of the colon and breast. *Br J Cancer*, 1973; 27: 167.

360 Armstrong BK, Doll R. Environmental factors and cancer incidence and mortality in different countries, with special reference to dietary practices. *Int J Cancer*, 1975; 15: 616.

361 Phillips RL, Garfinkel L, Kuzma JW *et al*. Cancer mortality among California Seventh-Day Adventists for selective cancer sites. *J Natl Cancer Inst*, 1980; 65: 1097.

362 Phillips RL, Snowdon DA. Dietary relationships with fatal colorectal cancer among Seventh-Day Adventists. *J Natl Cancer Inst*, 1985; 74: 307.

363 Smith AN, Pearce NE, Joseph JG. Major colorectal cancer aetiological hypotheses do not explain mortality trends among Maori and non-Maori New Zealanders. *Int J Epidemiol*, 1985; 14: 79.

364 Drasar BS, Jenkins DJA. Bacteria, diet and large bowel cancer. *Am J Clin Nutr*, 1976; 29: 1410.

365 Cruse JP, Lewin MR, Clark CG. Failure of bran to protect against experimental colon cancer in rats. *Lancet*, 1978; ii: 278.

366 Jass JR. Diet, butyric acid and differentiation of gastrointestinal tract tumours. *Med Hypotheses*, 1985; 18: 113.

367 Samelson SL, Nelson RL, Nyhus LM. Protective role of faecal pH in experimental colon carcinogenesis. *J R Soc Med*, 1985; 78: 230.

368 Thornton JR. High colonic pH promotes colorectal cancer. *Lancet*, 1981; i: 1091.

369 Alberts DS, Martínez ME, Roe DJ *et al*. Lack of effect of a high-fiber cereal supplement on the recurrence of colorectal adenomas. *N Engl J Med*, 2000; 342: 1156.

370 Schatzkin A, Lanza E, Corle D *et al*. Lack of effect of a low-fat, high-fiber diet on the recurrence of colorectal adenomas. *N Engl J Med*, 2000; 342: 1149.

371 Palmer RH. Bile acid heterogeneity and the gastrointestinal epithelium: from diarrhea to colon cancer. *J Lab Clin Med*, 1979; 94: 655.

372 Newmark HL, Wargovich MJ, Bruce WR. Colon cancer and dietary fat, phosphate and calcium: a hypothesis. *J Natl Cancer Inst*, 1984; 72: 1323.

373 Cruse JP, Lewin MR, Clark CG. An investigation into the mechanism of co-carcinogenesis of dietary cholesterol during the introduction of colon cancer in rats by 1,2 dimethylhydrazine. *Clin Oncol*, 1984; 10: 213.

374 Thomas MG, Thomson JPS, Williamson RCN. Oral calcium inhibits rectal epithelial proliferation in familial adenomatous polyposis. *Br J Surg*, 1993; 80: 499.

375 Weisgerber UM, Boeing H, Owen RW *et al*. Effect of longterm placebo controlled calcium supplementation on sigmoidal cell proliferation in patients with sporadic adenomatous polyps. *Gut*, 1996; 38: 396.

376 Bristol JB, Emmett PM, Heaton KW, Williamson RCN. Sugar, fat and the risk of colorectal cancer. *Br Med J*, 1985; 291: 1467.

377 Macquart-Moulin G, Riboli E, Cornée J, Kaaks R, Berthézene P. Colorectal polyps and diet: a case control study in Marseilles. *Int J Cancer*, 1987; 40: 179.

378 Wattenberg LW. Studies of polycyclic hydrocarbon hydroxylases of the intestine possibly related to cancer. *Cancer*, 1971; 28: 99.

379 Shamberger RJ. Relation of selenium to cancer. I. Inhibitory effect of selenium on carcinogenesis. *J Natl Cancer Inst*, 1970; 44: 931.

380 Soullier BK, Wilson PS, Nigro ND. Effect of selenium on azoxymethane-induced intestinal cancer in rats fed with high fat diet. *Cancer Lett*, 1981; 12: 343.

381 Virtamo J, Valkeila E, Alfthan G *et al*. Serum selenium and risk of cancer. A prospective follow up to 9 years. *Cancer*, 1987; 60: 145.

382 Honjo S, Kono S, Shinchi K *et al*. The relation of smoking, alcohol use and obesity to risk of sigmoid colon and rectal adenomas. *Jpn J Cancer Res*, 1995; 86: 1019.

383 Boutron MC, Faivre J, Dop MC, Quipourt V, Senesse P. Tobacco, alcohol, and colorectal tumors: a multistep process. *Am J Epidemiol*, 1995; 141: 1038.

384 Heineman EF, Zahm SH, Mclaughlin JK, Vaught JB. Increased risk of colorectal cancer among smokers: Results of a 26-year follow-up of US veterans and a review. *Int J Cancer*, 1994; 59: 728.

385 Newcomb PA, Storer BE, Marcus PM. Cigarette smoking in relation to risk of large bowel cancer in women. *Cancer Res*, 1995; 55: 4906.

386 Thun MJ, Namboodiri MM, Heath CW. Aspirin use and reduced risk of fatal colon cancer. *N Engl J Med*, 1991; 325: 1593.

387 Giovannucci E, Rimm EB, Stampfer MJ *et al*. Aspirin use and the risk for colorectal cancer and adenoma in male health professionals. *Ann Intern Med*, 1994; 121: 241.

388 Davidson M, Yoshizawa CN, Kolonel LN. Do sex hormones affect colorectal cancer? *Br Med J*, 1985; 290: 1868.

389 Agrez MV, Spencer RJ. Estrogen receptor protein in adenomas of the large bowel. *Dis Colon Rectum*, 1982; 25: 348.

390 Potter JD, McMichael AJ. Large bowel cancer in women in relation to reproductive and hormonal factors: a case control study. *J Natl Cancer Inst*, 1983; 71: 703.

391 Klein I, Parveen G, Gavaler JS, Vanthiel DH. Colonic polyps in patients with acromegaly. *Ann Intern Med*, 1982; 97: 27.

392 Wigley CB, Paraskeva C, Coventry R. Elevated production of

growth factor by human premalignant colon adenomas and a derived cell line. *Br J Cancer*, 1986; 54: 799.

393 Guo YS, Jin GF, Townsend CM *et al.* Insulin-like growth factor-II expression in carcinoma in colon cell lines: Implications for autocrine actions. *J Am Coll Surg*, 1995; 181: 145.

394 Saeki T, Salomon DS, Gullick WJ *et al.* Expression of cripto-1 in human colorectal adenomas and carcinomas is related to the degree of dysplasia. *Int J Oncol*, 1994; 5: 445.

395 Lothe RA, Peltomaki P, Meling GI *et al.* Genomic instability in colorectal cancer: relationship to clinicopathological variables and family history. *Cancer Res*, 1993; 53: 5849.

396 Liu B, Nicolaides NC, Markowitz S *et al.* Mismatch repair gene defects in sporadic colorectal cancers with microsatellite instability. *Nat Genet*, 1995; 9: 48.

397 Cunningham JM, Christensen ER, Tester DJ *et al.* Hypermethylation of the *hMLH1* promoter in colon cancer with microsatellite instability. *Cancer Res*, 1998; 58: 3455.

398 Jeevaratnam P, Cottier DS, Browett PJ *et al.* Familial giant hyperplastic polyposis predisposing to colorectal cancer: a new hereditary bowel cancer syndrome. *J Pathol*, 1996; 179: 20.

399 Thomas HJW, Whitelaw SC, Cottrell SE *et al.* Genetic mapping of the hereditary mixed polyposis syndrome to chromosome 6q. *Am J Hum Genet*, 1996; 58: 770.

400 Tomlinson I, Rahman N, Frayling I *et al.* Inherited susceptibility to colorectal adenomas and carcinomas: evidence for a new predisposition gene on 15q14-q22. *Gastroenterology*, 1999; 116: 789.

401 Laken SJ, Petersen GM, Gruber SB *et al.* Familial colorectal cancer in Ashkenazim due to a hypermutable tract in APC. *Nat Genet*, 1997; 17: 79.

402 Cannon-Albright LA, Skolnick MH, Bishop T, Lee RG, Burt RW. Common inheritance of susceptibility to colonic adenomatous polyps and associated colorectal cancers. *N Engl J Med*, 1988; 319: 533.

403 Burt RW, Bishop T, Cannon LA *et al.* Dominant inheritance of adenomatous colonic polyps and colorectal cancer. *N Engl J Med*, 1985; 312: 1540.

404 Boutron M-C, Faivre J, Quipourt V, Senesse P, Michiels C. Family history of colorectal tumours and implications for the adenoma–carcinoma sequence: a case control study. *Gut*, 1995; 37: 830.

405 Vasen HFA, Taal BG, Griffioen G *et al.* Clinical heterogeneity of familial colorectal cancer and its influence on screening protocols. *Gut*, 1994; 35: 1262.

406 Jass JR, Pokos V, Arnold JL *et al.* Colorectal neoplasms detected colonoscopically in at-risk members of colorectal cancer families stratified according to the finding of familial cancers with DNA microsatellite instability. *J Mol Med*, 1996; 74: 547.

407 Lang NP, Chu DZJ, Hunter CF *et al.* Role of aromatic amine acetyltransferase in human colorectal cancer. *Arch Surg*, 1986; 121: 1259.

408 Ilett KF, David BM, Detchon P, Castleden WM, Kwa R. Acetylation phenotype in colorectal carcinoma. *Cancer Res*, 1987; 47: 1466.

409 Shibuta K, Nakashima T, Able M *et al.* Molecular genotyping for N-acetylation polymorphism in Japanese patients with colorectal cancer. *Cancer*, 1994; 74: 3108.

410 Little J, Faivre J. Family history, metabolic gene polymorphism, diet and risk of colorectal cancer. *Eur J Cancer Prev*, 1999; 8: S61.

411 Bell DA, Stephens EA, Castranio T *et al.* Polyadenylation polymorphism in the acetyltransferase 1 gene (NAT1) increases risk of colorectal cancer. *Cancer Res*, 1995; 55: 3537.

412 Strange RC, Matharoo B, Faulder GC *et al.* The human glutathione S-transferases: a case-control study of the incidence of the GST1 0 phenotype in patients with adenocarcinoma. *Carcinogenesis*, 1991; 12: 25.

413 Szarka CE, Pfeiffer GR, Hum ST *et al.* Glutathione S-transferase activity and glutathione S-transferase mu expression in subjects with risk for colorectal cancer. *Cancer Res*, 1995; 55: 2789.

414 Chenevix-Trench G, Young J, Coggan M, Board P. Glutathione S-transferase M1 and T1 polymorphisms: susceptibility to colon cancer and age of onset. *Carcinogenesis*, 1995; 16: 1655.

415 Goelz SE, Vogelstein B, Hamilton SR, Feinberg AP. Hypomethylation of DNA from benign and malignant human colon neoplasms. *Science*, 1988; 228: 187.

416 Chen J, Giovannucci E, Kelsey K *et al.* A methylenetetrahydrofolate reductase polymorphism and the risk of colorectal cancer. *Cancer Res*, 1996; 56: 4862.

417 Ma J, Stampfer MJ, Giovannucci E *et al.* Methylenetetrahydrofolate reductase polymorphism, dietary interactions, and risk of colorectal cancer. *Cancer Res*, 1997; 57: 1098.

418 Kervinen K, Södervik H, Mäkelä J *et al.* Is the development of adenoma and carcinoma in proximal colon related to apolipoprotein E phenotype? *Gastroenterology*, 1996; 110: 1785.

419 Sivaraman L, Leatham MP, Yee J *et al.* CYP1A1 genetic polymorphisms and in situ colorectal cancer. *Cancer Res*, 1994; 54: 3692.

420 Jass JR, Constable L, Sutherland R *et al.* Adenocarcinoma of colon differentiating as dome epithelium of gut-associated lymphoid tissue. *Histopathology*, 2000; 36: 116.

421 Ming-Chai C, Chi-Yuan C, Pei YuC, Jen-Chun H. Evolution of colorectal cancer in schistosomiasis: transitional changes adjacent to large intestinal carcinoma in colectomy specimens. *Cancer*, 1980; 46: 1661.

422 Hamilton S. Colorectal carcinoma in patients with Crohn's disease. *Gastroenterology*, 1985; 89: 398.

423 Qizilbash AH. Radiation induced carcinoma of the rectum: a late complication of pelvic irradiation. *Arch Pathol*, 1974; 98: 118.

424 Rotmensch S, Avigad I, Soffer EE *et al.* Carcinoma of the large bowel after a single massive dose of radiation in healthy teenagers. *Cancer*, 1986; 57: 728.

425 Chu DZJ, Giacco G, Martin RG, Guinee VF. The significance of synchronous carcinoma and polyps in the colon and rectum. *Cancer*, 1986; 57: 445.

426 Kronborg O, Hage E, Fenger C, Deichgraeber E. Do synchronous adenomas influence prognosis after radical surgery for colorectal carcinoma? A prospective study. *Int J Colorectal Dis*, 1986; 1: 99.

427 Horii A, Han HJ, Shimada M *et al.* Frequent replication errors at microsatellite loci in tumors of patients with multiple primary cancers. *Cancer Res*, 1994; 54: 3373.

428 Cawkwell L, Li D, Lewis FA *et al.* Microsatellite instability in colorectal cancer: improved assessment using fluorescent polymerase chain reaction. *Gastroenterology*, 1995; 109: 465.

429 Heald RJ, Bussey HJR. Clinical experience at St. Mark's Hospital with multiple synchronous cancers of the colon and rectum. *Dis Colon Rectum*, 1975; 18: 6.

430 Copeland EM, Jones RS, Miller LD. Multiple colon neoplasms. *Arch Surg*, 1969; 98: 141.

431 Moertel CG, Bargen JA, Dockerty MB. Multiple carcinomas of the large intestine. *Gastroenterology*, 1958; 34: 85.
432 Schottenfeld D, Berg JW, Vitsky B. Incidence of multiple primary cancers. II. Index cancers arising in the stomach and lower digestive system. *J Natl Cancer Inst*, 1969; 43: 77.
433 Langevin JH, Nivatongs S. The true incidence of synchronous cancer of the large bowel. A prospective study. *Am J Surg*, 1984; 147: 330.
434 Cunliffe WJ, Hasleton PS, Tweedle DEF, Schofield PF. Incidence of synchronous and metachronous colorectal carcinoma. *Br J Surg*, 1984; 71: 941.
435 Fenoglio CM, Kaye GI, Lane N. Distribution of human colonic lymphatics in normal, hyperplastic and adenomatous tissue. *Gastroenterology*, 1973; 64: 51.
436 Cuthbertson AM, Hughes ESR, Pihl E. Metastatic 'early' colorectal cancer. *Aust N Z J Surg*, 1984; 54: 549.
437 Morson BC, Bussey HJR, Samoorian S. Policy of local excision for early cancer of the colorectum. *Gut*, 1977; 18: 1045.
438 Morson BC. Histological criteria for local excision. *Br J Surg*, 1985; 72: 953.
439 Morson BC, Whiteway JE, Jones EA, Macrae FA, Williams CB. Histopathology and prognosis of malignant colorectal polyps treated by endoscopic polypectomy. *Gut*, 1984; 25: 437.
440 Cooper HS. Surgical pathology of endoscopically removed malignant polyps of the colon and rectum. *Am J Surg Pathol*, 1983; 7: 613.
441 Volk EE, Goldblum JR, Petras RE, Carey WD, Fazio VW. Management and outcome of patients with invasive carcinoma arising in colorectal polyps. *Gastroenterology*, 1995; 109: 1801.
442 Cooper HS, Deppisch LM, Gourley WK *et al*. Endoscopically removed malignant colorectal polyps: clinicopathologic correlations. *Gastroenterology*, 1995; 108: 1657.
443 Muller S, Chesner IM, Igan MA *et al*. Significance of venous and lymphatic invasion in malignant polyps of the colon and rectum. *Gut*, 1990; 30: 1385.
444 Geraghty JM, Williams CB, Talbot IC. Malignant colorectal polyp: venous invasion and successful treatment by endoscopic polypectomy. *Gut*, 1991; 32: 774.
445 Haggitt RC, Glotzbach RE, Soffer EE, Wruble LD. Prognostic factors in colorectal carcinomas arising in adenomas: implications for lesions removed by endoscopic polypectomy. *Gastroenterology*, 1985; 89: 328.
446 Whiteway J, Nicholls RJ, Morson BC. The role of surgical local excision in the treatment of rectal cancer. *Br J Surg*, 1985; 72: 694.
447 Banerjee AK, Jehle EC, Shorthouse AJ, Buess G. Local excision of rectal tumours. *Br J Surg*, 1995; 82: 1165.
448 Shirouzu K, Isomoto H, Morodomi T. *et al*. Primary linitis plastica carcinoma of the colon and rectum. *Cancer*, 1994; 74: 1863.
449 Jass JR, Atkin WS, Cuzick J *et al*. The grading of rectal cancer: historical perspectives and a multivariate analysis of 447 cases. *Histopathology*, 1986; 10: 437.
450 Klappenbach RS, Kurman RJ, Sinclair CF, James LP. Composite carcinoma-carcinoid tumours of the gastrointestinal tract. *Am J Clin Pathol*, 1985; 84: 437.
451 Sundblad AS, Paz RA. Mucinous carcinomas of the colon and rectum and their relation to polyps. *Cancer*, 1982; 50: 2504.
452 Sasaki O, Atkin WS, Jass JR. Mucinous carcinoma of the rectum. *Histopathology*, 1987; 11: 259.
453 Symonds DA, Vickery AL. Mucinous carcinoma of the colon and rectum. *Cancer*, 1976; 37: 1891.
454 Jones EA, Morson BC. Mucinous adenocarcinoma in anorectal fistulae. *Histopathology*, 1984; 8: 279.
455 Biemer-Hüttman A-E, Walsh MD, McGuckin MA. *et al*. Mucin core protein expression in colorectal cancers with high levels of microsatellite instability indicates a novel pathway of morphogenesis. *Clin Cancer Res*, 2000; 6: 1909.
456 Pihl E, Nairn RC, Hughes ESR, Cuthbertson AM, Rollo AJ. Mucinous colorectal carcinoma: immunopathology and prognosis. *Pathology*, 1980; 12: 439.
457 Ajioka Y, Allison LJ, Jass JR. Significance of MUC1 and MUC2 mucin expression in colorectal cancer. *J Clin Pathol*, 1996; 49: 560.
458 van den Ingh HF, Ruiter DJ, Griffioen G, van Muijen GNP, Ferrone S. HLA antigens in colorectal tumours—low expression of HLA class I antigens in mucinous colorectal carcinomas. *Br J Cancer*, 1987; 55: 125.
459 Messerini L, Vitelli F, de Vitis LR *et al*. Microsatellite instability in sporadic mucinous colorectal carcinomas: relationship to clinico-pathological variables. *J Pathol*, 1997; 182: 380.
460 Connelly JH, Robey-Cafferty SS, El-Naggar AK, Cleary KR. Exophytic signet-ring cell carcinoma of the colorectum. *Arch Pathol Lab Med*, 1991; 115: 134.
461 Gibbs NM. Undifferentiated carcinoma of the large intestine. *Histopathology*, 1977; 1: 77.
462 Al-Sam SZ, Davies JD, Gibbs NM. Anomalous functional and behavioural characteristics of undifferentiated carcinomas of the large bowel. *J Pathol*, 1986; 148: 119.
463 Rüschoff J, Dietmaier W, Lüttges J. *et al*. Poorly differentiated colonic adenocarcinoma, medullary type: clinical, phenotypic, and molecular characteristics. *Am J Pathol*, 1997; 150: 1815.
464 Mills SE, Allen MS Jr, Cohen AR. Small cell undifferentiated carcinoma of the colon. *Am J Surg Pathol*, 1983; 7: 643.
465 Schwartz AM, Ornstein JM. Small-cell undifferentiated carcinoma of the rectosigmoid colon. *Arch Pathol Lab Med*, 1985; 109: 629.
466 Wick MR, Weatherby RP, Weiland LH. Small cell neuroendocrine carcinoma of the colon and rectum: clinical, histologic and ultrastructural study and immunohistochemical comparison with cloacogenic carcinoma. *Hum Pathol*, 1987; 18: 9.
467 Rubio CA. Clear cell adenocarcinoma of the colon. *J Clin Pathol*, 1995; 48: 1142.
468 Stenzel P, Sauer D. Clear cell change in metastatic colonic adenocarcinoma. *Histopathology*, 2000; 36: 471.
469 Hocking GR, Shembrey M, Hay D, Ostor AG. Alpha-fetoprotein-producing adenocarcinoma of the sigmoid colon with possible hepatoid differentiation. *Pathology*, 1995; 27: 277.
470 Yu Y-Y, Ogino T, Okada S. An alpha-fetoprotein-producing carcinoma of the rectum. *Acta Pathol Jpn*, 1992; 42: 684.
471 Yang AH, Chen WYK, Chiang H. Malignant rhabdoid tumour of the colon. *Histopathology*, 1994; 24: 89.
472 Chetty R, Bhathal PS. Caecal adenocarcinoma with rhabdoid phenotype: an immunohistochemical and ultrastructural analysis. *Virchows Arch A*, 1993; 422: 179.
473 Roncaroli F, Montironi R, Feliciotti F, Losi L, Eusebi V. Sarcomatoid carcinoma of the anorectal junction with neuroendocrine and rhabdomyoblastic features. *Am J Surg Pathol*, 1995; 19: 217.

474 Rognum TO, Fausa O, Brandtzaeg P. Immunohistochemical evaluation of carcinoembryonic antigen, secretory component and epithelial IgA in tubular and villous large-bowel adenomas with different grades of dysplasia. *Scand J Gastroenterol*, 1982; 17: 341.
475 Dukes CE. The classification of cancer of the rectum. *J Pathol Bacteriol*, 1932; 35: 323.
476 Thomas GDH, Dixon MF, Smeeton NC, Williams NS. Observer variation in the histological grading of rectal carcinoma. *J Clin Pathol*, 1983; 36: 385.
477 Tytgat KMAJ, Büller HA, Opdam FJM *et al*. Biosynthesis of human colonic mucin: MUC2 is the prominent secretory mucin. *Gastroenterology*, 1994; 107: 1352.
478 Reid PE, Culling CFA, Dunn WL, Ramey CW, Clay MG. Chemical and histochemical studies of normal and diseased human gastrointestinal tract. I. A comparison between histologically normal colon, colonic tumours, ulcerative colitis and diverticular disease of the colon. *Histochem J*, 1984; 16: 235.
479 Katsuyama T, Ono K, Nakayama J, Akamatsu T. Mucosubstance histochemistry of the normal mucosa and carcinoma of the large intestine. Galactose oxidase–Schiff reaction and lectin stainings. *Acta Pathol Jpn*, 1985; 35: 1409.
480 Lev R, Lance P, Camara P. Histochemical and morphologic studies of mucosa bordering rectosigmoid carcinomas: comparisons with normal, diseased, and malignant colonic epithelium. *Hum Pathol*, 1985; 16: 151.
481 Jass JR, Allison LJ, Edgar SG. Distribution of sialosyl Tn and Tn antigens within normal and malignant colorectal epithelium. *J Pathol*, 1995; 176: 143.
482 Cooper HS. Peanut lectin binding sites in large bowel carcinoma. *Lab Invest*, 1982; 47: 383.
483 Ogata S, Ho I, Chen A *et al*. Tumor-associated sialylated antigens are constitutively expressed in normal human colonic mucosa. *Cancer Res*, 1995; 55: 1869.
484 Blaszczyk M, Pak KY, Herlyn M, Sears HF, Steplewski Z. Characterization of Lewis antigens in normal colon and gastrointestinal adenocarcinomas. *Proc Natl Acad Sci USA*, 1985; 82: 3552.
485 Yuan M, Itzkowitz SH, Palekar A *et al*. Distribution of blood group antigens A, B, H, Lewis^a, and Lewis^b in human normal, fetal, and malignant colonic tissue. *Cancer Res*, 1985; 45: 4499.
486 Sakamoto J, Furukawa K, Cordon-Cardo C *et al*. Expression of lewis^a, lewis^b, x, and y blood group antigens in human colonic tumors and normal tissue and in human tumor-derived cell lines. *Cancer Res*, 1986; 46: 1553.
487 Cordon-Cardo C, Lloyd KO, Sakamoto J *et al*. Immunohistologic expression of blood-group antigens in normal human gastrointestinal tract and colonic carcinoma. *Int J Cancer*, 1986; 37: 667.
488 Schoentag R, Primus FJ, Kuhns W. ABH and Lewis blood group expression in colorectal carcinoma. *Cancer Res*, 1987; 47: 1695.
489 Itzkowitz SH, Yuan M, Fukushi Y *et al*. Lewis^x- and sialylated lewis^x-related antigen expression in human malignant and nonmalignant colonic tissues. *Cancer Res*, 1986; 46: 2627.
490 Gold P, Freeman SO. Specific carcinoembryonic antigens of the human digestive system. *J Exp Med*, 1965; 122: 467.
491 Buckley CH, Fox H. An immunohistochemical study of the significance of HCG secretion by large bowel adenocarcinomata. *J Clin Pathol*, 1979; 32: 368.
492 Bara J, André J, Gautier R, Burtin P. Abnormal pattern of mucus-associated MI antigens in histological normal mucosa adjacent to colonic adenocarcinomas. *Cancer Res*, 1984; 44: 4040.
493 Jothy S, Brazinsky SA, Chin-A-Loy M *et al*. Characterization of monoclonal antibodies to carcinoembryonic antigen with increased tumor specificity. *Lab Invest*, 1986; 54: 108.
494 Ma J, De Boer WGRM, Ward HA, Nairn RC. Another oncofetal antigen. *Br J Cancer*, 1980; 41: 325.
495 Pilbrow SJ, Hertzog PJ, Linnane AW. The adenoma–carcinoma sequence in the colorectum—early appearance of a hierarchy of small intestinal mucin antigen (SIMA) epitopes and correlation with malignant potential. *Br J Cancer*, 1992; 66: 748.
496 Zweibaum A, Hauri H-P, Sterchi E *et al*. Immunohistological evidence, obtained with monoclonal antibodies, of small intestinal brush border hydrolases in human colon cancers and foetal colons. *Int J Cancer*, 1984; 34: 591.
497 Young GP, MaCrae FA, Gibson PR, Alexeyeff M, Whitehead RH. Alimentary tract and pancreas: brush border hydrolases in normal and neoplastic colonic epithelium. *J Gastroenterol Hepatol*, 1992; 7: 347.
498 Heyderman E, Steele K, Ormerod M. A new antigen on the epithelial membrane: its immunoperoxidase localisation in normal and neoplastic tissues. *J Clin Pathol*, 1979; 32: 35.
499 Gendler SJ, Lancaster CA, Taylor-Papadimitriou J *et al*. Molecular cloning and expression of human tumour associated polymorphic epithelial mucin. *J Biol Chem*, 1990; 265: 15286.
500 Makin CA, Bobrow LG, Bodmer WF. Monoclonal antibody to cytokeratin for use in routine histopathology. *J Clin Pathol*, 1984; 37: 975.
501 Brown DT, Anderton BH, Wylie CC. The organisation of intermediate filaments in normal human colonic epithelium and colon carcinoma cells. *Int J Cancer*, 1983; 32: 163.
502 Pignatelli M. Models of colorectal tumour differentiation. *Cancer Surv*, 1993; 16: 3.
503 Gagliardi G, Kandemir O, Liu D *et al*. Changes in E-cadherin immunoreactivity in the adenoma–carcinoma sequence of the large bowel. *Virchows Arch*, 1995; 426: 149.
504 Koretz K, Schlag P, Boumsell L, Moller P. Expresssion of VLA-a6, and VLA-b1 chains in normal mucosa and adenomas of the colon, and in colon carcinomas and their liver metastases. *Am J Pathol*, 1991; 138: 741.
505 Stallmach A, v Lampe B, Matthes H, Bornhoft G, Riecken EO. Diminished expression of integrin adhesion molecules on human colonic epithelial cells during the benign to malign tumour transformation. *Gut*, 1992; 33: 342.
506 Ohannesian DW, Lotan D, Thomas P *et al*. Carcinoembryonic antigen and other glycoconjugates act as ligands for galectin-3 in human colon carcinoma cells. *Cancer Res*, 1995; 55: 2191.
507 Mulder JWR, Kruyt PM, Sewnath M *et al*. Colorectal cancer prognosis and expression of exon-v6-containing CD44 proteins. *Lancet*, 1994; 344: 1470.
508 Takeuchi K, Yamaguchi A, Urano T *et al*. Expression of CD44 variant exons 8–10 in colorectal cancer and its relationship to metastasis. *Jpn J Cancer Res*, 1995; 86: 292.
509 Filipe MI. Value of histochemical reactions for mucosubstances in the diagnosis of certain pathological conditions of the colon and rectum. *Gut*, 1969; 10: 577.
510 Filipe MI, Branfoot AC. Abnormal patterns of mucus secretion in

apparently normal mucosa of large intestine with cancer. *Cancer*, 1974; 34: 282.
511 Reid PE. Owen DA, Dunn WL *et al.* Chemical and histochemical studies of normal and diseased human gastrointestinal tract. III. Changes in the histochemical and chemical properties of the epithelial glycoproteins in the mucosa close to colonic tumours. *Histochem J*, 1985; 17: 171.
512 Culling CFA, Reid PE, Worth AJ, Dunn WL. A new histochemical technique of use in the interpretation and diagnosis of adenocarcinoma and villous lesions in the large intestine. *J Clin Pathol*, 1977; 30: 1056.
513 Sugihara K, Jass JR. Colorectal goblet cell sialomucin heterogeneity: its relation to malignant disease. *J Clin Pathol*, 1986; 39: 1088.
514 Hutchins JT, Reading CL, Giavazzi R, Hoaglund J, Jessup JM. Distribution of mono-, di-, and tri-O-acetylated sialic acids in normal and neoplastic colon. *Cancer Res*, 1988; 48: 483.
515 Dawson PA, Filipe MI. An ultrastructural and histochemical study of the mucous membrane adjacent to and remote from carcinoma of the colon. *Cancer*, 1976; 37: 2388.
516 Dawson PA, Filipe MI. Uptake of [^{35}S] sulphate in human colonic mucosa associated with carcinoma: an auto-radiographic analysis at the ultrastructural level. *Histochem J*, 1983; 15: 3.
517 Pilbrow SJ, Hertzog PJ, Pinczower GD, Linnane AW. Expression of a novel family of epitopes on small intestinal mucins in colorectal cancers, adjacent and remote mucosa. *Tumor Biol*, 1992; 13: 251.
518 Isaacson P, Attwood PRA. Failure to demonstrate specificity of the morphological and histochemical changes in mucosa adjacent to colonic carcinoma (transitional mucosa). *J Clin Pathol*, 1979; 32: 214.
519 Williams GT. Commentary: transitional mucosa of the large intestine. *Histopathology*, 1985; 9: 1237.
520 Lanza GJ, Altavilla G, Cavazzini L, Negrini R. Colonic mucosa adjacent to adenomas and hyperplastic polyps—a morphological and histochemical study. *Histopathology*, 1985; 9: 857.
521 Pilbrow SJ, Hertzog PJ, Linnane AW. Differentiation-associated changes in mucin glycoprotein antigenicity in mucosa adjacent to rare gastrointestinal tract tumours of non-mucosal origin. *J Pathol*, 1993; 169: 259.
522 Dawson PM, Habib NA, Rees HC, Williamson RCN, Wood CB. Influence of sialomucin at the resection margin on local tumour recurrence and survival of patients with colorectal cancer: a multivariate analysis. *Br J Surg*, 1987; 74: 366.
523 Dukes CE. Histological grading of rectal cancer. *Proc R Soc Med*, 1937; 30: 371.
524 Blenkinsopp WK, Stewart-Brown S, Blesovsky L, Kearney G, Fielding LP. Histopathology reporting in large bowel carcinoma. *J Clin Pathol*, 1981; 34: 509.
525 Whittaker MA, Carr NJ, Midwinter MJ, Badham DP, Higgins B. Acinar morphology in colorectal cancer is associated with survival but is not an independent prognostic variable. *Histopathology*, 2000; 36: 439.
526 Phillips SF. Functions of the large bowel: an overview. In: Polak JM, Bloom SR, Wright NA, Butler AG, eds. *Basic Science in Gastroenterology. Physiology of the Gut*. Glaxo Group Research Ltd 283: Royal Postgraduate Medical School, 1984.
527 Freedman LS, Macaskill P, Smith AN. Multivariate analysis of prognostic factors for operable rectal cancer. *Lancet*, 1984; ii: 733.
528 Chapuis PH, Dent OF, Fisher R *et al.* A multivariate analysis of clinical and pathological variables in prognosis after resection of large bowel carcinoma. *Br J Surg*, 1985; 72: 698.
529 Arends JW, Wiggers T, Thijs CT *et al.* The value of secretory component (SC) immunoreactivity in diagnosis and prognosis of colorectal cancers. *Am J Clin Pathol*, 1984; 82: 267.
530 Wiggers T, Arends JW, Schutte B, Volovics L, Bosman FT. A multivariate analysis of pathologic prognostic indicators in large bowel cancer. *Cancer*, 1988; 61: 386.
531 Itzkowitz SH, Bloom EJ, Kokal WA *et al.* A novel mucin antigen associated with prognosis in colorectal cancer patients. *Cancer*, 1990; 66: 1960.
532 Andersen SN, Rognum TO, Lund E, Meling GI, Hauge S. Strong HLA-DR expression in large bowel carcinomas is associated with good prognosis. *Br J Cancer*, 1993; 68: 80.
533 Stein B, Momburg F, Schwarz V *et al.* Reduction or loss of HLA-A, B, C antigens in colorectal carcinoma appears not to influence survival. *Br J Cancer*, 1988; 57: 364.
534 Moller P, Momburg F, Koretz K *et al.* Influence of major histocompatibility complex class I and II antigens on survival in colorectal carcinoma. *Cancer Res*, 1991; 51: 729.
535 Forster SJ, Talbot IC, Critchley DR. Laminin and fibronectin in rectal adenocarcinoma: relationship to tumour grade, stage and metastasis. *Br J Cancer*, 1984; 50: 51.
536 Dorudi S, Hanby AM, Poulsom R, Northover J, Hart IR. Level of expression of E-cadherin mRNA in colorectal cancer correlates with clinical outcome. *Br J Cancer*, 1995; 71: 614.
537 Teixeira CR, Tanaka S, Haruma K *et al.* Carcinoembryonic antigen staining patterns at the invasive tumor margin predict the malignant potential of colorectal carcinoma. *Oncology*, 1994; 51: 230.
538 Campo E, Munoz J, Miquel R *et al.* Cathepsin B expression in colorectal carcinomas correlates with tumor progression and shortened patient survival. *Am J Pathol*, 1994; 145: 301.
539 Jeziorska M, Haboubi NY, Schofield PF *et al.* Distribution of gelatinase B (MMP-9) and type IV collagen in colorectal carcinoma. *Int J Colorect Dis*, 1994; 9: 141.
540 Newell KJ, Witty JP, Rodgers WH, Matrisian LM. Expression and localization of matrix-degrading metalloproteinases during colorectal tumorigenesis. *Mol Carcinog*, 1994; 10: 199.
541 Quirke P, Dixon MF, Clayden AD. Prognostic significance of DNA aneuploidy and cell proliferation on rectal adenocarcinomas. *J Pathol*, 1987; 151: 285.
542 Shepherd NA, Richman PI, England J. Ki-67 derived proliferative activity in colorectal adenocarcinoma with prognostic correlations. *J Pathol*, 1988; 155: 213.
543 Mayer A, Takimoto M, Fritz E *et al.* The prognostic significance of proliferating cell nuclear antigen, epidermal growth factor receptor, and mdr gene expression in colorectal cancer. *Cancer*, 1993; 71: 2454.
544 Joyce WP, Fynes M, Moran KT *et al.* The prognostic value of nucleolar organiser regions in colorectal cancer: a 5-year follow-up study. *Ann R Coll Surg Engl*, 1990; 74: 172.
545 Ofner D, Riedmann B, Maier H *et al.* Standardized staining and analysis of argyrophilic nucleolar organizer region associated proteins (AgNORs) in radically resected colorectal adenocarcinoma—correlation with tumour stage and long-term survival. *J Pathol*, 1995; 175: 441.
546 Yamachika T, Nakanishi H, Inada K *et al.* A new prognostic factor

for colorectal carcinoma, thymidylate synthase, and its therapeutic significance. *Cancer*, 1998; 82: 70.

547 Moerkerk P, Arends JW, Vandriel M, Debruine A, Tenkate J. Type and number of Ki-ras point mutations relate to stage of human colorectal cancer. *Cancer Res*, 1994; 54: 3376.

548 Suchy B, Zietz C, Rabes HM. K-ras point mutations in human colorectal carcinomas: relation to aneuploidy and metastasis. *Int J Cancer*, 1992; 52: 30.

549 Kastrinakis WV, Ramchurren N, Rieger KM *et al*. Increased incidence of p53 mutations is associated with hepatic metastasis in colorectal neoplastic progression. *Oncogene*, 1995; 11: 647.

550 Kahlenberg MS, Stoler DL, Rodriguez-Bigas MA *et al*. p53 tumor suppressor gene mutations predict decreased survival of patients with sporadic colorectal carcinoma. *Cancer*, 2000; 88: 1814.

551 Sato K, Miyahara M, Saito T, Kobayashi M. c-myc mRNA overexpression is associated with lymph node metastasis in colorectal cancer. *Eur J Cancer*, 1994; 30A: 1113.

552 Smith DR, Myint T, Goh HS. Over-expression of the c-myc proto-oncogene in colorectal carcinoma. *Br J Cancer*, 1993; 68: 407.

553 Dix BR, Robbins P, Soong R *et al*. Common molecular genetic alterations in Dukes' B and C colorectal carcinomas are not short-term prognostic indicators of survival. *Int J Cancer*, 1994; 59: 747.

554 Purdie CA, O'Grady J, Piris J, Wyllie AH, Bird CC. p53 Expression in colorectal tumors. *Am J Pathol*, 1991; 138: 807.

555 Bosari S, Viale G, Bossi P *et al*. Cytoplasmic accumulation of p53 protein—an independent prognostic indicator in colorectal adenocarcinomas. *J Natl Cancer Inst*, 1994; 86: 681.

556 Sun X-F, Carstensen JM, Zhang H *et al*. Prognostic significance of cytoplasmic p53 oncoprotein in colorectal adenocarcinoma. *Lancet*, 1992; 340: 1369.

557 Remvikos Y, Thominaga O, Hammel P *et al*. Increased p53 protein content of colorectal tumours correlates with poor survival. *Br J Cancer*, 1992; 66: 758.

558 Poller DN, Baxter KJ, Shepherd NA. Bcl-2 gene protein expression in colorectal cancer: is it a useful prognostic factor? *J Pathol*, 1996; 178: 3A.

559 Manne U, Weiss HL, Myers RB *et al*. Nuclear accumulation of p53 in colorectal adenocarcinoma. *Cancer*, 1998; 83: 2456.

560 Ofner D, Riehemann K, Maier H *et al*. Immunohistochemistry detectable bcl-2 expression in colorectal carcinoma: correlation with tumour stage and patient survival. *Br J Cancer*, 1995; 72: 981.

561 Poller DN, Baxter KJ, Shepherd NA. p53 and RB1 gene proteins are not prognostic factors in colorectal cancer. *J Pathol*, 1995; 175: 103A.

562 Fukuda K, Monden T, Yamamoto H *et al*. Immunohistochemical study of retinoblastoma gene expression in colorectal carcinomas. *Int J Oncol*, 1994; 4: 117.

563 Martinez JA, Prevot S, Nordlinger B *et al*. Overexpression of *nm*23-H1 and *nm*23-H2 genes in colorectal carcinomas and loss of *nm*23-H1 expression in advanced tumour stages. *Gut*, 1995; 37: 712.

564 Zeng ZS, Hsu S, Zhang ZF *et al*. High level of Nm23-H1 gene expression is associated with local colorectal cancer progression not with metastases. *Br J Cancer*, 1994; 70: 1025.

565 Heide I, Thiede C, Poppe K *et al*. Expression and mutational analysis of Nm23-H1 in liver metastases of colorectal cancer. *Br J Cancer*, 1994; 70: 1267.

566 Ofner D, Maier H, Riedmann B *et al*. Immunohistochemically detectable p53 and mdm-2 oncoprotein expression in colorectal carcinoma: prognostic significance. *J Clin Pathol Mol Pathol*, 1995; 48: M12.

567 Loda M, Cukor B, Tam SW *et al*. Increased proteasome-dependent degradation of the cyclin-dependent kinase inhibitor p27 in aggressive colorectal carcinomas. *Nat Med*, 1997; 3: 231.

568 Hamilton SR. Molecular genetic alterations as potential prognostic indicators in colorectal carcinoma. *Cancer*, 1992; 69: 1589.

569 Khine K, Smith DR, Goh HS. High frequency of allelic deletion on chromosome 17p in advanced colorectal cancer. *Cancer*, 1994; 73: 28.

570 Takanishi DM, Angriman I, Yaremko ML *et al*. Chromosome 17p allelic loss in colorectal carcinoma: clinical significance. *Arch Surg*, 1995; 130: 585.

571 Ishimaru G, Ookawa K, Yamaguchi N *et al*. Allelic losses associated with the metastatic potential of colorectal carcinoma. *Int J Oncol*, 1994; 5: 267.

572 Jen J, Kim H, Piantadosi S *et al*. Allelic loss of chromosome 18q and prognosis in colorectal cancer. *N Engl J Med*, 1994; 331: 213.

573 Halling KC, French AJ, McDonell SK *et al*. Microsatellite instability and 8p allelic imbalance in stage B2 and C colorectal cancers. *J Natl Cancer Inst*, 1999; 91: 1295.

574 Wright CM, Dent OF, Barker M *et al*. The prognostic significance of extensive microsatellite instability in sporadic clinicopathologic stage C colorectal cancer. *Br J Surg*, 2000; 87: 1197.

575 Jass JR. Lymphocytic infiltration and survival in rectal cancer. *J Clin Pathol*, 1986; 39: 585.

576 Csiba A, Whitwell HL, Moore M. Distribution of histocompatibility and leucocyte differentiation antigens in normal human colon and in benign and malignant colonic neoplasms. *Br J Cancer*, 1984; 50: 699.

577 Umpleby HC, Heinemann D, Symes MO, Williamson RCN. Expression of histocompatibility antigens and characterization of mononuclear cell infiltrates in normal and neoplastic colorectal tissues of humans. *J Natl Cancer Inst*, 1985; 74: 1161.

578 Lampert IA, Kirkland S, Farrell S, Borysiewicz LK. HLA-DR expression in a human colon carcinoma cell line. *J Pathol*, 1985; 146: 337.

579 O'Connell J, O'Sullivan GC, Collins JK, Shanahan F. The Fas counterattack: Fas-mediated T cell killing by colon cancer cells expressing Fas ligand. *J Exp Med*, 1996; 184: 1075.

580 Ghosh AK, Moore M, Street AJ, Howat JMT, Schofield PF. Expression of HLA-D sub-region products in human colorectal carcinoma. *Int J Cancer*, 1986; 38: 459.

581 Monson JRT, Ramsden CW, Giles GR, Brennan TG, Guillou PJ. Lymphokine activated killer (LAK) cells in patients with gastrointestinal cancer. *Gut*, 1987; 28: 1420.

582 Tartter PI, Steinberg B, Barron DM, Martinelli G. The prognostic significance of natural killer cytotoxicity in patients with colorectal cancer. *Arch Surg*, 1987; 122: 1264.

583 Ogata S, Maimonis PJ, Itzkowitz SH. Mucins bearing the cancer-associated sialosyl-Tn antigen mediate inhibition of natural killer cell cytotoxicity. *Cancer Res*, 1992; 52: 4741.

584 Jerome KR, Brand DL, Bendt KM *et al*. Cytotoxic T-lymphocytes derived from patients with breast adenocarcinoma recognize an epitope present on the protein core of a mucin molecule

preferentially expressed by malignant cells. *Cancer Res*, 1991; 51: 2908.

585 Hamada Y, Yamamura M, Hioki K *et al*. Immunohistochemical study of carcino-embryonic antigen in patients with colorectal cancer. Correlation with plasma carcinoembryonic antigen levels. *Cancer*, 1985; 55: 136.

586 O'Brien MJ, Zamcheck N, Burke B *et al*. Immunocytochemical localization of carcinoembryonic antigen in benign and malignant colorectal tissues: assessment of diagnostic value. *Am J Clin Pathol*, 1981; 75: 283.

587 Arends JW, Wiggers T, Verstijnen C, Hilgers J, Bosman FT. Gastrointestinal cancer-associated antigen (GICA) immunoreactivity in colorectal carcinoma in relation to patient survival. *Int J Cancer*, 1984; 34: 193.

588 Durdey P, Cooper JC, Switala S, King RFGJ, Williams NS. The role of peptidases in cancer of the rectum and sigmoid colon. *Br J Surg*, 1985; 72: 378.

589 Gelister JSK, Mahmoud M, Lewin MR, Gaffney PJ, Boulos PB. Plasminogen activators in human colorectal neoplasia. *Br Med J*, 1986; 293: 728.

590 Gelister JSK, Jass JR, Mahmoud M, Gaffney PJ, Boulos PB. Role of urokinase in colorectal neoplasia. *Br J Surg*, 1987; 74: 460.

591 Coffey RJ, Shipley GD, Moses HL. Production of transforming growth factors by human colon cancer lines. *Cancer Res*, 1986; 46: 1164.

592 Adenis A, Peyrat JP, Hecquet B *et al*. Type I insulin-like growth factor receptors in human colorectal cancer. *Eur J Cancer*, 1995; 31A: 50.

593 Deans GT, Williamson K, Hamilton P *et al*. DNA densitometry of colorectal cancer. *Gut*, 1993; 34: 1566.

594 Jass JR, Mukawa K, Goh HS, Love SB, Capellaro D. Clinical importance of DNA content in rectal cancer measured by flow cytometry. *J Clin Pathol*, 1989; 42: 254.

595 Kouri M, Pyrhonen S, Mecklin J-P *et al*. The prognostic value of DNA-ploidy in colorectal carcinoma: a prospective study. *Br J Cancer*, 1990; 62: 976.

596 Tang R, Ho Y-S, You YT *et al*. Prognostic evaluation of DNA flow cytometric and histopathologic parameters of colorectal cancer. *Cancer*, 1995; 76: 1724.

597 Quirke P, Dyson DED. Flow cytometry: methodology and applications in pathology. *J Pathol*, 1986; 149: 79.

598 Goh HS, Jass JR, Atkin WS, Cuzick J, Northover JMA. Value of flow cytometric determination as a guide to prognosis in operable rectal cancer: a multivariate analysis. *Int J Colorect Dis*, 1987; 2: 17.

599 Carder PJ, Cripps KJ, Morris R *et al*. Mutation of the p53 gene precedes aneuploid clonal divergence in colorectal carcinoma. *Br J Cancer*, 1995; 71: 215.

600 Ahnen DJ, Feigl P, Quan G *et al*. Ki-ras mutation and p53 overexpression predict the clinical behavior of colorectal cancer: a Southwest Oncology Group study. *Cancer Res*, 1998; 58: 1149.

601 Lukish JR, Muro K, DeNobile J *et al*. Prognostic significance of DNA replication errors in young patients with colorectal cancer. *Ann Surg*, 1998; 227: 51.

602 Astler VB, Coller FA. The prognostic significance of direct extension of carcinoma of the colon and rectum. *Ann Surg*, 1954; 139: 846.

603 Newland RC, Chapuis PH, Smyth EJ. The prognostic value of substaging colorectal carcinoma. A prospective study of 1117 cases with standardized pathology. *Cancer*, 1987; 60: 852.

604 Hermanek P, Guggenmoos-Holzmann I. Prognostic factors in rectal carcinoma. A contribution to the further development of tumor classification. *Dis Colon Rectum*, 1989; 32: 593.

605 Compton C, Fenoglio-Preiser CM, Pettigrew N, Fielding LP. American Joint Committee on Cancer Prognostic Factors Consensus Conference. *Cancer*, 2000; 88: 1739.

606 Jass JR, Morson BC. Reporting colorectal cancer. *J Clin Pathol*, 1987; 40: 1016.

607 Sheffield JP, Talbot IC. Gross examination of the large intestine. *J Clin Pathol*, 1992; 45: 751.

608 Chan KW, Boey J, Wong SKC. A method of reporting radial invasion and surgical clearance of rectal carcinoma. *Histopathology*, 1985; 9: 1319.

609 Quirke P, Dixon MF, Durdey P, Williams NS. Local recurrence of rectal adenocarcinoma due to inadequate surgical resection. Histopathological and study of lateral tumour spread and surgical excision. *Lancet*, 1986; ii: 996.

610 MacFarlane JK, Ryall RDH, Heald RJ. Mesorectal excision for rectal cancer. *Lancet*, 1993; 341: 457.

611 Grinnell RS. Lymphatic block with atypical retrograde lymphatic metastases and spread in carcinoma of the colon and rectum. *Ann Surg*, 1966; 163: 272.

612 Phillips RKS, Hittinger R, Blesovsky L, Fry JS, Fielding LP. Large bowel cancer: surgical pathology and its relationship to survival. *Br J Surg*, 1984; 71: 604.

613 Wolmark N, Fisher B, Wieand HS. The prognostic value of the modifcations of the Dukes' C class of colorectal cancer. *Ann Surg*, 1986; 203: 115.

614 Sobin LH, Wittekind C. *TNM Classification of Malignant Tumours*. New York: Wiley-Liss, 1997.

615 Harrison JC, Dean PJ, El-zeky F, Vander Zwaag R. From Dukes through Jass: Pathological prognostic indicators in rectal cancer. *Hum Pathol*, 1994; 25: 498.

616 Jeffers MD, O'Dowd GM, Mulcahy H *et al*. The prognostic sigificance of immunohistochemically detected lymph node micrometastases in colorectal carcinoma. *J Pathol*, 1994; 172: 183.

617 Cutait R, Alves VA, Lopes LC *et al*. Restaging of colorectal cancer based on the identification of lymph node micrometastases through immunoperoxidase staining of CEA and cytokeratins. *Dis Colon Rectum*, 1991; 34: 917.

618 Adell G, Boeryd B, Franlung B, Sjodahl R, Hanansson L. Occurrence and prognostic importance of micrometastases in regional nodes in Dukes' B colorectal carcinoma: an immunohistochemical study. *Eur J Surg*, 1996; 162: 637.

619 Liefers G-J, Cleton-Jansen A-M, van de Velde CJH *et al*. Micrometastases and survival in stage II colorectal cancer. *N Engl J Med*, 1998; 339: 223.

620 Yamamoto N, Kato Y, Yanagisawa A *et al*. Predictive value of genetic diagnosis for cancer micrometastasis. *Cancer*, 1997; 80: 1393.

621 Greenson JK, Isenhart CE, Rice R *et al*. Identification of occult micrometastases in pericolic lymph nodes of Dukes' B colorectal cancer patients using monoclonal antibodies against cytokeratin and CC49. Correlation with long-term survival. *Cancer*, 1994; 73: 563.

622 Brynes RK, Hunter RL, Vellios F. Immunomorphologic changes in regional lymph nodes associated with cancer. *Arch Pathol Lab Med*, 1983; 107: 217.

623 Murphy J, Pocard M, O'Sullivan G *et al*. Causes and prognostic significance of variable lymph node retrieval in Dukes' B rectal carcinoma. *Gut*, 1999; 44: A84.
624 Pihl E, Nairn R, Milne BJ *et al*. Lymphoid hyperplasia: a major prognostic feature in 519 cases of colorectal carcinoma. *Am J Pathol*, 1980; 100: 469.
625 Jass JR, Love SB. Prognostic value of direct spread in Dukes C cases of rectal cancer. *Dis Colon Rectum*, 1989; 32: 477.
626 Talbot IC, Ritchie S, Leighton M *et al*. Invasion of veins by carcinoma of rectum: method of detection, histological features and significance. *Histopathology*, 1981; 5: 141.
627 Beskin C, Attwood W. Peripheral bone metastasis from carcinoma of the rectum. *Surgery*, 1952; 31: 273.
628 Dionne L. Pattern of blood-borne metastases from carcinoma of the rectum. *Cancer*, 1965; 18: 775.
629 Russell AH, Pelton J, Reheis CE *et al*. Adenocarcinoma of the colon: an autopsy study with implications for new therapeutic strategies. *Cancer*, 1985; 56: 1446.
630 Weiss L, Grundmann E, Torhorst J *et al*. Haematogenous metastatic patterns in colonic carcinoma: an analysis of 1541 necropsies. *J Pathol*, 1986; 150: 195.
631 Schulz W, Hagen C, Hort W. The distribution of liver metastases from colonic cancer. *Virchows Arch A*, 1985; 406: 279.
632 Chapman R. Spontaneous rupture of the spleen infiltrated by secondary carcinoma. *Br Med J*, 1962; i: 1319.
633 Reingold IM. Cutaneous metastases from internal carcinoma. *Cancer*, 1966; 19: 162.
634 Harcourt KF, Dennis DL. Laparotomy for 'ovarian tumours' in unsuspected carcinoma of the colon. *Cancer*, 1968; 21: 1244.
634a Chu P, Wu E, Weiss LM. Cytokeratin 7 and cytokeratin 20 expression in epithelial neoplasms: a survey of 435 cases. *Mod Pathol* 2000; 13: 962.
635 Matt SJ. Metastatic carcinoma of the penis secondary to carcinoma of the rectum. *J Urol*, 1960; 83: 163.
636 Drury BJ. Adenocarcinoma of the rectum with metastasis to the nailbed of the finger. *Calif Med*, 1959; 91: 35.
637 Shepherd NA, Baxter KJ, Love SB. Influence of local peritoneal involvement on pelvic recurrence and prognosis in rectal cancer. *J Clin Pathol*, 1995; 48: 849.
638 Shepherd NA, Baxter KR, Love SB. The prognostic importance of peritoneal involvement in colonic cancer: a prospective evaluation. *Gastroenterology*, 1997; 112: 1096.
639 Lash RH, Hart WR. Intestinal adenocarcinomas metastatic to the ovaries. A clinicopathological evaluation of 22 cases. *Am J Surg Pathol*, 1987; 11: 114.
640 Boreham P. Implantation metastases from cancer of the large bowel. *Br J Surg*, 1958; 46: 103.
641 Fermor B, Umpleby HC, Lever JV, Symes MO, Williamson RCN. Proliferative and metastatic potential of exfoliated colorectal cancer cells. *J Natl Cancer Inst*, 1986; 76: 347.
642 LeQuesne LP, Thomson AD. Implantation recurrence of carcinoma of the rectum and colon. *N Engl J Med*, 1988; 258: 578.
643 Dockerty MB. Pathologic aspects in the control of spread of colonic carcinoma. *Proc Staff Meet Mayo Clin*, 1958; 33: 157.
644 Goligher JC, Dukes CE, Bussey HJR. Local recurrence after sphincter-saving excisions for carcinoma of the rectum and rectosigmoid. *Br J Surg*, 1951; 39: 155.
645 Keynes WM. Implantation from the bowel lumen in cancer of the large intestine. *Ann Surg*, 1961; 153: 357.
646 Gricouroff G. Pathogenesis of recurrences on the suture line following surgical resection for carcinoma of the colon. *Cancer*, 1967; 20: 673.
647 Morson BC, Vaughan EG, Bussey HJR. Pelvic recurrence after excision of rectum for carcinoma. *Br Med J*, 1963; ii: 13.
648 Jass JR, Chapuis PH, Dixon MF *et al*. Staging of colorectal cancer. *Int J Colorect Dis*, 1987; 2: 123.
649 Adam IJ, Mohamdee MO, Martin IG *et al*. Role of circumferential margin involvement in the local recurrence of rectal cancer. *Lancet*, 1994; 344: 707.
650 Finlay IG, McArdle CS. Occult hepatic metastases in colorectal carcinoma. *Br J Surg*, 1986; 73: 732.
651 Jass JR, Love SB, Northover JMA. A new prognostic classification of rectal cancer. *Lancet*, 1987; i: 1303.
652 Muir FG, Bell AJY, Barlow KA. Multiple primary carcinomata of the colon, duodenum and larynx associated with keratoacanthoma of the face. *Br J Surg*, 1967; 54: 191.
653 Sanders GB, Hagen WH, Kinnaird DW. Adult intussusception and carcinoma of the colon. *Ann Surg*, 1958; 147: 796.
654 Miln DC, McLaughlin IS. Carcinoma of the proximal large bowel associated with acute appendicitis. *Br J Surg*, 1969; 56: 143.
655 Glotzer DJ. Colonic ulceration proximal to obstructing carcinoma. *Surgery*, 1964; 56: 950.
656 Rosato FE, Shelly WB, Fitts WT, Miller LD. Non-metastatic cutaneous manifestations of cancer of the colon. *Am J Surg*, 1969; 117: 277.
657 Sontag SJ, Schnell TG, Chejfec G *et al*. Barrett's oesophagus and colonic tumours. *Lancet*, 1985; i: 946.
658 Tripp MR, Sampliner RE, Kogan FJ, Morgan TR. Colorectal neoplasms and Barrett's esophagus. *Am J Gastroenterol*, 1986; 81: 1063.
659 Gardiner GW, Goldberg R, Currie D, Murray D. Colonic carcinoma associated with an abnormal collagen table. *Cancer*, 1984; 54: 2973.
660 Katayama Y, Kimura M, Konn M. Cronkhite–Canada syndrome associated with a rectal cancer and adenomatous changes in colonic polyps. *Am J Surg Pathol*, 1985; 9: 65.
661 Wheeler JMD, Warren BF, Jones AC, Mortensen NJM. Preoperative radiotherapy for rectal cancer: implications for surgeons, pathologists and radiologists. *Br J Surg*, 1999; 86: 1108.
662 Fu CG, Tominaga O, Nagawa H *et al*. Role of p53 and p21/WAF1 detection in patient selection for preoperative radiotherapy in rectal cancer patients. *Dis Colon Rectum*, 1998; 41: 68.
663 Modlin IM, Sandor A. An analysis of 8305 cases of carcinoid tumors. *Cancer*, 1997; 79: 813.
664 Berardi RS. Carcinoid tumors of the colon (exclusive of the rectum). *Dis Colon Rectum*, 1972; 15: 383.
665 O'Briain DS, Dayal Y, DeLellis RA *et al*. Rectal carcinoids as tumours of the hindgut endocrine cells. A morphological and immunohistochemical analysis. *Am J Surg Pathol*, 1983; 6: 131.
666 Federspiel BH, Burke AP, Sobin LH, Shekitka KM. Rectal and colonic carcinoids: a clinicopathologic study of 84 cases. *Cancer*, 1990; 65: 135.
667 Fiocca R, Rindi G, Capella C *et al*. Glucagon, glicentin, proglucagon, PYY, PP and pro-PP-icosapeptide immunoreactivities of rectal carcinoid tumours and related nontumor cells. *Regul Pept*, 1987; 29: 9.
668 Koura AN, Giacco GG, Curley SA, Skibber JM, Feig BW, Ellis LM. Carcinoid tumors of the rectum. Effect of size, histopathology,

and surgical treatment on metastasis free survival. *Cancer*, 1997; 79: 1294.

669 Shousha S. Signet-ring cell adenocarcinoma of rectum: a histological, histochemical and electron microscopic study. *Histopathology*, 1982; 6: 341.

670 Gledhill A, Hall PA, Cruse JP, Pollock DJ. Enteroendocrine cell hyperplasia, carcinoid tumours and adenocarcinoma in long-standing ulcerative colitis. *Histopathology*, 1986; 10: 501.

671 Miller RA, Hatton WS. Argyrophilic cell hyperplasia and an atypical carcinoid tumour complicating chronic ulcerative colitis. *Cancer*, 1982; 50: 2920.

672 Minkowitz S. Primary squamous cell carcinoma of the rectosigmoid portion of the colon. *Arch Pathol*, 1967; 84: 77.

673 Gaston EA, Wilde WL. Epidermoid carcinoma arising in a pilonidal sinus. *Dis Colon Rectum*, 1965; 8: 343.

674 Cabrera A, Pickren JW. Squamous metaplasia and squamous cell carcinoma of rectosigmoid. *Dis Colon Rectum*, 1967; 10: 288.

675 Mir-Madjlessi SH, Farmer RG. Squamous cell carcinoma of the rectal stump in a patient with ulcerative colitis. *Cleve Clin Q*, 1985; 52: 257.

676 Hall-Craggs M, Toker C. Basaloid tumour of the sigmoid colon. *Hum Pathol*, 1982; 13: 497.

677 Indinnimeo M, Cicchini C, Stazi A, Limiti MR, Ghini C. An unusual location of cloacogenic carcinoma. *Int Surg*, 1998; 83: 343.

678 Cerezo L, Alvarez M, Edwards W, Price G. Adenosquamous carcinoma of the colon. *Dis Colon Rectum*, 1985; 28: 597.

679 Weidner N, Zekan P. Carcinosarcoma of the colon. Report of a unique case with light and immunohistochemical studies. *Cancer*, 1986; 58: 1126.

680 Klein MS, Sherlock P. Gastric and colonic metastases from breast cancer. *Am J Dig Dis*, 1972; 17: 881.

681 Rees BI, Okwonga W, Jenkins IL. Intestinal metastases from carcinoma of the breast. *Clin Oncol*, 1976; 1: 113.

682 Davis JM. Carcinoma of the prostate presenting as disease of the rectum. *Br J Urol*, 1960; 32: 197.

683 Olsen BS, Carlisle RW. Adenocarcinoma of the prostate simulating primary rectal malignancy. *Cancer*, 1970; 25: 219.

684 Shoemaker CP, Hoyle CL, Levine SB, Farman J. Late solitary colonic recurrence of renal carcinoma. *Am J Surg*, 1970; 120: 99.

685 Fraser AM, Naunton Morgan M. Secondary carcinoma from the cervix involving the large bowel. *Br J Surg*, 1969; 56: 317.

686 Christodouloppoulos JB, Papaioannou AN, Drakopoulou EP, Kontos EK, Razis DV. Carcinoma of the cervix presenting with rectal symptomatology: report of three cases. *Dis Colon Rectum*, 1972; 15: 373.

687 Dukes CE. The significance of the unusual in the pathology of intestinal tumours. *Ann R Coll Surg*, 1949; 4: 90.

688 Drennan JM, Falconer CWA. Malignant leukoplakia of the rectum: metaplastic baso-squamous carcinoma of the rectal mucosa. *J Clin Pathol*, 1959; 12: 175.

39 Non-epithelial tumours of the large intestine

Tumours of lymphoid tissue

The large intestine is well endowed with lymphoid tissue and the prevalence and distribution of lymphoid tumours within the colorectum reflects the physiological distribution of lymphoid tissue [1,2]. Thus the caecum and anorectum are the commonest sites for primary lymphomas of the large bowel. The plentiful lymphoid tissue in the lower rectum and anus has resulted in the epithets of rectal and anal tonsil. Hyperplasia of this lymphoid tissue leads to polypoid lesions, usually solitary. Throughout the colorectum are numerous lymphoid aggregates, positioned in the lower mucosa and extending across the muscularis mucosae into the upper submucosa [3]. These lymphoglandular complexes (LGCs) may become hyperplastic and polypoid in several situations. In children hyperplasia causes the dramatic colonoscopic appearances of benign lymphoid polyposis. In adults, polypoid lymphoid hyperplasia occurs usually in response to chronic inflammatory conditions, especially ulcerative colitis, which may be accompanied by prominent lymphoid follicular hyperplasia [4], principally in the rectum, and diversion proctocolitis, which is characterized by lymphoid follicular hyperplasia, producing the highly distinctive endoscopic nodularity [5]. Furthermore, lymphocyte homing mechanisms of mantle cells ensure that LGCs are the site of tumescence for mantle cell lymphoma affecting the gut, causing the characteristic macroscopic pathology of lymphomatous polyposis [6].

Benign lymphoid polyps

Isolated benign lymphoid polyps, representing a localized exaggerated lymphoid response to a largely unrecognized antigenic stimulus, are almost entirely confined to the rectum and around the anorectal junction: such polyps elsewhere in the colon are exceptional [7]. They present as smooth, round tumours in the lower third of the rectum [8]. They are usually sessile but occasionally pedunculated (Fig. 39.1). Most are single but occasionally up to five polypoid nodules are seen. Multiplicity of lymphoid polyps, especially if involving more proximal large bowel, should always raise suspicions of lymphoma, unless the patient is a child, in which case benign lymphoid polyposis is the most likely diagnosis. Furthermore low-grade lymphomas of MALT (mucosa-associated lymphoid tissue) type can be polypoid and can mimic benign lymphoid polyps histologically [9].

Benign lymphoid polyps are slightly commoner in men in the third and fourth decades. They are usually asymptomatic, being found incidentally during examination for other conditions. They vary in size from a few millimetres to 5 cm in diameter and only rarely ulcerate [7]. Histologically, benign lymphoid polyps show an intact surface mucosa, either rectal or anal canal type, although this may be compressed or attenuated by the submucosal mass. The body of the polyp within the submucosa is composed of hyperplastic lymphoid tissue with multiple enlarged, geographical, lymphoid centres with prominent germinal centres (Fig. 39.1). The appearances are not dissimilar to those of a reactive lymph node apart from the lack of a capsule and sinuses. Sarcoid-like granulomas are sometimes present. Involvement of the muscularis propria is exceptional.

Benign lymphoid polyps show no increased risk of malignant lymphoma. Excision is curative although many regress without resort to excision. On biopsy, differentiation from malignant lymphoma, especially that deriving from mucosa-associated lymphoid tissue ('MALToma'), may be difficult. Any diagnostic doubt should encourage excision biopsy to fully refute the diagnosis of lymphoma. Helpful discriminative features of benign lymphoid polyp include its relatively small size, circumscription of the lesion, non-involvement of the muscularis propria, lack of ulceration and an absence of positive features of lymphoma, notably infiltration and destruction of epithelial structures ('lymphoepithelial lesions') and infiltration by cleaved lymphoid cells of germinal centres.

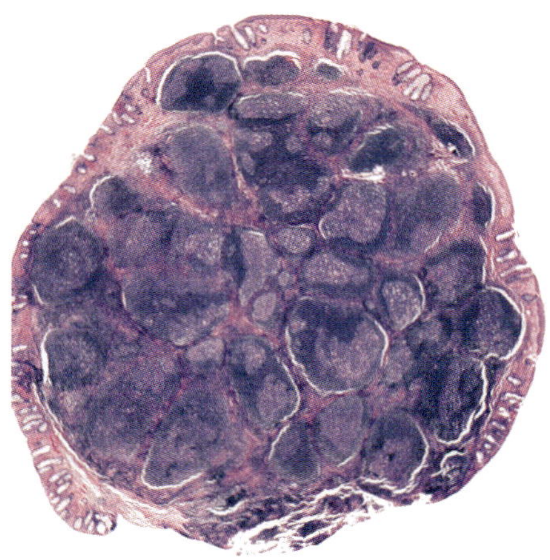

Fig. 39.1 Histology of a benign lymphoid polyp of the rectum. The lesion appears pedunculated and is characterized by lymphoid follicular hyperplasia in the submucosa. The overlying mucosa is intact.

On occasion molecular analysis may be required to demonstrate the lack of clonal immunoglobulin gene rearrangement, the characteristic molecular finding in B-cell lymphomas of the gut.

Benign lymphoid polyposis

Benign lymphoid polyposis is a loosely defined condition characterized by multiple lymphoid polyps with benign histological features. In adults a lymphoid polyposis may be due to hyperplastic LGCs, especially in ulcerative colitis and diversion proctocolitis. For the purpose of this discussion, the term is only applied to a rare condition of children in which LGCs show marked hyperplasia and present as a diffuse polyposis of the colorectum. Although the cause is not always known or suspected in individual cases, there is evidence that the polyposis is an exaggerated response to viral infection, especially echovirus and adenovirus [10]. A familial trait has been described [11] and the condition may also occur in immunodeficiency syndromes [12]. At colonoscopy, innumerable polyps festoon the intestinal mucosa. They consist of grey nodules measuring 0.3–0.6 cm in diameter. The polyps show an intact surface mucosa with prominent reactive lymphoid tissue in the underlying submucosa and often extending into the deep mucosa, as do physiological lymphoglandular complexes.

In children with colorectal benign lymphoid polyposis, response to steroid therapy is often dramatic, although the condition may regress without specific treatment. There is no propensity for malignant change and therefore major surgical resection is not indicated [13]. Apart from being a possible indicator of immunodeficiency and/or viral infection, the disease's main significance lies in its potential mimicry of other polyposis syndromes, most notably familial adenomatous polyposis (FAP). Cases have been recorded in which colectomy has been carried out for this condition in the erroneous belief that multiple polyps equated with FAP [14]. The importance of adequate histological sampling of polyposis syndromes cannot be overemphasized. In adults, a lymphoid polyposis should always raise suspicions of malignant (multiple) lymphomatous polyposis.

Malignant lymphoma of the large intestine

Malignant lymphoma occurring in the large bowel is usually the result of secondary spread from nodal disease. This is certainly the case in clinical and autopsy studies but in surgical pathology practice primary disease becomes more common [15]. There remain controversies about the definition of primary lymphoma of the gastrointestinal tract: the interested reader is referred to the general discussion concerning the definition and classification of primary gastrointestinal lymphoma (see p. 196) and to specialist texts [16]. For the purposes of this discussion, the REAL classification [17] has been used, with updated Kiel equivalents [18], with a reorganization of the REAL classification to reflect the occurrence and prevalence of these diseases in the large bowel.

Primary lymphoma of the colon and rectum represents only 0.2–0.5% of primary malignant neoplasms at this site but it does represent between 5% and 10% of primary gastrointestinal lymphomas [1]. As would be expected from the distribution of lymphoid tissue within the large intestine, the commonest sites of lymphoma are the caecum and the rectum (Fig. 39.2) [19]. The spectrum of disease is somewhat different from primary lymphoma affecting the stomach and small bowel, although the rarity of the disease means that there has been less accurate disease classification compared to counterparts in the stomach and small bowel. In the large bowel, as in the stomach, primary B-cell mucosa-associated lymphoid tissue (MALT) lymphoma is the commonest lymphoma type but, unlike in the stomach, low- and high-grade MALT-type tumours are about equal in incidence. However mantle cell lymphoma comprises about one-quarter of all cases of primary lymphoma of the colorectum [2]. Other lymphoma subtypes affecting this part of the alimentary system are distinctly unusual.

Localized primary lymphoma of the large intestine is a recognized complication of both major types of chronic inflammatory bowel disease [20]. Those lymphomas complicating ulcerative colitis show a spectrum of low- and high-grade MALT-type B-cell lymphomas; as with carcinoma complicating ulcerative colitis, extent and longevity of disease appear to be the major risk factors [20]. Colorectal lymphoma complicating Crohn's disease is less common than either that complicating ulcerative colitis or small bowel lymphoma in Crohn's disease. These lymphomas represent a disparate group of B-cell and T-cell lymphomas [20]. Anorectal lymphoma is a not uncommon complication of the acquired immune deficiency syndrome (AIDS), whilst radiation, ureterosigmoidostomy and renal transplantation have all been complicated by malignant lymphoma of the large bowel [21–24].

Primary B-cell MALT lymphoma of the large intestine

Localized B-cell MALT-type lymphoma comprises the majority of primary lymphomas of the large intestine. They are most conveniently divided into low- and high-grade lesions, although this division is arbitrary and is associated with some controversy. Tumours comprising more than 20% blast cells have been considered high-grade tumours [2]. MALT-type lymphoma is by its nature polymorphic and this highly characteristic cellular polymorphism accounts for some of the difficulties and controversies in lymphoma grading. Associations between gastric *Helicobacter pylori* (HP) infection and lymphoma have been described, with evidence of regression of MALT-type colorectal lymphoma after antibiotic treatment for HP [25]. It remains uncertain how strong the relationship is between colorectal lymphoma and gastric HP. Furthermore type B Epstein–Barr virus (EBV) has been demonstrated by *in situ* hybridization in high-grade lymphomas of the colorectum [26]. It seems likely that the genesis of colorectal lymphoma is multifactorial as HP, EBV and chronic inflammation (especially ulcerative colitis) have all been implicated.

Low-grade lymphomas tend to be less infiltrative and more superficial and may remain localized for long periods. Most commonly these lesions present as annular or plaque-like thickenings of the large intestine, although many are exophytic and polypoid. High-grade lymphomas of MALT type are more likely to be aggressive infiltrative tumours showing long segment involvement, multicentricity and advanced stage (Fig. 39.2). Very occasional cases of proven MALT-type lymphoma present with multifocal polyposis-like involvement of the colorectum, masquerading as malignant lymphomatous polyposis of mantle cell type [27,28].

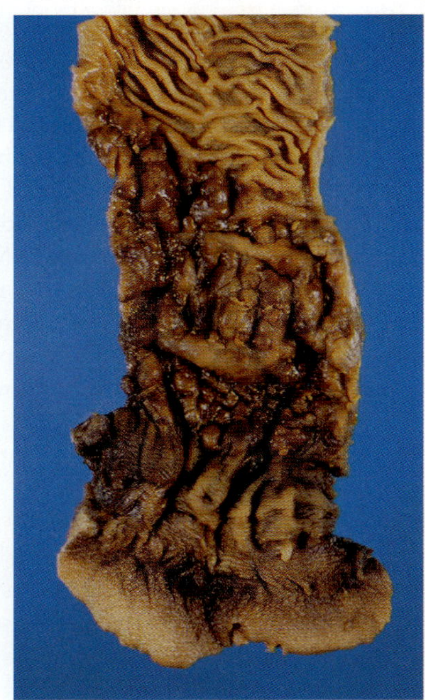

Fig. 39.2 A high-grade B-cell lymphoma of the rectum. There is characteristic diffuse, long segment involvement of the rectum, lower sigmoid colon and upper anal canal with extensive ulceration. The tumour showed massive involvement of local mesorectal lymph nodes.

As with MALT-type tumours elsewhere in the gut, these lymphomas show characteristic microscopic appearances. Low-grade lesions are characterized by large reactive germinal centres, surrounded by the lymphomatous cells. The commonest cells show the morphology of marginal zone lymphocytes, with features unfortunately similar to those of both mantle cells and follicle centre cells, the centrocytes. However, polymorphism, with prominent plasma cell differentiation and an admixture of blast cells, helps to differentiate this tumour from other lymphoma subtypes. If blast cells are numerous, making up more than 20% of the total, then a high-grade designation is appropriate [2].

Infiltration and destruction of the reactive germinal centres and of the mucosal epithelium of the colorectum comprise two morphological diagnostic discriminators for MALT-type lymphoma. The infiltration by, and destruction of, epithelium produces the characteristic lymphoepithelial lesion (LEL) (Fig. 39.3). These are not seen as often in intestinal MALT-type lymphoma as in their gastric counterpart. Also, lesions mimicking LELs do occur in other intestinal lymphomas, especially malignant lymphomatous polyposis (see below). Immunohistochemistry will demonstrate the B-cell nature of the tumour.

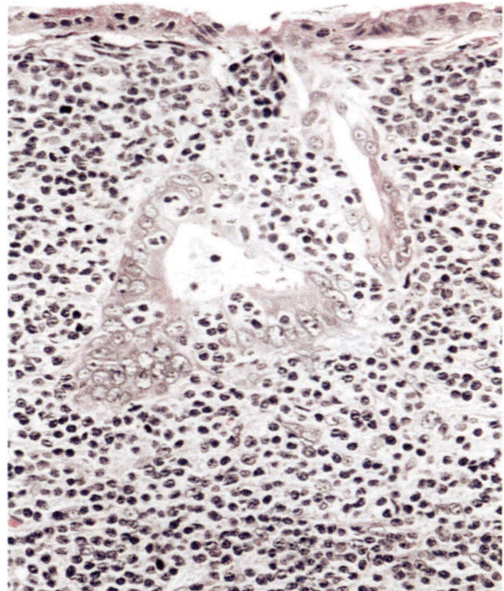

Fig. 39.3 Low-grade B-cell lymphoma of the colon. The central crypt is extensively infiltrated by lymphoid cells, producing the distinctive lymphoepithelial lesion.

As with MALT-type tumours elsewhere, often the most useful immunohistochemical marker is cytokeratin, as this will enhance the demonstration of epithelial destruction and LELs. There have been few formal studies of the molecular pathology of MALT-type lymphoma of the large intestine, because of the rarity of these lesions: a t(11;18) translocation with trisomy 3 has been described [29].

Low-grade tumours are, in general, amenable to local surgery and this may well be curative, if staging parameters are favourable. In general grade, stage and resectability determine the clinical behaviour and prognosis of these lymphomas [2,19]. Although low-grade lymphomas may show deep infiltration and local lymph node involvement, this is more common in high-grade lymphomas, and such staging may in turn preclude resection. Five-year survival rates for low-grade lymphoma are approximately 50%, with this figure falling to about 30% for high-grade tumours [2]. The efficacy of chemotherapy for these tumours remains marginal and its indications uncertain [19].

Malignant lymphomatous polyposis (mantle cell lymphoma)

This distinctive and relatively well characterized form of lymphoma represents about one-quarter of primary lymphomas of the colorectum [2,6,30]. Although it tends to present with large intestinal disease, the lymphoma also extensively involves the small bowel [6,30]. Gastric involvement is less pronounced, presumably because of the lack of lymphoid tissue in the normal stomach. The neoplasm usually presents with the physical effects of multiple polypoid masses in the intestine [30]. Thus mucous diarrhoea, steatorrhoea, protein-losing enteropathy or colopathy, abdominal pain and melaena are all recognized presentations. The lymphoma is a tumour of mantle cells, B-cell lymphocytes deriving from the mantle region, immediately adjacent to the germinal centre within lymphoid follicles. Also known as mantle cell lymphoma in the REAL classification, the tumour was originally termed multiple lymphomatous polyposis, a name that is still in regular usage. As polyposis implies the presence of multiple polyps, we believe this term should be discouraged because of tautology: malignant lymphomatous polyposis or simply lymphomatous polyposis would seem, to us, more appropriate.

Malignant lymphomatous polyposis (MLP) is exclusively a disease of adults, with a median age at presentation of 50 years. The condition is sporadic and no familial tendency has been recorded. Macroscopically the large intestinal mucosa shows innumerable relatively well circumscribed polypoid masses (Fig. 39.4). These are particularly found in the ileocaecal region (Fig. 39.4) [30]. Indeed the disease may present with an obstructing large mass, centred on the terminal ileum, and the involvement of the distal colon may only be detected subsequently. The lymphomatous polyps derive from pre-existing lymphoid aggregates and hence Peyer's patches of the small bowel and caecal and rectal LGCs are especially infiltrated by the neoplastic mantle cells. In advanced disease, most of the small and large bowel is involved (Fig. 39.4). The

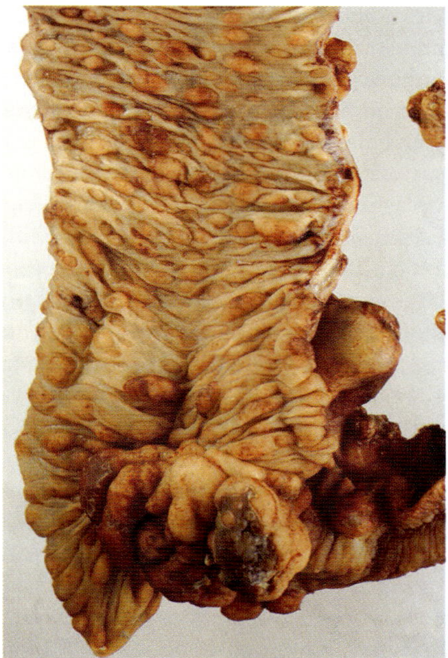

(a)

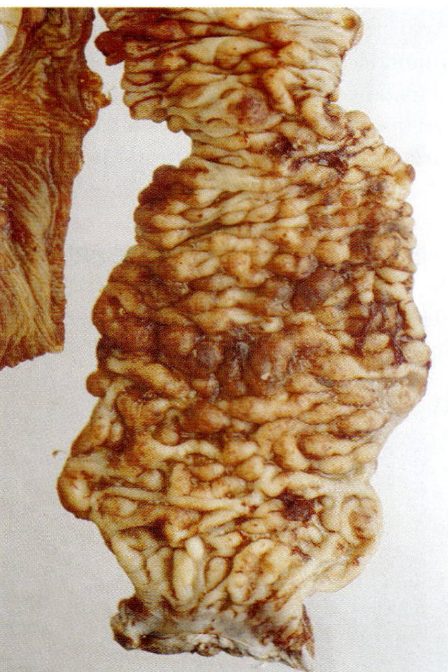

(b)

Fig. 39.4 Malignant lymphomatous polyposis of the colon and rectum: (a) the right colon demonstrating a mass lesion in the region of the terminal ileum and caecum with numerous polyps in the proximal colon and local lymph node involvement (at right); (b) the left colon and rectum from the same specimen showing massive polypoid rectal involvement.

polyps of MLP appear smooth because of the intact overlying mucosa, and usually measure between 0.5 cm and 1 cm. The endoscopic appearances are not unlike those of FAP.

Low-power microscopy reveals a characteristic nodular pattern: involvement is primarily in the lower mucosa and upper submucosa (Fig. 39.5). In smaller (and hence earlier) lesions, neoplastic mantle cells surround surviving germinal centres [6]. As the lesions become larger, the nodulation may be lost and the diffuse nature of the infiltrate becomes more apparent. High-power microscopy shows the relative monotonous infiltrate of small to intermediate-sized lymphoid cells with cleaved nuclei, inconsequential nucleoli and modest amounts of cytoplasm. These have a morphology, confusingly, like centrocytes of the germinal centre, and in the Kiel classification these tumours were known as diffuse centrocytic lymphoma [18]. Collections of epithelioid histiocytes, sometimes forming defined granulomas, are not uncommon. There is a variant of mantle cell lymphoma with larger blastoid cells: such cells are occasionally predominant in MLP.

Differentiation from low-grade malignant lymphoma of mucosa-associated lymphoid tissue may be difficult, especially on biopsy material. Whilst the morphological heterogeneity of MALT-type lymphoma and the presence of lymphoepithelial lesions (LELs) may be helpful, these are not specific. For instance, epithelial destruction in MLP often produces lesions that cannot be distinguished from classical LELs [6]. The relative paucity of blast cells in MLP may be helpful. However, the endoscopic appearances are usually the most helpful diagnostic indicator, although immunohistochemistry and even molecular analysis are required to fully substantiate the diagnosis of MLP. Mantle cell lymphoma is characterized by B lymphocytes that express CD5 and also cyclin-D1, neither of which is seen in MALT-type lymphoma, and hence these are useful discriminators of these diseases. The molecular basis of cyclin-D1 overexpression is a t(11,14) translocation in which the cyclin-D1 gene (on chromosome 11) is translocated to the immunoglobulin IgH gene on chromosome 14 [31]. MLP also shows bcl-1 gene rearrangement, further supporting the view that it is a gastrointestinal manifestation of mantle cell lymphoma [31].

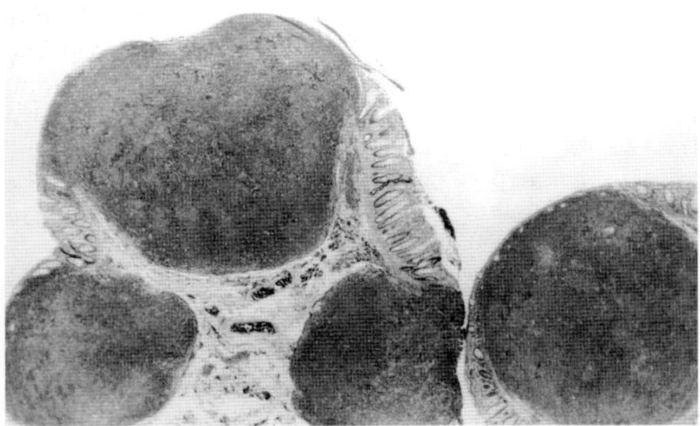

Fig. 39.5 Malignant lymphomatous polyposis. Circumscribed nodules of tumour are limited to the mucosa and submucosa.

Mantle cell lymphoma in general has a poor prognosis and MLP represents a relatively advanced and certainly multifocal stage of the lymphoma [2,30]. Bone marrow involvement is usually present at presentation: systemic disease and leukaemia are characteristic late features of MLP [6,30]. Because of its multifocal nature, major surgery is usually contraindicated although we have seen a case where the symptoms of colonic involvement (notably excessive mucus loss and electrolyte deficiency) necessitated emergency colectomy. Treatment is primarily by chemotherapy and the prognosis poor. In one series the majority of patients were dead in 5 years, despite treatment, with a mean survival of 3 years [32].

Other primary malignant lymphomas of the large intestine

MALT-type lymphoma and MLP make up the great majority of primary lymphomas in the large bowel. Burkitt-type lymphoma can involve the right colon in children, but this tumour is primarily of terminal ileal origin and is considered elsewhere (p. 380). Anorectal lymphoma is a recognized complication of AIDS. Most of these tumours are of high-grade type and show the features of diffuse large B-cell lymphoma or lymphoblastic lymphoma [33]. There is good evidence that these tumours are driven by EBV infection [34]. Despite the high-grade nature of these tumours, they are often confined to the anorectal region at presentation [35]. Nevertheless, as with extranodal lymphoma complicating AIDS at other sites, the prognosis is extremely poor [36]. T-cell lymphoma is relatively common in the small intestine but is distinctly unusual in the large bowel. There are isolated case reports of T-cell lymphomas, including one complicating Crohn's disease [20,37,38]. We have seen two examples of epitheliotropic T-cell lymphoma presenting in the large intestine, but these tumours more commonly affect the stomach and small intestine. Multifocality is a particular property of T-cell lymphomas in the gut, and rarely T-cell lymphoma can mimic MLP when involving the colon [39]. There are isolated reports of plasmacytomas in the large bowel and myelomatous involvement can lead to tumorous masses closely mimicking low- and high-grade lymphoma [40,41]. Large cell anaplastic lymphoma, primary to the rectum, has been described [42]. Curiously, follicular lymphoma is an extreme rarity in the large bowel. Reports of primary Hodgkin's disease of the large bowel should be treated with extreme scepticism. Many recorded cases of primary gastrointestinal Hodgkin's disease have been subsequently demonstrated to represent non-Hodgkin's lymphoma, often of T-cell phenotype.

The biopsy diagnosis of lymphoid tumours of the colorectum

The differentiation of benign lymphoid polyp/polyposis from malignant lymphoma is of critical importance. Endoscopic appearances and size are useful discriminators between benign and malignant lesions. However, low-grade lymphomas of MALT type in the rectum can be small and polypoid; they may also mimic benign lymphoid polyps histologically [9]. Ulceration is generally only a feature of lymphomas, which are usually appreciably larger than their benign counterparts. If the lesion is relatively small, then excisional biopsy will provide a fully representative, undistorted and well orientated specimen. The morphological discriminators of MALT-type lymphoma and MLP have been previously described but it is as well to emphasize the mimicry of MALT-type lymphoma by MLP histologically. Both lymphomas are characterized by a predominance of cells with centrocyte-like morphology and both may show lymphomatous destruction of epithelium. Their division, on biopsy material, can be difficult and all attention should paid to the clinical and colonoscopic features. Even then occasional cases of MALT-type tumour can manifest as polyposis [27,28]. With the ready availability of immunohistochemistry, it is advisable to perform this on all such cases: CD5 and cyclin-D1 immunohistochemistry will provide diagnostic results in nearly all cases. As favourable-stage MALT-type lymphoma is most appropriately treated by excisional surgery with or without chemotherapy and surgery is generally contraindicated in MLP, the importance of this distinction is indisputable.

Leukaemia in the large intestine

Acute myeloblastic leukaemia may cause tumorous masses in the large bowel. On occasion such granulocytic sarcomas may be the presenting feature of the disease, before the leukaemic phase [43]. The tumour cells have relatively plentiful eosinophilic cytoplasm, often with an eccentric nucleus. The cells themselves may mimic plasma cells or other primitive lymphoid cells and may lead to an erroneous diagnosis of malignant lymphoma, plasmacytoma or myelomatous involvement of the gut. Demonstration of chloroacetate esterase activity and lysozyme immunohistochemistry serve to confirm the diagnosis.

Connective tissue tumours

Despite the amount of connective tissue in the large bowel, these tumours are relatively unusual compared with their counterparts in other parts of the gut and with epithelial tumours of the colorectum. Lipomas are undoubtedly the commonest in the large bowel but they are usually discovered incidentally and do not, on the whole, cause symptoms. Most other connective tissue tumours present with the symptoms and signs of a mass effect in the colorectum. Of these gastrointestinal stromal tumours (GISTs) are the commonest but even these are unusual compared with GISTs arising in the stomach and small bowel.

Gastrointestinal stromal tumours

The concept of stromal tumours of the gut has undergone a radical overhaul in the last decade and we believe it is now apposite to consider most, if not all, tumours, with a spindle cell morphology and without identifying features indicating an origin from specific connective cells, as gastrointestinal stromal tumours (GISTs). This rethink has been prompted by the ready availability of immunohistochemistry for CD34 and c-kit and by molecular evidence [44,45]. It is not appropriate to recapitulate a comprehensive account of the histogenesis and the morphological features of gastrointestinal stromal tumours here as this subject has been dealt with elsewhere (p. 204). Although some have suggested that stromal tumours of the oesophagus and the colorectum, especially the rectum, are more likely to demonstrate specific features of smooth muscle tumours and should be largely considered as such [46,47], in general we prefer the broader brush approach (for the intestines at least) and to refer to all of these tumours, whatever their site of origin and their morphology, as GISTs. In this treatise, therefore, tumours that do not have the morphological features of specific entities such as neurilemmoma, neurofibroma or granular cell tumour have been regarded as GISTs. We do not deny that, rarely, tumours indistinguishable from leiomyomas elsewhere (e.g. in the uterus) do occur in the large bowel, specifically the rectum, but it is abundantly clear that such tumours are very rare in the colon and the majority of these tumours are therefore most conveniently regarded as GISTs.

GISTs are rare in the colon, compared with their gastric and small intestinal counterparts. For this reason, there is relatively little data on their histogenetic features, their behaviour and prognosis. Most studies indicate that the large bowel accounts for less than 10%, often less than 5%, of all GISTs [46–49]. Larger series of colonic spindle cell tumours predate the GIST concept and it is difficult to extract useful data from them [50–52]. Of particular importance is the fact that there is a much higher proportion of malignant GISTs, amongst colonic tumours, compared with GISTs elsewhere in the gut. Some show an epithelioid cell morphology, and some show the microscopic features of gastrointestinal autonomic nerve tumours (GANTs) (see p. 384).

It would appear that the ascending colon and transverse colon are the commonest sites for colonic GISTs and that most are large intramural masses, usually more than 5 cm in diameter and often in excess of 10 cm. Although some of these tumours share the morphological features of the apparently benign tumours, more characteristic of the stomach and small intestine, it is notoriously difficult to predict likely behaviour in these tumours. Time-honoured macroscopic and morphological features may be helpful. Size, the presence of necrosis, cellularity and tumour necrosis may be of some help. However, as with GISTs elsewhere, the mitotic rate supplies the most useful guide to likely behaviour and in its presence other parameters appear not to provide additional prognostic information. A rate of more than 10 mitoses per 10 high-power fields (hpf) will identify GISTs of high-grade malignancy [53,54]. Intermediate mitotic rates (between 1 and 3 mitoses per 30 hpf) have earned the appellation of borderline GIST [54] but there are effectively no data on this tumour, when in the colon, in the literature. Although pleomorphic sarcomas are relatively common amongst this group of tumours, occasional bizarre cells with grossly enlarged nuclei do occur in otherwise benign tumours and some care is advisable in assessing tumours with such cells, especially if they have low mitotic activity.

Frankly malignant GISTs, often termed pleomorphic sarcomas, are particularly aggressive, with high rates of metastatic disease (Fig. 39.6) [50–52]. These tumours characteristically cause blood-borne metastases; local lymph node involvement is an unusual feature [55]. One feature of such tumours which is relatively specific to the colon is that they may grow as confluent nodules in a longitudinal fashion, with a dominant mass and multinodular thickening of the adjacent colonic wall, a feature that is virtually never seen elsewhere in the gut [56]. This appearance is different from so-called leiomyomatosis of the colon, in which there are well separated nodules of spindle cell tumour [57], a lesion that is also seen in the oesophagus. Whether this extremely rare lesion is truly of smooth muscle derivation remains uncertain.

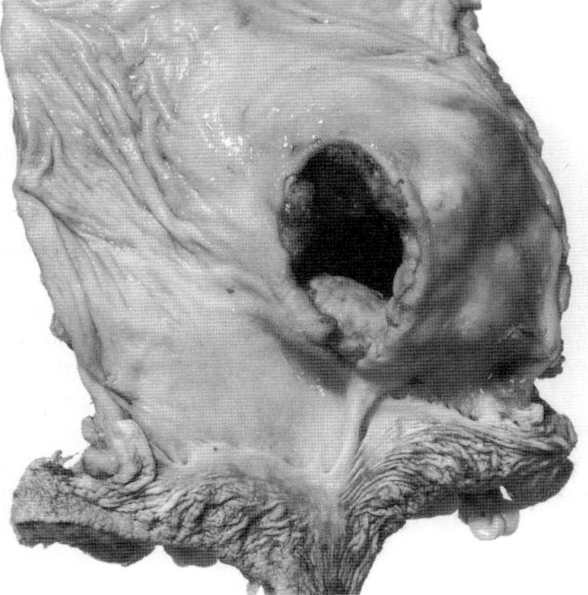

Fig. 39.6 A deep stromal tumour of the rectum. Although originally termed a leiomyosarcoma, this tumour has now been reclassified as a deep stromal tumour of the rectum. Its size with extensive ulceration and central necrosis presage a particularly aggressive behaviour.

The most significant features of GISTs, specific to the colon, are their rarity, their high malignant likelihood and their poorly defined management strategies. We cannot overemphasize the lack of predictability of many of these lesions: cases of small tumours with low mitotic activity have been described which have subsequently metastasized, often many years after the primary tumour has been excised. We would regard any colonic GIST as a potentially malignant lesion and would generally advise relatively radical surgery, if clinically indicated.

Stromal tumours in the rectum

Despite the concept of GISTs and the intentions of many to regard all spindle cells tumours of the gastrointestinal tract within this broad umbrella term, there is evidence that primary smooth muscle tumours do occur in the large bowel and that these are almost entirely restricted to the rectum and distal sigmoid colon [56]. The majority of tumours showing such definitive evidence of smooth muscle derivation derive from the muscularis mucosae. Indeed the rectum is the only part of the gut where tumours arise from the muscularis mucosae with any frequency [56]. These leiomyomas present as small intramucosal and submucosal nodules visible to the endoscopist as a small elevation [58]. They are usually incidental findings, only about 5 mm in diameter, although occasionally they may reach a size of 15 mm [58]. Whilst these occur at any age, they are slightly commoner in men with a male : female ratio of 1.8 : 1 [58]. Apart from the oesophageal leiomyoma, this rectal lesion is the only tumour of the gut characterized by morphologically typical (albeit apparently hypertrophic) smooth muscle cells with the typical bundling morphology [56]. They are almost universally benign [56,58].

Whilst the leiomyomatous polyp, arising from the muscularis mucosae, is undoubtedly the commonest spindle cell tumour of the rectum, there is a further spindle cell tumour of the lower rectum and anus with distinctive features. This tumour has become known as the deep intramural stromal tumour of the rectum [56,59]. It arises from the deep tissues of the rectum and anal canal and appears to derive from the muscularis propria (Fig. 39.6). Local recurrence is a characteristic feature of this tumour (in about half of cases) and late metastatic disease is also a considerable problem. It is possible that the high rate of metastatic disease, often after a considerable time period since primary surgery, relates to the inadequacy of that surgery, for this tumour is often treated initially by local excision only [55,58,59].

Deep intramural stromal tumours of the rectum are usually moderately large at presentation, because of their deep position in the anorectal wall, and often measure in excess of 5 cm

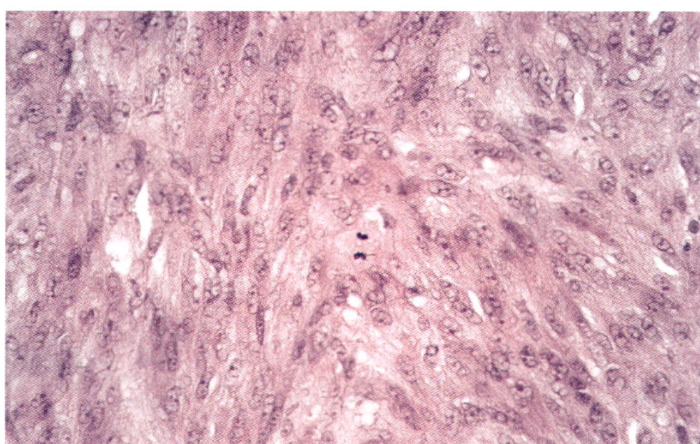

Fig. 39.7 A deep stromal tumour of the rectum. The tumour is spindle celled but with marked nuclear anaplasia and a high mitotic activity. The tumour recurred after local excision and ultimately the patient died of metastatic disease.

in diameter. Histologically they tend to be composed of relatively regular spindle cells with darkly staining nuclei in a fascicular pattern (Fig. 39.7) [56]. Those tumours that locally recur, or metastasize, are more cellular, with very closely packed spindle cells, and have the higher mitotic activity. These tumours should be treated aggressively because of their propensity for local recurrence. However, reports would suggest that, whilst radicality may prevent local recurrence, it may not materially affect the potential for metastatic disease and overall survival [56,58].

Tumours of adipose tissue

Lipoma

Whilst clinically significant lipomas are uncommon, small submucosal lipomas are not so very unusual as an incidental finding at colonoscopy. The right side of the colon is the commonest site (Fig. 39.8) [60,61]. Such lesions are seen at colonoscopy or in resection specimens as small (usually less than 2 cm) yellow circumscribed nodules with an intact overlying mucosa. Only in larger lesions is there surface ulceration: this may be a mechanical effect and does not imply, necessarily, any malignant likelihood (Fig. 39.8). Much larger lesions, especially in the right colon, may present because of a mass lesion, or characteristically with intussusception (Fig. 39.8). We have seen several examples of large bowel obstruction with intussusception caused by a large proximal colonic lipoma. The angiographic mimicry of angiodysplasia (angioectasia) of the proximal colon by lipoma has been described as lipomas have a large feeder vessel and produce a blush of smaller vessels like that seen in angiodysplasia [61].

Colorectal lipomas are usually single but are on occasion multiple. The term lipomatosis infers the presence of multiple lipomas. There are occasional case reports of lipomatosis

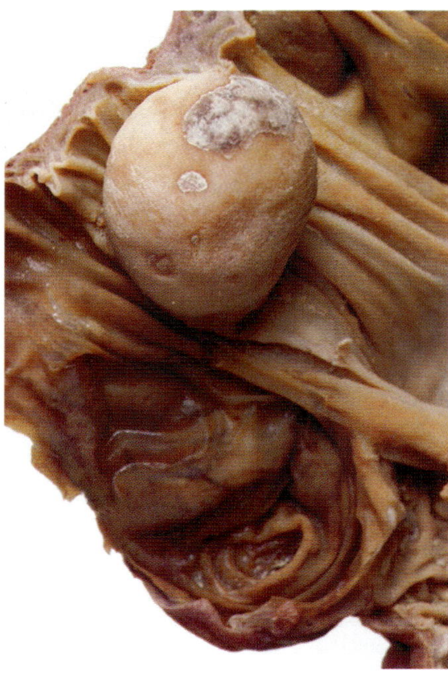

Fig. 39.8 A right hemicolectomy specimen demonstrating an intussuscepted lipoma of the proximal colon. The surface ulceration is a mechanical effect and does not indicate malignancy in this case.

occurring in the colonic submucosa [62,63], also involving the small bowel [64], in the appendices epiploicae [63] and in the pelvic connective tissues [65]. Such lipomatosis can result in multiple polyps in the colon and has been referred to as lipomatous polyposis [66]. As with other rare polyposis syndromes, there is potential mimicry of the more common and significant polyposis syndromes. It is probable that multiplicity of these fatty tumours is a hamartomatous phenomenon rather than a neoplastic one: there is no malignant potential of either solitary lipomas or lipomatosis.

Microscopically, the appearances of lipoma are those of simple adipose tissue, with circumscribed masses of adipocytes compressing the adjacent muscularis mucosae (Fig. 39.9) and, sometimes, the underlying muscularis propria. Necrosis and haemorrhage may occur if there are secondary mechanical effects, such as intussusception. Some lesions in this situation show much granulation tissue formation and this can be superficially disconcerting to the diagnostic pathologist. Atypical features, akin to those seen in lipomas of the subcutis, can be seen; these lesions have been termed atypical lipoma [67]. However frank liposarcoma is an extreme rarity in the colon and should only be diagnosed when lipoblasts are definitively demonstrated [67].

Lipohyperplasia of the ileocaecal valve

This condition, also known as lipomatosis and lipomatous hypertrophy of the ileocaecal valve, is characterized by an

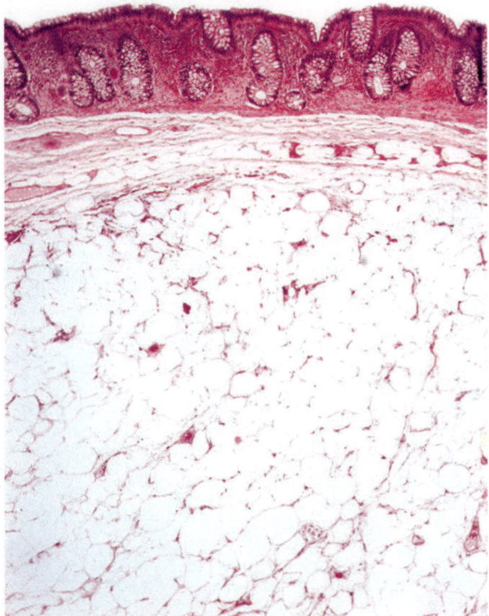

Fig. 39.9 A colonic lipoma showing the typical submucosal position with the compressed but otherwise normal overlying mucosa.

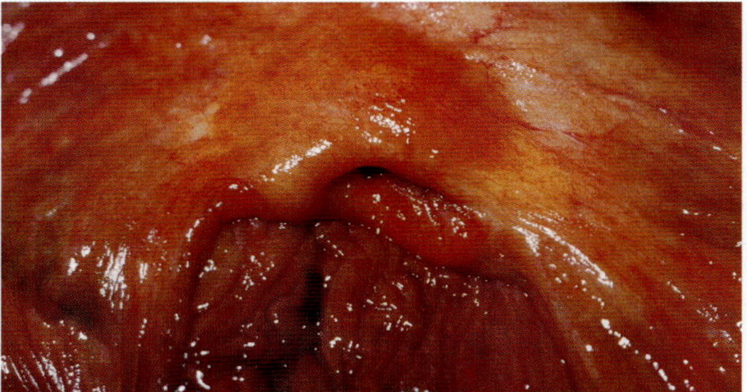

Fig. 39.10 Lipohyperplasia of the ileocaecal valve. The appearance has been likened to a pouting cervix uteri.

excess of adipose tissue in the submucosa of the ileocaecal valve producing thickening and pouting of the valve which protrudes into the caecum [68,69]. The thickening of the valve may produce narrowing of the lumen and the appearances of the valve have been likened to those of prolapsed haemorrhoids or a pouting cervix uteri (Fig. 39.10). In our experience mild lipohyperplasia of the ileocaecal valve is extremely common. Less commonly, especially in association with prolapse into the caecal lumen, the neoplasm-like prominence of the valve can masquerade as a malignant tumour on barium enema. Right hemicolectomy has been performed, on occasion, in the mistaken belief that a malignant tumour had been demonstrated radiologically. It may give rise, rarely, to symptoms of subacute obstruction and is but one cause of the ileocaecal valve syndrome [70].

The condition is, unsurprisingly, closely associated with obesity and histological examination reveals an excess of histologically normal adipose tissue in the submucosa. This accumulation is not encapsulated and gradually diminishes on either side of the valve. Occasionally the adipotic valve becomes congested and eroded with ulceration and bleeding. The lesion, which we believe is best termed lipohyperplasia as it is simply an increase in fatty tissue within the valve, should not be confused with lipoma or with true intestinal lipomatosis.

Vascular tumours of the large intestine

Haemangiomas

Most 'haemangiomas' are not true neoplasms at all but are merely malformations or hamartomas. Nevertheless they may present as mass lesions and are appropriately considered here. They usually present with rectal bleeding or with mechanical effects such as intussusception. Most haemangiomas of the large bowel are of the extensive cavernous type [71], most often in the sigmoid colon and/or rectum. Here they may involve a relatively long segment whilst involvement of the whole colon has been reported [72]. The angiomatous abnormality involves the entire blood supply, including perirectal or pericolic tissues as well as vessels within the bowel wall. We have seen cases where there is also extensive involvement of the ischiorectal fossa and the musculature of the buttock, unilaterally. Such involvement makes surgical treatment very difficult. Angiographic embolization has been attempted with some success, although there are dangers of causing necrosis of the bowel wall and other important structures.

Macroscopically, the colonic or rectal mucosa has a plum-coloured appearance but is intact and otherwise normal. Huge, tortuous vascular spaces can be seen in the bowel wall and adjacent tissues. These often contain easily recognizable phleboliths that show up radiographically and are a useful diagnostic sign. The microscopical appearance is like that of haemangiomas elsewhere, often with intravascular thrombosis as a prominent feature.

Multiplicity of haemangiomas can be seen in several conditions, some well defined and others less so. The blue rubber bleb naevus syndrome [73] is associated with cutaneous vascular naevi and prominent, often life-threatening gastrointestinal haemorrhage. The lesions are small (less than 0.5 cm) and have a blue wrinkled surface. In the colon, the haemangiomas are more likely to be left-sided and in the rectum. The Klippel–Trenaunay–Weber syndrome associates soft tissue and bone hypertrophy, varicose veins and port wine haemangiomas with vascular malformations of the gut. An apparent *forme fruste* of Peutz–Jeghers syndrome, due to incomplete penetrance of the gene, may result in multiple intestinal haemangiomas [73]. Histological assessment of these lesions, unless at the time of colonic resection, is not usually undertaken due to the considerable risks of inducing severe haemorrhage. Most of these lesions simply show the features of cavernous haemangiomas [74].

Other vascular tumours of the large intestine

Haemangiopericytomas [75] and glomus tumours [56] do occur in the colon and rectum but both are distinctly unusual. They show similar macroscopic and microscopic pathology to those seen elsewhere. We have seen one example of an angiosarcoma affecting the colon but meaningful discussion is not appropriate, as this malignancy is so rare in the colon. Much more common, in the context of AIDS, is Kaposi's sarcoma of the colon, rectum and anus. In the gut, small intestinal involvement is commonest in autopsy practice but gastric and colorectal involvement is more likely to be seen in clinical practice [76]. The disease is often multifocal and affects several parts of the gut. The presence of Kaposi's sarcoma in the intestines reflects advanced immune suppression. The disease itself does not necessarily imply a poor prognosis but the advanced immunosuppression that it is a marker of may do so [76,77].

Approximately one-quarter of AIDS sufferers will have Kaposi's sarcoma and about 40–50% of these will show gastrointestinal involvement [76,77]. It is almost exclusively a disease of homosexual men with AIDS. It presents colonoscopically in diverse forms. It may appear as a macular bluish lesion but polypoid, eruptive and papular variants are also described [76,78]. Kaposi's sarcoma masquerading as ulcerative colitis is also well recognized [79]. The neoplasm, now convincingly linked to human herpes virus 8 (HHV8) [80], is characterized histologically by pleomorphic spindle cells with adjacent clefts in which red cells are enmeshed. Haemorrhage, both old and recent, is usually demonstrated and hyaline droplets are characteristic features within the cytoplasm of the tumour cells.

Lymphangioma

Lymphangiomas of the colon and rectum are very uncommon and are usually found incidentally during investigations for unassociated symptomatology [81]. There is a confusing plethora of terminology, including lymphatic cyst, mesenteric cyst and cystic hygroma, which all probably represent the same spectrum of pathology. Along with haemangioma in the intestines, it is likely that lymphangioma is not a true neoplasm at all but rather a developmental abnormality or acquired as a hamartoma-like lesion. Lymphangiomas are more likely to involve the mesenteric tissues rather than the bowel wall itself. They may occur as polypoid lesions of the colonic submucosa, on a broad base, although more often they are ill-defined diffuse lesions in the colonic wall [81]. Their cut surfaces show cystic spaces from which lymph may exude. Histologically they are composed of widely dilated lymphatic spaces within which lymphocytes can be identified. These lesions should not be confused with lymphangiectasia, a condition that much more diffusely involves the intestinal mucosa and submucosa. Whilst lymphangiectasia is usually small intestinal and associated with protein-losing enteropathy, colonic variants have been rarely described [82,83].

Neurogenic tumours

Before initiating discussion on neurogenic tumours of the large intestine, it is appropriate to reaffirm the concept of gastrointestinal stromal tumours (GISTs). It is possible that GISTs in the large bowel, especially the colon, whether benign or malignant, may show some evidence of neural differentiation, particularly by immunohistochemistry. If such lesions conform to the general morphological descriptions of GISTs given elsewhere (see pp. 204, 383 and 615), then such lesions are appropriately considered as GISTs with their attendant (often uncertain) management strategies and prognosis. This section will consider those tumours with definitive morphological and immunohistochemical evidence of an origin in neural tissue within the large bowel.

Solitary benign neurofibroma of the rectum or colon is very rare as an isolated lesion. They usually present incidentally as small submucosal tumours that may diffusely involve the overlying mucosa (Fig. 39.11). This is not a feature, *per se*, to indicate any aggressive behaviour, but is more part of the character of diffuse-type neurofibromas seen elsewhere. The appearance has been likened to that of an early juvenile polyp in the colonic mucosa [56]. Even a solitary neurofibroma in the rectum may yet presage the presence of von Recklinghausen's disease [84] and it is wise to always raise this possibility when reporting such lesions. Gastrointestinal involvement is common in von Recklinghausen's disease [85], although the colon seems to be involved less frequently than the small intestine [86]. To add to the confusion concerning neurogenic differen-

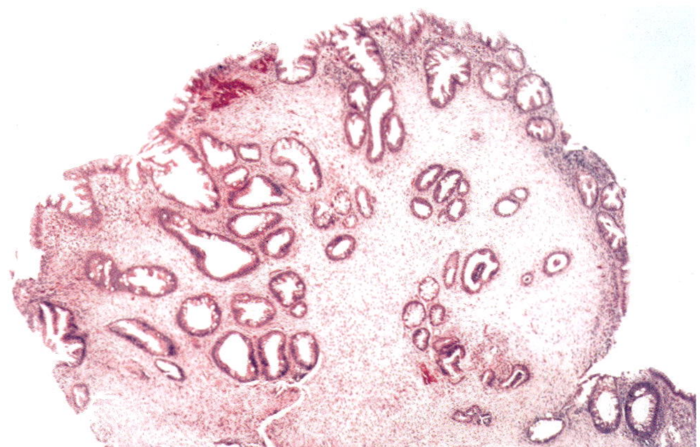

Fig. 39.11 A colonic neurofibroma. There is diffuse involvement of the overlying mucosa, a feature of no sinister significance. Curiously the surface of the mucosa shows metaplastic-type change.

tiation and GISTs, tumours with the morphological features of GISTs are relatively common features of von Recklinghausen's disease [86]. The neurofibromas of von Recklinghausen's disease may present either with obstruction or, more commonly, bleeding [87,88]. Carcinoid tumours and spindle cell sarcomas are both recognized complications of colorectal neurofibromatosis [86,89]. Neurilemmoma (schwannoma) appears to be excessively rare in the large intestine.

Ganglioneuroma and ganglioneuromatosis represent the ends of a spectrum of neurogenic lesions that contain Schwann cell, ganglion cell and neurite derivatives. Solitary ganglioneuroma of the colorectum is very rare and is much more likely to be seen in the retroperitoneum. It has been confusingly described as localized ganglioneuromatosis [90]. Ganglioneuromatosis itself represents a spectrum of disease from diffuse colorectal involvement to disease that is predominantly submucosal and results in polypoid masses in the large bowel. Diffuse intestinal ganglioneuromatosis, medullary carcinoma of the thyroid, phaeochromocytoma and multiple mucosal neuromas together comprise the inherited syndrome now known as multiple endocrine neoplasia (MEN) type IIb [90,91]. Although phaeochromocytoma and von Recklinghausen's disease frequently coexist, the neural tumours in neurofibromatosis and MEN-IIb differ in their distribution and histological appearances. Neurofibromas are made up of loose fibrous tissue with cells having their characteristic wavy appearance interspersed with occasional nerve fibres. The absence of ganglion cells would be consistent with a defect involving the sympathetic nerve supply to the gut. Diffuse ganglioneuromatosis, on the other hand, involves the nerves and the nerve cell bodies (ganglion cells) of the nerve plexuses and has no connective tissue component. The defect here may involve the parasympathetic nerve supply or non-adrenergic, non-cholinergic enteric nerves. Polypoid ganglioneuromatosis differs from diffuse intestinal ganglioneuromatosis in that the neural proliferation lies within the lamina propria and gives rise to mucosal polyps. There are recognized associations between polypoid ganglioneuromatosis on the one hand and juvenile polyposis and Cowden's syndrome on the other [92–94]. This demonstrates that the genetic defects associated with these polyposis syndromes affect many tissue types other than epithelium.

Submucosal, myenteric and subserosal neuronal hyperplasia is a common accompaniment of Crohn's disease, and the disorganized proliferation of several connective tissue elements, including nerves, ganglia, blood vessels, adipose tissue and smooth muscle has been likened to a hamartomatous lesion [95]. On occasion traumatic neuroma may be seen after previous surgery in the colon [96]. Granular cell tumours, now compellingly demonstrated to be tumours of nerve sheath origin, are an excessively rare lesion in the large intestine [97–99]. They show morphological identity to their more common counterparts in the skin and at other sites. It is likely that primary neurofibrosarcomas of the large bowel do exist but it is probable that such tumours have been, and will be, regarded as malignant GISTs unless evidence of their neural derivation is compelling.

Miscellaneous tumours of the colorectum and the retrorectal space

Very rarely other sarcomas have been described in the colon and rectum, including fibrosarcoma and rhabdomyosarcoma, but it is likely that many of these represent secondary involvement of the large bowel. Tumours arising in the retrorectal space may manifest as anorectal masses. Benign lesions include retrorectal cystic hamartomas (tailgut cysts) (see p. 664) and benign cystic teratomas. Chordoma and myxopapillary ependymoma, arising in or close to the sacrum, may secondarily involve the rectum. The 'Ivalon tumour' produces confounding histological appearances to the unwary [100]. Rectopexy, performed for rectal prolapse, using Ivalon, a sponge-like material, may result in a mass effect, often several years after the primary surgery. Removal of the mass and submission for histopathology has confused many a pathologist. This is because the Ivalon itself has an appearance not unlike osteoid and the incitement of a histiocytic and giant cell reaction, the latter resembling osteoclasts, further emphasizes the mimicry of a bone tumour. Viewing the lesion under cross-polarized light identifies the foreign material within the lesion and prevents the dispatching of a potentially embarrassing pathology report.

References

1 Richards MA. Lymphoma of the colon and rectum. *Postgrad Med J*, 1986; 62: 615.
2 Shepherd NA, Hall PA, Coates PJ, Levison DA. Primary malignant lymphoma of the colon and rectum. A histopathological and immunohistochemical analysis of 45 cases with clinicopathological correlations. *Histopathology*, 1988; 12: 235.
3 O'Leary AD, Sweeney EC. Lymphoglandular complexes of the colon: structure and distribution. *Histopathology*, 1986; 10: 267.
4 Flejou JF, Potet F, Bogomoletz WV *et al*. Lymphoid follicular proctitis. A condition different from ulcerative proctitis? *Dig Dis Sci*, 1988; 33: 314.
5 Yeong ML, Bethwaite PB, Prasad J, Isbister WH. Lymphoid follicular hyperplasia—a distinctive feature of diversion colitis. *Histopathology*, 1991; 19: 55.
6 Lavergne A, Brouland JP, Launay E, Nemeth J, Ruskone-Fourmestraux A, Galian A. Multiple lymphomatous polyposis of the gastrointestinal tract. An extensive histopathologic and immunohistochemical study of 12 cases. *Cancer*, 1994; 74: 3042.
7 Cornes JS, Wallace MH, Morson BC. Benign lymphomas of the rectum and anal canal. *J Pathol Bacteriol*, 1961; 82: 371.
8 Lloyd J, Darzi A, Teare J, Goldin RD. A solitary benign lymphoid polyp of the rectum in a 51 year old woman. *J Clin Pathol*, 1997; 50: 1034.

9 Schmid C, Vazquez JJ, Diss TC, Isaacson PG. Primary B-cell mucosa-associated lymphoid tissue lymphoma presenting as a solitary colorectal polyp. *Histopathology*, 1994; 24: 357.

10 Atwell JD, Burge D, Wright D. Nodular lymphoid hyperplasia of the intestinal tract in infancy and childhood. *J Pediatr Surg*, 1985; 20: 25.

11 Louw JH. Polypoid lesions of the large bowel in children with particular reference to benign lymphoid polyposis. *J Pediatr Surg*, 1968; 3: 195.

12 Shaw EB, Hennigar GR. Intestinal lymphoid polyposis. *Am J Clin Pathol*, 1974; 61: 417.

13 Benchimol D, Frileux P, Herve de Sigalony JP, Parc R. Benign lymphoid polyposis of the colon. Report of a case in an adult. *Int J Colorectal Dis*, 1991; 6: 165.

14 Berk T, Cohen Z, McLeod RS, Cullen JB. Surgery based on misdiagnosis of adenomatous polyposis. The Canadian Polyposis Registry experience. *Dis Colon Rectum*, 1987; 30: 588.

15 Crump M, Gospodarowicz M, Shepherd FA. Lymphoma of the gastrointestinal tract. *Semin Oncol*, 1999; 26: 324.

16 Isaacson PG, Norton AJ. *Extranodal Lymphomas*. Edinburgh: Churchill Livingstone, 1994: 15.

17 Isaacson PG. The revised European-American lymphoma (REAL) classification [editorial]. *Clin Oncol (R Coll Radiol)* 1995; 7: 347.

18 Stansfeld AG, Diebold J, Noel H *et al*. Updated Kiel classification for lymphomas. *Lancet*, 1988; 1: 292.

19 Zighelboim J, Larson MV. Primary colonic lymphoma. Clinical presentation, histopathologic features, and outcome with combination chemotherapy. *J Clin Gastroenterol*, 1994; 18: 291.

20 Shepherd NA, Hall PA, Williams GT *et al*. Primary malignant lymphoma of the large intestine complicating chronic inflammatory bowel disease. *Histopathology*, 1989; 15: 325.

21 Sibly TF, Keane RM, Lever JV, Southwood WF. Rectal lymphoma in radiation injured bowel. *Br J Surg*, 1985; 72: 879.

22 Coggon DN, Rose DH, Ansell ID. A large bowel lymphoma complicating renal transplantation. *Br J Radiol*, 1981; 54: 418.

23 Ghanem AN, Perry KC. Malignant lymphoma as a complication of ureterosigmoidostomy. *Br J Surg*, 1985; 72: 559.

24 Fan CW, Chen JS, Wang JY, Fan HA. Perforated rectal lymphoma in a renal transplant recipient: report of a case. *Dis Colon Rectum*, 1997; 40: 1258.

25 Matsumoto T, Iida M, Shimizu M. Regression of mucosa-associated lymphoid-tissue lymphoma of rectum after eradication of *Helicobacter pylori*. *Lancet*, 1997; 350: 115.

26 Kim YS, Kim JB, Kang YK, Nam ES, Park SH, Kim I. Viral genotypes and p53 expression in Epstein–Barr virus-associated primary malignant lymphomas of the intestines. *Hum Pathol*, 1999; 30: 1146.

27 Yatabe Y, Nakamura S, Nakamura T *et al*. Multiple polypoid lesions of primary mucosa-associated lymphoid-tissue lymphoma of colon. *Histopathology*, 1998; 32: 116.

28 Breslin NP, Urbanski SJ, Shaffer EA. Mucosa-associated lymphoid tissue (MALT) lymphoma manifesting as multiple lymphomatosis polyposis of the gastrointestinal tract. *Am J Gastroenterol*, 1999; 94: 2540.

29 Hosaka S, Akamatsu T, Nakamura S *et al*. Mucosa-associated lymphoid tissue (MALT) lymphoma of the rectum with chromosomal translocation of the t(11;18)(q21;q21) and an additional aberration of trisomy 3. *Am J Gastroenterol*, 1999; 94: 1951.

30 Isaacson PG, MacLennan KA, Subbuswamy SG. Multiple lymphomatous polyposis of the gastrointestinal tract. *Histopathology*, 1984; 8: 641.

31 Kumar S, Krenacs L, Otsuki T *et al*. bcl-1 rearrangement and cyclin D1 protein expression in multiple lymphomatous polyposis. *Am J Clin Pathol*, 1996; 105: 737.

32 Ruskone-Fourmestraux A, Aegerter P, Delmer A, Brousse N, Galian A, Rambaud JC. Primary digestive tract lymphoma: a prospective multicentric study of 91 patients. Groupe d'Etude des Lymphomes Digestifs. *Gastroenterology*, 1993; 105: 1662.

33 Reynolds P, Saunders LD, Layefsky ME, Lemp GF. The spectrum of acquired immunodeficiency syndrome (AIDS)-associated malignancies in San Francisco, 1980–1987. *Am J Epidemiol*, 1993; 137: 19.

34 Levine AM. AIDS-associated malignant lymphoma. *Med Clin North Am*, 1992; 76: 253.

35 Ioachim HL, Weinstein MA, Robbins RD, Sohn N, Lugo PN. Primary anorectal lymphoma. A new manifestation of the acquired immune deficiency syndrome (AIDS). *Cancer*, 1987; 60: 1449.

36 Cappell MS, Botros N. Predominantly gastrointestinal symptoms and signs in 11 consecutive AIDS patients with gastrointestinal lymphoma: a multicenter, multiyear study including 763 HIV-seropositive patients. *Am J Gastroenterol*, 1994; 89: 545.

37 Nagai T, Koyama R, Sasagawa Y *et al*. Diffuse infiltrating T-cell lymphoma of the colon associated with polyclonal hypergammaglobulinemia and hepatocellular carcinoma: report of a case. *Jpn J Med*, 1991; 30: 57.

38 Son HJ, Rhee PL, Kim JJ *et al*. Primary T-cell lymphoma of the colon. *Korean J Intern Med*, 1997; 12: 238.

39 Hirakawa K, Fuchigami T, Nakamura S *et al*. Primary gastrointestinal T-cell lymphoma resembling multiple lymphomatous polyposis. *Gastroenterology*, 1996; 111: 778.

40 Baumgartner BR, Hartmann TM. Extramedullary plasmacytoma of the colon. *Am J Gastroenterol*, 1985; 80: 1017.

41 Griffiths AP, Shepherd NA, Beddall A, Williams JG. Gastrointestinal tumour masses due to multiple myeloma: a pathological mimic of malignant lymphoma. *Histopathology*, 1997; 31: 318.

42 Morphopoulos G, Pitt MA, Bisset DL. Primary anaplastic large cell lymphoma of the rectum. *Histopathology*, 1995; 26: 190.

43 Catalano MF, Levin B, Hart RS, Troncoso P, DuBrow RA, Estey EH. Granulocytic sarcoma of the colon. *Gastroenterology*, 1991; 100: 555.

44 Miettinen M, Sarlomo-Rikala M, Lasota J. Gastrointestinal stromal tumors: recent advances in understanding of their biology. *Hum Pathol*, 1999; 30: 1213.

45 Chan JK. Mesenchymal tumors of the gastrointestinal tract: a paradise for acronyms (STUMP, GIST, GANT, and now GIPACT), implication of c-kit in genesis, and yet another of the many emerging roles of the interstitial cell of Cajal in the pathogenesis of gastrointestinal diseases? *Adv Anat Pathol*, 1999; 6: 19.

46 Miettinen M, Sarlomo RM, Lasota J. Gastrointestinal stromal tumours. *Ann Chir Gynaecol*, 1998; 87: 278.

47 Ueyama T, Guo KJ, Hashimoto H, Daimaru Y, Enjoji M. A clinicopathologic and immunohistochemical study of gastrointestinal stromal tumors. *Cancer*, 1992; 69: 947.
48 Erlandson RA, Klimstra DS, Woodruff JM. Subclassification of gastrointestinal stromal tumors based on evaluation by electron microscopy and immunohistochemistry. *Ultrastruct Pathol*, 1996; 20: 373.
49 Rudolph P, Bonichon F, Gloeckner K *et al*. Comparative analysis of prognostic indicators for sarcomas of the soft parts and the viscerae. *Verh Dtsch Ges Pathol*, 1998; 82: 246.
50 Tang CK, Melamed MR. Leiomyosarcoma of the colon exclusive of the rectum. *Am J Gastroenterol*, 1975; 64: 376.
51 Meijer S, Peretz T, Gaynor JJ *et al*. Primary colorectal sarcoma. A retrospective review and prognostic factor study of 50 consecutive patients. *Arch Surg*, 1990; 125: 1163.
52 Moyana TN, Friesen R, Tan LK. Colorectal smooth-muscle tumors. A pathobiologic study with immunohistochemistry and histomorphometry. *Arch Pathol Lab Med*, 1991; 115: 1016.
53 Evans HL. Smooth muscle tumors of the gastrointestinal tract. A study of 56 cases followed for a minimum of 10 years. *Cancer*, 1985; 56: 2242.
54 Newman PL, Wadden C, Fletcher CD. Gastrointestinal stromal tumours: correlation of immunophenotype with clinicopathological features. *J Pathol*, 1991; 164: 107.
55 Akwari OE, Dozois RR, Weiland LH, Beahrs OH. Leiomyosarcoma of the small and large bowel. *Cancer*, 1978; 42: 1375.
56 Appelman HD. Mesenchymal tumors of the gastrointestinal tract. In: Ming S, Goldman H, eds. *Pathology of the Gastrointestinal Tract*. Baltimore: Williams & Wilkins, 1998: 361.
57 Freni SC, Keeman JN. Leiomyomatosis of the colon. *Cancer*, 1977; 39: 263.
58 Walsh TH, Mann CV. Smooth muscle neoplasms of the rectum and anal canal. *Br J Surg*, 1984; 71: 597.
59 Haque S, Dean PJ. Stromal neoplasms of the rectum and anal canal. *Hum Pathol*, 1992; 23: 762.
60 Michowitz M, Lazebnik N, Noy S, Lazebnik R. Lipoma of the colon. A report of 22 cases. *Am Surg*, 1985; 51: 449.
61 Ryan J, Martin JE, Pollock DJ. Fatty tumours of the large intestine: a clinicopathological review of 13 cases. *Br J Surg*, 1989; 76: 793.
62 Ling CS, Leagus C, Stahlgren LH. Intestinal lipomatosis. *Surgery*, 1959; 46: 1054.
63 Swain VA, Young WF, Pringle EM. Hypertrophy of the appendices epiploicae and lipomatous polyposis of the colon. *Gut*, 1969; 10: 587.
64 Climie AR, Wylin RF. Small-intestinal lipomatosis. *Arch Pathol Lab Med*, 1981; 105: 40.
65 Jones DJ, Dharmeratnam R, Langstaff RJ. Large bowel obstruction due to pelvic lipomatosis. *Br J Surg*, 1985; 72: 309.
66 Yatto RP. Colonic lipomatosis. *Am J Gastroenterol*, 1982; 77: 436.
67 Snover DC. Atypical lipomas of the colon. Report of two cases with pseudomalignant features. *Dis Colon Rectum*, 1984; 27: 485.
68 Elliott GB, Sandy JT, Elliott KA, Sherkat A. Lipohyperplasia of the ileocecal valve. *Can J Surg*, 1968; 11: 179.
69 Boquist L, Bergdahl L, Andersson A. Lipomatosis of the ileocecal valve. *Cancer*, 1972; 29: 136.
70 Gazet JC. The ileocaecal valve syndrome. *Br J Surg*, 1964; 51: 371.
71 Mills CS, Lloyd TV, Van Aman ME, Lucas J. Diffuse hemangiomatosis of the colon. *J Clin Gastroenterol*, 1985; 7: 416.
72 Westerholm P. A case of diffuse haemangiomatosis of the colon and rectum. *Acta Chir Scand*, 1966; 109: 173.
73 Camilleri M, Chadwick VS, Hodgson HJ. Vascular anomalies of the gastrointestinal tract. *Hepatogastroenterology*, 1984; 31: 149.
74 Boley SJ, Brandt LJ, Mitsudo SM. Vascular lesions of the colon. *Adv Intern Med*, 1984; 29: 301.
75 Genter B, Mir R, Strauss R *et al*. Hemangiopericytoma of the colon: report of a case and review of literature. *Dis Colon Rectum*, 1982; 25: 149.
76 Parente F, Cernuschi M, Orlando G, Rizzardini G, Lazzarin A, Bianchi PG. Kaposi's sarcoma and AIDS: frequency of gastrointestinal involvement and its effect on survival. A prospective study in a heterogeneous population. *Scand J Gastroenterol*, 1991; 26: 1007.
77 Friedman SL. Kaposi's sarcoma and lymphoma of the gut in AIDS. *Baillieres Clin Gastroenterol*, 1990; 4: 455.
78 Weprin L, Zollinger R, Clausen K, Thomas FB. Kaposi's sarcoma: endoscopic observations of gastric and colon involvement. *J Clin Gastroenterol*, 1982; 4: 357.
79 Weber JN, Carmichael DJ, Boylston A *et al*. Kaposi's sarcoma of the bowel—presenting as apparent ulcerative colitis. *Gut*, 1985; 26: 295.
80 Strickler HD, Goedert JJ, Bethke FR *et al*. Human herpesvirus 8 cellular immune responses in homosexual men. *J Infect Dis*, 1999; 180: 1682.
81 Nakagawara G, Kojima Y, Mai M, Akimoto R, Miwa K. Lymphangioma of the transverse colon treated by transendoscopic polypectomy: report of a case and review of literature. *Dis Colon Rectum*, 1981; 24: 291.
82 Schaefer JW, Griffen WO Jr. Colonic lymphangiectasis associated with a potassium depletion syndrome. *Gastroenterology*, 1968; 55: 515.
83 Ivey K, DenBesten L, Kent TH, Clifton JA. Lymphangiectasia of the colon with protein loss and malabsorption. *Gastroenterology*, 1969; 57: 709.
84 Grodsky L. Neurofibroma of the rectum in a patient with von Recklinghausen's disease. *Am J Surg*, 1958; 95: 474.
85 Raszkowski HJ, Hufner RF. Neurofibromatosis of the colon: a unique manifestation of von Recklinghausen's disease. *Cancer*, 1971; 27: 134.
86 Fuller CE, Williams GT. Gastrointestinal manifestations of type 1 neurofibromatosis (von Recklinghausen's disease). *Histopathology*, 1991; 19: 1.
87 Petersen JM, Ferguson DR. Gastrointestinal neurofibromatosis. *J Clin Gastroenterol*, 1984; 6: 529.
88 Waxman BP, Buzzard AJ, Cox J, Stephens MJ. Gastric and intestinal bleeding in multiple neurofibromatosis with cardiomyopathy. *Aust N Z J Surg*, 1986; 56: 171.
89 Hough DR, Chan A, Davidson H. Von Recklinghausen's disease associated with gastrointestinal carcinoid tumors. *Cancer*, 1983; 51: 2206.
90 Shekitka KM, Sobin LH. Ganglioneuromas of the gastrointestinal tract. Relation to Von Recklinghausen disease and other multiple tumor syndromes. *Am J Surg Pathol*, 1994; 18: 250.
91 Carney JA, Go VL, Sizemore GW, Hayles AB. Alimentary-tract ganglioneuromatosis. A major component of the syndrome of multiple endocrine neoplasia, type 2b. *N Engl J Med*, 1976; 295: 1287.

92 Mendelsohn G, Diamond MP. Familial ganglioneuromatous polyposis of the large bowel. Report of a family with associated juvenile polyposis. *Am J Surg Pathol*, 1984; 8: 515.

93 Weidner N, Flanders DJ, Mitros FA. Mucosal ganglioneuromatosis associated with multiple colonic polyps. *Am J Surg Pathol*, 1984; 8: 779.

94 Lashner BA, Riddell RH, Winans CS. Ganglioneuromatosis of the colon and extensive glycogenic acanthosis in Cowden's disease. *Dig Dis Sci*, 1986; 31: 213.

95 Shepherd NA, Jass JR. Neuromuscular and vascular hamartoma of the small intestine: is it Crohn's disease? *Gut*, 1987; 28: 1663.

96 Chandrasoma P, Wheeler D, Radin DR. Traumatic neuroma of the intestine. *Gastrointest Radiol*, 1985; 10: 161.

97 Johnston J, Helwig EB. Granular cell tumors of the gastrointestinal tract and perianal region: a study of 74 cases. *Dig Dis Sci*, 1981; 26: 807.

98 Weitzner S, Lockard VG, Nascimento AG. Granular-cell myoblastoma of the cecum: report of a case. *Dis Colon Rectum*, 1976; 19: 675.

99 Cohen RS, Cramm RE. Granular-cell myoblastoma—an unusual rectal neoplasm. Report of a case. *Dis Colon Rectum*, 1969; 12: 120.

100 Jass JR, Shepherd NA, Maybee J. Tumours of the retrorectal space. In: Jass JR, Shepherd NA, Maybee J, eds. *Atlas of Surgical Pathology of the Colon, Rectum and Anus*. Edinburgh: Churchill Livingstone, 1989: 220.

40 Tumour-like lesions of the large intestine

Hyperplastic (metaplastic) polyp

The fundamental nature of this common epithelial polyp remains unresolved. The term 'hyperplastic' reflects the generally held view that the lesion is non-neoplastic. This is supported by the fact that the proliferative compartment remains limited to the crypt base [1,2], the polyps are generally only a few millimetres in diameter and malignant progression is described in rare case reports only [3]. Recent molecular insights challenge this view. K-*ras* mutation occurs in some hyperplastic polyps [4,5] and in microscopic hyperplastic foci (aberrant crypt foci) showing no evidence of dysplasia [6,7]. Clonal chromosomal changes implicating chromosome 1 (also characteristic of colorectal adenoma) have been documented within hyperplastic polyps [8,9]. Additional evidence of clonality is furnished by the demonstration of DNA microsatellite instability [10,11]. Cell kinetic studies have demonstrated hyperproliferation followed by a slowing in upward migration and delayed shedding of the surface epithelium that becomes hypermature [2]. An interesting relationship with the ulcer-associated cell lineage has been suggested [12]. The nature of the hyperplastic polyp is not adequately explained by any single term such as hyperplasia, neoplasia or metaplasia (see below). The lesion is likely to represent an epithelial response to a variety of stimuli, both genetic and environmental.

Hyperplastic polyps are unique amongst gastrointestinal polyps in being limited to the large intestine and appendix, with the majority occurring in the rectum and sigmoid colon. A small colonic polyp found proximal to the sigmoid colon is more likely to be an adenoma. Proximally located hyperplastic polyps may occur in association with colorectal cancer, in the condition hyperplastic polyposis (see below) or as a sporadic finding, particularly in females [13]. Hyperplastic polyps often cluster in large numbers around a cancer, particularly in lower sigmoid colon and rectum. They have been stated to outnumber adenomas by a factor of 10 : 1 [14]. This estimate originates from the pre-endoscopy era and does not accord with autopsy data [13]. It is interesting that the hyperplastic polyp to adenoma ratio is highest in populations at high risk for colorectal cancer, but falls to below unity in low-risk populations [13]. Migration from a low-risk to a high-risk area results in an increased frequency of hyperplastic polyps [15]. Hyperplastic polyps are detected more frequently in subjects with adenomas, and the finding of a distal hyperplastic polyp has been demonstrated to serve as a marker for a proximal adenoma, even if the clinical importance of this observation is disputed [16–22]. These data indicate that hyperplastic polyps may be caused by factors that are also implicated in the aetiology of colorectal neoplasia [23]. In fact hyperplastic polyps do share lifestyle risk factors with colorectal adenoma and carcinoma including low intake of dietary fibre, dietary calcium and non-steroidal anti-inflammatory drugs, increased intake of total fat and alcohol, an increased body mass index and a history of smoking [24,25]. Hyperplastic polyps are uncommon before the fifth decade, but do not show an obvious age relationship beyond the age of 50 years [13].

Hyperplastic polyps present as pale, sessile nodules that are usually sited upon mucosal folds (Fig. 40.1). They rarely exceed 5 mm in diameter. Large pedunculated examples have been described and may be mistaken for adenomas [26]. Examination of the surface topography (by dissecting microscope or *in vivo* stereomicroscopy) demonstrates the characteristically serrated or asteroid crypt openings [27]. Histological examination reveals a slightly thickened mucosa. The crypts show little branching or budding, but growth is probably achieved by crypt fission [28]. The cells lining the proliferative compartment in the crypt base often show enlarged, vesicular nuclei with prominent nucleoli. The nuclear membrane is delicate and there is no hyperchromatism. Mitoses may be frequent, but are limited to the crypt base though proliferation markers may persist in the upper crypt and surface epithelium [29]. Multinucleation and atypical mitoses may occur [30]. Endocrine cells are represented within

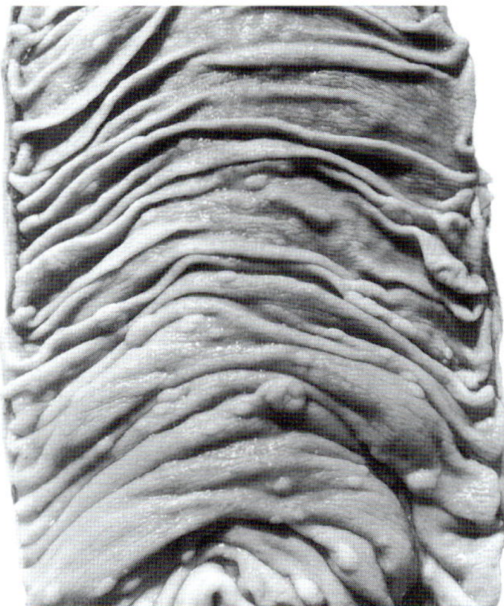

Fig. 40.1 Multiple hyperplastic polyps of the rectum.

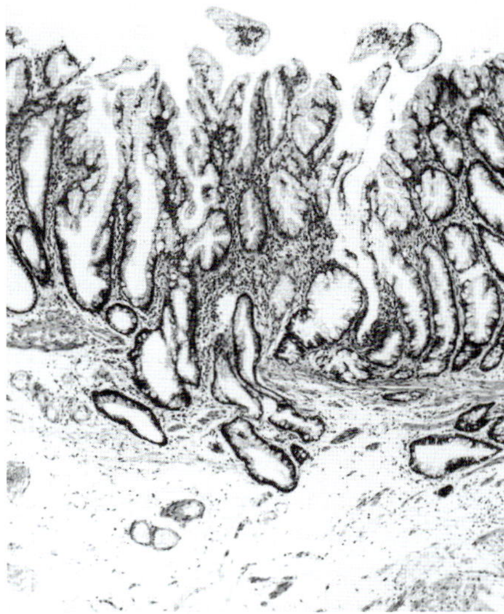

Fig. 40.2 Hyperplastic (metaplastic) polyp showing pseudoinvasion across the muscularis mucosae.

the basal epithelium. There may be pseudoinvasion with disruption of the muscularis mucosae (Fig. 40.2). The cytological appearances, in combination with pseudoinvasion, may deceive the unwary histopathologist into diagnosing carcinomatous invasion [31]. This appearance has also been described as inverted hyperplastic polyp [32] and is observed in the context of hyperplastic polyposis [33]. Above the proliferative zone the crypts become serrated and are lined by goblet cells and columnar cells (Fig. 40.3). The columnar cells differ from absorptive colonocytes in showing mucin secretion at the ultrastructural level [1]. The secretory nature of the columnar cell population is reinforced by the immunohistochemical demonstration of MUC2 goblet cell mucin (Fig. 40.4) and gastric

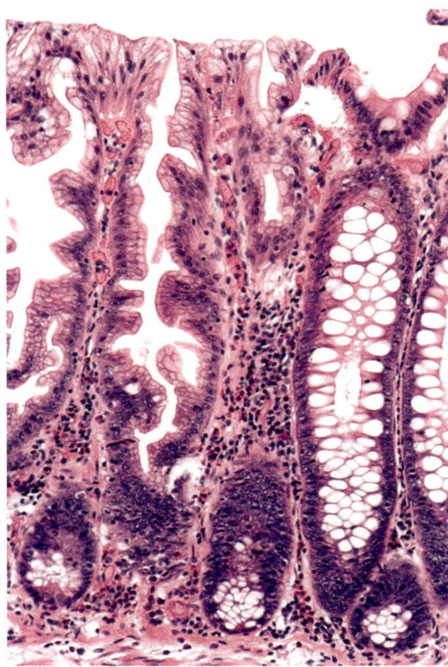

Fig. 40.3 Histology of hyperplastic polyp with normal crypts to the right.

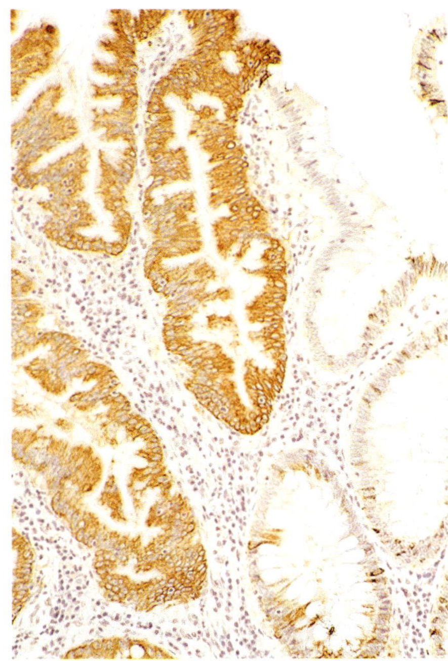

Fig. 40.4 Hyperplastic polyp showing increased MUC2 or goblet cell apomucin expression within the cytoplasm of 'columnar' cells (immunoperoxidase).

mucin MUC5AC [34]. Cytoplasm is relatively abundant, pale and eosinophilic.

The mucus in both goblet cells and columnar cells is more PAS positive than normal goblet cell mucus [35,36] and is also

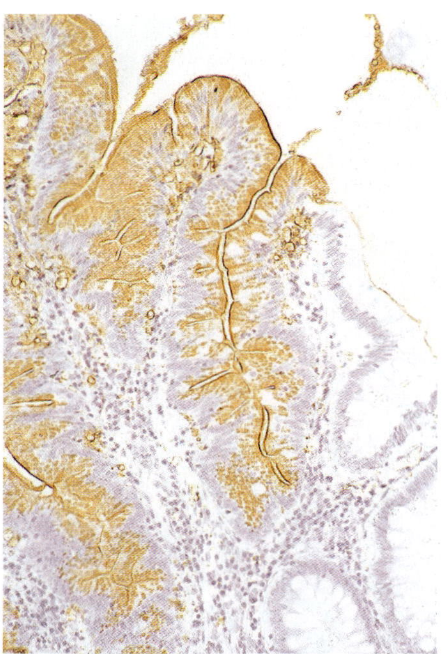

Fig. 40.5 Hyperplastic polyp showing up-regulation of the 'cancer-associated' marker SLe^x (immunoperoxidase).

positive with mild PAS, which is specific for non-O-acetyl sialic acid. Since non-O-acetyl sialic acid is digested by neuraminidase, alcianophilia is reduced following such treatment. This switch to a small intestinal type of sialic acid modifies the antigenicity of various sialylated carbohydrates. For example, the 'tumour-associated' sialylated structures STn and SLe^x (Fig. 40.5) are expressed (or rendered non-cryptic) in hyperplastic polyps [37].

The enzyme histochemistry of the hyperplastic polyp also reveals differences from normal colorectal mucosa. The hydrolytic enzymes esterase, acid phosphatase and ATPase and the respiratory enzyme succinic dehydrogenase all show reduced activity [38,39]. Diaphorases are not reduced and NADP diaphorase may show slightly increased activity [39]. It is interesting that colorectal carcinomas show similar alterations of sialic acid structure and enzyme histochemistry [35,38,39]. If one adds increased carcinoembryonic antigen (CEA) expression [35], reduced staining for secretory component and epithelial immunoglobulin A (IgA) [40] and loss of cytokeratin 20 [41] to the long list of phenotypes shared by hyperplastic polyps and colorectal cancer, the possibility of a relationship between these lesions receives considerable support. Nevertheless, the histochemical overlap is not exact. Hyperplastic polyps do not show the anomalous blood group antigen expression that is associated with neoplasms [42,43]. Furthermore, the increased binding by peanut agglutinin (PNA) [44] is limited to the Golgi zone [36,45]. The diffuse cytoplasmic binding by PNA that is observed in neoplasms may only be demonstrated in hyperplastic polyps following neuraminidase digestion.

Hyperplastic-type serrated crypts may occur within a variety of conditions or lesions including juvenile polyps, colorectal mucosal prolapse syndromes, the mucosa adjacent to colorectal cancer, and ulcerative colitis. These observations indicate that hyperplastic polyps may be initiated by a variety of stimuli. Increased lamina propria inflammation may drive epithelial hyperplasia through cytokine release [46]. Similarly, activated pericryptal myofibroblasts produce cytokines and growth factors and are known to proliferate in response to mucosal prolapse [47].

Hyperplastic polyposis

In this disorder, hyperplastic polyps are distributed throughout the large intestine and are notable for their size (often in excess of 1 cm) as well as number (sufficient to generate confusion with familial adenomatous polyposis) and occurrence in young subjects [3,26,48,49]. The association with colorectal cancer [3,26,50,51] is unlikely to be coincidental as indicated by the young age at onset of cancer [49], the occurrence of mixed polyps showing both hyperplastic and adenomatous features (see below) and descriptions of familial colorectal cancer in association with hyperplastic polyposis [11,52].

The frequency of K-*ras* mutation is low in hyperplastic polyposis and in large hyperplastic polyps, whereas loss of chromosome 1p is associated with a family history of hyperplastic polyposis [52]. Cancer in hyperplastic polyposis may be either DNA microsatellite stable or show DNA microsatellite instability at low (MSI-L) or high (MSI-H) levels [53]. There is evidence that the transition from hyperplasia to dysplasia in mixed polyps is driven by genetic instability, in turn due to inactivation of the DNA mismatch repair gene *hMLH1* through methylation and silencing of its promoter region [52–54]. There is a report describing regression of hyperplastic polyposis following treatment of rectal cancer [55]. It is likely that some instances of hyperplastic polyposis are explained by reversible mechanisms whereas others are not. Large but not necessarily numerous hyperplastic polyps occurring in the proximal colon may be a biomarker for the CpG island methylator phenotype (CIMP) known to be associated with colorectal cancer showing DNA microsatellite instability [56].

Typical adenomas may be found in subjects with hyperplastic polyposis. These would contribute to the increased risk of cancer and pose a management problem in light of the difficulty of distinguishing adenomas from large hyperplastic polyps during endoscopic examination. It is now appreciated that coexisting adenomas are not the exclusive explanation for an increased cancer risk [52,53]. Indeed, the fact that co-existing typical-appearing adenomas may show MSI-H

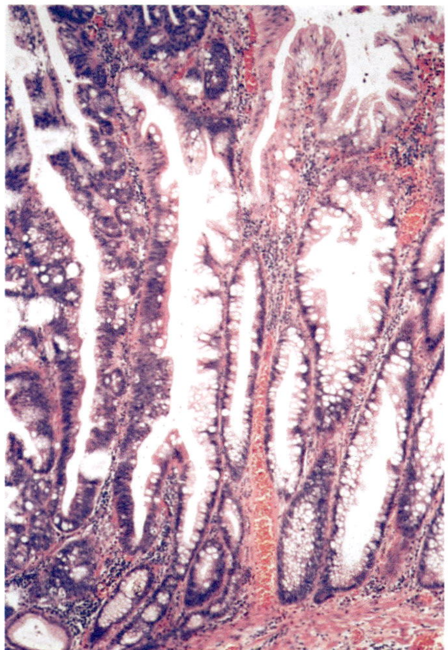

Fig. 40.6 Mixed adenoma (left) and hyperplastic polyp (right).

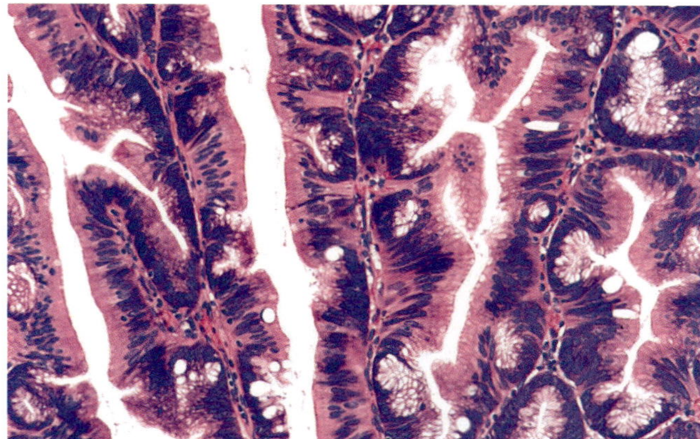

Fig. 40.7 Serrated adenoma.

suggests an origin from within a pre-existing hyperplastic polyp since MSI-H is rarely found in sporadic adenomas [53].

The highly variable phenotype, occasional finding of a positive family history and the demonstration of different molecular pathways of neoplastic evolution within the same patient all underline the difficulty of achieving a working definition of hyperplastic polyposis. A minimum of 20 hyperplastic polyps has been suggested [52], but large and proximally located hyperplastic polyps (in relatively small numbers) may be important biomarkers of increased cancer risk [53]. It is very likely, however, that as a precancerous condition, hyperplastic polyposis will turn out to be an example of an uncommon disorder that sheds considerable light on the nature and evolution of commonly occurring colorectal cancer.

Admixed hyperplastic polyp/adenoma and serrated adenoma

The admixed hyperplastic polyp/adenoma (Fig. 40.6) has been described as a collision of classical hyperplastic polyp and classical adenoma [57]. Serrated adenoma (Fig. 40.7) is considered to be an adenoma displaying a superficial architectural similarity to the hyperplastic polyp [57]. However, the resemblance to the hyperplastic polyp is not necessarily superficial. Serrated adenomas display the histochemical profile of the hyperplastic polyp [34,36] and the proliferative compartment is retained within the basal epithelium as in the hyperplastic polyp [58]. A proportion shows contiguity with a typical hyperplastic polyp. An origin within the latter is supported by the demonstration of shared mutations in DNA microsatellite markers [59]. Serrated adenomas occur in hyperplastic polyposis, prompting the renaming of this condition as serrated adenomatous polyposis [60]. There is surely a histogenetic link between hyperplastic polyp and serrated adenoma, but where should the line be drawn between the two? If, as noted above, some hyperplastic polyps are clonal, show neoplasia-associated genetic changes and are capable of growth through crypt fission, is there a need to draw a firm line at all? Clinical experience indicates that the majority of hyperplastic polyps have little, if any, malignant potential, whereas serrated adenomas do have significant malignant potential [57]. Typical, diminutive hyperplastic polyps of the distal colon and rectum should continue to be regarded as innocuous. Large, proximal hyperplastic polyps may warrant increased clinical concern [61]. Serrated polyps considered to be adenomatous or to include a dysplastic component should be managed as adenomas. Serrated adenomas are considered in more detail in Chapter 38.

A mixed polyposis family has been described [62]. The polyps showed mixed juvenile, adenomatous and hyperplastic features and could be a variant of juvenile polyposis (see below).

Juvenile polyp

This is a non-neoplastic epithelial polyp composed of tissues indigenous to the site of origin, but arranged in a haphazard manner. Most are found in young children and they may also occur in adults and as multiple familial lesions in association with various congenital defects [63]. These findings suggest that the juvenile polyp is a hamartoma rather than an acquired inflammatory lesion. However, inflammatory polyps may show a similar appearance [64]. It is possible that the lamina propria in affected individuals is especially prone to overgrowth at a particular developmental stage. This overgrowth

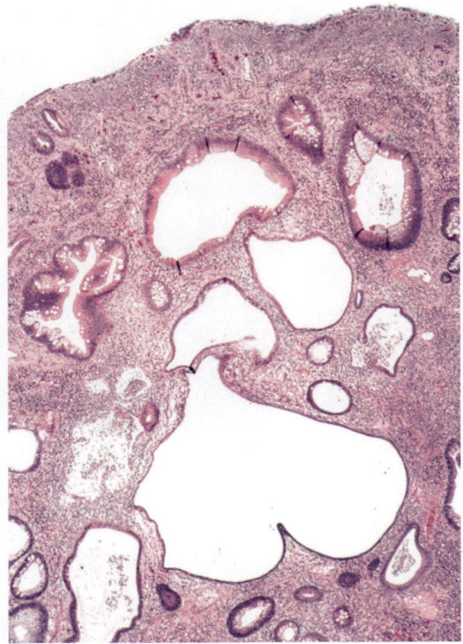

Fig. 40.8 Juvenile polyp with irregular and cystic glands separated by an abundant lamina propria.

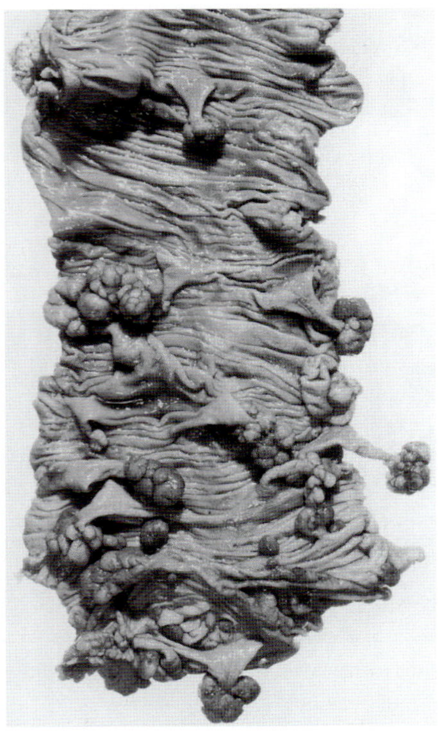

Fig. 40.9 Rounded lobulated polyps in juvenile polyposis.

might be caused by a relatively trivial inflammatory stimulus. The earliest lesions may be seen when colectomy is performed for the condition juvenile polyposis. They appear as foci of oedematous lamina propria with overlying epithelial ulceration.

The usual childhood lesion is solitary, but several may be present. Most occur in the rectum and present between the ages of 1 and 10 (peak at 4–5). Males and females are affected equally. Bleeding is the most common symptom, but some may autoamputate or prolapse through the anus. Macroscopically the typical lesion has a smooth spherical, red head and a narrow stalk. The cut surface shows cysts filled with mucin. The thin stalk lacks a muscularis mucosae and the polyp is liable to torsion, venous congestion, haemorrhage and infection.

Microscopically the polyp consists of epithelial tubules, which may be dilated or cystic, embedded in an excess of lamina propria (Fig. 40.8). The tubules are lined by an essentially normal epithelium. The surface is frequently ulcerated and there may be purulent inflammation of the lamina propria. There may occasionally be stromal metaplasia to cartilage or even bone. Muscularis mucosae is not included within the stroma. Solitary lesions are not thought to have a significant malignant potential, but rare examples of malignant change have been described [65,66]. Dysplasia has also been documented in a solitary polyp [67]. In the presence of inflammation, the epithelium not infrequently shows reactive changes that are easily confused with dysplasia. Crypts are replaced by eosinophilic columnar cells secreting small amounts of mucus. However, the nuclei are small and basally sited. Crypts may also assume a serrated contour reminiscent of the hyperplastic polyp.

Juvenile polyposis

In this condition numerous polyps of juvenile type are found in the large bowel (Fig. 40.9) and sometimes in the small bowel and stomach [68]. One rare form occurs in infancy and is associated with diarrhoea, haemorrhage, malnutrition, intussusception and death at an early age [69]. No family history is found. Remaining cases vary in their age of onset and may be either familial or sporadic. Sporadic cases are more likely to be associated with congenital defects including abnormalities of the cranium and heart, cleft palate, polydactyly and malrotations. Familial cases have been reported in three generations, indicative of autosomal dominant inheritance [70]. A germline mutation of *DPC4/SMAD4* has been reported in a proportion of juvenile polyposis families [71]. There is often a significant excess of colorectal cancer in these families and the number of reports of patients with both juvenile polyposis and cancer of the colon or rectum has risen in recent years [68–74]. The cumulative risk of colorectal cancer has been estimated as 68% by 60 years of age [72]. Of 85 patients with histologically proven juvenile polyposis known to the St Mark's Hospital Polyposis Registry, 16 have developed colorectal cancer [73]. Most of the cancers have occurred in patients between the ages of 20 and 40 (mean 34 years). These observations suggest that juvenile polyposis families should be managed like families with familial adenomatous polyposis.

The polyps in juvenile polyposis may adopt an atypical appearance with marked papillary infolding, a relative reduction in the amount of lamina propria and absence of surface ulceration [73]. Polyps of this type are more prone to the development of dysplasia and this probably accounts for their increased propensity for malignant change [73]. In the St Mark's series of polyps (over 1000) from juvenile polyposis patients, such atypical forms accounted for 17% of the total; 30% had foci of mild dysplasia, 15% had foci of moderate dysplasia and 2% had foci of severe dysplasia. In the remaining more typical juvenile polyps, only 7% had foci of mild dysplasia, 1% had foci of moderate dysplasia. There were only 21 typical adenomas in this series [73]. Juvenile polyposis has been described in association with ganglioneuromatous polyposis [74,75].

Peutz–Jeghers polyps

The Peutz–Jeghers syndrome has been discussed on p. 394. In about half of all cases one or more small polyps are found in the colon and rectum. These are rarely of clinical significance. However, there are recent reports of colorectal cancer arising in association with the Peutz–Jeghers syndrome [76–78]. Occasionally one or more polyps of Peutz–Jeghers type are found in the colon or rectum without any evidence of polyps in the stomach or small intestine (Fig. 40.10). Such tumours show a typical tree-like branching of smooth muscle derived from the muscularis mucosae and are covered by an entirely normal colorectal epithelium. Grossly, they may mimic adenoma and the correct diagnosis depends upon microscopic examination.

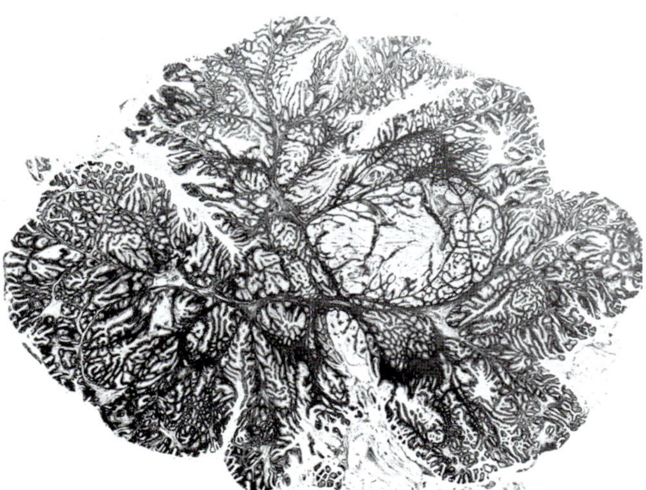

Fig. 40.10 Colonic polyp of Peutz–Jeghers type. The branching bands of smooth muscle are covered by an excess of normal colonic epithelium.

Cowden's syndrome (multiple hamartoma syndrome)

This rare condition, named after the family in which it was first described, is characterized by the presence of gastrointestinal, oral and cutaneous hamartomas and neoplasms of the breast and thyroid [79–81]. Inheritance is autosomal dominant and families have germline mutations of *PTEN* on chromosome 10q21–23 [82]. Gastrointestinal polyps have been described as hamartomatous (Fig. 40.11), inflammatory and occasionally adenomatous [83]. The hamartomas are often characterized by a myofibroblastic stroma [83]. The risk of colorectal cancer appears to be low, with breast and thyroid being the major sites of malignancy.

Bannayan–Riley–Ruvalcaba syndrome

This genetic disorder presents in childhood with macrocephaly and genital pigmentation. Mutations are found in *PTEN* (as for Cowden's syndrome) [84,85], and subjects may develop multiple hamartomas (lipomas and haemangiomas), thyroid neoplasms and autoimmune thyroiditis, as well as gastrointestinal hamartomas [86].

Inflammatory polyps

Non-neoplastic proliferations of either mucosa or granulation tissue may be due to various injuries of the colorectal

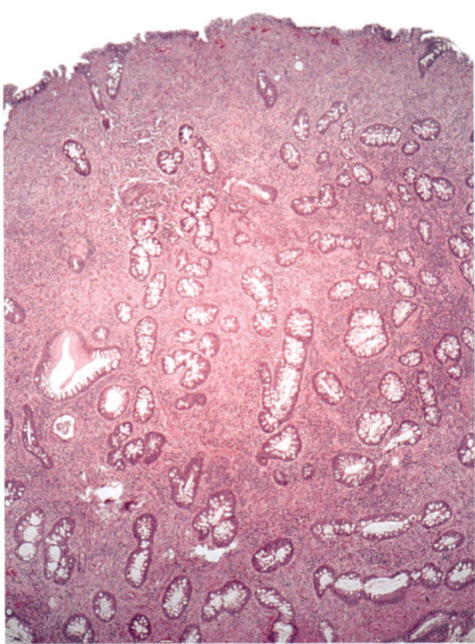

Fig. 40.11 Hamartomatous polyp in a subject with Cowden's syndrome.

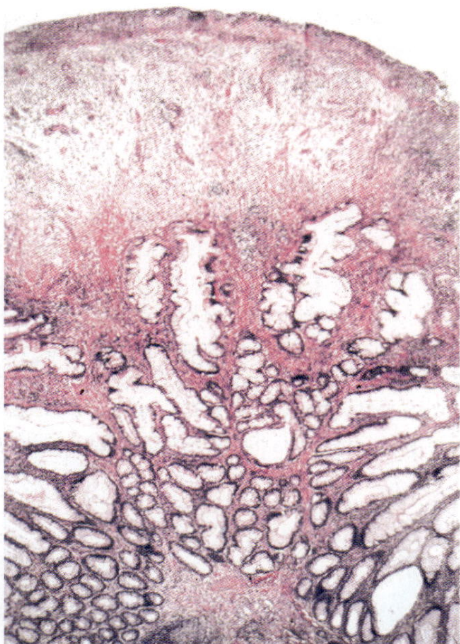

Fig. 40.12 Inflammatory 'cap' polyp. Elongated tortuous glands merge into a 'cap' of inflammatory granulation tissue.

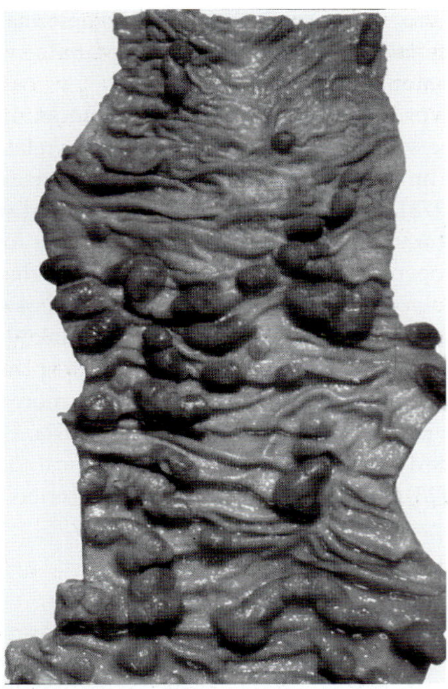

Fig. 40.13 Cap polyposis. There are multiple, sessile dark polyps resembling slugs that are situated on the apices of exaggerated mucosal folds.

epithelium. The most frequent cause is ulcerative colitis, but others include Crohn's disease, ischaemic bowel disease and schistosomiasis. Pseudopolyposis is an alternative but less satisfactory term. Radiologists may use the term pseudopolyposis to describe surviving mucosal islands visualized in double-contrast barium enemas. The polyps range in their gross appearance from finger-like projections to rounded masses. Finger-like polyps are often fused or bifid, giving rise to bizarre shapes. Bridges, through which a probe can be passed, may be formed. Inflammatory polyps are usually multiple. Variable amounts of inflammatory and granulation tissue are seen on microscopy. Cystic dilatation of glands may produce an appearance resembling the juvenile polyp. However, juvenile and inflammatory polyps are distinguished by the appearance of the surrounding mucosa and the clinical history. Furthermore, it is unusual to observe an oedematous lamina propria throughout the substance of an inflammatory polyp. Bizarre or giant pseudopolyposis is discussed on p. 511.

Ureterosigmoidostomy predisposes to the formation of inflammatory polyps. These lesions show an increased potential for neoplastic transformation; both dysplasia and carcinoma have been observed [87,88].

'Cap' polyps [89], eroded polypoid hyperplasia [90], polypoid prolapsing folds [91] and inflammatory myoglandular polyps [92] may be included under this general heading. Found mainly in the rectosigmoid region, these polyps comprise elongated, tortuous and distended crypts and are covered by a cap of inflammatory granulation tissue (Fig. 40.12). The stroma contains proliferated smooth muscle. In one series of 15 patients, cap polyps numbered between one and 70 [89]. They are dark red, sessile and usually located on the crest of a mucosal fold (Fig. 40.13). Mucosal prolapse and ischaemia may play a role in their causation (see p. 465) and some are related to diverticular disease [91]. Patients usually present with mucous diarrhoea, tenesmus or rectal bleeding and the condition may mimic inflammatory bowel disease. An association with protein-losing enteropathy has been described [93].

Cronkhite–Canada syndrome

This rare form of gastrointestinal polyposis presents with alopecia, skin pigmentation, nail atrophy, diarrhoea, malabsorption, protein-losing enteropathy and severe electrolyte disturbances [94,95]. The clinical symptoms may mimic inflammatory bowel disease [96]. It is often fatal. The cause is unknown and there is no evidence of a familial tendency. Severe juvenile polyposis presenting in infancy is sometimes described (incorrectly) as infantile Cronkhite–Canada syndrome.

The macroscopic and microscopic pathology is distinctive and the changes are the same throughout the gastrointestinal tract. The mucosa is diffusely thickened with superimposed polypoid hypertrophy without ulceration. Microscopically, the epithelial tubules may (as in juvenile polyps) show cystic dilatation and epithelial flattening. The lamina propria is expanded and oedematous, but shows little or no increase in inflammatory cell content. The appearance has some resemblance to 'colitis cystica superficialis', a complication of pellagra. The diagnosis can be made by rectal, gastric or jejunal biopsy.

Inflammatory fibroid polyp

Inflammatory fibroid polyp occurs in the colon but is much rarer here than in the stomach and small intestine [97–99]. The pathological features are identical to tumours arising at these latter sites (see pp. 219 and 397).

References

1 Kaye GI, Fenoglio CM, Pascal RR, Lane N. Comparative electron microscopic features of normal, hyperplastic and adenomatous human colonic epithelium. *Gastroenterology*, 1973; 64: 926.

2 Hayashi T, Yatani R, Apostol J, Stemmermann GN. Pathogenesis of hyperplastic polyps of the colon. A hypothesis based on ultrasturcture and in vitro kinetics. *Gastroenterology*, 1974; 66: 347.

3 Teoh HH, Delahunt B, Isbister WH. Case report. Dysplastic and malignant areas in hyperplastic polyps of the large intestine. *Pathology*, 1989; 21: 138.

4 Otori K, Oda Y, Sugiyama K *et al*. High frequency of K-*ras* mutations in human colorectal hyperplastic polyps. *Gut*, 1997; 40: 660.

5 Uchida H, Ando H, Maruyama K *et al*. Genetic alterations of mixed hyperplastic adenomatous polyps in the colon and rectum. *Jpn J Cancer Res*, 1998; 89: 299.

6 Jen J, Powell SM, Papadopoulos N *et al*. Molecular determinants of dysplasia in colorectal lesions. *Cancer Res*, 1994; 54: 5523.

7 Yamashita N, Minamoto T, Ochiai A, Onda M, Esumi H. Frequent and characteristic K-*ras* activation and absence of p53 protein accumulation in aberrant cyrpt foci of the colon. *Gastroenterology*, 1995; 108: 434.

8 Bardi G, Pandis N, Fenger C. *et al*. Deletion of 1p36 as a primary chromosomal aberration in intestinal tumorigenesis. *Cancer Res*, 1993; 53: 1895.

9 Bomme L, Bardi G, Pandis N *et al*. Clonal karyotypic abnormalities in colorectal adenomas: clues to the early genetic events in the adenoma-carcinoma sequence. *Genes Chromosomes Cancer*, 1994; 10: 190.

10 Lothe RA, Anderson SN, Hofstad B *et al*. Deletion of 1p loci and microsatellite instability in colorectal polyps. *Genes Chromosomes Cancer*, 1995; 14: 182.

11 Jeevaratnam P, Cottier DS, Browett PJ *et al*. Familial giant hyperplastic polyposis predisposing to colorectal cancer: a new hereditary bowel cancer syndrome. *J Pathol*, 1996; 179: 20.

12 Hanby AM, Poulsom R, Singh S *et al*. Hyperplastic polyps: a cell lineage which both synthesizes and secretes trefoil-peptides and has phenotypic similarity with the ulcer-associated cell lineage. *Am J Pathol*, 1993; 142: 663.

13 Jass JR, Young PJ, Robinson EM. Predictors of presence, multiplicity, size and dysplasia of colorectal adenomas. A necropsy study in New Zealand. *Gut*, 1992; 33: 1508.

14 Fenoglio CM, Lane N. The anatomical precursor of colorectal carcinoma. *Cancer*, 1974; 34: 918.

15 Stemmermann GN, Yatani R. Diverticulosis and polyps of the large intestine. A necropsy study of Hawaii Japanese. *Cancer*, 1973; 31: 1260.

16 Naveau S, Brajer S, Bedossa P, Poynard T, Chaput J-C. Hyperplastic colonic polyps as a marker for adenomas colonic polyps. *Eur J Gastroenterol Hepatol*, 1991; 3: 57.

17 Provenzale D, Martin ZZ, Holland KL, Sandler RS. Colon adenomas in patients with hyperplastic polyps. *J Clin Gastroenterol*, 1988; 10: 46.

18 Provenzale D, Garrett JW, Condon SE, Sandler RS. Risk for colon adenomas in patients with rectosigmoid hyperplastic polyps. *Ann Intern Med*, 1990; 113: 760.

19 Ansher AF, Lewis JH, Fleischer DE *et al*. Hyperplastic colonic polyps as a marker of adenomatous colonic polyps. *Am J Gastroenterol*, 1989; 84: 113.

20 Kellokumpu I, Kyllonen L. Multiple adenomas and synchronous hyperplastic polyps: predictors of metachronous colorectal adenomas. *Ann Chir Gynaecol*, 1991; 80: 30.

21 Opelka FG, Timmcke AE, Gathright JB, Ray JE, Hicks TC. Diminutive colonic polyps: an indication for colonoscopy. *Dis Colon Rectum*, 1992; 35: 178.

22 Imperiale TF, Wagner DR, Lin CY *et al*. Risk of advanced proximal neoplasms in asymptomatic adults according to the distal colorectal findings. *N Engl J Med*, 2000; 343: 169.

23 Jass JR. Relation between metaplastic polyp and carcinoma of the colorectum. *Lancet*, 1983; i: 28.

24 Martínez ME, McPherson RS, Levin B, Glober GA. A case-control study of dietary intake and other lifestyle risk factors for hyperplastic polyps. *Gastroenterology*, 1997; 113: 423.

25 Potter JD, Bigler J, Fosdick L *et al*. Colorectal adenomatous and hyperplastic polyps: smoking and N-acetyltransferase 2 polymorphisms. *Cancer Epidemiol Biomarkers Prev*, 1999; 8: 69.

26 Sumner HW, Wasserman NF, McClain CJ. Giant hyperplastic polyposis of the colon. *Dig Dis Sci*, 1981; 26: 85.

27 Tada S, Iida M, Yao T *et al*. Stereomicroscopic examination of surface morphology in colorectal epithelial tumors. *Hum Pathol*, 1993; 24: 1243.

28 Araki K, Ogata T, Kobayashi M, Yatani R. A morphological study on the histogenesis of human colorectal hyperplastic polyps. *Gastroenterology*, 1995; 109: 1468.

29 Carr NJ, Monihan JM, Nzeako UC, Murakata LA, Sobin LH. Expression of proliferating cell nuclear antigen in hyperplastic polyps, adenomas and inflammatory cloagenic polyps of the large intestine. *J Clin Pathol*, 1995; 48: 46.

30 Jass JR, Cottier DS, Pokos V, Parry S, Winship IM. Mixed epithelial polyps in association with hereditary non-polyposis colorectal cancer providing an alternative pathway of cancer histogenesis. *Pathology*, 1997; 29: 28.

31 Whittle TS, Varner W, Brown FM. Giant hyperplastic polyps of the colon simulating adenocarcinoma. *Am J Gastroenterol*, 1978; 69: 105.

32 Sobin LH. Inverted hyperplastic polyps of the colon. *Am J Surg Pathol*, 1985; 9: 265.

33 Shepherd NA. Inverted hyperplastic polyposis of the colon. *J Clin Pathol*, 1993; 46: 56.

34 Biemer H, Hüttmann A-E, Walsh MD *et al*. Immunohistochemical staining patterns of MUC1, MUC2, MUC4, and MUC5AC mucins in hyperplastic polyps, serrated adenomas, and traditional adenomas of the colorectum. *J Histochem Cytochem*, 1999; 47: 1039.

35 Jass JR, Filipe MI, Abbas E *et al*. A morphologic and histochemical study of metaplastic polyps of the colorectum. *Cancer*, 1984; 53: 510.

36 Jass JR, Smith M. Sialic acid and epithelial differentiation in colorectal polyps and cancer—a morphological, mucin and lectin histochemical study. *Pathology*, 1992; 24: 233.

37 Yuan M, Itzkowitz SH, Ferrell LD *et al*. Expression of lewis[x] and sialylated lewis[x] antigens in human colorectal polyps. *J Natl Cancer Inst*, 1987; 78: 479.

38 Wattenberg LW. A histochemical study of five oxidative enzymes in carcinoma of the large intestine in man. *Am J Pathol*, 1959; 35: 113.

39 Czernobilsky B, Tsou K-C. Adenocarcinoma, adenomas and polyps of the colon. Histochemical study. *Cancer*, 1968; 21: 165.

40 Jass JR, Faludy J. Immunohistochemical demonstration of IgA and secretory component in relation to epithelial cell differentiation in normal colorectal mucosa and metaplastic polyp: a semiquantitative study. *Histochem J*, 1985; 17: 373.

41 Ban S-I. Small hyperplastic polyps of the colorectum showing deranged cell organization: a lesion considered to be a serrated adenoma? *Am J Surg Pathol*, 1999; 23: 1158.

42 Vowden P, Lowe A, Lennox ES, Bleehen NM. Colonic polyp epithelial ABH blood group isoantigen (BGI) expression related to histological type and size. *Br J Surg*, 1984; 71: 906.

43 Cooper HS, Marshall C, Ruggerio F, Steplewski Z. Hyperplastic polyps of the colon and rectum. An immunohistochemical study with monoclonal antibodies against blood groups antigens (sialosyl-Le[a], Le[b], Le[x], Le[y], A, B, H). *Lab Invest*, 1987; 57: 421.

44 Boland CR, Montgomery CK, Kim YS. A cancer-associated mucin alteration in benign colonic polyps. *Gastroenterology*, 1982; 82: 664.

45 Cooper HS, Reuter VE. Peanut lectin-binding sites in polyps of the colon and rectum. *Lab Invest*, 1983; 49: 655.

46 Higaki S, Akazawa A, Nakamura H *et al*. Metaplastic polyp of the colon develops in response to inflammation. *J Gastroenterol Hepatol*, 1999; 14: 709.

47 Powell DW, Mifflin RC, Valentich JD *et al*. Myofibroblasts. II. Intestinal subepithelial myofibroblasts. *Am J Physiol*, 1999; 277: C183.

48 Williams GT, Arthur JF, Bussey HJR, Morson BC. Metaplastic polyps and polyposis of the colorectum. *Histopathology*, 1980; 4: 155.

49 Bengoechea O, Martinez-Penuela JM, Larrinaga B *et al*. Hyperplastic polyposis of the colorectum and adenocarcinoma in a 24 year old man. *Am J Surg Pathol*, 1987; 11: 323.

50 Warner AS, Glick ME, Fogt F. Multiple large hyperplastic polyps of the colon coincident with adenocarcinoma. *Am J Gastroenterol*, 1994; 89: 123.

51 McCann BG. A case of metaplastic polyposis of the colon associated with focal adenomatous change and metachronous adenocarcinomas. *Histopathology*, 1988; 13: 700.

52 Rashid A, Houlihan S, Booker S *et al*. Phenotypic and molecular characteristics of hyperplastic polyposis. *Gastroenterology*, 2000; 119: 323.

53 Jass JR, Iino H, Ruszkiewicz A *et al*. Neoplastic progression occurs through mutator pathways in hyperplastic polyposis of the colorectum. *Gut*, 2000; 47: 43.

54 Hawkins NJ, Gorman P, Tomlinson IP, Bullpitt P, Ward RL. Colorectal carcinomas arising in the hyperplastic polyposis syndrome progress through the chromosomal instability pathway. *Am J Pathol*, 2000; 157: 385.

55 Kusunoki M, Fujita S, Sakanoue Y *et al*. Disappearance of hyperplastic polyposis after resection of rectal cancer: report of two cases. *Dis Colon Rectum*, 1991; 34: 829.

56 Toyota M, Ahuja N, Ohe-Toyota M *et al*. CpG island methylator phenotype in colorectal cancer. *Proc Natl Acad Sci*, 1999; 96: 8681.

57 Longacre TA, Fenoglio-Preiser CM. Mixed hyperplastic adenomatous polyps/serrated adenomas. A distinct form of colorectal neoplasia. *Am J Surg Pathol*, 1990; 14: 524.

58 Rubio CA, Kato Y, Hirota T, Muto T. Flat serrated adenomas of the colorectal mucosa in Japanese patients. *In Vivo*, 1996; 10: 339.

59 Iino H, Jass JR, Simms LA *et al*. DNA microsatellite instability in hyperplastic polyps, serrated adenomas, and mixed polyps: a mild mutator pathway for colorectal cancer? *J Clin Pathol*, 1999; 52: 5.

60 Torlakovic E, Snover DC. Serrated adenomatous polyposis in humans. *Gastroenterology*, 1996; 110: 748.

61 Rothstein RD, Kochman M. Large hyperplastic polyps of the right colon. *Gastrointest Endosc*, 1998; 47: 211.

62 Thomas HJW, Whitelaw SC, Cottrell SE *et al*. Genetic mapping of the hereditary mixed polyposis syndrome to chromosome 6q. *Am J Hum Genet*, 1996; 58: 770.

63 Bussey HJR. Gastro-intestinal polyposis. *Gut*, 1970; 11: 970.

64 Franzin G, Zamboni G, Dina R, Scarpa A, Fratton A. Juvenile and inflammatory polyps of the colon—a histological and histochemical study. *Histopathology*, 1983; 7: 719.

65 Tung-hua L, Min-chang C, Hsien-chiu T. Malignant change of juvenile polyp of colon. A case report. *Chinese Med J*, 1978; 4: 434.

66 Jones MA, Hebert JC, Trainer TD. Juvenile polyp with intramucosal carcinoma. *Arch Pathol Lab Med*, 1987; 111: 200.

67 Friedman CJ, Fechner RE. A solitary juvenile polyp with hyperplastic and adenomatous glands. *Dig Dis Sci*, 1982; 27: 946.

68 McColl I, Bussey HJR, Veale AMC, Morson BC. Juvenile polyposis coli. *Proc R Soc Med*, 1964; 57: 896.

69 Sachatello CR, Hahn IS, Carrington CB. Juvenile gastrointestinal polyposis in a female infant. Report of a case and a review of the literature of a recently recognised syndrome. *Surgery*, 1974; 75: 107.

70 Smilow PC, Pryor CA, Swinton NW. Juvenile polyposis coli. A report of three patients in three generations of one family. *Dis Colon Rectum*, 1966; 9: 896.

71 Howe JR, Roth S, Ringold JC *et al*. Mutations in the *SMAD4/DPC4* gene in juvenile polyposis. *Science*, 1998; 280: 1086.

72 Murday V, Slack J. Inherited disorders associated with colorectal cancer. *Cancer Surv*, 1989; 8: 139.

73 Jass JR, Williams CB, Bussey HJR, Morson BC. Juvenile polyposis—a precancerous condition. *Histopathology*, 1988; 13: 619.

74 Mendelsohn G, Diamond MP. Familial ganglioneuromatous polyposis of the large bowel. Report of a family with associated juvenile polyposis. *Am J Surg Pathol*, 1984; 8: 515.

75 Weidner N, Flanders DJ, Mitros FA. Mucosal ganglioneuromatosis associated with multiple colonic polyps. *Am J Surg Pathol*, 1984; 8: 779.

76 Stockdale AD, Ashford RFU, Leader M. Gastrointestinal malignancy in association with Peutz–Jeghers syndrome—three further cases. *Clin Oncol*, 1984; 10: 299.

77 Tweedie JH, McCann BG. Peutz–Jeghers syndrome and metastasising colonic adenocarcinoma. *Gut*, 1984; 25: 1118.

78 Konishi F, Wyse NE, Muto F *et al*. Peutz–Jeghers polyposis associated with carcinoma of the digestive organs. *Dis Colon Rectum*, 1987; 30: 790.

79 Entius MM, Westerman AM, van Velthuysen ML *et al*. Molecular and phenotypic markers of hamartomatous polyposis syndromes in the gastrointestinal tract. *Hepatogastroenterology* 1999; 46: 661.

80 Thyresson HN, Doyle JA. Cowden's disease (multiple hamartoma syndrome). *Mayo Clin Proc*, 1981; 56: 179.

81 Haggitt RC, Reid BJ. Hereditary gastrointestinal polyposis syndrome. *Am J Surg Pathol*, 1986; 10: 871.

82 Nelen MR, Padberg GW, Peeters EAJ *et al*. Localization of the gene for Cowden disease to chromosome 10q22–23. *Nature Genet*, 1996; 13: 114.

83 Carlson GJ, Nivatvongs S, Snover DC. Colorectal polyps in Cowden's disease (multiple hamartoma syndrome). *Am J Surg Pathol*, 1984; 8: 763.

84 Arch EM, Goodman BK, Van Wesep RA *et al*. Deletion of *PTEN* in a patient with Bannayan–Riley–Ruvalcaba syndrome suggests allelism with Cowden disease. *Am J Med Genet*, 1997; 71: 489.

85 Marsh DJ, Dahia PLM, Zheng Z *et al*. Germline mutations in *PTEN* are present in Bannayan–Zonana syndrome. *Nature Genet*, 1997; 16: 333.

86 Gorlin RJ, Cohen JMM, Condon LM, Burke BA. Bannayan–Riley–Ruvalcaba syndrome. *Am J Med Genet*, 1992; 44: 307.

87 Ansell ID, Vellacott KD. Colonic polyps complicating ureterosigmoidoscopy. *Histopathology*, 1980; 4: 429.

88 Cipolla R, Garcia RL. Colonic polyps and adenocarcinoma complicating ureterosigmoidostomy: a report of a case. *Am J Gastroenterol*, 1984; 79: 453.

89 Williams GT, Bussey HJR, Morson BC. Inflammatory 'cap' polyps of the large intestine. *Br J Surg*, 1985; 72: 133.

90 Burke AP, Sobin LH. Eroded polypoid hyperplasia of the rectosigmoid. *Am J Gastroenterol*, 1990; 85: 975.

91 Kelly JK. Polypoid prolapsing mucosal folds in diverticular disease. *Am J Surg Pathol*, 1991; 15: 871.

92 Nakamura S-I, Kino I, Akagi T. Inflammatory myoglandular polyps of the colon and rectum. A clinicopathological study of 32 pedunculated polyps, distinct from other types of polyps. *Am J Surg Pathol*, 1992; 16: 772.

93 Oshitani N, Moriyama Y, Matsumoto T, Kobayashi K, Kitano A. Protein-losing enteropathy from cap polyposis. *Lancet*, 1995; 346: 1567.

94 Cronkhite LW, Canada WJ. Generalised gastrointestinal polyposis. An unusual syndrome of polyposis, pigmentation, alopecia and onychotrophia. *N Engl J Med*, 1955; 252: 1011.

95 Kindblom L, Angervall L, Santesson R, Selander S. Cronkhite–Canada syndrome: case report. *Cancer*, 1977; 39: 2651.

96 Ryall RJ. Polypoid hypertrophy of the gastrointestinal mucosa, presenting as ulcerative colitis. *Proc R Soc Med*, 1966; 59: 614.

97 Lifschitz O, Lew S, Witz M, Reiss R, Griffel B. Inflammatory fibroid polyp of sigmoid colon. *Dis Colon Rectum*, 1979; 22: 575.

98 Gooszen AW, Tjon ATR, Veselic M, Bolk JH, Lamers CB. Inflammatory fibroid polyp simulating malignant tumor of the colon in a patient with multiple hamartoma syndrome (Cowden's disease). *AJR*, 1995; 165: 1012.

99 Aubert A, Cazier A, Baglin AC *et al*. Inflammatory fibroid polyps of the colon. *Gastroenterol Clin Biol*, 1998; 22: 1106.

41 Miscellaneous conditions of the large intestine

Amyloid

Amyloid is an abnormally folded fibrillar protein that on structural examination is represented by the beta-pleated sheet, a complex network of fibrils varying in diameter from 7.5 to 10 nm that can be identified by electron microscopy. In routine diagnostic biopsies light microscopic examination will show amyloid deposition when stained with haematoxylin and eosin (H&E) either as an eosinophilic thickening of vessel walls or as an eosinophilic deposit in the extracellular matrix. The special staining characteristics of amyloid when examined histochemically are conveyed by the coupling of amyloid to glycoproteins. Congo Red stains these amyloid-associated glycoproteins (and other proteins) red, and the specificity for amyloid is given by the added apple-green birefringence that is found when the sections are viewed in polarized light. About 20 different unrelated proteins can form amyloid fibrils *in vivo*. Some of these are natural wild-type proteins that are inherently amyloidogenic and cause amyloidosis in old age or if present for long periods at abnormally high concentration, while others are acquired or inherited variants that aggregate into amyloid deposits [1]. In addition to the fibrils, amyloid deposits always contain the non-fibrillar pentraxin plasma protein, serum amyloid P component (SAP) that probably stabilizes amyloid fibrils by retarding their clearance. While Congo Red staining remains the most useful and cost-efficient diagnostic technique, histological diagnosis and classification of amyloid is greatly facilitated by the use of immunohistochemistry using antibodies directed at SAP (as a 'general' marker of amyloid) and the different possible protein components.

Amyloid deposition in the gastrointestinal tract is most commonly found in systemic type AA (reactive) amyloidosis that complicates a range of chronic inflammatory disorders such as rheumatoid arthritis, chronic infections such as tuberculosis and certain malignant tumours of different lineages [2]. Occasionally the underlying disease itself is centred on the gastrointestinal tract, for example, Crohn's disease. The commonest sites for AA amyloid deposition are the blood vessels, particularly in the submucosa, and the lamina propria of the mucosa [3]. Systemic AL amyloid, due to proliferative abnormalities of B cells and plasma cells, is more often found in the muscular layers of the bowel wall, although it is also frequently deposited in vessel walls. Senile amyloidosis, due to fibrillary deposits of transthyretin, is typically found in vessels and in the submucosa [4], while dialysis-associated amyloidosis due to β_2-microglobulin shows particularly heavy deposition in the submucosa and muscularis propria [5,6]. However, these patterns of amyloid deposition should in no way be considered exclusive for any one form of disease, and are no substitute for immunohistochemical characterization in the classification of the disease. Involvement of the gastrointestinal tract by hereditary systemic amyloidosis is extremely rare but may occur in some non-neuropathic (Ostertag-type) forms [1]. Generally speaking, amyloid deposition in systemic amyloidosis is more prevalent in the stomach and duodenum than the large bowel, and upper gastrointestinal biopsy is likely to be a more sensitive method of diagnosing amyloidosis than rectal biopsy [3], although rectal biopsy is more convenient.

Amyloid deposition localized to the gastrointestinal tract is uncommon. It may occasionally be found in the elderly [4], and there are case reports of localized amyloid tumours (amyloidomas) within the gastrointestinal tract [7,8]. In the latter the deposited protein frequently induces a foreign body-type giant cell reaction.

The clinical effects of amyloid deposition depend mainly on where the amyloid is deposited within the bowel. While most patients with gastrointestinal amyloidosis are asymptomatic, severe haemorrhage may result when fragile amyloid-infiltrated blood vessels rupture. Discrete ulcers and masses (amyloidoma) are commoner in the stomach and the colon than in the small bowel, which may be affected by a protein-losing enteropathy. Focal ulcers, sometimes leading to perforation, may occur in any part of the gastrointestinal tract and often represent multifocal localized ischaemia due to vascular deposition of amyloid in the submucosa and deeper in the bowel wall. Abnormalities of gut motility may result from amyloid within the muscularis propria and within the nerves of the myenteric plexus. This may result in pyloric obstruction, small intestinal stasis with bacterial overgrowth and malabsorption, large intestinal pseudo-obstruction or severe constipation.

A number of conditions enter the differential diagnosis of amyloidosis in the large bowel and it is prudent to use the Congo Red stain (or immunostaining for SAP) whenever an eosinophilic vascular or connective tissue deposit is encountered. Subepithelial deposition of amyloid may be confused with a thickened subepithelial collagen plate in collagenous colitis (see p. 523). The latter is 'fenestrated' by lymphocytes and capillaries and often shows a characteristic artefact where the surface epithelium appears to peel off the underlying subepithelial collagen band; features that are not usually seen in association with subepithelial amyloid deposition. Occasionally eosinophilic arteriosclerotic changes and fibrin may present diagnostic difficulty, especially following radiotherapy (see p. 519), while eosinophilic collagen deposition within the muscularis propria in systemic sclerosis or in familial visceral myopathies can cause confusion in full-thickness biopsies taken for the evaluation of intestinal pseudo-obstruction.

Endometriosis

Endometriosis of the large bowel is not uncommon. It is one of the commonest extragenitourinary sites of involvement, occurring in 15–20% of cases [9–11]. Despite this, bowel symptoms are relatively uncommon and most cases are discovered as incidental histological findings in colorectal specimens resected for other reasons. Symptoms of colorectal endometriosis when present are a frequent source of confusion with more serious colorectal conditions. They include bleeding, pain and obstruction. Bleeding and pain is classically cyclical, giving a clue towards the diagnosis. Endometriotic lesions almost never ulcerate, and when ulceration is seen, it is usually a consequence of repeated mucosal biopsies. Most endometriotic lesions are on the left side of the colon. Occasional caecal endometriomas have been associated with intussusception [12].

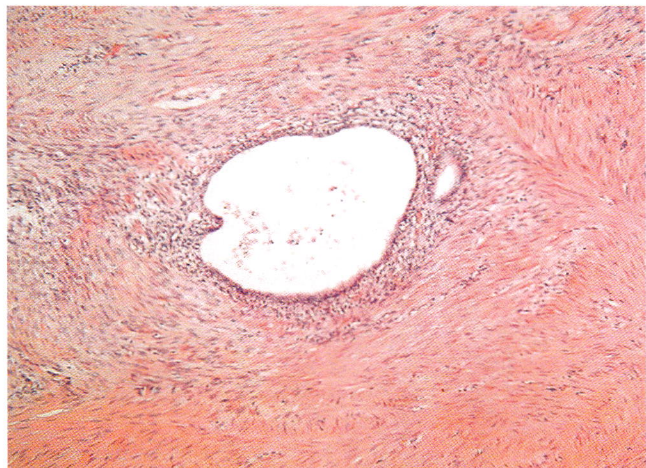

Fig. 41.1 Endometriotic gland and endometriotic stroma within the muscularis propria in endometriosis of the sigmoid colon.

It is often not appreciated clinically that endometriosis may occur in postmenopausal women, especially in those receiving sex hormone replacement therapy. This may cause clinical and histological confusion. We have seen a number of cases of colorectal adenocarcinoma accompanied by endometriosis within the bowel wall and subserosa that had led to radiological and macroscopic overstaging of the carcinoma. The histological diagnosis of endometriosis depends on the finding of both endometrial glands and endometrial-type stroma (Fig. 41.1).

Melanosis coli

Melanosis coli describes an accumulation of a brown granular pigment within histiocytes in the lamina propria of the colorectum (Fig. 41.2). It is closely related to increased epithelial cell apoptosis, both in laboratory animals and in humans [13,14]. Melanosis coli resembles lipofuscin in its staining characteristics and shows positivity with both periodic acid–Schiff (PAS) and the Masson–Hamperl reaction [15]. Autopsy studies have revealed a prevalence of up to 60%, but it is our impression that the condition is decreasing in frequency in the UK. Melanosis coli affects the right side of the colon more than the left, and it is seen in the appendix but not in the terminal ileum [16,17]. The lymphoid follicles in the colonic mucosa are not affected and may stand out as pale spots, although pigment-containing histiocytes may be found in the sinuses of lymph nodes draining an area of melanosis coli [18].

The important histological differential diagnosis is mucosal haemosiderosis, a feature of ischaemic colitis, and Perls' stain is often useful in the distinction. Whilst melanosis coli remains an important marker for anthraquinone laxative abuse, it has to be remembered that it is an end-product of apoptosis, and

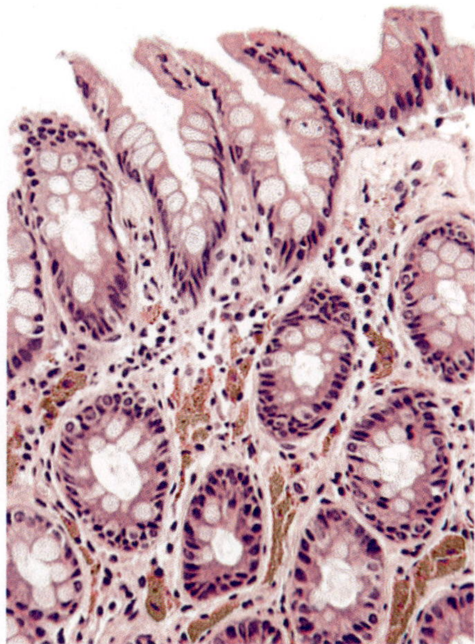

Fig. 41.2 Mucosal biopsy of melanosis coli showing pigment-containing histiocytes within the lamina propria.

several other drugs cause excess apoptosis and melanosis coli. The most frequent of these are non-steroidal anti-inflammatory drugs [14,19]. On the other hand, not all conditions characterized by increased apoptosis are associated with melanosis coli—it is not seen in graft-versus-host disease and human immunodeficiency virus (HIV) colitis. This may imply that a long-standing (rather than acute) increase in apoptotic activity is necessary in the aetiology of melanosis coli. Melanosis is also seen in some patients with ulcerative colitis [20]. Some such patients with distal ulcerative colitis present with constipation, and the melanosis may represent laxative use in some of these. In other patients with ulcerative colitis, active disease is associated with increased epithelial cell and lymphocyte apoptosis [20]. Another possible explanation is the use of sulphasalazine, which induces microscopic colitis (and presumed increased epithelial apoptosis) in a small number of patients.

Muciphages

Muciphages were first described as mucin-containing macrophages in the colorectal lamina propria by Azzopardi and Evans in 1966 [21]. They may occur in normal and abnormal colorectal mucosal biopsies [22] and they are not regarded as pathological in themselves; they can be found in up to 50% of rectal biopsies [21]. Muciphages are probably related to previous epithelial damage, usually subtle and clinically insignificant, that releases mucin into the lamina propria. They must not be mistaken for the characteristic macrophages of Whipple's disease [23] or metastatic malignant cells [24] or macrophages containing *Mycobacterium avium-intracellulare* (MAI). MAI-containing PAS-positive macrophages may be distinguished from PAS-positive muciphages by the use of a Ziehl–Neelsen stain. Table 41.1 highlights the range of conditions that enter the differential diagnosis of colorectal muciphages.

Pseudolipomatosis

This is a mucosal accumulation of microscopic gas bubbles, manifested as multiple spherical empty spaces of variable size in the lamina propria that resemble fat cells in paraffin sections. There is no epithelial or histiocytic lining to the spaces, and some are seen within lymphoid aggregates [26]. Large amounts result in a typical appearance endoscopically resembling 'muciphage mucosa' [26]. Pseudolipomatosis may be seen in association with pneumatosis coli [27,28]. The gas spaces are thought to arise usually as a consequence of air entering the lamina propria through minute breaches in the surface epithelium during insufflation at endoscopy. While this may sometimes occur in normal mucosa, it may be that atrophic mucosa, such as that found in inactive long-standing inflammatory bowel disease, is more susceptible. Pseudolipomatosis has also been described following inadequate washing of endoscopes following hydrogen peroxide endoscope disinfecting, when residual peroxide reacts with normal tissues to release oxygen [27,29].

Stercoral ulceration

Stercoral ulcers result from pressure of abnormally hard faecal masses on the mucosa of the large bowel, most commonly at the rectosigmoid junction where there is a narrow lumen whose expansion is restricted by the presence of neighbouring structures. They are usually a consequence of intractable constipation and are an uncommon cause of perforation and faecal peritonitis, which may be initiated with straining at stool. Non-absorbable antacids containing aluminium salts and cation exchange resins used to treat hyperkalaemia in renal patients appear to be contributory [30,31]. Stercoral ulcers appear as well demarcated, irregular longitudinal tears and perforations through which hard stool may be seen to protrude. The adjacent tissues appear necrotic or gangrenous. Histologically the appearances are of ulceration with focal ischaemic features and intense acute and chronic inflammation penetrating the bowel wall [32].

Gas cysts—pneumatosis coli

This condition in the colon is identical to pneumatosis cys-

Table 41.1 Mucosal accumulations in the colorectum. Modified from [25] with permission.

	Cytoplasmic composition	Diagnostic features	Clinical significance
Muciphages	Mucin	Tinctorial properties of mucin, CD68+	None
Melanosis coli	Lipofuscin-like pigment	PAS+, Masson–Hamperl+	Drug ingestion
Pseudolipomatosis	Gas	No histiocytic lining to gas cysts	Effects of endoscopy
Pneumatosis intestinalis*	Gas	Histiocytic and giant cell lining to gas cysts	Association with psychiatric and chronic lung diseases
Haemosiderosis	Iron-related compounds	Perls+	Marker of ischaemia, torsion and trauma
Barium granuloma*	Barium sulphate	Refractile crystals	Previous barium studies with mucosal rupture
Whipple's disease	*Tropheryma whippeii* bacteria	PAS+, bacilli on EM, PCR positive	Multi-system disorder
Signet ring cell carcinoma	Mucin	Tinctorial properties of mucin, cytokeratin+	Primary or metastatic carcinoma
Atypical mycobacteriosis	*Mycobacterium avlum intracellulare*	PAS+ but ZN reveals numerous acid fast bacilli	Immunosuppression, especially AIDS
Malakoplakia*	Michaelis-Gutmann (MG) bodies and lysosomes	MG bodies are Alcian blue/PAS and von Kossa+	May accompany other conditions, especially colorectal cancer
Langerhans cell histiocytosis *	Lysosomes	Normal properties of histiocytes, especially EM	Multi-system disorder
Chronic granulomatous disease	Lipofuscin-like pigment	PAS+, lipid+	Multi-system disorder in children
Glycolipid storage diseases	Varlous lipids	Dependent on disorder type	Multi-system disorders

* These diseases are primarily submucosal accumulations but may be seen within the lamina propria.
EM, electron microscopy; PCR, polymerase chain reaction; ZN, Ziehl–Neilson.

toides intestinalis of the small intestine and the aetiology is discussed in Chapter 27 (p. 402). It is characterized by gas cysts in the submucosal and subserosal layers of the large bowel wall and can affect the entire colon and rectum or just one part [33]. The disease is often symptomless but can present with diarrhoea, rectal bleeding due to mucosal erosion over the cysts, or rarely pneumoperitoneum from rupture of a gas cyst into the peritoneal cavity.

The macroscopic appearances are characteristic. The mucosal surface has a coarse cobblestone appearance due to large numbers of submucosal cysts, the apices of which may show intramucosal haemorrhage. The gas seems to be under some pressure, because rupture of the cysts during endoscopic biopsy or in fresh surgical specimens may cause a popping sound. The biopsy appearances are distinctive. Cystic spaces in the submucosa are lined by endothelial cells, macrophages and multinucleate macrophage giant cells with eosinophilic cytoplasm (Fig. 41.3). The connective tissue between the cysts, which are often multilocular, shows little inflammation. The covering mucosa is attenuated and sometimes contains small haemorrhages. The appearances are most likely to be confused with lymphangioma (see p. 620) or oleogranuloma (see p. 669).

Graft-versus-host disease

Graft-versus-host disease occurs when donor lymphocytes bearing different human leucocyte antigen (HLA) types from the host are given to an immunosuppressed individual, usually in the context of bone marrow transplantation. The large bowel (along with the skin, the remainder of the gastrointestinal tract and the biliary system) is a well recognized site of involvement in affected individuals, usually resulting in watery diarrhoea or rectal bleeding, and rectal biopsy is often used as a convenient method of confirming the clinical diagnosis. General features of the pathology of the condition are described in Chapter 17 (see p. 230).

The histological hallmark of graft-versus-host disease in the colorectum is increased apoptosis of the epithelial cells in the proliferative zone at the base of crypts [34,35]. In early cases this may be the only abnormality, and because it may be patchy several levels taken through the biopsy may be necessary to identify it with confidence. Typically the apoptotic cells are seen within lacunae along the crypt basement membrane (Fig. 41.4a) There may also be more overt epithelial cell necrosis in

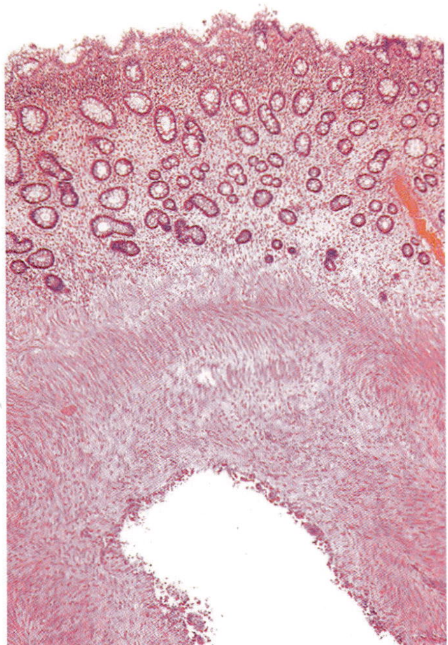

Fig. 41.3 Large bowel biopsy showing gas-filled spaces lined by histiocytes and giant cells in the submucosa.

the upper reaches of the crypt and on the luminal surface, which may result in crypts lined by flattened degenerate cells and distended by necrotic cells. This may induce an acute neutrophil infiltrate, and in florid acute graft-versus-host disease there may be total mucosal loss and ulceration. Chronic inflammatory cells in the lamina propria may be slightly increased, but this is rarely pronounced.

As the disease progresses towards chronic graft-versus-host disease the crypts whose stem cells have been damaged by the immunological attack become wiped out, leaving only 'gravestones' composed of isolated clusters of epithelial cells in the lamina propria. These clusters are often composed entirely of endocrine cells, probably reflecting the slow turnover of this cell population in comparison with colonocytes and goblet cells [36]. Residual crypts undergo regeneration by epithelial proliferation and crypt fission, resulting in a markedly distorted mucosal architecture (Fig. 41.4b) that may suggest long-standing inactive chronic ulcerative colitis. However, in chronic graft-versus-host disease it is generally accompanied by fibrosis of the lamina propria, an unusual feature of ulcerative colitis, and this, the increased apoptotic activity, and the clinical history serve to make the distinction. Conditions that are more important in the differential diagnosis are cytomegalovirus colitis, which is also common in immunosuppressed patients and which may also give rise to increased epithelial apoptosis, and the effects of pre-bone marrow transplant chemotherapy conditioning regimes, that may produce virtually identical histological changes to acute graft-versus-host disease during the first 3 weeks following the transplant. Confident histological diagnosis is virtually impossible during this time frame. Increased epithelial apoptosis is also a feature of HIV infection (see p. 474) and some forms of drug-induced colitis (see p. 514).

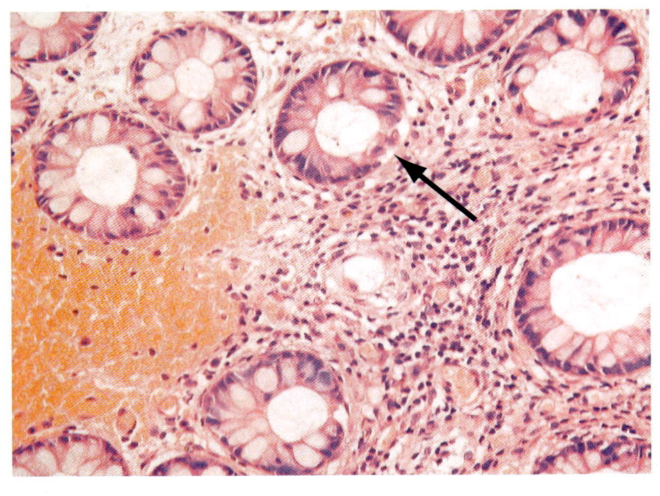

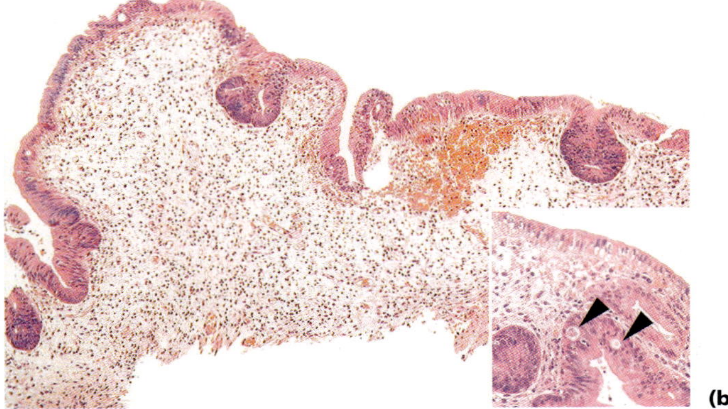

Fig. 41.4 Graft-versus-host disease: (a) a rectal biopsy with early subtle changes of focal apoptosis in occasional crypt bases (arrow) and a degenerate crypt in the centre of the field; (b) late in the history with extensive crypt drop-out and crypt distortion, but focal apoptosis is still seen (inset).

Chronic graft-versus-host disease may also give rise to submucosal and even transmural fibrosis of the intestinal wall, and can lead to bowel strictures.

Effects of bowel preparation

Old fashioned hyperosmolar bowel preparations for colonoscopy have been reported to cause considerable oedema and mucin depletion in the absence of inflammation [37]. The newer ones may cause focal acute colitis in the proximal colon leading to an erroneous diagnosis of Crohn's disease [38–41].

Appendices epiploicae

Appendices epiploicae come to the notice of histopathologists when they undergo torsion. This results in infarction and haemorrhage, occasionally with resolution; there may be intestinal stenosis, but this is rare. They may also autoamputate and present as peritoneal loose bodies. Fat necrosis, hyalinization and calcification are seen histologically.

Barium granuloma

Barium granulomas result from extravasation of radiological contrast material into the bowel wall via mucosal tears or diverticula. They may present as polypoid or ulcerated lesions that can closely mimic a tumour endoscopically, especially when they are not discovered until some considerable time after the causative barium enema examination. The rectum is most commonly involved, and macroscopically the raised lesions may vary from white to grey-pink in colour, and may be ulcerated with yellow plaque-like areas. On rare occasions they may penetrate into the bowel wall resulting in barium abscesses and barium peritonitis. Barium granulomas are comprised of macrophages containing light green/grey barium sulphate crystals that may vary in size and shape from small granular crystals to large rhomboidal forms. They are anisotropic in polarized light and may be identified histochemically by the Rhodizonate method and characterized further by energy-dispersive X-ray analysis [42].

Malakoplakia

Malakoplakia involving the large intestine may be seen in association with ulcerative colitis, in patients with coexisting debilitating illnesses or malignancy, or rarely in isolation. It may present as ulcers with sentinel polyps, as a tumour-like mass, or even as diffuse thickening of the bowel wall. Histologically malakoplakia is composed of sheets of large macrophages with eosinophilic granular cytoplasm (Hansemann cells) containing characteristic PAS-positive iron-containing calculospherules (Michaelis–Gutmann bodies) [43,44].

Scorpion and snake bites

Scorpion bites are a cause of acute pancreatitis beloved of examination candidates and rare in life. Scorpion bites may also result in haemorrhagic ischaemic colitis, as may rattlesnake bites. These are toxin-mediated colitides [45].

References

1 Pepys MB. Pathogenesis, diagnosis and treatment of systemic amyloidosis. *Philos Trans R Soc Lond B Biol Sci*, 2001; 356: 203.

2 Tan SY, Pepys MB. Amyloidosis. *Histopathology*, 1994; 25: 403.

3 Yamada M, Hatakeyama S, Tsukagoshi H. Gastrointestinal amyloid deposition in AL (primary or myeloma-associated) and AA (secondary) amyloidosis. *Hum Pathol*, 1985; 16: 1206.

4 Rocken C, Saeger W, Linke RP. Gastrointestinal amyloid deposits in old age. *Pathol Res Pract*, 1994; 190: 641.

5 Borczuk A, Mannion C, Dickson D, Alt E. Intestinal pseudoobstruction and ischemia secondary to both 2-microglobulin and serum A amyloid deposition. *Mod Pathol*, 1995; 8: 577.

6 Jimenez RE, Price DA, Pinkus GS *et al*. Development of gastrointestinal beta2-microglobulin amyloidosis correlates with time on dialysis. *Am J Surg Pathol*, 1998; 22: 729.

7 Senapati A, Fletcher C, Bultitude MI, Jackson BT. Amyloid tumour of the rectum. *J R Soc Med*, 1995; 88: 48.

8 Deans GT, Hale RJ, McMahon RFT, Brough WA. Amyloid tumour of the colon. *J Clin Pathol*, 1995; 48: 592.

9 Tagart REB. Endometriosis of the large intestine. *Br J Surg*, 1959; 47: 27.

10 Spjut HJ, Perkins DE. Endometriosis of the sigmoid colon and rectum. *Am J Roentgenol*, 1969; 82: 1070.

11 Davis C, Alexander RW, Buenger EG. Surgery of endometrioma of the ileum and colon. *Am J Surg*, 1963; 105: 250.

12 Fujimoto A, Osuga Y, Tsutsumi O, Fuji T, Okagaki R, Taketani Y. Successful laparoscopic treatment of ileo-cecal endometriosis producing large bowel obstruction. *J Obstet Gynaecol Res*, 2001; 27: 221.

13 Walker NI, Smith MM, Smithers BM. Ultrastructure of human melanosis coli with reference to its pathogenesis. *Pathology*, 1993; 25: 120.

14 Byers RJ, Marsh P, Parkinson D, Haboubi NY. Melanosis coli is associated with an increase in colonic epithelial apoptosis and not with laxative abuse. *Histopathology*, 1997; 30: 160.

15 Walker NI, Bennett RE, Axelsen RA. Melanosis coli. A consequence of anthraquinone-induced apoptosis of colonic epithelial cells. *Am J Pathol*, 1988; 131: 465.

16 Ming SC, Goldman H. Disorders common to the gastrointestinal tract. In: *Pathology of the Gastrointestinal Tract*, 2nd edn. Baltimore: Williams & Wilkins, 1998: 410.

17 Rutty GN, Shaw PA. Melanosis of the appendix: prevalence, distribution and review of the pathogenesis of 47 cases. *Histopathology*, 1997; 30: 319.

18 Hall M, Eusebi V. Yellow-brown spindle bodies in mesenteric lymph nodes: a possible relationship with melanosis coli. *Histopathology*, 1978; 2: 47.

19 Lee FD. The importance of apoptosis in the histopathology of drug related lesions of the large intestine. *J Clin Pathol*, 1993; 46: 118.

20 Pardi DS, Tremaine WJ, Rothenberger HJ, Batts KP. Melanosis coli in inflammatory bowel disease. *J Clin Gastroenterol*, 1998; 26: 167.

21 Azzopardi JG, Evans DJ. Mucoprotein containing histiocytes (muciphages) in the rectum. *J Clin Pathol*, 1966; 19: 368.

22 Salto-Tellez M, Price AB. What is the significance of muciphages in colorectal biopsies? *Histopathology*, 2000; 36: 556.

23 Caravati CM, Litch M, Weisiger BB *et al*. Diagnosis of Whipple's disease by rectal biopsy with report of 3 additional cases. *Ann Intern Med*, 1963; 58: 166.

24 Talbot IC, Price AB. Assessment of abnormalities: diagnostic signposts. In: *Biopsy Pathology in Colorectal Disease*. London: Chapman & Hall, 1995: 54.

25 Shepherd NA. Muciphages and other accumulations in the colorectal mucosa. *Histopathology*, 2000; 36: 559.

26 Snover DC, Sandstad J, Hutton S. Mucosal pseudolipomatosis of the colon. *Am J Clin Pathol*, 1985; 84: 575.

27 Waring JP, Manne RK, Wadas DD, Sanowski RA. Mucosal pseudolipomatosis: an air pressure related colonoscopy complication. *Gastrointest Endosc*, 1989; 35: 93.

28 Gagliardi G, Thompson IW, Hershman MJ, Forbes A, Hawley PR, Talbot IC. Pneumatosis coli: a proposed pathogenesis based on study of 25 cases and review of the literature. *Int J Colorect Dis*, 1996; 11: 111.

29 Ryan CK, Potter GD. Disinfectant colitis. Rinse as well as you wash. *J Clin Gastroenterol*, 1995; 21: 6.

30 Aquilo JJ, Zinche H, Woods JE, Buckingham JM. Intestinal perforation due to faecal impaction after renal transplantation. *J Urol*, 1976; 116: 153.

31 Archibald SD, Jirsch DW, Bear RA. Gastrointestinal complications of renal transplantation: 2 the colon. *Can Med Assoc J*, 1978; 119: 1301.

32 Huttunen R, Heikkinen E, Larmi TKI. Stercoraceous and idiopathic perforations of the colon. *Surg Gynecol Obstet*, 1975; 140: 756.

33 Galandiuk S, Fazio VW. Pneumatosis cystoides intestinalis. *Dis Colon Rectum*, 1986; 29: 358.

34 Bombi JA, Nadal A, Carreras E *et al*. Assessment of histopathologic changes in the colonic biopsy in acute graft-versus-host disease. *Am J Clin Pathol*, 1995; 103: 690.

35 Snover DC. Graft versus host disease of the gastrointestinal tract. *Am J Surg Pathol*, 1991; 14 (Suppl 1): 101.

36 Lampert IA, Thorpe P, van Noorden S *et al*. Selective sparing of enterochromaffin cells in graft versus host disease affecting the colonic mucosa. *Histopathology*, 1985; 9: 875.

37 Leriche M, Devroede G, Sanchez G *et al*. Changes in the rectal mucosa induced by hypertonic enemas. *Dis Colon Rectum*, 1978; 21: 227.

38 Saunders DR, Sillery J, Rachmilewitz D *et al*. Effect of Bisacodyl on the structure and function of rodent and human intestine. *Gastroenterology*, 1977; 72: 849.

39 Meisel JI, Bergman D, Graney D *et al*. Human rectal mucosa: proctoscopic and morphological changes caused by laxatives. *Gastroenterology*, 1977; 72: 1274.

40 Pockros RJ, Foroozan P. Golytely lavage versus a standard colonoscopy preparation: effect on a normal colonic mucosal histology. *Gastroenterology*, 1985; 88: 545.

41 Pike BF, Phillipi PJ, Lawson EH. Soap colitis. *N Engl J Med*, 1971; 285: 217.

42 Levison DA, Crocker PR, Smith A, Blackshaw AJ, Bartram CI. Varied light and scanning electron microscopic appearances of barium sulphate in smears and histological sections. *J Clin Pathol*, 1984; 37: 481.

43 Lewin K, Harell J, Lee A, Crowley L. An electron microscopic study: demonstration of bacilliform organisms in malakoplakic macrophages. *Gastroenterology*, 1974; 66: 28.

44 Radin DR, Chandrosoma P, Halls JM. Colonic malakoplakia. *Gastrointest Radiol*, 1984; 9: 359.

45 Wallace JF. Disorders caused by venoms, bites and stings. In: Petersdorf RG, Adams RD, Brauwald E *et al*., eds. *Harrison's Principles of Internal Medicine*, 10th edn. New York: McGraw-Hill, 1983: 1241.

PART

7 Anal region

42 Normal anal region

Anatomy

The anal canal is an anteroposterior slit 3–4 cm in length situated between the rectum above and the perianal skin below [1]. Different workers use different anatomical landmarks to define its precise upper and lower limits; for example, pathologists tend to use the upper and lower borders of the internal anal sphincter [2], the definition which will be used in this account; while clinicians usually quote the level of the levator ani muscle (the site of the so-called anorectal angle) for the upper limit and the anal orifice for the lower; and anatomists frequently use the levels of the anal valves (see below) and the anal orifice, respectively [3]. The anal canal is separated posteriorly from the tip of the coccyx by a mass of fibromuscular tissue (the anococcygeal ligament), and anteriorly from the membranous part of the urethra and the bulb of the penis in the male, or the lower end of the vagina in the female, by the perineal body. On each side lies an ischiorectal fossa.

The mucosal lining of the upper half of the anal canal is thrown into some six to 12 vertical folds (Fig. 42.1). These are the *anal columns*, whose lower ends are joined together, at a level about midway down the internal sphincter, by the anal valves, small transverse crescentic folds of mucosa which mark the position of the *pectinate* or *dentate line*. Small recesses immediately proximal to the anal valves, within which faecal material may become lodged giving rise to inflammation, are termed the *anal sinuses*. Below the dentate line the mucosal lining of the anal canal is smooth and this zone is sometimes called the pecten (Fig. 42.1). The submucous connective tissue of the upper anal canal is loose, but in the pecten denser fibroelastic tissue anchors down the epithelium firmly to the underlying superficial part of the internal sphincter, creating a submucosal barrier at the dentate line which is important in limiting the spread of cancer in this region.

Beneath the mucosa of the upper two-thirds or so of the anal canal, within the connective tissue, is the internal rectal venous plexus that gives the overlying mucosa a plum-coloured or bluish appearance. Moreover, in the left lateral, right anterior and right posterior zones of the anal canal this plexus is modified into three specialized vascular *anal cushions* [4] consisting of submucosal anastomosing networks of arterioles and venules, with arteriovenous communications, which have a certain resemblance to erectile tissue [5]. These cushions bulge into the lumen of the anal canal, possibly playing a role in the maintenance of normal anal continence [6]. Secondary folds often intersect the cushions to a variable degree, and longitudinal clefts in the cushions give rise to the anal columns. When they become engorged and prolapsed downwards, they give rise to haemorrhoids (see p. 669). Another plexus, the external rectal venous plexus, lies beneath the mucosa of the lower part of the pecten and the skin of the anal margin.

The arterial supply of the anal canal comes from the superior, middle and inferior rectal arteries, but there is great individual variation of anatomical detail [4]. The venous drainage of the anal canal is the subject of some controversy. Many older texts state that the internal rectal plexus drains into the portal system via the superior rectal vein while the external venous plexus drains into the systemic venous circulation via the inferior rectal vein, and that the connections between the portal and systemic circulations in this area are very poor. However, more recent injection studies [4] suggest that there are usually free communications between the superior, middle and inferior rectal veins and that the venous drainage from the anal cushions, although anatomically closely related to the internal plexus, is primarily to the systemic circulation. The lymphatic drainage of the anal canal above the dentate line goes to the superior rectal group of lymph nodes, whereas the superficial inguinal glands drain the tissues below this line.

The dentate line itself was formerly considered to represent the site of the anal membrane in the fetus, that is, the junction of the endodermally derived cloaca and the ectodermal proctodaeum or anal pit. Furthermore, the anal papillae, small projections on the edges of the anal valves, were considered to be remnants of this anal membrane. However, more recent studies [7] of developing human embryos have challenged this view, proposing that the anal membrane is represented in the adult by the whole of the so-called transitional zone of the anal canal, a histologically distinct area usually extending proximally from the dentate line over a distance of about 1 cm (see below), rather than by the narrow dentate line itself. Whatever the precise embryological origin of this zone of the anal canal there are quite marked changes in the nervous in-

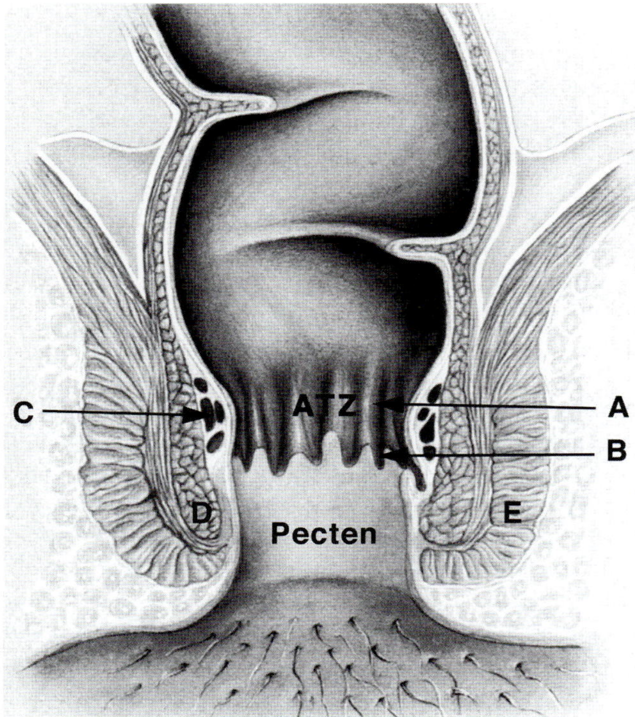

Fig. 42.1 Diagram of the normal anatomy of the anorectal region. ATZ, anal transitional zone; A, anal columns; B, dentate line; C, submucosal vascular cushions; D, internal sphincter; and E, external sphincter.

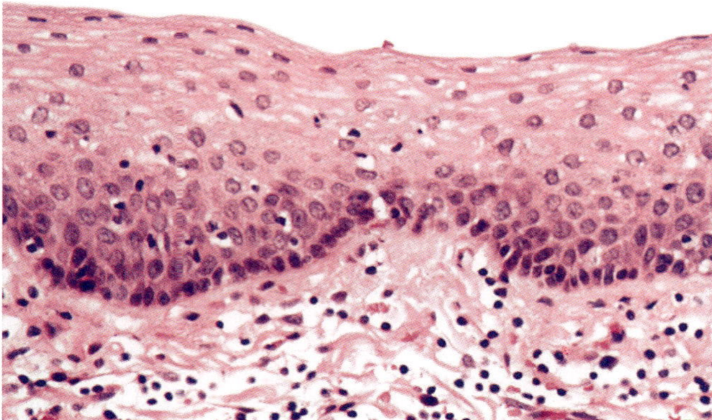

Fig. 42.2 Squamous zone of anal canal.

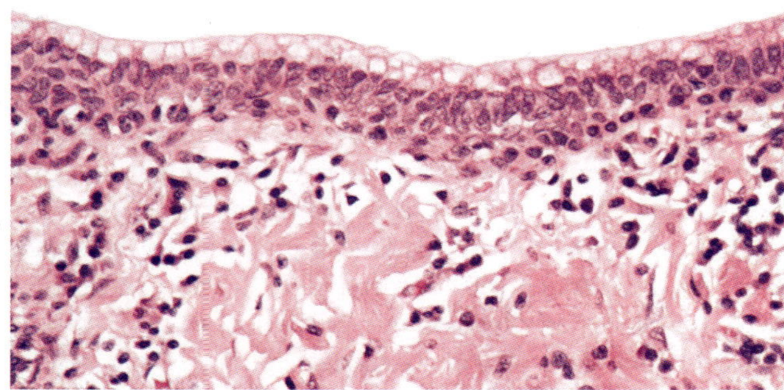

Fig. 42.3 Anal transitional zone epithelium with pseudostratified columnar surface cells containing small amounts of mucin.

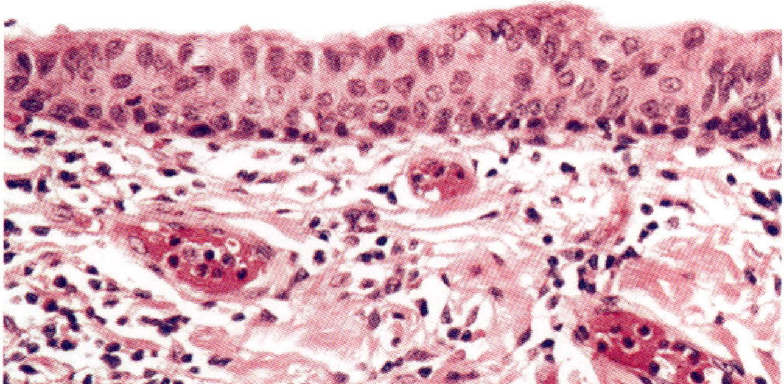

Fig. 42.4 Urothelial-like variant of anal transitional zone epithelium.

nervation at or close to the dentate line. Below this, the lining of the anal canal possesses a somatic type of nerve supply, in keeping with an ectodermal origin. This area is therefore extremely sensitive to touch and pain. The mucosa above the dentate line, on the other hand, is insensitive, being supplied by autonomic nerves typical of endodermally derived structures.

The internal anal sphincter is composed of smooth muscle (involuntary) fibres and is really only an enlarged portion of the circular muscle of the rectum, with which it is continuous (Fig. 42.1). The external anal sphincter is composed of striated (voluntary) muscle and is often said to have three parts, subcutaneous, superficial and deep, although in reality these are scarcely separable from one another. Both internal and external sphincters are notable for the fact that they are muscles which have a continuous resting tone, a phenomenon shared with the other skeletal muscles of the pelvic floor but which is most unusual in skeletal muscles elsewhere in the body. Nevertheless, the anal sphincters do not appear to be of prime importance in the maintenance of normal faecal continence, as shown by the fact that major functional deficit does not result from their division, for example in the treatment of anal fistula. It is the tonic contraction of the puborectalis muscle which, by virtue of the fact that it forms a sling around the lower rectum, pulls it upwards and anteriorly to form and maintain the anorectal angle, which is the prime factor controlling continence [8]. The internal sphincter appears to be chiefly responsible for the finer degrees of control, i.e. for flatus and loose stool, while the role of the external sphincter is to maintain continence under 'emergency conditions' such as coughing, sneezing or during diarrhoeal illnesses.

Histology

The anal canal can be divided into three zones on the basis of the histological appearance of its mucosal lining [2,9]. The upper *colorectal zone* is covered by large intestinal-type mucosa, which differs from normal colorectal mucosa only in that the goblet cells of the crypts contain a predominance of sialomucins over sulphomucins, and in that the smooth muscle fibres of the muscularis mucosae frequently appear splayed with occasional fibres extending upwards into the lamina propria in between the crypts. In the more proximal rectum these two features are frequently associated with pathological mucosal prolapse (see p. 464) but in the colorectal zone of the anal canal they are sufficiently common to be regarded as normal, probably because minor degrees of prolapse of this mucosa, which is poorly anchored by fibrous tissue to the underlying internal sphincter, is common during normal defecation. The lowest part of the anal canal is the *squamous zone* (Fig. 42.2), which is lined by non-keratinizing squamous epithelium devoid of specialized sweat glands or pilosebaceous structures. At the lower border of the internal sphincter this merges into the true perianal skin, which does possess hair follicles, sweat and apocrine glands.

In between the colorectal and squamous zones is the *anal transitional zone*, which is covered for the most part by a stratified epithelium with varying patterns of differentiation. Columnar cells, often producing small quantities of mucin, are frequent (Fig. 42.3), but polygonal cells (Fig. 42.3) or more flattened cells may also be found, the latter giving the mucosa an appearance that is very reminiscent of urothelium [2] (Fig. 42.4). Occasional melanocytes may be found in the mucosa of both the transitional and squamous zones, and are often abundant in the adjacent perianal skin [10].

The relationship between the histological zones of the anal canal and the gross anatomical landmarks is not entirely uniform, due to some individual variation both in the width of the transitional zone and in the contours of its upper and lower margins. Mucin staining of whole specimens has shown that the lower limit of the transitional zone usually coincides with the anatomical dentate line and extends proximally over a distance of about 1 cm. The lower pecten of the anal canal corresponds with the histological squamous zone. However, in about 10% of cases the transitional zone has a higher (entirely above the dentate line) or lower (straddling the dentate line) location while in a small minority it appears to be completely absent or restricted to one segment of the circumference of the anal canal [11].

Arising from the mucosa of the anal transitional zone, with their orifices opening behind the cusps of the anal valves, are the *anal glands*, six to 10 in number (Fig. 42.5). These are branching ducts that pass downwards and outwards through the submucosa, often extending into, or even through, the muscle of the internal anal sphincter [12]. They act as a channel through which infection can reach the perianal tissues and ischiorectal fossa. Their lining epithelium is identical to the stratified columnar epithelium of the anal transitional zone, but tiny intraepithelial microcysts are a frequent finding [2]. The ducts of the anal glands are sometimes surrounded by lymphoid tissue.

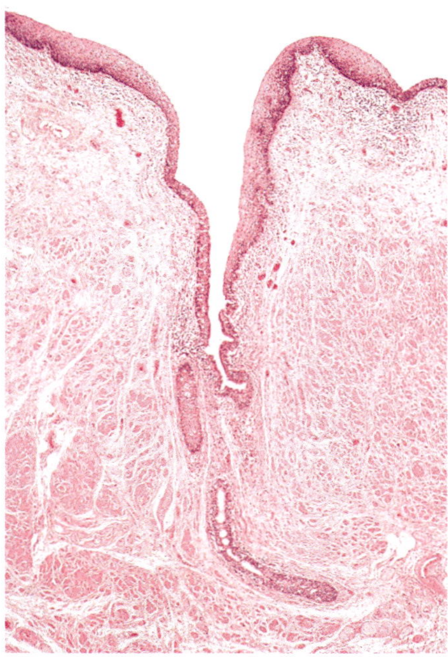

Fig. 42.5 Normal anal crypt lined by transitional epithelium, and an anal duct lined by stratified columnar epithelium.

Epithelial mucins produced by the columnar cells of both the anal transitional zone and the anal glands are similar. They are a mixture of sulphomucins and sialomucins, but unlike those of the large bowel mucosa, they are not O-acetylated [13]. Endocrine cells are also present in these epithelia, usually with argyrophil but non-argentaffin granules [10].

References

1 Parks AG. Modern concepts of the anatomy of the ano-rectal region. *Postgrad Med J*, 1958; 34: 360.
2 Fenger C. The anal transitional zone. *Acta Pathol Microbiol Scand [A]*, 1987; 95: 1.
3 Nivatvongs S, Stern HS, Fryd DS. The length of the anal canal. *Dis Colon Rectum*, 1981; 24: 600.
4 Thomson WHF. The nature of haemorrhoids. *Br J Surg*, 1975; 62: 542.
5 Stelzner F. Die Hamorrhoiden und andere Krankheiten des Corpus cavernosum recti und des Analkanals. *Dtsch Med Wochenschr*, 1963; 88: 689.
6 Gibbons CP, Trowbridge EA, Bannister JJ, Read NW. Role of anal cushions in maintaining continence. *Lancet*, 1986; i: 886.

7 Nobles VP. The development of the human anal canal. *J Anat*, 1984; 138: 575.
8 Parks AG. Anorectal incontinence. *Proc R Soc Med*, 1975; 68: 681.
9 Fenger C. Histology of the anal canal. *Am J Surg Pathol*, 1988; 12: 41.
10 Fenger C, Lyon H. Endocrine cells and melanin-containing cells in the anal canal epithelium. *Histochem J*, 1982; 14: 631.
11 Fenger C. The anal transitional zone. Location and extent. *Acta Pathol Microbiol Scand [A]*, 1979; 87: 379.
12 McColl I. The comparative anatomy and pathology of anal glands. *Ann R Coll Surg*, 1967; 40: 36.
13 Fenger C, Nielsen VT. Dysplastic changes in the anal canal epithelium in minor surgical specimens. *Acta Pathol Microbiol Immunol Scand [A]*, 1981; 89: 463.

43 Inflammatory disorders of the anal region

Anal fissure

The typical anal fissure is found in the midline posteriorly and is very infrequent in other quadrants of the anal canal. It forms an elongated triangular ulcer in the squamous mucous membrane of the lower anal canal overlying the internal sphincter and the subcutaneous part of the external sphincter. The pathogenesis of anal fissure is not clear. Predisposing causes include loss of the normal elasticity and mobility of the mucosa due usually to fibrosis accompanying chronic infection, and it is probable that trauma by the passage of hard faecal masses may be a precipitating factor. There is an increase in the resting pressures of the internal sphincter [1] in patients with anal fissures but this could be a secondary effect [2]. Furthermore, there is poor support of the internal sphincter in the posterior midline and the mucosa may therefore be more susceptible to damage. Superficial fissures may heal spontaneously but more often the condition becomes chronic, probably because associated muscle spasm and constant exposure to infection interfere with healing [3]. Microscopic appearances are those of non-specific inflammation. The edges of chronic fissures are often thickened and somewhat undermined, and the tissues immediately adjacent are oedematous and heavily infiltrated by lymphocytes and plasma cells. The oedematous skin at the lower end of the fissure may form a little polypoid projection, the 'sentinel tag', in a proportion of cases.

Fissures are commonly classified into acute and chronic, primary or secondary [4]. Secondary fissures are linked with known disorders such as Crohn's disease, leukaemia, primary syphilis or a squamous carcinoma. They can also be the result of damage from childbirth and previous anal surgery. In children, fissures can be a common cause of minor rectal bleeding and are often lateral rather than posterior [5].

Anal fistula and anal abscess

An anorectal fistula or abscess usually begins with an infection of the anal glands [6]. These lie in the submucosa of the anal canal but branches penetrate through the internal sphincter to the potential space between it and the external sphincter. Their ducts open into the anal crypts at the level of the dentate line. In many cases the glands can penetrate into and through the external sphincter. Infection within these glands can track in several directions dependent on the complexity of the branching. The classification of anal fistula is based on knowledge of the anatomy of these anal glands. The main anatomical varieties of fistula are [7,8]:

1 *Intersphincteric*. The track runs between the internal and external sphincteric muscle. It is deemed low if it runs distally to the skin and high if it runs proximally to open into the rectum.
2 *Transphincteric*. In this variety the track runs through the external sphincter and through the ischiorectal fossa to the perianal skin.
3 *Suprasphincteric*. Here the track passes upwards into the intersphincteric space, above the external sphincter and back into the ischiorectal fossa to the perianal skin.
4 *Extrasphincteric*. This is secondary to pelvic sepsis rather than anal gland infection and discharges through the ischiorectal fossa to the skin.

The relative frequency of the various types among 769 fistulae seen at St Mark's Hospital was intersphincteric 55.9%, transphincteric 21.3%, suprasphincteric 3.4% and extrasphincteric 3.0%; 16.4% were classified superficial in association with chronic anal fissures and sentinel tags [9].

Pathogenesis

Infection of the glands is probably the most common cause [6]. Various authors have demonstrated infection in and around the glands in cases of fistulae and have suggested that the chronicity of the condition is due to persistence of the anal gland epithelium in the part of the tract adjoining the internal opening, the presence of this persisting epithelium keeping the opening patent and preventing healing [10]. Infection does not of itself explain the persistence of anal fistula [11].

The anal glands may be regarded as diverticula of the anal canal. As in the case of any diverticulum of the alimentary tract, including the appendix, the contents of the glands are subject to stasis and secondary infection. Thus, bacteria will multiply in a gland that has been obstructed by faecal material, foreign bodies or as a result of trauma. Those glands that pass right through the internal sphincter, moreover, will not be able to discharge their contents readily, for the tone of the muscle will tend to compress their lumen. Thus, cystic dilatation of the gland occurs. In fact, a fistula *in ano* is virtually a sinus secondary to disease of the anal gland, and this view fits with the practical observation that there is no clinically detectable internal opening in about half the cases. The condition in such cases is a sinus rather than a true fistula for one end is blind. A fistula, by definition, is open at both ends. It seems likely that stasis and secondary infection of the gland are generally due to obstruction resulting from inflammation: the most common cause is probably an anal fissure.

The ducts of normal anal glands are often surrounded by well developed lymphoid tissue, forming the so-called anal 'tonsils' [12]. It is believed that this lymphoid tissue may become the focus of inflammation, specific or non-specific, and of local or blood-borne origin. Certainly the midportion of the anal canal shows a special liability to intramural hyperplasia of the lymphoid tissue comparable to the hyperplasia of the lymphoid tissues of the oropharyngeal and ileocaecal region.

Histology

During the exploration and surgical treatment of anal fistula and abscesses it is important that representative pieces of tissue from the track should be sent for histological examination, particularly to exclude carcinoma. Various patterns can be seen (Fig. 43.1). In the great majority of cases sections will show an ordinary pyogenic type of inflammatory reaction. Attention, however, must be given to the cellular infiltrate as in one series 6% of subjects with leukaemia had anal lesions, and in 20% of these cases the anal lesions were the initial presentation [13]. Giant cells of the foreign body type are frequently encountered; presumably they are a reaction to the presence within the fistulous track of material derived from the faeces (Fig. 43.1a). An oleogranulomatous reaction is occasionally present (Fig. 43.1b) and is probably due to treatment of the condition with vaseline-impregnated gauze, or the escape into the fistula of oily substances used for softening the faeces. It is important that a foreign body reaction should be distinguished from tuberculosis or the granulomatous (sarcoid) type of response seen in Crohn's disease. The most valuable distinguishing feature is the presence of discrete, compact, epithelioid granulomas in Crohn's disease (Fig. 43.1c). Confluent epithelioid granulomas as opposed to discrete ones suggest tuberculosis, as does caseous necrosis (Fig. 43.1d) and miliary tuberculosis can present as an anal abscess [14]. The spread of infection in and around fistulous tracks can provoke tissue damage such as fat necrosis, secondary vasculitis and degenerative changes in striated muscle with the formation of giant hyperchromatic nuclei. Bearing in mind what has already been said about the pathogenesis of anal fistulae, some surgeons during the course of a 'lay-open' operation will excise what they believe to be the intersphincteric abscess or infected anal gland. This tissue may be sent for histological examination, in which case it should be possible to identify the anal gland as it passes through the internal sphincter to communicate with an abscess cavity or fistulous track in the intersphincteric plane. Occasionally *Trichuris* and *Enterobius vermicularis* may be the cause of an anal canal abscess [15,16] and there is a report describing actinomycosis occurring as a secondary infection [17].

Crohn's disease

The importance of the anal manifestations of Crohn's disease was discussed on p. 506 [18]. The frequency of anal lesions in Crohn's disease varies from 25 to 80% [19,20]. This range reflects the site of primary involvement, it being more common the more distal the disease. However, some 5% of patients will not have proximal lesions [21] and up to 10 years can elapse before intestinal involvement is manifest. Another reason for the wide variation in incidence of perianal disease is because of changing definitions of what constitutes Crohn's disease. For example, patients with terminal ileal disease may have diarrhoea and perianal skin irritation. If this is scored as a perianal complication of Crohn's disease, naturally high figures will occur. The diagnosis of Crohn's disease can be made by histological examination of pieces of tissue taken for biopsy or during surgical treatment of the anal lesion. It will only be helpful in those 60% of cases of Crohn's disease in which sarcoid-like granulomas are present. In patients without such a tissue response the diagnosis rests on the clinical appearance of the anal lesion together with any evidence of intestinal involvement. The anal lesions may be fissures, skin tags, cavitating ulcers, fistulae, strictures or abscesses. In 5% of cases they are sufficiently debilitating to warrant rectal excision [22].

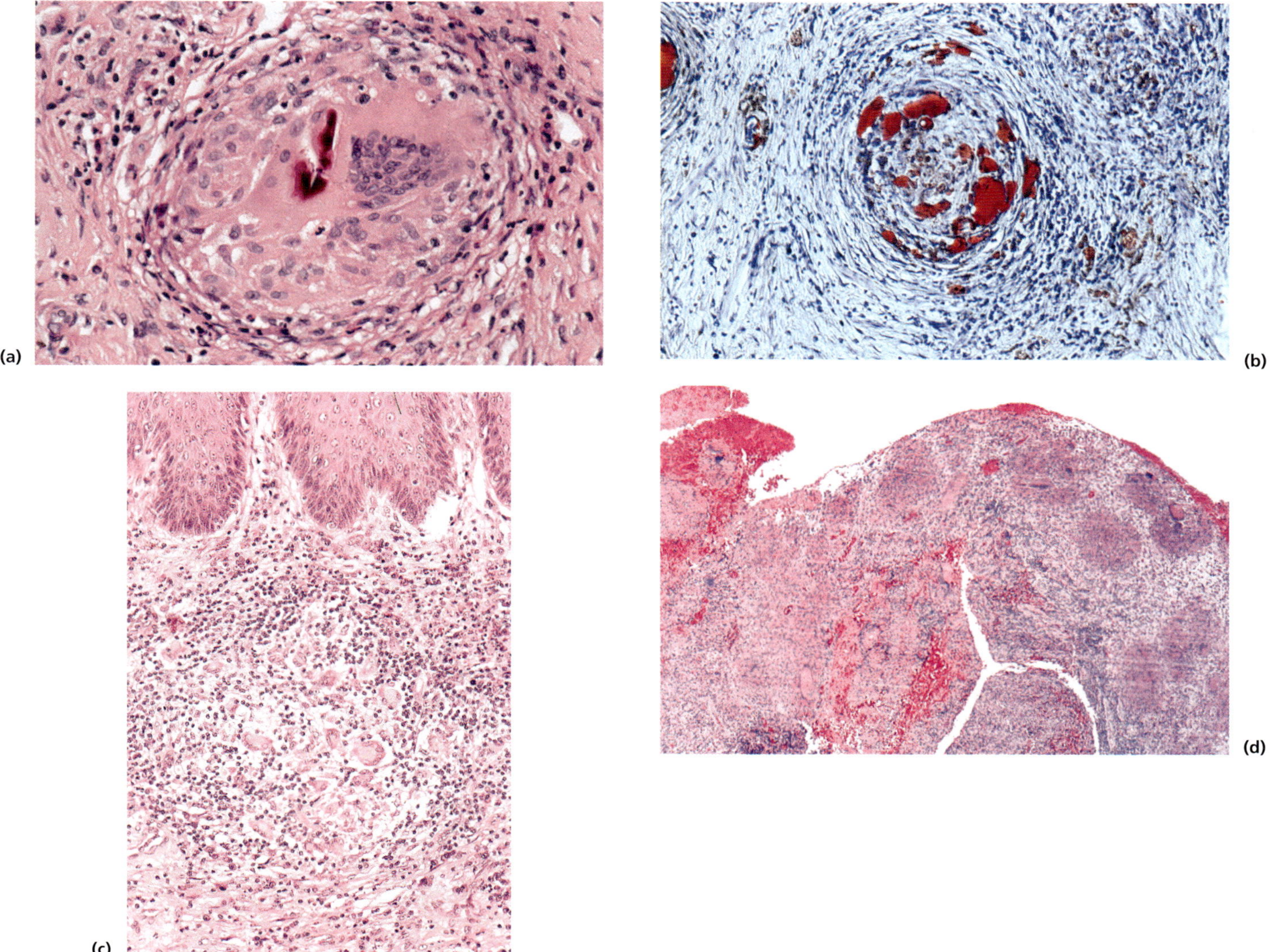

Fig. 43.1 (a) Foreign body giant cell reaction in an anal fistula. (b) Oleogranulomatous reaction in an anal fistula. (c) Histology of an anal lesion of Crohn's disease showing a sarcoid granuloma beneath the perianal skin. (d) Tuberculous anal fistula showing granulomatous reaction with caseation.

Because the clinical features are not always distinctive and a granulomatous histology is absent from some 40% of cases, it is probable that anal lesions due to Crohn's disease will continue to remain unrecognized until the abdominal disease becomes manifest. Apart from lack of characteristic clinical and histological features, the failure to biopsy all anal lesions at the time of surgical treatment must be a frequent cause of failure to recognize the pathology. It is probable that Crohn's disease so often affects the anus because of the aggregations of lymphoid tissue around the anal glands [12], in the same way that the disorder commonly affects the terminal ileum because of the great amount of lymphoid tissue there.

A sarcoid reaction is a purely descriptive term applicable to any collection of epithelioid cells, sometimes with giant cells, without central caseation, although a little central necrosis with preservation of the reticulin pattern is permissible. In some cases of Crohn's disease of the anus, the granulomas are few in number and are very sparsely distributed. In other cases the tissues of the dermis, subcutaneous fat and fistulous track are riddled with lesions. The chances of finding granulomas are dependent on the amount of tissue available for examination. For this reason small biopsies are often inadequate.

A confident distinction between the sarcoid reaction due to Crohn's disease, sarcoidosis or tuberculosis is impossible on histological evidence alone. The presence of caseation is suggestive of tuberculosis, but examination by Ziehl–Neelsen staining is often negative and culture or molecular diagnostic approaches to the diagnosis should be considered in suspicious cases.

Giant cells of the foreign body type are commonly seen in tissue removed from anal fistulae. They usually appear spherical, with a tendency for their many nuclei to be centrally placed, in contrast to the peripheral position of the nuclei in Langhans giant cells. They are isolated or grouped in small numbers, and may be placed around foreign matter such as vegetable material derived from the faeces. However, many seem to be regenerating myoblasts following the inflammatory destruction of striated muscle cells. Epithelioid cells are not a feature of an ordinary foreign body reaction. Their absence provides a useful, if arbitrary, distinction from the sarcoid type of tissue response.

There is a well documented association between perianal Crohn's disease and carcinomas in this region. Adenocarcinomas may arise in the glandular epithelium of the anorectal junction or in association with fistulae [23]. Squamous cell carcinomas of the anal canal have been described also [23,24].

Anorectal tuberculosis

Tuberculosis of the anorectal region is now a rare disease in Western countries, having steadily declined over the past 50 years [25]. However, it still occurs in those countries where pulmonary and intestinal tuberculosis are common. There are two different clinical types. First, there are those presenting with anal ulceration who usually have active pulmonary tuberculosis; acid-fast bacilli can be readily demonstrated in smears from the surface of the ulcer or in biopsy material [26,27]. Second, there are those who have anal fissures, fistulae or chronic anorectal abscesses. The fistulae are often anatomically complex and may be associated with stricture of the lower rectum. There is a history of pulmonary tuberculosis in most cases, but this is often of a mild or chronic character. The histological diagnosis can be difficult, especially the distinction from Crohn's disease (Fig. 43.1c,d). The only certain way to establish it is by demonstrating the acid-fast bacilli in biopsy material, by *Mycobacterium tuberculosis*-specific polymerase chain reaction, or by culture of fresh tissue from the anal lesion.

Ulcerative colitis

Although anal lesions do occur in patients with ulcerative colitis, they are less frequent than, and have a different character from, the anal lesions of Crohn's disease. Ordinary anal and rectovaginal fistulae are seen, but the inflammatory changes in the anal canal and anal margin are usually more superficial, presenting as an acute anal fissure or excoriation of the skin around the anus. Whereas chronic anal lesions are characteristic of Crohn's disease, acute perianal or ischiorectal abscesses are more frequent in ulcerative colitis. The histology shows no specific features.

Histoplasmosis

We know of one case report of disseminated histoplasmosis that presented with granulomatous lesions in the tongue and anal region [28]. In a review of 77 cases of reported gastrointestinal histoplasmosis none involved the anus [29].

Venereal infection

Infection of the anal region is a common complication of anal intercourse, and syphilis, chancroid, herpes simplex, lymphogranuloma venereum, granuloma inguinale and amoebiasis may all present as anal ulceration [30].

Syphilis

The primary lesion of anal syphilis can be easily confused with anal lesions due to other causes, in particular simple anal fissure [31]. The clinical distinction from carcinoma, the anal lesions of Crohn's disease and tuberculous ulcer can also be difficult. It must be remembered that the clinical appearance of primary syphilis of the anus more often resembles one of the above, particularly fissure *in ano*, than the typical penile type of sore [31,32].

The technique of diagnosis is exactly the same as for a penile sore except that if the ulcer has been covered with even the smallest quantity of lubricant during examination, study of material from its surface is compromised. Even the gentlest wiping is often painful for the patient. Moreover, the ulcer readily bleeds and blood hinders the detection of spirochaetes. If an anal lesion gives rise to suspicion of primary syphilis, the surface of the ulcer must not be exposed to any lubricant until relevant examinations have been completed. Another cause of difficulty is the recent application of antiseptic and antibiotic ointment. The diagnosis of anal syphilis should always be confirmed by the appropriate serological tests. The organisms may also be demonstrated in the tissue by means of immunofluorescence.

Manifestations of secondary syphilis can also be seen in the anal region. They include dermatitis of the perianal skin and, at a latter stage, condylomas. The latter are moist, reddened hypertrophic papules and are distinguishable clinically from condyloma acuminata (viral warts), although both types can be present together.

Granuloma inguinale

This condition, which is not to be confused with lymphogranuloma venereum, is a venereal disease characterized by a slowly progressive ulceration of the tissues in the genital and perianal region. It is widespread in the tropics [33] and is a chronic granulomatous condition caused by *Calymmatobacterium granulomatis*.

Macroscopically there are ulcerated areas of varying size. On microscopic examination a well circumscribed mass of chronic inflammatory cells is seen, with infiltration mainly by polymorphs and plasma cells. Amongst these are a few lymphocytes and occasionally large round macrophages in which the diagnostic Donovan bodies can be demonstrated by Leishman, Giemsa or Warthin–Starry stains. Adjacent squamous epithelium may show pseudoepitheliomatous hyperplasia.

Lymphogranuloma venereum

This usually presents as a proctitis and has already been considered on p. 480. The anal manifestations include confluent nodules with fissuring, multiple anal fistulae and perianal elephantiasis.

Chancroid

This condition, which is rare in developed countries, is caused by *Haemophilus ducreyii* and can produce multiple painful perianal ulcers with abscesses in the draining lymph nodes. The diagnosis is made from identification of typical organisms in a swab of the ulcer and by subsequent culture.

Hidradenitis suppurativa

This is a chronic inflammatory condition that affects the skin and subcutaneous tissues of those parts of the integument where apocrine sweat glands are found, namely the axilla, areola of the breast, umbilicus, genitalia and perianal area. Perianal hidradenitis is an uncommon condition that is more frequent in males than females. The affected area of skin has a red and white blotchy appearance and is thickened and oedematous with watery pus draining from multiple openings of sinus tracks. The persistent chronic nature of the disease leads to ulceration and scarring [34]. Lesions can be localized or involve large areas of perianal skin extending onto the buttocks and differ from fistulae by being superficial to the sphincteric muscle and not connected to the intersphincteric plane [34]. Microscopic examination of excised specimens shows an inflammatory exudate consisting of plasma cells, lymphocytes and occasional giant cells of the foreign body type, with formation of sinus tracks. Epithelioid granulomas are very seldom seen and if present should raise the possibility of perianal Crohn's disease [35]. The latter become lined by squamous epithelium by downgrowth from the surface skin. The fact that the disease occurs in sites that include apocrine glands has led to the view that hidradenitis suppurativa results from a primary infection of apocrine glands. Other studies, however, indicate that these glands are infected secondarily to keratin plugging of hair follicles and a pilosebaceous folliculitis and that hidradenitis can affect skin in sites other than apocrine gland-bearing areas [36]. The cause of the disease is not understood but, like acne, it seems to have some relationship to hormonal activity. Other aetiological factors suggested include excessive local moisture in apposing skin surfaces and the difficulty of maintaining cleanliness in the regions involved. Malignant change has been reported [37].

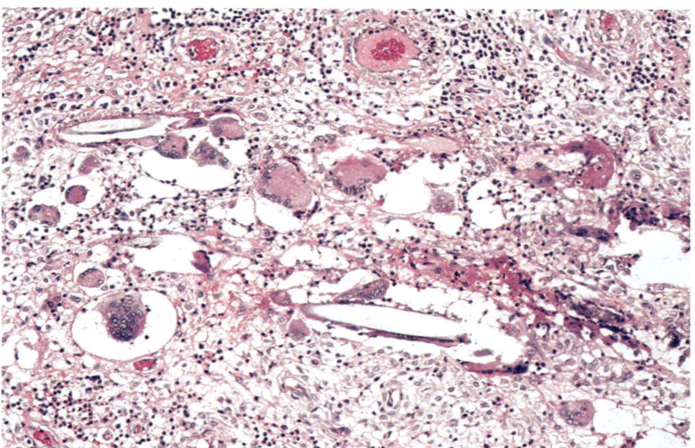

Fig. 43.2 Histology of a pilonidal sinus. Hair shafts embedded in granulation tissue.

Pilonidal sinus

A pilonidal sinus consists of single or multiple pits typically in the skin crease of the natal cleft which extend into subcutaneous abscess tracks lined by granulation tissue containing a mass of loose hair. The tracks branch, most often in a cephalad direction and laterally into the buttocks, but occasionally towards the anus. Pilonidal sinuses are most common in young adults, mostly men. Hirsutism, chronic irritation and intertrigo are precipitating factors. It now seems certain that pilonidal sinuses are caused by puncture of the skin of the natal cleft by ingrowing hair shafts [38]. An inflammatory reaction results, leading to the formation of a pit lined by squamous epithelium into which more hair and skin debris penetrates. Further secondary infection causes the formation of subcutaneous abscess tracks. Microscopic examination of surgically excised pilonidal sinuses shows chronic inflammatory granulation tissue lining abscess tracks, which usually, though not invariably, contain numerous hair shafts around which there is a florid foreign body giant cell reaction (Fig. 43.2). They occur at any site of hair growth and have been described in the anal canal [39,40]. Malignant change to squamous cell carcinoma has been reported [41,42].

References

1 Hancock BD. The internal sphincter and anal fissure. *Br J Surg*, 1977; 64: 92.

2 Kuypers HC. Is there really sphincter spasm in anal fissure? *Dis Colon Rectum*, 1983; 26: 493.

3 Shafik A. A new concept of the anatomy of the anal sphincter. Mechanism and the physiology of defecation. *Am J Surg*, 1982; 144: 262.

4 Crapp AR, Alexander-Williams J. Fissure-in-ano and anal stenosis. *Clin Gastroenterol*, 1975; 43: 619.

5 Kleinhaus S. Miscellaneous anal disorders. In: Ravitch MM, ed. *Paediatric Surgery*, 3rd edn. Chicago: Year Book Medical Publishers, 1979: 1078.

6 Parks AG. Pathogenesis and treatment of fistula-in-ano. *Br Med J*, 1961; 1: 463.

7 Parks AG, Gordon PH, Hardcastle JD. A classification of fistula-in-ano. *Br J Surg*, 1976; 63: 1.

8 Fazio VW. Complex anal fistulae. *Gastroenterol Clin North Am*, 1987; 16: 93.

9 Marks CG, Ritchie JK. Anal fistulae at St Mark's Hospital. *Br J Surg*, 1977; 64: 84.

10 Hawley PR. Anorectal fistula. *Clin Gastroenterol*, 1975; 4: 635.

11 Lunniss PJ, Faris B, Rees HC, Heard S, Phillips RKS. Histological and microbiological assessment of the role of microorganisms in chronic anal fistula. *Br J Surg*, 1993; 80: 1072.

12 Parks AG, Morson BC. Fistula-in-ano. *Proc R Soc Med*, 1962; 55: 751.

13 Vanheuverzwyn R, Delannoy A, Michaux JL, Dive C. Anal lesions in haematologic disease. *Dis Colon Rectum*, 1980; 23: 310.

14 O'Donohue MK, Waldron RP, O'Malley E. Miliary tuberculosis presenting as an acute perianal abscess. *Dis Colon Rectum*, 1987; 30: 697.

15 Mortensen NJ, Thompson JP. Perianal abscess due to *Enterobius vermicularis*. *Dis Colon Rectum*, 1984; 27: 677.

16 Feigen GM. Suppurative anal cryptitis associated with *Trichuris trichuria*. *Dis Colon Rectum*, 1987; 30: 620.

17 Alvarado-Cerna R, Bracho-Riquelme R. Perianal actinomycosis—a complication of a fistula-in-ano. Report of a case. *Dis Colon Rectum*, 1994; 37: 378.

18 Cohen Z, McLeod RS. Perianal Crohn's disease. *Gastroenterol Clin North Am*, 1987; 16: 175.

19 Fielding JF. Perianal lesions in Crohn's disease. *J R Coll Surg*, 1972; 17: 32.

20 Lockhart-Mummery HE, Morson BC. Crohn's disease of the large intestine. *Gut*, 1964; 5: 493.

21 Lockhart-Mummery HE. Crohn's disease: anal lesions. *Dis Colon Rectum*, 1975; 18: 200.

22 Buchmann P, Keighley MRB, Allan RN, Thompson H, Alexander-Williams J. Natural history of perianal Crohn's disease. *Am J Surg*, 1980; 140: 642.

23 Connell WR, Sheffield JP, Kamm MA *et al*. Lower gastrointestinal malignancy in Crohn's disease. *Gut*, 1994; 35: 347.

24 Lumley JW, Stitz RW. Crohn's disease and anal carcinoma: an association? A case report and review of the literature. *Aust N Z J Surg*, 1991; 61: 76.

25 Logan St VCD. Anorectal tuberculosis. *Proc R Soc Med*, 1969; 62: 1227.

26 Ahlberg JL, Bergstrand O, Holmstrom B, Ullman J, Wallberg P. Anal tuberculosis. A report of two cases. *Acta Chir Scand*, 1980; 50: 45.

27 Whalen TV, Kovakik PJ, Old WL. Tuberculosis anal ulcer. *Dis Colon Rectum*, 1980; 23: 54.

28 Earle JHO, Highman JH, Lockey E. A case of disseminated histoplasmosis. *Br Med J*, 1960; i: 607.

29 Cappell MS, Mandell W, Grimes MM, Neu HC. Gastrointestinal histoplasmosis. *Dig Dis Sci*, 1988; 33: 353.

30 McMillan A, Smith IW. Painful anal ulceration in homosexual men. *Br J Surg*, 1984; 71: 215.

31 Samenius B. Primary syphilis of the anorectal region. *Dis Colon Rectum*, 1968; 11: 462.

32 Quinn TC, Lukehart SA, Goodell S *et al*. Rectal mass caused by *Treponema pallidum*: confirmation by immunofluorescent staining. *Gastroenterology*, 1982; 82: 135.

33 Greenblatt RB, Dienst RB, Baldwin KR. Lymphogranuloma venereum and granuloma inguinale. *Med Clin N Am*, 1959; 43: 1493.

34 Culp CE. Chronic hidradenitis suppurativa of the anal canal. *Dis Colon Rectum*, 1983; 26: 669.

35 Attanoos RL, Appleton MAC, Hughes LE *et al*. Granulomatous hidradenitis suppurativa and cutaneous Crohn's disease. *Histopathology*, 1993; 23: 111.

36 Anderson MJ, Dockerty MB. Perianal hidradenitis suppurativa. *Dis Colon Rectum*, 1958; 1: 23.

37 Humphrey LJ, Playforth H, Leavell VW. Squamous cell carcinoma arising in hidradenitis suppurativum. *Arch Dermatol*, 1969; 100: 59.

38 Weale FE. A comparison of Barber's and post-anal pilonidal sinuses. *Br J Surg*, 1964; 51: 513.

39 Ortiz H, Marti J, DeMiguel M, Carmona A, Cabanas IP. Hair-containing lesions within the anal canal. *Int J Colorectal Dis*, 1987; 2: 153.

40 Taylor BA, Hughes LE. Circumferential perianal pilonidal sinuses. *Dis Colon Rectum*, 1984; 27: 120.

41 Gaston EA, Wilde WL. Epidermoid carcinoma arising in a pilonidal sinus. *Dis Colon Rectum*, 1965; 8: 343.

42 Lineaweaver WC, Brumsom MB, Smith JF, Franzini DA, Rumley TO. Squamous carcinoma arising in a pilonidal sinus. *J Surg Oncol*, 1984; 27: 239.

44 Tumours and tumour-like lesions of the anal region

Epithelial tumours of the anal canal are all uncommon and represent a diverse collection of histological types. This reflects the many different varieties of epithelium seen in this area. A detailed knowledge of the histology of the epithelial lining of the anorectal region is an essential prerequisite to the classification of anorectal tumours.

A distinction should be made between malignant tumours of the anal canal and the anal margin. The former are mostly non-keratinizing variants of squamous cell carcinoma arising from the mucous membrane. The latter are keratinizing squamous cell carcinomas of the perianal skin with a generally better prognosis and requiring less aggressive treatment. Apart from the exceptional occurrence of lymphomas and connective tissue tumours in the anorectal region, consideration must also be given to tumours of the ischiorectal fossae and to presacral tumours.

Benign epithelial tumours and precancerous lesions of the anorectal region

This section encompasses a heterogeneous group of lesions, some arising in the anal canal, some in the perianal skin and some within both sites. Squamous cell papillomas arising from the epithelium of the anal canal, both below and above the dentate line, are encountered only rarely. They may be related to viral warts even when human papillomavirus (HPV) immunohistochemistry is negative.

Fibroepithelial polyp

Also known as skin tags, these common lesions have been viewed as burnt-out, thrombosed haemorrhoids but may represent a primary hyperplasia of the subepithelial connective tissue of the anal mucosa [1]. The polyps consist of a myxoid or collagenous stroma covered by squamous epithelium (Fig. 44.1). The stromal fibroblasts or myofibroblasts may be multinucleated and may occasionally show atypical nuclear features [1]. The same cells may be found in normal subepithelial connective tissue of the anal canal mucosa. Mast cells are also present and may be implicated in the pathogenesis of these lesions through the production of fibrogenic factors [1]. Vacuolation of the superficial keratinocytes is another feature of these lesions [2].

Inflammatory cloacogenic polyp

This is an example of the polypoid variant of the solitary ulcer/mucosal prolapse syndrome (p. 464). The polyps are covered with a combination of colorectal and transitional zone epithelium [3,4]. There is superficial ulceration and the epithelium shows florid regenerative hyperplasia, mimicking an adenoma (Fig. 44.2). The lamina propria contains increased amounts of smooth muscle. Prolapsing haemorrhoids may show similar epithelial changes [5]. Inflammatory cloacogenic polyps have been described in children [6].

Squamous hyperplasia (leucoplakia)

A variety of pathological lesions may present clinically as a white plaque. A common cause is squamous metaplasia and hyperkeratosis of the transitional mucosa at the lower pole of prolapsing internal haemorrhoids or upgrowth of thickened squamous mucosa from the anal canal over ulcerating haem-

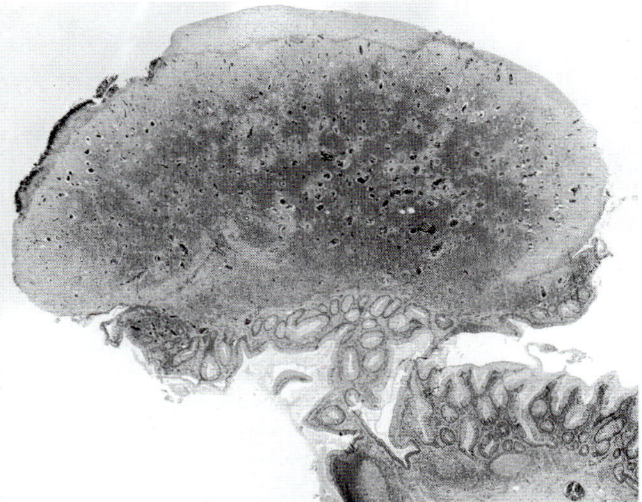

Fig. 44.1 Fibroepithelial polyp of the anal canal composed of a connective tissue core that is partly covered by squamous epithelium with superficial ulceration.

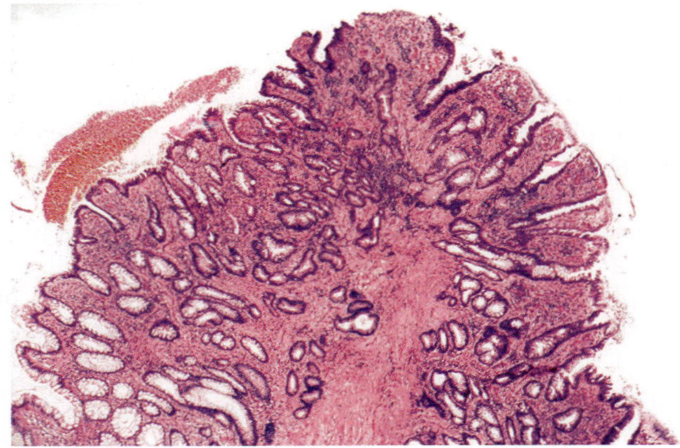

Fig. 44.2 Inflammatory cloacogenic polyp.

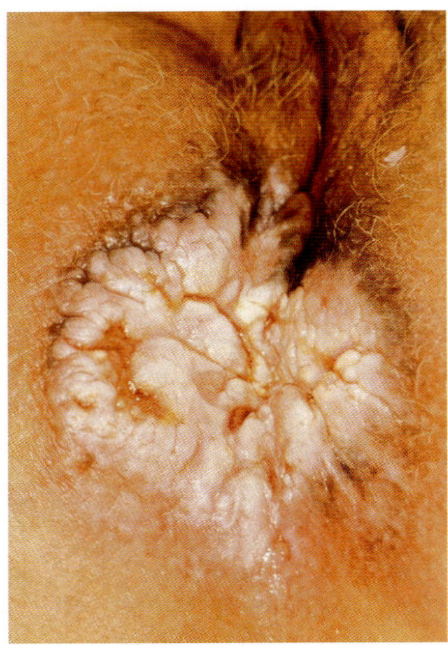

Fig. 44.3 Anal leucoplakia.

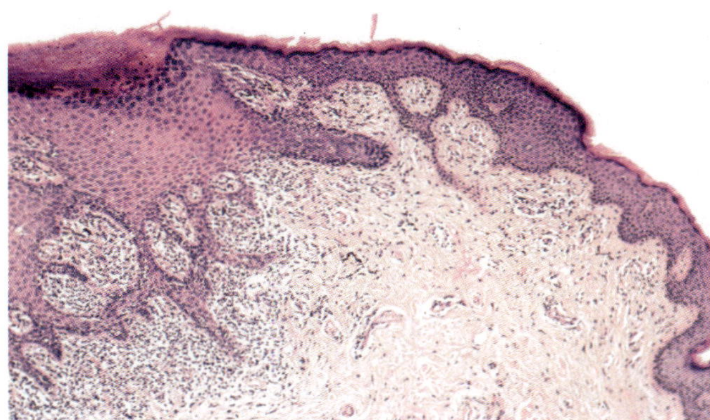

Fig. 44.4 Anal leucoplakia (left of field).

orrhoids. There is no evidence that such white plaques are precancerous. However, precancerous epithelial dysplasia may present as a white plaque in the anal canal. Specific dermatological conditions such as lichen planus and lichen sclerosus (et atrophicus), may affect lower anal canal and perianal skin and present clinically as a white plaque. Any prolonged irritation in the perianal region may lead to a chronic, non-specific dermatitis characterized histologically by hyperkeratosis and chronic inflammatory cell infiltration of the dermis.

When the above causes of white plaque are excluded, there remains a specific condition occurring in the lower anal canal and perianal skin. The term leucoplakia is no longer acceptable as a histopathological diagnosis and the following lesion, analogous to terminology applied to the vulva, is described as anal hyperplasia (generally without dysplasia). Clinical inspection discloses a white, thickened and sometimes circumferential anal lesion (Fig. 44.3). Microscopically, there is hyperkeratosis, focal parakeratosis and acanthosis. Wispy spikes of epithelium project into the underlying connective tissue in which there is a dense lymphocytic and plasma cell infiltrate. The infiltrate often follows the sawtooth contour of the dermoepidermal junction in a band-like manner and invades the lower epidermis (Fig. 44.4). The appearances thereby closely mimic lichen planus, except for the greater degree of acanthosis and the presence of parakeratosis. Epithelial dysplasia is seen in a minority of cases only. At St Mark's Hospital, patients have been treated by local excision, which in some instances has required skin grafting [7]. The lesion has been observed to recur, and progression to malignancy has been recorded, the cancers generally being well differentiated squamous cell carcinomas. In other patients squamous hyperplasia and carcinoma have been synchronous presentations. One patient was treated by excision of the rectum and developed recurrent disease around the colostomy. The lesion is therefore a distinct clinicopathological entity with a definite risk of cancer, but the aetiology remains obscure.

Dysplasia and carcinoma *in situ* or anal intraepithelial neoplasia

Dysplasia or anal intraepithelial neoplasia (AIN) of the anal canal is found in the transitional epithelium above the dentate line more frequently than in the squamous mucous membrane of the lower anal canal [8–10]. This observation corresponds with the relative incidence of invasive carcinoma above and below the dentate line (see p. 659). In a meticulous examination of a consecutive series of minor surgical specimens, dysplasia was an incidental finding in 2.3%, but was severe in only one out of 306 cases [11]. Patients with dysplasia were younger than a corresponding series of patients with established anal canal carcinoma. In a systematic examination of the anal region in 139 surgical specimens for anal cancer, rectal cancer or inflammatory bowel disease, 16 squamous cell carcinomas of the anal canal were discovered. Severe dysplasia was present in 13 of these, but in none of the other specimens. Dysplasia occurred patchily and away from the cancers as well as in the immediately adjacent epithelium [12]. Such observations give strong support to the concept that anal cancer frequently develops in a background of epithelial dysplasia and that the risk of cancer is greatest for severe dysplasia (or AIN III) amounting to carcinoma *in situ*. The natural history of low-grade AIN is uncertain, but progression of AIN III to carcinoma has been observed [13].

Histological examination reveals a thickened epithelium in which undifferentiated cells with a high nucleocytoplasmic ratio extend from their usual basal position towards the mucosal surface (Fig. 44.5). Varying degrees of nuclear pleomorphism and increased mitotic activity are also present. The histopathology of anal canal dysplasia is similar to cervical dysplasia or intraepithelial neoplasia (usually the non-keratinizing small cell or basaloid type) and it now seems likely that the same group of sexually transmitted agents is implicated in both disorders. This is supported by observations of concomitant genital and anal neoplasia [14], similar epidemiology of anal and genital neoplasia [15,16], and the association between anal cancer and homosexual activity or anal intercourse [17,18]. The principal contender for a role in such transmission is the group of small DNA viruses known collectively as human papillomavirus (HPV). Indeed, AIN may show squamous maturation, individual cell dyskeratosis and koilocytosis, histopathological features that are indicative of HPV infection (Fig. 44.6). There is often concomitant hyperkeratosis and the lesion then presents as a white plaque. The grading of AIN is subject to considerable interobserver variation. It has been suggested that only two grades (low and high) should be used [19].

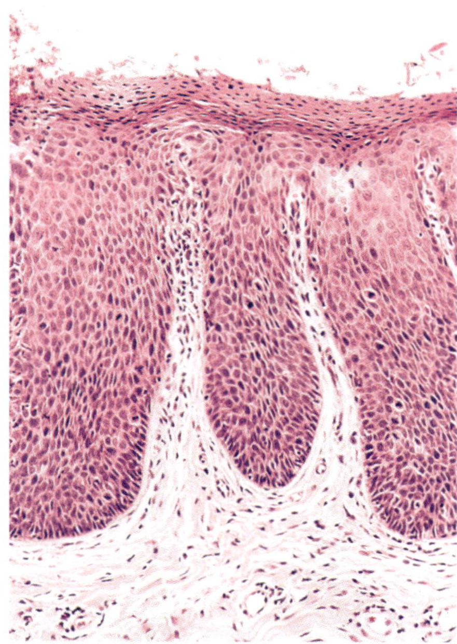

Fig. 44.5 Severe dysplasia or grade III intraepithelial neoplasia of the anal canal.

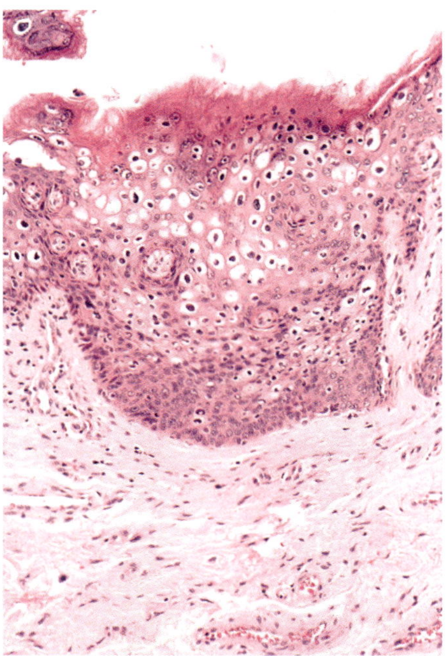

Fig. 44.6 Koilocytosis within grade I anal intraepithelial neoplasia.

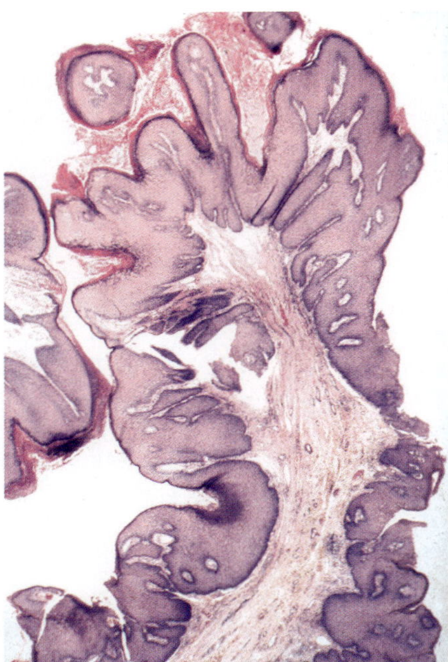

Fig. 44.7 Condyloma acuminatum or viral wart.

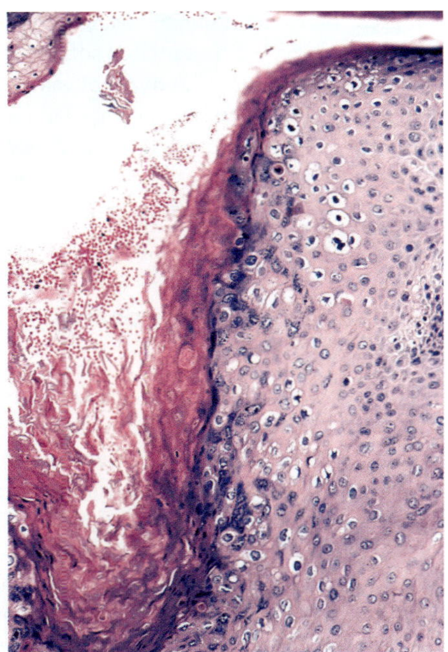

Fig. 44.8 Koilocytosis in condyloma acuminatum.

Viral warts (condylomata acuminata)

These papilliferous, warty growths are found in the perianal region as well as other parts of the perineum, the vulva and penis. They are often multiple, covering a wide area of perianal skin and may extend into the anal canal but do not involve rectal mucosa. They are caused by members of the HPV family, of which over 50 types have now been identified [20]. Types 6 and 11 have been implicated in the aetiology of anogenital warts, whereas types 16 and 18 (sometimes in association with 6 and 11) are associated with anogenital squamous carcinoma [21]. Genital warts are being seen with increasing frequency, and anal warts are especially common in male homosexuals and females who practise anal intercourse. Anal dysplasia and carcinoma are also being described in male homosexuals, both with and without the acquired immune deficiency syndrome (AIDS) [19,22,23]. Such observations as well as reports of malignant transformation within viral warts [24,25] strongly support the concept of an oncogenic role for particular HPV types.

Low-power microscopy reveals the characteristic acuminate or sawtooth outline that is due to marked papillomatosis involving a thickened or acanthotic epithelium (Fig. 44.7). Other features include hyperplasia of the prickle cells, parakeratosis, hyperkeratosis and an underlying chronic inflammatory cell infiltrate. The most notable feature is vacuolation or koilocytosis of cells in the upper layers of the epidermis (Fig. 44.8). The nuclei of these cells give a positive immunohistochemical reaction with HPV antibodies (Fig. 44.9). The occasional dyskeratotic cell is seen, especially if the wart has been treated with podophyllin. This should not be equated with dysplasia.

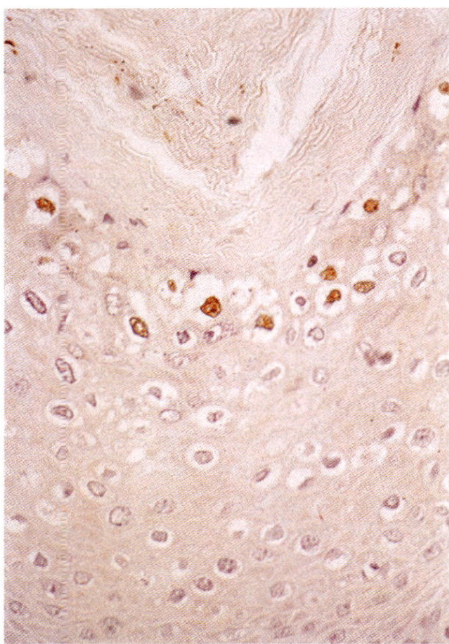

Fig. 44.9 Wart virus coat antigen within nuclei of vacuolated cells (immunoperoxidase).

Giant condyloma and verrucous carcinoma

These lesions are considered together because if they are not

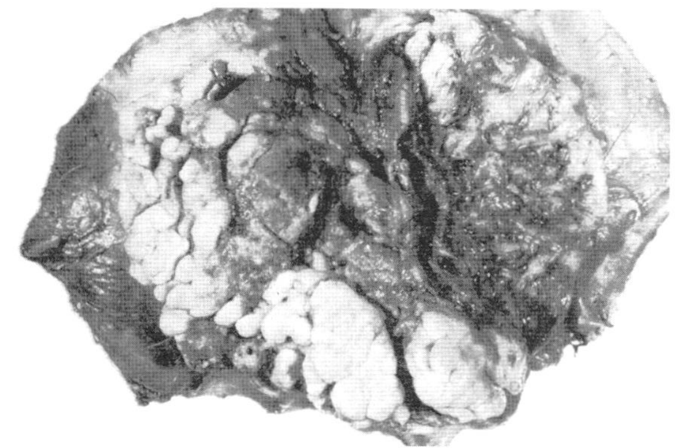

Fig. 44.10 Giant condyloma.

identical, they certainly share several aetiological, pathological and clinical features. In the past, the term verrucous carcinoma has been employed in two ways: one to describe the lesion under discussion and the other to describe the well differentiated end of the spectrum of squamous cell carcinoma. The latter use has been a source of confusion and should not be continued.

Giant condyloma (of Buschke and Loewenstein) is a rare penile or vulval lesion which presents as a large warty, cauliflower-like growth (Fig. 44.10) and characteristically penetrates and burrows into the deeper tissues. Similar lesions occur even more rarely in the perianal and anorectal region [25–30]. Cases have been described showing extensive erosion of the soft tissues around the anus with invasion of the ischiorectal fossae, perirectal tissues and even the pelvic cavity [31]. These tumours may not only become ulcerated but be complicated by the formation of fistulous tracks and sinuses. The lesion is resistant to treatment with podophyllin. In spite of its locally aggressive behaviour, giant condyloma shows limited metastatic potential. Lymph node metastases have been described following transformation to a conventional squamous cell carcinoma [32]. Total excision is therefore usually curative, but this may only be achieved by abdominoperineal excision (and sometimes more radical surgery) in advanced cases [31,33]. Lesions are generally insensitive to radiotherapy, but useful tumour shrinkage may be produced by means of preoperative chemoradiotherapy [34]. There is no evidence that radiotherapy can transform giant condyloma/verrucous carcinoma into a more aggressive tumour. The microscopic features are similar to those of the typical anal wart, including the presence of vacuolated cells [25]. The major difference is the presence of endophytic or downward growth by giant condyloma. However, the advancing tongues of epithelium are bulbous and pushing, with an intact basement membrane. HPV types 6 and 11 are found in giant condyloma/verrucous carcinoma, as in simple viral warts. Subtypes of HPV6 with variations in non-coding (regulatory) DNA may account for the differing behaviour of giant condyloma [35,36]. The progression to dysplasia and squamous cell carcinoma has been documented [25]. In a review of 33 cases, 14 (42%) were considered to show malignant transformation [33]. The molecular basis for this transformation is unknown. Additional infection with HPV16 or 18 could be one mechanism.

Keratoacanthoma

This is not a premalignant lesion, but is mentioned at this juncture because an incision biopsy can easily be misdiagnosed as a well differentiated squamous cell carcinoma. Its rare occurrence in the perianal region should therefore be appreciated [37]. The pilar tumour, more usually associated with the scalp, can be mistaken for both keratoacanthoma and squamous cell carcinoma, but is an extremely rare occurrence in the perianal skin.

Bowen's disease

This is essentially a form of carcinoma *in situ* that typically affects the skin of the head and neck and the upper and lower limbs, but is very rarely found in the perianal skin [38–40]. When occurring in the anogenital region, Bowen's disease is sometimes termed erythroplasia. It presents as a red, encrusted plaque with irregular edges. The lesions can be multiple. The presence of ulceration usually indicates that invasive carcinoma has developed. Microscopically the changes are no different from those found in the common sites of Bowen's disease. Dyskeratotic and mitotically active cells with large, atypical nuclei are seen within an acanthotic epithelium, sometimes showing hyperkeratosis and parakeratosis. Whilst Bowen's disease is not generally caused by HPV (usually actinic or rarely arsenic induced), HPV type 16 has been detected in anal Bowen's disease [41,42]. Clearly Bowen's disease is not a single clinical entity [43,44].

Bowenoid papulosis

This presents as a papular eruption in the anogenital region, usually in young to middle-aged adults. The histology somewhat resembles Bowen's disease, but the scattered dyskeratotic cells are set against a background of near-normal epithelial maturation. A 'salt and pepper' effect is imparted by a random scattering of dyskeratotic and mitotically active cells (Fig. 44.11). Unlike Bowen's disease, bowenoid papulosis apparently shows no propensity for malignant invasion and no association with internal malignancy [45] and is therefore controlled by conservative means. The lesions may regress spontaneously. Although bowenoid papulosis is a distinct clinical entity, several HPV types are implicated in its aetiology: 16, 18, 31, 32, 34, 35, 39, 42, 48 and 51–54 [46,47]. Recurrence has been described [48].

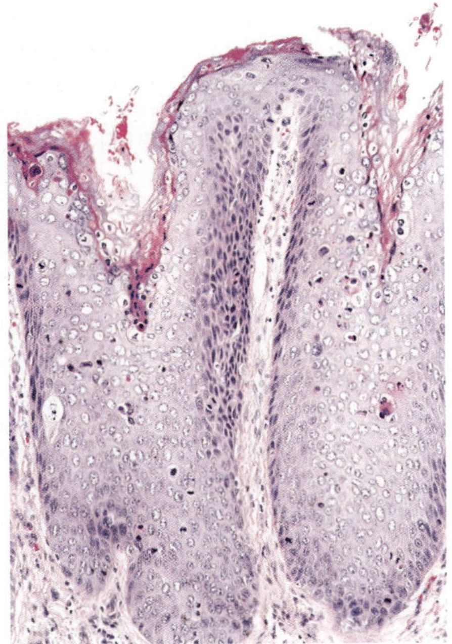

Fig. 44.11 Bowenoid papulosis.

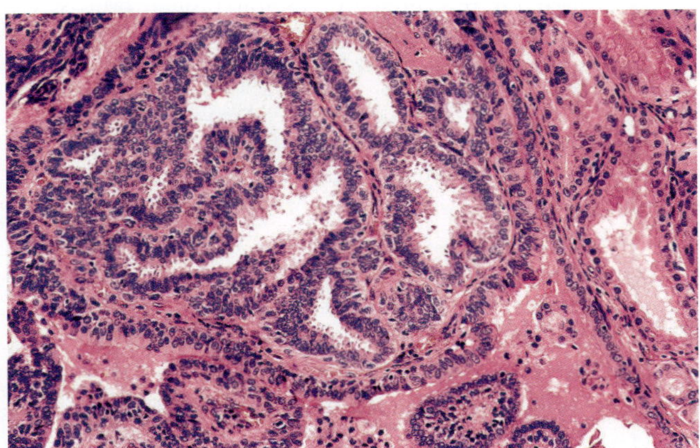

Fig. 44.12 Hidradenoma papilliferum.

Sweat gland tumours

The least rare is the benign hidradenoma papilliferum, derived from apocrine sweat glands [49]. The lesion usually occurs in middle-aged women and presents as a circumscribed, firm nodule rarely greater than 1 cm in diameter. On section it is often cystic. Microscopically the tumour shows a papillary pattern in which two cell types can be discerned. A columnar cell layer with apical blebs rests upon a layer of cuboidal cells with eosinophilic cytoplasm (Fig. 44.12). The latter contain periodic acid–Schiff (PAS)-positive, diastase-resistant material. Apocrine metaplasia may occur.

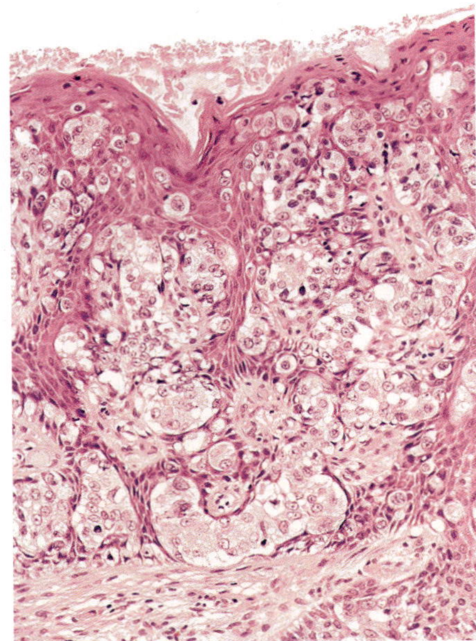

Fig. 44.13 Paget's disease of perianal skin. The epidermis is infiltrated by clear Paget cells with a vesicular nucleus.

Extramammary Paget's disease

Paget's disease of the perianal skin is a rare neoplastic condition which presents clinically as a slightly raised, red, scaly and moist area [50–53]. The condition affects elderly persons of either sex and is indistinguishable histologically from Paget's disease of the breast [54]. The diagnosis is established by biopsy which reveals the characteristic Paget cells in an epidermis that may show pseudoepitheliomatous hyperplasia. The cells occur singly or in small groups and are concentrated mainly within the basal region of the epidermis. They may invade the ducts of sweat glands or the epithelium lining hair follicles. The typical Paget cell is large with foamy, vacuolated cytoplasm and a vesicular nucleus which is sometimes displaced towards the periphery of the cell (Fig. 44.13). The cells secrete mucus that is diastase–PAS and alcian blue positive.

The histogenesis of perianal Paget's disease is not fully understood, but ultrastructural and immunohistochemical studies have helped to clarify the debate [55,56]. As well as secreting mucus, Paget cells express other glandular phenotypes including epithelial membrane antigen [56], carcinoembryonic antigen [55–57] and low molecular weight cytokeratins [55–58]. These findings highlight the differences between Paget cells and squamous epithelium and are consistent with the concept that Paget cells originate within glandular skin appendages. An alternative hypothesis implicating pluripotential intraepidermal cells cannot be excluded [59], but firm evidence for such a histogenesis is lacking. Immunohistochemical studies have indicated similar antigenic profiles between perianal and mammary Paget's disease, notably the expression of human milk fat globule glycoprotein antigens [56], casein [59], and gross cystic disease fluid protein [55,56,60]. However, higher expression of c-erb B-2 and nm23 oncoproteins is seen in mammary Paget's disease [60]. Perianal Paget's disease (unlike mammary but like other forms of extramammary Paget's disease occurring in the vulva, axilla, eyelid, external ear and oesophagus) is not usually associated with an underlying malignancy.

It has been suggested that extramammary Paget cells arise from the ducts of apocrine glands and show selective diffuse infiltration of the adjoining squamous epithelium by virtue of their extraordinary epidermotropism. The widespread or multifocal nature of the disease means that local excision is often followed by recurrence [61]. Conceivably this might be prevented by wide local excision with frozen section control.

Some cases of perianal Paget's disease are associated with an underlying malignancy [50], but the latter is usually a mucin-secreting adenocarcinoma rather than a typical apocrine malignancy [62]. In this context it is important to distinguish between genuine Paget's disease and downward pagetoid spread by signet ring cells from a primary anorectal adenocarcinoma [63]. Signet ring cells usually secrete more mucus than Paget cells and invade the epidermis singly and diffusely with no predilection for the basal zone. Unfortunately, many of the markers expressed by Paget cells of putative apocrine origin are also expressed by signet ring cell carcinomas of the large bowel [63]. A useful exception is the specific apocrine marker gross cystic disease fluid protein [63–66]. On the other hand, the existing markers will ably distinguish epithelial Paget cells from pagetoid melanotic malignant melanoma and Bowen's disease of the perianal skin, both of which may mimic Paget's disease histologically.

Malignant epithelial tumours of the anal canal

Squamous cell carcinoma of the anal canal

Cancer of the anal region is uncommon in England and Wales, probably being responsible for no more than 100 deaths per annum. It is impossible to be precise because cancer of the anal margin is registered with other malignant neoplasms of the skin and many deaths from anal carcinoma are probably registered under rectal cancer. A better picture of the incidence is obtained from the study of surgical patients, in whom anal cancer as a whole comprises only 3% of all anorectal cancers [67]. Anal cancer is being seen with increasing frequency amongst male homosexuals, both with and without AIDS [18,22,23]. Sexually transmitted HPV has been implicated in the aetiology of anal neoplasia in male homosexuals [68]. HPV types 16 and 18 have been identified within squamous cell carcinoma of the anus [21,69–71]. These types are associated with E6 and E7 proteins having a high binding affinity for tumour suppressor gene products (retinoblastoma and p53) [72–74]. Immunosuppression associated with the AIDS epidemic is likely to be an important cofactor, accounting, at least in part, for the increasing incidence [23,75]. Anal cancers in immunosuppressed subjects are more likely to be multifocal, persistent, recurrent and aggressive [76,77]. Interestingly, AIDS and anal warts appear to be independent risk factors in relation to risk of AIN [75]. Screening for precursor lesions has been advocated in human immunodeficiency virus (HIV)-infected male homosexuals in view of their considerably increased risk [16,78,79]. The possible role of chronic inflammation associated with Crohn's disease [80] and such venereal diseases as syphilis and lymphogranuloma venereum should not be forgotten. Minor inflammatory lesions probably play little part in the causation of anal cancer [81].

Squamous cell carcinoma of the anal margin is relatively common in parts of South America and the Indian subcontinent where conditions of extreme poverty are found. Under these circumstances carcinoma of the penis, vulva and cervix, as well as of the anus, are more prevalent.

The importance of distinguishing between squamous carcinoma of the anal canal and anal margin was emphasized many years ago [82]. These two types of cancer differ in their epidemiology, pathology and behaviour. Anal canal carcinoma is nearly three times more common than cancer of the anal margin in the population of England and Wales. The age incidence is the same (average 57 years), but anal canal cancer is more common in women than men (3:2), whereas anal margin carcinoma is more frequent in men (4:1) [83].

Site

The majority of squamous carcinomas of the anal canal arise above, or mainly above, the dentate line (Figs 44.14 & 44.15) and within the region of the transitional zone [83,84]. Probably only about one-quarter arise from the squamous mucous membrane of the lower anal canal. Moreover, direct spread in continuity is preferentially upwards in the submucosal plane because downward spread is limited by the way in which the dentate line is tethered to the underlying internal sphincter, thus obliterating the submucosal layer. This also explains why most anal canal cancers present clinically as tumours of the lower rectum.

Histology

Squamous carcinomas of the anal canal show a diversity of histological structure which reflects the variability and instability

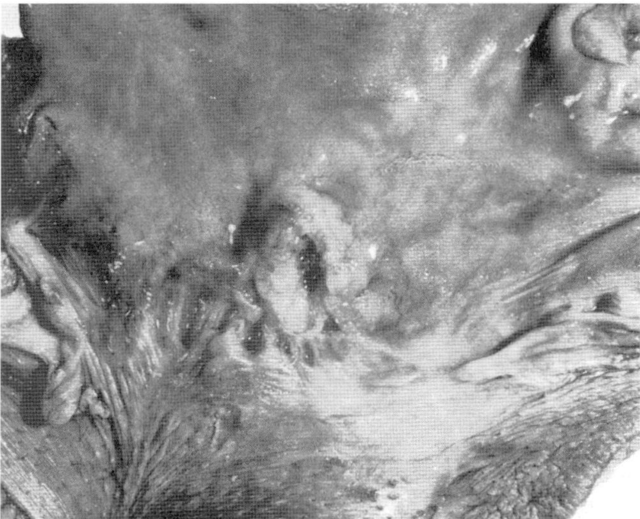

Fig. 44.14 Small ulcerating squamous cell carcinoma lying just above the dentate line of the anal canal.

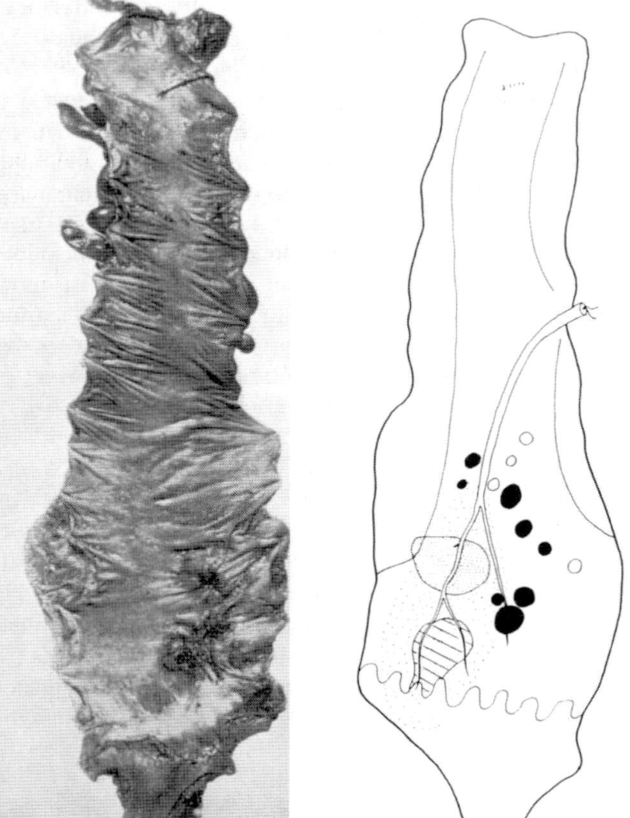

Fig. 44.15 (a) Squamous cell carcinoma of the anal canal with preferential upward spread in continuity with tumour re-erupting through the mucosa of the middle third of the rectum. (b) Chart of (a) showing position of primary growth just above the dentate line, growth re-erupting through the rectal wall and involvement of haemorrhoidal lymph nodes.

of the epithelium in this area. They have been divided into two principal types which occur with roughly equal frequency. The first has been given a variety of names: 'basaloid', 'cloacogenic', 'transitional' or the more descriptive term 'non-keratinizing, small cell squamous carcinoma' [8,85–87]. This tumour is found in the upper anal canal and arises from the epithelium of the junctional or cloacogenic zone. Second is the ordinary or large cell squamous cell carcinoma. This may show some keratinization, but extensively keratinizing squamous cell carcinomas are more common in the perianal skin. Mucoepidermoid carcinoma of the upper anal canal has been described, but is rare [88,89]. Careful histological examination will show that most, if not all, can be distinguished from salivary gland mucoepidermoid carcinoma and would be better designated as squamous carcinoma with mucinous microcysts [90]. This pattern has also been described as ductal differentiation [83].

The distinction between basaloid and squamous cell carcinoma is subjective [83]. Mixed types commonly occur and the clinical outcome for the two types is the same [91–94]. Pure basaloid carcinomas appear to be uncommon [83]. Some find the presence of HPV not to be correlated with histological type [69], but others associate prominent basaloid features with high-risk HPV subtypes [95]. Keratin expression matches the morphological heterogeneity, with both simple and keratinocyte keratins occurring in the same lesion [83]. In view of the preceding points it is recommended that basaloid and squamous cell carcinoma should not be regarded as distinct entities. The generic term 'squamous cell carcinoma' should be employed and qualified by a description of the histopathological features [96]. However, it is important to appreciate the range of histological types of squamous cell carcinoma that may be encountered in the anal canal so that they can be distinguished from other malignancies arising in the anorectal region. The most important differential diagnoses are small and large cell undifferentiated carcinoma of rectal origin (see p. 580), malignant melanoma (p. 661), basal cell carcinoma of the anal margin (p. 663), endocrine tumours and direct spread from a primary tumour of the female genital tract.

Squamous cell carcinomas showing basaloid features may resemble basal cell carcinoma of hairbearing skin. Features common to both include the formation of islands of small cells with basophilic cytoplasm and a distinctive pattern of nuclear palisading at the periphery of the clumps of tumour cells (Fig. 44.16). There may be some differentiation towards squamous cells in small concentric whorls, and sharply defined plugs of keratin may be scattered throughout the tumour. One feature unlike basal cell carcinoma is the presence of masses of eosinophilic necrosis surrounded by a relatively narrow rim of tumour cells giving a 'Swiss cheese' appearance under the low power of the microscope. In occasional cases there can be a striking likeness to transitional cell carcinoma of the bladder.

Because anal cancer is rare, most series have been retrospec-

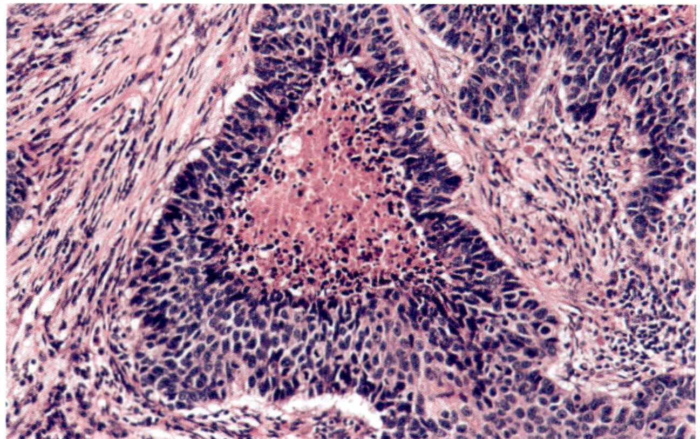

Fig. 44.16 Basaloid or small cell, non-keratinizing squamous carcinoma of the anal canal. Peripheral nuclear palisading and a central necrotic zone are typical findings.

tive and relatively small. The majority of reports have stated that poor differentiation influences prognosis adversely [8,97,98], but this effect is insignificant in the presence of variables relating to tumour stage [97,99]. However, radiotherapy and chemoradiotherapy are becoming the preferred primary forms of treatment [40,100–102]; detailed pathological staging then, of course, becomes impossible. Under these circumstances the main role of the pathologist is to establish the correct diagnosis and comment on the type and grade of the tumour as obtained by an incisional biopsy. This information may not only be useful for stratifying patients in therapeutic trials, but may have a direct bearing on management. For example, sphincter-saving local excision is the treatment of choice for tumours less than 2 cm in diameter, but is inappropriate if the carcinoma is poorly differentiated [97]. A particular type of poorly differentiated squamous cell carcinoma is characterized by small cells, nuclear moulding, a high mitotic rate and diffuse infiltration [99]. Squamous cell carcinoma with mucinous microcysts is also associated with a poor prognosis [99]. Nevertheless, a superficial biopsy may not always be representative of the tumour as a whole. DNA aneuploidy as demonstrated by flow cytometry has been shown to be an independent prognostic factor [99]. Aneuploidy and proliferation are both correlated with the presence of HPV [20]. The small cell undifferentiated ('oat cell') carcinoma is rare, but it is important that this entity is recognized when it occurs. Radical surgery invariably fails because, like the pulmonary counterpart, the disease is generalized at the time of diagnosis [97].

Cytogenetics and molecular pathology

Deletion of chromosomes 11q and 3p are described in anal canal squamous cell carcinoma [103]. Immunohistochemical evidence of p53 overexpression was demonstrated in AIN as well as invasive cancer and did not correlate with HPV type [104]. However, mutant p53 is more common in actinic-related squamous cell carcinoma [105]. K-*ras* mutations are uncommon in anal cancer and limited to those that are non-HPV associated [106]. The role of E6 and E7 HPV proteins is noted above.

Spread and prognosis

Squamous cell carcinoma of the anal canal shows preferential direct spread upwards into the lower third of the rectum, which explains why many squamous carcinomas (and giant condylomas) of the anal canal present clinically as tumours of the lower rectum. This is probably because the least line of resistance is upwards in the submucous layer. Anal canal carcinoma also spreads to the superior haemorrhoidal lymph nodes and to nodes on the lateral wall of the pelvis as well as to the inguinal glands. Haemorrhoidal lymph node involvement has been found in about 43% of major operation specimens of anal cancer seen at St Mark's Hospital. Clinical and pathological evidence of inguinal gland metastases is recorded in about 36% of cases. There is clinical evidence that in anal canal carcinoma the inguinal nodes are involved at a later stage than the haemorrhoidal glands, the malignant cells possibly spreading backwards from within the pelvis [84,98,107]. The presence of lymph node metastases has an important adverse effect upon prognosis as does the size of the growth and the depth of invasion [92]. Measurements of depth of invasion should be made using the easily identified outer border of the internal anal sphincter as a point of reference. Chemoradiotherapy is now the primary treatment of choice for anal canal squamous carcinoma that is not amenable to local excision [108]. Local excision is performed only for tumours less than 2 cm in diameter [100]. Detailed pathological staging will obviously be impossible for patients treated by modalities other than radical surgery, and there is a need for an internationally agreed system of clinicopathological staging so that the results of therapeutic trials performed in different centres can be compared.

Most surgical series report corrected 5-year survival rates of between 50 and 65% [98]. The results of radiotherapy appear to be equally good [93] and patients treated by this modality are of course spared both the trauma of radical surgery and the need for a permanent colostomy.

Malignant melanoma

Malignant melanoma of the anal canal is uncommon, one case presenting for eight squamous cell carcinomas of this region and one for every 250 rectal adenocarcinomas [109]. Only 1.5% of malignant melanomas develop in this site, a proportion that is likely to decrease as the number of solar-associated cutaneous melanomas goes on increasing. The age incidence is about the same as for cancer of the rectum and the sexes are affected equally [110–114]. Patients present with bleeding or an

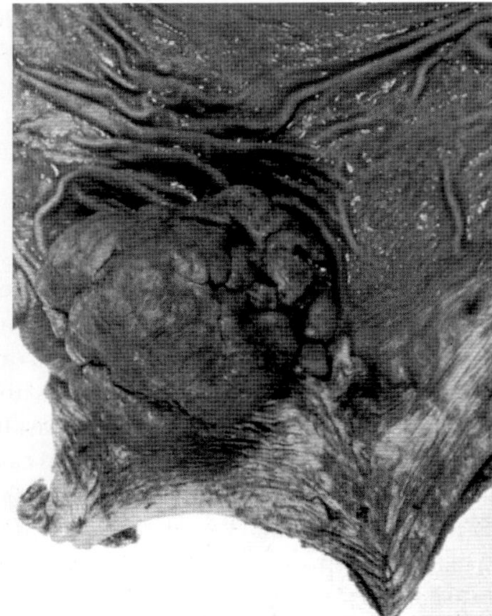

Fig. 44.17 Polypoid malignant melanoma of anal canal.

altered bowel habit and a protuberant or polypoid mass is seen in the lower rectum, anal canal and sometimes projecting downwards beyond the anal verge (Fig. 44.17). The lesion can resemble thrombosed piles, especially if pigment is present. However, pigment is not always obvious on macroscopic observation. An association with neurofibromatosis type 1 has been reported [115].

Malignant melanoma invariably arises from the transitional zone above the dentate line. Melanocytes are normally found in this location and the tumour is therefore classified among the melanomas of mucous membranes. The diagnosis is made by biopsy, but the distinction from lymphoma, undifferentiated carcinoma of the rectum and poorly differentiated squamous carcinoma of the anal canal can be difficult unless obvious pigmentation is present. The microscopic appearances are variable [116]. The tumours are often very invasive with a marked degree of pleomorphism and large numbers of mitotic figures. One of the most common appearances is that of polygonal cells with eosinophilic cytoplasm, each with a large slightly eccentric nucleus and prominent single nucleolus. The cells are arranged in packets or more diffuse sheets. Spindle cell forms occur also, requiring careful distinction from spindle cell squamous carcinoma (pseudosarcoma) of the anal canal [117]. Sometimes the appearance may closely mimic carcinoid tumours. Tumour giant cells, when present, are a helpful indication towards the correct diagnosis and the presence of junctional change, which may present at the lower pole of the growth, will facilitate the diagnosis. However, areas of junctional change are often destroyed by ulceration. Pigmentation can be found in about half of all cases if searched for carefully. Silver staining methods, the immunohistochemical demonstration of S-100 protein and the identification of melanosomes at the ultrastructural level are useful special techniques.

Malignant melanoma of the anal canal spreads rapidly in the anorectal tissues and may even ulcerate onto the perianal skin through the ischiorectal fossae. The superior haemorrhoidal group of lymph nodes is involved early in the course of the disease with later spread to the glands on the lateral wall of the pelvis, the para-aortic nodes and the inguinal glands. Death occurs from widespread blood-borne metastases, mostly to the liver and lungs. The survival rate after surgical excision is measured in months rather than years, although there is one report of survival for over 5 years before the patient died from generalized metastases [118].

Adenocarcinoma

Columnar epithelium lines the transitional zone of the anal canal and must obviously be prone to neoplastic change. However, because all malignancies in this site invade upwards and present as rectal tumours, there is no way of distinguishing adenocarcinoma of the anal canal from adenocarcinoma of the lower rectum. For this reason all typical adenocarcinomas of the anorectal region are grouped as cancers of the lower third of the rectum at St Mark's Hospital. However, two special forms of adenocarcinoma peculiar to this region deserve special mention: adenocarcinoma of the anal ducts or glands, and mucinous adenocarcinoma associated with anorectal fistulae [119].

Adenocarcinoma of anal ducts and glands

Acceptable examples of adenocarcinoma of anal ducts or glands are extremely rare [120,121]. These tumours are flat, mainly submucosal growths which tend to spread widely within the tissues of the anal canal producing stenosis. Microscopically they are adenocarcinomas in which the epithelium lining the glands bears a close resemblance to normal anal ducts. There may be associated pagetoid spread [122]. For the diagnosis to be established for certain it is necessary to demonstrate a transition from anal canal duct epithelium to carcinoma through an *in situ* stage. Otherwise the distinction from adenocarcinoma of the rectum, squamous cell carcinoma of the anal canal with mucinous microcysts (glandular differentiation) and apocrine carcinoma of the perianal skin can be difficult if not impossible. Anal duct carcinomas should be separated from mucinous carcinomas arising in anorectal fistulae (see below). There is evidence that mucin histochemistry may be useful in distinguishing between anal duct or gland carcinoma and other adenocarcinomas of the anorectal region. Goblet cells of the rectum and anal canal transitional zone secrete O-acetyl sialomucin and this type of mucus is at least partially retained in adenocarcinomas of the lower rectum. On the other hand, sialomucin in anal gland adenocarcinomas lacks O-acetyl groups. O-acetyl groups can be demonstrated indi-

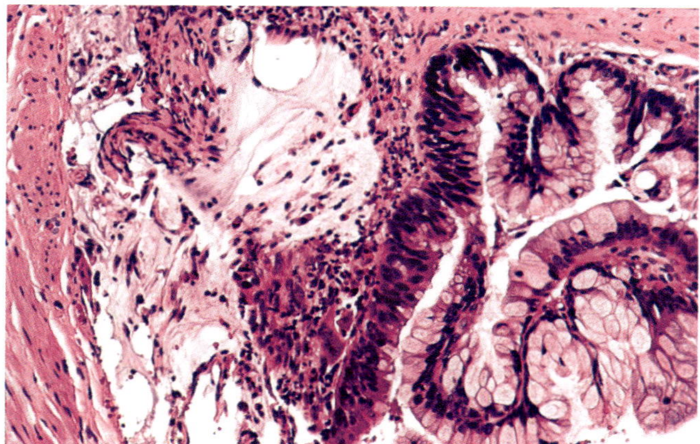

Fig. 44.18 Well differentiated mucinous adenocarcinoma within anorectal fistula.

rectly through the acquisition of PAS reactivity that accompanies their removal following saponification with potassium hydroxide. Such a test is positive for rectal and negative for anal gland adenocarcinoma [123].

Mucinous adenocarcinoma in anorectal fistulae

In this condition patients present with anorectal fistulae or recurrent abscesses around the anus. Mucus can sometimes be clearly seen within abscesses or fistulous tracks but there is no visible mucosal lesion within the rectum. Microscopic examination of biopsies obtained during surgical treatment shows fragments of mucinous carcinoma that may be so well differentiated that the diagnosis of adenocarcinoma is not even considered (Fig. 44.18). Awareness of the condition is important because the diagnosis may be otherwise unsuspected by both clinician and pathologist.

It has been suggested that these unusual tumours arise in duplications of the lower end of the hindgut [124]. Support for this view is provided by the fact that some of the fistulous tracks are lined by entirely normal rectal mucosa including muscularis mucosae [124]. Furthermore, it may be possible to demonstrate that rectal mucosa lines the upper part of the track, giving way to squamous epithelium at the appropriate line of the anal valves. Others suggest that these tumours arise in pre-existing anal sinuses or fistulae [125]. Examples of this condition have been observed in association with Crohn's disease [80,126].

The tumours are well differentiated and characterized by the presence of pools of mucin which dissect and infiltrate the stromal tissues of the perianal and perirectal regions. There are two important differential diagnoses. Anal fistulae can sometimes be lined by essentially normal rectal mucosa. Innocent misplacement of this epithelium may occur, closely mimicking a well differentiated mucinous carcinoma. Misplacement of epithelium may also complicate solitary ulcer syndrome ('colitis cystica profunda'). The clinical setting should help in the differentiation of these conditions.

Malignant epithelial tumours of the anal margin

Squamous cell carcinoma of the anal margin

Squamous cell carcinomas of the anal margin mostly arise at the junction of the squamous mucous membrane of the lower end of the anal canal with the hairbearing perianal skin [127]. This junctional origin, the appearance of the tumours, their histology and behaviour suggest a comparison with squamous carcinoma of the lip. At both sites one usually encounters a slowly growing, keratinizing squamous cell carcinoma which metastasizes to regional lymph nodes at a late stage in its natural history.

Squamous cell carcinoma is about one-third as frequent as anal canal carcinoma [84,128]. It is more common in men than women (4:1), but there is no significant difference in age incidence compared with adenocarcinoma of the rectum or squamous cell carcinoma of the anal canal. There are case reports of squamous cell carcinoma arising in the anal skin tags of a patient with Crohn's disease [129] and in association with perianal hidradenitis suppurativa [130]. Verrucous carcinoma arising in a pilonidal sinus has been described [131]. Macroscopically, the lesion presents either as an ulcer or a cauliflower-like growth (Fig. 44.15). Microscopically it is usually a well differentiated, keratinizing squamous cell carcinoma [107]. Poorly differentiated tumours are very rare.

Inguinal lymph node metastases are found in about 20% of cases [100]. The majority of anal margin cancers are treated by local excision of the primary tumour. In advanced cases that have been treated by radical removal of the rectum, involvement of the haemorrhoidal group of lymph nodes is exceptional. Advanced disease would today be treated by radiotherapy in most centres.

The 5-year survival figures for anal margin cancer show the prognosis to be more favourable than for disease of the anal canal [98]. This is despite the fact that the former were mainly treated by local excision and the latter by radical excision of rectum and anus. Size, extensive local invasion (T3 or T4) and inguinal lymph node involvement are adverse prognostic features [100].

Basal cell carcinoma

Basal cell carcinoma of the perianal skin is rare and accounts for only 0.2% of tumours in the anorectal region [132]. In a series of 34 patients the median age was 68 (range 43–86) and the sexes were affected equally [132]. The macroscopic and microscopic features are no different from those seen in rodent ulcers occurring elsewhere. It is important to distinguish basal cell carcinoma from basaloid squamous cell carcinoma of the anal canal. Histological features that would support a diagnosis of basal cell carcinoma include prominent nuclear palisading, formation of a characteristic stroma, clefting between the epithelial islands and surrounding stroma, low invasiveness and little nuclear pleomorphism. The macroscopic appearances, including the difference in location, will also be important guides to the correct diagnosis. In the series referred to above, the death rate was not higher than the normal population of the same age and sex and in fact no death was due to basal cell carcinoma [132].

Miscellaneous tumours

We have seen a few examples of adenocarcinoma of the perianal apocrine glands without any evidence of extramammary Paget's disease. They were ulcerating growths and microscopic examination showed glands lined by columnar epithelium containing PAS-positive apical secretions.

Smooth muscle tumours arising from the internal sphincter are very rare. Perianal rhabdomyosarcoma has been reported [133–135], and a rhabdomyoma has been described in a neonate [136]. Benign lymphoid polyps are not infrequently found in the upper anal canal just above the dentate line, though they are more common in rectal mucosa. Malignant lymphoma of the anal canal is rare [137,138], but it is not uncommon for perianal abscess to be a presenting sign of leukaemia [139]. There has been a recent increase in anorectal B-cell lymphoma in subjects with AIDS, particularly in male homosexuals [140,141]. There is a report of a cutaneous T-cell lymphoma presenting initially as a perianal lesion [142]. Langerhans cell histiocytosis has been reported in children [143,144] and an adult [145]. Perianal Kaposi's sarcoma has been described in HIV-infected persons [146]. In a series of 74 cases of benign granular cell 'myoblastoma' of the gastrointestinal tract, 16 were reported to occur in the perianal region [147]. Lipoma, liposarcoma, fibrosarcoma and aggressive angiomyxoma [148] are seen in the ischiorectal fossa. Secondary carcinoma can occasionally present in the anal canal as a manifestation of spread by implantation from an adenocarcinoma of the colon or rectum (see p. 588). The internal haemorrhoidal plexus is a rare site of metastatic spread from a primary growth in the lung [149].

Presacral tumours

A wide variety of conditions can present as a presacral tumour. Most of them fall into one of four categories: congenital abnormalities, bone tumours, neurogenic tumours and a miscellaneous group of lesions including secondary carcinoma and connective tissue tumours. Among the congenital anomalies dermoid cysts, teratomas, meningocoele and pelvic kidney can be included. Among bone and connective tissue tumours found at this site are chordoma, osteochondroma, giant cell tumour, Ewing's sarcoma and myeloma. Neurofibroma, schwannoma, ependymoma and primitive neuroectodermal tumours are also seen [150,151].

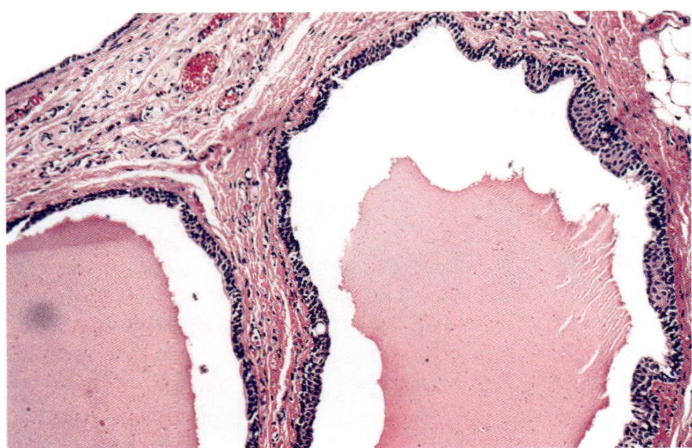

Fig. 44.19 Retrorectal cyst hamartoma.

Rectrorectal cyst hamartoma

This rare condition may be discovered incidentally or present in a variety of ways including large bowel obstruction, abscesses and recurrent fistulae due to complicating infection, or with complaints such as pain and tenesmus [152,153]. It is unclear whether the condition is acquired as a result of cystic change and misplacement of anal gland epithelium following an episode of inflammation or whether it represents a congenital anomaly. It is possible that small examples discovered incidentally are acquired, whereas the larger presacral masses are congenital defects arising from remnants of the embryonic postanal segment or tailgut [152]. The latter hypothesis receives support from the fact that the lesion arises in the posterior midline of the anococcygeal and rectrorectal areas. Specimens comprise multilocular cysts lined by squamous, transitional and columnar epithelium (Fig. 44.19). Bundles of smooth muscle occupy the surrounding connective tissue. The differential diagnosis includes simple anal gland cysts, teratoma, dermoid cyst, duplication cysts of the rectum and well differentiated adenocarcinoma of the anal glands. There are reports of adenocarcinoma developing in rectrorectal cyst hamartoma [154], emphasizing the need to achieve complete surgical removal.

References

1 Groisman GM, Polak-Charcon S. Fibroepithelial polyps of the anus. A histologic, immunohistochemical, and ultrastructural study, including comparison with the normal anal subepithelial layer. *Am J Surg Pathol*, 1998; 22: 70.

2 Beer TW, Carr NJ. Fibroepithelial polyps of the anus with epithelial vacuolation. *Am J Surg Pathol*, 1999; 23: 488.
3 Lobert PF, Appelman HD. Inflammatory cloacogenic polyp. A unique inflammatory lesion of the anal transitional zone. *Am J Surg Pathol*, 1981; 5: 761.
4 Chetty R, Bhathal PS, Slavin JL. Prolapse-induced inflammatory polyps of the colorectum and anal transitional zone. *Histopathology*, 1993; 23: 63.
5 Kaftan SM, Haboubi NY. Histopathological changes in haemorrhoid associated mucosa and submucosa. *Int J Colorect Dis*, 1995; 10: 15.
6 Bass J, Soucy P, Walton M, Nizalik E. Inflammatory cloacogenic polyps in children. *J Pediatr Surg*, 1995; 30: 585.
7 Donaldson DR, Jass JR, Mann CV. Anal leukoplakia. *Gut*, 1987; 28: A1368.
8 Klotz RG, Pamukcoglu T, Souillard H. Transitional cloacogenic carcinoma of the anal canal. *Cancer*, 1967; 20: 1727.
9 Grodsky L. Current concepts on cloacogenic transitional cell anorectal cancer. *JAMA*, 1969; 207: 2057.
10 Foust RL, Dean PJ, Stoler MH, Moinuddin SM. Intraepithelial neoplasia of the anal canal in hemorrhoidal tissue: a study of 19 cases. *Hum Pathol*, 1991; 22: 528.
11 Fenger C, Nielsen VT. Dysplastic changes in the anal canal epithelium in minor surgical specimens. *Acta Pathol Microbiol Immunol Scand [A]*, 1981; 89: 463.
12 Fenger C, Nielsen VT. Precancerous changes in the anal canal epithelium in resection specimens. *Acta Pathol Microbiol Immunol Scand [A]*, 1986; 94: 63.
13 Scholefield JH, Ogunbiyi OA, Smith JHF, Rogers K, Sharp F. Treatment of anal intraepithelial neoplasia. *Br J Surg*, 1994; 81: 1238.
14 Schlaerth JB, Morrow CP, Nalick RH, Gaddis O. Anal involvement by carcinoma *in situ* of the perineum in women. *Obstet Gynecol*, 1984; 64: 406.
15 Peters RK, Mark TM. Patterns of anal carcinoma by gender in Los Angeles County. *Br J Cancer*, 1983; 48: 629.
16 Melbye M, Rabkin C, Frisch M, Biggar RJ. Changing patterns of anal cancer incidence in the United States, 1940–1989. *Am J Epidemiol*, 1994; 139: 772.
17 Peters RK, Mack TM, Bernstein L. Parallels in the epidemiology of selected anogenital carcinomas. *J Natl Cancer Inst*, 1984; 72: 609.
18 Daling JR, Weiss NS, Klopfenstein LL *et al*. Correlates of homosexual behaviour and the incidence of anal cancer. *JAMA*, 1982; 247: 1988.
19 Carter PS, Sheffield JP, Shepherd N *et al*. Interobserver variation in the reporting of the histopathological grading of anal intraepithelial neoplasia. *J Clin Pathol*, 1994; 47: 1032.
20 Noffsinger AE, Hui YZ, Suzuk L *et al*. The relationship of human papillomavirus to proliferation and ploidy in carcinoma of the anus. *Cancer*, 1995; 75: 958.
21 Palmer JG, Scholefield JH, Coates PJ *et al*. Anal cancer and human papillomaviruses. *Dis Colon Rectum*, 1989; 32: 1016.
22 Croxson T, Chabon B, Rorat E, Barash M. Intraepithelial carcinoma of the anus in homosexual men. *Dis Colon Rectum*, 1984; 27: 325.
23 Breese PL, Judson FN, Penley KA, Douglas JM. Anal human papillomavirus infection among homosexual and bisexual men: prevalence of type-specific infection and association with human immunodeficiency virus. *Sex Transm Dis*, 1995; 22: 7.
24 Lee SH, McGregor DH, Kuziez MN. Malignant transformation of perianal condyloma acuminatum: a case report with review of the literature. *Dis Colon Rectum*, 1981; 24: 462.
25 Bogomoletz WV, Potet F, Molas G. Condylomata acuminata, giant condyloma acuminatum (Buschke–Lowenstein tumour) and verrucous squamous cell carcinoma of the perianal and anorectal region: a continuous precancerous spectrum? *Histopathology*, 1985; 9: 1155.
26 Knoblich R, Failing JF. Condyloma acuminatum (Buschke–Lowenstein tumour) of the rectum. *Am J Clin Pathol*, 1967; 48: 389.
27 Judge JR. Giant condyloma acuminatum involving vulva and rectum. *Arch Pathol*, 1969; 88: 46.
28 Gingrass PJ, Bubrick MP, Hitchcock CR, Strom RL. Anorectal verrucose squamous cell carcinoma; report of two cases. *Dis Colon Rectum*, 1978; 21: 210.
29 Elliot MS, Werner ID, Immelman EJ, Harrison AC. Giant condyloma acuminatum (Buschke–Lowenstein tumour) of the anorectum. *Dis Colon Rectum*, 1979; 22: 497.
30 Drut R, Ontiveros S, Cabral DH. Perianal verrucose carcinoma spreading to the rectum. *Dis Colon Rectum*, 1975; 18: 516.
31 Grassegger A, Hopfl R, Hussl H, Wicke K, Fritsch P. Buschke–Loewenstein tumour infiltrating pelvic organs. *Br J Dermatol*, 1994; 130: 221.
32 Marsh RW, Agaliotis D, Killeen RJ. Treatment of invasive squamous cell carcinoma complicating anal Buschke–Lowenstein tumor: a case history. *Cutis*, 1995; 55: 358.
33 Bertram P, Treutner KH, Rubben A, Hauptmann S, Schumpelick V. Invasive squamous-cell carcinoma in giant anorectal condyloma (Buschke–Lowenstein tumor). *Langenbecks Arch Chir*, 1995; 380: 115.
34 Hyacinthe M, Karl R, Coppola D *et al*. Squamous-cell carcinoma of the pelvis in a giant condyloma acuminatum: use of neoadjuvant chemoradiation and surgical resection. *Dis Colon Rectum*, 1998; 41: 1450.
35 Boshart M, zur Hausen H. Human papillomaviruses in Buschke–Lowenstein tumors: physical state of the DNA and identification of a tandem duplication in the noncoding region of a human papillomavirus 6 subtype. *J Virol*, 1986; 58: 963.
36 Rando RF, Sedlacek T, Hunt J *et al*. Verrucous carcinoma of the vulva associated with an unusual type 6 human papillomavirus. *Obstet Gynecol*, 1986; 67: 708.
37 Elliot GB, Fisher BK. Perianal keratoacanthoma. *Arch Dermatol*, 1967; 95: 81.
38 Grodsky L. Bowen's disease of the anal region (squamous cell carcinoma-*in-situ*): report of three cases. *Am J Surg*, 1954; 88: 710.
39 Scoma JA, Levy EI. Bowen's disease of the anus. *Dis Colon Rectum*, 1975; 18: 137.
40 Beck DE, Karulf RE. Combination therapy for epidermoid carcinoma of the anal canal. *Dis Colon Rectum*, 1994; 37: 1118.
41 Bensaude A, Parturier-Albot M. Anal localization of Bowen's disease. *Proc R Soc Med*, 1971; 64: 3.
42 Ikenberg H, Gissmann L, Gross G *et al*. Human papillomavirus type 16-related DNA in genital Bowen's disease and in bowenoid papulosis. *Int J Cancer*, 1983; 32: 563.
43 Marchesa P, Fazio VW, Oliart S, Goldblum JR, Lavery C. Perianal

Bowen's disease: a clinicopathologic study of 47 patients. *Dis Colon Rectum*, 1997; 40: 1286.

44 Sarmiento JM, Wolff BG, Burgart LJ, Frizelle FA, Illstrup DM. Perianal Bowen's disease: associated tumors, human papillomavirus, surgery, and other controversies. *Dis Colon Rectum*, 1997; 40: 912.

45 Patterson JW, Kao GF, Graham JH, Helwig EB. Bowenoid papulosis. A clinicopathologic study with ultrastructural observations. *Cancer*, 1986; 57: 823.

46 Cobb MW. Human papillomavirus infection. *J Am Acad Dermatol*, 1990; 22: 547.

47 Rudlinger R, Grob R, Yu YX *et al*. Human papillomavirus-35-positive bowenoid papulosis of the anogenital area and concurrent human papillomavirus-35-positive verruca with bowenoid dysplasia of the periungual area. *Arch Dermatol*, 1989; 125: 655.

48 Grussendorf CE. Anogenital premalignant and malignant tumors (including Buschke–Lowenstein tumors). *Clin Dermatol*, 1997; 15: 377.

49 Meeker JH, Neubecker RD, Helwig EB. Hidradenoma papilliferum. *Am J Clin Pathol*, 1962; 37: 182.

50 Helwig EB, Graham JH. Anogenital (extramammary) Paget's disease. *Cancer*, 1963; 16: 387.

51 Grodsky L. Extramammary Paget's disease of the perianal region. *Dis Colon Rectum*, 1960; 3: 502.

52 Linder JM, Myers RT. Perianal Paget's disease. *Am Surg*, 1970; 36: 342.

53 Goldman S, Ihre T, Lagerstedt U, Svensson C. Perianal Paget's disease: report of five cases. *Int J Colorect Dis*, 1992; 7: 167.

54 Potter B. Extramammary Paget's disease. *Acta Derm Venereol*, 1967; 47: 259.

55 Mazoujian G, Pinkus GS, Haagensen DE. Extramammary Paget's disease—evidence for an apocrine origin. An immunoperoxidase study of gross cystic disease fluid protein-15, carcinoembryonic antigen and keratin proteins. *Am J Surg Pathol*, 1984; 8: 43.

56 Ordonez NG, Awalt H, Mackay B. Mammary and extramammary Paget's disease. An immunocytochemical and ultrastructural study. *Cancer*, 1987; 59: 1173.

57 Kariniemi A-L, Forsman L, Wahlstrom T, Vesterinen E, Andersson L. Expression of differentiation antigens in mammary and extramammary Paget's disease. *Br J Dermatol*, 1984; 110: 203.

58 Nagle RB, Lucas DO, McDaniel KM, Clark VA, Schmalzel GM. Paget's cells. New evidence linking mammary and extramammary Paget cells to a common cell phenotype. *Am J Clin Pathol*, 1985; 83: 431.

59 Bussolati G, Pich A. Mammary and extramammary Paget's disease. An immunocytochemical study. *Am J Pathol*, 1975; 80: 117.

60 Nakamura G, Shikata N, Shoji T *et al*. Immunohistochemical study of mammary and extramammary Paget's disease. *Anticancer Res*, 1995; 15: 467.

61 Marchesa P, Fazio VW, Oliart S *et al*. Long-term outcome of patients with perianal Paget's disease. *Ann Surg Oncol*, 1997; 4: 475.

62 Sasaki M, Terada T, Nakanuma Y *et al*. Anorectal mucinous adenocarcinoma associated with latent perianal Paget's disease. *Am J Gastroenterol*, 1990; 85: 199.

63 Armitage NR, Jass JR, Richman PI, Thomson JPS, Phillips RKS. Paget's disease of the anus: a clinicopathological study. *Br J Surg*, 1989; 76: 60.

64 Battles OE, Page DL, Johnson JE. Cytokeratins, CEA, and mucin histochemistry in the diagnosis and characterization of extramammary Paget's disease. *Am J Clin Pathol*, 1997; 108: 6.

65 Goldblum JR, Hart WR. Perianal Paget's disease: a histologic and immunohistochemical study of 11 cases with and without associated rectal adenocarcinoma. *Am J Surg Pathol*, 1998; 22: 170.

66 Nowak MA, Guerriere KP, Pathan A, Campbell TE, Deppisch LM. Perianal Paget's disease: distinguishing primary and secondary lesions using immunohistochemical studies including gross cystic disease fluid protein-15 and cytokeratin 20 expression. *Arch Pathol Lab Med*, 1998; 122: 1077.

67 Morson BC. The polyp–cancer sequence in the large bowel. *Proc R Soc Med*, 1974; 67: 451.

68 Frazer IH, Medley G, Crapper RM, Brown TC, Mackay IR. Association between anorectal dysplasia, human papillomavirus, and human immunodeficiency virus infection in homosexual men. *Lancet*, 1986; ii: 657.

69 Shroyer KR, Brookes CG, Markham NE, Shroyer AL. Detection of human papillomavirus in anorectal squamous cell carcinoma. Correlation with basaloid pattern of differentiation. *Am J Clin Pathol*, 1995; 104: 299.

70 Noffsinger A, Witte D, Fenoglio-Preiser CM. The relationship of human papillomaviruses to anorectal neoplasia. *Cancer*, 1992; 70: 1276.

71 Zaki SR, Judd R, Coffield LM *et al*. Human papillomavirus infection and anal carcinoma. Retrospective analysis by in situ hybridization and the polymerase chain reaction. *Am J Pathol*, 1992; 140: 1345.

72 Dyson H, Howley PM, Munger K, Harlow E. The human papillomavirus-16 E7 oncoprotein is able to bind to the retinoblastoma gene product. *Science*, 1989; 243: 934.

73 Munger K, Werness BA, Dyson N *et al*. Complex formation of human papillomavirus E7 proteins with the retinoblastoma tumor suppessor gene product. *EMBO J*, 1989; 8: 4099.

74 Werness BA, Levine AJ, Howley PM. Association of human papillomaviorus type 16 and 18, E6 proteins with p53. *Science*, 1990; 248: 76.

75 Carter PS, de Ruiter A, Whatrup C *et al*. Human immunodeficiency virus infection and genital warts as risk factors for anal intraepithelial neoplasia in homosexual men. *Br J Surg*, 1995; 82: 474.

76 McMillan A, Bishop PE. Clinical course of anogenital warts in men infected with human immunodeficiency virus. *Genitourin Med*, 1989; 65: 225.

77 Sillman FH, Sedlis A. Anogenital papillomavirus infection and neoplasia in immunodeficient women: an update. *Dermatol Clin*, 1991; 9: 353.

78 Goldie SJ, Kuntz KM, Weinstein MC *et al*. The clinical effectiveness and cost-effectiveness of screening for anal squamous intraepithelial lesions in homosexual and bisexual HIV-positive men. *JAMA*, 1999; 281: 1822.

79 Palefsky JM, Holly EA, Ralston ML *et al*. High incidence of anal high-grade squamous intra-epithelial lesions among HIV-positive and HIV-negative homosexual and bisexual men. *AIDS*, 1998; 12: 495.

80 Connell WR, Sheffield JP, Kamm MA *et al*. Lower gastrointestinal malignancy in Crohn's disease. *Gut*, 1994; 35: 347.

81 Frisch M, Olsen JH, Bautz A, Melbye M. Benign anal lesions and the risk of anal cancer. *N Engl J Med*, 1994; 331: 300.

82 Gabriel WB. Squamous cell carcinoma of the anus and anal canal. An analysis of 55 cases. *Proc R Soc Med*, 1941; 34: 139.

83 Williams GR, Talbot IC. Anal carcinoma—a histological review. *Histopathology*, 1994; 25: 507.

84 Morson BC. The pathology and results of treatment of squamous cell carcinoma of the anal canal and anal margin. *Proc R Soc Med*, 1960; 53: 416.

85 Lone F, Berg JW, Stearns MW. Basaloid tumours of the anus. *Cancer*, 1960; 13: 907.

86 Pang LSC, Morson BC. Basaloid carcinoma of the anal canal. *J Clin Pathol*, 1967; 20: 28.

87 Jass JR, Sobin LH. *Histological typing of intestinal tumours. WHO International Classification of Tumours*. Berlin: Springer-Verlag, 1989.

88 Berg JW, Lone F, Stearns MW. Mucoepidermoid anal cancer. *Cancer*, 1960; 13: 914.

89 Morson BC, Volkstadt H. Mucoepidermoid tumours of the anal canal. *J Clin Pathol*, 1963; 16: 200.

90 Dougherty BG, Evans HL. Carcinoma of the anal canal: a study of 69 cases with special attention to histologic grading. *Am J Clin Pathol*, 1984; 81: 696.

91 Clark J, Petrelli N, Herrera L, Mittelman A. Epidermoid carcinoma of the anal canal. *Cancer*, 1986; 57: 400.

92 Frost DB, Richards PC, Montague ED, Giacco GG, Martin RG. Epidermoid cancer of the anorectum. *Cancer*, 1984; 53: 1285.

93 Salmon RJ, Zafrani B, Labib A, Asselain B, Girodet J. Prognosis of cloacogenic and squamous cancers of the anal canal. *Dis Colon Rectum*, 1986; 29: 336.

94 Greenall MJ, Quan SHQ, De Cosse JJ. Epidermoid cancer of the anus. *Br J Surg*, 1985; 72: 97.

95 Frisch M, Fenger C, van-den-Brule AJ *et al*. Variants of squamous cell carcinoma of the anal canal and perianal skin and their relation to human papillomaviruses. *Cancer Res*, 1999; 59: 753.

96 Fenger C, Frisch M, Jass JR, Williams GT, Hilden J. Anal cancer subtype reproducibility study. *Virchows Arch*, 2000; 436: 229.

97 Boman BM, Moertel CG, O'Connell MJ *et al*. Carcinoma of the anal canal. A clinical and pathologic study of 188 cases. *Cancer*, 1984; 54: 114.

98 Hardcastle JD, Bussey HJR. Results of surgical treatment of squamous cell carcinoma of the anal canal and anal margin seen at St. Mark's Hospital 1928 66. *Proc R Soc Med*, 1968; 61: 27.

99 Shepherd NA, Scholefield JH, Love SB, England J, Northover JMA. Prognostic factors in anal squamous carcinoma: a multivariate analysis of clinical, pathological and flow cytometric parameters in 235 cases. *Histopathology*, 1990; 16: 545.

100 Deans GT, McAleer JJA, Spence RAJ. Malignant anal tumours. *Br J Surg*, 1994; 81: 500.

101 Touboul E, Schlienger M, Buffat L *et al*. Epidermoid carcinoma of the anal margin: 17 cases treated with curative-intent radiation therapy. *Radiother Oncol*, 1995; 34: 195.

102 Schlag PM, Hunerbein M. Anal cancer: multimodal therapy. *World J Surg*, 1995; 19: 282.

103 Muleris M, Salmon R-J, Girodet J, Zafrani B, Dutrillaux B. Recurrent deletions of chromosomes 11q and 3p in anal canal carcinoma. *Int J Cancer*, 1987; 39: 595.

104 Walts AE, Koeffler HP, Said JW. Localization of p53 protein and human papillomavirus in anogenital squamous lesions: immunohistochemical and in situ hybridization studies in benign, dysplastic, and malignant epithelia. *Hum Pathol*, 1993; 24: 1238.

105 Coulter LK, Wolber R, Tron VA. Site-specific comparison of p53 immunostaining in squamous cell carcinomas. *Hum Pathol*, 1995; 26: 531.

106 Hiorns LR, Scholefield JH, Palmer JG, Shepherd NA, Kerr IB. Ki-ras oncogene mutations in non-HPV-associated anal carcinoma. *J Pathol*, 1990; 161: 99.

107 Morson BC, Pang LSC. Pathology of anal cancer. *Proc R Soc Med*, 1968; 61: 623.

108 UKCCCR Anal Cancer Trial Working Party. Epidermoid anal cancer: results from the UKCCCR randomised trial of radiotherapy alone versus radiotherapy, 5-fluorouracil, and mitomycin. *Lancet*, 1996; 348: 1049.

109 Morson BC, Volkstadt H. Malignant melanoma of the anal canal. *J Clin Pathol*, 1963; 16: 126.

110 Bolivar JC, Harris JW, Branch W, Sherman RT. Melanoma of the anorectal region. *Surg Gynecol Obstet*, 1982; 154: 337.

111 Quan SHQ, White JE, Deddish MR. Malignant melanoma of the anorectum. *Dis Colon Rectum*, 1959; 2: 275.

112 Brady MS, Kavolius JP, Quan SH. Anorectal melanoma. A 64-year experience at Memorial Sloan-Kettering Cancer Center. *Dis Colon Rectum*, 1995; 38: 146.

113 Konstadoulakis MM, Ricaniadis N, Walsh D, Karakousis CP. Malignant melanoma of the anorectal region. *J Surg Oncol*, 1995; 58: 118.

114 Goldman S, Glimelius B, Pahlman L. Anorectal malignant melanoma in Sweden. Report of 49 patients. *Dis Colon Rectum*, 1990; 33: 874.

115 Ben-Izhak O, Groisman GM. Anal malignant melanoma and soft-tissue malignant fibrous histiocytoma in neurofibromatosis type 1. *Arch Pathol Lab Med*, 1995; 119: 285.

116 Mason JK, Helwig EB. Anorectal melanoma. *Cancer*, 1966; 19: 39.

117 Kalogeropoulous NK, Antonakopoulos GN, Agapitos MB, Papacharalampous NX. Spindle cell carcinoma (pseudosarcoma) of the anus: a light electron microscopic and immunocytochemical study of a case. *Histopathology*, 1985; 9: 987.

118 Berkley JL. Melanoma of the anal canal: report of a case of five-year survival after abdominoperineal resection. *Dis Colon Rectum*, 1960; 3: 159.

119 Tarazi R, Nelson RL. Anal adenocarcinoma: a comprehensive review. *Semin Surg Oncol*, 1994; 10: 235.

120 Basik M, Rodriguez-Bigas MA, Penetrante R, Petrelli NJ. Prognosis and recurrence patterns of anal adenocarcinoma. *Am J Surg*, 1995; 169: 233.

121 Wellman KF. Adenocarcinoma of anal duct origin. *Can J Surg*, 1962; 5: 311.

122 Wong AY, Rahilly MA, Adams W, Lee CS. Mucinous anal gland carcinoma with perianal Pagetoid spread. *Pathology*, 1998; 30: 1.

123 Fenger C, Filipe MI. Mucin histochemistry of the anal canal epithelium. Studies of normal mucosa and mucosa adjacent to carcinoma. *Histochem J*, 1981; 13: 921.

124 Jones EA, Morson BC. Mucinous adenocarcinoma in anorectal fistulae. *Histopathology*, 1984; 8: 279.

125 Anthony T, Simmang C, Lee EL, Turnage RH. Perianal mucinous adenocarcinoma. *J Surg Oncol*, 1997; 64: 218.

126 Ky A, Sohn N, Weinstein MA, Korelitz BI. Carcinoma arising in anorectal fistulas of Crohn's disease. *Dis Colon Rectum*, 1998; 41: 992.

127 Greenall MJ, Quan SHQ, Stearns MW, Urmacher C, DeCosse JJ. Epidermoid cancer of the anal margin. Pathologic features, treatment and clinical results. *Am J Surg*, 1985; 149: 95.

128 Kuehn PG, Beckett R, Eisenberg H, Reed JF. Epidermoid carcinoma of the perianal skin and anal canal. A review of 157 cases. *N Engl J Med*, 1964; 270: 614.

129 Somerville KW, Langman MJS, Da Cruz DJ, Balfour TW, Sully L. Malignant transformation of anal skin tags in Crohn's disease. *Gut*, 1984; 25: 1124.

130 Shukla VK, Hughes LE. A case of squamous cell carcinoma complicating hidradenitis suppurativa. *Eur J Surg Oncol*, 1995; 21: 106.

131 Anscombe AM, Isaacson P. An unusual variant of squamous cell carcinoma (inverted verrucous carcinoma) arising in a pilonidal sinus. *Histopathology*, 1983; 7: 123.

132 Nielsen OV, Jensen SL. Basal cell carcinoma of the anus—a clinical study of 34 cases. *Br J Surg*, 1981; 68: 856.

133 Fagundes LA. Embryonal rhabdomysarcoma (sarcoma botryoides) of the anus. *Gastroenterology*, 1963; 44: 351.

134 Raney RB, JrCrist W, Hays D *et al.* Soft tissue sarcoma of the perineal region in childhood. A report from the Intergroup Rhabdomyosarcoma Studies I and II, 1972 through 1984. *Cancer*, 1990; 65: 2787.

135 Kessler KJ, Kerlakian GM, Welling RE. Perineal and perirectal sarcomas: report of two cases. *Dis Colon Rectum*, 1996; 39: 468.

136 Lapner PC, Chou S, Jimenez C. Perianal fetal rhabdomyoma: case report. *Pediatr Surg Int*, 1997; 12: 544.

137 Steele RJC, Eremin O, Krajewski AS, Ritchie GL. Primary lymphoma of the anal canal presenting as perianal suppuration. *Br Med J*, 1985; 291: 311.

138 Porter AJ, Meagher AP, Sweeney JL. Anal lymphoma presenting as a perianal abscess. *Aust N Z J Surg*, 1994; 64: 279.

139 Kott I, Urca I. Perianal abscess as a presenting sign of leukaemia. *Dis Colon Rectum*, 1969; 11: 213.

140 Heise W, Arasteh K, Mostertz P *et al.* Malignant gastrointestinal lymphomas in patients with AIDS. *Digestion*, 1997; 58: 218.

141 Ioachim HL, Antonescu C, Giancott F, Dorsett B, Weinstein MA. EBV-associated anorectal lymphomas in patients with acquired immune deficiency syndrome. *Am J Surg Pathol*, 1997; 21: 997.

142 Hill VA, Hall-Smith P, Smith NP. Cutaneous T-cell lymphoma presenting with atypical perianal lesions. *Dermatology*, 1995; 190: 313.

143 Grapin C, Audry G, Josset P *et al.* Histiocytosis X revealed by complex anal fistula. *Eur J Pediatr Surg*, 1994; 4: 184.

144 Kader HA, Ruchelli E, Maller ES. Langerhans' cell histiocytosis with stool retention caused by a perianal mass. *J Pediatr Gastroenterol Nutr*, 1998; 26: 226.

145 Conias S, Strutton G, Stephenson G. Adult cutaneous Langerhans cell histiocytosis. *Australas J Dermatol*, 1998; 39: 106.

146 Barrett WL, Callahan TD, Orkin BA. Perianal manifestations of human immunodeficiency virus infection: experience with 260 patients. *Dis Colon Rectum*, 1998; 41: 606.

147 Johnston J, Helwig EB. Granular cell tumors of the gastrointestinal tract and perianal region. *Dig Dis Sci*, 1981; 26: 807.

148 Fetsch JF, Laskin WB, Lefkowitz M, Kindblom LG, Meis KJ. Aggressive angiomyxoma: a clinicopathologic study of 29 female patients. *Cancer*, 1996; 78: 79.

149 Ger R, Reuben J. Squamous cell carcinoma of the anal canal: a metastatic lesion. *Dis Colon Rectum*, 1968; 11: 213.

150 Genna M, Leopardi F, Fambri P, Postorino A. Neurogenic tumors of the ano-rectal region. *Ann Ital Chir*, 1997; 68: 351.

151 Webber EM, Fraser RB, Resch L, Giacomantonio M. Perianal ependymoma presenting in the neonatal period. *Pediatr Pathol Lab Med*, 1997; 17: 283.

152 Edwards M. Multilocular retrorectal cystic disease—cyst-hamartoma. *Dis Colon Rectum*, 1961; 4: 103.

153 Mills SE, Walker AN, Stallings RG, Allen S. Retrorectal cyst hamartoma. *Arch Pathol Lab Med*, 1984; 108: 737.

154 Marco V, Autonell J, Farre J, Fernandez-Layos M, Doncel F. Retrorectal cyst hamartomas. Report of two cases with adenocarcinoma developing in one. *Am J Surg Pathol*, 1982; 6: 707.

45 Miscellaneous conditions of the anal region

Haemorrhoids

Haemorrhoids are caused by prolapse of the vascular anal cushions that lie in the submucosa at the anorectal junction [1,2]. These cushions are normal structures made up of arterioles, venules and arteriovenous communications which are situated in the left lateral, right anterior and right posterior parts of the anal canal—the three anatomical positions at which haemorrhoids usually occur. Previous suggestions that haemorrhoids represent varicosities of the inferior rectal veins resulting from venous hypertension have now been discounted and there is no evidence that they occur with increased frequency in patients with portal hypertension [2,3]. Haemorrhoids may occur at any time during adult life although they present most commonly in the third decade. The factors leading to prolapse of the anal cushions and the development of haemorrhoids are not well understood. Many affected patients give a history of straining at defecation due to constipation, and while this alone may sometimes be sufficient to push the cushions out of the anal canal it also causes venous engorgement of the cushions, making their displacement during defecation more likely [1]. Chronic straining may also cause stretching, and later disruption, of the surrounding supporting tissues, so that while prolapse of the anal cushions may be intermittent at first, it is permanent later [4]. The association of haemorrhoids with a low dietary fibre intake [5] is probably a consequence of the straining required to expel the small, hard faeces that occur with low-fibre diets. The development of haemorrhoids in pregnancy may be related to raised intra-abdominal pressure and pelvic venous engorgement. Spasm of the anal sphincters [6], heredity and the erect posture may be contributory factors, while infrequently haemorrhoids may be the first manifestation of a rectal tumour or develop during an episode of severe diarrhoea.

Once they have prolapsed, the venous drainage from the anal cushions is impeded, so that haemorrhoids become progressively engorged. This leads to complications that include bleeding, thrombosis, strangulation or infection. Bleeding from haemorrhoids is usually of arteriolar origin. It is only rarely profuse, but nevertheless may give rise to chronic anaemia. Some examples of the fibroepithelial polyp of the anal canal may be the end-result of thrombosis and organization of the internal haemorrhoid.

Microscopic examination of excised haemorrhoids shows a plexus of dilated vascular spaces, some of which have rather more smooth muscle in their walls than would be expected for ordinary veins of the same size. Varying degrees of haemorrhage and thrombosis are seen and the overlying mucous membrane is thickened. There may be squamous metaplasia of the overlying transitional zone. The whole appearance can have a close resemblance to a cavernous haemangioma. It is advisable to examine haemorrhoidal specimens histologically as this may disclose the presence of unsuspected lesions, notably dysplasia of the overlying squamous or transitional epithelium.

Perianal haematoma

This presents as a tender lump beneath the skin of the anal verge, and is due to rupture and thrombosis of the perianal vein. It is a painful but harmless condition that is unrelated to so-called internal haemorrhoids.

Oleogranuloma

This is a foreign body reaction to non-absorbable oily substances in the tissues. The usual cause of anorectal oleogranuloma is oil used as a vehicle in the injection treatment of haemorrhoids [7,8]. The degree of reaction depends upon the type of oil used. Vegetable oils produce the least severe reaction, followed by animal fats, with mineral oils causing the most extensive changes. Oleogranuloma can present as a rounded submucous tumour in the anal canal just above the dentate line, but annular and even ulcerating lesions have been described [9,10]. Unless biopsy is performed in such cases the clinical diagnosis of carcinoma may be made, leading to unnecessary radical excision of the rectum [11]. Oleogranulomatous inflammation can be found in any part of the rectum and even as high as the rectosigmoid junction, presumably

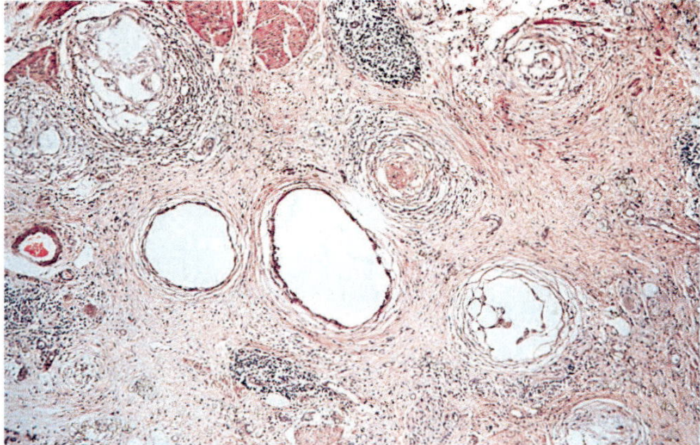

Fig. 45.1 Oleogranulomatous inflammation. Chronic inflammatory reaction, showing numerous histiocytes around oil-containing spaces.

because the injected oil can track upwards in the submucosal layer. Sometimes the reaction may extend into the other layers of the rectal wall as well as into the perirectal fat.

The histology of oleogranuloma is characteristic (Fig. 45.1). In the early stages there is an acute inflammatory response, including many eosinophils. This is followed by increasing fibrosis and a variable degree of inflammation that subsides with increasing age of the lesion. Rounded spaces lined by large mononuclear or multinucleate histiocytes are scattered throughout. These spaces contained the oil which is removed from the tissues during the course of histological preparation but can be demonstrated in frozen sections of formalin-fixed material. The histological appearance can be confused with lymphangioma [12] or with cystic pneumatosis (see p. 636).

Anal incontinence

The major elements that maintain anal continence in the normal subject are the internal and external anal sphincters and the musculature of the pelvic floor [13]. Of these, it has been claimed that the most important is the puborectalis muscle which forms a muscular sling around the rectum. By its continued tonic contraction, which pulls the rectum forwards, this muscle maintains the normal anorectal angle and creates a flutter valve which only opens when the puborectalis relaxes during defecation [14]. The role of the external anal sphincter, which also consists of voluntary skeletal muscle in a continuous state of partial tonic contraction, is more controversial [15].

Some authors suggest that its role is only to give fine control of continence, especially when there are sudden increases in intra-abdominal pressure such as during coughing and sneezing, but others give it much greater importance [16]. The internal sphincter is made up of involuntary smooth muscle. Its contraction maintains closure of the anal canal into an antero-posterior slit and is believed to play an important role in controlling continence to flatus and fluid faeces [15]. Although most accounts stress the roles of these muscular elements in maintaining normal continence, other factors are undoubtedly of importance. These include rectal and anal sensation, the consistency of the stools and the capacity of the rectum.

Most patients with anal incontinence have an underlying disorder of the large intestine: inflammatory bowel disease or tumours of the rectum are the most common. In elderly subjects with chronic constipation, rectal distension due to faecal impaction may result in reflex relaxation of the internal sphincter, causing 'overflow' leakage of fluid faeces around the impacted stool—this is usually remedied by removal of the obstructing faecal bolus. Other causes of incontinence are pelvic trauma, including surgical and obstetric trauma, and neurological lesions, usually of the spinal cord, cauda equina or lumbosacral roots [17].

When these 'secondary' types of anal incontinence are excluded, there remains a significant number of patients, the great majority of them females, with so-called 'primary' or 'idiopathic' faecal incontinence. A considerable proportion of these have coexisting rectal prolapse or 'perineal descent' (see p. 466) and recent physiological and histopathological studies indicate that a significant proportion have dysfunction of the pelvic floor musculature and external anal sphincter due to neuropathic damage to these skeletal muscles [18,19]. Affected patients usually give a long history of constipation and prolonged straining at defecation and the development of incontinence is often gradual, initially occurring only on coughing or sneezing but in severe cases progressing to complete incontinence even when standing or sitting. Clinical examination reveals a patulous anal sphincter which fails to contract either voluntarily or reflexly, and usually there is impaired anorectal sensation. Histological examination of the external sphincter and puborectalis muscles shows a variable degree of atrophy with fatty or fibrous replacement and the surviving fibres show fibre type grouping, indicative of denervation, with secondary myopathic changes. Similar, but less marked, changes are found in the levator ani muscle. Careful examination of the small intramuscular nerve branches supplying the external sphincter shows endoneurial fibrosis [18,19].

These findings suggest that in many patients the pathogenesis of idiopathic incontinence is neuropathic damage to the puborectalis and external sphincter muscles, which leads to a failure to maintain the normal anorectal angle and failure of tonic anal sphincter contraction. Damage to the peripheral nerve supply of the pelvic flow musculature, mainly from the pudendal nerves, would therefore appear to be the underlying abnormality. This could occur in a number of ways. Obstetric or other forms of pelvic trauma might be involved in some patients, while in others the chronic straining at defecation which is a frequent precursor to the development of incontinence might cause repeated stretch injury to the pudendal nerves by producing perineal descent or frank rectal prolapse. It has been suggested that entrapment of these nerves in the pelvis, under the sacrospinous ligaments, may be important in some cases [19].

References

1 Thomson WHF. The nature of haemorrhoids. *Br J Surg*, 1975; 62: 542.
2 Bernstein WC. What are haemorrhoids and what is their relationship to the portal venous system? *Dis Colon Rectum*, 1983; 26: 829.
3 Weinshel E, Chen W, Falkenstein DB, Kessler R, Raicht RF. Hemorrhoids or rectal varices: defining the cause of massive rectal hemorrhage in patients with portal hypertension. *Gastroenterology*, 1986; 90: 744.
4 Haas PA, Fox TA, Haas GP. The pathogenesis of hemorrhoids. *Dis Colon Rectum*, 1984; 27: 442.
5 Burkitt DP. Varicose veins, DVT and haemorrhoids; epidemiology and suggested aetiology. *Br Med J*, 1972; ii: 556.
6 Hancock BD. The internal sphincter and anal fissure. *Br J Surg*, 1977; 64: 92.
7 Susnow DA. Oleogranuloma of the rectum. *Am J Surg*, 1952; 83: 496.
8 Graham-Stewart CW. Injection treatment of haemorrhoids. *Br Med J*, 1962; i: 213.
9 Webb AJ. Oleocysts presenting as rectal tumours. *Br J Surg*, 1966; 53: 410.
10 Hernandez V, Hernandez IA, Berthrong M. Oleo-granuloma simulating carcinoma of the rectum. *Dis Colon Rectum*, 1967; 10: 205.
11 Symmers WSC. Simulation of cancer by oil granulomas of therapeutic origin. *Br Med J*, 1955; ii: 1536.
12 Dalton ML, Gronvall JA. Lymphangioma of the rectum. *Dis Colon Rectum*, 1963; 6: 385.
13 Duthie HL. Progress report: anal continence. *Gut*, 1971; 12: 844.
14 Parks AG. Anorectal incontinence. *Proc R Soc Med*, 1975; 68: 681.
15 Henry MM. Current concepts in anorectal physiology. *Br J Hosp Med*, 1986; 35: 238.
16 Bartolo DCC, Read NW, Jarratt JA *et al*. Differences in anal sphincter function and clinical presentation in patients with pelvic floor descent. *Gastroenterology*, 1983; 85: 68.
17 Butler ECB. Complete rectal prolapse following removal of tumours of the cauda equina. *Proc R Soc Med*, 1954; 47: 521.
18 Parks AG, Swash M, Urich H. Sphincter denervation in anorectal incontinence and rectal prolapse. *Gut*, 1977; 18: 656.
19 Swash M. Idiopathic faecal incontinence: histopathological evidence on pathogenesis. *Clin Gastroenterol*, 1980; 1: 71.

Index

Page numbers in *italics* refer to pages on which figures appear.
'*vs.*' denotes differential diagnosis